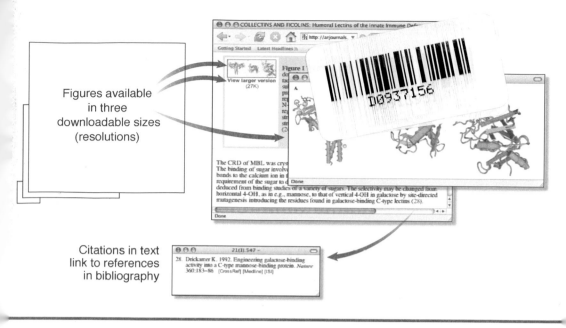

Figures available
in three
downloadable sizes
(resolutions)

Citations in text
link to references
in bibliography

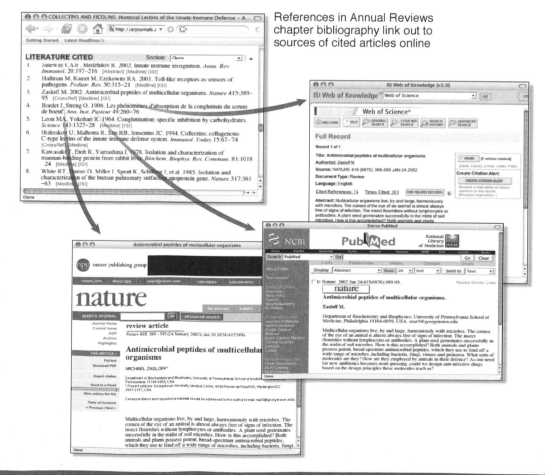

References in Annual Reviews
chapter bibliography link out to
sources of cited articles online

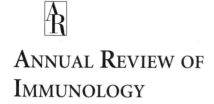

ANNUAL REVIEW OF
IMMUNOLOGY

ANNUAL REVIEW OF IMMUNOLOGY

VOLUME 23, 2005

WILLIAM E. PAUL, *Editor*
National Institutes of Health, Bethesda, Maryland

C. GARRISON FATHMAN, *Associate Editor*
Stanford University, Stanford, California

LAURIE H. GLIMCHER, *Associate Editor*
Harvard University School of Public Health

www.annualreviews.org science@annualreviews.org 650-493-4400

ANNUAL REVIEWS
4139 El Camino Way • P.O. Box 10139 • Palo Alto, California 94303-0139

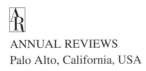

ANNUAL REVIEWS
Palo Alto, California, USA

International Standard Serial Number: 0732-0582
International Standard Book Number: 0-8243-3023-4

All Annual Reviews publication titles are registered trademarks of Annual Reviews.

∞ The paper used in this publication meets the minimum requirements of American
National Standards for Information Sciences—Permanence of Paper for Printed Library
Materials, ANSI Z39.48-1992.

Annual Reviews and the Editors of its publications assume no responsibility for the
statements expressed by the contributors to this *Annual Review*.

TYPESET BY TECHBOOKS, FAIRFAX, VA
PRINTED AND BOUND BY CAPITAL CITY PRESS, MONTPELIER, VT

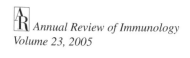
Annual Review of Immunology
Volume 23, 2005

CONTENTS

INDEXES

ERRATA
An online log of corrections to *Annual Review of Immunology* chapters
may be found at http://immunol.annualreviews.org/errata.shtml

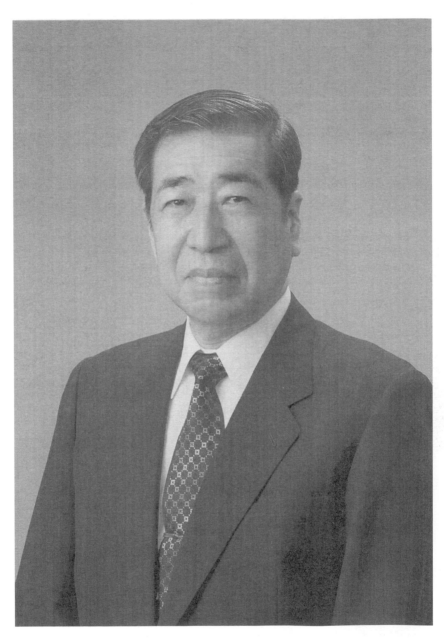

Annu. Rev. Immunol. 2005. 23:1–21
doi: 10.1146/annurev.immunol.23.021704.115806
First published online as a Review in Advance on September 10, 2004

INTERLEUKIN-6: From Basic Science to Medicine—40 Years in Immunology

Tadamitsu Kishimoto

*Graduate School of Frontier Bioscience, Osaka University, Osaka 565-0871,
Japan; email: kishimot@imed3.med.osaka-u.ac.jp*

Key Words   antibody production, B cell differentiation, cytokine, signal
transduction, anticytokine receptor therapy

■ **Abstract**   This essay summarizes my 40 years of research in immunology. As a
young physician, I encountered a patient with Waldenström's macroglobulinemia, and
this inspired me to study the structure of IgM. I began to ask how antibody responses are
regulated. In the late 1960s, the essential role of T cells in antibody production had been
reported. In search of molecules mediating T cell helper function, I discovered activities
in the culture supernatant of T cells that induced proliferation and differentiation of B
cells. This led to my life's work: studying one of those factors, interleukin-6 (IL-6).
To my surprise, IL-6 turned out to play additional roles, including myeloma growth
factor and hepatocyte-stimulating factor activities. More importantly, it was involved
in a number of diseases, such as rheumatoid arthritis and Castleman's disease. I feel
exceptionally fortunate that my work not only revealed the framework of cytokine
signaling, including identification of the IL-6 receptor, gp130, NF-IL6, STAT3, and
SOCS-1, but also led to the development of a new therapy for chronic inflammatory
diseases.

EARLY DAYS

I was born in Japan in 1939, in the southern, rural part of Osaka prefecture. Being
an only child, my parents cherished me too much, turning me into a spoiled child:
You can perhaps trace this element in me even now! In 1946, I entered primary
school near our home and remained in my hometown until graduating from high
school at the age of 18. School was peaceful and idyllic, with plenty of freedom
and no competition.

What first sparked my interest in medicine? It was Dr. Hideyo Noguchi. As a
child, I read his biography and was very impressed by his life and achievements.
I dreamed of becoming a medical researcher in the United States like him. After
finishing at the local high school, I entered Osaka University Medical School,
whose hospital had a strong reputation within Osaka prefecture.

ENCOUNTER WITH MY MENTOR

After a two-year premedical course at Osaka University, I joined the medical school in 1960. I found the lectures in basic medicine, such as anatomy, biochemistry, and pharmacology, boring; they only mentioned facts that we had to memorize. There was certainly no scientific pursuit involved, no question "Why?"

In my fifth year at medical school, Professor Yuichi Yamamura, a professor of biochemistry at Kyushu University, was appointed chairman of the department of medicine at Osaka University. He had graduated from Osaka University Medical School during World War II and served as a doctor in the navy. He discovered that dead mycobacterium could induce cavities in the lungs of rabbits that had been sensitized with BCG, the first demonstration of the involvement of delayed-type hypersensitivity in tuberculosis cavity formation. He went on to identify several cell surface components responsible for the induction of delayed-type hypersensitivity. This led to his life's work: cancer immunotherapy using cellular components of mycobacterium, and from there, the study of innate immunity.

I was excited by Professor Yamamura's lecture on immunological diseases, such as systemic lupus erythematosus. It prompted me to consider many interesting problems. Why does the immune system produce antibodies against the body's own DNA? Why do patients show such a wide variety of symptoms? In response to his lecture, I decided to enter his department and engage in immunology research. It was not only the contents of the lecture that influenced me; I also began to regard Professor Yamamura as my lifetime mentor in medicine.

STUDIES ON IgM

In a ward of the hospital, I met a patient with Waldenström's macroglobulinemia, a disease characterized by increased levels of monoclonal IgM. This prompted me to investigate the molecular structure of IgM. In the mid-1960s, one of the hottest topics in immunology was the structure and function of immunoglobulin molecules. IgM was one of the molecules that particularly attracted immunologists' attention because it loses antibody activities such as hemagglutination upon reduction and alkylation. At that time, Metzger and Small had just published papers claiming that IgM was composed of five subunits with two heavy chains and two light chains (1, 2). In contrast, studies by my supervisor, Dr. Kaoru Onoue, suggested instead that IgM antibody had only five high-affinity antigen-binding sites and each subunit had only one high-affinity site (3).

I purified human IgM from a patient's serum and analyzed its structure by papain and pepsin digestions. I obtained ten Fab papain fragments as well as five $(Fab')^2$ peptic fragments. By employing activated papain without reducing reagents, I succeeded in isolating large Fc fragments with molecular mass of 320 kDa, in which five Fc fragments were linked together with disulfide bridges (4). These results confirmed that IgM was composed of five IgG-like subunits, linked together by disulfide binds between the Fc portions. All these features were later confirmed directly when IgM was visualized by electron microscopy (5). By employing monoclonal IgM with anti-DNP activity, Ashman and Metzger detected ten antigen-binding sites per IgM molecule. With hindsight, the detection of only five binding sites by Onoue was due to heterogeneous affinity of antibody molecules.

Several years ago, I gave a lecture on IL-6 at a medical school in the United States. A graduate student approached me afterwards and said, "I read a paper on molecular structure of IgM in the 1960s authored by T. Kishimoto. Is he your father?" I was pleased to hear this, realizing over again that my research in immunology has spanned 40 years.

B CELL GROWTH AND DIFFERENTIATION FACTORS

In 1970, I went to the United States as a postdoctoral fellow in Dr. K. Ishizaka's laboratory at Johns Hopkins University in Baltimore. It was my first visit to the United States. In the early 1970s, there were still enormous differences between Japan and the United States in every aspect of life. For instance, one dollar was worth 360 yen at that time. My stipend as a "joshu" (equivalent to postdoc in the United States) at the university was 58,000 yen (less than $200) per month. But in the United States, I earned $1000 per month, five times more than the amount I was used to in Japan. There were also big differences in equipment and laboratory instruments. Over the past 30 years, this situation has completely changed. In some cases, the stipend of a postdoctoral fellow in Japan is better than in the United States, and in the leading laboratories, the equipment and instruments are often of higher quality, too. As a result, the younger generation of Japanese students is not as eager to study abroad as my own generation. It is a pity that our young people tend to be less academically "hungry." When I was in the United States, the young Asian scientists there were mostly Japanese, and I think Japanese scientists made a major contribution to the development of the life sciences in America in the 1960s.

In 1967, Dr. Ishizaka identified a new immunoglobulin, IgE, which mediates allergic reactions (6). Johns Hopkins invited him from Children's Asthma Research Institute in Denver, and I joined his group, first as a postdoctoral fellow and later as an assistant professor in 1970. In 1968, interactions between T and B cells in the antibody production were made clear by J.F.A.P. Miller and H. Claman (7, 8). Immunology was rapidly moving from immunochemistry toward cellular immunology. Dr. Ishizaka and I both decided to turn in this direction. We had research backgrounds in immunochemistry, and Dr. Ishizaka was interested in the regulation of IgE production. We thus tried to develop an in vitro culture system in which IgE was produced, as well as IgG and IgM. We measured the amounts of antibodies quantitatively using the immunochemical method. For this purpose we chose rabbit lymphocytes because we were both familiar with rabbit immunoglobulins from our previous studies on IgM and IgE. This system had two disadvantages. First, inbred strains were not available. Second, identification and separation of T and B cells were very difficult, even though anti-Ig columns could be applied for the separation of B cells. Nevertheless, an advantage with the rabbit system was that it was easy to establish an in vitro system for IgE antibody production using the Marbrook method. By using mesenteric lymph node cells primed with DNP-conjugated Ascaris antigen or ragweed antigen, we succeeded in inducing in vitro anti-DNP IgE as well as IgG antibody production by stimulating a DNP-homologous carrier (9).

Armed with this in vitro system, we went on to demonstrate the presence of soluble factors that enhance antibody production. When DNP-Asc primed lymphocytes were cultured with a DNP-heterologous carrier, such as DNP-bovine γ-globulin (DNP-BGG), there was little or no induction of anti-DNP IgG and IgE. By adding the culture supernatants obtained from Asc-primed lymphocytes stimulated with Asc antigen, IgG and IgE antibody production was augmented, which indicated to us the presence of factors responsible for B cell stimulation. Schimpl & Wecker (10) reported the presence of similar factors from alloantigen-stimulated murine T cells. They called these factors T cell replacing factor (TRF).

Dr. Ishizaka and I reported these results in 1973 (11–13). It was a memorable paper for me, because it set me on my life's work studying IL-6. The paper also contained the important suggestion that the factor(s) that enhance the IgE response might be different from those enhancing the IgG response. Culture supernatants from lymphocytes primed with BGG in complete Freund's adjuvant (CFA) augmented the IgG response but not IgE, whereas supernatants from cells primed with ragweed antigen in aluminum hydroxide gel, a very good adjuvant for the IgE response, could induce very high IgE production. Today, every immunologist would interpret this result as Th1 versus Th2 and γ-interferon (IFN) from Th1 versus IL-4 from Th2. In 1973, however, we could not offer a plausible explanation. Speculating that the factor(s) might have Ig-binding activity, we tried to absorb the activity by Ig-conjugated column but were unsuccessful. I am just happy now that our early experimental results in the 1970s already suggested the presence of isotype-specific factors.

In the 1970s, nobody working in immunology was interested in antigen nonspecific factors, or so-called cytokines. People even neglected any activities (or what was going on) in the culture "soup." At that time, most immunologists were instead attracted by so-called "antigen-specific factors." Many experimental results showed that the factors had H-2 restriction and their activity was absorbed with anti-H-2 antibody or antigenic determinants. Now we know this is not true. History teaches us the importance of accurate experiments: We should not be biased by the fashionable ideas of influential scientists.

At that time, I did not believe in the presence of so-called antigen-specific helper or suppressor factors. In fact, I was confident that even the antigen-specific response of lymphocytes would follow the standard theory of cell biology. In the early 1970s, Ishizaka's group elucidated the triggering mechanism of histamine release from basophils: The crosslinkage of high-affinity IgE receptors activates the signal cascade of mast cells (14). I thought that this principle could be applied to the B cell responses; the crosslinkage of antigen receptors on the surface might activate B cells to become responsive to nonspecific T cell factors. My hypothesis was this: The interaction and crosslinkage of antigen receptors of B cells with antigens should be antigen-specific, whereas the factors could be antigen-nonspecific.

To prove this hypothesis, I attempted to induce Ig-production in B cells with anti-Ig and T cell factor(s). It was successful (15). Once again, I owed this success to the use of rabbit lymphocytes. In murine lymphocytes, negative signals through Fc receptors were strong, and Ig-production could not be induced. In the 1970s and 1980s, only studies with murine lymphocytes were widely accepted, so our studies were not generally appreciated. But later, Parker et al. managed to induce Ig in murine B cells by employing anti-Ig-conjugated beads that block negative signals through Fc receptors (16). With this event, our own studies were finally recognized and cited in the field.

The experimental design using anti-Ig plus T cell factor was also used to great effect by W.E. Paul's group (17, 18). This led them to the discovery of BSF-1, later renamed IL-4.

DISCOVERY OF IL-6

After my four years of study in the United States, I returned to the department of medicine in Osaka University chaired by Professor Yamamura, and began to investigate B cell growth and differentiation factors, which led to my life's work, IL-6. At this point, we switched our experimental system from rabbit lymphocytes to human cells for two reasons: (a) Monoclonal and homogeneous cells, such as transformed B cell lines or leukemic cells, were available; and (b) we could easily separate T and B cells by exploiting cell surface markers. We established an in vitro culture system of human peripheral lymphocytes in which polyclonal IgM and IgG production was induced by pokeweed mitogen (PWM) stimulation. We demonstrated that T cell factor(s) released from mitogen-stimulated T cells reconstitute Ig production in PWM-stimulated B cells (19). This confirmed the presence of factors that affect the antibody production of human B cells, just as previously observed in rabbit lymphocytes.

Fortunately, we happened to meet a chronic B cell leukemia (B-CLL) patient whose leukemic cells were responsive to anti-Ig and a cell-free supernatant of PHA-stimulated T cells (PHA-sup). Neither anti-Ig nor PHA-sup alone induced any IgM secretion (20). This confirmed our previous finding with rabbit lymphocytes, i.e., that two signals, crosslinkage of Ig receptors and T cell factor(s), are required for the activation and differentiation of B cells into antibody producing cells. Further characterization of the factors raised the possibility that at least two distinct kinds of factor(s) were present: one for growth of anti-Ig-stimulated B-CLL cells, and the other for differentiation into Ig-producing cells.

While we were studying human T cell factors, Morgan and colleagues (21) reported that a cell-free supernatant from PHA-stimulated T cells induces continuous growth of human T cells. On the basis of this result, Gillis & Smith (22) succeeded in the long-term propagation of human and murine cytotoxic T cells. In light of this, it was clear that we should next test whether all these factors reported on B cells and cytotoxic T cells were the same or different from each other.

In 1976, Dr. R.A. Good, president of the Sloan-Kettering Cancer Institute, visited Osaka for an annual meeting of the Japanese Cancer Association. I took Dr. and Mrs. Good to Kyoto for some sightseeing. During the short visit, Dr. Good appeared more interested in my ongoing experiments than in sightseeing! He kindly invited me to spend a couple of months every summer at the Sloan-Kettering. This gave me a great opportunity to screen a number of transformed or neoplastic B and T cell lines that were available at the Sloan-Kettering: B cell lines responsive to T cells factors, and T cell lines that secrete T cell factors. During my stay at the Sloan-Kettering, I identified several transformed B cell lines that produced Igs responding to T cell factor(s). One of these was the famous CESS cell line, which was later used as the indicator cells in the cloning of IL-6. I also found a subclone of a T cell line, CEM, which could be used as parental cells for generation of human T cell hybridomas. By establishing T cell hybridomas, we demonstrated the presence of two different kinds of B cell stimulatory factors: one for the growth of anti-Ig-stimulated B-CLL cells, and the other for Ig-induction in B-CLL cells or CESS cells (23).

Using murine lymphocytes, W.E. Paul, M. Howard, and their colleagues (24) suggested the presence of a B cell–specific growth factor (BCGF). They used a short-term B cell costimulator assay with anti-IgM. In their study, proliferation of anti-IgM-stimulated B cells was augmented by adding a culture supernatant of a mitogen-stimulated murine thymoma cell line (EL-4). They showed that this activity is different from IL-2 because it was not absorbed by an IL-2-dependent cytotoxic T cell line. The factor was later purified to homogeneity by their group as BSF-1, and its cDNA was cloned by Dr. T. Honjo's group. It is now called IL-4. The presence of a second BCGF activity was also reported by several groups, including K. Takatsu's and S. Swain's (25, 26). This factor, which they called B151 TRF or (DL)BCGF, induced growth and IgM production in the murine B cell line, BCL_1. Later, this factor was cloned and named IL-5.

From the late 1970s to the early 1980s, a number of factors were reported, but none of them were purified and their cDNAs were not cloned. Many questions were waiting to be answered. For instance (*a*) Do B cell–specific growth and differentiation factors really exist that are distinct from the growth factor for cytotoxic T cells (IL-2)? (*b*) If they do, how many factors are there? (*c*) Is B cell–specific growth factor different from B cell differentiation factor? In the early 1980s, the field of immunology was flooded with, and hampered by, complicated nomenclatures. It was evident that there were more names than factors to be named!

Under such circumstances, Dr. W.E. Paul and I organized a meeting to consider the nomenclature of these substances when the International Congress of

Immunology was held in Kyoto in August 1983. At the meeting, participants agreed that factors that had been functionally and chemically well characterized should be given a formal designation, namely B cell stimulatory factor (BSF) followed by a consecutive number (i.e., BSF-1, BSF-2. . .). On the basis of the available data, the 20 kDa mouse BCGF, studied by W.E. Paul's group, was designated BSF-1, while our human B cell differentiation factor (BCDF), which induces Ig-induction in CESS cells and B-CLL cells, was named BSF-2. However, these designations did not last long, because within a few years all the cDNAs encoding BSFs were cloned. In 1985, I wrote a review article for the *Annual Review of Immunology* entitled "Factors Affecting B Cell Growth and Differentiation" (27). In the conclusion, I wrote, "The isolation of several B cell stimulatory factors and the cloning and sequencing of their genes should be accomplished in the near future. And the activation mechanism of B cells may be revealed at molecular level by employing theoretically pure recombinant BSFs." Within a year, in 1986, the cDNAs encoding BSFs had been cloned. This led me to an entirely new world, which I had never expected. BSFs were not merely B cell stimulatory factors!

INTO MOLECULAR IMMUNOLOGY

Cloning of IL-6

In early 1980s, my mentor, Professor Yamamura, was elected president of Osaka University. He established the Institute for Molecular and Cellular Biology as a research center for molecular biology, and he invited Professor Yoshio Okada, who discovered cell fusion by Sendai virus in the 1950s, to be a director of the Institute. I joined him in 1983. This move enabled me to accomplish more molecular-oriented research into B cell factors. We invited Dr. Tadatsugu Taniguchi from Tokyo to the institute as a professor. At that time, he was only 35 years old and the youngest professor at Osaka University. He had succeeded in cloning the cDNA for IL-2 in 1983 (28), in the face of tough international competition. This was the first cloning of a cDNA for an interleukin. The field of "factor(s)" was heading inexorably to the molecular level. Because I was trained as a medical doctor, I had no background in molecular biology, having never been involved in cDNA cloning or DNA sequencing. The early 1980s were therefore difficult years for us.

T. Honjo, who had done beautiful work on Ig isotype switching in the 1970s, moved into the field of interleukins. At a meeting held in late 1985 in Japan, he reported that his group had succeeded in isolating the cDNA encoding BSF-1, later called IL-4. The paper was published in early 1986 (29). I was very much surprised and shocked. Indeed, I felt that I had been completely defeated. Dr. Honjo also reported, together with Dr. Takatsu, the cloning of the cDNA for (B151) TRF, later called IL-5, at the International Congress of Immunology in Toronto in the summer of 1986.

It was really hard for us to isolate a cDNA for BCDF/BSF-2 because we did not have experience in the field of molecular biology. After several years of struggling with repeated failures, I, together with T. Hirano and colleagues, finally obtained what we wanted in June 1986: the cDNA for BSF-2, later called IL-6 (30). I appreciated the technical assistance and advice of Dr. T. Taniguchi. We submitted a paper to *Nature*, but at that time I was worried that our molecule might be the same as T. Honjo's TRF/BCGF II, and hence our paper would be rejected. In spite of my worry, both papers, his and ours, were published in the same issue of *Nature* in November (31). The two molecules were fortunately different from each other.

While trying to isolate the cDNA for BSF-2, we noticed that the same activity was observed in cardiac myxoma cells (32, 33). Cardiac myxoma is a benign heart tumor originating from the atrium. Patients with cardiac myxoma exhibit a wide variety of autoimmune and inflammatory symptoms, including autoantibodies, fever, joint pains, and anemia. All these symptoms disappear after surgical removal of the tumors. We found that cardiac myxoma cells produced a large amount of BSF-2 detectable by our antibody against purified BSF-2. With this result, I thought the molecule we were studying might contribute to the pathology of autoimmune diseases and play an important role not only in B cell immunology but also in various diseases. Perhaps I could attribute this kind of instinct to my medical training.

Biology of IL-6

Cloning of the BSF-2/IL-6 cDNA revealed that this molecule had in fact been studied under several different names by numerous labs. It seemed that IL-6 might have various interesting biological activities not limited to B cell immunology. It had been regarded as a novel interferon, but studies with recombinant IL-6 and anti-IL-6 antibody demonstrated that this was not the case (34).

As mentioned earlier, structural studies of immunoglobulin (Ig) molecules were hot topics in immunology in the 1950s and 1960s. Every immunologist wanted to have murine monoclonal Igs. M. Potter succeeded in generating murine plasmacytomas by simply injecting mineral oil into the peritoneal cavities of BALB/c mice (35). This achievement accelerated the structural and genetic studies on immunoglobulins. Intraperitoneal injection of mineral oil induced granulomas that produced plasmacytoma growth factor. One year after IL-6 was cloned, the partial amino acid sequence of plasmacytoma growth factor was determined, and it turned out to be mouse IL-6 (36). Indeed, transgenic expression of IL-6 in BALB/c mice induced monoclonal, transplantable plasmacytomas (37), confirming that IL-6 functions as a plasmacytoma growth factor. In addition, it turned out that human myeloma cells were responsive to IL-6, and some myeloma cells also produced IL-6. In most cases, bone marrow stromal cells produced a large amount of IL-6, which might be responsible for the generation and expansion of multiple myelomas in the bone marrow (38). I remember vividly how much I was excited by the fact that IL-6 functioned as a myeloma/plasmacytoma growth factor.

Another excitement for me at that time was the discovery that IL-6 functions as a hepatocyte stimulating factor (HSF) (39, 40). It was already known that acute inflammation is accompanied by changes in concentration of many plasma proteins, a decrease in albumin and increased levels of many so-called acute phase proteins, including C-reactive protein (CRP), fibrinogen, serum amyloid protein, and haptoglobin. Indeed, this observation had been applied to various laboratory tests for the diagnosis of disease. Because inflammation, injury, or cancer in other parts of the body results in the increased synthesis of acute phase proteins in the liver, some had suggested the existence of hormone-like mediators, termed HSF. Using recombinant IL-6 and anti-IL-6 antibody, Gauldie, Heinrich, and colleagues (39, 40) confirmed that HSF was in fact IL-6. This opened up a new field studying cytokines and disease. Later, generation of IL-6 knockout mice by G. Köhler and his group showed that IL-6 was an essential molecule for antiviral antibody responses, as well as for the induction of acute phase reaction (41). We were getting almost daily requests for IL-6 cDNA protein and antibody from immunologists all over the world, and most weeks we learned fascinating new information about IL-6 function.

IL-6 Receptor and gp130

Despite this excitement, I decided not to expand our studies on the activities of IL-6 on various tissues and cells but moved directly to the subcellular level: receptors, signaling molecules, and gene expression. At that time, absolutely nothing was known about cytokine signal transduction. I particularly wanted to reveal the signaling pathway of cytokines "from surface to nucleus" by using IL-6 as a model. In the mid-1980s, none of the cytokine receptors, except for IL-2 receptor α chain (TAC), had been identified at the molecular level. The number of cytokine receptors on the cell surface is usually on the order of 10^2 to 10^3, a hundred times less than that of hormone or growth factor receptors. Seed & Aruffo (42) developed a high efficiency COS cell expression vector, and shortly afterward we succeeded in isolating the cDNA for IL-6 receptor by employing this method. This was the first example of the cloning of a cytokine receptor. It had an Ig-like domain at the N-terminal but no unique sequences in any other portions. It had a very short intracytoplasmic portion and did not have kinase domains. These features made it unlike an authentic "receptor" at that time, and *Nature* did not want to publish it, but *Science* kindly accepted it in 1988 (43). In the following two years, most cytokine receptors, including interferon receptors, IL-2 receptor β chain, and erythropoietin receptor, were isolated using the same or similar methods. The results were very interesting. They each showed very similar tertiary structures and thus comprised a large family of cytokine receptors. Even receptors for growth hormone and prolactin belong to this family.

Our excitement continued. We prepared an antibody against IL-6 receptor which could precipitate the 80 kDa protein. Interestingly, when T. Taga precipitated the IL-6 receptor following IL-6 stimulation of cells, another protein of 130 kDa was always coprecipitated (44). Without stimulation, only the 80 kDa band could be detected. I was thrilled with this result and speculated that the IL-6 receptor consisted of two polypeptide chains, 80 kDa and 130 kDa, and that IL-6 stimulation would trigger association of the two chains. As the 80 kDa IL-6 receptor had a very short intracytoplasmic portion without any unique sequence, it was reasonable for us to speculate that the 130 kDa chain was responsible for signal transduction. We called this molecule simply gp130, because it was a cell surface glycoprotein of 130 kDa. Fortunately, in less than a year, we isolated a cDNA for gp130 by using anti-gp130 antibody (45).

Our excitement still continued. When we examined the expression pattern of gp130, we found it was expressed ubiquitously in all tissues, even in cells that lacked detectable expression of the 80 kDa IL-6 receptor (45). This result suggested to me that gp130 was not merely a component of the IL-6 receptor; perhaps it functioned as a common signal transducer for various cytokines. If many different cytokines shared the same receptor component, then we could easily explain the redundant activity of several cytokines.

This prediction turned out to be true. In the following years, we and others, including Dr. Yancopoulos, Dr. Metcalf, and colleagues, reported that ciliary neurotropic factor (CNTF), leukemia inhibitory factor (LIF), oncostatin M (OM), IL-11, and cardiotropin-1 (CT-1) all used gp130 as a component of their receptors (46–50). This explained why these cytokines had very similar activities. IL-6 was shown to inhibit the growth of a murine leukemic cell line, M1, and to induce differentiation into macrophages. Sachs and Metcalf also reported on factors called MGI-2 and LIF, respectively (51, 52), which exert a similar activity on M1 cells. MGI-2 turned out to be identical to IL-6, although LIF remained a distinct molecule. It became clear that LIF used gp130 as its receptor component, which explained why IL-6 and LIF show similar biological activities. The principle that cytokine receptors consist of two polypeptide chains, namely a specific receptor for each cytokine and a common signal transducer, turned out to be applicable to other cytokine receptor systems, too. For example, IL-3, IL-5, and GM-CSF use a common β component as their receptors. Interleukins for the growth and development of lymphocytes, IL-2, IL-4, IL-7, IL-9, and IL-15, use a common γ-component that was originally identified as a component of IL-2 receptor. I think the discovery of gp130 may be one of my most important achievements, for it introduced a completely new concept into the cytokine receptor field.

MAP Kinase-NF-IL6 Pathway

IL-6 is produced not only by T cells, but also by a panoply of cells including macrophages, fibroblasts, synovial cells, endothelial cells, glia cells, and keratinocytes. IL-6 expression was induced by a variety of stimuli, including cytokines such as IL-1, tumor necrosis factor (TNF), and platelet-derived growth factor (PDGF). Bacterial and viral infection and microbial components such as lipopolysaccharide (LPS) were also potent inducers of IL-6.

All the above findings led me to study the mechanisms of the IL-6 gene expression. One year after the isolation of the IL-6 cDNA, S. Akira and his colleagues cloned the IL-6 gene and searched the promoter regions of the gene responsible for the regulation of IL-6 expression. We determined a novel 14 bp dyad sequence motif in the IL-6 promoter region that conferred IL-1-induced IL-6 expression. Next, we identified a nuclear factor binding to this motif, NF-IL6 (53). The cDNA of NF-IL6 was cloned, and shortly afterwards it became clear that it contains a region highly homologous to C/EBP, a rat liver nuclear factor with a leucine zipper structure.

Interestingly, although C/EBP was constitutively expressed, NF-IL6 was only expressed upon stimulation with various inflammatory signals such as LPS, IL-1, TNF, and even IL-6. Particularly in the liver, various stimuli, including IL-6, strongly induced NF-IL6 but not IL-6. This indicated that NF-IL6 might be responsible for the induction of acute phase proteins. Indeed, NF-IL6 was bound to the IL-6-responsive elements in the promoter regions of acute phase genes. These results showed that C/EBP and NF-IL6 were involved in negative and positive acute phase reactions, respectively: C/EBP is constitutively expressed and regulates the albumin gene, whereas NF-IL6, which is induced by inflammatory signals including IL-6, positively regulates the expression of the acute phase genes. We studied the transcriptional activation of NF-IL6 to elucidate the signal transduction pathway through gp130. Phosphorylation of NF-IL6 at threonine 235 by a Ras-dependent MAP kinase was shown to be essential for transcription factor activity (54). Although we had clearly identified one of the pathways of signal transduction through gp130, this was not so exciting because a Ras/MAP kinase cascade had been already described in the signaling of various growth factors.

JAK-STAT Pathway

As mentioned above, none of the cytokine receptors have tyrosine kinase domains in their cytoplasmic regions. Nevertheless, dimerization of the receptors can activate tyrosine kinase activity in cells. We had previously noticed that various members of the cytokine receptor family contain similar sequences of about 60 amino acids in their membrane-proximal cytoplasmic regions. In particular, 8 amino acid stretches in these regions were strongly conserved. We termed these stretches Box1, and speculated that they might bind specific intracytoplasmic tyrosine kinases (55, 56). Although we searched extensively for tyrosine kinases that would bind to the dimerized gp130, we were beaten in this race by J. Ihle's group (57–59). They identified JAK family tyrosine kinases as the major players downstream of the receptor in cytokine signal transduction.

Acute phase gene expression is the most suitable model for the study of signal transduction through gp130. Two types of IL-6 responsive element, type 1 and type 2, were present in the promoter regions of the acute phase genes. Type 1 IL-6 responsive element bound members of the C/EBP family, including NF-IL6 that we had already identified (53). A nuclear factor, which bound to Type 2 IL-6 responsive element, was identified by P. Heinrich and colleagues (60). They called this nuclear factor acute phase responsive factor (APRF). IL-6 stimulation induced tyrosine phosphorylation of APRF within minutes, and the phosphorylated APRF was translocated into the nucleus. This process was strongly reminiscent of the activation of interferon-stimulated gene factor 3 (ISGF3) following IFN stimulation. Therefore, we hypothesized that APRF was a target of JAK tyrosine kinases and an important downstream component of signal transduction through gp130. S. Akira and his colleagues set out to clone the cDNA for APRF. It was a tough competition with P. Heinrich. I thought that Heinrich's group had almost done it. However, Akira's group succeeded in isolating the cDNA sooner than I had expected. They injected recombinant IL-6 into mice intravenously and isolated livers within minutes. They used approximately 8000 mice and a large amount of recombinant IL-6. These reagents would have cost about $2 million if we had purchased them commercially, but instead they were kindly donated by Ajinomoto Co. Ltd.

Our cloning of APRF revealed that it had a high degree of homology to the p91 subunit of the ISGF3 family involved in IFN signaling (61). APRF was tyrosine phosphorylated and translocated to the nucleus in response to IL-6 in hepatocytes. Tyrosine phosphorylation of APRF was also observed in response to other cytokines (LIF, OM, CNTF, CT-1, and IL-11) whose receptors share gp130, but not in response to IFN. In contrast, p91 was not phosphorylated in response to IL-6. From these results, we surmised that several different p91-related factors were present, and selective activation of those factors might explain the diversity of cellular responses to different cytokines. Later this was confirmed by the isolation of different p91-related factors, now called STATs (from STAT1 to STAT6). In February 1994, just after cloning the APRF cDNA, I went to the United States and learned that J. Darnell's group had already cloned a novel p91-related factor named STAT3 and submitted the paper to *Science*. We submitted our paper to *Cell*, asking the editor to publish it simultaneously with Darnell's paper in *Science*. Fortunately, both their paper and ours appeared in April 1994 in *Science* and *Cell*, respectively (61, 62).

Negative Feedback Pathway, SOCS

After the isolation of STAT3, we were naturally led to search for other members of the STAT family. Using the monoclonal antibody that we had generated against a sequence motif found in the SH2 domain of STAT3, we screened a murine thymus cDNA library and isolated about 20 new genes. One of them encoded the molecule that we originally called SSI-1 (STAT-induced STAT inhibitor) (63). Dominant-negative STAT3 could inhibit the IL-6- or LIF-induced SSI-1 expression, indicating that this was one of the target genes of STAT3. Moreover, overexpression of SSI-1 could inhibit LIF- or IL-6-induced M1 differentiation. When SSI-1 and JAK-1 were coexpressed in COS cells, SSI-1 interacted with JAK-1 and inhibited its kinase activity. We concluded that SSI-1 must be involved in the negative feedback regulation of cytokine signals. At that time, the Hilton, Nicola, and Metcalf group at the Walter and Eliza Hall Institute and Yoshimura at Kurume University each cloned the same gene, and the three papers were published together in the same issue of *Nature* in June 1997 (64, 65). An Australian group named it SOCS, for suppressor of cytokine signals. Because this terminology represents the biological nature of this molecule more exactly than SSI, it has become the widely used nomenclature.

My investigation into how IL-6 signals are transmitted and regulated from "cell surface to the nucleus" is now almost complete. Our group has identified almost all the signaling components except for JAK tyrosine kinase, including IL-6, IL-6 receptor, gp130, NF-IL6, STAT3 (APRF), and SOCS (SSI). Our group at Institute for Cellular and Molecular Biology at Osaka University was most active in the late 1980s and early 1990s. In those times, more than 30 students and research fellows were working there, and interesting results emerged almost weekly. Indeed, someone in the United States once commented, "We can never compete with Kishimoto's Army!"

Other Projects Besides IL-6

Besides IL-6-related studies, several interesting projects were going on in our laboratory at that time. H. Kikutani's group was studying IgE binding receptors, and they identified the B cell marker CD23 as FcεRII (66, 67). At that time, the existence of many B cell markers, such as CD19, CD20, and CD21, were known, but their function or natural ligands were not. An exception was CD21, which functioned as receptor for a complement fragment, C3d and Epstein-Barr virus. Thus, CD23 was the second marker whose function was disclosed. Moreover, they identified two different species of FcεRII, i.e., FcεRIIa and IIb, which had different structures in their N-terminal intracytoplasmic portions. Interestingly, FcεRIIa expression was limited to a certain stage of B cells, but FcεRIIb was expressed on B cells, monocytes, and eosinophils, and their expression was regulated by IL-4 (68).

T. Nagasawa and H. Kikutani identified a new cytokine involved in pre–B cell development, called PBSF (SDF-1) (69). The essential role of PBSF/SDF-1 in B lymphopoiesis was confirmed by the preparation of the gene-deficient mice (70). An interesting story emerged when Nagasawa isolated a receptor for PBSF/SDF1 (CXCR4) (71). He noticed that its sequence was a murine homolog of fusin, the human immunodeficiency virus I entry coreceptor. This suggested to us that inhibitors of CXCR4 might be created as efficient drugs for AIDS. However, when he generated the CXCR4 knockout mice (72), they were embryonic lethal, raising potential safety problems with such drugs. Interestingly, these mice were defective in the large vessels supplying the gastrointestinal tract, indicating the existence of a new signaling system for organ vascularization.

We also identified a novel molecule for bone development (73). Komori, in our laboratory, was also studying B lymphopoiesis. To see how a transcription factor, cbf1, would function in the lymphoid development, he prepared the knockout mice as usual. To our surprise, knockout mice died just after birth without breathing.

He noticed that the mice did not have any bone, completely lacking ossification. In other words, cbf1 plays an essential role in osteogenesis. The result contributed to the subsequent identification of the gene responsible for a dominantly inherited disease, cleidocranial dysplasia. Komori went into the field of bone research and has been publishing interesting papers ever since.

BENCH TO BEDSIDE

In 1991, when the activities of our laboratory at the Institute for Cellular and Molecular Biology were at their peak, I was asked to be chairman of the department of medicine. My mentor, Professor Yamamura, who used to hold the post, had passed away in 1990. Having entered that department in 1965 after graduating from the medical school, I had a nostalgic feeling toward the department, but I initially declined the invitation, wanting to continue my basic studies. However, the medical school faculty persisted in their attempts to persuade me, and finally I accepted the invitation. In an article that appeared in *Science* in 1990, I read an impressive passage: "With science having largely demystified the 'witchcraft' of immune response, immunologists are turning to the next challenge: putting their new knowledge to clinical use in taming pathological immune responses. Successes are still mostly on the horizon." I felt it was the appropriate time to try to apply our basic studies on IL-6 to human disease.

I had been at a similar crossroads one year earlier. I was invited to Harvard Medical School, which offered me a chaired professorship in the department of medicine. Professor Tosteson, dean of the school, said to me, "The most excellent graduate students and postdoctoral fellows come to Harvard from all over the world, and you can do your research with them. You may not be able to make such an environment in Osaka." While I was wavering between going to Boston and staying in Osaka, Professor Yamamura, who was seriously sick at the time, told me not to go. He urged me instead to work for Japanese science and young Japanese scientists. So, after experiencing several difficult choices in my life, I finally moved to the department of medicine as chairman.

While studying IL-6, I had noticed that this molecule is involved in various diseases, including chronic inflammation and hemopoietic malignancies. For example, cardiac myxoma cells produce large amounts of IL-6, which explains various symptoms of the patients. In 1988, we reported the constitutive overproduction of IL-6 by synovial tissues of rheumatoid patients (74). This well explains all the symptoms seen in patients. We also found an abnormal overproduction of IL-6 in patients with Castleman's disease (75). Affected lymph node cells overproduced IL-6, which explained symptoms such as high fever, anemia, acute phase reactions, hyper γ-globulinemia, secondary amyloidosis, and massive plasma cell infiltration into affected lymph nodes. Later, it turned out that a Kaposi's sarcoma associated herpesvirus [Human Herpes Virus 8 (HHV-8)] was a causative agent, and a viral genome could be detected in Castleman's lymph nodes (76). The HHV-8 genome encoded a viral IL-6 that directly binds human gp130 to stimulate the production of endogenous IL-6 (77). From these findings in patients with cardiac myxomas, rheumatoid arthritis, and Castleman's disease, we expected that the blockade of IL-6 and its receptor interactions would provide a new therapy for these diseases.

On the basis of these experimental and clinical results, we started to develop an anti-IL6 receptor blockade therapy. Together with Chugai Pharmaceutical Co. Ltd. and the MRC Collaborative Center in London, mouse monoclonal antibody binding human IL-6 receptor was humanized by complementarity-determing region (CDR) grafting. This antibody was applied to treat seven patients with multicentric Castleman's disease, with the approval of our institute's ethical committee and the patients' consent (78). Immediately after administering the antibody, fever and fatigue disappeared, while anemia, as well as serum levels of C-reactive protein, fibrinogen, and albumin started to improve. After three months of treatment, hyper γ-globulinemia and lymphadenopathy were remarkably alleviated, as were renal function abnormalities in patients with amyloidosis. The pathophysiologic significance of IL-6 in Castleman's disease was thus confirmed, and blockade of IL-6 signal by anti-IL-6 receptor antibody was shown to be a potential new therapy for IL-6-related diseases. The phase II clinical trial with 28 Castleman's patients was done in 2002, and the antibody showed a significant effect on all patients. As Castleman's disease is an orphan disease, the antibody for this disease will be on the market in the beginning of 2005.

After the successful experimental therapy of Castleman's patients, we tried to apply the same antibody for the treatment of rheumatoid patients. To investigate the direct role of IL-6 in the development of rheumatoid arthritis, IL-6-deficient mice were backcrossed for eight generations into C57BL/6 mice, and histological manifestations were compared between wild-type and IL-6-deficient mice following the induction of antigen-induced arthritis (79). Wild-type mice developed severe arthritis, whereas IL-6-deficient mice displayed little or no arthritis. The expression of TNF mRNA in the synovial tissues in IL-6-deficient mice was comparable to that of wild-type mice, even though no arthritis was observed in the former. Recently, S. Sakaguchi and colleagues reported that deleting the IL-6 gene in his SKG mice, which develop rheumatoid arthritis owing to the mutation of the T cell signaling pathway, resulted in the complete protection from the development of the disease, whereas 20% of TNF-α-deficient SKG mice still developed the disease (80). All these basic studies encouraged me to apply anti-IL-6 receptor therapy to patients with rheumatoid arthritis.

In 2001 and 2002, phase II trials had been completed in Japan with 164 patients, and in Europe with 359 patients. The results were comparable with or better than anti-TNF antibody or soluble TNF receptor therapies (81). The incidence of a 20% improvement in disease activity according to the American College of Rheumatology criteria (ACR20) was 78% in the Japanese phase II trial. The incidences of 50% and 70% improvement in disease activity (ACR50 and ACR70) were 40% and 16%, respectively. In long-term trials of over 15 months, ACR20, 50, and 70 reached 88%, 67%, and 42%, respectively. After long-term administration, the serum IL-6 level gradually decreased and reached an undetectable level in some patients, which suggested that anti-IL-6 receptor therapy was not simply anti-inflammatory but might affect the fundamentals of the immune system. At present, large-scale phase III trials are being carried out in Japan by Chugai Pharma Co. Ltd. and in Europe and the United States by Roche Co. Ltd. The results of these trials will be available in 2005 and 2007, respectively.

Another exciting clinical result was observed in the treatment of systemic onset juvenile idiopathic arthritis (sJIA). sJIA is a severe multi-organ disease, which is accompanied by symptoms such as spiking fever, skin rash, arthritis, pericarditis, hepatosplenomegaly and growth retardation. A high dose of corticosteroids is the only medication that suppresses the disease activity, and anti-TNF therapy is not very effective. Phase I/II trials of 11 children were carried out by Professor Yokota in Yokohama City University. After administration of the antibody, high-grade or quotidian fever subsided and arthritis improved quickly in all the children, accompanied by the normalization of all the laboratory tests, including CRP. Eighteen months after treatment, we observed that one of the children grew taller by 18 cm. IL-6 inhibits the signaling pathway provided by growth hormone, and so the result confirmed that the growth retardation observed in sJIA was due to the overproduction of IL-6. Long-term administration normalized the serum IL-6 levels in several children, which again indicated that IL-6 might fundamentally restore the immune disorders in sJIA. At the moment, we do not understand the pathogenesis of sJIA. Because the effects of our antibody treatment on sJIA patients were so dramatic, further studies into changes in immune function and gene expression in the patients before and after treatment might provide important insights into the pathogenesis of the disease. If so, our studies "from laboratory to clinic" will again move "from clinic to basic studies."

FROM UNIVERSITY PRESIDENT TO COUNCIL FOR SCIENCE AND TECHNOLOGY POLICY

In June 1997, I was elected president of Osaka University. I felt greatly honored to be president of my alma mater, one of the most prestigious universities in Japan. However, for a while I could not decide whether to accept the position, for several reasons. A big research grant ($3 million per year for five years) had recently been awarded to my laboratory in April. At that time, I really wanted to concentrate on my research because it was getting very exciting. I agreed to be president on the condition that I could still be involved in research. But I soon realized that it was almost impossible to combine the two roles. Our studies on SOCS were lagging very much behind those of the Melbourne group. I realized that good research required concentration. As president, I devoted myself to the development of Osaka University as a more internationally competitive research-oriented university. I had established two new graduate schools, for frontier bioscience and information science. All ten faculties, including natural as well as social and human sciences, had been reorganized as graduate schools, to which undergraduate courses were attached. The annual budget reached almost $1 billion, and the quantity of competitive research grants was increased.

My six-year term as a president ended in August 2003, and I was very much looking forward to being back in the laboratory. I thought that I might still catch up with the front line. I was donated $5 million by Chugai Pharma Co. Ltd. to establish my laboratory in the graduate school of frontier biosciences. As a professor of immunology, I restarted my laboratory with several faculty, fellows, and graduate students. Our aims are to reveal the mechanism whereby blockade of IL-6 signaling could show such a significant curable effect on JIA or RA. It was not due to a simple anti-inflammatory effect, as I have already discussed. My studies originated in B cell immunology, developed into molecular immunology, and moved into clinical medicine, and are once again going back to basic immunology and molecular biology.

When I had just restarted my laboratory, I was asked to be a member of the Council for Science and Technology Policy in the Japanese government, chaired by the prime minister. Again, I hesitated to accept but was persuaded that it was a very important task upon which the future of Japanese science depended. I am now mainly working at the cabinet office in Tokyo, three or four days a week, with one or two days in my laboratory at Osaka University. I would be happy if I could devote myself to creating better environments for young talented scientists in Japan.

Here I am closing the story of my 40-year history as a basic immunologist, a chairman of internal medicine, a university president and a policy maker in Japanese science. I think I was very lucky as a researcher because I found an interesting molecule, IL-6, with pleiotropic activity and an involvement in the pathogenesis of several diseases. Now, the results are going to be applied to patients with otherwise incurable diseases. Through these studies, many young scientists were trained to become internationally highly regarded researchers, including Drs. T. Hirano, H. Kikutani, S. Akira, and T. Taga. If I were embarking on my career again today, I think I would hesitate to follow the same path: 1 may not be so fortunate the next time!

The *Annual Review of Immunology* is online at http://immunol.annualreviews.org

LITERATURE CITED

1. Miller F, Metzger H. 1965. Characterization of a human macroglobulin. II. Distribution of the disulfide bonds. *J. Biol. Chem.* 240:4740–45

2. Lamm ME, Small PA Jr. 1966. Polypeptide chain structure of rabbit immunoglobulins. II. γM-immunoglobulin. *Biochemistry* 5:267–76

3. Onoue K, Kishimoto T, Yamamura Y. 1968. Structure of human immunoglobulin M.

II. Isolation of a high molecular weight Fc fragment of IgM composed of several Fc subunits. *J. Immunol.* 100:238–44

4. Kishimoto T, Onoue K, Yamamura Y. 1968. Structure of human immunoglobulin M. 3. Pepsin fragmentation of IgM. *J. Immunol.* 100:1032–40

5. Svehag SE, Chesebro B, Bloth B. 1967. Ultrastructure of γM immunoglobulin and

α macroglobulin: electron-microscopic study. *Science* 158:933–36

6. Ishizaka K, Ishizaka T, Terry WD. 1967. Antigenic structure of γE-globulin and reaginic antibody. *J. Immunol.* 99:849–58

7. Miller JF, Mitchell GF. 1968. Cell to cell interaction in the immune response. I. Hemolysin-forming cells in neonatally thymectomized mice reconstituted with thymus or thoracic duct lymphocytes. *J. Exp. Med.* 128:801–20

8. Claman HN, Chaperon EA, Selner JC. 1968. Thymus-marrow immunocompetence. 3. The requirement for living thymus cells. *Proc. Soc. Exp. Biol. Med.* 127:462–66

9. Ishizaka K, Kishimoto T. 1972. Regulation of antibody response in vitro. II. Formation of rabbit reaginic antibody. *J. Immunol.* 109:65–73

10. Schimpl A, Wecker E. 1973. Studies on the source and action of the T-cell replacing factor (TRF). *Adv. Exp. Med. Biol.* 29:179–82

11. Kishimoto T, Ishizaka K. 1973. Regulation of antibody response in vitro. VII. Enhancing soluble factors for IgG and IgE antibody response. *J. Immunol.* 111:1194–205

12. Kishimoto T, Ishizaka K. 1973. Regulation of antibody response in vitro. VI. Carrier-specific helper cells for IgG and IgE antibody response. *J. Immunol.* 111:720–32

13. Kishimoto T, Ishizaka K. 1973. Regulation of antibody response in vitro. V. Effect of carrier-specific helper cells on generation of hapten-specific memory cells of different immunoglobulin classes. *J. Immunol.* 111:1–9

14. Ishizaka T, Tomioka H, Ishizaka K. 1971. Degranulation of human basophil leukocytes by anti-γE antibody. *J. Immunol.* 106:705–10

15. Kishimoto T, Miyake T, Nishizawa Y, Watanabe T, Yamamura Y. 1975. Triggering mechanism of B lymphocytes. I. Effect of anti-immunoglobulin and enhancing soluble factor on differentiation and proliferation of B cells. *J. Immunol.* 115:1179–84

16. Parker DC, Wadsworth DC, Schneider GB. 1980. Activation of murine B lymphocytes by anti-immunoglobulin is an inductive signal leading to immunoglobulin secretion. *J. Exp. Med.* 152:138–50

17. Howard M, Paul WE. 1983. Regulation of B-cell growth and differentiation by soluble factors. *Annu. Rev. Immunol.* 1:307–33

18. Nakanishi K, Howard M, Muraguchi A, Farrar J, Takatsu K, et al. 1983. Soluble factors involved in B cell differentiation: identification of two distinct T cell–replacing factors (TRF). *J. Immunol.* 130:2219–24

19. Hirano T, Kuritani T, Kishimoto T, Yamamura Y. 1977. In vitro immune response of human peripheral lymphocytes. I. The mechanism(s) involved in T cell helper functions in the pokeweed mitogen-induced differentiation and proliferation of B cells. *J. Immunol.* 119:1235–41

20. Yoshizaki K, Nakagawa T, Kaieda T, Muraguchi A, Yamamura Y, Kishimoto T. 1982. Induction of proliferation and Ig production in human B leukemic cells by anti-immunoglobulins and T cell factors. *J. Immunol.* 128:1296–301

21. Ruscetti FW, Morgan DA, Gallo RC. 1977. Functional and morphologic characterization of human T cells continuously grown in vitro. *J. Immunol.* 119:131–38

22. Gillis S, Smith KA. 1977. Long term culture of tumour-specific cytotoxic T cells. *Nature* 268:154–56

23. Kishimoto T, Hirano T, Kuritani T, Yamamura Y, Ralph P, Good RA. 1978. Induction of IgG production in human B lymphoblastoid cell lines with normal human T cells. *Nature* 271:756–58

24. Howard M, Farrar J, Hilfiker M, Johnson B, Takatsu K, et al. 1982. Identification of a T cell–derived B cell growth factor distinct from interleukin 2. *J. Exp. Med.* 155:914–23

25. Takatsu K, Tominaga A, Hamaoka T. 1980. Antigen-induced T cell–replacing factor (TRF). I. Functional characterization of a TRF-producing helper T cell subset and

genetic studies on TRF production. *J. Immunol.* 124:2414–22

26. Swain SL, Dutton RW. 1982. Production of a B cell growth-promoting activity, (DL)BCGF, from a cloned T cell line and its assay on the BCL1 B cell tumor. *J. Exp. Med.* 156:1821–34

27. Kishimoto T. 1985. Factors affecting B-cell growth and differentiation. *Annu. Rev. Immunol.* 3:133–57

28. Taniguchi T, Matsui H, Fujita T, Takaoka C, Kashima N, et al. 1983. Structure and expression of a cloned cDNA for human interleukin-2. *Nature* 302:305–10

29. Noma Y, Sideras P, Naito T, Bergstedt-Lindquist S, Azuma C, et al. 1986. Cloning of cDNA encoding the murine IgG1 induction factor by a novel strategy using SP6 promoter. *Nature* 319:640–46

30. Hirano T, Yasukawa K, Harada H, Taga T, Watanabe Y, et al. 1986. Complementary DNA for a novel human interleukin (BSF-2) that induces B lymphocytes to produce immunoglobulin. *Nature* 324:73–76

31. Kinashi T, Harada N, Severinson E, Tanabe T, Sideras P, et al. 1986. Cloning of complementary DNA encoding T-cell replacing factor and identity with B-cell growth factor II. *Nature* 324:70–73

32. Hirano T, Taga T, Nakano N, Yasukawa K, Kashiwamura S, et al. 1985. Purification to homogeneity and characterization of human B-cell differentiation factor (BCDF or BSFp-2). *Proc. Natl. Acad. Sci. USA* 82:5490–94

33. Jourdan M, Bataille R, Seguin J, Zhang XG, Chaptal PA, Klein B. 1990. Constitutive production of interleukin-6 and immunologic features in cardiac myxomas. *Arthritis Rheum.* 33:398–402

34. Hirano T, Matsuda T, Hosoi K, Okano A, Matsui H, Kishimoto T. 1988. Absence of antiviral activity in recombinant B cell stimulatory factor 2 (BSF-2). *Immunol. Lett.* 17:41–45

35. Potter M, Boyce CR. 1962. Induction of plasma-cell neoplasms in strain BALB/c mice with mineral oil and mineral oil adjuvants. *Nature* 193:1086–87

36. Nordan RP, Pumphrey JG, Rudikoff S. 1987. Purification and NH2-terminal sequence of a plasmacytoma growth factor derived from the murine macrophage cell line P388D1. *J. Immunol.* 139:813–17

37. Suematsu S, Matsusaka T, Matsuda T, Ohno S, Miyazaki J, et al. 1992. Generation of plasmacytomas with the chromosomal translocation t(12;15) in interleukin 6 transgenic mice. *Proc. Natl. Acad. Sci. USA* 89:232–35

38. Kawano M, Hirano T, Matsuda T, Taga T, Horii Y, et al. 1988. Autocrine generation and requirement of BSF-2/IL-6 for human multiple myelomas. *Nature* 332:83–85

39. Gauldie J, Richards C, Harnish D, Lansdorp P, Baumann H. 1987. Interferon β_2/B-cell stimulatory factor type 2 shares identity with monocyte-derived hepatocyte-stimulating factor and regulates the major acute phase protein response in liver cells. *Proc. Natl. Acad. Sci. USA* 84:7251–55

40. Andus T, Geiger T, Hirano T, Northoff H, Ganter U, et al. 1987. Recombinant human B cell stimulatory factor 2 (BSF-2/IFN-β2) regulates β-fibrinogen and albumin mRNA levels in Fao-9 cells. *FEBS Lett.* 221:18–22

41. Kopf M, Baumann H, Freer G, Freudenberg M, Lamers M, et al. 1994. Impaired immune and acute-phase responses in interleukin-6-deficient mice. *Nature* 368:339–42

42. Seed B, Aruffo A. 1987. Molecular cloning of the CD2 antigen, the T-cell erythrocyte receptor, by a rapid immunoselection procedure. *Proc. Natl. Acad. Sci. USA* 84:3365–69

43. Yamasaki K, Taga T, Hirata Y, Yawata H, Kawanishi Y, et al. 1988. Cloning and expression of the human interleukin-6 (BSF-2/IFN β2) receptor. *Science* 241:825–28

44. Taga T, Hibi M, Hirata Y, Yamasaki K, Yasukawa K, et al. 1989. Interleukin-6 triggers the association of its receptor with a possible signal transducer, gp130. *Cell* 58:573–81

45. Hibi M, Murakami M, Saito M, Hirano T, Taga T, Kishimoto T. 1990. Molecular cloning and expression of an IL-6 signal transducer, gp130. *Cell* 63:1149–57

46. Ip NY, Nye SH, Boulton TG, Davis S, Taga T, et al. 1992. CNTF and LIF act on neuronal cells via shared signaling pathways that involve the IL-6 signal transducing receptor component gp130. *Cell* 69:1121–32

47. Gearing DP, Comeau MR, Friend DJ, Gimpel SD, Thut CJ, et al. 1992. The IL-6 signal transducer, gp130: an oncostatin M receptor and affinity converter for the LIF receptor. *Science* 255:1434–37

48. Liu J, Modrell B, Aruffo A, Marken JS, Taga T, et al. 1992. Interleukin-6 signal transducer gp130 mediates oncostatin M signaling. *J. Biol. Chem.* 267:16763–66

49. Yin T, Taga T, Tsang ML, Yasukawa K, Kishimoto T, Yang YC. 1993. Involvement of IL-6 signal transducer gp130 in IL-11-mediated signal transduction. *J. Immunol.* 151:2555–61

50. Pennica D, Shaw KJ, Swanson TA, Moore MW, Shelton DL, et al. 1995. Cardiotrophin-1. Biological activities and binding to the leukemia inhibitory factor receptor/gp130 signaling complex. *J. Biol. Chem.* 270:10915–22

51. Shabo Y, Lotem J, Rubinstein M, Revel M, Clark SC, et al. 1988. The myeloid blood cell differentiation-inducing protein MGI-2A is interleukin-6. *Blood* 72:2070–73

52. Hilton DJ, Nicola NA, Gough NM, Metcalf D. 1988. Resolution and purification of three distinct factors produced by Krebs ascites cells which have differentiation-inducing activity on murine myeloid leukemic cell lines. *J. Biol. Chem.* 263:9238–43

53. Akira S, Isshiki H, Sugita T, Tanabe O, Kinoshita S, et al. 1990. A nuclear factor for IL-6 expression (NF-IL6) is a member of a C/EBP family. *EMBO J.* 9:1897–906

54. Nakajima T, Kinoshita S, Sasagawa T, Sasaki K, Naruto M, et al. 1993. Phosphorylation at threonine-235 by a ras-dependent mitogen-activated protein kinase cascade is essential for transcription factor NF-IL6. *Proc. Natl. Acad. Sci. USA* 90:2207–11

55. Murakami M, Narazaki M, Hibi M, Yawata H, Yasukawa K, et al. 1991. Critical cytoplasmic region of the interleukin 6 signal transducer gp130 is conserved in the cytokine receptor family. *Proc. Natl. Acad. Sci. USA* 88:11349–53

56. Murakami M, Hibi M, Nakagawa N, Nakagawa T, Yasukawa K, et al. 1993. IL-6-induced homodimerization of gp130 and associated activation of a tyrosine kinase. *Science* 260:1808–10

57. Silvennoinen O, Witthuhn BA, Quelle FW, Cleveland JL, Yi T, Ihle JN. 1993. Structure of the murine Jak2 protein-tyrosine kinase and its role in interleukin 3 signal transduction. *Proc. Natl. Acad. Sci. USA* 90:8429–33

58. Watling D, Guschin D, Muller M, Silvennoinen O, Witthuhn BA, et al. 1993. Complementation by the protein tyrosine kinase JAK2 of a mutant cell line defective in the interferon-γ signal transduction pathway. *Nature* 366:166–70

59. Silvennoinen O, Ihle JN, Schlessinger J, Levy DE. 1993. Interferon-induced nuclear signalling by Jak protein tyrosine kinases. *Nature* 366:583–85

60. Wegenka UM, Buschmann J, Lutticken C, Heinrich PC, Horn F. 1993. Acute-phase response factor, a nuclear factor binding to acute-phase response elements, is rapidly activated by interleukin-6 at the posttranslational level. *Mol. Cell Biol.* 13:276–88

61. Akira S, Nishio Y, Inoue M, Wang XJ, Wei S, et al. 1994. Molecular cloning of APRF, a novel IFN-stimulated gene factor 3 p91-related transcription factor involved in the gp130-mediated signaling pathway. *Cell* 77:63–71

62. Zhong Z, Wen Z, Darnell JE Jr. 1994. Stat3: a STAT family member activated by tyrosine phosphorylation in response to epidermal growth factor and interleukin-6. *Science* 264:95–98

63. Naka T, Narazaki M, Hirata M, Matsumoto T, Minamoto S, et al. 1997. Structure and function of a new STAT-induced STAT inhibitor. *Nature* 387:924–29

64. Starr R, Willson TA, Viney EM, Murray LJ, Rayner JR, et al. 1997. A family of cytokine-inducible inhibitors of signalling. *Nature* 387:917–21

65. Endo TA, Masuhara M, Yokouchi M, Suzuki R, Sakamoto H, et al. 1997. A new protein containing an SH2 domain that inhibits JAK kinases. *Nature* 387:921–24

66. Kikutani H, Suemura M, Owaki H, Nakamura H, Sato R, et al. 1986. Fcε receptor, a specific differentiation marker transiently expressed on mature B cells before isotype switching. *J. Exp. Med.* 164:1455–69

67. Kikutani H, Inui S, Sato R, Barsumian EL, Owaki H, et al. 1986. Molecular structure of human lymphocyte receptor for immunoglobulin E. *Cell* 47:657–65

68. Yokota A, Kikutani H, Tanaka T, Sato R, Barsumian EL, et al. 1988. Two species of human Fcε receptor II (Fcε RII/CD23): tissue-specific and IL-4-specific regulation of gene expression. *Cell* 55:611–18

69. Nagasawa T, Kikutani H, Kishimoto T. 1994. Molecular cloning and structure of a pre-B-cell growth-stimulating factor. *Proc. Natl. Acad. Sci. USA* 91:2305–9

70. Nagasawa T, Hirota S, Tachibana K, Takakura N, Nishikawa S, et al. 1996. Defects of B-cell lymphopoiesis and bone-marrow myelopoiesis in mice lacking the CXC chemokine PBSF/SDF-1. *Nature* 382:635–38

71. Nagasawa T, Nakajima T, Tachibana K, Iizasa H, Bleul CC, et al. 1996. Molecular cloning and characterization of a murine pre-B-cell growth-stimulating factor/stromal cell-derived factor 1 receptor, a murine homolog of the human immunodeficiency virus 1 entry coreceptor fusin. *Proc. Natl. Acad. Sci. USA* 93:14726–29

72. Tachibana K, Hirota S, Iizasa H, Yoshida H, Kawabata K, et al. 1998. The chemokine receptor CXCR4 is essential for vascularization of the gastrointestinal tract. *Nature* 393:591–94

73. Komori T, Yagi H, Nomura S, Yamaguchi A, Sasaki K, et al. 1997. Targeted disruption of Cbfa1 results in a complete lack of bone formation owing to maturational arrest of osteoblasts. *Cell* 89:755–64

74. Hirano T, Matsuda T, Turner M, Miyasaka N, Buchan G, et al. 1988. Excessive production of interleukin 6/B cell stimulatory factor-2 in rheumatoid arthritis. *Eur. J. Immunol.* 18:1797–801

75. Yoshizaki K, Matsuda T, Nishimoto N, Kuritani T, Taeho L, et al. 1989. Pathogenic significance of interleukin-6 (IL-6/BSF-2) in Castleman's disease. *Blood* 74:1360–67

76. Soulier J, Grollet L, Oksenhendler E, Cacoub P, Cazals-Hatem D, et al. 1995. Kaposi's sarcoma-associated herpesvirus-like DNA sequences in multicentric Castleman's disease. *Blood* 86:1276–80

77. Chatterjee M, Osborne J, Bestetti G, Chang Y, Moore PS. 2002. Viral IL-6-induced cell proliferation and immune evasion of interferon activity. *Science* 298:1432–35

78. Nishimoto N, Sasai M, Shima Y, Nakagawa M, Matsumoto T, et al. 2000. Improvement in Castleman's disease by humanized anti-interleukin-6 receptor antibody therapy. *Blood* 95:56–61

79. Ohshima S, Saeki Y, Mima T, Sasai M, Nishioka K, et al. 1998. Interleukin 6 plays a key role in the development of antigen-induced arthritis. *Proc. Natl. Acad. Sci. USA* 95:8222–26

80. Hata T, Sakaguchi N, Yoshitomi H, Iwakura Y, Sekikawa K, et al. 2004. Distinct contribution of IL-6, TNF-α, IL-1, and IL-10 to T cell–mediated spontaneous autoimmune arthritis in mice. *J. Clin. Invest.* 114:582–88

81. Nishimoto N, Yoshizaki K, Miyasaka N, Yamamoto K, Kawai S, et al. 2004. Treatment of rheumatoid arthritis with humanized anti-interleukin-6 receptor antibody: a multicenter, double-blind, placebo-controlled trial. *Arthritis Rheum.* 50:1761–69

Annu. Rev. Immunol. 2005. 23:23–68
doi: 10.1146/annurev.immunol.23.021704.115839
First published online as a Review in Advance on September 16, 2004

TNF/TNFR Family Members in Costimulation of T Cell Responses

Tania H. Watts

Department of Immunology, University of Toronto, Toronto, Ontario,
M5S 1A8, Canada; email: tania.watts@utoronto.ca

Key Words   survival signaling, T effector cell, T cell memory

■ **Abstract**   Several members of the tumor necrosis factor receptor (TNFR) family function after initial T cell activation to sustain T cell responses. This review focuses on CD27, 4-1BB (CD137), OX40 (CD134), HVEM, CD30, and GITR, all of which can have costimulatory effects on T cells. The effects of these costimulatory TNFR family members can often be functionally, temporally, or spatially segregated from those of CD28 and from each other. The sequential and transient regulation of T cell activation/survival signals by different costimulators may function to allow longevity of the response while maintaining tight control of T cell survival. Depending on the disease condition, stimulation via costimulatory TNF family members can exacerbate or ameliorate disease. Despite these complexities, stimulation or blockade of TNFR family costimulators shows promise for several therapeutic applications, including cancer, infectious disease, transplantation, and autoimmunity.

INTRODUCTION

The specificity of T cell responses is controlled by the antigen-specific T cell receptor (TCR).[1] However, full T cell activation is generally achieved only in the presence of additional receptor-ligand interactions. When these interactions take place at the same time as TCR engagement and allow T cells to make IL-2 and survive, they are referred to as "costimulatory" signals. It is well established that engagement of CD28 by its ligands B7.1 or B7.2 lowers the threshold for activation of T cells and provides key costimulatory signals to allow high-level IL-2 production and survival of naive T cells (1, 2). The T cell response is not a single event. T cells first recognize antigen-MHC on an antigen-presenting cell (APC) and, in their first few hours of activation, commit to programmed expansion (3, 4). Initial activation is usually dependent on CD28-B7 interaction. Subsequently, T cells go on to differentiate into effector cells, which can interact with B cells in germinal centers and/or migrate out of the lymphoid organs and carry out their effector functions

---

[1]See Appendix for a full list of abbreviations used.

in the peripheral tissues. Although the majority of T effector cells are short-lived, some antigen-experienced cells remain as long-lived memory cells (5). T cells receive activation or survival signals at each stage of the response, including naive, effector, and memory stages. Members of the TNFR family are emerging as key mediators of survival signaling in T cells subsequent to the initial effects of CD28-B7 interaction.

TNFR/TNF family interactions can influence T cell responses in a number of ways. They can influence inflammation and innate immunity (6), lymphoid organization (7, 8), or activation of APCs (9–11), or they can provide direct signals to T cells (12). CD40 may function as a master switch for T cell costimulation because of its ability to induce B7 family ligands as well as several TNF family ligands on dendritic cells (DCs) (1, 13–18). TNFR2 can augment T cell proliferation and thus may also provide a costimulatory signal for T cells (see 19 and references cited therein). However, as reviewed elsewhere (6, 7), TNF and its receptors have a diverse and complex set of interactions with the immune system and are not discussed in detail here. This review focuses on several members of the TNFR/TNF ligand superfamily that play a direct role in T cell responses subsequent to initial T cell activation, namely CD27/CD70, CD134 (OX40)/OX40L, CD137 (4-1BB)/4-1BBL, HVEM/LIGHT, CD30/CD30L, and GITR/GITRL (Figure 1).

SIGNALING BY COSTIMULATORY TNFR FAMILY MEMBERS

TNFR family members fall into three groups, death domain (DD)–containing receptors, decoy receptors, and TNF receptor-associated factor (TRAF) binding receptors (20–22). DD-containing TNFRs (such as FAS, TNFRI, and DR3) can activate caspase cascades via DD-containing signaling intermediates, leading to apoptosis. TRAF binding receptors, such as TNFR2, lack DDs but contain motifs of 4–6 amino acids that function to recruit TRAF proteins (23). TRAF binding receptors, including the six that are the focus of this review, are associated with cellular activation, differentiation, and survival signaling.

Figure 2 summarizes the signaling pathway for 4-1BB. This signaling pathway recapitulates the signaling pathway first defined for TNFR2 and is similar to that of other costimulatory TNFR family members (reviewed in 22). Six mammalian TRAF proteins have been identified to date (21). All the costimulatory members of the TNFR family can recruit TRAF2 to their signaling complexes, but they show differences in recruitment of other TRAF proteins (22, 24) (Figure 1). Peptides derived from the cytoplasmic tails of TNFR family members have widely divergent affinities for TRAF2 (25), so there may be differences in the efficiency of TRAF recruitment by the different TNFR family members in vivo.

Both TRAF2 and 5, when over-expressed, induce activation of nuclear factor κB (NF-κB), a family of transcription factors that induce genes associated with cell

Ligands

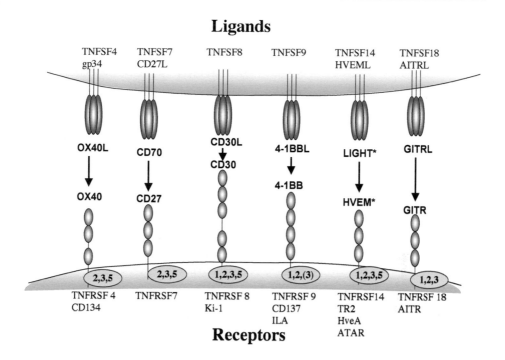

Receptors

(1,2,3,5) TNFR associated factors   ⬮ Cysteine-rich domain

Figure 1 Costimulatory TNFR/TNF family members. Common (in bold) and standardized TNFR/TNF family nomenclature (http://www.gene.ucl.ac.uk/nomenclature/genefamily/tnftop.html) are provided, as well as alternative names for receptors and ligands. *LIGHT also interacts with LTβR and the decoy receptor DcR3/TR6; HVEM also interacts with LTα3. The costimulatory TNFR family members are type I transmembrane proteins, characterized by cysteine-rich motifs in their extracellular domains (20). The ligands for the costimulatory TNFR family members are type II cell surface glycoproteins. The cytoplasmic domains of costimulatory TNFR family members contain TRAF2 binding motifs consisting of the major conserved motif, (P/S/A/T)x (Q/E)E, or the minor motif, PxQxxD (307). TRAF trimers are recruited to TNFRs upon receptor ligation (307). The TRAF proteins that interact with each receptor are indicated in the figure; references for these TRAF associations are as follows: OX40 (29, 30); CD27 (27, 28, 43); CD30 (33–36); 4-1BB (24, 31, 50); HVEM (38); GITR (39, 40). Note that TRAF3 association is observed with human but not mouse 4-1BB.

survival, including TRAF1, cellular inhibitors of apoptosis (cIAP1 and 2), Bcl-X_L and c-flip (26). All the TRAF2-binding costimulatory TNFR family members activate NF-κB (27–42). Aggregation of TRAF2 upon receptor ligation also results in recruitment and activation of mitogen activated protein (MAP) 3 kinases or MAP4 kinases, thereby linking TRAF2 to the jun-N-terminal kinase/stress-activated

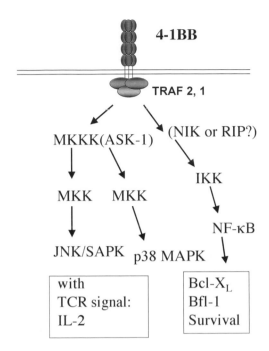

Figure 2   Signaling by 4-1BB and related TNFR family members. TRAFs 1 and 2 were initially identified in immunoprecipitates of TNFR2 (308), and the signaling pathway delineated for 4-1BB to date recapitulates that determined for TNFR2 (22). TRAF2 links TNFR family members to downstream signaling pathways, whereas TRAF1 acts as a modulator of TRAF2 signaling (22, 46). 4-1BB signaling is TRAF2-dependent (30, 31, 50). The role of apoptosis inducing kinase (ASK)–1 in linkage of TRAF2 to JNK and p38 MAPK signaling, as well as the potential role of NF-κB inducing kinase (NIK) in linking TRAF2 to the inhibitor of κB kinase (IKK) complex, were determined by overexpressing dominant negative (DN) forms (31, 44, 45). Thus, the particular kinases linking 4-1BB/TRAF2 to downstream signaling pathways in primary T cells are unknown. Once 4-1BB is induced on the cell surface, 4-1BB-dependent JNK and p38 activation are independent of TCR signaling, but a TCR signal is required for 4-1BB to costimulate IL-2 production. There are two pathways of NF-κB activation: (*a*) The classical pathway activated by TNF and TLR ligands induces the activation of the IKK complex and degradation of IκB; (*b*) the alternate pathway of NF-κB activation involves processing the p100 precursor to create p52 and is used by LTβR and BAFFR (26). For GITR signaling, there is evidence that the classical NF-κB pathway is activated (42).

protein kinase (JNK/SAPK) and p38 MAPK cascades (reviewed in 21, 22). CD27, 4-1BB, and GITR have also been shown to activate p38 and JNK in primary cells (36, 43–45).

TRAF1, which lacks the RING finger domain required for NF-κB activation, functions to sustain TRAF2 signaling in the CD40 signaling pathway (46) and is also required for maximal 4-1BB-dependent signaling in T cells (C. Srokowski, G. Pulle-Stadt, E. Tsitsikov & T.H. Watts, manuscript in preparation). In contrast, TRAF3 antagonizes the effects of TRAF2 in NF-κB activation by OX40, CD27, and CD30 (27, 29, 30, 34).

The importance of TRAF proteins for signaling by TNFR family members has been tested using gene-targeted or transgenic mice (47–49). Truncation of the RING finger domain of TRAF2 and 5 converts them into dominant negative (DN) proteins. Primary T cells lacking TRAF2 or expressing dominant negative TRAF2 (TRAF2.DN) show defects in p38 activation and cytokine production in response to 4-1BB or CD30 signaling (36, 45, 50). TRAF2.DN expression in T cells greatly reduces anti-OX40-induced survival and longevity of T cells in vivo (51). In contrast, the absence of TRAF5 in T cells had no impact on the ability of T cells to produce IL-2 or proliferate. However, TRAF5$^{-/-}$ T cells produced higher levels of cytokines, with a more pronounced effect on Th2 cytokines, and TRAF5$^{-/-}$ mice were more prone to Th2-driven allergic inflammation (52). TRAF5$^{-/-}$ mice showed impaired proliferative responses to anti-CD3 plus transfected CD70; however, no defects in NF-κB or JNK activation were observed (53). Taken together, it appears that TRAF2 or the TRAF2 binding site is critical for TNFR superfamily mediated-survival signaling as well as induction of cytokines in T cells, whereas TRAF5 may modulate OX40 and CD27 signaling, leading to alterations in cytokine production and/or proliferation.

OX40 signaling sustains the expression of anti-apoptotic Bcl-2 family members, Bcl-2 and Bcl-X$_L$, following CD28 signaling (54). More recently, Song et al. (55) demonstrated that OX40 signaling can maintain the active form of protein kinase B (PKB) following CD28 signaling. In the CD28 signaling pathway, the phosphatidylinositol 3-kinase (PI-3K)-dependent activation of PKB is important in CD28-mediated upregulation of Bcl-X$_L$ levels and T cell survival (56). The link between OX40 and PI-3K-dependent PKB activation and its relation to the TRAF2-IKK-NF-κB-mediated pathway of survival signaling (Figure 2) is unknown. OX40 ligation on pre-activated T cells leads to rapid activation of PKB, suggesting a relatively direct effect (55). However, OX40-induced downregulation of the inhibitory receptor CTLA-4 may also contribute to OX40-induced maintenance of CD28-dependent survival signaling (51). In contrast, 4-1BB-mediated induction of Bcl-X$_L$ message or protein was not blocked by PI-3K inhibitors but was sensitive to inhibitors of NF-κB, suggesting that 4-1BB-induced survival is independent of the PI-3K-PKB pathway (32).

In addition to TRAFs, CD27 and GITR can associate in cell lines with Siva-1, a protein linked to apoptosis when overexpressed in leukemic T cell lines (57–59). The relevance of this interaction for primary T cell responses is unclear, given the evidence that these receptors are usually associated with activation and survival rather than apoptosis. Murine 4-1BB also associates with p56lck, through a consensus lck binding motif (60). However, this sequence is altered in human 4-1BB, and its significance is again unclear.

In summary, costimulatory TNFR family members are linked via TRAF proteins to NF-κB and stress kinase signaling, which in turn results in enhancement of survival signaling, cytokine production, and cellular proliferation. There is some evidence for associations of costimulatory TNFR family members with additional signaling molecules, but the significance of such associations to biological function is unknown.

CD27/CD70

Expression

CD27 and its ligand, CD70, have been characterized in both human and mouse where CD27 is expressed on natural killer (NK) cells, B cells, and naive CD4 and CD8 T cells (reviewed in 61). In humans, CD27 expression increases transiently with activation (62, 63) and is subsequently downregulated on T effector cells after several rounds of cell division. This loss of CD27 correlates with high levels of effector function (see 64 and references therein). CD27$^-$ CD8 effector cells are observed in human cytomegalovirus infection but are notably decreased in HIV-specific CD8 T cell responses (65, 66), where the lack of CD27$^-$ effector cells is associated with poor control of viral infection (67, 68). CD27 is also downregulated on effector T cells in mice: Effector-memory lymphocytic choriomeningitis virus (LCMV)-specific CD8 T cells are CD27$^{lo/int.}$, whereas central memory T cells are CD27$^+$ (69). After influenza infection of mice, CD27$^-$ CD8 effector T cells are found primarily in blood, lung, and spleen but are absent from lymph nodes (P.A. Baars, R. van Lier, personal communication). CD27 is also expressed on thymocytes, and anti-CD27 treatment of mice initially suggested a role for CD27 in T cell development (70). However, these effects were not borne out in the CD27$^{-/-}$ mice, which have normal numbers of mature and immature T cells (71).

CD70 is found on activated T cells, B cells, and DCs (16, 72–75). CD70 is induced on mouse B cells and DC by anti-CD40 or LPS and on DC by GM-CSF (18). CD70 is also expressed on activated T cells but at lower levels than on activated B cells (18). Following intranasal (i.n.) infection of mice with influenza virus, CD70 is detected on T cells and B cells in the draining lymph nodes. CD70 is also expressed on T cells in the lung but is largely intracellular, suggesting that CD70 is regulated posttranslationally as well as transcriptionally (18). The expression pattern of CD27 and CD70 suggests that CD27 on T cells may receive signals by binding CD70 on activated B cells, DCs, or through T-T interaction.

CD27 Function In Vitro

Engagement of CD27 with antibody or ligand can enhance CD4 or CD8 T cell proliferation and cytokine production when given in the presence of other costimulatory signals, such as PHA or IL-2 (61, 72, 76–80). CD27 engagement does not costimulate high-level IL-2 production by T cells, but it induces TNF at comparable levels to that induced by CD28 engagement, promotes development of cytotoxic T lymphocyte (CTL) effectors, and enhances T cell survival (71, 78). CD27 is not a costimulatory molecule in the strict sense of the definition, but it enhances responses by increasing T cell expansion. Whereas CD28 promotes cell division, CD27 appears to promote T cell expansion by allowing T cells to survive through successive divisions, without influencing the rate of cell division (81). The finding that CD27 is downregulated on effector cells suggests that CD27-mediated effects take place relatively early in a response. Although not the subject of this review, CD27 signaling in B cells also plays a direct role in B cell memory commitment and differentiation and contributes to germinal center formation (see 82–84 and references therein).

In Vivo Models of CD27/CD70 Function

Transgenic mice expressing CD70 under the control of the CD19 promoter show normal T cell development but accumulate increased numbers of CD4 and CD8 T cells with an effector phenotype by 4 weeks of age (85). Furthermore, the mice show a progressive decline in mature B cells, dependent on the presence of T cell–expressed CD27 and secretion of IFN-γ by T cells (85). Young CD70-transgenic mice show enhanced CD8 T cell responses to influenza virus, as well as enhanced clearance of tumors (86, 309). These effects are due to increased numbers of effector cells as well as increased effector function per cell (killing, IFN-γ levels) (86). Transient administration of soluble CD70 protein (sCD70) together with antigen causes greater expansion of T cells than Ag plus LPS, also consistent with a role for CD70 in T cell expansion. Furthermore, co-administration of sCD70 with Ag replaces the requirement for adjuvant and prevents the tolerance induction that is otherwise observed with administration of antigen alone (87).

Although CD70 transgenic mice have increased numbers of CD4 and CD8 effector T cells and initially show increased T effector responses to influenza virus, by 6 months of age the mice succumb to opportunistic infections with *Pneumocystis carinii* (309). This immunodeficiency is attributed to an antigen-dependent progressive conversion of the naive T cells to T effector cells over time, thereby depleting the naive T cell pool. This finding may explain the tight regulation of CD70 expression observed in vivo (18).

Conversely, mice lacking CD27 show reduced numbers of CD4 and CD8 T cells in the lung and spleen following primary and secondary infection with influenza A delivered intranasally (71). The effects on Ag-specific CD8 T cells are even larger in the secondary response than in the primary response, and effects on numbers of cells in the lung are more substantial than those in the spleen, suggesting a preferential defect in accumulation of T cells at sites of effector T cell activity (71). To further delineate effects of CD27 on the primary and secondary phase of the immune response, Hendricks et al. (81) analyzed mice lacking both CD27 and CD28. Given the role of CD28 in the primary response, it was not surprising that CD8 T cell responses in lung, spleen, and draining lymph node (DLN) were severely impaired in the double knock-out animals (81). Hendricks et al. went on to dissect the individual contributions of CD27 and CD28 by analyzing TCR transgenic influenza-specific CD8 T cells lacking CD27 or CD28, adoptively transferred into WT mice. During primary responses to influenza, CD28 had the greatest impact on Ag-specific CD8 T cell numbers in the spleen, whereas CD27 deficiency had the largest impact on the number of CD8 T cells accumulating in the lung and DLN (81). Thus, both CD27 and CD28 on T cells play a role in T cell expansion, but with different precise roles: (a) CD28 influences cell division and perhaps initial survival in the lymphoid organs, and (b) CD27 signaling maintains T cell survival and enhances T cell accumulation in the peripheral tissues (81). The greater effects of CD27 on memory responses may be due to lack of survival of T cells in the primary response and/or due to effects of CD27 in the secondary response.

CD27 and Disease

Anti-CD70 antibodies can prevent experimental autoimmune encephalomyelitis (EAE) in mice. This effect of CD70 blockade on EAE is not due to impaired T cell priming, but may be due to inhibition of TNF induction (88). A number of studies have shown that CD27/CD70 can enhance tumor or graft rejection, with CD70 transfection enhancing both NK-dependent and T cell–dependent mechanisms of tumor elimination (86, 89–93).

OX40/OX40L

Expression

Originally identified as a molecule expressed on activated T cells from rat (94), OX40 has since been characterized in mouse and human, where its expression is also restricted to activated T cells (reviewed in 95, 96). OX40 is also the receptor for feline immunodeficiency virus (97). OX40 is preferentially expressed on activated CD4 rather than CD8 T cells under a number of conditions (95, 98), suggesting a more prominent role for OX40 on CD4 T cells. However, under conditions of strong antigenic stimulation, OX40 can also be induced on CD8 T cells (99–102). In the gut, OX40 and OX40L are inducible on the CD8 intraepithelial lymphocyte (IEL) population by anti-CD3, and OX40 expression is associated with cytotoxic effector function of IELs (103). OX40 expression on T cells peaks at 48 hr following in vitro activation, declining again between 72 and 96 hr (104). Although CD28 is not essential for OX40 expression, engagement of CD28 can enhance the kinetics and level of OX40 expression on T cells (54, 105). OX40 is preferentially expressed on Th2 cells in some models (106, 107), but it can also be expressed on Th1 cells (104, 107, 108) and can play a role in both Th1 and Th2 responses (to be discussed below). In vivo, OX40-expressing CD4 T cells are found in close proximity to antigen-activated B cells in the spleen (107, 109).

Whereas OX40 expression appears to be restricted to T cells, OX40L is expressed on a number of cell types. First identified as a molecule induced by HTLV-1 infection of T cells (110, 111), OX40L is expressed on activated B cells (15, 112–114), and reverse signaling via OX40L can enhance B cell proliferation/differentiation (113). OX40L is also expressed on activated T cells (111), CD40-ligand-activated DCs (115–117), IL-3-treated plasmacytoid DCs (118), human vascular epithelial cells (119, 120), and a novel $CD4^+CD3^-B220^-MHC$ $II^+B7^{lo}OX40L^{hi}CD30L^{hi}$ accessory cell in the T cell–B cell contact area of the spleen (107). OX40 and its ligand can be expressed for prolonged periods during chronic infection (75) and are observed in the central nervous system of mice with EAE (121), as well as in inflamed tissues in a number of autoimmune and inflammatory diseases in mouse (122–124) and human (125–129).

Role of OX40 in CD4 T Cell Expansion, Survival, Th1 and Th2 Responses

Initial studies using OX40L or anti-OX40 antibody to mediate T cell activation showed that OX40 signaling on T cells can enhance cytokine production and proliferation of CD4 T cells (reviewed in 95), an effect that can occur in the absence of CD28 (114). Although most evidence suggests a role for OX40 primarily on CD4 T cells, agonistic anti-OX40 antibodies can enhance the expansion of both CD4 and CD8 T cells in vivo (101, 130–132). Many studies have shown an important or preferential role for OX40 in Th2 responses (75, 99, 105, 107, 115, 133–139). However, it is clear that OX40 can contribute to Th1 responses (104, 122, 140, 141). Thus, OX40 does not appear to play a role in determining whether a response becomes Th1 or Th2 (104, 116, 142); rather, it can contribute to ongoing Th1 or Th2 responses and may have greater effects on Th2 responses owing to the higher levels of OX40 on Th2 cells.

Although a TCR plus OX40 signal alone can induce some IL-2 production, OX40 does not replace CD28 or influence the initial rate of cell division, but OX40 does allow recovery of greater numbers of T cells later in the response (54, 55, 104, 130). Systemic administration of agonistic anti-OX40 antibodies in the presence of LPS enhances T cell survival following superantigen administration in vivo (143). As discussed above, OX40 signaling sustains the expression of anti-apoptotic Bcl-2 family members, Bcl-2 and $Bcl-X_L$, consistent with its role in T cell survival (54, 55).

Analysis of OX40/OX40L Function Using Gene-Targeted and Transgenic Mice

Mice lacking OX40 or its ligand show defects in CD4 T cell proliferative responses to viruses and protein antigens, with no obvious skewing toward Th1 or Th2 responses, no defect in germinal center formation, and either no defect or a partial defect in antibody responses (15, 116, 144, 145). CD8 T cell responses to viruses were unimpaired in OX40$^{-/-}$ or OX40L$^{-/-}$ mice (116, 144), whereas there were small defects in alloantigen or contact sensitivity–induced CD8 T cell responses in the absence of OX40L (15, 116). The effects of OX40 on CD8 T cells in these studies may be due to indirect effects of OX40 on CD4 T cell help. OX40- or OX40L-deficient mice also show reduced graft-versus-host disease (GVHD), with a much greater effect on MHC class II– versus MHC class I–restricted responses (146). Thus, OX40 plays a clear role in CD4 T cell responses in vivo but is dispensable for CD8 T cell responses in vivo.

Transgenic overexpression of OX40L in DC results in increased CD4 but not CD8 T cell accumulation in the B cell follicles (147). On T cells, constitutive over-expression of OX40L results in accumulation of CD4 effector T cells, increased CD4 T cell responses, as well as an autoimmune phenotype characterized by in-flammation of the lung and intestine, with no change in CD8 populations (148). Thus, both gene-targeted and transgenic mice support a role for OX40 primarily on CD4 T cells.

There are conflicting data on the effect of OX40 or OX40L deficiency on B cell responses in mice. Three studies showed no defect in antibody responses to both protein and infectious agents (KLH, VSV, influenza virus, L. Major, *N. brasiliensis*) in OX40- or OX40L-deficient mice (116, 144, 145). In contrast, three other studies showed decreased IgG responses to KLH or alloantigen in the absence of OX40 or OX40L (15, 107, 149). Differences in route of immunization, antigen dose, or adjuvant do not appear to explain the discrepant results. However, the requirement for OX40 ligation for maximal IgG production was most apparent after multiple immunizations, consistent with a role for OX40/OX40L in sustaining the ability of T cells to maintain memory B cell responses (107, 149).

Role of OX40L on Different Cell Types In Vivo

OX40L is found on a number of cell types, and evidence suggests that there may be sequential effects of OX40L expressed by different APC subsets. OX40L on DC can contribute to CD4 T cell expansion (116, 117). This likely takes place at about 48 hr after initial activation, the time at which OX40 is induced on TCR/CD28-activated T cells. OX40L on B cells can sustain CD4 TCR transgenic T cells 3–4 days after activation (136), and memory B cell defects are detected under condi-tions where only B cells lack OX40L, again supporting a functional role for OX40L on B cells (149). A novel accessory cell that is CD3$^-$CD4$^+$CD11c$^-$B220$^-$MHCII$^+$ B7^{lo}OX40L$^+$CD30L$^+$ associates with OX40$^+$ but not OX40$^-$ CD4 T cells several weeks after immunization, and this association correlates with the preferential survival of OX40$^{+/+}$ T cells in vivo (107). Thus CD4$^+$CD3$^-$OX40L$^+$CD30L$^+$ accessory cells appear to provide survival signals to primed and memory CD4 T cells weeks after activation.

Role of OX40/OX40L in Primary Versus Memory Responses

Several lines of evidence show that OX40 can play a role in both primary and secondary responses. Provision of agonistic anti-OX40 antibodies can clearly augment primary expansion and survival of CD4 T cells in vivo, and naive OX40$^{-/-}$ T cells show decreased proliferation in vitro (130, 131, 143, 145). In several models, OX40-OX40L interaction was found to affect T cell recall responses, although it was not always clear in these studies if these effects were on initial priming, survival of memory cells or secondary expansion (15, 135, 144). Transfer of a 1:1 mixture of OX40$^{+/+}$ and OX40$^{-/-}$ T cells into recombinase activating gene (RAG)– deficient mice followed by immunization results in a nearly 3:1 ratio of OX40$^+$ to OX40$^-$ T cells by 4 weeks post transfer, consistent with a role for OX40L in long-term T cell survival in vivo (107). In support of the role of OX40L in memory responses, we found that transfer of Ag-specific CD4 TCR transgenic T cells into OX40L$^{-/-}$ mice, followed by sequential immunizations at days 1 and 22 posttransfer, showed a profound defect on secondary expansion of the CD4 T cells in OX40L$^{-/-}$ mice under conditions in which OX40 deficiency had a negligible effect on primary T cell expansion (149a). These data suggest that under conditions of limiting Ag stimulation, OX40L has a more important role in T cell memory.

Does OX40 Play a Role in T Cell Migration?

OX40/OX40L can influence the number of T cells accumulating in B cell follicles by a factor of two- to threefold (117, 147), and OX40$^{-/-}$ mice exhibit two- to threefold decreases in accumulation of CD4 T cells in the BAL following i.n. infection with influenza virus (144). Effects on T cell numbers at particular sites could be due to a number of factors, including an influence of OX40/OX40L on initial expansion of the T cells prior to their migration; an influence of OX40/OX40L on migration of CD4$^+$ T cells into B cell follicles or inflammatory sites; effects of OX40/OX40L on continued proliferation or survival of T cells; or an influence of OX40/OX40L signals on retention of cells at the site of infection. These effects can be difficult to dissect in vivo. Evidence that OX40 could directly influence migration comes from studies showing that OX40L expression on DCs induces increased CXCR5 expression by T cells (105). Conversely, blockade of OX40L using OX40-Ig is associated with a decrease in CXCR5 expression by CD4$^+$ T cells and amelioration of chronic colitis (150). OX40 binding to OX40L expressed on human vascular endothelial cells can induce the endothelial cells to produce the CC chemokine Rantes/CCL5 by reverse signaling, raising the possibility that OX40-OX40L interactions during T cell–endothelial cell contact result in enhanced T cell recruitment to inflammatory sites (151).

Manipulation of OX40/OX40L During the
Immune Response to Infection

In several infectious disease models, OX40 functions to enhance immune responses, which can be beneficial or detrimental for disease outcome, depending on the infection and predominance of a Th1 versus Th2 response. Treatment of BALB/c mice with OX40-Ig (an OX40L-blocking reagent) ameliorates lung pathology and cachexia following influenza infection of mice, consistent with a role for OX40L in accumulation of T cells at sites of infection/inflammation (152). Increasing OX40 signaling via systemic administration of a soluble form of OX40L results in increased CD4 Th1 responses in the lung, increased pathogen clearance, and decreased eosinophilia in response to i.n. infection with *Cryptococcus neoformans* (141). Similarly, treatment of C57BL/6 mice with soluble OX40L enhanced granuloma formation and control of *L. donovani* (153).

Manipulation of OX40-OX40L interactions in Leishmaniasis has different outcomes depending on the model. In BALB/c mice, blockade or deficiency in OX40L ameliorates progressive Leishmaniasis induced by *Leishmania major*, an effect attributed to suppression of the Th2 response (75, 138). Conversely, transgenic expression of OX40L in C57BL/6 mice, which normally control *Leishmania*, resulted in an elevated Th2 response and decreased parasite clearance (138).

Role of OX40/OX40L in Autoimmune
and Inflammatory Reactions

A large body of evidence suggests that OX40-OX40L interactions play a role in autoimmunity and inflammation. OX40-OX40L interaction is required for the induction of EAE in mice, and depletion of OX40[+] T cells or preventing OX40-OX40L interactions ameliorates disease (121, 129, 154, 155). Conversely, triggering OX40 signaling exacerbates EAE (140, 156). In mice, blockade or deficiency in OX40/OX40L reduces the severity of collagen-induced arthritis (122), chronic and adoptive transfer models of colitis (123, 150, 157, 158), contact hypersensitivity reactions (116, 124), airway inflammation in mouse asthma models (135, 137, 139, 142), and diabetes incidence (159). OX40L can also be detected in human airway smooth muscle (ASM) of healthy controls as well as of asthma patients, but asthma patients' ASM cells show greater induction of IL-6 in response to OX40L ligation than do healthy donor ASM cells, suggesting a pathogenic role for OX40L in asthma. This study provides another example of reverse signaling by OX40L (160).

The absence of OX40 does not in itself appear to induce tolerance (159). However, provision of agonistic anti-OX40 can reverse T cell anergy induced in vivo by peptide administration (161). Interestingly, transfer of self-specific CD4 T cells into recipient mice induces expansion of T cells, which remain anergic. However, concomitant administration of agonistic anti-OX40 antibodies relieves these self-specific T cells from their anergic state, resulting in autoimmunity and death of the anti-OX40-treated recipient mice (162). Taken together, the above studies suggest an important role for OX40 in maintenance of inflammatory and autoimmune diseases and support the idea that OX40/OX40L is an important therapeutic target (96).

Role of OX40 in Alloresponses and Cancer

Deficiency in OX40 or OX40L does not alter T cell proliferation in a mixed lymphocyte reaction (MLR) (116, 145) but OX40L$^{-/-}$ DC induce less effector cytokines than WT APC (116) and induce weaker allo-CTL responses (15), consistent with earlier evidence that OX40 is important in alloresponses (163). Similarly, administration of blocking antibodies to OX40L can ameliorate lethal GVHD in mice (164). OX40 deficiency on T cells has a much greater impact on CD4 T cell–mediated GVHD, with CD8-mediated GVHD largely independent of OX40 (146). OX40 blockade can also delay allograft rejection by CD28/CD40L doubly deficient mice under conditions in which anti-CD70, anti-ICOSL, and anti-4-1BBL had no effect (165). Conversely, there is evidence that OX40L transduction of tumor cells (166, 167) or anti-OX40 stimulation can enhance antitumor responses (98, 168–170).

4-1BB/4-1BBL

Expression

4-1BB and its ligand have been characterized in both mouse and human (reviewed in 171). 4-1BB was originally identified as a molecule expressed on activated T cells (172). In vitro, 4-1BB expression on T cells peaks at about 48 hr of primary T cell activation and declines again by 4–5 days (100, 171, 173). In vivo analysis of 4-1BB expression shows that its expression can be earlier and more transient than observed in vitro (174), with 4-1BB expression coinciding with expression of the early T cell activation antigen CD69 at 12–36 hr postimmunization and preceding the transition to the CD44^{hi} state (175). Both CD8 and CD4 T cells, including Th1 and Th2 cells, can express 4-1BB (16); however, at least in some circumstances, CD8 T cells can upregulate 4-1BB more rapidly and to higher levels than CD4 T cells (98, 176). With nonreplicating antigens, 4-1BB expression is rapid and transient; however, its expression can be sustained under conditions of graft rejection or persistent infection (177, 178). Interestingly, the 4-1BB sequence in NOD mice shows several amino acid differences from the sequence of 4-1BB in B10 mice, and 4-1BB is a candidate gene for *idd9.3*, a locus that controls diabetes progression (179).

In addition to its well-established role as an inducible costimulatory receptor on T cells (171, 180), 4-1BB has been found on a number of other cell types. 4-1BB is expressed on a subset of splenic DCs, where it is downregulated by CD40 signaling (16). Low levels of 4-1BB are found on BM-derived DCs, and expression is increased by LPS stimulation (181). 4-1BB is also constitutively expressed on human monocytes (182), follicular dendritic cells (183), cytokine-treated NK cells (184), as well as activated eosinophils (185) and microglia (186). On DC, engagement of 4-1BB can induce IL-6 and IL-12 production (16, 181), whereas on NK cells, agonistic anti-4-1BB antibody induces IFN-γ production, and this in turn can augment CD8 T cell responses (184). In vivo treatment of RAG mice with anti-4-1BB leads to a small increase in the activity of the DC in subsequent T cell proliferation assays ex vivo. These data suggest that, independently of any effects on lymphocytes, 4-1BB signaling in DC may impact the immune response (181).

4-1BBL is expressed on activated macrophages, DC, and B cells (16, 17, 187–189). CD40 is a major regulator of 4-1BBL expression on B cells and DC (13, 16, 17). At sites of inflammation, 4-1BBL is also expressed on other cell types, including cardiac myocytes (190), human neurons (186), and aortic tissue (191). 4-1BBL does not appear to be expressed on resting or activated murine T cells (16). Thus, direct T cell activation through 4-1BB signaling most likely results from interaction of 4-1BB on activated T cells with 4-1BBL on activated APC. Engagement of 4-1BBL on mouse B cells or human monocytes with 4-1BB fusion proteins has also been shown to induce reverse signaling in B cells and monocytes through 4-1BBL (183, 192–194). Although 4-1BB can clearly have a direct role on T cells, the possibility of 4-1BB signaling on multiple cell types as well as evidence for reverse signaling by 4-1BBL complicates the interpretation of studies involving in vivo manipulation of 4-1BB/4-1BBL signaling.

Analysis of 4-1BB Function on Mouse T Cells

Initial analysis of 4-1BB on mouse T cells indicated that 4-1BB can augment T cell proliferation (reviewed in 171). 4-1BBL can costimulate both Th1 and Th2 cytokine production and as such does not appear to play a role in determining cytokine profile or level of cytokines produced; rather, it regulates the number of cytokine-producing cells (173, 195). Isolated T cells from CD28$^{-/-}$ mice can proliferate and make cytokines in response to anti-CD3 and 4-1BBL alone (50), and anti-4-1BB can replace CD28 signals for early CD8 T cell expansion in vivo (196). When signals through the TCR are strong, costimulation with 4-1BBL can induce similar levels of IL-2 as CD28-mediated costimulation. However, under conditions of limited antigenic stimulation, 4-1BBL is not as effective as B7-CD28 interaction (50), consistent with its physiological role following CD28 signaling (197, 198). In vitro, 4-1BBL can activate both CD4 and CD8 T cells (100, 173, 195, 199). In contrast, agonistic anti-4-1BB antibodies show a preferential effect on CD8 T cells (200). Although 4-1BBL can replace CD28 in allowing cell division and IL-2 production by resting T cells, a major effect of 4-1BB appears to be on T cell survival. 4-1BB engagement prevents activation-induced cell death in T cells (201), and in vivo administration of agonistic anti-4-1BB during superantigen treatment of mice prolonged T cell survival, with greater effects on CD8 T cells (174). This effect of 4-1BBL on T cell survival is dependent on NF-κB activation

(32), which in turn induces Bcl-X_L and Bfl-1, two pro-survival members of the Bcl-2 family. Taken together, the data suggest that 4-1BB signaling can impact both cell division and survival of CD4 and CD8 T cells, particularly in the absence of CD28 (100, 199, 202). However, in other studies, the effect of 4-1BB ligation appears to be mainly on cell survival (17, 203).

4-1BBL Stimulation of Human T Cells

As is the case with mouse T cells, both CD4 and CD8 T cells in human respond to 4-1BBL stimulation (176, 204, 205). Evidence to date has primarily shown a role for human 4-1BBL in augmenting Th1 cytokines (176, 205). Modification of monocytes with a recombinant adenovirus vector expressing 4-1BBL resulted in up to a 100-fold lowering of the effective peptide dose required for expansion of memory CD8 T cells compared with monocytes modified with vector alone (206). 4-1BBL can also costimulate cord blood T cells, but only after pre-activation with antigen or cytokines (207, 208). 4-1BBL stimulation of human CD8 T cells results in enhanced expansion as well as upregulation of effector molecules, including perforin, granzyme A, and cytokines (202, 206). In comparison to B7-mediated costimulation, 4-1BBL seems to be more effective in driving CD8 memory T cells toward a fully differentiated CD27$^-$ effector state (206). This contrasts with mouse CD8 T cells, where 4-1BBL appears to control cell number rather than effector function per T cell (197, 199). 4-1BBL also upregulates Bcl-X_L expression by human T cells (198, 202, 206, 207). Inclusion of 4-1BBL stimulation in cultures of anti-CD3/CD28-stimulated T cells results in substantial increases in recovery of T cells at 12–25 days of culture with minor effects on cell recoveries before 10 days (198). Thus 4-1BB ligation appears to be an important mediator of human CD8 T cell survival in vitro. Humans accumulate CD28$^-$ CD8 T cells with age or chronic infection (see references cited in 202), and human CD28$^-$ T cells are able to expand, develop effector function, and upregulate Bcl-X_L in response to 4-1BBL costimulation (202, 208). Thus, 4-1BBL may be an effective costimulator for enhancing T cell responses in the aged or in chronically infected individuals. In support of this idea, systemic treatment with agonistic anti-4-1BB rescues otherwise defective T cell priming observed with T cells from aged mice (209).

Effects of 4-1BB Engagement with Agonistic Anti-4-1BB Antibodies In Vivo

Agonistic antibodies specific for 4-1BB were found to greatly enhance the expansion of CD8 T cells, with more modest effects on CD4 T cells (200, 210). In general, the agonistic anti-4-1BB antibodies that had been shown to preferentially activate CD8 T cells in vitro had stimulatory effects on CD8 T cell responses to tumors and viruses, as well as in MHC class I– and MHC class II–restricted GVHD models (17, 98, 196, 200, 203, 210–212). Systemic delivery of agonistic anti-4-1BB prevents and even reverses anergy induced by soluble antigens (213). As discussed above, it is difficult in these models to determine which cell types are directly responding to 4-1BB because of the possibility of 4-1BB signaling on DC and NK cells in addition to the direct effects on T cells. In some tumor models, effects of anti-4-1BB clearly require the presence of CD4, CD8, and NK cells (214, 215), whereas in other models the response to anti-4-1BB is retained after CD4 T cell and NK cell depletion (216). Further resolution of the relative role of anti-4-1BB on T cells versus non–T cells requires testing of anti-4-1BB in models in which only the T cells or non–T cells express 4-1BB.

In contrast to the stimulatory effects of anti-4-1BB on CD8 T cell responses to tumors, alloantigen, or viral antigens, several studies have shown that the same stimulatory antibodies inhibit humoral immunity and can block or reverse autoimmunity in mouse models of lupus or EAE (217–221). In the EAE model, anti-4-1BB initially resulted in CD4 T cell expansion, but CD4 T cells disappeared at later time points (219). Anti-4-1BB therapy of MRL/lpr mice appears to induce deletion of B cells via an IFN-γ-dependent mechanism (218). A similar effect on progressive depletion of B cells is seen in mice constitutively expressing 4-1BBL under the control of an MHC class II promoter (222) or in mice expressing a CD70 transgene (85). These findings suggest that too much costimulation, particularly under conditions of chronic stimulation, can lead to the production of cytokines such as IFN-γ at levels that inhibit cell proliferation. In support of this idea, Myers et al. (223) found that anti-4-1BB stimulation of adoptively transferred CD8 T cells in the presence of Toll-receptor triggering (LPS) resulted in profound expansion of CD8 T cells, which in turn led to suppression of CD4 T cell proliferation by a TGF-β-dependent mechanism. Follow-up experiments also show that this effect is Ag-specific and IFN-γ-dependent (L. Myers & A. Vella, manuscript in preparation). The finding that anti-4-1BB can have apparently inhibitory or stimulatory effects depending on the disease and/or level of immune response means that one should exercise caution in applying anti-4-1BB therapeutically.

Studies of 4-1BB/4-1BBL Using Gene-Targeted Mice

In general, mice lacking 4-1BB or 4-1BBL show defects in CD8 T cell responses to viruses, with no defects in antibody or CD4 T cell responses to vesicular stomatitis virus (VSV), LCMV, or influenza virus (224–226). However, the anti-phosphorylcholine antibody response to *S. pneumoniae* was decreased in 4-1BBL$^{-/-}$ mice, although the anti–pneumococcal surface protein A (PspA) antibody response was not (221). Although the CD8 T cell response to VSV is decreased in 4-1BB$^{-/-}$ mice, the ex vivo responses of T cells to anti-CD3 are higher in the absence of 4-1BB, although the mechanism for this effect is unknown (226).

With strongly replicating pathogens, such as *Listeria* and LCMV, CD8 T cell responses in the absence of 4-1BBL show rather minor defects, and these were observed already by day 7–8 of priming (225, 227). In contrast, 4-1BBL$^{-/-}$ mice primed with a weak antigen, an LCMV peptide, failed to survive lethal challenge with a virulent strain of LCMV, suggesting a role for 4-1BBL in CD8 T cell memory (228). With influenza delivered intraperitoneally, which results in very limited viral replication, the effects of CD28 and 4-1BBL are temporally segregated. Not surprisingly, CD28 deficiency results in greatly reduced primary expansion of CD8 T cells. In contrast, the absence of 4-1BBL had no impact on the initial expansion or contraction of the response but resulted in decreases in CD8 T cell numbers at 3–6 weeks after influenza infection and decreased recall CD8 responses (197). Analysis of the effects of 4-1BBL deficiency on influenza-specific responses following i.n. infection is required to determine whether these defects are also observed under more physiological conditions.

In 4-1BBL$^{-/-}$ mice, adoptively transferred OVA-specific CD8 T cells show normal initial expansion and contraction. However, they show defects in T cell survival late in the primary response as well as in secondary expansion to OVA/LPS (175), and thus recapitulate the results seen with influenza infection of these mice (197). The different timing of when defects are observed in the gene-targeted mice analyzed with LCMV versus influenza virus or ovalbumin may reflect differences in Ag load, which in turn may affect how efficiently and when the 4-1BB receptor and ligand are induced.

Interestingly, a single dose of agonistic anti-4-1BB antibody, delivered at the time of initial influenza virus infection, can partially restore the primary expansion of CD28$^{-/-}$ CD8 T cells and result in a wild-type-level secondary response in the absence of further administration of antibody. In contrast, agonistic anti-4-1BB antibody had only a transient effect during priming of 4-1BBL$^{-/-}$ mice and failed to correct the secondary response defect unless added at the time of challenge (211). These studies show that signals through 4-1BB are transient and may be required at later times in the T cell response to maintain T cell numbers. In contrast, CD28 signals appear to be dispensable after initial priming. This raises the question of what induces 4-1BB and its ligand weeks after the initial viral infection has been cleared.

Although CD28 and 4-1BBL show distinct effects during immune responses to influenza, they show redundant effects on skin allograft rejection, with only doubly deficient CD28$^{-/-}$4-1BBL$^{-/-}$ mice showing delayed graft rejection (224). Skin allografts, with a high density of alloantigen-expressing cells, represent a very strong immunological stimulus, and in this case sufficient 4-1BB and 4-1BBL may be induced to allow full rejection in the absence of CD28.

In contrast to the studies with LCMV and influenza virus, which show a predominant effect of 4-1BB on CD8 T cells (197, 225), MHC class I– versus MHC class II–restricted GVHD models are similarly impaired in 4-1BB$^{-/-}$ or 4-1BBL$^{-/-}$ mice (212). Similarly, transfer of CD4 or CD8 Ag-specific T cells into 4-1BBL$^{+/+}$ or 4-1BBL$^{-/-}$ mice followed by immunization with Ag/LPS showed that 4-1BBL affects the secondary response of both CD4 and CD8 T cells (175). In a model of herpes-induced stromal keratitis, in which Th1 T cells are considered to be the major mediators of disease, 4-1BB deficiency was found to prevent disease by influencing the number of T cells infiltrating the eye (178). Whether this is due to a trafficking defect rather than effects on activation of T cells in the LN or survival at the site is difficult to distinguish.

Taken together, studies with 4-1BBL$^{-/-}$ and 4-1BB$^{-/-}$ mice suggest a predominant role for 4-1BB on CD8 recall responses, with effects temporally segregated with respect to CD28-mediated effects. However, effects on CD4 T cell responses are clearly observed in some models.

4-1BB in Cancer Therapy

The finding that agonistic antibodies can greatly enhance the expansion of CD8 T cells in vivo (200, 210) raised interest in 4-1BB as a therapeutic target, particularly for cancer therapy (12). Significant improvements in antitumor responses have been observed in mice using transfected or adenovirus-delivered 4-1BBL (229–232) or using anti-4-1BB antibodies delivered systemically or expressed on tumors as a single chain Fv (17, 98, 203, 210, 233). In general, CD28 signaling is also required for these effects (17, 234). It is assumed that anti-4-1BB is directly expanding CD8 T cells in many of these models; however, there is also the possibility for effects of anti-4-1BB on NK cells and DC (215). In humans, the finding that 4-1BBL allows much better expansion of CD8 T cells than anti-CD3/CD28 alone (198) suggests that 4-1BBL stimulation will be useful in adoptive immunotherapy of cancer (235).

HVEM/LIGHT

The TNFR family member herpes virus entry mediator (HVEM) was first isolated as the receptor for herpes simplex virus 1 (HSV-1) (236). HVEM binds to two TNF family ligands, Ltα3 and LIGHT (see Appendix) (237). LIGHT binds to three receptors: HVEM, LTβ receptor (LTβR), and the decoy receptor DcR3/TR6 (237–239). The possibility of multiple receptor-ligand interactions on different cells complicates the interpretation of experiments involving manipulation of HVEM-LIGHT interactions (reviewed in 7, 240). LIGHT is closely linked with CD70 and 4-1BBL on human chromosome 19/mouse chromosome 17 (241), consistent with related functions of these TNF family ligands. This discussion focuses on the activation of T cells via direct HVEM-LIGHT interactions.

Expression of HVEM/LIGHT

HVEM is expressed on resting T cells, monocytes, and immature DC, whereas LIGHT is induced upon activation of CD4 and CD8 T cells, monocytes, and NK cells and is also found on immature but not mature DC (37, 237, 240, 242, 243). HVEM is downregulated upon T cell activation, and LIGHT binding to HVEM also induces its further downregulation on T cells (242) and DC (244). This reciprocal expression of HVEM and LIGHT on T cells (242) and the downregulation of LIGHT upon DC maturation (243) means that there is only a narrow window of time in the first few hours after initial T cell activation in which HVEM-LIGHT interactions can occur. Nevertheless, both LIGHT and HVEM mRNA and LIGHT expression on infiltrating mononuclear cells can be detected at 3 and 7 days posttransplant in cardiac allografts, suggesting that in vivo both receptors and ligands can be simultaneously expressed (245).

HVEM-LIGHT Interactions on T Cells In Vitro

Evidence that LIGHT binding to HVEM on T cells provides a costimulatory signal via HVEM signaling comes from several in vitro studies in which recombinant LIGHT protein or anti-HVEM immobilized with a suboptimal dose of anti-CD3 allows T cell proliferation, NF-κB activation, and/or cytokine production (37, 238, 243, 246, 247). Because the LTβR is absent from T cells, these effects of LIGHT can be attributed to LIGHT-HVEM interaction. Costimulatory effects of LIGHT on purified T cells are independent of CD28 signaling (246).

Blocking of HVEM-LIGHT interaction using HSV-1 glycoprotein D, anti-HVEM, or HVEM-Ig inhibits the proliferation of purified T cells responding to anti-CD3 or anti-CD3/CD28 (248–250). Furthermore, two studies showed that purified LIGHT$^{-/-}$ T cells have decreased responses to anti-CD3 alone, consistent with HVEM-LIGHT interactions during T-T interaction enhancing proliferation (251, 252). Although a third study did not show any defect in proliferation of LIGHT$^{-/-}$ T cells (253), this may reflect lower cell densities in the cultures leading to less efficient T-T contact.

In addition to effects of LIGHT on T cell signaling via HVEM, LIGHT can also contribute to T cell activation indirectly by inducing DC maturation (244), an effect that is enhanced in the presence of CD40L. Addition of anti-LIGHT antibodies to cultures of T cells and DC inhibits T cell–induced IL-12 production by DC (254), suggesting a role for LIGHT in T-DC interactions. Whether this effect is due to T-T activation leading to activated T-DC interaction or to a direct effect of LIGHT binding to DC, and whether this involves LTβR or HVEM signals, is not clear. Evidence also suggests that reverse signaling through LIGHT in T cells can contribute to T cell activation (255–257). Thus, the possibility of LIGHT/HVEM binding to more than one receptor/ligand, the possibility of direct signaling in T cells versus effects on DC maturation/activation, as well as reverse signaling by the ligand complicate the interpretation of these studies.

In Vivo Manipulation of HVEM-LIGHT Interactions

Overexpression of LIGHT under control of the lck or CD2 promoter in mice results in an autoimmune phenotype, with splenomegaly, lymphadenopathy, severe inflammation in the intestine, expanded populations of CD4 and CD8 T cells, and abnormalities in lymphoid tissues (241, 258, 259). These studies suggest that LIGHT is an important regulator of T cell activation, particularly in mucosal tissues (241, 258). However, recent evidence suggests that IgA nephropathy and intestinal inflammation caused by transgenic expression of LIGHT is dependent on signaling through LTβR, rather than HVEM (260).

Mice expressing LIGHT under control of the proximal lck promoter show enhanced negative selection of thymocytes (261), and blockade with HVEM-Ig or

LTβR-Ig also suggested a role for LIGHT in negative selection (310). However, thymi from LIGHT$^{-/-}$ mice had normal cellularity and cell subsets, arguing against a major role for LIGHT in T cell development (251–253).

Although the interaction of LIGHT with LTβR led to the expectation that LIGHT$^{-/-}$ mice would have lymphoid abnormalities, there were no defects in lymph node numbers or architecture in the absence of LIGHT alone. However, effects of LIGHT on controlling numbers of mesenteric lymph nodes could be observed in mice lacking both LIGHT and LTβ (7, 252).

Deficiency in LIGHT preferentially affects CD8 T cell proliferation compared with CD4 T cell proliferation to anti-CD3 (251) or in an MLR (252). Similarly, after superantigen administration in vivo, LIGHT$^{-/-}$ mice show defects in CD8 T cell survival but not in CD4 T cell survival (253). However, LIGHT can also influence CD4 T cell responses, as CD4 IL-2 production was decreased in an MLR in which both the stimulators and responders lacked LIGHT (252). There are conflicting data on whether LIGHT$^{-/-}$ T cells show defects in survival or cell division (251, 252). The response of LIGHT$^{-/-}$ T cells to anti-CD3 alone results in decreased T cell survival, with no defect in cell division (252). Conversely, LIGHT$^{-/-}$ T cell responses to anti-CD3 plus anti-CD28 showed defects in CD8 T cell division, a defect attributed to decreased IL-2R surface expression (251).

LIGHT$^{-/-}$ mice show decreased CTL recall responses after immunization with a papilloma virus peptide (253). However, no defect in antibody responses or in the ex vivo CTL activity were observed following VSV-infection of LIGHT$^{-/-}$ mice (252). Thus, there does not appear to be a major requirement for LIGHT in primary antiviral immunity, although this should be further analyzed with other infectious models, particularly at mucosal sites.

Role of LIGHT in Allorecognition

Several studies have shown that LIGHT pathway blockers, including HVEM-Ig, anti-HVEM, and DcR3, block MLRs (243, 250, 262). Investigators obtained different results when analyzing alloresponses in the absence of LIGHT, depending on whether the T cells or the APC lack LIGHT. In an MLR, the complete absence of LIGHT in both responders and stimulators resulted in defects in CD8 T cell proliferation as well as CD4 T cell IL-2 production (252). Similarly LIGHT$^{-/-}$ CD8 T cells showed a decreased MLR to allogeneic P815 mastocytoma target cells (251). In contrast, WT T cells showed no defect in response to allogeneic LIGHT$^{-/-}$ stimulators (253). Thus, in the MLR, LIGHT seems to be more important on responding T cells than on the stimulators, consistent with a role for LIGHT in T-T interaction. Whether T-T interactions via LIGHT-HVEM are important in vivo has been difficult to ascertain.

Several studies suggest a role for LIGHT in allorecognition in vivo. Administration of LTβR-Ig can block GVHD in mice in a model in which T cells lack LTα, thus pointing to a role for LIGHT in GVHD (246). Combining LTβR-Ig with an anti-CD40L-blocking antibody resulted in complete prevention of GVHD (263). LIGHT$^{-/-}$ mice reject skin allografts, as rapidly as WT mice; however, LIGHT$^{-/-}$CD28$^{-/-}$ mice (252) show a delay of skin allograft rejection, similar to the delay in graft rejection seen in 4-1BBL$^{-/-}$CD28$^{-/-}$ mice (224). The absence of LIGHT has only a modest effect on survival of cardiac allografts in mice; however, cyclosporin A–treated LIGHT$^{-/-}$ mice show prolonged graft survival (245). Taken together, these studies show a clear role for LIGHT in graft rejection. However, the relative importance of HVEM-LIGHT versus LTβR-LIGHT interactions in allorecognition in vivo is not known.

LIGHT and Antitumor Immunity

Soluble LIGHT can cause apoptosis of tumors in vitro, and LIGHT transfection allows tumor regression in a nude mouse model (37, 238, 239). The effect of LIGHT on tumor death is independent of HVEM and occurs via an LTβR-TRAF3-dependent death pathway (264). Injection of LIGHT cDNA directly into tumor nodules results in regression of tumors, with maximal effects requiring both CD4 and CD8 T cells (246). LIGHT-induced tumor regression correlates with increased CTL activity against the tumors, suggesting that LIGHT can act as a costimulator for T cells in this system. More recently, transfection of LIGHT into tumors highlighted the dual role of LIGHT in tumor rejection: interaction of LIGHT with LTβR on the stroma induces production of chemokines, including CCL21, which attracts T cells, which in turn can respond to costimulation by LIGHT expressed on the tumor cells (247).

In summary, although the effects of LIGHT are complex and pleiotropic, LIGHT-HVEM interaction has a clear role in CD28-independent T cell activation in vitro, with preferential effects on CD8 T cells in some but not all models. LIGHT plays a role in allorecognition, particularly when other costimulatory signals are limiting. In these aspects, LIGHT appears similar to 4-1BBL. However, in contrast to the role of 4-1BBL in CD8 T cell memory to viruses, evidence to date has not shown a major effect of LIGHT on antiviral responses. Further work is required to assess the role of HVEM/LIGHT in primary and memory T cell responses and to pinpoint which in vivo effects of LIGHT can be attributed specifically to interactions with HVEM.

CD30/CD30L

CD30 was originally discovered on Hodgkin's lymphoma and Reed-Sternberg cells (265), where overexpression of CD30 results in ligand-independent NF-κB activation and is thereby thought to contribute to malignancy (266). The release of soluble CD30 from activated cells is associated with a number of diseases, including neoplasia, viral infection, and various autoimmune disorders (reviewed in 267). This discussion focuses on the role of CD30 on normal T cells.

Expression

CD30 is expressed on activated α/β as well as γ/δ T cells, on virally infected T cells, B cells, and NK cells (267, 268), and on eosinophils (269). Although CD30 is found in the thymus, its expression is confined to the medulla (270). Initial analysis suggested that CD30 was preferentially expressed on Th2 cells (267, 271). However, CD30 can also be expressed on Th0 and Th1 cells (267, 272). CD30 is inducible by TCR signaling, in a CD28-dependent manner, or by IL-4 (267, 273, 274). In terms of its preferential expression on Th2 cells, CD30 is similar to OX40. However, CD30 expression is more dependent on Th2 cytokines than is OX40 (274), and CD30 expression differs from OX40 in its dependence on STAT6, a critical mediator of IL-4-mediated signaling (274).

CD30L is expressed on resting B cells (275) as well as on activated T cells, where reverse signaling via CD30L can occur (276, 277). CD30L is also observed in inflamed tissues, including cardiac myocytes of mice and humans with myocarditis (190, 278). As is the case with OX40L, CD30L is found in areas of T cell–B cell contact and is expressed together with OX40L on a unique accessory cell that appears to maintain survival of primed and memory T cells (107).

Function of CD30 on T Cells In Vitro

As is the case with other costimulatory TNFR family members, engagement of CD30 together with the TCR can result in enhancement of proliferation and cytokine production (36, 267, 279, 280). Although CD30L induces enhanced proliferation of anti-CD3-treated primary T cells, it can cause death or inhibitory effects on some lymphoma cell lines (279, 281, 282). When overexpressed in human embryonic kidney 293 cells, CD30 can potentiate TNFR-I-induced death by sequestering TRAF2 and promoting its degradation (283). However, there is no evidence that it functions in this way in primary T cells. Stimulation with agonistic anti-CD30 antibodies or blockade with anti-CD30L antibodies led to the suggestion that CD30 promotes Th2-type responses in humans (284). However, as discussed above, CD30 can also be found on activated CD8 and Th1 cells and can also enhance IFN-γ production by Ag-specific T cells previously grown in IL-4 to induce CD30 expression (36).

In addition to its costimulatory effects, anti-CD30 treatment of primed murine T cells in the absence of TCR stimulation leads to IL-13 production (36). CD30-induced IL-13 induction is dependent on TRAF2 and p38 activation, but it is independent of NF-κB (36). Because IL-13 can contribute to parasite clearance as well as eosinophilia in the lung (285), this effect of anti-CD30 is consistent with a role for CD30 in Th2 responses.

Analysis of CD30 Function Using Gene-Targeted Mice

CD30$^{-/-}$ mice have normal numbers and subsets of LN, spleen, and bone marrow cells. Primary CD8 T cell responses to VSV as well as anti-VSV antibody production and class switch are unaffected by CD30 deficiency (286). CD30-deficient T cells proliferate normally to anti-CD3 or superantigen, arguing against a major role for CD30-CD30L interactions by T-T interaction (286). Although initial analysis of CD30$^{-/-}$ mice suggested a partial defect in negative selection of T cells (286), this was not borne out in later studies (287). The different results observed in the initial studies are unexplained but might be due to insufficient backcrossing of the mice. The finding that OX40 and CD30 have in common the expression of their ligands on accessory cells at sites of T-B interaction (107) and an association with Th2 responses (95, 267) raises the issue of whether they might have similar functions in the immune response in vivo. However, in studies of experimental Leishmaniasis in BALB/c mice, blockade of CD30L had no effect under conditions in which anti-OX40L abrogated disease (75). There is a preliminary report that there is decreased and delayed expansion of adoptively transferred Ag-specific CD8 T cells in CD30L$^{-/-}$ mice compared with WT mice, and upon reimmunization the CD8$^+$ T cells in CD30L$^{-/-}$ mice failed to re-expand (288). These data suggest that CD30 may be important in T cell memory. To date, CD30$^{-/-}$ and CD30L$^{-/-}$ mice have not been carefully examined for defects in primary or secondary CD4 responses, which might be expected based on the similarity of CD30 and OX40 expression and function.

CD30 in Diabetes

Conflicting roles for CD30 have been suggested in diabetes. CD30 was identified as a candidate gene for *idd9.2*, a gene controlling diabetes progression, and there are several sequence differences between CD30 in NOD versus B10 mice (179, 289). Anti-CD30L neutralizing antibodies block spontaneous diabetes development in NOD mice and prevent islet-cell-specific T cell proliferation ex vivo (290). In contrast, in an adoptive transfer model of diabetes that is CD8$^+$ T cell mediated, the absence of CD30 on the T cells resulted in exacerbated disease (291). Although the latter study was interpreted as indicating a negative role for CD30 in T cell responses, the complexity of the model, conflicting data in other models of diabetes, and the lack of lymphoproliferative disorders in CD30$^{-/-}$ mice argues against a predominant role for CD30 in inhibition of T cell responses.

GITR/GITRL

Expression

Glucocorticoid-induced TNFR family related gene (GITR) was first identified as a dexamethasone-inducible molecule on a murine T cell hybridoma (292). The human equivalent of GITR, also known as AITR, was identified by its homology to the extracellular domain of TNFR family members (39, 40). GITR is expressed only at low levels on resting mouse and human T cells, but it is upregulated upon activation of CD4 and CD8 T cells, with peak expression at 24 hr and greater induction in the presence of CD28 signaling (39, 42, 292, 293). In addition to its expression on activated T cells, a substantial level of GITR is constitutively expressed on $CD4^+CD25^+$ regulatory T cells (Tregs) (294, 295).

Human GITRL was first cloned from cultured human umbilical vein endothelial cells, which show low levels of surface GITRL (39, 40). Several groups have recently cloned mouse GITRL (41, 293, 296, 297). GITRL is expressed at low levels on B cells, macrophages and BM-derived DC (297, 298). In mouse, GITRL expression is controlled by the transcription factor NF-1 (297). GITRL is transiently upregulated on APC by TLR stimulation but is downregulated by 48 hr (293, 297). GITRL is absent from resting T cells, although there are conflicting data on whether GITRL is present on activated T cells (293, 297). Thus, its expression pattern suggests that GITR on activated T cells most likely receives signals from GITRL on APCs, early after initial T cell activation.

Function of GITR as a Costimulator of Conventional T Cells

Evidence for a costimulatory role for GITR on T cells comes from studies of GITRL or anti-GITR stimulation of T cells. Anti-GITR or GITRL can costimulate proliferation of naive, Th1, or Th2 CD4 T cells and CD8 T cells in the presence of suboptimal concentrations of anti-CD3 (41, 42, 295, 297, 299, 300). GITRL is also costimulatory for $CD28^{-/-}$ T cells (295). In addition to increased proliferation, GITR ligation in the presence of a TCR signal upregulates IL-2Rα, IFN-γ, IL-2, IL-4, and IL-10, and it enhances killing in a redirected lysis assay (42, 299). Effects of GITR on induction of proliferation and survival seen on conventional T cells are also seen on Tregs (discussed further below) (41, 42, 299).

Initial analysis of $GITR^{-/-}$ mice showed no abnormalities in lymphocyte numbers or subsets (301). However, T cells from $GITR^{-/-}$ mice showed hyperresponsiveness to immobilized anti-CD3, raising the possibility that GITR is a negative regulator of T cell responses. However, subsequent analysis of $GITR^{+/+}$ versus $GITR^{-/-}$ T cell responses to anti-CD3 plus GITRL clearly show a costimulatory role for GITR-GITRL interaction (293, 299).

Role of GITR in Preventing Suppression Induced by $CD25^+$ Regulatory T Cells

Tregs, a subset of $CD4^+$ T cells often characterized by surface expression of CD25 in the absence of overt activation, suppress T cell responses in vivo (reviewed in 302). Two strategies led to the finding that GITR is constitutively expressed on Tregs: (a) GITR-specific monoclonal antibodies were identified in a screen for antibodies raised against $CD25^+$ Tregs that could block T suppression (295), and (b) gene array analysis of $CD25^+$ Tregs compared with their $CD25^-$ counterparts revealed that Tregs constitutively expressed high levels of GITR, with further induction upon activation (294). Addition of anti-GITR to co-cultures of Tregs and CD25$^-$ T cells results in a loss of suppression, whereas antibodies to other TNFR family members such as CD27, CD30, OX40, and CD40 did not have the same effect (294, 295). Subsequent work showed that Tregs, isolated on the basis of constitutive GITR expression, regardless of expression of CD25, could prevent development of colitis in an adoptive transfer model, whereas addition of anti-GITR antibodies led to induction of disease (303). This study suggested that GITR might be a better marker of Tregs than CD25. However, as pointed out by Gavin & Rudensky (302), because GITR, like CD25, is induced on conventional T cells upon activation, there are limitations to its use as a marker of Tregs.

GITR does not play a role in the development or basal function of Tregs, as Tregs from GITR$^{-/-}$ or GITR$^{+/+}$ mice show similar suppressive activity in the absence of GITR ligation, and similar numbers of Tregs are found in the thymus of both types of mice (293, 299). However, GITR$^{-/-}$ mice have 33% fewer CD25$^+$CD4$^+$ T cells in spleen and LN, suggesting a possible role of GITR in maintaining Treg numbers in the periphery (293). The finding that GITR regulates NF-κB activation is consistent with a role for GITR in controlling T cell survival (39–41).

Because Tregs constitutively express GITR, and because anti-GITR can induce autoimmunity, researchers concluded that GITR controls T suppressor function (295, 303). The initial interpretation of these studies was that GITR engagement on the Tregs allows them to proliferate, overcome their anergic state, and lose their suppressor function (294, 295, 303). However, preincubation of the CD25$^+$ or CD25$^-$ T cells with anti-GITR did not lead to subsequent loss of suppression (294, 295), so determining which population of T cells was directly responding to anti-GITR was difficult. GITR is rapidly induced upon activation of CD4 effector T cells, and GITR ligation can enhance conventional T cell responses (41, 42, 295, 297, 299), including those of autoreactive CD4$^+$ effector T cells (300). Thus, it is possible that effects of GITR on both Tregs and T effectors contribute to its abrogation of suppression. The assumption that anti-GITR acts as an agonist is supported by data showing that soluble GITRL has a similar function in abrogating T cell suppression as anti-GITR (41).

To delineate the relative importance of GITR signaling on CD25$^+$CD4$^+$ Tregs compared with its effects on CD4$^+$ effector T cells in abrogation of suppression, Stephens et al. (293) used coculture of CD25$^+$ or CD25$^-$cells from GITR$^{+/+}$ and GITR$^{-/-}$ mice. They found that the presence of GITR on the CD25$^-$CD4$^+$ effector T cells, rather than on the CD25$^+$ suppressor cells, was critical for the reversal of suppression by anti-GITR. In this study, GITR$^{+/+}$ and GITR$^{-/-}$ T cells had similar responses to stimulation in the absence of Tregs, suggesting that the main effect of GITR ligation on T effector cells is to allow them to resist the effects of T suppressor cells. GITRL is present on resting APC, upregulated transiently upon TLR activation, and then downregulated within 48 hr (293, 297). This leads to a model in which binding of GITRL on APC to GITR on recently activated T cells allows them to resist the effects of T suppressor cells. Binding of GITRL to T suppressors can also allow their expansion. Later in the response, when GITRL becomes limiting, the Tregs would then dominate and limit the response (293, 297).

Other Costimulatory TNFR Family Members and Tregs

CD25$^+$CD4$^+$ Tregs have a number of markers of activated T cells, and they also express 4-1BB and OX40. Initial reports indicated that ligation of these and other TNFR family molecules fails to abrogate suppression by Tregs (294, 295). In contrast, two recent reports have shown effects of anti-4-1BB (304) or anti-OX40 (305) on counteracting Treg function. The difference between these and earlier studies remains to be resolved. Because CD28 can overcome the anergic state of Tregs, other costimulatory molecules may substitute a similar costimulatory signal under some circumstances. On the basis of the knowledge of GITR signaling to date, it is not immediately obvious why GITR signals, as opposed to signals from other costimulatory TNFR family members, are particularly good at rendering T effectors resistant to the effects of suppressor cells.

SUMMARY AND CONCLUSIONS

There is general consensus that the costimulatory TNFR family members function to sustain T cell numbers after initial CD28-dependent T cell activation, in a TRAF2-dependent manner. The ability of several different TNFR family members to transiently control T cell activation/survival at distinct stages in the response may be important in providing multiple points to fine-tune the response. Many effects of TNFR family members observed in gene-targeted mice are not "all or nothing," but rather appear to affect T cell survival quantitatively, with quite subtle effects in some models. Given their similarities in function and signaling pathways, the different family members may have some redundancy that will be revealed when mice lacking more than one receptor or ligand are analyzed. However, an initial analysis of mice lacking both OX40L and 4-1BBL suggests that these two costimulatory ligands act independently and non-redundantly with respect to CD4 and CD8 T cell activation (149a). Further work is required to determine which distinct effects of the TNF family costimulators can be attributed to distinct downstream signaling and which simply reflect the availability of the different ligands and receptors with common signaling pathways on particular cells at particular stages of activation.

Table 1 summarizes the most prominent effects of costimulatory TNFR family members on T cell responses. As discussed elsewhere, major questions remain with respect to the location and timing of these interactions in vivo (306). The expression of CD27 and HVEM on resting T cells and the induction of their ligands shortly after activation suggests that they may function by T-T or T-APC interaction relatively early after TCR/CD28 signals. OX40 and 4-1BB signals on T cells are delayed with respect to initial activation and likely occur through interaction with

TABLE 1   Some key features of TNFR costimulatory receptors on T cells

Receptor	Function on T cells
CD27	Expansion of CD4 and CD8 T cells Acts after CD28 to sustain T effector cell survival Affects T cell accumulation in lung more than in spleen Influences secondary responses more than primary responses
OX40	Predominant effect on CD4 T cells Contributes to ongoing Th1 or Th2 responses, Th2 more than Th1 Functions after CD28 to sustain CD4 T cell survival Important for CD4 T cell memory Important target in autoimmunity
4-1BB	Greater effect on CD8 than CD4 T cells in antiviral immunity In GVHD, both CD4 and CD8 T cells affected Functions after CD28 to sustain T cell survival Important for T cell memory Promising results in cancer therapy models
HVEM	T cell costimulator T-T interaction Limited analysis of HVEM effects in vivo
CD30	T cell costimulator: Affects Th2 more than Th1 (?) Affects CD8 T cell memory (?) Limited analysis of effects in vivo
GITR	Costimulatory for CD25$^-$ and CD25$^+$ T cells Allows proliferation of Tregs, releases Tregs from anergy Renders T effectors resistant to effects of Tregs

ligands on activated APC. OX40 shows preferential effects on CD4 T cells, whereas 4-1BB can act on CD4 and CD8 T cells but shows preferential effects on CD8 T cells in some models. Mice deficient in the OX40, CD27, or 4-1BB costimulatory pathway all show greater defects in secondary responses compared with primary responses, consistent with their role in maintenance of memory T cells. Although OX40 can function to modulate ongoing Th1 and Th2 responses, OX40 and CD30 show higher expression on Th2 cells in some circumstances and thus may have larger effects on Th2 responses. GITR can play a costimulatory role on most T cell subsets, but a major function of GITR appears to be to allow T effectors to resist the effects of T suppressor cells.

Several costimulatory TNFR family members show promise for manipulation of host response to disease. However, ligation of TNFR family members can be protective or harmful, depending on how they are manipulated and the degree of inflammation. Transient stimulation through costimulatory TNFR family members can enhance antiviral and anticancer responses in vivo, and blockade of these costimulatory pathways can be beneficial for autoimmunity and transplantation. In contrast, the use of agonistic antibodies that stimulate anticancer or antiviral responses under conditions of strong immune or inflammatory conditions leads to suppression of responses, apparently by induction of inhibitory cytokines. Similarly, constitutive expression of the costimulatory ligands tends to have devastating consequences in mice, with autoimmunity or profound immunosuppression the result. Thus, care must be used in the application of costimulatory TNF family members to human disease.

APPENDIX

Abbreviations used: APC, antigen-presenting cell; ASM, airway smooth muscle; BAL, bronchial alveolar lavage; CTL, cytotoxic T lymphocyte; DC, dendritic cell; DcR3, decoy receptor 3; DD, death domain; DLN, draining lymph node; DN, dominant negative; EAE, experimental autoimmune encephalomyelitis; GITR, glucocorticoid-induced TNFR family related gene; GM-CSF, granulocyte macrophage colony stimulating factor; GVHD, graft-versus-host disease; HIV, human immunodeficiency virus; HSV-1, herpes simplex virus-1; HTLV, human T cell leukemia virus; HVEM, herpes virus entry mediator; IEL, intraepithelial lymphocytes; i.n., intranasal; JNK/SAPK, jun-N-terminal kinase/stress-activated protein kinase; KLH, keyhole limpet hemocyanin; LCMV, lymphocytic choriomeningitis virus; LIGHT, lymphotoxin-like, exhibits inducible expression, and competes with HSV glycoprotein D for HVEM, a receptor expressed by T lymphocytes; LPS, lipopolysaccharide; LT, lymphotoxin; MAPK, mitogen activated protein kinase; MHC, major histocompatibility complex; MLR, mixed lymphocyte reaction; NF-κB, nuclear factor κB; NK, natural killer; NOD, nonobese diabetic; PI-3K, phosphatidylinositol 3-kinase; PKB, protein kinase B; PspA, pneumococcal surface protein A; RAG, recombinase activating gene; RING, really interesting new gene; TCR, T cell receptor; TLR, Toll-like receptor; TRAF, TNFR receptor-associated factor; TNF, tumor necrosis factor; TNFR, TNF receptor; Treg, regulatory T cell; VSV, vesicular stomatitis virus.

ACKNOWLEDGMENTS

The literature search for this article was completed in June 2004. Thanks to Jannie Borst, Anthony Vella, Rene van Lier, Mick Croft, and Ethan Shevach for providing preprints and/or helpful discussion. Thanks to Jennifer Gommerman and Lena Serghides for critical reading of the manuscript. Figure 1 was adapted from a figure provided by Linh Nguyen. Funding for my research in T cell costimulation was provided by the Canadian Institutes of Health Research, the National Cancer Institute of Canada, the Arthritis Society of Canada, and CANVAC, the Canadian Network for Vaccines and Immunotherapeutics.

The *Annual Review of Immunology* is online at http://immunol.annualreviews.org

LITERATURE CITED

1. Lenschow DJ, Walunas TL, Bluestone JA. 1996. CD28/B7 system of T cell co-stimulation. *Annu. Rev. Immunol.* 14: 233–58

2. Sharpe AH, Freeman GJ. 2002. The B7-CD28 superfamily. *Nat. Rev. Immunol.* 2:116–26

3. Wong P, Pamer EG. 2003. CD8 T cell responses to infectious pathogens. *Annu. Rev. Immunol.* 21:29–70

4. Lee WT, Pasos G, Cecchini L, Mittler JN. 2002. Continued antigen stimulation is not required during CD4+ T cell clonal expansion. *J. Immunol.* 168:1682–89

5. Sprent J, Surh CD. 2002. T cell memory. *Annu. Rev. Immunol.* 20:551–79

6. Kollias G, Kontoyiannis D. 2002. Role of TNF/TNFR in autoimmunity: Specific TNF receptor blockade may be advantageous to anti-TNF treatments. *Cytokine Growth Factor Rev.* 13:315–21

7. Pfeffer K. 2003. Biological functions of tumor necrosis factor cytokines and their receptors. *Cytokine Growth Factor Rev.* 14:185–91

8. Gommerman JL, Browning JL. 2003. Lymphotoxin/light, lymphoid microenvironments and autoimmune disease. *Nat. Rev. Immunol.* 3:642–55

9. Josien R, Li HL, Ingulli E, Sarma S, Wong BR, et al. 2000. TRANCE, a tumor necrosis factor family member, enhances the longevity and adjuvant properties of dendritic cells in vivo. *J. Exp. Med.* 191:495–502

10. Bachmann MF, Wong BR, Josien R, Steinman RM, Oxenius A, Choi Y. 1999. TRANCE, a tumor necrosis factor family member critical for CD40 ligand–independent T helper cell activation. *J. Exp. Med.* 189:1025–31

11. Quezada SA, Jarvinen LZ, Lind EF, Noelle RJ. 2004. CD40/CD154 interactions at the interface of tolerance and immunity. *Annu. Rev. Immunol.* 22:307–28

12. Croft M. 2003. Co-stimulatory members of the TNFR family: keys to effective T-cell immunity? *Nat. Rev. Immunol.* 3:609–20

13. DeBenedette MA, Shahinian A, Mak TW, Watts TH. 1997. Costimulation of CD28− lymphocytes by 4-1BB ligand. *J. Immunol.* 158:551–59

14. Ohshima Y, Tanaka Y, Tozawa H, Takahashi Y, Maliszewski C, Delespesse G. 1997. Expression and function of OX40 ligand on human dendritic cells. *J. Immunol.* 159:3838–48

15. Murata K, Ishii N, Takano H, Miura S, Ndhlovu LC, et al. 2000. Impairment of antigen-presenting cell function in mice lacking expression of OX40 ligand. *J. Exp. Med.* 191:365–74

16. Futagawa T, Akiba H, Kodama T, Takeda K, Hosoda Y, et al. 2002. Expression and function of 4-1BB and 4-1BB ligand on murine dendritic cells. *Int. Immunol.* 14:275–86

17. Diehl L, van Mierlo GJ, den Boer AT, van der Voort E, Fransen M, et al. 2002. In vivo triggering through 4-1BB enables Th-independent priming of CTL in the presence of an intact CD28 costimulatory pathway. *J. Immunol.* 168:3755–62

18. Tesselaar K, Xiao Y, Arens R, van Schijndel GM, Schuurhuis DH, et al. 2003. Expression of the murine CD27 ligand CD70 in vitro and in vivo. *J. Immunol.* 170:33–40

19. Kim EY, Teh HS. 2001. TNF type 2 receptor (p75) lowers the threshold of T cell activation. *J. Immunol.* 167:6812–20

20. Locksley RM, Killeen N, Lenardo MJ. 2001. The TNF and TNF receptor superfamilies: integrating mammalian biology. *Cell* 104:487–501

21. Dempsey PW, Doyle SE, He JQ, Cheng

G. 2003. The signaling adaptors and pathways activated by TNF superfamily. *Cytokine Growth Factor Rev.* 14:193–209

22. Aggarwal BB. 2003. Signalling pathways of the TNF superfamily: a double-edged sword. *Nat. Rev. Immunol.* 3:745–56

23. Chung JY, Park YC, Ye H, Wu H. 2002. All TRAFs are not created equal: common and distinct molecular mechanisms of TRAF-mediated signal transduction. *J. Cell Sci.* 115:679–88

24. Arch RH, Gedrich RW, Thompson CB. 1998. Tumor necrosis factor receptor-associated factors (TRAFs)—a family of adapter proteins that regulates life and death. *Genes Dev.* 12:2821–30

25. Ye H, Wu H. 2000. Thermodynamic characterization of the interaction between TRAF2 and tumor necrosis factor receptor peptides by isothermal titration calorimetry. *Proc. Natl. Acad. Sci. USA* 97:8961–66

26. Karin M, Lin A. 2002. NF-κB at the crossroads of life and death. *Nat. Immunol.* 3:221–27

27. Yamamoto H, Kishimoto T, Minamoto S. 1998. NF-κB activation in CD27 signaling: involvement of TNF receptor-associated factors in its signaling and identification of functional region of CD27. *J. Immunol.* 161:4753–59

28. Akiba H, Nakano H, Nishinaka S, Shindo M, Kobata T, et al. 1998. CD27, a member of the tumor necrosis factor receptor superfamily, activates NF-κB and stress-activated protein kinase/c-Jun N-terminal kinase via TRAF2, TRAF5, and NF-$\kappa\beta$-inducing kinase. *J. Biol. Chem.* 273:13353–58

29. Kawamata S, Hori T, Imura A, Takaori-Kondo A, Uchiyama T. 1998. Activation of OX40 signal transduction pathways leads to tumor necrosis factor receptor-associated factor (TRAF) 2- and TRAF5-mediated NF-κB activation. *J. Biol. Chem.* 273:5808–14

30. Arch RH, Thompson CB. 1998. 4-1BB and Ox40 are members of a tumor necrosis factor (TNF)-nerve growth factor receptor subfamily that bind TNF receptor-associated factors and activate nuclear factor κB. *Mol. Cell. Biol.* 18:558–65

31. Jang IK, Lee ZH, Kim YJ, Kim SH, Kwon BS. 1998. Human 4-1BB (CD137) signals are mediated by TRAF2 and activate nuclear factor-κB. *Biochem. Biophys. Res. Comm.* 242:613–20

32. Lee HW, Park SJ, Choi BK, Kim HH, Nam KO, Kwon BS. 2002. 4-1BB promotes the survival of CD8$^+$ T lymphocytes by increasing expression of Bcl-x_L and Bfl-1. *J. Immunol.* 169:4882–88

33. Ansieau S, Scheffrahn I, Mosialos G, Brand H, Duyster J, et al. 1996. Tumor necrosis factor receptor-associated factor (TRAF)-1, TRAF-2, and TRAF-3 interact in vivo with the CD30 cytoplasmic domain; TRAF-2 mediates CD30-induced nuclear factor kappa B activation. *Proc. Natl. Acad. Sci. USA* 93:14053–58

34. Duckett CS, Gedrich RW, Gilfillan MC, Thompson CB. 1997. Induction of nuclear factor κB by the CD30 receptor is mediated by TRAF1 and TRAF2. *Mol. Cell. Biol.* 17:1535–42

35. Aizawa S, Nakano H, Ishida T, Horie R, Nagai M, et al. 1997. Tumor necrosis factor receptor-associated factor (TRAF) 5 and TRAF2 are involved in CD30-mediated NF-κB activation. *J. Biol. Chem.* 272:2042–45

36. Harlin H, Podack E, Boothby M, Alegre ML. 2002. TCR-independent CD30 signaling selectively induces IL-13 production via a TNF receptor-associated factor/p38 mitogen-activated protein kinase-dependent mechanism. *J. Immunol.* 169:2451–59

37. Harrop JA, McDonnell PC, Brigham-Burke M, Lyn SD, Minton J, et al. 1998. Herpesvirus entry mediator ligand (HVEM-L), a novel ligand for HVEM/TR2, stimulates proliferation of

T cells and inhibits HT29 cell growth. *J. Biol. Chem.* 273:27548–56

38. Marsters SA, Ayres TM, Skubatch M, Gray CL, Rothe M, Ashkenazi A. 1997. Herpesvirus entry mediator, a member of the tumor necrosis factor receptor (TNFR) family, interacts with members of the TNFR-associated factor family and activates the transcription factors NF-κB and AP-1. *J. Biol. Chem.* 272:14029–32

39. Kwon B, Yu KY, Ni J, Yu GL, Jang IK, et al. 1999. Identification of a novel activation-inducible protein of the tumor necrosis factor receptor superfamily and its ligand. *J. Biol. Chem.* 274:6056–61

40. Gurney AL, Marsters SA, Huang RM, Pitti RM, Mark DT, et al. 1999. Identification of a new member of the tumor necrosis factor family and its receptor, a human ortholog of mouse GITR. *Curr. Biol.* 9:215–18

41. Ji HB, Liao G, Faubion WA, Abadia-Molina AC, Cozzo C, et al. 2004. Cutting edge: the natural ligand for glucocorticoid-induced TNF receptor-related protein abrogates regulatory T cell suppression. *J. Immunol.* 172:5823–27

42. Kanamaru F, Youngnak P, Hashiguchi M, Nishioka T, Takahashi T, et al. 2004. Costimulation via glucocorticoid-induced TNF receptor in both conventional and CD25+ regulatory CD4+ T cells. *J. Immunol.* 172:7306–14

43. Gravestein LA, Amsen D, Boes M, Calvo CR, Kruisbeek AM, Borst J. 1998. The TNF receptor family member CD27 signals to Jun N-terminal kinase via Traf-2. *Eur. J. Immunol.* 28:2208–16

44. Cannons JL, Hoeflich KP, Woodgett JR, Watts TH. 1999. Role of the stress kinase pathway in signaling via the T cell costimulatory receptor 4-1BB. *J. Immunol.* 163:2990–98

45. Cannons JL, Choi Y, Watts TH. 2000. Role of TNF receptor-associated factor 2 and p38 mitogen-activated protein kinase activation during 4-1BB-dependent immune response. *J. Immunol.* 165:6193–204

46. Arron JR, Pewzner-Jung Y, Walsh MC, Kobayashi T, Choi Y. 2002. Regulation of the subcellular localization of tumor necrosis factor receptor-associated factor (TRAF)2 by TRAF1 reveals mechanisms of TRAF2 signaling. *J. Exp. Med.* 196:923–34

47. Yeh WC, Shahinian A, Speiser D, Kraunus J, Billia F, et al. 1997. Early lethality, functional NF-κB activation, and increased sensitivity to TNF-induced cell death in TRAF2-deficient mice. *Immunity* 7:715–25

48. Lee SY, Reichlin A, Santana A, Sokol KA, Nussenzweig MC, Choi Y. 1997. TRAF2 is essential for JNK but not NF-κB activation and regulates lymphocyte proliferation and survival. *Immunity* 7:703–13

49. Tada K, Okazaki T, Sakon S, Kobarai T, Kurosawa K, et al. 2001. Critical roles of TRAF2 and TRAF5 in tumor necrosis factor-induced NF-κB activation and protection from cell death. *J. Biol. Chem.* 276:36530–34

50. Saoulli K, Lee SY, Cannons JL, Yeh WC, Santana A, et al. 1998. CD28-independent, TRAF2-dependent costimulation of resting T cells by 4-1BB ligand. *J. Exp. Med.* 187:1849–62

51. Prell RA, Evans DE, Thalhofer C, Shi T, Funatake C, Weinberg AD. 2003. OX40-mediated memory T cell generation is TNF receptor-associated factor 2 dependent. *J. Immunol.* 171:5997–6005

52. So T, Salek-Ardakani S, Nakano H, Ware CF, Croft M. 2004. TNF receptor-associated factor 5 limits the induction of Th2 immune responses. *J. Immunol.* 172:4292–97

53. Nakano H, Sakon S, Koseki H, Takemori T, Tada K, et al. 1999. Targeted disruption of Traf5 gene causes defects in CD40- and CD27-mediated lymphocyte

activation. *Proc. Natl. Acad. Sci. USA* 96:9803–8

54. Rogers PR, Song J, Gramaglia I, Killeen N, Croft M. 2001. OX40 promotes Bcl-x_L and Bcl-2 expression and is essential for long-term survival of CD4 T cells. *Immunity* 15:445–55

55. Song J, Salek-Ardakani S, Rogers PR, Cheng M, Van Parijs L, Croft M. 2004. The costimulation-regulated duration of PKB activation controls T cell longevity. *Nat. Immunol.* 5:150–56

56. Jones RG, Parsons M, Bonnard M, Chan VS, Yeh WC, et al. 2000. Protein kinase B regulates T lymphocyte survival, nuclear factor κB activation, and Bcl-X_L levels in vivo. *J. Exp. Med.* 191:1721–34

57. Prasad KV, Ao Z, Yoon Y, Wu MX, Rizk M, et al. 1997. CD27, a member of the tumor necrosis factor receptor family, induces apoptosis and binds to Siva, a proapoptotic protein. *Proc. Natl. Acad. Sci. USA* 94:6346–51

58. Spinicelli S, Nocentini G, Ronchetti S, Krausz LT, Bianchini R, Riccardi C. 2002. GITR interacts with the pro-apoptotic protein Siva and induces apoptosis. *Cell Death Differ.* 9:1382–84

59. Py B, Slomianny C, Auberger P, Petit PX, Benichou S. 2004. Siva-1 and an alternative splice form lacking the death domain, Siva-2, similarly induce apoptosis in T lymphocytes via a caspase-dependent mitochondrial pathway. *J. Immunol.* 172:4008–17

60. Kim YJ, Pollok KE, Zhou Z, Shaw A, Bohlen JB, et al. 1993. Novel T cell antigen 4-1BB associates with the protein tyrosine kinase p56lck1. *J. Immunol.* 151:1255–62

61. Lens SM, Tesselaar K, van Oers MH, van Lier RA. 1998. Control of lymphocyte function through CD27-CD70 interactions. *Semin. Immunol.* 10:491–99

62. Borst J, Sluyser C, De Vries E, Klein H, Melief CJ, Van Lier RA. 1989. Alternative molecular form of human T cell–specific antigen CD27 expressed upon T cell activation. *Eur. J. Immunol.* 19:357–64

63. de Jong R, Loenen WA, Brouwer M, van Emmerik L, de Vries EF, et al. 1991. Regulation of expression of CD27, a T cell–specific member of a novel family of membrane receptors. *J. Immunol.* 146:2488–94

64. Hamann D, Kostense S, Wolthers KC, Otto SA, Baars PA, et al. 1999. Evidence that human CD8$^+$CD45RA$^+$CD27$^-$ cells are induced by antigen and evolve through extensive rounds of division. *Int. Immunol.* 11:1027–33

65. Appay V, Dunbar PR, Callan M, Klenerman P, Gillespie GM, et al. 2002. Memory CD8$^+$ T cells vary in differentiation phenotype in different persistent virus infections. *Nat. Med.* 8:379–85

66. Kuijpers TW, Vossen MT, Gent MR, Davin JC, Roos MT, et al. 2003. Frequencies of circulating cytolytic, CD45RA$^+$CD27$^-$, CD8$^+$ T lymphocytes depend on infection with CMV. *J. Immunol.* 170:4342–48

67. van Baarle D, Kostense S, Hovenkamp E, Ogg G, Nanlohy N, et al. 2002. Lack of Epstein-Barr virus- and HIV-specific CD27$^-$ CD8$^+$ T cells is associated with progression to viral disease in HIV-infection. *AIDS* 16:2001–11

68. van Baarle D, Kostense S, van Oers MH, Hamann D, Miedema F. 2002. Failing immune control as a result of impaired CD8$^+$ T-cell maturation: CD27 might provide a clue. *Trends Immunol.* 23:586–91

69. Wherry EJ, Teichgraber V, Becker TC, Masopust D, Kaech SM, et al. 2003. Lineage relationship and protective immunity of memory CD8 T cell subsets. *Nat. Immunol.* 4:225–34

70. Gravestein LA, van Ewijk W, Ossendorp F, Borst J. 1996. CD27 cooperates with the pre–T cell receptor in the regulation of murine T cell development. *J. Exp. Med.* 184:675–85

71. Hendriks J, Gravestein LA, Tesselaar K, van Lier RAW, Schumacher TNM, Borst J. 2000. CD27 is required for generation and long-term maintenance of T cell immunity. *Nat. Immunol.* 1:433–40

72. Bowman MR, Crimmins MA, Yetz-Aldape J, Kriz R, Kelleher K, Herrmann S. 1994. The cloning of CD70 and its identification as the ligand for CD27. *J. Immunol.* 152:1756–61

73. Tesselaar K, Gravestein LA, van Schijndel GM, Borst J, van Lier RA. 1997. Characterization of murine CD70, the ligand of the TNF receptor family member CD27. *J. Immunol.* 159:4959–65

74. Oshima H, Nakano H, Nohara C, Kobata T, Nakajima A, et al. 1998. Characterization of murine CD70 by molecular cloning and mAb. *Int. Immunol.* 10:517–26

75. Akiba H, Miyahira Y, Atsuta M, Takeda K, Nohara C, et al. 2000. Critical contribution of OX40 ligand to T helper cell type 2 differentiation in experimental Leishmaniasis. *J. Exp. Med.* 191:375–80

76. Camerini D, Walz G, Loenen WA, Borst J, Seed B. 1991. The T cell activation antigen CD27 is a member of the nerve growth factor/tumor necrosis factor receptor gene family. *J. Immunol.* 147:3165–69

77. Goodwin RG, Alderson MR, Smith CA, Armitage RJ, VandenBos T, et al. 1993. Molecular and biological characterization of a ligand for CD27 defines a new family of cytokines with homology to tumor necrosis factor. *Cell* 73:447–56

78. Hintzen RQ, Lens SM, Lammers K, Kuiper H, Beckmann MP, van Lier RA. 1995. Engagement of CD27 with its ligand CD70 provides a second signal for T cell activation. *J. Immunol.* 154:2612–23

79. Gravestein LA, Nieland JD, Kruisbeek AM, Borst J. 1995. Novel mAbs reveal potent co-stimulatory activity of murine CD27. *Int. Immunol.* 7:551–57

80. Stuhler G, Zobywalski A, Grunebach F, Brossart P, Reichardt VL, et al. 1999. Immune regulatory loops determine productive interactions within human T lymphocyte–dendritic cell clusters. *Proc. Natl. Acad. Sci. USA* 96:1532–35

81. Hendriks J, Xiao Y, Borst J. 2003. CD27 promotes survival of activated T cells and complements CD28 in generation and establishment of the effector T cell pool. *J. Exp. Med.* 198:1369–80

82. Nagumo H, Agematsu K, Shinozaki K, Hokibara S, Ito S, et al. 1998. CD27/CD70 interaction augments IgE secretion by promoting the differentiation of memory B cells into plasma cells. *J. Immunol.* 161:6496–502

83. Raman VS, Akondy RS, Rath S, Bal V, George A. 2003. Ligation of CD27 on B cells in vivo during primary immunization enhances commitment to memory B cell responses. *J. Immunol.* 171:5876–81

84. Xiao Y, Hendriks J, Langerak P, Jacobs H, Borst J. 2004. CD27 is acquired by primed B cells at the centroblast stage and promotes germinal center formation. *J. Immunol.* 172:7432–41

85. Arens R, Tesselaar K, Baars PA, van Schijndel GM, Hendriks J, et al. 2001. Constitutive CD27/CD70 interaction induces expansion of effector-type T cells and results in IFNγ-mediated B cell depletion. *Immunity* 15:801–12

86. Arens R, Schepers K, Nolte MA, van Oosterwijk MF, van Lier RA, et al. 2004. Tumor rejection induced by CD70-mediated quantitative and qualitative effects on effector CD8+ T cell formation. *J. Exp. Med.* 199:1595–605

87. Rowley TF, Al-Shamkhani A. 2004. Stimulation by soluble CD70 promotes strong primary and secondary CD8+ cytotoxic T cell responses in vivo. *J. Immunol.* 172:6039–46

88. Nakajima A, Oshima H, Nohara C, Morimoto S, Yoshino S, et al. 2000. Involvement of CD70-CD27 interactions

in the induction of experimental autoimmune encephalomyelitis. *J. Neuroimmunol.* 109:188–96

89. Couderc B, Zitvogel L, Douin-Echinard V, Djennane L, Tahara H, et al. 1998. Enhancement of antitumor immunity by expression of CD70 (CD27 ligand) or CD154 (CD40 ligand) costimulatory molecules in tumor cells. *Cancer Gene Ther.* 5:163–75

90. Nieland JD, Graus YF, Dortmans YE, Kremers BL, Kruisbeek AM. 1998. CD40 and CD70 co-stimulate a potent in vivo antitumor T cell response. *J. Immunother.* 21:225–36

91. Lorenz MG, Kantor JA, Schlom J, Hodge JW. 1999. Anti-tumor immunity elicited by a recombinant vaccinia virus expressing CD70 (CD27L). *Hum. Gene Ther.* 10:1095–103

92. Wu T, Hering B, Kirchof N, Sutherland D, Yagita H, Guo Z. 2001. The effect of OX40/OX40L and CD27/CD70 pathways on allogeneic islet graft rejection. *Transplant Proc.* 33:217–18

93. Kelly JM, Darcy PK, Markby JL, Godfrey DI, Takeda K, et al. 2002. Induction of tumor-specific T cell memory by NK cell–mediated tumor rejection. *Nat. Immunol.* 3:83–90

94. Paterson DJ, Jefferies WA, Green JR, Brandon MR, Corthesy P, et al. 1987. Antigens of activated rat T lymphocytes including a molecule of 50,000 Mr detected only on CD4 positive T blasts. *Mol. Immunol.* 24:1281–90

95. Weinberg AD, Vella AT, Croft M. 1998. OX-40: life beyond the effector T cell stage. *Semin. Immunol.* 10:471–80

96. Sugamura K, Ishii N, Weinberg AD. 2004. Therapeutic targeting of the effector T-cell co-stimulatory molecule OX40. *Nat. Rev. Immunol.* 4:420–31

97. Shimojima M, Miyazawa T, Ikeda Y, McMonagle EL, Haining H, et al. 2004. Use of CD134 as a primary receptor by the feline immunodeficiency virus. *Science* 303:1192–95

98. Taraban VY, Rowley TF, O'Brien L, Chan HT, Haswell LE, et al. 2002. Expression and costimulatory effects of the TNF receptor superfamily members CD134 (OX40) and CD137 (4-1BB) and their role in the generation of antitumor immune responses. *Eur. J. Immunol.* 32:3617–27

99. Baum PR, Gayle RB III, Ramsdell F, Srinivasan S, Sorensen RA, et al. 1994. Molecular characterization of murine and human OX40/OX40 ligand systems: identification of a human OX40 ligand as the HTLV-1-regulated protein gp34. *EMBO J.* 13:3992–4001

100. Cannons JL, Lau P, Ghumman B, DeBenedette MA, Yagita H, et al. 2001. 4-1BBL induces cell division, sustains survival and enhances effector function of CD4 and CD8 T cells with similar efficacy. *J. Immunol.* 167:1313–24

101. Bansal-Pakala P, Halteman BS, Cheng MH, Croft M. 2004. Costimulation of CD8 T cell responses by OX40. *J. Immunol.* 172:4821–25

102. Kotani A, Ishikawa T, Matsumura Y, Ichinohe T, Ohno H, et al. 2001. Correlation of peripheral blood OX40$^+$(CD134$^+$) T cells with chronic graft-versus-host disease in patients who underwent allogeneic hematopoietic stem cell transplantation. *Blood* 98:3162–64

103. Wang HC, Klein JR. 2001. Multiple levels of activation of murine CD8$^+$ intraepithelial lymphocytes defined by OX40 (CD134) expression: effects on cell-mediated cytotoxicity, IFN-γ, and IL-10 regulation. *J. Immunol.* 167:6717–23

104. Gramaglia I, Weinberg AD, Lemon M, Croft M. 1998. OX-40 ligand: a potent costimulatory molecule for sustaining primary CD4 T cell responses. *J. Immunol.* 161:6510–17

105. Walker LS, Gulbranson-Judge A, Flynn S, Brocker T, Raykundalia C, et al. 1999. Compromised OX40 function in

CD28-deficient mice is linked with failure to develop CXC chemokine receptor 5-positive CD4 cells and germinal centers. *J. Exp. Med.* 190:1115–22

106. Roos A, Schilder-Tol EJ, Weening JJ, Aten J. 1998. Strong expression of CD134 (OX40), a member of the TNF receptor family, in a T helper 2–type cytokine environment. *J. Leukoc. Biol.* 64: 503–10

107. Kim MY, Gaspal FM, Wiggett HE, McConnell FM, Gulbranson-Judge A, et al. 2003. CD4+CD3− accessory cells costimulate primed CD4 T cells through OX40 and CD30 at sites where T cells collaborate with B cells. *Immunity* 18: 643–54

108. Rogers PR, Croft M. 2000. CD28, Ox-40, LFA-1, and CD4 modulation of Th1/Th2 differentiation is directly dependent on the dose of antigen. *J. Immunol.* 164:2955–63

109. Stuber E, Strober W. 1996. The T cell–B cell interaction via OX40-OX40L is necessary for the T cell–dependent humoral immune response. *J. Exp. Med.* 183:979–89

110. Tanaka Y, Inoi T, Tozawa H, Yamamoto N, Hinuma Y. 1985. A glycoprotein antigen detected with new monoclonal antibodies on the surface of human lymphocytes infected with human T-cell leukemia virus type-I (HTLV-I). *Int. J. Cancer* 36:549–55

111. Miura S, Ohtani K, Numata N, Niki M, Ohbo K, et al. 1991. Molecular cloning and characterization of a novel glycoprotein, gp34, that is specifically induced by the human T-cell leukemia virus type I transactivator p40tax. *Mol. Cell. Biol.* 11:1313–25

112. Godfrey WR, Fagnoni FF, Harara MA, Buck D, Engleman EG. 1994. Identification of a human OX-40 ligand, a costimulator of CD4+ T cells with homology to tumor necrosis factor. *J. Exp. Med.* 180:757–62

113. Stuber E, Neurath M, Calderhead D, Fell HP, Strober W. 1995. Cross-linking of OX40 ligand, a member of the TNF/NGF cytokine family, induces proliferation and differentiation in murine splenic B cells. *Immunity* 2:507–21

114. Akiba H, Oshima H, Takeda K, Atsuta M, Nakano H, et al. 1999. CD28-independent costimulation of T cells by OX40 ligand and CD70 on activated B cells. *J. Immunol.* 162:7058–66

115. Ohshima Y, Yang LP, Uchiyama T, Tanaka Y, Baum P, et al. 1998. OX40 costimulation enhances interleukin-4 (IL-4) expression at priming and promotes the differentiation of naive human CD4+ T cells into high IL-4-producing effectors. *Blood* 92:3338–45

116. Chen AI, McAdam AJ, Buhlmann JE, Scott S, Lupher ML Jr, et al. 1999. Ox40-ligand has a critical costimulatory role in dendritic cell:T cell interactions. *Immunity* 11:689–98

117. Fillatreau S, Gray D. 2003. T cell accumulation in B cell follicles is regulated by dendritic cells and is independent of B cell activation. *J. Exp. Med.* 197:195–206

118. Ito T, Amakawa R, Inaba M, Hori T, Ota M, et al. 2004. Plasmacytoid dendritic cells regulate Th cell responses through OX40 ligand and type I IFNs. *J. Immunol.* 172:4253–59

119. Imura A, Hori T, Imada K, Ishikawa T, Tanaka Y, et al. 1996. The human OX40/gp34 system directly mediates adhesion of activated T cells to vascular endothelial cells. *J. Exp. Med.* 183:2185–95

120. Kunitomi A, Hori T, Imura A, Uchiyama T. 2000. Vascular endothelial cells provide T cells with costimulatory signals via the OX40/gp34 system. *J. Leukoc. Biol.* 68:111–18

121. Weinberg AD, Wegmann KW, Funatake C, Whitham RH. 1999. Blocking OX40/OX40 ligand interaction in vitro and in vivo leads to decreased T-cell

function and amelioration of EAE. *J. Immunol.* 162:1818–26

122. Yoshioka T, Nakajima A, Akiba H, Ishiwata T, Asano G, et al. 2000. Contribution of OX40/OX40 ligand interaction to the pathogenesis of rheumatoid arthritis. *Eur. J. Immunol.* 30:2815–23

123. Malmstrom V, Shipton D, Singh B, Al-Shamkhani A, Puklavec MJ, et al. 2001. CD134L expression on dendritic cells in the mesenteric lymph nodes drives colitis in T cell–restored SCID mice. *J. Immunol.* 166:6972–81

124. Sato T, Ishii N, Murata K, Kikuchi K, Nakagawa S, et al. 2002. Consequences of OX40-OX40 ligand interactions in Langerhans cell function: enhanced contact hypersensitivity responses in OX40L-transgenic mice. *Eur. J. Immunol.* 32:3326–35

125. Aten J, Roos A, Claessen N, Schilder-Tol EJ, Ten Berge IJ, Weening JJ. 2000. Strong and selective glomerular localization of CD134 ligand and TNF receptor-1 in proliferative lupus nephritis. *J. Am. Soc. Nephrol.* 11:1426–38

126. Tateyama M, Fujihara K, Ishii N, Sugamura K, Onodera Y, Itoyama Y. 2002. Expression of OX40 in muscles of polymyositis and granulomatous myopathy. *J. Neurol. Sci.* 194:29–34

127. Stuber E, Buschenfeld A, Luttges J, Von Freier A, Arendt T, Folsch UR. 2000. The expression of OX40 in immunologically mediated diseases of the gastrointestinal tract (celiac disease, Crohn's disease, ulcerative colitis). *Eur. J. Clin. Invest.* 30:594–99

128. Giacomelli R, Passacantando A, Perricone R, Parzanese I, Rascente M, et al. 2001. T lymphocytes in the synovial fluid of patients with active rheumatoid arthritis display CD134-OX40 surface antigen. *Clin. Exp. Rheumatol.* 19:317–20

129. Carboni S, Aboul-Enein F, Waltzinger C, Killeen N, Lassmann H, Pena-Rossi C. 2003. CD134 plays a crucial role in the pathogenesis of EAE and is upregulated in the CNS of patients with multiple sclerosis. *J. Neuroimmunol.* 145:1–11

130. Gramaglia I, Jember A, Pippig SD, Weinberg AD, Killeen N, Croft M. 2000. The OX40 costimulatory receptor determines the development of CD4 memory by regulating primary clonal expansion. *J. Immunol.* 165:3043–50

131. Evans DE, Prell RA, Thalhofer CJ, Hurwitz AA, Weinberg AD. 2001. Engagement of OX40 enhances antigen-specific CD4$^+$ T cell mobilization/memory development and humoral immunity: comparison of αOX-40 with αCTLA-4. *J. Immunol.* 167:6804–11

132. De Smedt T, Smith J, Baum P, Fanslow W, Butz E, Maliszewski C. 2002. Ox40 costimulation enhances the development of T cell responses induced by dendritic cells in vivo. *J. Immunol.* 168:661–70

133. Flynn S, Toellner KM, Raykundalia C, Goodall M, Lane P. 1998. CD4 T cell cytokine differentiation: The B cell activation molecule, OX40 ligand, instructs CD4 T cells to express interleukin 4 and upregulates expression of the chemokine receptor, Blr-1. *J. Exp. Med.* 188:297–304

134. Delespesse G, Ohshima Y, Yang LP, Demeure C, Sarfati M. 1999. OX40-mediated cosignal enhances the maturation of naive human CD4$^+$ T cells into high IL-4-producing effectors. *Int. Arch. Allergy Immunol.* 118:384–86

135. Jember AG, Zuberi R, Liu FT, Croft M. 2001. Development of allergic inflammation in a murine model of asthma is dependent on the costimulatory receptor OX40. *J. Exp. Med.* 193:387–92

136. Linton PJ, Bautista B, Biederman E, Bradley ES, Harbertson J, et al. 2003. Costimulation via OX40L expressed by B cells is sufficient to determine the extent of primary CD4 cell expansion and Th2 cytokine secretion in vivo. *J. Exp. Med.* 197:875–83

137. Hoshino A, Tanaka Y, Akiba H, Asakura Y, Mita Y, et al. 2003. Critical role

for OX40 ligand in the development of pathogenic Th2 cells in a murine model of asthma. *Eur. J. Immunol.* 33:861–69

138. Ishii N, Ndhlovu LC, Murata K, Sato T, Kamanaka M, Sugamura K. 2003. OX40 (CD134) and OX40 ligand interaction plays an adjuvant role during in vivo Th2 responses. *Eur. J. Immunol.* 33:2372–81

139. Salek-Ardakani S, Song J, Halteman BS, Jember AG, Akiba H, et al. 2003. OX40 (CD134) controls memory T helper 2 cells that drive lung inflammation. *J. Exp. Med.* 198:315–24

140. Kaleeba JA, Offner H, Vandenbark AA, Lublinski A, Weinberg AD. 1998. The OX-40 receptor provides a potent costimulatory signal capable of inducing encephalitogenicity in myelin-specific CD4$^+$ T cells. *Int. Immunol.* 10:453–61

141. Humphreys IR, Edwards L, Walzl G, Rae AJ, Dougan G, et al. 2003. OX40 ligation on activated T cells enhances the control of *Cryptococcus neoformans* and reduces pulmonary eosinophilia. *J. Immunol.* 170:6125–32

142. Arestides RS, He H, Westlake RM, Chen AI, Sharpe AH, et al. 2002. Costimulatory molecule OX40L is critical for both Th1 and Th2 responses in allergic inflammation. *Eur. J. Immunol.* 32:2874–80

143. Maxwell JR, Weinberg A, Prell RA, Vella AT. 2000. Danger and OX40 receptor signaling synergize to enhance memory T cell survival by inhibiting peripheral deletion. *J. Immunol.* 164:107–12

144. Kopf M, Ruedl C, Schmitz N, Gallimore A, Lefrang K, et al. 1999. OX40-deficient mice are defective in Th cell proliferation but are competent in generating B cell and CTL responses after virus infection. *Immunity* 11:699–708

145. Pippig SD, Pena-Rossi C, Long J, Godfrey WR, Fowell DJ, et al. 1999. Robust B cell immunity but impaired T cell proliferation in the absence of CD134 (OX40). *J. Immunol.* 163:6520–29

146. Blazar BR, Sharpe AH, Chen AI, Panoskaltsis-Mortari A, Lees C, et al. 2003. Ligation of OX40 (CD134) regulates graft-versus-host disease (GVHD) and graft rejection in allogeneic bone marrow transplant recipients. *Blood* 101: 3741–48

147. Brocker T, Gulbranson-Judge A, Flynn S, Riedinger M, Raykundalia C, Lane P. 1999. CD4 T cell traffic control: in vivo evidence that ligation of OX40 on CD4 T cells by OX40-ligand expressed on dendritic cells leads to the accumulation of CD4 T cells in B follicles. *Eur. J. Immunol.* 29:1610–16

148. Murata K, Nose M, Ndhlovu LC, Sato T, Sugamura K, Ishii N. 2002. Constitutive OX40/OX40 ligand interaction induces autoimmune-like diseases. *J. Immunol.* 169:4628–36

149. Kato H, Kojima H, Ishii N, Hase H, Imai Y, et al. 2004. Essential role of OX40L on B cells in persistent alloantibody production following repeated alloimmunizations. *J. Clin. Immunol.* 24:237–48

149a. Dawicki W, Bertram EM, Sharpe AH, Watts TH. 2004. 4-1BB and OX40 act independently to facilitate robust CD8 and CD4 recall responses. *J. Immunol.* 173:5944–51

150. Obermeier F, Schwarz H, Dunger N, Strauch UG, Grunwald N, et al. 2003. OX40/OX40L interaction induces the expression of CXCR5 and contributes to chronic colitis induced by dextran sulfate sodium in mice. *Eur. J. Immunol.* 33:3265–74

151. Kotani A, Hori T, Matsumura Y, Uchiyama T. 2002. Signaling of gp34 (OX40 ligand) induces vascular endothelial cells to produce a CC chemokine RANTES/CCL5. *Immunol. Lett.* 84:1–7

152. Humphreys IR, Walzl G, Edwards L, Rae A, Hill S, Hussell T. 2003. A critical role for OX40 in T cell–mediated immunopathology during lung viral infection. *J. Exp. Med.* 198:1237–42

153. Zubairi S, Sanos SL, Hill S, Kaye PM. 2004. Immunotherapy with OX40L-Fc

or anti-CTLA-4 enhances local tissue responses and killing of *Leishmania donovani. Eur. J. Immunol.* 34:1433–40

154. Weinberg AD, Bourdette DN, Sullivan TJ, Lemon M, Wallin JJ, et al. 1996. Selective depletion of myelin-reactive T cells with the anti-OX-40 antibody ameliorates autoimmune encephalomyelitis. *Nat. Med.* 2:183–89

155. Ndhlovu LC, Ishii N, Murata K, Sato T, Sugamura K. 2001. Critical involvement of OX40 ligand signals in the T cell priming events during experimental autoimmune encephalomyelitis. *J. Immunol.* 167:2991–99

156. Weinberg AD, Lemon M, Jones AJ, Vainiene M, Celnik B, et al. 1996. OX-40 antibody enhances for autoantigen specific Vβ8.2+ T cells within the spinal cord of Lewis rats with autoimmune encephalomyelitis. *J. Neurosci. Res.* 43:42–49

157. Higgins LM, McDonald SA, Whittle N, Crockett N, Shields JG, MacDonald TT. 1999. Regulation of T cell activation in vitro and in vivo by targeting the OX40-OX40 ligand interaction: amelioration of ongoing inflammatory bowel disease with an OX40-IgG fusion protein, but not with an OX40 ligand-IgG fusion protein. *J. Immunol.* 162:486–93

158. Totsuka T, Kanai T, Uraushihara K, Iiyama R, Yamazaki M, et al. 2003. Therapeutic effect of anti-OX40L and anti-TNF-α MAbs in a murine model of chronic colitis. *Am. J. Physiol. Gastrointest. Liver Physiol.* 284:G595–603

159. Martin-Orozco N, Chen Z, Poirot L, Hyatt E, Chen A, et al. 2003. Paradoxical dampening of anti-islet self-reactivity but promotion of diabetes by OX40 ligand. *J. Immunol.* 171:6954–60

160. Burgess JK, Carlin S, Pack RA, Arndt GM, Au WW, et al. 2004. Detection and characterization of OX40 ligand expression in human airway smooth muscle cells: a possible role in asthma? *J. Allergy Clin. Immunol.* 113:683–89

161. Bansal-Pakala P, Jember AG, Croft M. 2001. Signaling through OX40 (CD134) breaks peripheral T-cell tolerance. *Nat. Med.* 7:907–12

162. Lathrop SK, Huddleston CA, Dullforce PA, Montfort MJ, Weinberg AD, Parker DC. 2004. A signal through OX40 (CD134) allows anergic, autoreactive T cells to acquire effector cell functions. *J. Immunol.* 172:6735–43

163. Stuber E, von Freier A, Marinescu D, Folsch UR. 1998. Involvement of OX40-OX40L interactions in the intestinal manifestations of the murine acute graft-versus-host disease. *Gastroenterology* 115:1205–15

164. Tsukada N, Akiba H, Kobata T, Aizawa Y, Yagita H, Okumura K. 2000. Blockade of CD134 (OX40)-CD134L interaction ameliorates lethal acute graft-versus-host disease in a murine model of allogeneic bone marrow transplantation. *Blood* 95:2434–39

165. Demirci G, Amanullah F, Kewalaramani R, Yagita H, Strom TB, et al. 2004. Critical role of OX40 in CD28 and CD154-independent rejection. *J. Immunol.* 172:1691–98

166. Gri G, Gallo E, Di Carlo E, Musiani P, Colombo MP. 2003. OX40 ligand-transduced tumor cell vaccine synergizes with GM-CSF and requires CD40-Apc signaling to boost the host T cell antitumor response. *J. Immunol.* 170:99–106

167. Yanagita S, Hori T, Matsubara Y, Ishikawa T, Uchiyama T. 2004. Retroviral transduction of acute myeloid leukaemia-derived dendritic cells with OX40 ligand augments their antigen presenting activity. *Br. J. Haematol.* 124:454–62

168. Weinberg AD, Rivera MM, Prell R, Morris A, Ramstad T, et al. 2000. Engagement of the OX-40 receptor in vivo enhances antitumor immunity. *J. Immunol.* 164:2160–69

169. Gerloni M, Xiong S, Mukerjee S, Schoenberger SP, Croft M, Zanetti M.

2000. Functional cooperation between T helper cell determinants. *Proc. Natl. Acad. Sci. USA* 97:13269–74

170. Pan PY, Zang Y, Weber K, Meseck ML, Chen SH. 2002. OX40 ligation enhances primary and memory cytotoxic T lymphocyte responses in an immunotherapy for hepatic colon metastases. *Mol. Ther.* 6:528–36

171. Vinay DS, Kwon BS. 1998. Role of 4-1BB in immune responses. *Semin. Immunol.* 10:481–89

172. Kwon BS, Weismann SM. 1989. cDNA sequences of two inducible T-cell genes. *Proc. Natl. Acad. Sci. USA* 86:1963–67

173. Gramaglia I, Cooper D, Miner KT, Kwon BS, Croft M. 2000. Co-stimulation of antigen-specific CD4 T cells by 4-1BB ligand. *Eur. J. Immunol.* 30:392–402

174. Takahashi C, Mittler RS, Vella AT. 1999. Cutting edge: 4-1BB is a bona fide CD8 T cell survival signal. *J. Immunol.* 162:5037–40

175. Dawicki W, Watts TH. 2004. Expression and function of 4-1BB during CD4 versus CD8 T cell responses in vivo. *Eur. J. Immunol.* 34:743–51

176. Wen T, Bukczynski J, Watts TH. 2002. 4-1BB ligand-mediated costimulation of human T cells induces CD4 and CD8 T cell expansion, cytokine production and the development of cytolytic effector function. *J. Immunol.* 168:4897–906

177. Tan JT, Ha J, Cho HR, Tucker-Burden C, Hendrix RC, et al. 2000. Analysis of expression and function of the costimulatory molecule 4-1BB in alloimmune responses. *Transplantation* 70:175–83

178. Seo SK, Park HY, Choi JH, Kim WY, Kim YH, et al. 2003. Blocking 4-1BB/4-1BB ligand interactions prevents herpetic stromal keratitis. *J. Immunol.* 171:576–83

179. Lyons PA, Hancock WW, Denny P, Lord CJ, Hill NJ, et al. 2000. The NOD *Idd9* genetic interval influences the pathogenicity of insulitis and contains

molecular variants of Cd30, Tnfr2, and Cd137. *Immunity* 13:107–15

180. Watts TH, DeBenedette MA. 1999. T cell costimulatory molecules other than CD28. *Curr. Opin. Immunol.* 11:286–93

181. Wilcox RA, Chapoval AI, Gorski KS, Otsuji M, Shin T, et al. 2002. Cutting edge: expression of functional CD137 receptor by dendritic cells. *J. Immunol.* 168:4262–67

182. Kienzle G, von Kempis J. 2000. CD137 (ILA/4-1BB), expressed by primary human monocytes, induces monocyte activation and apoptosis of B lymphocytes. *Int. Immunol.* 12:73–82

183. Pauly S, Broll K, Wittmann M, Giegerich G, Schwarz H. 2002. CD137 is expressed by follicular dendritic cells and costimulates B lymphocyte activation in germinal centers. *J. Leukoc. Biol.* 72:35–42

184. Wilcox RA, Tamada K, Strome SE, Chen L. 2002. Signaling through NK cell–associated CD137 promotes both helper function for CD8[+] cytolytic T cells and responsiveness to IL-2 but not cytolytic activity. *J. Immunol.* 169:4230–36

185. Heinisch IV, Bizer C, Volgger W, Simon HU. 2001. Functional CD137 receptors are expressed by eosinophils from patients with IgE-mediated allergic responses but not by eosinophils from patients with non-IgE-mediated eosinophilic disorders. *J. Allergy Clin. Immunol.* 108:21–28

186. Reali C, Curto M, Sogos V, Scintu F, Pauly S, et al. 2003. Expression of CD137 and its ligand in human neurons, astrocytes, and microglia: modulation by FGF-2. *J. Neurosci. Res.* 74:67–73

187. Goodwin RG, Din WS, Davis-Smith T, Anderson DM, Gimpel SD, et al. 1993. Molecular cloning of a ligand for the inducible T cell gene 4-1BB: a member of an emerging family of cytokines with homology to tumor necrosis factor. *Eur. J. Immunol.* 23:2631–41

188. Summers KL, Hock BD, McKenzie JL,

Hart DN. 2001. Phenotypic characterization of five dendritic cell subsets in human tonsils. *Am. J. Pathol.* 159:285–95

189. Laderach D, Wesa A, Galy A. 2003. 4-1BB-ligand is regulated on human dendritic cells and induces the production of IL-12. *Cell Immunol.* 226:37–44

190. Seko Y, Takahashi N, Oshima H, Shimozato O, Akiba H, et al. 2001. Expression of tumour necrosis factor (TNF) ligand superfamily co-stimulatory molecules CD30L, CD27L, OX40L, and 4-1BBL in murine hearts with acute myocarditis caused by Coxsackievirus B3. *J. Pathol.* 195:593–603

191. Seko Y, Sugishita K, Sato O, Takagi A, Tada Y, et al. 2004. Expression of costimulatory molecules (4-1BBL and Fas) and major histocompatibility class I chain-related A (MICA) in aortic tissue with Takayasu's arteritis. *J. Vasc. Res.* 41:84–90

192. Langstein J, Michel J, Fritsche J, Kreutz M, Andreesen R, Schwarz H. 1998. CD137 (ILA/4-1BB), a member of the TNF receptor family, induces monocyte activation via bidirectional signaling. *J. Immunol.* 160:2488–94

193. Langstein J, Schwarz H. 1999. Identification of CD137 as a potent monocyte survival factor. *J. Leukoc. Biol.* 65:829–33

194. Pollok KE, Kim Y-J, Hurtado J, Zhou Z, Kim KK, Kwon BS. 1994. 4-1BB T cell antigen binds to mature B cells and macrophages, and costimulates anti-μ-primed splenic B cells. *Eur. J. Immunol.* 24:367–74

195. Chu NR, DeBenedette MA, Stiernholm BJ, Barber BH, Watts TH. 1997. Role of IL-12 and 4-1BB ligand in cytokine production by CD28$^+$ and CD28$^-$ T cells. *J. Immunol.* 158:3081–89

196. Halstead ES, Mueller YM, Altman JD, Katsikis PD. 2002. In vivo stimulation of CD137 broadens primary antiviral CD8$^+$ T cell responses. *Nat. Immunol.* 3:536–41

197. Bertram EM, Lau P, Watts TH. 2002. Temporal segregation of CD28 versus 4-1BBL-mediated costimulation: 4-1BBL influences T cell numbers late in the primary response and regulates the size of the memory response following influenza infection. *J. Immunol.* 168:3777–85

198. Maus MV, Thomas AK, Leonard DG, Allman D, Addya K, et al. 2002. Ex vivo expansion of polyclonal and antigen-specific cytotoxic T lymphocytes by artificial APCs expressing ligands for the T-cell receptor, CD28 and 4-1BB. *Nat. Biotechnol.* 20:143–48

199. Cooper D, Bansal-Pakala P, Croft M. 2002. 4-1BB (CD137) controls the clonal expansion and survival of CD8 T cells in vivo but does not contribute to the development of cytotoxicity. *Eur. J. Immunol.* 32:521–29

200. Shuford WW, Klussman K, Tritchler DD, Loo DT, Chalupny J, et al. 1997. 4-1BB costimulatory signals preferentially induce CD8$^+$ T cell proliferation and lead to the amplification in vivo of cytotoxic T cell responses. *J. Exp. Med.* 186:47–55

201. Hurtado JC, Kim YJ, Kwon BS. 1997. Signals through 4-1BB are costimulatory to previously activated splenic T cells and inhibit activation-induced cell death. *J. Immunol.* 158:2600–9

202. Bukczynski J, Wen T, Watts TH. 2003. Costimulation of human CD28$^-$ T cells by 4-1BB ligand. *Eur. J. Immunol.* 33:446–54

203. May KF Jr, Chen L, Zheng P, Liu Y. 2002. Anti-4-1BB monoclonal antibody enhances rejection of large tumor burden by promoting survival but not clonal expansion of tumor-specific CD8$^+$ T cells. *Cancer Res.* 62:3459–65

204. Alderson MR, Smith CA, Tough TW, Davis-Smith T, Armitage RJ, et al. 1994. Molecular and biological characterization of human 4-1BB and its ligand. *Eur. J. Immunol.* 24:2219–27

205. Kim YJ, Kim SH, Mantel P, Kwon BS. 1998. Human 4-1BB regulates CD28 co-stimulation to promote Th1 cell responses. *Eur. J. Immunol.* 28:881–90

206. Bukczynski J, Wen T, Ellefsen K, Gauldie J, Watts TH. 2004. Costimulatory ligand 4-1BBL (CD137L) as an efficient adjuvant for human antiviral cytotoxic T cell responses. *Proc. Natl. Acad. Sci. USA* 101:1291–96

207. Laderach D, Movassagh M, Johnson A, Mittler RS, Galy A. 2002. 4-1BB costimulation enhances human CD8$^+$ T cell priming by augmenting the proliferation and survival of effector CD8$^+$ T cells. *Int. Immunol.* 14:1155–67

208. Kim YJ, Brutkiewicz RR, Broxmeyer HE. 2002. Role of 4-1BB (CD137) in the functional activation of cord blood CD28$^-$ CD8$^+$ T cells. *Blood* 100:3253–60

209. Bansal-Pakala P, Croft M. 2002. Defective T cell priming associated with aging can be rescued by signaling through 4-1BB (CD137). *J. Immunol.* 169:5005–9

210. Melero I, Shuford WW, Newby SA, Aruffo A, Ledbetter JA, et al. 1997. Monoclonal antibodies against the 4-1BB T-cell activation molecule eradicate established tumors. *Nat. Med.* 3:682–85

211. Bertram EM, Dawicki W, Sedgmen B, Bramson JL, Lynch DH, Watts TH. 2004. A switch in costimulation from CD28 to 4-1BB during primary versus secondary CD8 T cell response to influenza in vivo. *J. Immunol.* 172:981–88

212. Blazar BR, Kwon BS, Panoskaltsis-Mortari A, Kwak KB, Peschon JJ, Taylor PA. 2001. Ligation of 4-1BB (CDw137) regulates graft-versus-host disease, graft-versus-leukemia, and graft rejection in allogeneic bone marrow transplant recipients. *J. Immunol.* 166:3174–83

213. Wilcox RA, Tamada K, Flies DB, Zhu G, Chapoval AI, et al. 2004. Ligation of CD137 receptor prevents and reverses established anergy of CD8$^+$ cytolytic T

lymphocytes in vivo. *Blood* 103:177–84

214. Melero I, Johnston JV, Shufford WW, Mittler RS, Chen L. 1998. NK1.1 cells express 4-1BB (CDw137) costimulatory molecule and are required for tumor immunity elicited by anti-4-1BB monoclonal antibodies. *Cell. Immunol.* 190:167–72

215. Pan PY, Gu P, Li Q, Xu D, Weber K, Chen SH. 2004. Regulation of dendritic cell function by NK cells: mechanisms underlying the synergism in the combination therapy of IL-12 and 4-1BB activation. *J. Immunol.* 172:4779–89

216. Miller RE, Jones J, Le T, Whitmore J, Boiani N, et al. 2002. 4-1BB-specific monoclonal antibody promotes the generation of tumor-specific immune responses by direct activation of CD8 T cells in a CD40$^-$ dependent manner. *J. Immunol.* 169:1792–800

217. Mittler RS, Bailey TS, Klussman K, Trailsmith MD, Hoffmann MK. 1999. Anti-4-1BB monoclonal antibodies abrogate T cell–dependent humoral immune responses in vivo through the induction of helper T cell anergy. *J. Exp. Med.* 190:1535–40

218. Sun Y, Chen HM, Subudhi SK, Chen J, Koka R, Chen L, Fu YX. 2002. Costimulatory molecule-targeted antibody therapy of a spontaneous autoimmune disease. *Nat. Med.* 8:1405–13

219. Sun Y, Lin X, Chen HM, Wu Q, Subudhi SK, et al. 2002. Administration of agonistic anti-4-1BB monoclonal antibody leads to the amelioration of experimental autoimmune encephalomyelitis. *J. Immunol.* 168:1457–65

220. Foell J, Strahotin S, O'Neil SP, McCausland MM, Suwyn C, et al. 2003. CD137 costimulatory T cell receptor engagement reverses acute disease in lupus-prone NZB x NZW F1 mice. *J. Clin. Invest.* 111:1505–18

221. Wu ZQ, Khan AQ, Shen Y, Wolcott KM, Dawicki W, et al. 2003. 4-1BB

(CD137) differentially regulates murine in vivo protein- and polysaccharide-specific immunoglobulin isotype responses to *Streptococcus pneumoniae*. *Infect. Immun.* 71:196–204

222. Zhu G, Flies DB, Tamada K, Sun Y, Rodriguez M. 2001. Progressive depletion of peripheral B lymphocytes in 4-1BB (CD137) ligand/I-Eα-transgenic mice. *J. Immunol.* 167:2671–76

223. Myers L, Takahashi C, Mittler RS, Rossi RJ, Vella AT. 2003. Effector CD8 T cells possess suppressor function after 4-1BB and Toll-like receptor triggering. *Proc. Natl. Acad. Sci. USA* 100:5348–53

224. DeBenedette MA, Wen T, Bachmann MF, Ohashi PS, Barber BH, et al. 1999. Analysis of 4-1BB ligand-deficient mice and of mice lacking both 4-1BB ligand and CD28 reveals a role for 4-1BB ligand in skin allograft rejection and in the cytotoxic T cell response to influenza virus. *J. Immunol.* 163:4833–41

225. Tan JT, Whitmire JK, Ahmed R, Pearson TC, Larsen CP. 1999. 4-1BB ligand, a member of the TNF family, is important for the generation of antiviral CD8 T cell responses. *J. Immunol.* 163:4859–68

226. Kwon BS, Hurtado JC, Lee ZH, Kwack KB, Seo SK, et al. 2002. Immune responses in 4-1BB (CD137)-deficient mice. *J. Immunol.* 168:5483–90

227. Shedlock DJ, Whitmire JK, Tan J, MacDonald AS, Ahmed R, Shen H. 2003. Role of CD4 T cell help and costimulation in CD8 T cell responses during Listeria monocytogenes infection. *J. Immunol.* 170:2053–63

228. Tan JT, Whitmire JK, Murali-Krishna K, Ahmed R, Altman JD, et al. 2000. 4-1BB costimulation is required for protective anti-viral immunity after peptide vaccination. *J. Immunol.* 164:2320–25

229. Melero I, Bach N, Hellstrom KE, Aruffo A, Mittler RS, Chen L. 1998. Amplification of tumor immunity by gene transfer of the co-stimulatory 4-1BB ligand: synergy with the CD28 co-stimulatory pathway. *Eur. J. Immunol.* 28:1116–21

230. Guinn BA, DeBenedette MA, Watts TH, Berinstein NL. 1999. 4-1BBL cooperates with B7-1 and B7-2 in converting a B cell lymphoma cell line into a longlasting antitumor vaccine. *J. Immunol.* 162:5003–10

231. Martinet O, Ermekova V, Qiao JQ, Sauter B, Mandeli J, et al. 2000. Immunomodulatory gene therapy with interleukin 12 and 4-1BB ligand: long-term remission of liver metastases in a mouse model. *J. Natl. Cancer Inst.* 92:931–36

232. Wiethe C, Dittmar K, Doan T, Lindenmaier W, Tindle R. 2003. Enhanced effector and memory CTL responses generated by incorporation of receptor activator of NF-κB (RANK)/RANK ligand costimulatory molecules into dendritic cell immunogens expressing a human tumor-specific antigen. *J. Immunol.* 171:4121–30

233. Ye Z, Hellstrom I, Hayden-Ledbetter M, Dahlin A, Ledbetter JA, Hellstrom KE. 2002. Gene therapy for cancer using single-chain Fv fragments specific for 4-1BB. *Nat. Med.* 8:343–48

234. Guinn BA, Bertram EM, DeBenedette MA, Berinstein NL, Watts TH. 2001. 4-1BBL enhances anti-tumor responses in the presence or absence of CD28 but CD28 is required for protective immunity against parental tumors. *Cell Immunol.* 210:56–65

235. Vonderheide RH, June CH. 2003. A translational bridge to cancer immunotherapy: exploiting costimulation and target antigens for active and passive T cell immunotherapy. *Immunol. Res.* 27:341–56

236. Montgomery RI, Warner MS, Lum BJ, Spear PG. 1996. Herpes simplex virus-1 entry into cells mediated by a novel member of the TNF/NGF receptor family. *Cell* 87:427–36

237. Mauri DN, Ebner R, Montgomery RI, Kochel KD, Cheung TC, et al. 1998.

LIGHT, a new member of the TNF super-family, and lymphotoxin α are ligands for herpesvirus entry mediator. *Immunity* 8:21–30

238. Zhai Y, Guo R, Hsu TL, Yu GL, Ni J, et al. 1998. LIGHT, a novel ligand for lymphotoxin β receptor and TR2/HVEM induces apoptosis and suppresses in vivo tumor formation via gene transfer. *J. Clin. Invest.* 102:1142–51

239. Yu KY, Kwon B, Ni J, Zhai Y, Ebner R, Kwon BS. 1999. A newly iden-tified member of tumor necrosis fac-tor receptor superfamily (TR6) sup-presses LIGHT-mediated apoptosis. *J. Biol. Chem.* 274:13733–36

240. Granger SW, Rickert S. 2003. LIGHT-HVEM signaling and the regulation of T cell–mediated immunity. *Cytokine Growth Factor Rev.* 14:289–96

241. Granger SW, Ware CF. 2001. Turning on LIGHT. *J. Clin. Invest.* 108:1741–42

242. Morel Y, Schiano de Colella JM, Har-rop J, Deen KC, Holmes SD, et al. 2000. Reciprocal expression of the TNF family receptor herpes virus entry mediator and its ligand LIGHT on activated T cells: LIGHT down-regulates its own receptor. *J. Immunol.* 165:4397–404

243. Tamada K, Shimozaki K, Chapoval AI, Zhai Y, Su J, et al. 2000. LIGHT, a TNF-like molecule, costimulates T cell prolif-eration and is required for dendritic cell–mediated allogeneic T cell response. *J. Immunol.* 164:4105–10

244. Morel Y, Truneh A, Sweet RW, Olive D, Costello RT. 2001. The TNF superfamily members LIGHT and CD154 (CD40 lig-and) costimulate induction of dendritic cell maturation and elicit specific CTL activity. *J. Immunol.* 167:2479–86

245. Ye Q, Fraser CC, Gao W, Wang L, Busfield SJ, et al. 2002. Modulation of LIGHT-HVEM costimulation prolongs cardiac allograft survival. *J. Exp. Med.* 195:795–800

246. Tamada K, Shimozaki K, Chapoval AI, Zhu G, Sica G, et al. 2000. Modula-tion of T-cell-mediated immunity in tu-mor and graft-versus-host disease mod-els through the LIGHT co-stimulatory pathway. *Nat. Med.* 6:283–89

247. Yu P, Lee Y, Liu W, Chin RK, Wang J, et al. 2004. Priming of naive T cells in-side tumors leads to eradication of estab-lished tumors. *Nat. Immunol.* 5:141–49

248. La S, Kim J, Kwon BS, Kwon B. 2002. Herpes simplex virus type 1 glycopro-tein D inhibits T-cell proliferation. *Mol. Cells* 14:398–403

249. Wang J, Lo JC, Foster A, Yu P, Chen HM, et al. 2001. The regulation of T cell homeostasis and autoimmunity by T cell–derived LIGHT. *J. Clin. Invest.* 108:1771–80

250. Harrop JA, Reddy M, Dede K, Brigham-Burke M, Lyn S, et al. 1998. Antibodies to TR2 (herpesvirus entry mediator), a new member of the TNF receptor super-family, block T cell proliferation, expres-sion of activation markers, and produc-tion of cytokines. *J. Immunol.* 161:1786–94

251. Liu J, Schmidt CS, Zhao F, Okragly AJ, Glasebrook A, et al. 2003. LIGHT-deficiency impairs CD8$^+$ T cell expan-sion, but not effector function. *Int. Im-munol.* 15:861–70

252. Scheu S, Alferink J, Potzel T, Barchet W, Kalinke U, Pfeffer K. 2002. Targeted disruption of LIGHT causes defects in costimulatory T cell activation and re-veals cooperation with lymphotoxin β in mesenteric lymph node genesis. *J. Exp. Med.* 195:1613–24

253. Tamada K, Ni J, Zhu G, Fiscella M, Teng B, et al. 2002. Cutting edge: selective impairment of CD8$^+$ T cell function in mice lacking the TNF superfamily mem-ber LIGHT. *J. Immunol.* 168:4832–35

254. Morel Y, Truneh A, Costello RT, Olive D. 2003. LIGHT, a new TNF superfam-ily member, is essential for memory T helper cell–mediated activation of den-dritic cells. *Eur. J. Immunol.* 33:3213–19

255. Shi G, Wu Y, Zhang J, Wu J. 2003. Death

decoy receptor TR6/DcR3 inhibits T cell chemotaxis in vitro and in vivo. *J. Immunol.* 171:3407–14

256. Shi G, Luo H, Wan X, Salcedo TW, Zhang J, Wu J. 2002. Mouse T cells receive costimulatory signals from LIGHT, a TNF family member. *Blood* 100:3279–86

257. Wan X, Zhang J, Luo H, Shi G, Kapnik E, et al. 2002. A TNF family member LIGHT transduces costimulatory signals into human T cells. *J. Immunol.* 169:6813–21

258. Shaikh RB, Santee S, Granger SW, Butrovich K, Cheung T, et al. 2001. Constitutive expression of LIGHT on T cells leads to lymphocyte activation, inflammation, and tissue destruction. *J. Immunol.* 167:6330–37

259. Wang J, Lo JC, Foster A, Yu P, Chen HM, et al. 2001. The regulation of T cell homeostasis and autoimmunity by T cell-derived LIGHT. *J. Clin. Invest.* 108:1771–80

260. Wang J, Anders RA, Wu Q, Peng D, Cho JH, et al. 2004. Dysregulated LIGHT expression on T cells mediates intestinal inflammation and contributes to IgA nephropathy. *J. Clin. Invest.* 113:826–35

261. Wang J, Fu YX. 2003. LIGHT (a cellular ligand for herpes virus entry mediator and lymphotoxin receptor)-mediated thymocyte deletion is dependent on the interaction between TCR and MHC/self-peptide. *J. Immunol.* 170:3986–93

262. Kwon BS, Tan KB, Ni J, Oh KO, Lee ZH, et al. 1997. A newly identified member of the tumor necrosis factor receptor superfamily with a wide tissue distribution and involvement in lymphocyte activation. *J. Biol. Chem.* 272:14272–76

263. Tamada K, Tamura H, Flies D, Fu YX, Celis E, et al. 2002. Blockade of LIGHT/LTβ and CD40 signaling induces allospecific T cell anergy, preventing graft-versus-host disease. *J. Clin. Invest.* 109:549–57

264. Rooney IA, Butrovich KD, Glass AA, Borboroglu S, Benedict CA, et al. 2000. The lymphotoxin-β receptor is necessary and sufficient for LIGHT-mediated apoptosis of tumor cells. *J. Biol. Chem.* 275:14307–15

265. Schwab U, Stein H, Gerdes J, Lemke H, Kirchner H, et al. 1982. Production of a monoclonal antibody specific for Hodgkin and Sternberg-Reed cells of Hodgkin's disease and a subset of normal lymphoid cells. *Nature* 299:65–67

266. Horie R, Higashihara M, Watanabe T. 2003. Hodgkin's lymphoma and CD30 signal transduction. *Int. J. Hematol.* 77:37–47

267. Horie R, Watanabe T. 1998. CD30: expression and function in health and disease. *Semin. Immunol.* 10:457–70

268. Biswas P, Rovere P, De Filippi C, Heltai S, Smith C, et al. 2000. Engagement of CD30 shapes the secretion of cytokines by human γδ T cells. *Eur. J. Immunol.* 30:2172–80

269. Matsumoto K, Terakawa M, Miura K, Fukuda S, Nakajima T, Saito H. 2004. Extremely rapid and intense induction of apoptosis in human eosinophils by anti-CD30 antibody treatment in vitro. *J. Immunol.* 172:2186–93

270. Romagnani P, Annunziato F, Manetti R, Mavilia C, Lasagni L, et al. 1998. High CD30 ligand expression by epithelial cells and Hassal's corpuscles in the medulla of human thymus. *Blood* 91:3323–32

271. Romagnani S, Del Prete G, Maggi E, Chilosi M, Caligaris-Cappio F, Pizzolo G. 1995. CD30 and type 2 T helper (Th2) responses. *J. Leukoc. Biol.* 57:726–30

272. Tarkowski M. 2003. Expression and a role of CD30 in regulation of T-cell activity. *Curr. Opin. Hematol.* 10:267–71

273. Gilfillan MC, Noel PJ, Podack ER, Reiner SL, Thompson CB. 1998. Expression of the costimulatory receptor CD30 is regulated by both CD28 and cytokines. *J. Immunol.* 160:2180–87

274. Toennies HM, Green JM, Arch RH. 2004. Expression of CD30 and Ox40 on T lymphocyte subsets is controlled by distinct regulatory mechanisms. *J. Leukoc. Biol.* 75:350–57

275. Younes A, Consoli U, Zhao S, Snell V, Thomas E, et al. 1996. CD30 ligand is expressed on resting normal and malignant human B lymphocytes. *Br. J. Haematol.* 93:569–71

276. Wiley SR, Goodwin RG, Smith CA. 1996. Reverse signaling via CD30 ligand. *J. Immunol.* 157:3635–39

277. Shimozato O, Takeda K, Yagita H, Okumura K. 1999. Expression of CD30 ligand (CD153) on murine activated T cells. *Biochem. Biophys. Res. Commun.* 256:519–26

278. Seko Y, Ishiyama S, Nishikawa T, Kasajima T, Hiroe M, et al. 2002. Expression of tumor necrosis factor ligand superfamily costimulatory molecules CD27L, CD30L, OX40L and 4-1BBL in the heart of patients with acute myocarditis and dilated cardiomyopathy. *Cardiovasc. Pathol.* 11:166–70

279. Smith CA, Gruss HJ, Davis T, Anderson D, Farrah T, et al. 1993. CD30 antigen, a marker for Hodgkin's lymphoma, is a receptor whose ligand defines an emerging family of cytokines with homology to TNF. *Cell* 73:1349–60

280. Bowen MA, Lee RK, Miragliotta G, Nam SY, Podack ER. 1996. Structure and expression of murine CD30 and its role in cytokine production. *J. Immunol.* 156:442–49

281. Gruss HJ, Boiani N, Williams DE, Armitage RJ, Smith CA, Goodwin RG. 1994. Pleiotropic effects of the CD30 ligand on CD30-expressing cells and lymphoma cell lines. *Blood* 83:2045–56

282. Muta H, Boise LH, Fang L, Podack ER. 2000. CD30 signals integrate expression of cytotoxic effector molecules, lymphocyte trafficking signals, and signals for proliferation and apoptosis. *J. Immunol.* 165:5105–11

283. Duckett CS, Thompson CB. 1997. CD-30-dependent degradation of TRAF2: implications for negative regulation of TRAF signaling and the control of cell survival. *Genes Dev.* 11:2810–21

284. Del Prete G, De Carli M, D'Elios MM, Daniel KC, Almerigogna F, et al. 1995. CD30-mediated signaling promotes the development of human T helper type 2–like T cells. *J. Exp. Med.* 182:1655–61

285. Wynn TA. 2003. IL-13 effector functions. *Annu. Rev. Immunol.* 21:425–56

286. Amakawa R, Hakem A, Kundig TM, Matsuyama T, Simard JJ, et al. 1996. Impaired negative selection of T cells in Hodgkin's disease antigen CD30-deficient mice. *Cell* 84:551–62

287. DeYoung AL, Duramad O, Winoto A. 2000. The TNF receptor family member CD30 is not essential for negative selection. *J. Immunol.* 165:6170–73

288. Podack ER, Strbo N, Sotosec V, Muta H. 2002. CD30—governor of memory T cells? *Ann. NY Acad. Sci.* 975:101–13

289. Siegmund T, Armitage N, Wicker LS, Peterson LB, Todd JA, Lyons PA. 2000. Analysis of the mouse CD30 gene: a candidate for the NOD mouse type 1 diabetes locus Idd9.2. *Diabetes* 49:1612–16

290. Chakrabarty S, Nagata M, Yasuda H, Wen L, Nakayama M, et al. 2003. Critical roles of CD30/CD30L interactions in murine autoimmune diabetes. *Clin. Exp. Immunol.* 133:318–25

291. Kurts C, Carbone FR, Krummel MF, Koch KM, Miller JF, Heath WR. 1999. Signalling through CD30 protects against autoimmune diabetes mediated by CD8 T cells. *Nature* 398:341–44

292. Nocentini G, Giunchi L, Ronchetti S, Krausz LT, Bartoli A, et al. 1997. A new member of the tumor necrosis factor/nerve growth factor receptor family inhibits T cell receptor–induced apoptosis. *Proc. Natl. Acad. Sci. USA* 94:6216–21

293. Stephens GL, McHugh RS, Whitters MJ, Young DA, Collins M, Shevach EM.

2004. Engagement of GITR on effector T cells by its ligand mediates resistance to suppression by CD4+CD25+ T cells. *J. Immunol.* 173:5008–20

294. McHugh RS, Whitters MJ, Piccirillo CA, Young DA, Shevach EM, et al. 2002. CD4+CD25+ immunoregulatory T cells: gene expression analysis reveals a functional role for the glucocorticoid-induced TNF receptor. *Immunity* 16:311–23

295. Shimizu J, Yamazaki S, Takahashi T, Ishida Y, Sakaguchi S. 2002. Stimulation of CD25+CD4+ regulatory T cells through GITR breaks immunological self-tolerance. *Nat. Immunol.* 3:135–42

296. Kim JD, Choi BK, Bae JS, Lee UH, Han IS, et al. 2003. Cloning and characterization of GITR ligand. *Genes Immun.* 4:564–69

297. Tone M, Tone Y, Adams E, Yates SF, Frewin MR, et al. 2003. Mouse glucocorticoid-induced tumor necrosis factor receptor ligand is costimulatory for T cells. *Proc. Natl. Acad. Sci. USA* 100:15059–64

298. Yu KY, Kim HS, Song SY, Min SS, Jeong JJ, Youn BS. 2003. Identification of a ligand for glucocorticoid-induced tumor necrosis factor receptor constitutively expressed in dendritic cells. *Biochem. Biophys. Res. Commun.* 310:433–38

299. Ronchetti S, Zollo O, Bruscoli S, Agostini M, Bianchini R, et al. 2004. GITR, a member of the TNF receptor superfamily, is costimulatory to mouse T lymphocyte subpopulations. *Eur. J. Immunol.* 34:613–22

300. Kohm AP, Williams JS, Miller SD. 2004. Cutting edge: Ligation of the glucocorticoid-induced TNF receptor enhances autoreactive CD4+ T cell activation and experimental autoimmune encephalomyelitis. *J. Immunol.* 172:4686–90

301. Ronchetti S, Nocentini G, Riccardi C, Pandolfi PP. 2002. Role of GITR in acti-

vation response of T lymphocytes. *Blood* 100:350–52

302. Gavin M, Rudensky A. 2003. Control of immune homeostasis by naturally arising regulatory CD4+ T cells. *Curr. Opin. Immunol.* 15:690–96

303. Uraushihara K, Kanai T, Ko K, Totsuka T, Makita S, et al. 2003. Regulation of murine inflammatory bowel disease by CD25+ and CD25− CD4+ glucocorticoid-induced TNF receptor family-related gene⁺ regulatory T cells. *J. Immunol.* 171:708–16

304. Choi BK, Bae JS, Choi EM, Kang WJ, Sakaguchi S, et al. 2004. 4-1BB-dependent inhibition of immunosuppression by activated CD4+CD25+ T cells. *J. Leukoc. Biol.* 75:785–91

305. Takeda I, Ine S, Killeen N, Ndhlovu LC, Murata K, et al. 2004. Distinct roles for the OX40-OX40 ligand interaction in regulatory and nonregulatory T cells. *J. Immunol.* 172:3580–89

306. Bertram EM, Dawicki W, Watts TH. 2004. Role of T cell costimulation in anti-viral immunity. *Semin. Immunol.* 16:185–96

307. Ye H, Park YC, Kreishman M, Kieff E, Wu H. 1999. The structural basis for the recognition of diverse receptor sequences by TRAF2. *Mol. Cell* 4:321–30

308. Rothe M, Pan MG, Henzel WJ, Ayres TM, Goeddel DV. 1995. The TNFR2-TRAF signaling complex contains two novel proteins related to baculoviral inhibitor of apoptosis proteins. *Cell* 83:1243–52

309. Tesselaar K, Arens R, van Schijndel GM, Baars PA, van der Valk MA, et al. 2003. Lethal T cell immunodeficiency induced by chronic costimulation via CD27-CD70 interactions. *Nat. Immunol.* 4:49–54

310. Wang J, Chun T, Lo JC, Wu Q, Wang Y, et al. 2001. The critical role of LIGHT, a TNF family member, in T cell development. *J. Immunol.* 167:5099–105

Annu. Rev. Immunol. 2005. 23:69–99
doi: 10.1146/annurev.immunol.23.021704.115638
First published online as a Review in Advance on September 22, 2004

DEVELOPMENT AND REGULATION OF CELL-MEDIATED IMMUNE RESPONSES TO THE BLOOD STAGES OF MALARIA: Implications for Vaccine Research

Michael F. Good, Huji Xu, Michelle Wykes, and Christian R. Engwerda

The Queensland Institute of Medical Research, Brisbane, 4029, Australia; email: michaelG@qimr.edu.au

Key Words   malaria, CD4 cells, cytokines, apoptosis

■ **Abstract**   The immune response to the malaria parasite is complex and poorly understood. Although antibodies and T cells can control parasite growth in model systems, natural immunity to malaria in regions of high endemicity takes several years to develop. Variation and polymorphism of antibody target antigens are known to impede immune responses, but these factors alone cannot account for the slow acquisition of immunity. In human and animal model systems, cell-mediated responses can control parasite growth effectively, but such responses are regulated by parasite load via direct effects on dendritic cells and possibly on T and B cells as well. Furthermore, high parasite load is associated with pathology, and cell-mediated responses may also harm the host. Inflammatory cytokines have been implicated in the pathogenesis of cerebral malaria, anemia, weight loss, and respiratory distress in malaria. Immunity without pathology requires rapid parasite clearance, effective regulation of the inflammatory antiparasite effects of cellular responses, and the eventual development of a repertoire of antibodies effective against multiple strains. Data suggest that this may be hastened by exposure to malaria antigens in low dose, leading to augmented cellular immunity and rapid parasite clearance.

INTRODUCTION

Malaria remains one of the world's greatest public health challenges. Although first visualized microscopically by Laveran more than 120 years ago, the parasite has resisted all efforts to control it, despite a century of medical achievements against a range of serious human pathogens, most notably the development of vaccines and the discovery of antibiotics. Today, an estimated 40% of the world's population remains at risk of malaria, with 500 million cases annually, resulting

0732-0582/05/0423-0069$14.00

in 1–2 million deaths, mostly of young children, each year. Ninety percent of the deaths occur in sub-Saharan Africa, but all tropical poor countries are affected. The disease is transmitted by female mosquitoes of the *Anopheles* genus, and transmission was once common in more temperate zones (where these mosquito species still exist) before economic development, mosquito control programs, and effective use of antimalarial chemotherapy. The development of widespread resistance to relatively inexpensive drugs (such as chloroquine), the difficulty of controlling highly efficient mosquito vectors (such as *A. gambiae*), and poor economic growth of many countries (whose current GDP per capita is sometimes 20–50 times lower than the wealthiest countries) have meant that poorer tropical countries have been unable to control malaria. The disease itself has contributed significantly to economic stagnation and its own perpetuation. The development of an effective and inexpensive vaccine is thus a major focus of research. This represents a significant scientific challenge, however, because the organism has a complex life cycle and has developed many immunological defense strategies (1).

Because the organism spends a significant proportion of its life cycle history within red blood cells (RBCs) and thus is not contained within a specific tissue site, immune mechanisms directed against the parasite can readily affect many host organs (discussed below). It is thus critical to understand not only how immune mechanisms can kill the parasite, but how they affect host tissues and how they are regulated. This review focuses on cellular immune responses to the blood stage of the parasite's life cycle, their ability to kill the parasite and to contribute to host pathology, and factors that modulate this balance. Strategies for applying this knowledge to vaccine development are then addressed.

Infection of the human host commences when a female anopheline mosquito injects micron-sized haploid sporozoites during a blood meal (Figure 1). Following infection with *Plasmodium falciparum*, the most deadly of the human parasites, those sporozoites that travel to the liver and invade hepatocytes (typically 1–10 in number) develop over a period of about one week into an exoerythrocytic schizont containing approximately 30,000 merozoites. For two of the four human species (*P. vivax*, *P. ovale*), dormant hypnozoite forms can develop (leading to delayed clinical attacks months or years later), but for *P. falciparum*, there are no dormant forms and merozoites are released from infected hepatocytes and then invade RBCs. There follows a 48 h cycle during which a single invaded merozoite develops into a "ring" trophozoite, a mature trophozoite, and finally a schizont, which gives rise to approximately 16 new merozoites. This occurs within a parasitophorous vacuole in the RBC. The parasite dramatically alters the physiological and biochemical processes of its host RBC (2) and adorns its surface with parasite-encoded molecules that further affect the RBC's mobility and trafficking within the body. The parasite biomass increases very rapidly and activates innate immune mechanisms, some of which researchers have more clearly defined (3), including natural killer (NK) cells and $\gamma\delta$ T cells. At about this time, parasitized RBCs (pRBC) are detectable microscopically, and symptoms of disease first occur,

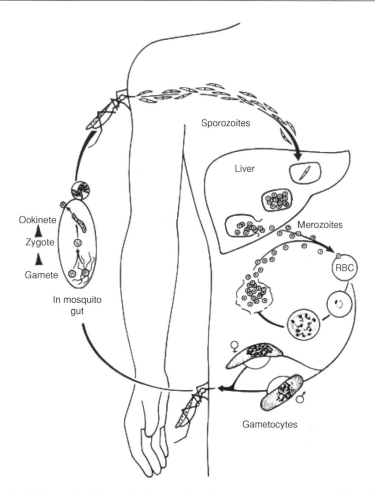

Figure 1   Life cycle of the malaria parasite. Sporozoites are inoculated by a female anopheline mosquito and then travel to the liver. After about one week, parasites have multiplied intracellularly and merozoites rupture from infected hepatocytes to invade red blood cells (RBCs). For *P. falciparum*, the RBC life cycle lasts 48 h, during which time merozoites multiply and approximately 16 new merozoites are released to invade fresh cells. Gametocytes develop within red cells and are taken up by the mosquito to fertilize in the mosquito's gut and produce zygotes, ookinetes, and then sporozoites. Figure from Miller et al. (181).

characterized by fever, chills, headache, lassitude, and gastro-intestinal symptoms. In the naive, untreated individual, these can rapidly escalate into cerebral malaria, anemia, severe organ failure, and death. In a semi-immune individual, or during the first six months of life in a malaria-endemic community where the mother has developed immunity, parasite growth is attenuated. To complete the life cycle in the human host, sexual forms (gametocytes) develop within the RBCs. These are taken up by the mosquito during a blood meal, and in the mosquito gut, where the temperature is lower, male and female gametes emerge from the infected RBCs in a process referred to as exflagellation. The gametes fertilize in the gut, give rise to ookinetes that burrow into the gut wall, and develop into oocysts containing immature sporozoites. These travel to the salivary gland of the mosquito to continue the life cycle.

Within the human host, immune responses can develop to all stages of the parasite. In different model systems (animal models and in vitro human systems), these immune responses have been shown to be capable of killing parasites (4). These observations have provided the foundations for vaccine strategies aimed at sporozoites, liver stage forms, blood stage forms, and sexual forms (5–12).

IMMUNE RESPONSES TO THE BLOOD STAGES

Malaria parasites develop within RBCs, which do not express MHC molecules. However, RBCs do express parasite-encoded antigens on their surface, the most important of which are the variant surface antigens (VSAs). The best characterized of these is PfEMP1 (13–15), for which approximately 60 variant gene copies occur in each parasite. Each parasite expresses one of these at a time. PfEMP1 has a complex structure and through different domains is able to mediate binding of the pRBC to different host tissues via different host receptors, including CD36, ICAM-1, chondroitic sulfate A, and hyaluronic acid. Binding to the small venules in different host tissues results in sequestration of the mature stages of the parasite (the forms that express PfEMP1). This results in local pathology (see below) and also interferes with the ability of the spleen to clear parasites from the blood.

Clearance of a parasite clone appears to follow the development of a VSA-specific antibody response (16). Parasites that have switched expression to a different VSA survive and multiply. The new clone may have a slightly different phenotype in terms of tissue adhesion, resulting in different pathology (17, 18). This process continues, resulting in sequential peaks of parasite density in the blood (19). Over time, the heights of the peaks gradually diminish, indicating that factors other than the repertoire of VSA-specific antibodies are contributing to parasite clearance. Antibodies to the merozoite surface appear to constitute one important factor; cell-mediated immunity (CMI) may be another. Merozoite surface proteins (MSPs) exhibit polymorphisms, but each parasite clone expresses only one allele of each MSP, indicating that a clone cannot escape immune surveillance by simply switching expression to a different variant form. Furthermore, limited data suggest that target antigens of CMI are conserved. It is thus of considerable interest as to why these immune responses cannot rapidly control parasite growth. Data summarized below suggest that the parasite can effectively suppress both T and B cell responses to itself.

Regulation of Immune Responses to Merozoite Antigens

There are many merozoite surface proteins (20, 21). Study of MSP-specific immune responses has focused on MSP1. Evidence to date suggests that antibodies to this protein contribute more significantly to parasite control than antibodies to other proteins, at least in terms of its ability to block merozoite invasion of RBCs (22).

MSP1 is a large protein (molecular mass 200 kDa) expressed on the surface of merozoites and attached to the cell membrane by a GPI anchor (23). MSP1 contains conserved regions and dimorphic regions, which exist in one of two forms. During the process of merozoite invasion of RBCs, MSP1 is processed in two proteolytic steps such that only the carboxyl terminal 19 kDa tail, $MSP1_{19}$, is carried into the new RBC (24). Although different regions of MSP1 have been studied with respect to vaccine development and have shown promise (25), $MSP1_{19}$ and the larger $MSP1_{42}$ fragments (consisting of $MSP1_{19}$ plus an amino-terminal portion, $MSP1_{33}$) represent the most promising regions of the molecule (26–30). Most immunological analyses have been undertaken with $MSP1_{19}$. Although $MSP1_{19}$ is one of the conserved regions of the protein, researchers have identified seven polymorphic amino acid positions for *P. falciparum* (31, 32). The ability of these polymorphisms to abrogate immunological recognition has not been defined; however, antibodies can discriminate between allelic forms of $MSP1_{19}$ from the rodent parasite, *P. yoelii* (33).

Investigators have know for more than 10 years that vaccination of mice with recombinant $MSP1_{19}$ from *P. yoelii* can lead to protection from blood and sporozoite challenge (26–28, 34). Studies by different groups have shown that a critical factor for protection is the induction of a very high titer antibody response. B cell–deficient mice are not protected by $MSP1_{19}$ vaccination, and $MSP1_{19}$-specific Th1 cells cannot adoptively transfer protection (35). Only those vaccination regimens that induce a high titer antibody response in normal mice result in protection. $MSP1_{19}$ antibodies per se, however, are not sufficient for protection. An active immune response that occurs postinfection is critical (27, 36). The importance of this response has been shown by the inability of $MSP1_{19}$ antibodies, even in high titer, to passively transfer complete resistance to immunodeficient mice (nude, μMT, SCID, $CD4^+$ T cell–depleted) while being able to transfer resistance to immunocompetent animals. When transferred into immunodeficient mice that are then infected with *P. yoelii*, antibodies can significantly delay the appearance of microscopic parasitemia for several days. When parasites appear, however, they grow rapidly and the mice succumb to infection. These data suggest that passive antibodies alone can clear most, but not all, parasites, which grow quickly when antibody levels decline. The active immune response that develops postinfection and that is required to eradicate parasites is $CD4^+$ T cell– and B cell–dependent. The specificities of these responses have not been defined, but data suggest that $MSP1_{19}$ itself needs not be a target antigen (36). Thus, although vaccine-induced immunity to $MSP1_{19}$ is largely antibody dependent, cell-mediated and other antibody responses are likely to be involved.

MSP1$_{19}$ is a small molecule, and as such MHC genes play an important role in regulating immunological responsiveness (37, 38). Two recombinant forms of MSP1$_{19}$ have been studied, one a GST fusion protein and the other a histidine-tagged protein. Immunological responsiveness mapped to different H-2 genes for these two constructs, which contained the same malaria-specific sequences, indicating that nonmalaria sequence elements were critical to the regulation of immunological responsiveness. However, helper T cell epitopes also reside with the MSP1$_{19}$ sequence itself (35) which suggests that infection could boost a vaccine-induced immune response. However, given that an active immune response after primary infection is required to eliminate all parasites (as described above), one might expect that this active immune response per se would also be able to control subsequent infections.

Another factor relevant to whether vaccine-induced immunity will provide protection against subsequent infections is the durability of immunological B cell memory to MSP1$_{19}$. Recent data suggest that MSP1$_{19}$-specific memory B cells alone provide no protection against infection and, furthermore, that during infection nearly all such cells undergo apoptotic deletion (M. Wykes, Y. Zhou, X.Q. Liu, M.F. Good, manuscript submitted). By contrast, these cells do not undergo apoptosis, but rather are activated and proliferate when stimulated with recMSP1$_{19}$.

The critical factor central to regulation of long-term immunity may be the magnitude of the antibody response following vaccination and the ability of long-lived plasma cells to maintain high antibody levels until first infection. A high (but not a low or moderate) antibody response will eliminate nearly all parasites. The remaining parasites are unlikely to lead to apoptosis of MSP1$_{19}$-specific memory B cells and will themselves initiate an active immune response that will clear all remaining parasites. The magnitude of a parasite-induced CMI response is inversely related to the parasite load initiating the response (see below), and if most parasites have been removed by antibody, CMI responses will be high. However, if the initial antibody response is not sufficiently high there will be a high, residual parasite load that is likely to lead to apoptosis of memory B cell responses and much diminished CMI. The regulation of the active immune response by the parasite load is described in more detail below.

Regulation of CMI to Malaria

Investigators have known for more than 20 years that CD4$^+$ T cells, independent of antibody, can limit parasite growth. Early studies using "μ-suppressed" mice (39), which have been repeated using mice genetically incapable of making B cells (40, 41), have shown that protective immunity can develop following infection in such mice. Furthermore, parasite-specific CD4$^+$ T cells can adoptively transfer protection (42–44), and investigators have defined target antigens/epitopes for some protective CD4$^+$ T cells (45, 46). Some transfer experiments have been performed using SCID recipients, thus indicating that no additional T or B cell responses from the recipients were contributing to parasite control. These rodent experiments give hope that vaccine-induced CMI in humans might provide an additional vaccine strategy. Some key events in the development of CMI during malaria defined in both human and rodent studies are summarized in Figure 2.

There is some doubt, however, as to the role of CMI in naturally acquired immunity in humans. This comes from examining the effect of HIV infection on malaria risk. A number of studies (e.g., 47) have failed to demonstrate an association between HIV status and malaria. However, a major recent study did show an inverse relationship between parasite load and $CD4^+$ T cell numbers in HIV-infected individuals (48): Other studies have been more consistent in identifying a link between HIV status and malaria symptoms rather than with parasite load (49, 50). The studies of parasite load have involved adults, and it is not known what effect HIV infection of children would have on induction of CMI. One of the difficulties in interpretation of the malaria-HIV coinfection studies is that it is not possible to attribute any loss of antiparasite or antidisease immunity to $CD4^+$ T cells acting independently of antibody. Thus, the human data have not been particularly helpful in identifying the role of human CMI in controlling parasite burden. Some studies have shown that human $CD4^+$ T cells can kill malaria parasites in vitro (51, 52) and others that the parasite-specific in vitro lymphoproliferative responses of malaria endemic residents were predictive of resistance to clinical malaria (53). Although these studies do not prove that human CMI plays a protective role, they together with the murine data lend support to an important role that human $CD4^+$ T cells, independently of antibody, might play in controlling parasite growth.

If CMI can reduce or eliminate infection, at least in experimental models, the question must be asked as to why it takes several years of endemic exposure to develop protective immunity. As mentioned above, although parasite density has sequential peaks following exposure, the height of the peaks gradually diminishes. Although CMI may contribute to this decline in peak parasite loads, it is unclear why this process takes so long. Regulation of dendritic cell (DC) function and parasite-induced apoptosis of effector cells may be two important regulatory factors.

Although DCs play a crucial role in priming T cell responses (Figure 2), there are data to suggest that in human and rodent malaria, DC function can be modulated by pRBC, including inhibition of DC maturation (54, 55), as well as decreased IL-12 and increased IL-10 production by *P. yoelii*–pRBC (55). Ligation of CD36 and/or CD51 on human DCs mimics the inhibition of DCs by pRBC (56), suggesting that these receptors mediate the delivery of negative-regulatory signals to DCs. However, other studies in rodent malaria found no such inhibition of DC maturation (57, 58), although DCs exposed to pRBC inhibited T cell proliferation and IL-2 production (58), suggesting these important aspects of DC function were inhibited by pRBC. Despite these studies on DC-pRBC interactions, the receptors used by these DCs to recognize pRBC, the way they capture and process malaria antigens, the tissue sites where *Plasmodium*-specific T cell responses are primed, and the molecules involved in this process are unknown. These gaps in our knowledge remain a bottleneck in the development of a successful vaccine to induce CMI and

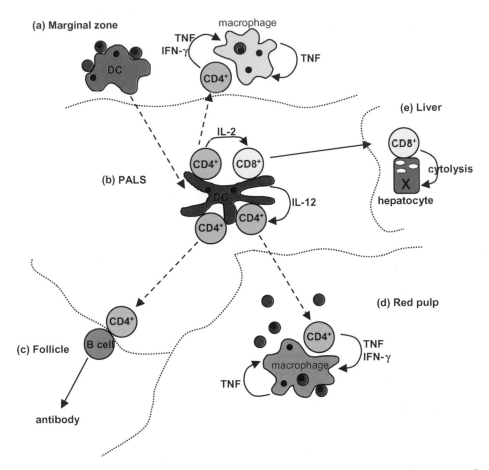

Figure 2 CMI in malaria. (*a*) Parasite antigen is likely to be captured by DC in or around the marginal zone (MZ) by mechanisms that have yet to be defined. (*b*) DCs migrate to the periarteriolar lymphoid sheath (PALS), where they can prime antigen-specific CD4+ T cells via antigen presented in association with MHC class II and costimulation provided by accessory molecules. These T cells may provide help in the form of IL-2 for parasite-specific CD8+ T cells also primed by DC via antigen on MHC class I molecules. (*c*) Activated CD4+ T cells can migrate to the border of the PALS and B cell follicles and provide cytokine and costimulatory help for B cell parasite-specific antibody production. (*d*) Parasite-specific CD4+ T cells may migrate to the red pulp where pRBC are removed by resident macrophages. This process may also occur in the MZ (*a*). CD4+ T cells can recognize peptide antigen on MHC class II molecules on macrophages and help in the generation of microbocidal reactive oxygen intermediates (ROI) and reactive nitrogen intermediates (RNI) by these cells by providing proinflammatory cytokines such as tumor necrosis factor (TNF) and IFN-γ. (*e*) Parasite-specific CD8+ and CD4+ T cells can migrate to other organs where pRBC sequester (e.g., the brain) or exoerythrocytic life cycle stages exist, such as the liver.

protect against malaria because without this knowledge, the correct targeting of vaccine antigen and adjuvant to an appropriate DC subpopulation in the best tissue site for induction of effective antiparasitic CMI may not be possible.

A further immunoregulatory scenario that has recently been explored in a rodent model is that a parasite infection can cause apoptotic deletion of parasite-specific, but not nonspecific, Th1 CD4$^+$ T cells (59, 60). As was shown for effector CD4$^+$ T cells, parasite-specific CD4$^+$ T cells with a helper function were also shown to be depleted as a result of infection (61). The deletion of Th1 CD4$^+$ T cells negatively impacts the ability of CD4$^+$ T cells to subsequently control parasite burden. Investigators previously showed that cultured mononuclear cells from infected individuals exhibited higher rates of apoptosis in vitro (62), but they could not determine whether the cells undergoing apoptosis were specific for malaria. In the rodent study (60), neither Fas nor tumor necrosis factor (TNF) was shown to be involved, but apoptosis was prevented by treating the animals with anti-IFN-γ antibodies. An early nonmalaria study also postulated IFN-γ as a key factor responsible for the cell death of effector CD4$^+$ T cells and as a possible mechanism for self-tolerance (63). Moreover, recent studies have suggested that IFN-γ is responsible for eliminating responding CD4$^+$ T cells in several other systems by inducing apoptosis of activated CD4$^+$ T cells (64–66). Although IFN-γ is involved in the apoptosis of malaria parasite-specific cells, the observation that bystander CD4$^+$ Th1 cells are not deleted during infection suggests that cognate interaction between T cells and antigen-presenting cells is a critical step. Deletion of parasite-specific CD4$^+$ T cells as a result of infection could explain in large part why such cells, with demonstrated ability to kill parasites in model systems, fail to contribute to the rapid induction of long-term immunity.

CMI and Vaccine Approaches

All malaria antigens currently under consideration as vaccine candidates have been chosen on the ability of specific antibodies to inhibit parasite growth. They are located on the merozoite surface (such as MSP1, above) or on the surface of pRBC. Although such antigens might also stimulate antibody-independent CMI, their ability to stimulate CMI was not considered in their selection as possible vaccine candidates. Because T cells recognize antigen only after processing, any parasite protein could theoretically be a target of protective CD4$^+$ T cells. However, the only intracellular antigen identified as a possible target antigen is the enzyme hypoxanthine guanine xanthine phosphoribosyl transferase (HGXPRT), a purine salvage enzyme critical to parasite survival because the parasite cannot make purines de novo (45).

HGXPRT is a relatively abundant antigen in the parasite. It is located in electron-dense regions in merozoites and in vesicles in the red cell cytoplasm (67). Because of its location, it would be released into the serum at the time the infected red cell ruptures and might be expected to tolerize potentially reactive T cells (68). Although its sequence does differ from human HGPRT, it is not known whether malaria-exposed individuals contain HGXPRT-reactive T cells.

A Low-Dose Vaccine Strategy

As discussed above, some of the major obstacles to inducing a protective immune response to malaria include antigenic polymorphism, limited immunological recognition of individual target antigens/vaccine candidates, and inhibition of DC function and apoptosis of effector and memory T and B cells from antigen overload. An approach that could potentially nullify all these numerous obstacles would be to combine all parasite antigens (thus counteracting the first two obstacles) in an ultralow dose (counteracting the latter two obstacles). Two recent studies lend support to this concept. Pombo et al. (69) recently reported that a pulsed ultralow-dose infection of naive human volunteers induced a potent Th1 CMI response, and the few volunteers who were subsequently challenged demonstrated increased resistance to infection. In a recent study, mice immunized with subpatent pulsed *P. chabaudi* infection were protected against challenge with not only an homologous strain of parasite but with a heterologous strain as well (S. Elliott, R. Kuns, M.F. Good, manuscript submitted). The mice exhibited potent Th1 CMI responses. Low-dose immunization has previously been shown to induce protection against other organisms (70, 71). A live malaria infection is an impractical way to deliver a vaccine. Recently, however, dead antigen formulated with alum and IL-12 was shown to induce robust protection of mice against *P. chabaudi* (72). Although antigen dose was not small in this study, it is reasonable to expect that dead antigen in low dose, formulated with IL-12 or agents which direct a Th1 response might also protect. Preliminary murine data suggest this approach will induce protection (M.F. Good and V. McPhun, unpublished data).

IMMUNOPATHOLOGY

Although CMI responses can kill parasites, rodent studies clearly demonstrate that they can cause significant immunopathology, including cerebral malaria, anemia, and weight loss. These conditions are discussed below, but when considering vaccine approaches that induce CMI, strategies must also be considered to minimize the risk of associated pathology. Recent data suggest that induction of regulatory T cells might be critical to establishing the balance between a cellular response that kills parasites and one that damages host tissue (73). In the rodent model, *P. yoelii*, early IFN-γ and TNF responses are required to inhibit parasite growth, and these must be quelled to minimize risk to the host. The immune responses to a lethal strain of *P. yoelii* is characterized by high levels of circulating transforming growth factor (TGF)-β within 24 h and a blunting of the antiparasite Th1 response leading to rapid parasite growth and high mortality. Conversely, the immune responses to the nonlethal strain is characterized by a delay in the TGF-β response enabling the parasite load to be reduced prior to a downregulation of the Th1 response (73). Clearly, parasite factors regulated the timing of the TGF-β response in these studies, but these remain to be identified.

The extent of pathology caused in humans by a CMI response to malaria is unknown. Although investigators debate the significance of naturally acquired human CMI to control parasite growth, they know even less of the role of CMI in causing pathology in humans. Adults, and to a lesser extent children, have, before malaria exposure, circulating $CD4^+$ Th1 cells with an activated phenotype that react vigorously in vitro with malaria parasites (74, 75). Evidence suggests that these T cells are not responding to a malaria superantigen in vitro. The T cells express diverse TCRs and recognize parasite antigens in an HLA-restricted manner. The ability of parasite-specific T cell clones generated from nonexposed individuals to recognize various environmental antigens suggests that they have arisen because of exposure to these environmental organisms and antigens and are cross-reactive with the parasite. Because Th1 cytokines have been implicated in disease, researchers have hypothesized that such parasite cross-reactive cells could contribute to pathology upon first encounter with the parasite (74, 76). The ability of such cells, in the presence of adherent cells, to inhibit parasite growth by up to 90% also suggests that such cells, arising because of exposure to cross-reactive organisms, can contribute to controlling parasite growth in vivo. Adoptively transferred parasite-specific Th1 $CD4^+$ cells can reduce parasite load in mice but also cause severe pathology (77).

SEVERE MALARIA

Severe malaria encompasses the major life-threatening clinical syndromes in malaria patients and includes cerebral malaria, anemia, and respiratory distress syndrome. In this section, we review our current understanding of the pathology leading to these conditions and discuss some of the strategies being developed to prevent them.

Cerebral Malaria

Cerebral malaria (CM) is a syndrome defined by an unarousable coma, not attributable to other causes from clinical or cerebrospinal fluid analysis, with any level of *P. falciparum* parasitemia (78, 79). It is a major cause of death in people infected with *P. falciparum*, and approximately 1% of *P. falciparum* infections progress to CM (80, 81). The great majority of cases occur in young children in sub-Saharan Africa, and 10%–20% of children who develop CM die, and many survivors are left with permanent neurological damage (80, 81). Importantly, in terms of prevention (see below), high blood parasitemia is significantly correlated with risk of developing CM (82).

CM was long thought to result from blood vessel obstruction by pRBC, leading to ischemia and petechial hemorrhages. However, it is now clear that CM also involves systemic inflammation that includes the increased expression of adhesion molecules on cerebral microvascular endothelial cells (MVECs) leading to cytoadherance of pRBC, activated leukocytes and platelets, and subsequent damage to the blood-brain barrier. CM is also likely the common endpoint for several pathways leading to pathogenesis (see below).

CELLULAR SEQUESTRATION IN THE BRAIN DURING CM   A key feature of human CM is the sequestration of pRBC in the microvasculature of various organs, most notably in the brain (83). Sequestration is mediated by parasite molecules, such as PfEMP1 (84, 15), CLAG9 (85, 86), and RSP1/2 (87), expressed on knob-like protrusions found on pRBC (reviewed in 88). These molecules bind to a range of host receptors on MVECs, including CD36 (89), thrombospondin (90), ICAM-1 (CD54) (91), VCAM-1 (CD106) (92), CD62E (E-selectin) (92), CD62P (P-selectin) (93), $\alpha_v\beta_3$ integrin (94), chondroitin-4-sulfate (95), and hyaluronic acid (96), although the latter two are primarily involved in pRBC sequestration in the placenta during pregnancy. Despite many reports that cerebral sequestration of pRBCs, but not leukocytes, was typical during CM, other studies have shown these assumptions to be incorrect. Analysis of brain tissue from adult and childhood CM cases show the presence of sequestered leukocytes in the brain vasculature (97, 98). Therefore, the view that CM results primarily from blockage of cerebral vessels by pRBC leading to ischemia and petechial hemorrhages appears to be too simplistic. In a recent study on brain tissue from children that died with CM in Malawi, three patterns in the brain microvasculature emerged: (*a*) sequestration of pRBC only, (*b*) sequestration of pRBC with hemorrhages and accumulation of pigmented leukocytes, and (*c*) no sequestration (99). These distinct patterns led the authors to postulate the existence of different pathogenic mechanisms in human CM associated with pre- and postschizont rupture of RBC. This hypothesis is supported by the concept that host-derived inflammatory mediators play a key role in the pathogenesis of CM (100).

IMMUNOLOGICAL REGULATION OF HUMAN CM   Much of the data collected and analyzed in relation to CM derives from studies on peripheral blood. Studies on plasma collected from children in East Africa (101) and West Africa (102) with malaria showed a strong correlation between TNF levels and severity of disease. A similar association between serum TNF and malaria severity was also reported in nonimmune adults (103). The TNF receptor 2 (TNFR2; CD120b) complex has also been observed on the surface of brain MVECs in human CM (104, 105), and TNF protein and mRNA have been found in the brains of CM patients (106), suggesting that the TNF/TNFR2 pathway may be important in CM. However, blockade of this pathway using an anti-TNF monoclonal antibody (107) or Pentoxifylline (108) failed to improve survival of African children with CM.

Other cytokines elevated in patients with severe malaria include IL-1β (102), IL-6 (103), and IFN-γ (109, 110). Both IL-1β and IL-6 appear to be released along with TNF when mononuclear cells recognize parasite molecules released following schizont rupture of pRBC (111, 112). A major inducer of TNF and IL-1β release by macrophages is the glycosylphosphatidylinositol (GPI)-anchor molecule of

P. falciparum MSPs (113). This molecule is now a major target for antipathology strategies (see below). Elevated serum IFN-γ is likely to enhance the production of the above mononuclear cell-derived inflammatory cytokines (Figure 3). Studies in vitro have identified NK and $\gamma\delta$ T cells as potential sources of IFN-γ during *P. falciparum* infection (114–116), and parasite-specific CD4$^+$ T cells are also likely a significant source of this cytokine (117). A recent study in Gambia found that heterozygotes for an IFN-γR1 polymorphism had a lower incidence of CM and death from this condition (118), supporting a role for IFN-γ in the pathogenesis of CM.

Nitric oxide (NO) is a gas that can modulate antimicrobial activity, smooth muscle contraction, neurotransmission, cytokine production, and adhesion molecule expression on MVECs (119). High levels of inducible NO synthase 2 (NOS2) expression has been reported in brain tissue taken from fatal cases of CM (120), suggesting that NO may contribute to CM pathogenesis. It has been postulated that NO produced by cerebral MVECs in response to proinflammatory cytokines may cross the blood-brain barrier and disrupt neurotransmission during CM (100). However, others (121, 122) found low plasma arginine concentrations in Tanzanian children with CM, compared with healthy controls, leading to decreased NOS2 expression and low NO production. A similar finding was reported in adults from Indonesia (123). These investigators postulated that NO protects against CM by decreasing production of proinflammatory cytokines, reducing expression of cell surface endothelial molecules, and thereby preventing pRBC sequestration. The complex interaction between NO and the immune system may account for different roles ascribed to this molecule during CM. Furthermore, the site of NO production and surrounding immunological microenvironment may also determine the effects of this physiological modulator in malaria.

The generation of proinflammatory cytokines is often accompanied by production of anti-inflammatory cytokines in homeostatic processes that have evolved to limit tissue damage. However, there are few studies on anti-inflammatory cytokines in human CM. One study that analyzed plasma IL-10 and TNF in children from Gabon with malaria found a reduced ratio of IL-10:TNF in those with CM (124). However, another study in children from Ghana failed to find any such difference (125). In Vietnamese adults, plasma IL-10 levels were higher in those that died with severe malaria than those that survived, but CM victims had lower levels than others (126). TGF-β expression was detected in the brains of Malawian children who died with CM (106), while another study reported elevated levels of TGF-β in the brains of nonimmune European patients that died with CM (127). Therefore, there is little evidence at present that elevated levels of anti-inflammatory cytokines reduce the risk of CM in humans.

EXPERIMENTAL CM IN MICE   Although monkey, rat, and hamster models of CM have been studied, the vast majority of experimental data comes from *P. berghei* ANKA infection of mice. This model allows comparisons between resistant (e.g., BALB/c and A/J) and susceptible (e.g., C57BL/6 and CBA) strains of mice, as

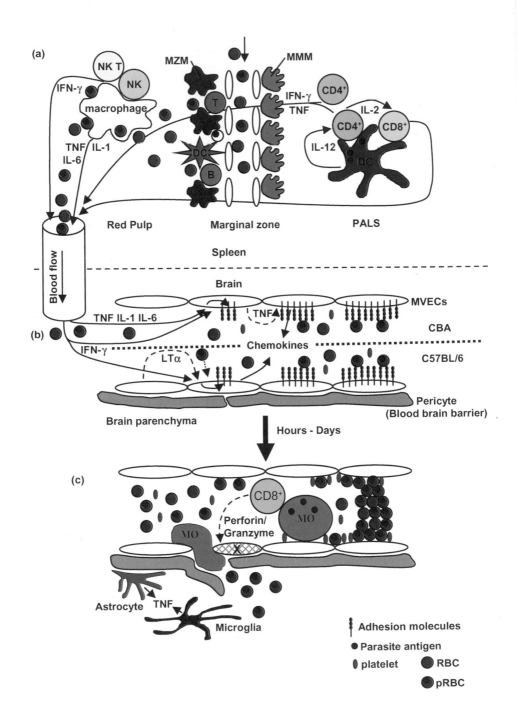

well as analysis of various gene knockout animals to define molecular pathways leading to pathogenesis. Not all features of human disease are represented in mice. However, this is not surprising given the emerging complexity of pathogenesis in human CM (see above). Nevertheless, susceptible mice do display ataxia, convulsions, and coma associated with sequestration of leukocytes and accumulation of pRBC in the brain microvasculature (128). Consequently, this model has provided important insights into the pathogenesis of CM and enabled potential targets for modulation to be identified for study in humans.

IMMUNOLOGICAL REGULATION OF MURINE CM   Both cellular and molecular components of the host immune immune response to *Plasmodium* parasites contribute to the pathogenesis of CM.

Cells   There is a clear role for T cells in the development of experimental CM (ECM). Early studies found that T cell–deficient nude mice were resistant to ECM (129). This finding was later supported by studies in T cell– and B cell–deficient RAG2$^{-/-}$ mice (130). Analysis of T cell subpopulations using depleting

---

Figure 3   The pathogenesis of experimental CM (ECM). (*a*) pRBC enter the spleen and are removed from the circulation by macrophages in the red pulp, and possibly the marginal zone (MZM). Parasite antigen is acquired by DCs that migrate into the PALS and prime antigen-specific CD4$^+$ and CD8$^+$ T cells. CD4$^+$ T cells provide help for CD8$^+$ T cells in the form of IL-2 and other costimulatory signals to DCs, as well as by producing and IFN-γ. NKT cells can be activated by DC or macrophages that present parasite antigens, such as GPIs, in association with CD1d. Macrophages in the red pulp can also produce proinflammatory cytokines such as TNF, IL-1, and IL-6 in response to signals from pRBC and IFN-γ, produced by CD4$^+$ T cells, NKT cells, or NK cells. The proinflammatory cytokines produced in the spleen have ready access to the blood supply. (*b*) In CBA mice (above dotted line), TNF, and possibly other proinflammatory cytokines, cause microvascular endothelial cells (MVECs) in the brain to express cell adhesion molecules, such as ICAM-1, VCAM-1, and PECAM-1. These activated endothelial cells can produce TNF and chemokines to further amplify this activation cascade. In C57BL/6 mice (below dotted line), lymphotoxin α (LTα) produced locally in the brain mediates expression of cell adhesion molecules on MVECs, possible acting with IFN-γ and/or parasite molecules in the local tissue microenvironment. (*c*) Leukocytes and pRBC bind adhesion molecules expressed on MVECs. This cellular accumulation is also mediated by platelets. The blockage of cerebral vessels may lead to hypoxic ischemia, and perforin and granzymes produced by activated CD8$^+$ T cells may damage the blood-brain barrier. The cytokine milieu in local tissue microenvironments may also modify endothelial tight junctions, leading to perivascular accumulation of pRBCs and leukocytes that can further damage the blood-brain barrier. Inflammatory mediators may also cross the blood-brain barrier and activate astrocytes and microglia that may themselves produce proinflammatory cytokines such as TNF.

antibodies have identified critical roles for CD4$^+$ T cells (131–133) and CD8$^+$ T cells in the pathogenesis of ECM in C57BL/6 mice (130, 132, 133). Furthermore, perforin-deficient C57BL/6 mice are resistant to ECM (130, 134), indicating that the perforin/granzyme cytolytic pathway may be a major pathogenic mechanism employed by CD8$^+$ T cells during ECM. Recently, blockade of the negative regulatory T cell costimulatory molecule CD152 (CTLA-4) was shown to enhance the development of ECM in C57BL/6 mice (135), providing evidence that modulation of T cell activation can have dramatic effects on the pathogenesis of ECM. This possibility must be given important consideration when vaccines containing *P. falciparum* T cell epitopes are tested in humans.

The spleen appears to be a key site for priming of *P. berghei* ANKA–specific T cell responses. Splenectomy is as effective at protecting mice from ECM as depletion of CD4$^+$ or CD8$^+$ T cells (136, 137). Therefore, *P. berghei* ANKA–specific T cells are apparently primed in the spleen by DC that have captured parasite antigen in the marginal zone or red pulp regions either directly, via exosomes, or indirectly, via cross-presentation by phagocytosis of macrophages containing pRBC or their remnants (Figure 3). This priming probably occurs in the periarteriolar lymphoid sheath (PALS) region in tightly regulated, sequential steps (138, 139). Data from T cell depletion studies indicate that CD4$^+$ T cells are required in the early stages of infection but that depletion closer to the onset of ECM symptoms does not alter the course of disease (133). In contrast, depletion of CD8$^+$ T cells either early in infection or around the time that ECM symptoms begin can prevent the onset of disease (130, 133). Hence, a model can be envisaged in which *P. berghei* ANKA–specific CD4$^+$ T cells are activated by DC and then provide help for *P. berghei* ANKA–specific CD8$^+$ T cell activation and expansion (Figure 3). Activated CD8$^+$ T cells are able to enter the circulation and adhere to MVECs in the brain and contribute to tissue pathology (130, 133).

NKT cells are a relatively small T cell subpopulation that express NK and T cell receptors and recognize glycolipids presented in association with CD1d molecules on antigen-presenting cells (140). Upon stimulation, they rapidly produce large amounts of IFN-γ and IL-4, and they can influence the balance of pro- and anti-inflammatory cytokine production during infectious disease (141). Two key pieces of data point to an important role for NKT cells in ECM pathogenesis. First, CD1d-restricted NKT cells recognize *Plasmodium* GPIs (142). Second, NKT cells from susceptible C57BL/6 mice produce IFN-γ and promote pathology following *P. berghei* ANKA infection, whereas in BALB/c mice they promote Th2 polarization and resistance to ECM (143). Attempts to prevent the activation of these cells by vaccinating against parasite GPIs are promising (see below) (144).

Other cells involved in ECM pathogenesis include macrophages (128, 145), neutrophils (146), platelets (147), and endothelial cells (147–149). Macrophages, neutrophils, and platelets accumulate in the brains of mice with ECM, and macrophages and neutrophils are capable of producing cytolytic molecules that can kill MVECs (145, 146), whereas platelets can promote interactions between inflammatory cells and MVECs in the brain (147–149). In addition, TNF activation of endothelial cells results in ICAM-1 upregulation (150), and LFA-1 expressed by leukocytes and platelets binds to ICAM-1, thereby mediating interactions between these cells and cerebral MVECs (147).

The modulation and/or damage of MVECs during *P. berghei* ANKA infection appears to be a critical event in ECM pathogenesis (147–149). However, the precise mechanisms that mediate these events remain unknown. Astrocytes and microglia also appear to contribute to the development of ECM. Although these cells are not in direct contact with pRBC, they are activated early in ECM pathogenesis (151), and both appear to produce TNF mRNA and protein following infection (152).

Cytokines and chemokines TNF appears to be a key mediator of ECM in CBA/Ca mice infected with *P. berghei* ANKA. These mice had elevated serum TNF following infection, and antibody blockade prevented the onset of ECM symptoms (145). In contrast, C57BL/6 mice had relatively low levels of serum TNF, and TNF blockade failed to prevent ECM (153). Furthermore, C57BL/6 mice lacking a functional TNF gene are as susceptible to ECM as control animals (154). However, in C57BL/6 mice, the closely related TNF family member lymphotoxin α (LTα) appears to be a key mediator of pathogenesis following infection. Mice lacking a functional LTα gene do not develop ECM and have reduced systemic inflammation, as indicated by decreased serum nitrate and IFN-γ, decreased expression of ICAM-1 on brain MVECs, and reduced recruitment of activated leukocytes to the brain (154). Interestingly, all these features observed in LTα-deficient mice during infection were also found in TNF-deficient mice, despite the fact that they died with ECM. The one feature that distinguished TNF- and LTα-deficient mice was the accumulation of pRBC in the cerebral microvasculature (154), indicating that this process is important in ECM pathogenesis in C57BL/6 mice. Significantly, this is also a major feature of human CM (see above), suggesting that TNF plays a limited role in the events that mediate the sequestration of pRBC to the cerebral microvasculature. In contrast, LTα appears to be critical to this process. The identification of the precise LTα signaling pathway that contributes to the binding of pRBC to cerebral MVECs may provide an opportunity to develop strategies to prevent this process and thereby prevent CM. Together, these data point toward at least two pathways of ECM pathogenesis, one that is TNF-dependent (represented in *P. berghei* ANKA–infected CBA mice), and another that is LTα-dependent (represented in *P. berghei* ANKA–infected C57BL/6 mice).

Other inflammatory cytokines and receptors have important roles in the pathogenesis of ECM. Neutralization of IFN-γ in CBA mice prevented the development of ECM (155), and mice deficient in IFN-γ (131) or IFN-γR (156) were also protected from this condition. In addition, mice deficient in TNFR2 (CD120b), but not TNFR1 (CD120a), were resistant to ECM (157). However, the use of 129/Sv and mixed C57BL/6 $\times$ 129/Sv mice in these cytokine- and receptor-knockout studies means that effects from genetic factors associated with 129/Sv mice cannot be excluded. Nevertheless, the IFN-γ neutralization data in CBA mice (155) support a model in which IFN-γ and TNF act on cerebral MVECs to upregulate expression of adhesion molecules that then mediate accumulation of activated leukocytes and pRBC in cerebral microvasculature (Figure 3). However, evidence for a role for IFN-γ in CM induction in C57BL/6 mice is unclear, although a recent microarray analysis of mRNA transcripts in the brain, spleen, and bone marrow of C57BL/6 mice following infection reported that IFN-γ-regulated gene transcripts were the most abundant of the inflammatory-related transcripts detected (158).

As with human CM, our understanding of the role of anti-inflammatory molecules in ECM is far less than that for proinflammatory cytokines. However, the administration of IL-10 to CBA mice gave some protection against ECM, whereas treatment with anti-IL-10 monoclonal antibody significantly increased the incidence of ECM in resistant BALB/c mice (159), suggesting that this cytokine may reduce the likelihood of ECM development. Roles for other anti-inflammatory cytokines in ECM, such as TGF-β, are unknown at present.

Chemokines play an essential role in the recruitment of leukocytes to all sites within the body. Therefore, they are integral to the pathogenesis mediated by CMI during CM. The presence of potentially pathogenic CD8$^+$ T cells in the cerebral microvasculature during ECM (130, 132, 133) led to a search for chemokines that mediate recruitment of this and other activated cell populations to the brain. Analysis of chemokine receptor mRNA accumulation in activated CD8$^+$ T cells isolated from *P. berghei* ANKA–infected mice with ECM revealed increased levels of CCR2, CCR5, CXCR3, and CXCR4, relative to naive CD8$^+$ T cells isolated from uninfected control mice (130). Subsequent studies in CCR5-deficient mice backcrossed onto the C57BL/6 background showed a small delay in the onset of ECM (130), whereas studies in CCR5-deficient mice on the mixed C57BL/6 × 129/Ola background found a more dramatic reduction in the incidence of ECM (up to 80%) (160). These results highlight potential differences in ECM development in mice from different genetic backgrounds, but they also indicate that there may be some redundancy in the chemokines that mediate recruitment of pathogenic CD8$^+$ T cells to the brain. Nevertheless, the identification of chemokines involved in the recruitment of CD8$^+$ T cells to the brain, as well as other potential pathogenic cells such as monocytes, neutrophils, and platelets, during CM could provide an opportunity to test reagents that block this recruitment and thereby prevent CM.

Anemia

Anemia is a significant complication of *P. falciparum* infection in malaria endemic regions, both in terms of morbidity and mortality. However, compared with our understanding of the pathogenesis of CM, relatively little is known about both host and parasite factors that contribute to malaria anemia. Children and pregnant women are especially susceptible to anemia during malaria infection (161). Several factors can contribute to severe anemia in malaria patients. First, increased blood parasitemia means there are fewer RBCs that are capable of efficiently transporting oxygen. Second, there is an increased rate of removal of uninfected RBCs from the circulation during malaria. Studies in Thailand have shown that pRBCs account for less than 10% of RBCs removed from the circulation of malaria patients (162). The lifespan of uninfected RBCs decreases during malaria infection (163), and decreasing levels of the complement regulatory proteins CR1 (CD35) and decay accelerating factor (CD55) on the surface of RBCs following *P. falciparum* infection allow immune complexes and C3b to bind RBCs, leading to destruction by phagocytosis and complement-mediated lysis (164). Third, erythropoiesis is suppressed in people infected with *P. falciparum*. The frequency of erythroid progenitors in the bone marrow of children with severe malaria was reduced compared with those with uncomplicated malaria (165). In mice, nonlethal infection with *P. chabaudi adami* led to decreased erythropoiesis in the bone marrow but an increase in the spleen (166). However, mice infected with *P. berghei* also showed decreased erythropoiesis in the spleen. Studies in *P. vinckei* (167) and *P. chabaudi* (168) infections of mice indicate that suppression of erythropoiesis is mediated by TNF production. Elevated plasma TNF levels have also been significantly associated with anemia in children in Zaire (now the Democratic Republic of Congo) and Kenya (169, 170). Low plasma IL-10 levels have also been found in malaria patients with severe anemia, but not in patients with CM or uncomplicated malaria (125). IL-10 and TNF counter-regulate each other's activity, and in malaria patients with severe anemia, this regulatory mechanism likely breaks down. Increased TNF levels suppress erythropoiesis as well as mediate sequestration of pRBC by stimulating the expression of adhesion molecules on endothelial cells in various tissue sites (see above). Therefore, a potential problem with generating CMI to *P. falciparum* is the associated production of proinflammatory cytokines that may cause complications such as anemia. However, it is anticipated that effective CMI will prevent significant blood parasitemia from developing, thereby limiting the scale of CMI response, and regulatory mechanisms will develop concurrently with CMI to limit pathogenic effects. The development of regulatory pathways that modulate CMI is a key event in any vaccine strategy, and one that has been studied in any detail only very recently. A safe vaccine that stimulates CMI to *P. falciparum* will also likely need to induce regulatory elements that prevent complications such as anemia.

Respiratory Distress Syndrome

Respiratory distress syndrome (RDS) is a feature of malaria in African children (171) and Asian adults (172). Again, the pathogenesis of RDS in malaria is poorly understood. RDS can be caused by injury to the lung microvascular endothelium and alveolar epithelium via proinflammatory mechanisms involving activated neutrophils and/or cytokines (173). However, although pulmonary edema is associated with RDS in malaria (172), it does not appear to be the basis of RDS in African children (171). RDS in malaria can be caused by heart failure, parasite sequestration in the lungs, or the increased requirement for respiration associated with CM (171). However, RDS is most often associated with metabolic acidosis, usually involving lactic acidemia (171, 172, 174), and this acidosis is a poor prognostic sign in children with severe malaria (175). The main clinical sign of RDS is deep breathing caused by attempts to release CO_2 to compensate for the acidosis (176). Several factors contribute to the accumulation of lactic acid in malaria patients, including: (*a*) reduced oxygen delivery to tissues as a result of anemia (see above), causing increased tissue production of lactate (171); (*b*) the production of lactate by *P. falciparum* itself, although this is likely to be minor (177); (*c*) reduced liver function in malaria resulting in decreased clearance of lactate (178); and (*d*) proinflammatory cytokines, such as TNF, contributing to increased lactate production (179). CMI generated against parasites is likely to contribute to this last factor. Therefore, concerns about generating CMI to *P. falciparum* and the production of proinflammatory cytokines causing complications such as anemia (see above) are also relevant for RDS. Nevertheless, one anti-disease vaccine approach that targets *P. falciparum* GPI (see below) has been shown to significantly reduce clinical signs of RDS in the mouse *P. berghei* ANKA model (144). Given the likely underestimates of the prevalence of RDS in malaria and associated mortality (171), understanding the pathogenesis of RDS in malaria remains an important goal for research aimed at developing treatments for severe malaria.

Approaches to Prevent and Treat Severe Malaria

At least three broad approaches are being considered to prevent or treat severe malaria: (*a*) vaccines aimed at reducing parasite burden, (*b*) vaccines that target parasite molecules capable of inducing significant inflammation, and (*c*) immunomodulation to block or dampen the activities of proinflammatory molecules that contribute to pathogenesis.

An effective vaccine that reduced blood parasitemia would reduce the incidence of severe malaria by reducing the risk of CM, preventing anemia by increasing numbers and survival time of uninfected RBCs, and minimizing the risk of metabolic acidosis and RDS. Such vaccines include those that stimulate *P. falciparum*–specific antibodies and CMI, which were discussed above. A promising approach to prevent CM is vaccination against *P. falciparum* molecules known to induce inflammatory responses. The prime candidate for such a vaccine strategy is *P. falciparum* GPI (144). Mice immunized with synthetic GPI glycan conjugated to keyhole limpet hemocyanin produced antibodies capable of recognizing native GPI in *P. falciparum* trophozoites and schizonts. These antibodies could also block GPI-induced TNF production by macrophages. Importantly, immunized mice were significantly protected (58%–75% survival) from ECM following *P. berghei* ANKA infection, compared with sham immunized mice and naive control mice (no survival) (144). However, although these data suggest a GPI vaccine for human CM may be possible, caution must be exercised in any human study because of the potential for *P. falciparum* GPI to skew immune responses toward either pro- or anti-inflammatory pathways via interactions with NKT cells (see above), depending on unknown host genetic factors. In addition, a major issue with such an antidisease vaccine is that it will mask symptoms of malaria and thereby foster much higher blood parasitemia, possibly leading to a delay in clinical symptoms rather than preventing them. The higher parasite burden in these individuals would also increase the likelihood of developing complications such as CM, anemia, or RDS.

Immunomodulation remains a major hope to treat severe malaria patients. Life-threatening disease can develop very rapidly, and once in hospital, 80% of deaths in African children occur within 24 hours of admission (82, 180). One of the biggest problems in attempting to treat severe malaria by immunomodulation is that many of the host factors associated with malaria pathogenesis, such as TNF, LTα, and IFN-γ, all play important roles in the generation of CMI against malaria parasites. Therefore, a major challenge is to devise strategies that limit pathology without substantially affecting the protective immune functions of these molecules. As mentioned above, attempts to neutralize TNF using antibodies or drugs and thereby prevent death from CM have failed. Nevertheless, targeting molecules such as LTα or IFN-γ for a limited time under controlled conditions to prevent severe malaria warrants further consideration. Whether this is performed using antibodies, soluble receptors, or drugs is an open question. Given the seriousness of severe malaria in many African communities, the development of effective immunomodulatory strategies could significantly impact mortality arising from malaria.

CONCLUDING REMARKS

In this review we have analyzed the contribution of cellular immune responses to both protection from malaria and pathogenesis. Although there is evidence from human and animal model systems that CMI can control parasite load, the factors that regulate CMI are poorly understood. DCs, central to the initiation of immune responses, are directly affected by pRBCs and high parasite density and can lead to apoptosis of effector and helper CD4$^+$ T cells as well as antibody-producing B cells. These regulatory mechanisms may have arisen to quell potentially harmful effects on host tissues, but the net result is often ineffective antiparasite immunity and significant host pathology. Recent attempts to boost antiparasite cellular immunity by exposure to ultralow-dose parasite loads may provide a more effective mechanism to kill parasites and subsequently limit host pathology.

ACKNOWLEDGMENTS

We thank Louis Miller and Eleanor Riley for reading this review and providing helpful comments. We also thank Joy Chapple and Tracey Checkley for assistance in preparing the manuscript. Research in the authors' laboratories is supported by the Australian National Health and Medical Research Council and the UNDP/World Bank/WHO Special Program for Research and Training in Tropical Diseases (TDR). C.R.E. and H.X. are Australian NHMRC Career Development Fellows.

The *Annual Review of Immunology* is online at http://immunol.annualreviews.org

LITERATURE CITED

1. Good MF, Stanisic DI, Xu H, Elliott S, Wykes M. 2004. The immunological challenge to developing a vaccine to the blood stages of malaria parasites. *Immunol. Rev.* In press
2. Kirk K. 2001. Membrane transport in the malaria-infected erythrocyte. *Physiol. Rev.* 81:495–537
3. Stevenson MM, Riley EM. 2004. Innate immunity to malaria. *Nat. Rev. Immunol.* 4:169–80
4. Hoffman SL, ed. 1996. *Malaria Vaccine Development: A Multi-Immune Response Approach*. Washington, DC: ASM Press
5. Chauhan VS, Bhardwaj D. 2003. Current status of malaria vaccine development. *Adv. Biochem. Eng. Biotechnol.* 84:143–82
6. Reeder JC. 2001. Towards a malaria vaccine for Papua New Guinea. *PNG Med. J.* 44:17–23
7. Wipasa J, Elliott S, Xu H, Good MF. 2002. Immunity to asexual blood stage malaria and vaccine approaches. *Immunol. Cell Biol.* 80:401–14
8. Moorthy V, Hill AV. 2002. Malaria vaccines. *Br. Med. Bull.* 62:59–72
9. Greenwood B, Alonso P. 2002. Malaria vaccine trials. *Chem. Immunol.* 80:366–95
10. Schofield L. 2002. Antidisease vaccines. *Chem. Immunol.* 80:322–42
11. Good MF. 2001. Towards a blood-stage vaccine for malaria: Are we following all the leads? *Nat. Rev. Immunol.* 1:117–25
12. Doolan DL, Hoffman SL. 2002. Nucleic acid vaccines against malaria. *Chem. Immunol.* 80:308–21
13. Baruch DI, Pasloske BL, Singh HB, Bi X, Ma XC, et al. 1995. Cloning the *P. falciparum* gene encoding PfEMP1, a malarial variant antigen and adherence receptor on the surface of parasitized human erythrocytes. *Cell* 82:77–87
14. Su XZ, Heatwole VM, Wertheimer SP, Guinet F, Herrfeldt JA, et al. 1995. The large diverse gene family var encodes proteins involved in cytoadherence and antigenic variation of *Plasmodium falciparum*–infected erythrocytes. *Cell* 82:89–100
15. Smith JD, Chitnis CE, Craig AG, Roberts DJ, Hudson-Taylor DE, et al. 1995. Switches in expression of *Plasmodium falciparum var* genes correlate with changes in antigenic and cytoadherent phenotypes of infected erythrocytes. *Cell* 82:101–10
16. Bull PC, Lowe BS, Kortok M, Molyneux CS, Newbold CI, Marsh K. 1998. Parasite antigens on the infected red cell surface are targets for naturally acquired immunity to malaria. *Nat. Med.* 4:358–60
17. Fried M, Nosten F, Brockman A, Brabin BJ, Duffy PE. 1998. Maternal antibodies block malaria. *Nature* 395:851–52
18. Jensen AT, Magistrado P, Sharp S, Joergensen L, Lavstsen T, et al. 2004. *Plasmodium falciparum* associated with severe childhood malaria preferentially expresses PfEMP1 encoded by group A *var* genes. *J. Exp. Med.* 199:1179–90
19. Miller LH, Good MF, Milon G. 1994. Malaria pathogenesis. *Science* 264:1878–83
20. Holder AA. 1994. Proteins on the surface of the malaria parasite and cell invasion. *Parasitology* 108(Suppl):S5–18
21. Berzins K. 2002. Merozoite antigens involved in invasion. *Chem. Immunol.* 80:125–43
22. O'Donnell RA, de Koning-Ward TF, Burt RA, Bockarie M, Reeder JC, et al. 2001. Antibodies against merozoite surface protein (MSP)-1_{19} are a major component of the invasion-inhibitory response in

individuals immune to malaria. *J. Exp. Med.* 193:1403–12

23. Holder AA, Guevara Patino JA, Uthaipibull C, Syed SE, Ling IT, et al. 1999. Merozoite surface protein 1, immune evasion, and vaccines against asexual blood stage malaria. *Parassitologia* 41:409–14

24. Blackman MJ, Heidrich HG, Donachie S, McBride JS, Holder AA. 1990. A single fragment of a malaria merozoite surface protein remains on the parasite during red cell invasion and is the target of invasion-inhibiting antibodies. *J. Exp. Med.* 172:379–82

25. Genton B, Betuela I, Felger I, Al-Yaman F, Anders RF, et al. 2002. A recombinant blood-stage malaria vaccine reduces *Plasmodium falciparum* density and exerts selective pressure on parasite populations in a phase 1-2b trial in Papua New Guinea. *J. Infect. Dis.* 185:820–27

26. Ling IT, Ogun SA, Holder AA. 1995. The combined epidermal growth factor-like modules of *Plasmodium yoelii* merozoite surface protein-1 are required for a protective immune response to the parasite. *Parasite Immunol.* 17:425–33

27. Daly TM, Long CA. 1995. Humoral response to a carboxyl-terminal region of the merozoite surface protein-1 plays a predominant role in controlling blood-stage infection in rodent malaria. *J. Immunol.* 155:236–43

28. Hirunpetcharat C, Tian JH, Kaslow DC, van Rooijen N, Kumar S, et al. 1997. Complete protective immunity induced in mice by immunization with the 19-kilodalton carboxyl-terminal fragment of the merozoite surface protein-1 (MSP1$_{19}$) of *Plasmodium yoelii* expressed in *Saccharomyces cerevisiae*: correlation of protection with antigen-specific antibody titer, but not with effector CD4$^+$ T cells. *J. Immunol.* 159:3400–11

29. Kumar S, Yadava A, Keister DB, Tian JH, Ohl M, et al. 1995. Immunogenicity and in vivo efficacy of recombinant *Plasmodium falciparum* merozoite surface protein-1 in Aotus monkeys. *Mol. Med.* 1:325–32

30. Tian JH, Kumar S, Kaslow DC, Miller LH. 1997. Comparison of protection induced by immunization with recombinant proteins from different regions of merozoite surface protein 1 of *Plasmodium yoelii*. *Infect. Immun.* 65:3032–36

31. Miller LH, Roberts T, Shahabuddin M, McCutchan TF. 1993. Analysis of sequence diversity in the *Plasmodium falciparum* merozoite surface protein-1 (MSP-1). *Mol. Biochem. Parasitol.* 59:1–14

32. Jongwutiwes S, Tanabe K, Kanbara H. 1993. Sequence conservation in the C-terminal part of the precursor to the major merozoite surface proteins (MSP1) of *Plasmodium falciparum* from field isolates. *Mol. Biochem. Parasitol.* 59:95–100

33. Burns JM Jr, Parke LA, Daly TM, Cavacini LA, Weidanz WP, Long CA. 1989. A protective monoclonal antibody recognizes a variant-specific epitope in the precursor of the major merozoite surface antigen of the rodent malarial parasite *Plasmodium yoelii*. *J. Immunol.* 142:2835–40

34. Renia L, Ling IT, Marussig M, Miltgen F, Holder AA, Mazier D. 1997. Immunization with a recombinant C-terminal fragment of *Plasmodium yoelii* merozoite surface protein 1 protects mice against homologous but not heterologous *P. yoelii* sporozoite challenge. *Infect. Immun.* 65:4419–23

35. Tian JH, Good MF, Hirunpetcharat C, Kumar S, Ling IT, et al. 1998. Definition of T cell epitopes within the 19 kDa carboxyl-terminal fragment of *Plasmodium yoelii* merozoite surface protein 1 (MSP1$_{19}$) and their role in immunity to malaria. *Parasite Immunol.* 20:263–78

36. Hirunpetcharat C, Vukovic P, Liu XQ, Kaslow DC, Miller LH, Good MF. 1999. Absolute requirement for an active immune response involving B cells and Th cells in immunity to *Plasmodium yoelii* passively acquired with antibodies to the

19-kDa carboxyl-terminal fragment of merozoite surface protein-1. *J. Immunol.* 162:7309–14

37. Tian JH, Miller LH, Kaslow DC, Ahlers J, Good MF, et al. 1996. Genetic regulation of protective immune response in congenic strains of mice vaccinated with a subunit malaria vaccine. *J. Immunol.* 157:1176–83

38. Stanisic DI, Martin LB, Liu XQ, Jackson D, Cooper J, Good MF. 2003. Analysis of immunological nonresponsiveness to the 19-kilodalton fragment of merozoite surface protein 1 of *Plasmodium yoelii*: rescue by chemical conjugation to diphtheria toxoid (DT) and enhancement of immunogenicity by prior DT vaccination. *Infect. Immun.* 71:5700–13

39. Grun JL, Weidanz WP. 1983. Antibody-independent immunity to reinfection malaria in B-cell-deficient mice. *Infect. Immun.* 41:1197–204

40. van der Heyde HC, Huszar D, Woodhouse C, Manning DD, Weidanz WP. 1994. The resolution of acute malaria in a definitive model of B cell deficiency, the JHD mouse. *J. Immunol.* 152:4557–62

41. von der Weid T, Honarvar N, Langhorne J. 1996. Gene-targeted mice lacking B cells are unable to eliminate a blood stage malaria infection. *J. Immunol.* 156:2510–16

42. Brake DA, Long CA, Weidanz WP. 1988. Adoptive protection against *Plasmodium chabaudi adami* malaria in athymic nude mice by a cloned T cell line. *J. Immunol.* 140:1989–93

43. Taylor-Robinson AW, Phillips RS, Severn A, Moncada S, Liew FY. 1993. The role of TH1 and TH2 cells in a rodent malaria infection. *Science* 260:1931–34

44. Amante FH, Good MF. 1997. Prolonged Th1-like response generated by a *Plasmodium yoelii*–specific T cell clone allows complete clearance of infection in reconstituted mice. *Parasite Immunol.* 19:111–26

45. Makobongo MO, Riding G, Xu H, Hirun-petcharat C, Keough D, et al. 2003. The purine salvage enzyme hypoxanthine guanine xanthine phosphoribosyl transferase is a major target antigen for cell-mediated immunity to malaria. *Proc. Natl. Acad. Sci. USA* 100:2628–33

46. Wipasa J, Hirunpetcharat C, Mahakunkijcharoen Y, Xu H, Elliott S, Good MF. 2002. Identification of T cell epitopes on the 33-kDa fragment of *Plasmodium yoelii* merozoite surface protein 1 and their antibody-independent protective role in immunity to blood stage malaria. *J. Immunol.* 169:944–51

47. Chandramohan D, Greenwood BM. 1998. Is there an interaction between human immunodeficiency virus and *Plasmodium falciparum*? *Int. J. Epidemiol.* 27:296–301

48. Whitworth J, Morgan D, Quigley M, Smith A, Mayanja B, et al. 2000. Effect of HIV-1 and increasing immunosuppression on malaria parasitaemia and clinical episodes in adults in rural Uganda: a cohort study. *Lancet* 356:1051–56

49. French N, Nakiyingi J, Lugada E, Watera C, Whitworth JA, Gilks CF. 2001. Increasing rates of malarial fever with deteriorating immune status in HIV-1-infected Ugandan adults. *AIDS* 15:899–906

50. Grimwade K, French N, Mbatha DD, Zungu DD, Dedicoat M, Gilks CF. 2003. Childhood malaria in a region of unstable transmission and high human immunodeficiency virus prevalence. *Pediatr. Infect. Dis. J.* 22:1057–63

51. Brown J, Greenwood BM, Terry RJ. 1986. Cellular mechanisms involved in recovery from acute malaria in Gambian children. *Parasite Immunol.* 8:551–64

52. Fell AH, Currier J, Good MF. 1994. Inhibition of *Plasmodium falciparum* growth in vitro by CD4$^+$ and CD8$^+$ T cells from non-exposed donors. *Parasite Immunol.* 16:579–86

53. Mshana RN, Boulandi J, Mayombo J, Mendome G. 1993. In vitro lymphoproliferative responses to malaria antigens: a

prospective study of residents of a holoen-demic area with perennial malaria transmission. *Parasite Immunol.* 15:35–45

54. Urban BC, Ferguson DJ, Pain A, Willcox N, Plebanski M, et al. 1999. *Plasmodium falciparum*–infected erythrocytes modulate the maturation of dendritic cells. *Nature* 400:73–77

55. Ocana-Morgner C, Mota MM, Rodriguez A. 2003. Malaria blood stage suppression of liver stage immunity by dendritic cells. *J. Exp. Med.* 197:143–51

56. Urban BC, Willcox N, Roberts DJ. 2001. A role for CD36 in the regulation of dendritic cell function. *Proc. Natl. Acad. Sci. USA* 98:8750–55

57. Seixas E, Cross C, Quin S, Langhorne J. 2001. Direct activation of dendritic cells by the malaria parasite, *Plasmodium chabaudi chabaudi. Eur. J. Immunol.* 31:2970–78

58. Luyendyk J, Olivas OR, Ginger LA, Avery AC. 2002. Antigen-presenting cell function during *Plasmodium yoelii* infection. *Infect. Immun.* 70:2941–49

59. Hirunpetcharat C, Good MF. 1998. Deletion of *Plasmodium berghei*–specific CD4+ T cells adoptively transferred into recipient mice after challenge with homologous parasite. *Proc. Natl. Acad. Sci. USA* 95:1715–20

60. Xu H, Wipasa J, Yan H, Zeng M, Makobongo MO, et al. 2002. The mechanism and significance of deletion of parasite-specific CD4+ T cells in malaria infection. *J. Exp. Med.* 195:881–92

61. Wipasa J, Xu H, Stowers A, Good MF. 2001. Apoptotic deletion of Th cells specific for the 19-kDa carboxyl-terminal fragment of merozoite surface protein 1 during malaria infection. *J. Immunol.* 167:3903–9

62. Toure-Balde A, Sarthou JL, Aribot G, Michel P, Trape JF, et al. 1996. *Plasmodium falciparum* induces apoptosis in human mononuclear cells. *Infect. Immun.* 64:744–50

63. Liu Y, Janeway CA Jr. 1990. Interferon γ plays a critical role in induced cell death of effector T cell: a possible third mechanism of self-tolerance. *J. Exp. Med.* 172:1735–39

64. Dalton DK, Haynes L, Chu CQ, Swain SL, Wittmer S. 2000. Interferon γ eliminates responding CD4 T cells during mycobacterial infection by inducing apoptosis of activated CD4 T cells. *J. Exp. Med.* 192:117–22

65. Chu CQ, Wittmer S, Dalton DK. 2000. Failure to suppress the expansion of the activated CD4 T cell population in interferon γ–deficient mice leads to exacerbation of experimental autoimmune encephalomyelitis. *J. Exp. Med.* 192:123–28

66. Scanga CA, Mohan VP, Yu K, Joseph H, Tanaka K, et al. 2000. Depletion of CD4+ T cells causes reactivation of murine persistent tuberculosis despite continued expression of interferon γ and nitric oxide synthase 2. *J. Exp. Med.* 192:347–58

67. Shahabuddin M, Gunther K, Lingelbach K, Aikawa M, Schreiber M, et al. 1992. Localisation of hypoxanthine phosphoribosyl transferase in the malaria parasite *Plasmodium falciparum. Exp. Parasitol.* 74:11–19

68. Mitchison NA. 1968. The dosage requirements for immunological paralysis by soluble proteins. *Immunology* 15:509–30

69. Pombo DJ, Lawrence G, Hirunpetcharat C, Rzepczyk C, Bryden M, et al. 2002. Immunity to malaria after administration of ultra-low doses of red cells infected with *Plasmodium falciparum. Lancet* 360:610–17

70. Bretscher PA, Wei G, Menon JN, Bielefeldt-Ohmann H. 1992. Establishment of stable, cell-mediated immunity that makes "susceptible" mice resistant to *Leishmania major. Science* 257:539–42

71. Shata MT, Tricoche N, Perkus M, Tom D, Brotman B, et al. 2003. Exposure to low infective doses of HCV induces cellular immune responses without consistently detectable viremia or seroconversion in chimpanzees. *Virology* 314:601–16

72. Su Z, Tam MF, Jankovic D, Stevenson MM. 2003. Vaccination with novel immunostimulatory adjuvants against blood-stage malaria in mice. *Infect. Immun.* 71:5178–87

73. Omer FM, de Souza JB, Riley EM. 2003. Differential induction of TGF-β regulates proinflammatory cytokine production and determines the outcome of lethal and non-lethal *Plasmodium yoelii* infections. *J. Immunol.* 171:5430–36

74. Currier J, Sattabongkot J, Good MF. 1992. 'Natural' T cells responsive to malaria: evidence implicating immunological cross-reactivity in the maintenance of TCR $\alpha\beta+$ malaria-specific responses from non-exposed donors. *Int. Immunol.* 4:985–94

75. Fell AH, Silins SL, Baumgarth N, Good MF. 1996. *Plasmodium falciparum*–specific T cell clones from non-exposed and exposed donors are highly diverse in TCR β chain V segment usage. *Int. Immunol.* 8:1877–87

76. Currier J, Beck HP, Currie B, Good MF. 1995. Antigens released at schizont burst stimulate *Plasmodium falciparum*–specific CD4$^+$ T cells from non-exposed donors: potential for cross-reactive memory T cells to cause disease. *Int. Immunol.* 7:821–33

77. Hirunpetcharat C, Finkelman F, Clark IA, Good MF. 1999. Malaria parasite-specific Th1-like T cells simultaneously reduce parasitemia and promote disease. *Parasite Immunol.* 21:319–29

78. Warrell D, Molyneux M, Beales P. 1990. Severe and complicated malaria. *Trans. R. Soc. Trop. Med. Hyg.* 84(Suppl.):1–65

79. Marsh K, Forster D, Waruiru C, Mwangi I, Winstanley M, et al. 1995. Indicators of life-threatening malaria in African children. *N. Engl. J. Med.* 332:1399–404

80. World Health Org. 2000. Roll back malaria: spotlight on Africa. *TDR News* 62:10, 15

81. Snow RW, Trape JF, Marsh K. 2001. The past, present and future of childhood malaria mortality in Africa. *Trends Parasitol.* 17:593–97

82. Molyneux ME, Taylor TE, Wirima JJ, Borgstein A. 1989. Clinical features and prognostic indicators in paediatric cerebral malaria: a study of 131 comatose Malawian children. *Q. J. Med.* 71:441–59

83. MacPherson GG, Warrell MJ, White NJ, Looareesuwan S, Warrell DA. 1985. Human cerebral malaria. A quantitative ultrastructural analysis of parasitized erythrocyte sequestration. *Am. J. Pathol.* 119:385–401

84. Roberts DJ, Craig AG, Berendt AR, Pinches R, Nash G, et al. 1992. Rapid switching to multiple antigenic and adhesive phenotypes in malaria. *Nature* 357:689–92

85. Gardiner DL, Holt DC, Thomas EA, Kemp DJ, Trenholme KR. 2000. Inhibition of *Plasmodium falciparum clag9* gene function by antisense RNA. *Mol. Biochem. Parasitol.* 110:33–41

86. Trenholme KR, Gardiner DL, Holt DC, Thomas EA, Cowman AF, Kemp DJ. 2000. *clag9*: a cytoadherence gene in *Plasmodium falciparum* essential for binding of parasitized erythrocytes to CD36. *Proc. Natl. Acad. Sci. USA* 97:4029–33

87. Pouvelle B, Buffet PA, Lepolard C, Scherf A, Gysin J. 2000. Cytoadhesion of *Plasmodium falciparum* ring-stage-infected erythrocytes. *Nat. Med.* 6:1264–68

88. Craig A, Scherf A. 2001. Molecules on the surface of the *Plasmodium falciparum* infected erythrocyte and their role in malaria pathogenesis and immune evasion. *Mol. Biochem. Parasitol.* 115:129–43

89. Oquendo P, Hundt E, Lawler J, Seed B. 1989. CD36 directly mediates cytoadherence of *Plasmodium falciparum* parasitized erythrocytes. *Cell* 58:95–101

90. Roberts DD, Sherwood JA, Spitalnik SL, Panton LJ, Howard RJ, et al. 1985. Thrombospondin binds falciparum malaria parasitized erythrocytes and may

mediate cytoadherence. *Nature* 318:64–66

91. Berendt AR, Simmons DL, Tansey J, Newbold CI, Marsh K. 1989. Intercellular adhesion molecule-1 is an endothelial cell adhesion receptor for *Plasmodium falciparum. Nature* 341:57–59

92. Ockenhouse CF, Tegoshi T, Maeno Y, Benjamin C, Ho M, et al. 1992. Human vascular endothelial cell adhesion receptors for *Plasmodium falciparum*-infected erythrocytes: roles for endothelial leukocyte adhesion molecule 1 and vascular cell adhesion molecule 1. *J. Exp. Med.* 176:1183–89

93. Ho M, Schollaardt T, Niu X, Looareesuwan S, Patel KD, Kubes P. 1998. Characterization of *Plasmodium falciparum*–infected erythrocyte and P-selectin interaction under flow conditions. *Blood* 91:4803–9

94. Siano JP, Grady KK, Millet P, Wick TM. 1998. Short report: *Plasmodium falciparum*: cytoadherence to $\alpha_v\beta_3$ on human microvascular endothelial cells. *Am. J. Trop. Med. Hyg.* 59:77–79

95. Fried M, Duffy PE. 1996. Adherence of *Plasmodium falciparum* to chondroitin sulfate A in the human placenta. *Science* 272:1502–4

96. Beeson JG, Rogerson SJ, Cooke BM, Reeder JC, Chai W, et al. 2000. Adhesion of *Plasmodium falciparum*–infected erythrocytes to hyaluronic acid in placental malaria. *Nat. Med.* 6:86–90

97. Porta J, Carota A, Pizzolato GP, Wildi E, Widmer MC, et al. 1993. Immunopathological changes in human cerebral malaria. *Clin. Neuropathol.* 12:142–46

98. Patnaik JK, Das BS, Mishra SK, Mohanty S, Satpathy SK, Mohanty D. 1994. Vascular clogging, mononuclear cell margination, and enhanced vascular permeability in the pathogenesis of human cerebral malaria. *Am. J. Trop. Med. Hyg.* 51:642–47

99. Taylor TE, Fu WJ, Carr RA, Whitten RO, Mueller JG, et al. 2004. Differentiating the pathologies of cerebral malaria by postmortem parasite counts. *Nat. Med.* 10:143–45

100. Clark IA, Rockett KA, Cowden WB. 1991. Proposed link between cytokines, nitric oxide and human cerebral malaria. *Parasitol. Today* 7:205–7

101. Grau GE, Taylor TE, Molyneux ME, Wirima JJ, Vassalli P, et al. 1989. Tumor necrosis factor and disease severity in children with falciparum malaria. *N. Engl. J. Med.* 320:1586–91

102. Kwiatkowski D, Hill AV, Sambou I, Twumasi P, Castracane J, et al. 1990. TNF concentration in fatal cerebral, non-fatal cerebral, and uncomplicated *Plasmodium falciparum* malaria. *Lancet* 336:1201–4

103. Kern P, Hemmer CJ, Van Damme J, Gruss HJ, Dietrich M. 1989. Elevated tumor necrosis factor alpha and interleukin-6 serum levels as markers for complicated *Plasmodium falciparum* malaria. *Am. J. Med.* 87:139–43

104. Hunt NH, Grau GE. 2003. Cytokines: accelerators and brakes in the pathogenesis of cerebral malaria. *Trends Immunol.* 24:491–99

105. Lou J, Lucas R, Grau GE. 2001. Pathogenesis of cerebral malaria: recent experimental data and possible applications for humans. *Clin. Microbiol. Rev.* 14:810–20

106. Brown H, Turner G, Rogerson S, Tembo M, Mwenechanya J, et al. 1999. Cytokine expression in the brain in human cerebral malaria. *J. Infect. Dis.* 180:1742–46

107. van Hensbroek MB, Palmer A, Onyiorah E, Schneider G, Jaffar S, et al. 1996. The effect of a monoclonal antibody to tumor necrosis factor on survival from childhood cerebral malaria. *J. Infect. Dis.* 174:1091–97

108. Di Perri G, Di Perri IG, Monteiro GB, Bonora S, Hennig C, et al. 1995. Pentoxifylline as a supportive agent in the treatment of cerebral malaria in children. *J. Infect. Dis.* 171:1317–22

109. Ho M, Sexton MM, Tongtawe P, Looareesuwan S, Suntharasamai P, Webster

HK. 1995. Interleukin-10 inhibits tumor necrosis factor production but not antigen-specific lymphoproliferation in acute *Plasmodium falciparum* malaria. *J. Infect. Dis.* 172:838–44

110. Ringwald P, Peyron F, Vuillez JP, Touze JE, Le Bras J, Deloron P. 1991. Levels of cytokines in plasma during *Plasmodium falciparum* malaria attacks. *J. Clin. Microbiol.* 29:2076–78

111. Clark IA, Virelizier JL, Carswell EA, Wood PR. 1981. Possible importance of macrophage-derived mediators in acute malaria. *Infect. Immun.* 32:1058–66

112. Kwiatkowski D, Cannon JG, Manogue KR, Cerami A, Dinarello CA, Greenwood BM. 1989. Tumour necrosis factor production in falciparum malaria and its association with schizont rupture. *Clin. Exp. Immunol.* 77:361–66

113. Schofield L, Hackett F. 1993. Signal transduction in host cells by a glycosylphosphatidylinositol toxin of malaria parasites. *J. Exp. Med.* 177:145–53

114. Goodier MR, Lundqvist C, Hammarstrom ML, Troye-Blomberg M, Langhorne J. 1995. Cytokine profiles for human $V\gamma9^+$ T cells stimulated by *Plasmodium falciparum*. *Parasite Immunol.* 17:413–23

115. Hensmann M, Kwiatkowski D. 2001. Cellular basis of early cytokine response to *Plasmodium falciparum*. *Infect. Immun.* 69:2364–71

116. Artavanis-Tsakonas K, Riley EM. 2002. Innate immune response to malaria: rapid induction of IFN-γ from human NK cells by live *Plasmodium falciparum*–infected erythrocytes. *J. Immunol.* 169:2956–63

117. Scragg IG, Hensmann M, Bate CA, Kwiatkowski D. 1999. Early cytokine induction by *Plasmodium falciparum* is not a classical endotoxin-like process. *Eur. J. Immunol.* 29:2636–44

118. Koch O, Awomoyi A, Usen S, Jallow M, Richardson A, et al. 2002. IFNGR1 gene promoter polymorphisms and susceptibility to cerebral malaria. *J. Infect. Dis.* 185:1684–87

119. MacMicking J, Xie QW, Nathan C. 1997. Nitric oxide and macrophage function. *Annu. Rev. Immunol.* 15:323–50

120. Maneerat Y, Viriyavejakul P, Punpoowong B, Jones M, Wilairatana P, et al. 2000. Inducible nitric oxide synthase expression is increased in the brain in fatal cerebral malaria. *Histopathology* 37:269–77

121. Anstey NM, Weinberg JB, Hassanali MY, Mwaikambo ED, Manyenga D, et al. 1996. Nitric oxide in Tanzanian children with malaria: inverse relationship between malaria severity and nitric oxide production/nitric oxide synthase type 2 expression. *J. Exp. Med.* 184:557–67

122. Lopansri BK, Anstey NM, Weinberg JB, Stoddard GJ, Hobbs MR, et al. 2003. Low plasma arginine concentrations in children with cerebral malaria and decreased nitric oxide production. *Lancet* 361:676–78

123. Boutlis CS, Tjitra E, Maniboey H, Misukonis MA, Saunders JR, et al. 2003. Nitric oxide production and mononuclear cell nitric oxide synthase activity in malaria-tolerant Papuan adults. *Infect. Immun.* 71:3682–89

124. May J, Lell B, Luty AJ, Meyer CG, Kremsner PG. 2000. Plasma interleukin-10: Tumor necrosis factor (TNF)-α ratio is associated with TNF promoter variants and predicts malarial complications. *J. Infect. Dis.* 182:1570–73

125. Kurtzhals JA, Adabayeri V, Goka BQ, Akanmori BD, Oliver-Commey JO, et al. 1998. Low plasma concentrations of interleukin 10 in severe malarial anaemia compared with cerebral and uncomplicated malaria. *Lancet* 351:1768–72

126. Day NP, Hien TT, Schollaardt T, Loc PP, Chuong LV, et al. 1999. The prognostic and pathophysiologic role of pro- and antiinflammatory cytokines in severe malaria. *J. Infect. Dis.* 180:1288–97

127. Deininger MH, Kremsner PG, Meyermann R, Schluesener HJ. 2000. Differential cellular accumulation of transforming

growth factor-β1, -β2, and -β3 in brains of patients who died with cerebral malaria. *J. Infect. Dis.* 181:2111–15

128. Rest JR. 1982. Cerebral malaria in inbred mice. I. A new model and its pathology. *Trans. R. Soc. Trop. Med. Hyg.* 76:410–15

129. Finley RW, Mackey LJ, Lambert PH. 1982. Virulent *P. berghei* malaria: prolonged survival and decreased cerebral pathology in cell-dependent nude mice. *J. Immunol.* 129:2213–18

130. Nitcheu J, Bonduelle O, Combadiere C, Tefit M, Seilhean D, et al. 2003. Perforin-dependent brain-infiltrating cytotoxic CD8$^+$ T lymphocytes mediate experimental cerebral malaria pathogenesis. *J. Immunol.* 170:2221–28

131. Yanez DM, Manning DD, Cooley AJ, Weidanz WP, van der Heyde HC. 1996. Participation of lymphocyte subpopulations in the pathogenesis of experimental murine cerebral malaria. *J. Immunol.* 157:1620–24

132. Hermsen C, van de Wiel T, Mommers E, Sauerwein R, Eling W. 1997. Depletion of CD4$^+$ or CD8$^+$ T-cells prevents *Plasmodium berghei* induced cerebral malaria in end-stage disease. *Parasitology* 114(Pt. 1):7–12

133. Belnoue E, Kayibanda M, Vigario AM, Deschemin JC, van Rooijen N, et al. 2002. On the pathogenic role of brain-sequestered $\alpha\beta$ CD8$^+$ T cells in experimental cerebral malaria. *J. Immunol.* 169:6369–75

134. Potter S, Chaudhri G, Hansen A, Hunt NH. 1999. Fas and perforin contribute to the pathogenesis of murine cerebral malaria. *Redox Rep.* 4:333–35

135. Jacobs T, Graefe SE, Niknafs S, Gaworski I, Fleischer B. 2002. Murine malaria is exacerbated by CTLA-4 blockade. *J. Immunol.* 169:2323–29

136. Curfs JH, Schetters TP, Hermsen CC, Jerusalem CR, van Zon AA, Eling WM. 1989. Immunological aspects of cerebral lesions in murine malaria. *Clin. Exp. Immunol.* 75:136–40

137. Hermsen CC, Mommers E, van de Wiel T, Sauerwein RW, Eling WM. 1998. Convulsions due to increased permeability of the blood-brain barrier in experimental cerebral malaria can be prevented by splenectomy or anti–T cell treatment. *J. Infect. Dis.* 178:1225–27

138. Van den Eertwegh AJ, Boersma WJ, Claassen E. 1992. Immunological functions and in vivo cell-cell interactions of T cells in the spleen. *Crit. Rev. Immunol.* 11:337–80

139. Jenkins MK, Khoruts A, Ingulli E, Mueller DL, McSorley SJ, et al. 2001. In vivo activation of antigen-specific CD4 T cells. *Annu. Rev. Immunol.* 19:23–45

140. Arase H, Arase N, Ogasawara K, Good RA, Onoc K. 1992. An NK1.1$^+$ CD4$^+$8$^-$ single-positive thymocyte subpopulation that expresses a highly skewed T-cell antigen receptor V$_\beta$ family. *Proc. Natl. Acad. Sci. USA* 89:6506–10

141. Yoshimoto T, Paul WE. 1994. CD4^{pos}, NK1.1^{pos} T cells promptly produce interleukin 4 in response to in vivo challenge with anti-CD3. *J. Exp. Med.* 179:1285–95

142. Schofield L, McConville MJ, Hansen D, Campbell AS, Fraser-Reid B, et al. 1999. CD1d-restricted immunoglobulin G formation to GPI-anchored antigens mediated by NKT cells. *Science* 283:225–29

143. Hansen DS, Siomos MA, Buckingham L, Scalzo AA, Schofield L. 2003. Regulation of murine cerebral malaria pathogenesis by CD1d-restricted NKT cells and the natural killer complex. *Immunity* 18:391–402

144. Schofield L, Hewitt MC, Evans K, Siomos MA, Seeberger PH. 2002. Synthetic GPI as a candidate anti-toxic vaccine in a model of malaria. *Nature* 418:785–89

145. Grau GE, Fajardo LF, Piguet PF, Allet B, Lambert PH, Vassalli P. 1987. Tumor necrosis factor (cachectin) as an essential mediator in murine cerebral malaria. *Science* 237:1210–12

146. Chen L, Zhang Z, Sendo F. 2000.

Neutrophils play a critical role in the pathogenesis of experimental cerebral malaria. *Clin. Exp. Immunol.* 120:125–33

147. Grau GE, Tacchini-Cottier F, Vesin C, Milon G, Lou JN, et al. 1993. TNF-induced microvascular pathology: active role for platelets and importance of the LFA-1/ICAM-1 interaction. *Eur. Cytokine Netw.* 4:415–19

148. Lou J, Donati YR, Juillard P, Giroud C, Vesin C, et al. 1997. Platelets play an important role in TNF-induced microvascular endothelial cell pathology. *Am. J. Pathol.* 151:1397–405

149. Combes V, Rosenkranz AR, Redard M, Pizzolato G, Lepidi H, et al. 2004. Pathogenic role of P-selectin in experimental cerebral malaria: importance of the endothelial compartment. *Am. J. Pathol.* 164:781–86

150. Grau GE, Pointaire P, Piguet PF, Vesin C, Rosen H, et al. 1991. Late administration of monoclonal antibody to leukocyte function-antigen 1 abrogates incipient murine cerebral malaria. *Eur. J. Immunol.* 21:2265–67

151. Medana IM, Hunt NH, Chan-Ling T. 1997. Early activation of microglia in the pathogenesis of fatal murine cerebral malaria. *Glia* 19:91–103

152. Medana IM, Hunt NH, Chaudhri G. 1997. Tumor necrosis factor-alpha expression in the brain during fatal murine cerebral malaria: evidence for production by microglia and astrocytes. *Am. J. Pathol.* 150:1473–86

153. Hermsen CC, Crommert JV, Fredix H, Sauerwein RW, Eling WM. 1997. Circulating tumour necrosis factor alpha is not involved in the development of cerebral malaria in *Plasmodium berghei*–infected C57Bl mice. *Parasite Immunol.* 19:571–77

154. Engwerda CR, Mynott TL, Sawhney S, De Souza JB, Bickle QD, Kaye PM. 2002. Locally up-regulated lymphotoxin α, not systemic tumor necrosis factor α, is the principle mediator of murine cerebral malaria. *J. Exp. Med.* 195:1371–77

155. Grau GE, Heremans H, Piguet PF, Pointaire P, Lambert PH, et al. 1989. Monoclonal antibody against interferon γ can prevent experimental cerebral malaria and its associated overproduction of tumor necrosis factor. *Proc. Natl. Acad. Sci. USA* 86:5572–74

156. Amani V, Vigario AM, Belnoue E, Marussig M, Fonseca L, Mazier D, Renia L. 2000. Involvement of IFN-γ receptor-mediated signaling in pathology and antimalarial immunity induced by *Plasmodium berghei* infection. *Eur. J. Immunol.* 30:1646–55

157. Lucas R, Juillard P, Decoster E, Redard M, Burger D, et al. 1997. Crucial role of tumor necrosis factor (TNF) receptor 2 and membrane-bound TNF in experimental cerebral malaria. *Eur. J. Immunol.* 27:1719–25

158. Sexton AC, Good RT, Hansen DS, D'Ombrain MC, Buckingham L, et al. 2004. Transcriptional profiling reveals suppressed erythropoiesis, up-regulated glycolysis, and interferon-associated responses in murine malaria. *J. Infect. Dis.* 189:1245–56

159. Kossodo S, Monso C, Juillard P, Velu T, Goldman M, Grau GE. 1997. Interleukin-10 modulates susceptibility in experimental cerebral malaria. *Immunology* 91:536–40

160. Belnoue E, Kayibanda M, Deschemin JC, Viguier M, Mack M, et al. 2003. CCR5 deficiency decreases susceptibility to experimental cerebral malaria. *Blood* 101:4253–59

161. Nagel RL. 2002. Malarial anemia. *Hemoglobin* 26:329–43

162. Price RN, Simpson JA, Nosten F, Luxemburger C, Hkirjaroen L, et al. 2001. Factors contributing to anemia after uncomplicated falciparum malaria. *Am. J. Trop. Med. Hyg.* 65:614–22

163. Looareesuwan S, Ho M, Wattanagoon

Y, White NJ, Warrell DA, et al. 1987. Dynamic alteration in splenic function during acute falciparum malaria. *N. Engl. J. Med.* 317:675–79

164. Stoute JA, Odindo AO, Owuor BO, Mibei EK, Opollo MO, Waitumbi JN. 2003. Loss of red blood cell-complement regulatory proteins and increased levels of circulating immune complexes are associated with severe malarial anemia. *J. Infect. Dis.* 187:522–25

165. Abdalla SH, Wickramasinghe SN. 1988. A study of erythroid progenitor cells in the bone marrow of Gambian children with falciparum malaria. *Clin. Lab. Haematol.* 10:33–40

166. Villeval JL, Lew A, Metcalf D. 1990. Changes in hemopoietic and regulator levels in mice during fatal or nonfatal malarial infections. I. Erythropoietic populations. *Exp. Parasitol.* 71:364–74

167. Clark IA, Chaudhri G. 1988. Tumour necrosis factor may contribute to the anaemia of malaria by causing dyscry-thropoiesis and erythrophagocytosis. *Br. J. Haematol.* 70:99–103

168. Yap GS, Stevenson MM. 1992. *Plasmodium chabaudi* AS: erythropoietic responses during infection in resistant and susceptible mice. *Exp. Parasitol.* 75:340–52

169. Shaffer N, Grau GE, Hedberg K, Davachi F, Lyamba B, et al. 1991. Tumor necrosis factor and severe malaria. *J. Infect. Dis.* 163:96–101

170. Nyakundi JN, Warn P, Newton C, Mumo J, Jephthah-Ochola J. 1994. Serum tumour necrosis factor in children suffering from *Plasmodium falciparum* infection in Kilifi District, Kenya. *Trans. R. Soc. Trop. Med. Hyg.* 88:667–70

171. Marsh K, English M, Crawley J, Peshu N. 1996. The pathogenesis of severe malaria in African children. *Ann. Trop. Med. Parasitol.* 90:395–402

172. White NJ. 1986. Pathophysiology. *Clin. Trop. Med. Commun. Dis.* 1:55–90

173. Ware LB, Matthay MA. 2000. The acute respiratory distress syndrome. *N. Engl. J. Med.* 342:1334–49

174. Krishna S, Waller DW, ter Kuile F, Kwiatkowski D, Crawley J, et al. 1994. Lactic acidosis and hypoglycaemia in children with severe malaria: pathophysiological and prognostic significance. *Trans. R. Soc. Trop. Med. Hyg.* 88:67–73

175. Taylor TE, Borgstein A, Molyneux ME. 1993. Acid-base status in paediatric *Plasmodium falciparum* malaria. *Q. J. Med.* 86:99–109

176. English M, Waruiru C, Amukoye E, Murphy S, Crawley J, et al. 1996. Deep breathing in children with severe malaria: indicator of metabolic acidosis and poor outcome. *Am. J. Trop. Med. Hyg.* 55:521–24

177. Jensen MD, Conley M, Helstowski LD. 1983. Culture of *Plasmodium falciparum*: the role of pH, glucose, and lactate. *J. Parasitol.* 69:1060–67

178. Molyneux ME, Looareesuwan S, Menzies IS, Grainger SL, Phillips RE, et al. 1989. Reduced hepatic blood flow and intestinal malabsorption in severe falciparum malaria. *Am. J. Trop. Med. Hyg.* 40:470–76

179. Clark IA, Rockett KA. 1994. The cytokine theory of human cerebral malaria. *Parasitol. Today* 10:410–12

180. Brewster DR, Kwiatkowski D, White NJ. 1990. Neurological sequelae of cerebral malaria in children. *Lancet* 336:1039–43

181. Miller LH, Howard RJ, Carter R, Good MF, Nussenzweig V, Nussenzweig RS. 1986. Research toward malaria vaccines. *Science* 234:1349–56

Annu. Rev. Immunol. 2005. 23:101–25
doi: 10.1146/annurev.immunol.23.021704.115625
Copyright © 2005 by Annual Reviews. All rights reserved
First published online as a Review in Advance on October 19, 2004

THE T CELL RECEPTOR: Critical Role of the Membrane Environment in Receptor Assembly and Function

Matthew E. Call and Kai W. Wucherpfennig

*Department of Cancer Immunology and AIDS, Dana-Farber Cancer Institute and Harvard Medical School, Boston, Massachusetts 02115;
email: kai_wucherpfennig@dfci.harvard.edu*

Key Word   antigen receptor, membrane protein oligomerization, lipid bilayer, signaling

■ **Abstract**   Recent studies have demonstrated that cell membranes provide a unique environment for protein-protein and protein-lipid interactions that are critical for the assembly and function of the T cell receptor (TCR)-CD3 complex. Highly specific polar interactions among transmembrane (TM) domains that are uniquely favorable in the lipid environment organize the association of the three signaling dimers with the TCR. Each of these three assembly steps depends on the formation of a three-helix interface between one basic and two acidic residues in the membrane environment. The same polar TM residues that drive assembly also play a central role in quality control and export by directing the retention and degradation of free subunits and partial complexes, while membrane proximal cytoplasmic signals control recycling and degradation of surface receptors. Recent studies also suggest that interactions between the membrane and the cytoplasmic domains of CD3 proteins may be important for receptor triggering.

INTRODUCTION

The T cell antigen receptor (TCR) delivers signals that are crucial at distinct stages of T cell development in the thymus, as well as for the activation and differentiation of mature T cells into effector and memory cells in the periphery. Although biophysical and biochemical studies have provided a wealth of information on the structure and function of the extracellular domains (1–6) and the intracellular signaling pathways initiated by receptor activation (7–10), some of the questions that are most important for a complete understanding of the TCR remain unanswered: What are the molecular mechanisms governing the assembly of this complex membrane receptor? What is the composition and structure of the complete multichain receptor? How does ligand binding by the extracellular domains result in receptor triggering? This review discusses recent work that has provided a new perspective on these issues through experimental approaches that consider the unique environment

0732-0582/05/0423-0101$14.00   **101** provided by the biological lipid bilayer. These studies have delineated specific protein-protein and protein-lipid interactions occurring within the membrane that are important for receptor assembly and function.

The T cell receptor was first molecularly defined by exploiting the differences in gene expression profiles between T and B lymphocytes (11, 12). The TCRα and TCRβ proteins encoded by these genes were shown to form a disulfide-linked heterodimer that is responsible for ligand recognition because transfection of TCRα and TCRβ cDNAs was sufficient to transfer the MHC-peptide specificity of one T cell to another (13, 14). A small subset of T cells was subsequently found to express a second type of antigen receptor composed of the TCRγ and TCRδ chains (15). The TCRδ chain has greater sequence homology to TCRα, whereas the TCRγ chain is more closely related to TCRβ (16, 17). During T cell development in the thymus, a third type of TCR is expressed in which the TCRβ chain is paired with the pTα chain that serves as a surrogate for TCRα at an early stage of thymocyte development before rearrangement at the TCRα locus (Figure 1b) (18). pTα differs from TCRα in that it has only a single extracellular Ig-domain and a larger cytoplasmic domain (19), features that are relevant for signaling via the pre-TCR (20, 21).

Experiments using antibodies raised against the receptor resulted in the identification of four distinct polypeptides that were noncovalently associated with the TCR heterodimer: the CD3γ, CD3δ, and CD3ε chains and the disulfide-linked homodimer of the ζ chain (22–27) (Figure 1a). Although the TCRα and TCRβ chains have very short cytoplasmic domains, the associated proteins all bear cytoplasmic tails with conserved tyrosine-based motifs that are phosphorylated upon receptor triggering and recruit a complex set of intracellular signaling molecules (28–30; reviewed in 7, 8, 10). Simultaneous transfection of cDNAs encoding all six proteins into non-T cells permitted surface expression of the receptor complex (31, 32), while the absence of any one subunit resulted in a loss of surface expression, as is also observed in T cells (24, 33–35). The TCR$\alpha\beta$, CD3$\gamma\delta\varepsilon$, and ζ chains are thus necessary and sufficient for surface expression in the absence of any other T cell–specific proteins.

VALENCY AND STOICHIOMETRY OF THE TCR-CD3 COMPLEX

The complexity of the receptor made a definitive assessment of its structure and composition a challenging task. Two related but distinct problems had to be addressed to resolve this issue: the valency (the number of ligand-binding TCR heterodimers per complex) and the stoichiometry of the complex (the molar ratios among the subunits). The first major advance in determining the subunit stoichiometry was the finding that each complex contained at least two CD3ε chains. Two groups came to this conclusion by examining T cell hybridomas (36) and primary T cells from transgenic mice (36, 37) that expressed both murine and

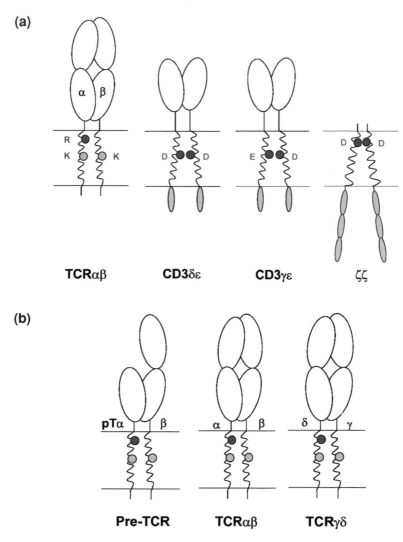

Figure 1   Ionizable residues located in the TM domains of the TCRαβ heterodimer and the CD3δε, CD3γε, and ζζ signaling dimers. (*a*) Three basic residues are located in the TM domains of the TCR heterodimer, and a pair of acidic residues is located in each of the three signaling dimers. The lysine residues in the TM of TCRα and β are positioned near the center of the predicted TM domains, like the pairs of acidic TM residues in CD3δε and CD3γε. The TM arginine of TCRα and the aspartic acid pair of the ζζ dimer are located in the N-terminal third of the respective TM domains. (*b*) The three basic TM residues are fully conserved in all TCR forms: the pre-TCR, TCRαβ, and TCRγδ.

human forms of the CD3ε chain. Using monoclonal antibodies specific for either murine or human CD3ε proteins, both forms were found to be present in the same receptor complex at the cell surface on the basis of coimmunoprecipitation and fluorescence resonance energy transfer (FRET) experiments. Transfection experiments in non–T cells demonstrated that CD3ε could form a stable heterodimer with either CD3γ or CD3δ, but that CD3γ and CD3δ proteins did not directly interact (32). The CD3 proteins therefore appeared to participate in the assembly of the TCR-CD3 complex in the form of two different heterodimers, CD3$\delta\varepsilon$ and CD3$\gamma\varepsilon$ (Figure 1a).

One of the most striking features of the TCR-CD3 subunits is the presence of three basic residues in the transmembrane (TM) regions of the TCR$\alpha\beta$ heterodimer, and of two acidic residues in each of the three different signaling dimers (Figure 1a). These potentially charged TM residues were proposed to drive the associations between TCR and CD3 components by forming pairwise ionic interactions similar to salt bridges commonly observed in soluble proteins (38, 39). Because six acidic residues are present in the TM domains of these signaling dimers (CD3$\delta\varepsilon$, CD3$\gamma\varepsilon$, $\zeta\zeta$), assembly of a TCR heterodimer with a single copy of each would result in a receptor complex with three basic and six acidic TM residues. This potential charge imbalance could be reconciled by postulating the existence of as yet undiscovered subunits bearing additional basic TM residues, or by proposing models in which the CD3 components associate with more than one TCR heterodimer within a single TCR-CD3 complex. The latter model carries with it the possibility that receptor triggering could occur via a conformational change within a preformed TCR dimer or multimer, as recently described for EpoR (40, 41) and other cytokine and hormone receptors (42, 43). On the basis of these considerations, investigators proposed two major groups of TCR-CD3 models, the first model holding that there is a single TCR heterodimer and one copy of each of the three signaling dimers per complex (32, 44–46), and the second set of models proposing that two or more TCR heterodimers are present per complex (47–50).

The simplest multivalent model consists of two TCR heterodimers and one copy of each of the three signaling dimers (Figure 2b). Two groups tested this model directly by analyzing T cells expressing two different TCR heterodimers or two distinct TCRβ chains. Singer and colleagues (44) crossed two TCR transgenic mouse strains expressing distinct receptors to obtain mice whose T cells expressed two TCRα and two TCRβ chains. These four TCR polypeptides could be distinguished on two-dimensional gels following deglycosylation. Immunoprecipitation of surface-expressed receptors labeled with [^{125}I] showed that an antibody to one TCRα chain did not coprecipitate the second TCRα chain, and the same result was obtained using antibodies to either TCRβ chain. The authors therefore concluded that the receptor complex contained only a single TCR heterodimer. However, using a similar experimental approach, de la Hera and colleagues (47) came to the opposite conclusion. This group analyzed T cells that expressed two different TCRβ chains with distinct Vβ sequences by immunoprecipitation with one Vβ chain antibody, followed by Western blotting with the second Vβ specificity.

(a)   Monovalent αβ TCR Model

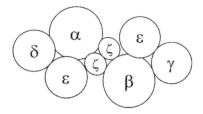

(b)   Bivalent αβ TCR Model

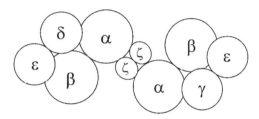

Figure 2   Monovalent and multivalent models of the TCR-CD3 complex. Shown here are two representative models of the TCR-CD3 complex that differ by the number of TCR heterodimers and the placement of the signaling dimers within the complex. The monovalent model was proposed by Punt et al. (44); the multivalent model was proposed by Fernandez-Miguel et al. (47).

They observed coprecipitation of the two TCRβ chains, but the T cells had not been surface-labeled prior to lysis, and this approach therefore did not distinguish intact surface-expressed complexes from assembly intermediates and potentially misfolded side products originating from intracellular compartments. Also, the major fraction of the coprecipitated β chain was not part of a disulfide-linked TCR heterodimer, and it was not established whether the complex containing the two TCRβ chains also contained any of the other subunits.

Exley et al. (50) proposed that the surface-expressed receptor has a multivalent structure, and they attempted to measure the molecular mass of detergent-solubilized TCR-CD3 complexes directly from surface-labeled cells by fractionation on sucrose gradients. Extracts from cells solubilized with low concentrations of nonionic detergents (0.2% digitonin with 0.04% Triton X-100) exhibited two broad, overlapping TCR-CD3 peaks, one of which was estimated to have a higher molecular weight than predicted for a monovalent TCR-CD3 complex. It is difficult, however, to exclude the presence of partially solubilized complexes and aggregates of membrane proteins under such conditions.

With conflicting reports supporting two different types of mutually exclusive TCR-CD3 models, the valency of the receptor remained controversial. An experimental approach was required that would allow the isolation of TCR-CD3 complexes in which all subunits were fully represented so that the number of TCR heterodimers per complex and the stoichiometric relationship among all subunits could be defined. Call et al. (46) designed a strategy to isolate intact radiolabeled TCR-CD3 complexes using a sequential nondenaturing immunoprecipitation (snIP) procedure based on specialized affinity tags that permitted elution under nondenaturing conditions. Proteins carrying the streptavidin (SA)-binding peptide (SBP; 46, 51) were specifically captured using SA and eluted by competition with free biotin under conditions that preserved the noncovalent interactions among receptor components. Subsequent capture of the eluted proteins with an antibody directed against a second tag attached to another subunit within the complex thus permitted isolation of only those complexes that contained both affinity tags as well as all associated proteins. These experiments were performed in an in vitro translation system (52–57) with endoplasmic reticulum (ER) microsomes from B cells, which are closely related to T cells but do not express any component of the TCR-CD3 complex (46). When the SBP and hemagglutinin (HA)-peptide tags were placed on CD3ε chains, or on the TCRβ and ζ chains, the snIP procedure resulted in recovery of intact radiolabeled complexes containing all subunits, validating the utility of the approach and confirming the incorporation of at least two CD3ε chains per complex (46).

The multivalent TCR-CD3 models were directly tested by performing the snIP analysis on reactions in which two copies of the TCRβ chain were equipped with SBP and HA tags. No radiolabeled proteins were recovered with this procedure (46), and the same result was obtained when the tags were placed on TCRα chains. The results were confirmed with a second human TCR$\alpha\beta$ and replacement of the second-step affinity tag (58). Because the SBP and HA affinity tags differ substantially in length, the two different TCR$\alpha\beta$ heterodimers formed in an assembly reaction containing both TCRβ chains were also clearly distinguishable by molecular weight under nonreducing conditions. Both TCRβ chains assembled equally well with TCRα, CD3, and ζ chains, but they were not coprecipitated in single-step immunoprecipitation experiments using antibodies to the first or the second tag. A similar analysis of TCR-CD3 complexes assembled in T cell–derived ER microsomes demonstrated that the presence of T cell–specific ER proteins did not change the outcome of the experiment.

Researchers had never made direct measurements of the stoichiometric relationships among all the TCR-CD3 components within a complex because of two fundamental problems: Any method of isolation targeting a single subunit would inevitably result in over-representation of that component relative to the others; and uniform radiolabeling of proteins in T cells could not be reliably achieved because the half-lives of the individual polypeptides vary widely. Over-representation of individual subunits was prevented with the snIP procedure by targeting both the TCRβ chain and the ζ protein, which is known to be the final component to join the complex. Direct measurements of the densitometric ratios among the components of fully assembled TCR-CD3 complexes isolated in this manner indicated a ratio of one TCR$\alpha\beta$ heterodimer, one $\zeta\zeta$ homodimer, two CD3ε chains, and one copy each of CD3γ and CD3δ (58). Analysis of key assembly intermediates lacking the ζ or CD3γ chains demonstrated that the stepwise association of a single TCR$\alpha\beta$ heterodimer with CD3$\delta\varepsilon$, CD3$\gamma\varepsilon$, and $\zeta\zeta$ dimers resulted in a monovalent TCR-CD3 structure, and this analysis also confirmed that the assembly process observed in the in vitro translation system was consistent with observations made in cellular systems (24, 45, 59).

PROTEIN INTERACTIONS IN THE MEMBRANE ENVIRONMENT IN THE ASSEMBLY OF THE TCR-CD3 COMPLEX

If a single TCR$\alpha\beta$ heterodimer assembles with all three signaling dimers within a TCR-CD3 complex, how do the three basic and six acidic TM residues participate in assembly and surface expression of the receptor? Using mutant T cells lacking TCRβ protein and therefore deficient in surface TCR expression, Morley et al. (60) and Alcover et al. (61) observed that surface TCR expression could be restored by transfection of the wild-type TCRβ chain, but not by transfection of a TCRβ chain with a mutation of the conserved lysine in the predicted TM domain. Blumberg et al. (62) used a TCRα-deficient T cell mutant to perform similar experiments and found that at least one of the two basic residues in the TCRα TM domain was required for surface TCR expression, but it appeared that either the lysine or the arginine was sufficient. The acidic residues in the signaling chains were also important, as mutation of these residues in CD3γ (63) or the ζ chain (64) resulted in a loss of TCR surface expression.

Klausner and colleagues (39) proposed that one-to-one pairing of basic and acidic residues leads to assembly of TCR and CD3 chains. When pairs of TCR and CD3 chains were transfected into COS cells, associations between TCRα and CD3δ or CD3ε were observed, as were interactions between TCRβ and CD3γ, CD3δ, or CD3ε (32, 39). The TM domain of TCRα alone was found to interact with CD3δ, even when fused to the ectodomain of CD4 (38) or Tac (CD25) (38, 39). Using such a Tac/α chimeric protein, Cosson et al. (39) observed an interaction between TCRα and CD3δ that involved the basic and acidic residues of the TM domains. Either the arginine at position five or the lysine at position ten in the TCRα TM domain was sufficient for association with CD3δ, but the interaction was lost when both basic residues or the CD3δ aspartic acid were mutated. When the basic and acidic residues were moved to different positions within their respective TM sequence, the association was maintained as long as the two remained at similar positions along the TM domain relative to one another and to the membrane (39). Formation of charge pairs therefore appeared to be responsible for the interaction between these two proteins, but how such a mechanism could achieve specificity in assembling the entire receptor was not evident. This model also failed to explain how the six acidic TM residues of CD3$\delta\varepsilon$, CD3$\gamma\varepsilon$ and $\zeta\zeta$ would interact with the three basic TM residues of the TCR.

Although the pairwise transfection experiments in non–T cells demonstrated that pairing of basic and acidic TM residues could result in an association between two polypeptides, the simplest assembly intermediates that were actually observed in T cells consisted of single TCR chains or a TCR$\alpha\beta$ dimer associated with a CD3$\gamma\varepsilon$ or CD3$\delta\varepsilon$ dimer (45). It was therefore not clear whether one-to-one TCR-CD3 interactions were relevant to the natural receptor assembly process. Definition of the interactions that result in the formation of this complex receptor structure thus required an approach in which the structural requirements for assembly could be systematically examined. Taking advantage of the fact that mutations in any or all subunits can be studied using the in vitro TCR-CD3 assembly system, Call et al. (46) examined the function of the three basic TCR TM residues in the context of physiologically relevant assembly intermediates. A complex of the CD3$\delta\varepsilon$ heterodimer with TCRα or with the TCR$\alpha\beta$ heterodimer has been observed as a very early intermediate in developing thymocytes (45). Examining the requirements for CD3$\delta\varepsilon$ assembly with TCR$\alpha\beta$, Call et al. (46) observed that mutations at the lysine residue in the TCRα TM sequence resulted in loss of CD3$\delta\varepsilon$ association, but that mutation of the other two basic residues had no effect. This interaction involved three chains because the TCRα-CD3$\delta\varepsilon$ complex was formed with equal efficiency in the absence of TCRβ or other receptor components and required only the TM domain of TCRα. A precise role could also be assigned to the other lysine located in the TM domain of TCRβ because mutation of this TM residue caused specific loss of CD3$\gamma\varepsilon$ but did not affect association of CD3$\delta\varepsilon$. Mutation of the arginine residue at position five in the TCRα TM domain had no effect on association of CD3$\delta\varepsilon$ or CD3$\gamma\varepsilon$, but it did cause specific loss of $\zeta\zeta$ association. Therefore, in a context in which all subunits were available, the three basic TM residues exhibited very specific and nonredundant roles in assembly (Figure 3).

These results clearly demonstrate that assembly of each of the three signaling dimers requires a single basic TM residue of the TCR and raise the question of whether one or both acidic residues of a given signaling dimer are essential for the creation of the proper protein-protein interface in the membrane. Alanine substitutions of the TM aspartic acid in either CD3δ or CD3ε resulted in a loss of TCRα association, indicating that this three-chain interaction requires the TM lysine of TCRα as well as both acidic TM residues of CD3$\delta\varepsilon$. Consistent with this model, conservative substitution of either aspartic acid to asparagine reduced association with TCRα by 70%–80% relative to wild-type, indicating that the two aspartic acids make similar contributions to assembly with TCRα. TCRα-CD3$\delta\varepsilon$ assembly requires a very specific steric arrangement among these three residues because exchanging the basic and acidic residues among the three TM regions, even while maintaining one lysine and two aspartic acids, was not tolerated. This assembly step is thus driven by an unusual interaction among one basic and two acidic residues located in the center of the TM domains within the

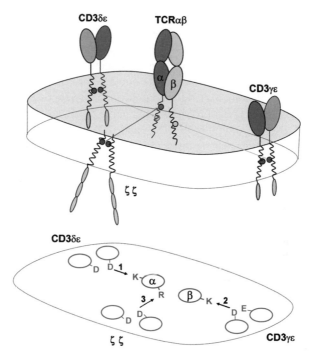

Figure 3   Organization of TCR-CD3 assembly based on the interaction of ionizable TM residues. Site-directed mutagenesis experiments demonstrated that each basic TCR TM residue serves a distinct role in the assembly process and provides an interaction site for one of the three signaling dimers (CD3$\delta\varepsilon$, CD3$\gamma\varepsilon$, $\zeta\zeta$). Each assembly step results in the formation of a three-helix interface in the membrane involving one basic TCR TM residue (*blue*) and a pair of acidic TM residues (*red*) from the interacting signaling dimer. Formation of the correct receptor structure thus requires proper placement of all nine basic/acidic TM residues.

lipid bilayer. Further experiments demonstrated that this surprising arrangement extends to the association of CD3$\gamma\varepsilon$ and $\zeta\zeta$ because each assembly step required both acidic residues in the signaling dimer but only one particular basic residue of the TCR. The formation of the complete TCR-CD3 complex is thus dependent on the specific coordination of nine ionizable residues within the lipid bilayer, and mutation of any one of these residues to alanine abrogates formation of the TCR-CD3 complex.

The three basic TCR TM residues are conserved in all TCR forms ($\alpha\beta$, $\gamma\delta$, and pre-TCR) and across species, suggesting that assembly of all TCRs is based on the same principal mechanism. Interestingly, although the assembly and surface expression of the $\alpha\beta$ TCR-CD3 complex absolutely requires all six polypeptides, the requirements for CD3 subunits appear to be somewhat different for $\gamma\delta$ TCR and pre-TCR assembly. In mice that lack expression of CD3δ, production of mature

$\alpha\beta$ T cells was predictably blocked owing to lack of surface TCR expression (35). However, early stages of thymic development depending on pre-TCR expression were normal, and development of mature $\gamma\delta$ T cells was unaffected. Conversely, CD3γ deficiency in mice resulted in a complete block of development in all T cell lineages (34). The differences in the outcome of CD3δ or CD3γ deficiency for $\alpha\beta$ versus $\gamma\delta$ T cells may reflect significant differences in the subunit composition of these two types of receptor. Brenner and colleagues (65) found that human $\gamma\delta$ TCR assembled with both CD3γ and CD3δ, as in $\alpha\beta$ T cells, but that CD3δ oligosaccharide processing differed in the two types of cells. However, Love and colleagues (66) reported that the TCR-CD3 complex on the surface of primary mouse $\gamma\delta$ T cells contained little or no CD3δ compared with that in $\alpha\beta$ T cells examined in parallel, despite the presence of abundant quantities of free CD3δ protein and CD3$\delta\varepsilon$ heterodimers in intracellular compartments. If the $\gamma\delta$ TCR-CD3 complex does not include the CD3$\delta\varepsilon$ heterodimer, then the TCRδ chain (which is homologous to TCRα) may instead assemble with CD3$\gamma\varepsilon$ and the $\gamma\delta$ TCR-CD3 complex may thus contain two copies of CD3$\gamma\varepsilon$ rather than one copy of each CD3$\gamma\varepsilon$ and CD3$\delta\varepsilon$. A similar arrangement may apply to the pre-TCR in CD3δ-deficient mice, but these notions have yet to be directly tested.

GENERAL SIGNIFICANCE OF ASSEMBLY MECHANISM

A wider significance of this receptor assembly mechanism is suggested by the presence of three other signaling dimers in different cell types of hematopoietic origin: FcRγ (67), DAP12 (68) and DAP10 (69–71). These three signaling dimers are similar to the ζ chain in that they carry acidic residues within the predicted TM portion of the molecule, a cytoplasmic domain with a tyrosine-based phosphorylation motif and only a short extracellular domain. The receptors with which they associate carry similarly situated basic TM residues, raising the possibility that the three-helix arrangement described above for the TCR also guides the assembly process for these receptor systems. The signaling protein DAP12 associates with several distinct activating natural killer (NK) cell receptors, including KIR2DS and NKG2C/CD94 (72–74). Preliminary mutagenesis studies indicate that for both KIR2DS and NKG2C, assembly with DAP12 is based on the creation of a three-helix interface in the membrane involving one basic and two acidic residues (J. Feng, D. Garrity & K.W. Wucherpfennig, unpublished data). Assembly based on the same mechanism is particularly significant considering that KIR2DS and NKG2C share no primary sequence homology, belong to different structural families, and adopt different TM topologies, since KIR2DS is a type I membrane protein while NKG2C is a type II membrane protein. The fact that such evolutionarily diverse receptors as KIR2DS and NKG2C share a common structural motif directing assembly with signaling partners suggests that this intramembrane arrangement is particularly advantageous. Assembly based on protein interactions in the membrane does not interfere with the interaction of extracellular domains with ligands or the formation of signaling complexes on phosphorylated cytoplasmic domains following receptor triggering. Given that exposure of three ionizable sidechains to the hydrophobic interior of the lipid bilayer would be energetically unfavorable, the three-helix arrangement may also provide an interaction between the ligand-binding subunit(s) and signaling dimer(s) that is extremely stable.

UNIQUE PROPERTIES OF THE MEMBRANE ENVIRONMENT FOR PROTEIN-PROTEIN INTERACTION

To understand how these interactions within the membrane result in specific assembly of these receptor complexes, one must consider the unique properties of the lipid bilayer environment for protein-protein interactions. Popot & Engelman (75) have published a comprehensive review on this topic containing a detailed discussion of many of the points touched on here. In this review, we consider two major features that dictate which protein-protein interactions arc favorable in the membrane environment: (*a*) The lipid as a solvent for proteins limits the structural diversity of membrane-spanning domains, and (*b*) the chemical composition of the lipid bilayer makes particular protein-protein interactions energetically favorable. These properties serve to explain the structural arrangement observed in the TCR-CD3 complex and other membrane protein complexes.

Cartoon depictions of the lipid bilayer commonly used to delineate cellular and organellar boundaries or to indicate the point of division between extracellular and cytoplasmic domains of membrane proteins are frequently misleading in terms of scale. The cellular membrane spans approximately 60 Å on average and is composed of two distinct regions: The hydrophobic core that is composed of semiordered hydrocarbon chains is approximately 30 Å in thickness and is flanked by the polar headgroup layers, each of which contributes about 15 Å. The hydrophobic interior, often represented as diminutively thin in comparison to the extramembrane domains of embedded proteins, actually corresponds roughly to the height of a single immunoglobulin domain. TM helices thus provide an extended surface for specific protein-protein interactions in an environment in which hydrogen-bonding and electrostatic interactions are much stronger than in the aqueous phase owing to the absence of competing water and ions. For the same reason, electrostatic attraction occurs over wider distances in biological membranes, an aspect that may be important for the assembly of the TCR-CD3 complex (88).

The membrane has been described as a two-dimensional fluid in which mobile lipid and protein molecules move within the plane of the membrane. Because of this organization, protein-protein, protein-lipid, and lipid-lipid interactions occur only laterally. The hydrophobic environment places severe restrictions on the type of secondary structures that can effectively span the bilayer. A linear polypeptide stretch of ∼15–25 amino acid residues bearing sidechains of sufficient average hydrophobicity spontaneously adopts an α-helical conformation in the lipid bilayer for two primary reasons: an α helix satisfies the hydrogen-bonding requirements of the polar backbone carbonyl and amide groups and simultaneously permits energetically favorable contacts between hydrophobic sidechains and the nonpolar solvent (76). Although other structures such as the beta-barrel have been described for proteins with multiple membrane-spanning segments, an α helix is the energetically most favorable structure for an individual TM domain (77, 78). The possible variations in structure are therefore relatively narrow compared with protein domains in an aqueous environment: For an ideal α helix to span the 30 Å hydrophobic interior, approximately 20 amino acids are required, according to the characteristic helical rise of 1.5 Å per residue. Longer hydrophobic stretches can be accommodated by increased helix tilt, but TM helices shorter than 15 residues are rare. The limited diversity in secondary structure and the strength of polar protein-protein interactions in the membrane thus require mechanisms that ensure specificity of assembly. For the TCR-CD3 complex, specificity results from the following features: (a) Formation of the individual TCR, CD3$\gamma\varepsilon$ and CD3$\delta\varepsilon$ heterodimers is based on interaction of the extracellular domains; (b) each higher-order assembly step involves creation of a three-helix rather than a two-helix interface in the membrane between the TCR and the respective signaling dimer; and (c) association of $\zeta\zeta$ requires prior assembly of both CD3$\delta\varepsilon$ and CD3$\gamma\varepsilon$ with TCR.

The membrane environment supports dimerization or multimerization based on polar and nonpolar protein interactions (Figure 4). The best-studied example of dimer formation based on nonpolar TM interactions is the glycophorin A (GpA) dimer. Mutagenesis of the TM region indicated that a motif of seven critical residues, LIxxGVxxGVxxT (Figure 4a), was responsible for the specific dimerization of the TM helices (79, 80). The solution nuclear magnetic resonance structure of the TM homodimer confirmed that these residues participated in close packing interactions at the interface, which contained a high degree of surface complementarity. A critical structural feature was the presence of two glycine residues spaced four residues apart because they allowed close interactions between the two monomers: The sidechains of the two valine residues in the GVxxGV motif formed a ridge that packed against the groove created by the two glycines of the opposing monomer (80a). Subsequent studies revealed that such a GxxxG motif alone can drive oligomerization of model TM α helices (81).

Although polar residues occur at greatly reduced frequencies within TM α helices compared with those in soluble proteins (about 5% versus 22%; Reference 78), they tend to be significantly more conserved than those found in soluble proteins (82). Recent work by two groups examining the effects of polar residues in the context of model TM α helices revealed that a single polar residue bearing a carboxylate (Asp, Glu; see Figure 4c) or carboxamide (Asn, Gln; see Figure 4d) sidechain placed within a generic hydrophobic TM sequence can induce oligomerization (83, 84). The acidic residues (Asp, Glu) in such dimers or trimers may be partially or completely protonated, which would remove the charge-charge repulsion and permit hydrogen-bonding interactions. Nuclear magnetic resonance studies of an asparagine-induced trimer supported the hypothesis that the

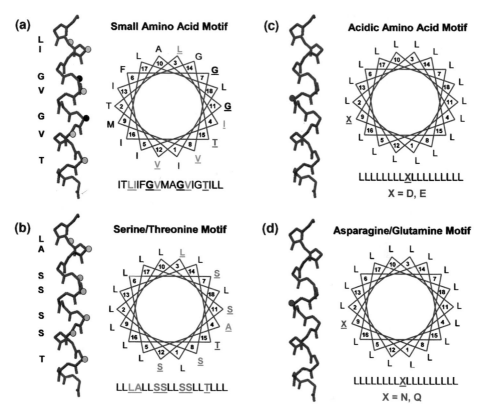

Figure 4 TM helix motifs that support specific protein-protein interactions in the membrane environment. (*a*) The small amino acid motif permits close packing interactions between two TM helices, as exemplified by the glycophorin A (GpA) structure. Polar residues can also support TM helix interactions, as exemplified by the three other motifs. (*b*) The contribution of a single serine/threonine to helix interactions is rather small, but dimerization can result from multiple serine/threonine residues appropriately spaced along TM helices. In contrast, (*c*) carboxyl (aspartic acid/glutamic acid) or (*d*) a single carboxamide (asparagine/glutamine) within a hydrophobic helix can be sufficient to drive formation of SDS-stable homodimers or homotrimers.

polar residues were buried at the trimer interface, where they participated in a hydrogen-bonding network (85). In the hydrophobic environment of the lipid bilayer interior, hydrogen-bonding interactions are expected to be especially favorable and significantly stronger than similar interactions in an aqueous environment owing to the absence of free ions, water molecules, and other polar groups that compete for hydrogen bonds (75). Single serine or threonine residues did not support TM helix oligomerization, possibly because the hydroxyl-containing sidechains of these residues can satisfy their hydrogen-bonding potential locally through intrahelical contacts to the i-3 or i-4 backbone carbonyl oxygen atoms (86). However, searching a library of synthetic TM sequences that was semirandomized at the positions of the seven critical residues in the GpA dimerization interface, Engelman and colleagues (87) found that motifs containing multiple serine and threonine residues were strongly favored to form helix dimers (Figure 4b). Thus, a cooperative network of hydrogen bonds along an extended interface of α helices could support dimer formation in a manner similar to the focused contacts among the more polar sidechains of aspartic acid, glutamic acid, asparagine, or glutamine residues.

The observation that packing of acidic sidechains at a protein interface can induce oligomerization in the membrane is surprising and raises the interesting question of whether the acidic amino acid pairs in the signaling dimers that are critical for TCR-CD3 assembly interact directly with each other before assembling with the third α helix bearing the basic TCR TM residue. Like GpA, formation of the ζ chain homodimer is driven by TM helix contacts (64). The interhelical disulfide bond is predicted to be at the second position of the membrane-spanning portion, and the aspartic acids are located at position six, approximately one turn down an α helix (3.6 residues per turn). The constraint of the interhelical disulfide bond therefore makes it likely that the aspartic acids are located at the $\zeta\zeta$ dimer interface. This conclusion is supported by the observation that substitution of the aspartic acid affects homodimer formation (46, 64). For example, replacement of aspartic acid by asparagine resulted in more efficient dimerization (46). In contrast to the studies on model TM helices discussed above in which the acidic residues were responsible for dimerization, a polar residue at this position was not essential: Although disulfide bond formation was adversely affected when the aspartic acid was mutated to alanine (64), dimer formation was still observed in two-step snIP experiments (M.E. Call, J. Pyrdol & K.W. Wucherpfennig, unpublished data). Interestingly, although changing one or both aspartic acids to asparagine increased disulfide-linked $\zeta\zeta$ dimer formation, these changes reduced association with TCR to 20% and 0%, respectively (46; M.E. Call, J. Pyrdol & K.W. Wucherpfennig, unpublished data). The required interaction partner for the TM arginine of TCRα is therefore likely to be a very specific site formed by the two TM aspartic acids at the interface of the $\zeta\zeta$ homodimer.

Despite the limited structural diversity of TM segments, the TM helix interactions required for TCR-CD3 assembly are thus highly specific, and the requirement for the formation of a three-helix interface contributes a significant degree of discrimination at each assembly step. Although pairwise association of TCRα with CD3δ displayed very loose requirements with respect to positioning of the polar TM residues (39), the requirements for formation of the TCRα-CD3$\delta\varepsilon$ trimer were specific because even minor changes in sidechain structure or sequence context interfered with assembly (46). The three-helix arrangement may also be the most effective structure for shielding the three polar residues from the lipid and may not result in a charge imbalance, depending on the ionization state of the basic and acidic sidechains (46, 88).

ROLE OF POLAR TM RESIDUES IN ER QUALITY CONTROL AND EXPORT

In addition to their critical role in organizing the TCR-CD3 assembly process, the polar TM residues also serve as signals for quality control in the ER. Klausner and colleagues (89, 90) demonstrated that the basic residues in the TCR TM domains promote degradation of TCR chains that fail to assemble. In T cells with mutations or deficiencies in one of the CD3 subunits, TCRα and TCRβ chains are retained in the ER and degraded with rapid kinetics (91–93). The TM sequence of TCRα alone was sufficient to induce ER retention and degradation when fused to the ectodomain of a type I membrane protein that is normally transported to the cell surface (Tac/CD25). This effect was entirely attributable to the presence of the two basic TM residues because replacement of both basic residues by leucine resulted in transport of the Tac/TCRα TM chimera to the cell surface with normal kinetics (90). The same observation was made in similar experiments examining the TCRβ TM sequence. When expressed together, TCRα and TCRβ formed a disulfide-linked heterodimer that was retained and degraded with kinetics similar to the individual chains. Interestingly, coexpression of CD3γε slowed degradation of TCR chains and resulted in the formation of TCR-CD3 complexes with a longer half-life (94). Sequestration of basic residues in the TCR TM domains at protein-protein interfaces therefore masks these degradation signals (Figure 5).

This effect was not unique to the basic TM residues: When individual CD3 proteins were expressed in the absence of other subunits, ER retention and rapid degradation was observed, and introduction of single acidic residues into the Tac TM sequence also caused retention, indicating that exposed basic or acidic residues result in a similar phenotype (90). These Tac chimeras carrying basic or acidic TM residues were properly targeted to the ER because they were glycosylated, but they remained largely susceptible to extraction with alkaline buffers, indicating that they were not stably embedded into the lipid bilayer. This effect was position-dependent and most pronounced when basic or acidic residues were introduced near the center of the TM segment, which corresponds to the placement of the basic and acidic residues involved in assembly of TCR with CD3δε and CD3γε. Interestingly, whereas CD3γ expressed alone was retained and rapidly degraded, coexpression with CD3ε resulted in the formation of stable, long-lived CD3γε heterodimers that resided in the ER (93). The assembly of CD3 heterodimers may therefore partially shield the acidic residues from the hydrophobic interior of the membrane at a protein-protein interface. Full shielding may result only when this dimer assembles with the appropriate TCR TM region.

The observation that both TCR-CD3 assembly as well as degradation of individual chains and partial complexes are dependent on ionizable TM residues can be explained by an assembly model in which the Sec61p channel plays an integral role. The Sec61p channel in the ER is the site of membrane protein integration (95, 96). Experimental evidence indicates that this protein complex allows the TM

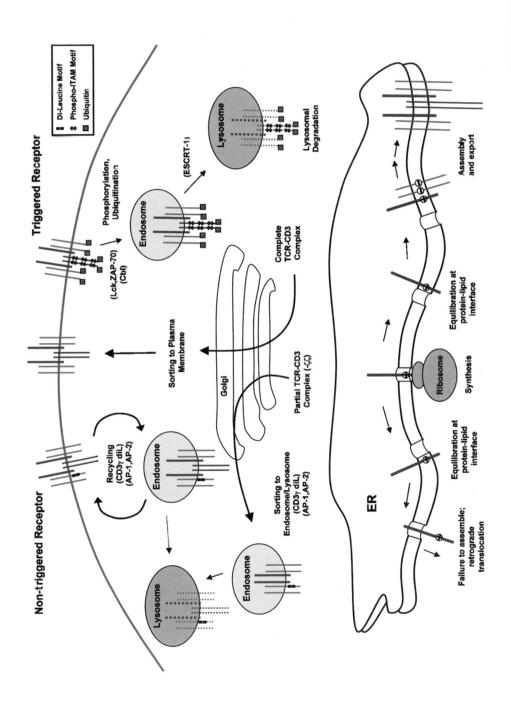

domain of a nascent polypeptide to equilibrate dynamically between the lipid and aqueous phases on the basis of the relative hydrophobicity of its sequence (97, 98). TM domains containing basic or acidic residues may not fully partition into the lipid bilayer but rather may be retained at water-lipid or protein-lipid interfaces in the vicinity of the protein channel. According to this model, only the sequestration of these highly polar residues at protein-protein interfaces by assembly with the appropriate TCR-CD3 subunits could fully shield them from the lipid and result in stable integration into the lipid bilayer. Conversely, polypeptides whose TM domains remain at the interface are subject to retrograde transport through Sec61p or other channel(s) into the cytosol, which is the first step in the degradation of ER proteins in the proteasome (99–102).

The dynamic equilibrium model gains experimental support from studies with a model type I membrane protein whose interaction with the Sec61p channel was studied by introduction of a photoreactive amino acid in the TM domain (98). During translocation of the polypeptide, transient interactions between the TM domain and the Sec61α and Sec61γ proteins were observed, and direct interaction of the TM domain with lipids could be visualized on the basis of lipid crosslinks. When an arginine was introduced into the TM sequence of this protein, ER targeting and glycosylation were normal, but a large fraction of the polypeptide remained alkaline extractable. The mutant exhibited stronger crosslinks to Sec61α and Sec61γ than to the wild-type sequence, and the mutant showed additional crosslinks to a channel-associated protein, the translocating chain-associating membrane (TRAM) protein (98). This effect was even more pronounced when two basic residues were placed into the TM region, but both mutant proteins maintained contact with surrounding lipids because lipid crosslinks were still observed. These observations indicate that although the wild-type protein rapidly exited the channel and became embedded in the lipid bilayer, the mutant proteins were retained at the interface of channel and surrounding lipid. The strong crosslinks to TRAM suggest that this protein may play a role in the retention of insufficiently hydrophobic TM sequences. The Sec61p channel and surrounding protein(s) therefore create an amphipathic environment in which TCR-CD3 components with exposed polar residues may exist

---

Figure 5   Assembly and intracellular targeting of the TCR-CD3 complex. The ionizable TM residues provide a quality control mechanism in the ER because free chains or certain assembly intermediates are retained and rapidly degraded in the proteasome following retrograde transport to the cytosol. Assembly shields the ionizable TM residues at protein-protein interfaces away from the hydrophobic interior of the membrane and permits export to the cell surface. The di-leucine motif in the cytoplasmic tail of CD3γ directs recycling of TCR-CD3 complexes from the cell surface through early endosomes, and it is also responsible for rapid redistribution of TCR-CD3 complexes to the immunological synapse following TCR triggering. Phosphorylated receptors can be ubiquitinated by Cbl and Cbl-b, resulting in sorting by the ESCRT-1 complex and degradation in lysosomes.

in a dynamic equilibrium between hydrophobic and hydrophilic environments until they properly assemble into a structure in which basic and acidic residues are effectively shielded.

TRAFFICKING OF TCR-CD3 COMPLEXES OUTSIDE THE ER

Sequestration of strongly polar TM residues at specific protein-protein interfaces not only results in the specific oligomerization of receptor components, but also serves as a quality control mechanism that leads to export of the correctly assembled structure as well as removal of unassembled receptor components. An ER retention signal in the cytoplasmic domain of CD3ε also contributes to quality control in ER (103), and other signals determine the fate of partial complexes outside the ER. The TCR$\alpha\beta$-CD3$\gamma\varepsilon$-CD3$\delta\varepsilon$ hexamer lacking $\zeta\zeta$ can be exported from the ER, but is sorted from the Golgi complex to the lysosomal pathway for degradation (24). This lysosomal sorting step depends on a di-leucine (di-L: SDxxxLL) motif in the membrane-proximal portion of the CD3γ cytoplasmic tail (104, 105) that is masked by assembly with the ζ chain (106). This motif permits binding of the adaptor proteins AP-1 and AP-2, which direct the formation of clathrin-coated sorting vesicles (107). The CD3γ di-L motif also directs constitutive internalization of TCR-CD3 complexes from the cell surface, the vast majority of which are rapidly recycled to the cell surface from early endosomal compartments (reviewed in 108). Activation of PKC by phorbol ester treatment or TCR ligation increases the rate of internalization and results in a rapid reduction of TCR-CD3 levels at the cell surface. This effect is due to PKC-mediated phosphorylation of a serine residue N-terminal to the aspartic acid residue in the di-L motif, which is thought to induce a conformational change that makes the di-L motif more accessible to the AP-1 and AP-2 complexes (105, 107). The di-L motif also provides a mechanism for rapid redistribution of TCRs following T cell activation because TCRs in transit through recycling endosomes are targeted to the immunological synapse (109).

In addition to the PKC dependent, di-L-mediated redistribution of receptors, T cell activation also induces degradation of triggered receptors (110). Ligand-induced receptor degradation does not depend on the CD3γ di-L motif, but it requires the activity of Lck, ZAP-70, and Cbl (108). The Cbl proteins (Cbl and Cbl-b) have E3 ubiquitin (Ub) ligase activity and transfer Ub molecules to the ε-amino group on lysine residues of target proteins (111). Cbl is one of the molecules recruited to phosphorylated ZAP-70 through its phosphotyrosine-binding SH2 domain (112). Because ZAP-70 binds to the phosphorylated immunoreceptor tyrosine-based activation motifs (ITAM) of triggered TCR-CD3 complexes, Cbl is locally available to ubiquitinate the CD3 and ζ cytoplasmic tails. Ubiquitination results in sorting of these complexes to lysosomes through recognition by Tsg101, a component of the endosomal sorting complex ESCRT-1 (113). These signals thus direct the trafficking, cycling, and degradation of receptor complexes, while the ionizable TM residues provide a quality control mechanism in the ER that distinguishes between correctly assembled complexes and assembly intermediates.

PROTEIN-LIPID INTERACTIONS AND TCR TRIGGERING

Structural and functional studies of membrane proteins still present a significant challenge because most techniques designed for studying protein-protein interactions have been developed for soluble proteins. Many of the studies that form the basis of our current understanding of the structure and function of the TCR have necessarily relied on the use of engineered protein fragments lacking the membrane-embedded domains. As discussed above, the TM domains of the TCR-CD3 components contain critical signals that direct the proper assembly and intracellular processing of the receptor. There is also evidence that interactions between the cytoplasmic domains of the signaling components and the plasma membrane may play an important role in TCR activation. Although the cytoplasmic domain of the ζ chain appears to be unstructured in aqueous solution, a recombinant ζ_{cyt} peptide exhibited a far-ultraviolet circular dichroism spectrum characteristic of α helical structures in the presence of lipid vesicles (114). Adoption of a helical conformation specifically depended on the presence of lipids with acidic head groups, which are naturally enriched in the inner leaflet of the plasma membrane. These in vitro studies may reflect a natural interaction between the ζ_{cyt} sequence and the cytoplasmic face of the plasma membrane. Interestingly, the α helical, lipid-bound conformation was resistant to tyrosine phosphorylation by Lck, whereas phosphorylation of the ζ_{cyt} peptide resulted in a loss of lipid binding. Stern and colleagues (114) therefore proposed a model of TCR-CD3 activation in which the cytoplasmic tail of the ζ chain is reversibly bound to the inner leaflet of the plasma membrane in an α helical conformation that sequesters the ITAM phosphorylation sites from Src kinases. Dislodging of the cytoplasmic domains from the membrane by ligand-induced receptor clustering could thus permit receptor phosphorylation and trigger the subsequent cascade of signaling events.

In summary, the studies discussed in this review establish the great importance of the membrane environment for the assembly and transport of TCR-CD3 complexes based on signals contained within the membrane-spanning and membrane-proximal domains. Experiments with the cytoplasmic domain of the ζ chain further suggest that direct interactions with the inner leaflet of the plasma membrane could be relevant for TCR signaling. The membrane environment must therefore be considered as a key element for the assembly, targeting, and function of this important receptor.

The *Annual Review of Immunology* is online at
http://immunol.annualreviews.org

LITERATURE CITED

1. Garcia KC, Degano M, Stanfield RL, Brunmark A, Jackson MR, et al. 1996. An $\alpha\beta$ T cell receptor structure at 2.5 Å and its orientation in the TCR-MHC complex. *Science* 274:209–19

2. Garboczi DN, Ghosh P, Utz U, Fan QR, Biddison WE, Wiley DC. 1996. Structure of the complex between human T-cell receptor, viral peptide and HLA-A2. *Nature* 384:134–41

3. Garcia KC, Teyton L, Wilson IA. 1999. Structural basis of T cell recognition. *Annu. Rev. Immunol.* 17:369–97

4. Davis MM, Krogsgaard M, Huppa JB, Sumen C, Purbhoo MA, et al. 2003. Dynamics of cell surface molecules during T cell recognition. *Annu. Rev. Biochem.* 72:717–42

5. Sun ZJ, Kim KS, Wagner G, Reinherz EL. 2001. Mechanisms contributing to T cell receptor signaling and assembly revealed by the solution structure of an ectodomain fragment of the CD3$\varepsilon\gamma$ heterodimer. *Cell* 105:913–23

6. Kjer-Nielsen L, Dunstone MA, Kostenko L, Ely LK, Beddoe T, et al. 2004. Crystal structure of the human T cell receptor CD3$\varepsilon\gamma$ heterodimer complexed to the therapeutic mAb OKT3. *Proc. Natl. Acad. Sci. USA* 101:7675–80

7. Weiss A, Littman DR. 1994. Signal transduction by lymphocyte antigen receptors. *Cell* 76:263–74

8. Cantrell DA. 1996. T cell antigen receptor signal transduction pathways. *Cancer Surv.* 27:165–75

9. Germain RN, Stefanova I. 1999. The dynamics of T cell receptor signaling: complex orchestration and the key roles of tempo and cooperation. *Annu. Rev. Immunol.* 17:467–522

10. Samelson LE. 2002. Signal transduction mediated by the T cell antigen receptor: the role of adapter proteins. *Annu. Rev. Immunol.* 20:371–94

11. Hedrick SM, Cohen DI, Nielsen EA, Davis MM. 1984. Isolation of cDNA clones encoding T cell-specific membrane-associated proteins. *Nature* 308:149–53

12. Yanagi Y, Yoshikai Y, Leggett K, Clark SP, Aleksander I, Mak TW. 1984. A human T cell-specific cDNA clone encodes a protein having extensive homology to immunoglobulin chains. *Nature* 308:145–49

13. Dembic Z, Haas W, Weiss S, McCubrey J, Kiefer H, et al. 1986. Transfer of specificity by murine α and β T-cell receptor genes. *Nature* 320:232–38

14. Saito T, Weiss A, Miller J, Norcross MA, Germain RN. 1987. Specific antigen-Ia activation of transfected human T cells expressing murine Ti $\alpha\beta$-human T3 receptor complexes. *Nature* 325:125–30

15. Brenner MB, McLean J, Dialynas DP, Strominger JL, Smith JA, et al. 1986. Identification of a putative second T-cell receptor. *Nature* 322:145–49

16. Chien YH, Iwashima M, Kaplan KB, Elliott JF, Davis MM. 1987. A new T-cell receptor gene located within the alpha locus and expressed early in T-cell differentiation. *Nature* 327:677–82

17. Saito H, Kranz DM, Takagaki Y, Hayday AC, Eisen HN, Tonegawa S. 1984. A third rearranged and expressed gene in a clone of cytotoxic T lymphocytes. *Nature* 312:36–40

18. Groettrup M, Ungewiss K, Azogui O, Palacios R, Owen MJ, et al. 1993. A novel disulfide-linked heterodimer on pre-T cells consists of the T cell receptor beta chain and a 33 kd glycoprotein. *Cell* 75:283–94

19. Saint-Ruf C, Ungewiss K, Groettrup M, Bruno L, Fehling HJ, von Boehmer H. 1994. Analysis and expression of a cloned pre-T cell receptor gene. *Science* 266:1208–12

20. Borowski C, Li X, Aifantis I, Gounari F, von Boehmer H. 2004. Pre-TCRα and TCRα are not interchangeable partners of TCRβ during T lymphocyte development. *J. Exp. Med.* 199:607–15

21. Aifantis I, Borowski C, Gounari F, Lacorazza HD, Nikolich-Zugich J, von Boehmer H. 2002. A critical role for the cytoplasmic tail of pTα in T lymphocyte development. *Nat. Immunol.* 3:483–88

22. van Agthoven A, Terhorst C, Reinherz E, Schlossman S. 1981. Characterization of T cell surface glycoproteins T1 and T3 present on all human peripheral T lymphocytes and functionally mature thymocytes. *Eur. J. Immunol.* 11:18–21

23. Borst J, Prendiville MA, Terhorst C. 1982. Complexity of the human T lymphocyte-specific cell surface antigen T3. *J. Immunol.* 128:1560–65

24. Sussman JJ, Bonifacino JS, Lippincott-Schwartz J, Weissman AM, Saito T, et al. 1988. Failure to synthesize the T cell CD3-zeta chain: structure and function of a partial T cell receptor complex. *Cell* 52:85–95

25. Samelson LE, Harford JB, Klausner RD. 1985. Identification of the components of the murine T cell antigen receptor complex. *Cell* 43:223–31

26. Clevers H, Alarcon B, Wileman T, Terhorst C. 1988. The T cell receptor/CD3 complex: a dynamic protein ensemble. *Annu. Rev. Immunol.* 6:629–62

27. Klausner RD, Lippincott-Schwartz J, Bonifacino JS. 1990. The T cell antigen receptor: insights into organelle biology. *Annu. Rev. Cell Biol.* 6:403–31

28. Reth M. 1989. Antigen receptor tail clue. *Nature* 338:383–84

29. Straus DB, Weiss A. 1992. Genetic evidence for the involvement of the lck tyrosine kinase in signal transduction through the T cell antigen receptor. *Cell* 70:585–93

30. Iwashima M, Irving BA, van Oers NS, Chan AC, Weiss A. 1994. Sequential interactions of the TCR with two distinct cytoplasmic tyrosine kinases. *Science* 263:1136–39

31. Hall C, Berkhout B, Alarcon B, Sancho J, Wileman T, Terhorst C. 1991. Requirements for cell surface expression of the human TCR/CD3 complex in non-T cells. *Int. Immunol.* 3:359–68

32. Manolios N, Letourneur F, Bonifacino JS, Klausner RD. 1991. Pairwise, cooperative and inhibitory interactions describe the assembly and probable structure of the T-cell antigen receptor. *EMBO J.* 10:1643–51

33. Geisler C. 1992. Failure to synthesize the CD3-γ chain. Consequences for T cell antigen receptor assembly, processing, and expression. *J. Immunol.* 148:2437–45

34. Haks MC, Krimpenfort P, Borst J, Kruisbeek AM. 1998. The CD3γ chain is essential for development of both the TCRαβ and TCRγδ lineages. *EMBO J.* 17:1871–82

35. Dave VP, Cao Z, Browne C, Alarcon B, Fernandez-Miguel G, et al. 1997. CD3δ deficiency arrests development of the αβ but not the γδ T cell lineage. *EMBO J.* 16:1360–70

36. Blumberg RS, Ley S, Sancho J, Lonberg N, Lacy E, et al. 1990. Structure of the T-cell antigen receptor: evidence for two CD3ε subunits in the T-cell receptor-CD3 complex. *Proc. Natl. Acad. Sci. USA* 87:7220–24

37. de la Hera A, Muller U, Olsson C, Isaaz S, Tunnacliffe A. 1991. Structure of the T cell antigen receptor (TCR): two CD3ε subunits in a functional TCR/CD3 complex. *J. Exp. Med.* 173:7–17

38. Manolios N, Bonifacino JS, Klausner RD. 1990. Transmembrane helical interactions and the assembly of the T cell receptor complex. *Science* 249:274–77

39. Cosson P, Lankford SP, Bonifacino JS,

Klausner RD. 1991. Membrane protein association by potential intramembrane charge pairs. *Nature* 351:414–16

40. Livnah O, Stura EA, Middleton SA, Johnson DL, Jolliffe LK, Wilson IA. 1999. Crystallographic evidence for preformed dimers of erythropoietin receptor before ligand activation. *Science* 283:987–90

41. Remy I, Wilson IA, Michnick SW. 1999. Erythropoietin receptor activation by a ligand-induced conformation change. *Science* 283:990–93

42. Carr PD, Gustin SE, Church AP, Murphy JM, Ford SC, et al. 2001. Structure of the complete extracellular domain of the common beta subunit of the human GM-CSF, IL-3, and IL-5 receptors reveals a novel dimer configuration. *Cell* 104:291–300

43. He X, Chow D, Martick MM, Garcia KC. 2001. Allosteric activation of a spring-loaded natriuretic peptide receptor dimer by hormone. *Science* 293:1657–62

44. Punt JA, Roberts JL, Kearse KP, Singer A. 1994. Stoichiometry of the T cell antigen receptor (TCR) complex: each TCR/CD3 complex contains one $TCR\alpha$, one $TCR\beta$, and two $CD3\varepsilon$ chains. *J. Exp. Med.* 180:587–93

45. Kearse KP, Roberts JL, Singer A. 1995. $TCR\alpha$-$CD3\delta\varepsilon$ association is the initial step in $\alpha\beta$ dimer formation in murine T cells and is limiting in immature $CD4^+$ $CD8^+$ thymocytes. *Immunity* 2:391–99

46. Call ME, Pyrdol J, Wiedmann M, Wucherpfennig KW. 2002. The organizing principle in the formation of the T cell receptor-CD3 complex. *Cell* 111:967–79

47. Fernandez-Miguel G, Alarcon B, Iglesias A, Bluethmann H, Alvarez-Mon M, et al. 1999. Multivalent structure of an $\alpha\beta$ T cell receptor. *Proc. Natl. Acad. Sci. USA* 96:1547–52

48. Jacobs H. 1997. Pre-TCR/CD3 and TCR/CD3 complexes: decamers with differential signalling properties? *Immunol. Today* 18:565–69

49. San Jose E, Sahuquillo AG, Bragado R, Alarcon B. 1998. Assembly of the TCR/CD3 complex: CD3 ε/δ and CD3 ε/γ dimers associate indistinctly with both $TCR\alpha$ and $TCR\beta$ chains. Evidence for a double TCR heterodimer model. *Eur. J. Immunol.* 28:12–21

50. Exley M, Wileman T, Mueller B, Terhorst C. 1995. Evidence for multivalent structure of T-cell antigen receptor complex. *Mol. Immunol.* 32:829–39

51. Wilson DS, Keefe AD, Szostak JW. 2001. The use of mRNA display to select high-affinity protein-binding peptides. *Proc. Natl. Acad. Sci. USA* 98:3750–55

52. Ribaudo RK, Margulies DH. 1992. Independent and synergistic effects of disulfide bond formation, beta 2-microglobulin, and peptides on class I MHC folding and assembly in an in vitro translation system. *J. Immunol.* 149:2935–44

53. Bijlmakers MJ, Neefjes JJ, Wojcik-Jacobs EH, Ploegh HL. 1993. The assembly of H2-Kb class I molecules translated in vitro requires oxidized glutathione and peptide. *Eur. J. Immunol.* 23:1305–13

54. Bijlmakers MJ, Benaroch P, Ploegh HL. 1994. Assembly of HLA DR1 molecules translated in vitro: binding of peptide in the endoplasmic reticulum precludes association with invariant chain. *EMBO J.* 13:2699–707

55. Ribaudo RK, Margulies DH. 1995. Polymorphism at position nine of the MHC class I heavy chain affects the stability of association with beta 2-microglobulin and presentation of a viral peptide. *J. Immunol.* 155:3481–93

56. Huppa JB, Ploegh HL. 1997. In vitro translation and assembly of a complete T cell receptor-CD3 complex. *J. Exp. Med.* 186:393–403

57. Hebert DN, Zhang JX, Helenius A. 1998. Protein folding and maturation in a cell-free system. *Biochem. Cell Biol.* 76:867–73

58. Call ME, Pyrdol J, Wucherpfennig KW. 2004. Stoichiometry of the T-cell receptor-CD3 complex and key intermediates

assembled in the endoplasmic reticulum. *EMBO J.* 23:2348–57

59. Wegener AM, Hou X, Dietrich J, Geisler C. 1995. Distinct domains of the CD3-γ chain are involved in surface expression and function of the T cell antigen receptor. *J. Biol. Chem.* 270:4675–80

60. Morley BJ, Chin KN, Newton ME, Weiss A. 1988. The lysine residue in the membrane-spanning domain of the beta chain is necessary for cell surface expression of the T cell antigen receptor. *J. Exp. Med.* 168:1971–78

61. Alcover A, Mariuzza RA, Ermonval M, Acuto O. 1990. Lysine 271 in the transmembrane domain of the T-cell antigen receptor beta chain is necessary for its assembly with the CD3 complex but not for α/β dimerization. *J. Biol. Chem.* 265:4131–35

62. Blumberg RS, Alarcon B, Sancho J, McDermott FV, Lopez P, et al. 1990. Assembly and function of the T cell antigen receptor. Requirement of either the lysine or arginine residues in the transmembrane region of the α chain. *J. Biol. Chem.* 265:14036–43

63. Dietrich J, Neisig A, Hou X, Wegener AM, Gajhede M, Geisler C. 1996. Role of CD3γ in T cell receptor assembly. *J. Cell Biol.* 132:299–310

64. Rutledge T, Cosson P, Manolios N, Bonifacino JS, Klausner RD. 1992. Transmembrane helical interactions: zeta chain dimerization and functional association with the T cell antigen receptor. *EMBO J.* 11:3245–54

65. Krangel MS, Bierer BE, Devlin P, Clabby M, Strominger JL, et al. 1987. T3 glycoprotein is functional although structurally distinct on human T-cell receptor γ T lymphocytes. *Proc. Natl. Acad. Sci. USA* 84:3817–21

66. Hayes SM, Love PE. 2002. Distinct structure and signaling potential of the $\gamma\delta$ TCR complex. *Immunity* 16:827–38

67. Ravetch JV, Bolland S. 2001. IgG Fc receptors. *Annu. Rev. Immunol.* 19:275–90

68. Lanier LL, Corliss BC, Wu J, Leong C, Phillips JH. 1998. Immunoreceptor DAP12 bearing a tyrosine-based activation motif is involved in activating NK cells. *Nature* 391:703–7

69. Wu J, Song Y, Bakker AB, Bauer S, Spies T, et al. 1999. An activating immunoreceptor complex formed by NKG2D and DAP10. *Science* 285:730–32

70. Diefenbach A, Raulet DH. 2003. Innate immune recognition by stimulatory immunoreceptors. *Curr. Opin. Immunol.* 15:37–44

71. Lanier LL. 2001. On guard—activating NK cell receptors. *Nat. Immunol.* 2:23–27

72. Wu J, Cherwinski H, Spies T, Phillips JH, Lanier LL. 2000. DAP10 and DAP12 form distinct, but functionally cooperative, receptor complexes in natural killer cells. *J. Exp. Med.* 192:1059–68

73. Vilches C, Parham P. 2002. KIR: diverse, rapidly evolving receptors of innate and adaptive immunity. *Annu. Rev. Immunol.* 20:217–51

74. Campbell KS, Colonna M. 1999. DAP12: a key accessory protein for relaying signals by natural killer cell receptors. *Int. J. Biochem. Cell Biol.* 31:631–36

75. Popot JL, Engelman DM. 2000. Helical membrane protein folding, stability, and evolution. *Annu. Rev. Biochem.* 69:881–922

76. White SH, Wimley WC. 1999. Membrane protein folding and stability: physical principles. *Annu. Rev. Biophys. Biomol. Struct.* 28:319–65

77. Curran AR, Engelman DM. 2003. Sequence motifs, polar interactions and conformational changes in helical membrane proteins. *Curr. Opin. Struct. Biol.* 13:412–17

78. Ubarretxena-Belandia I, Engelman DM. 2001. Helical membrane proteins: diversity of functions in the context of simple architecture. *Curr. Opin. Struct. Biol.* 11:370–76

79. Lemmon MA, Flanagan JM, Hunt JF,

Adair BD, Bormann BJ, et al. 1992. Glycophorin A dimerization is driven by specific interactions between transmembrane α-helices. *J. Biol. Chem.* 267:7683–89

80. Lemmon MA, Flanagan JM, Treutlein HR, Zhang J, Engelman DM. 1992. Sequence specificity in the dimerization of transmembrane α-helices. *Biochemistry* 31:12719–25

80a. MacKenzie KR, Prestegard JH, Engelman DM. 1997. A transmembrane helix dimer: structure and implications. *Science* 276:131–33

81. Russ WP, Engelman DM. 2000. The GxxxG motif: a framework for transmembrane helix-helix association. *J. Mol. Biol.* 296:911–19

82. Tourasse NJ, Li WH. 2000. Selective constraints, amino acid composition, and the rate of protein evolution. *Mol. Biol. Evol.* 17:656–64

83. Gratkowski H, Lear JD, DeGrado WF. 2001. Polar side chains drive the association of model transmembrane peptides. *Proc. Natl. Acad. Sci. USA* 98:880–85

84. Zhou FX, Merianos HJ, Brunger AT, Engelman DM. 2001. Polar residues drive association of polyleucine transmembrane helices. *Proc. Natl. Acad. Sci. USA* 98:2250–55

85. Zhou FX, Cocco MJ, Russ WP, Brunger AT, Engelman DM. 2000. Interhelical hydrogen bonding drives strong interactions in membrane proteins. *Nat. Struct. Biol.* 7:154–60

86. Ballesteros JA, Deupi X, Olivella M, Haaksma EE, Pardo L. 2000. Serine and threonine residues bend α-helices in the $\chi_1 = g^-$ conformation. *Biophys. J.* 79:2754–60

87. Dawson JP, Weinger JS, Engelman DM. 2002. Motifs of serine and threonine can drive association of transmembrane helices. *J. Mol. Biol.* 316:799–805

88. Engelman DM. 2003. Electrostatic fasteners hold the T cell receptor-CD3 complex together. *Mol. Cell* 11:5–6

89. Bonifacino JS, Cosson P, Klausner RD. 1990. Colocalized transmembrane determinants for ER degradation and subunit assembly explain the intracellular fate of TCR chains. *Cell* 63:503–13

90. Bonifacino JS, Cosson P, Shah N, Klausner RD. 1991. Role of potentially charged transmembrane residues in targeting proteins for retention and degradation within the endoplasmic reticulum. *EMBO J.* 10:2783–93

91. Minami Y, Weissman AM, Samelson LE, Klausner RD. 1987. Building a multichain receptor: synthesis, degradation, and assembly of the T-cell antigen receptor. *Proc. Natl. Acad. Sci. USA* 84:2688–92

92. Chen C, Bonifacino JS, Yuan LC, Klausner RD. 1988. Selective degradation of T cell antigen receptor chains retained in a pre-Golgi compartment. *J. Cell Biol.* 107:2149–61

93. Bonifacino JS, Suzuki CK, Lippincott-Schwartz J, Weissman AM, Klausner RD. 1989. Pre-Golgi degradation of newly synthesized T-cell antigen receptor chains: intrinsic sensitivity and the role of subunit assembly. *J. Cell Biol.* 109:73–83

94. Wileman T, Carson GR, Concino M, Ahmed A, Terhorst C. 1990. The γ and ε subunits of the CD3 complex inhibit pre-Golgi degradation of newly synthesized T cell antigen receptors. *J. Cell Biol.* 110:973–86

95. Gorlich D, Rapoport TA. 1993. Protein translocation into proteoliposomes reconstituted from purified components of the endoplasmic reticulum membrane. *Cell* 75:615–30

96. Matlack KE, Mothes W, Rapoport TA. 1998. Protein translocation: tunnel vision. *Cell* 92:381–90

97. Borel AC, Simon SM. 1996. Biogenesis of polytopic membrane proteins: membrane segments assemble within translocation channels prior to membrane integration. *Cell* 85:379–89

98. Heinrich SU, Mothes W, Brunner J, Rapoport TA. 2000. The Sec61p complex mediates the integration of a membrane

protein by allowing lipid partitioning of the transmembrane domain. *Cell* 102: 233–44

99. Wiertz EJ, Tortorella D, Bogyo M, Yu J, Mothes W, et al. 1996. Sec61-mediated transfer of a membrane protein from the endoplasmic reticulum to the proteasome for destruction. *Nature* 384:432–38

100. Plemper RK, Wolf DH. 1999. Retrograde protein translocation: ERADication of secretory proteins in health and disease. *Trends Biochem. Sci.* 24:266–70

101. Lilley BN, Ploegh HL. 2004. A membrane protein required for dislocation of misfolded proteins from the ER. *Nature* 429:834–40

102. Ye Y, Shibata Y, Yun C, Ron D, Rapoport TA. 2004. A membrane protein complex mediates retro-translocation from the ER lumen into the cytosol. *Nature* 429:841–47

103. Mallabiabarrena A, Fresno M, Alarcon B. 1992. An endoplasmic reticulum retention signal in the CD3ε chain of the T-cell receptor. *Nature* 357:593–96

104. Letourneur F, Klausner RD. 1992. A novel di-leucine motif and a tyrosine-based motif independently mediate lysosomal targeting and endocytosis of CD3 chains. *Cell* 69:1143–57

105. Dietrich J, Hou X, Wegener AM, Geisler C. 1994. CD3γ contains a phosphoserine-dependent di-leucine motif involved in down-regulation of the T cell receptor. *EMBO J.* 13:2156–66

106. Dietrich J, Geisler C. 1998. T cell receptor ζ allows stable expression of receptors containing the CD3γ leucine-based receptor-sorting motif. *J. Biol. Chem.* 273:26281–84

107. Dietrich J, Kastrup J, Nielsen BL, Odum N, Geisler C. 1997. Regulation and function of the CD3γ DxxxLL motif: a binding site for adaptor protein-1 and adaptor protein-2 in vitro. *J. Cell Biol.* 138:271–81

108. Geisler C. 2004. TCR trafficking in resting and stimulated T cells. *Crit. Rev. Immunol.* 24:67–86

109. Das V, Nal B, Dujeancourt A, Thoulouze MI, Galli T, et al. 2004. Activation-induced polarized recycling targets T cell antigen receptors to the immunological synapse; involvement of SNARE complexes. *Immunity* 20:577–88

110. Valitutti S, Muller S, Salio M, Lanzavecchia A. 1997. Degradation of T cell receptor (TCR)-CD3-ζ complexes after antigenic stimulation. *J. Exp. Med.* 185:1859–64

111. Joazeiro CA, Wing SS, Huang H, Leverson JD, Hunter T, Liu YC. 1999. The tyrosine kinase negative regulator c-Cbl as a RING-type, E2-dependent ubiquitin-protein ligase. *Science* 286:309–12

112. Lupher ML Jr, Reedquist KA, Miyake S, Langdon WY, Band H. 1996. A novel phosphotyrosine-binding domain in the N-terminal transforming region of Cbl interacts directly and selectively with ZAP-70 in T cells. *J. Biol. Chem.* 271:24063–68

113. Sundquist WI, Schubert HL, Kelly BN, Hill GC, Holton JM, Hill CP. 2004. Ubiquitin recognition by the human TSG101 protein. *Mol. Cell* 13:783–89

114. Aivazian D, Stern LJ. 2000. Phosphorylation of T cell receptor ζ is regulated by a lipid dependent folding transition. *Nat. Struct. Biol.* 7:1023–26

Annu. Rev. Immunol. 2005. 23:127–59
doi: 10.1146/annurev.immunol.23.021704.115628
First published online as a Review in Advance on October 11, 2004

CHEMOKINES, SPHINGOSINE-1-PHOSPHATE, AND CELL MIGRATION IN SECONDARY LYMPHOID ORGANS

Jason G. Cyster
Howard Hughes Medical Institute and Department of Microbiology and Immunology,
University of California, San Francisco, California 94143-0414;
email: cyster@itsa.ucsf.edu

Key Words CXCR5, CCR7, CXCR4, S1P, exit

■ **Abstract** Secondary lymphoid organs serve as hubs for the adaptive immune system, bringing together antigen, antigen-presenting cells, and lymphocytes. Two families of G protein–coupled receptors play essential roles in lymphocyte migration through these organs: chemokine receptors and sphingosine-1-phosphate (S1P) receptors. Chemokines expressed by lymphoid stromal cells guide lymphocyte and dendritic cell movements during antigen surveillance and the initiation of adaptive immune responses. S1P receptor-1 is required for lymphocyte egress from thymus and secondary lymphoid organs and is downregulated by the immunosuppressive drug FTY720. Here, we review the steps associated with the initiation of adaptive immune responses in secondary lymphoid organs, highlighting the roles of chemokines and S1P.

INTRODUCTION

That secondary lymphoid organs are sites for immune response initiation has long been known (1), and experiments in mice engineered to lack secondary lymphoid organs have established their critical role in mammalian adaptive immunity (2, 3). A feature unique to lymphoid tissues is the dependence of almost every aspect of their function on cell migration. Naive B and T lymphocytes continually enter secondary lymphoid organs from the blood and migrate within minutes to the juxtaposed B cell follicles and T cell zones, respectively (Figure 1). Within these compartments, B and T cells continue to migrate vigorously, surveying for antigen. Lymphoid follicles contain resident stromal cells, including follicular dendritic cells (FDC) that capture and display antigen on their surface for recognition by B cells, whereas T zones contain numerous bone marrow–derived dendritic cells (DC) that display MHC-peptide complexes to the migrating T cells.[1]

---

[1]See Appendix for a full list of abbreviations used.

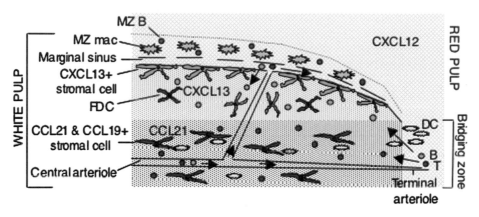

Figure 1   Organization of the splenic white pulp. The diagram represents a longitudinal cross-section of a white-pulp cord segment together with surrounding red pulp. The distribution of CCL21 (SLC) is shown in red shading and CXCL13 (BLC) in green shading, and these areas correspond to the T zone and follicles, respectively. Lymphoid stromal cells are shown in red or green to reflect their chemokine-producing activity. FDC, which may contribute to CXCL13 production, are shown in blue to highlight their unique antigen-capturing properties. Other cell types are as indicated. CXCL12 (SDF-1, *yellow shading*) is abundant in the red pulp. The central arteriole, typically located centrally in the white-pulp cord, gives rise to terminal arterioles, some of which end in the marginal sinus that surrounds the follicles while others pass through the bridging zone between white pulp and red pulp before terminating. B and T lymphocytes released from terminal arterioles migrate into the white-pulp cord, whereas other cell types (not depicted) pass out of the spleen through the red pulp. For simplicity, the heterogeneity of the T-zone DC and the marginal zone (MZ) macrophage populations and the cell types in the red pulp are not depicted. Although only small numbers of B and T cells are shown in follicles and the T zone, these compartments would be packed, membrane-to-membrane, with lymphocytes.

Secondary lymphoid organs are strategically positioned to sample antigens that enter through almost any body surface; the spleen filters antigens from the blood, lymph nodes (LNs) filter lymph draining from skin or mucosal surfaces, and Peyer's patches (PPs) obtain antigen by transepithelial transport from the intestinal lumen. Most naive lymphocytes that enter a lymphoid organ fail to detect their specific antigen and, after a period of about 12–18 h for T cells and 24 h for B cells, migrate out to return to circulation and go on to survey further lymphoid organs. Exit from LNs occurs through the medulla, which contains sinuses that connect to the efferent lymphatic vessel, and cells return to circulation via the thoracic duct. Exit from PPs also occurs via migration into lymphatic vessels, whereas egress from the spleen involves migration from the lymphoid regions (white-pulp cords) into the nonlymphoid red pulp and then into venous circulation.

Upon antigen encounter, cell migration within lymphoid organs undergoes rapid changes. Numerous antigen-presenting cells migrate into T zones and follicles, events induced by Toll-like receptor (TLR) signals and inflammatory cytokines. Antigen-reactive lymphocytes quickly shut down their exit program, ensuring that they remain within the antigen-bearing tissue. Within hours, antigen-engaged B cells migrate from follicles to the boundary of the T zone to interact with helper T cells. Antigen-specific T cells that have made initial recognition with antigen-bearing DC go on to make extended contacts with DC, and some CD4 T cells migrate to the follicle to interact with activated B cells. CD8 T cells and some of the CD4 T cells, after activation and several rounds of division, reacquire exit capability and migrate out of the lymphoid tissue, having undergone extensive changes in their cytokine and homing molecule expression that equip them to travel to inflamed tissue and carry out effector functions. Activated B cells become antibody-secreting plasma cells and migrate to the medulla of LNs or the red pulp of spleen, although some exit the lymphoid tissue to migrate to the bone marrow or epithelial surfaces. A small number of activated B cells in T-dependent responses take a different route, migrating back into the follicle to differentiate into germinal center (GC) cells. Further migration events occur within the GC during the processes of selection and affinity maturation.

Of the numerous molecules needed to guide cell movements during the initiation of adaptive immune responses, the chemotactic cytokines, or chemokines, have perhaps the most pervasive influence. The first sections of this review focus on the roles of chemokines in cell homing to lymphoid follicles and T cell zones, and in facilitating interactions between cells during the initiation of adaptive immunity. Although much has been learned about how cells enter lymphoid organs and home to their respective compartments, how they get out is poorly understood. The first molecular details of the egress process are emerging, facilitated by the discovery of an immunosuppressive molecule, termed FTY720, that blocks exit. This work is revealing the role of another type of soluble mediator, a lysophospholipid (sphingosine-1-phosphate, S1P), in lymphocyte trafficking. The second half of this review focuses on the information emerging on the requirements for cell egress from secondary lymphoid organs and thymus.

THE CHEMOKINE FAMILY

Chemokines constitute a family of over 40 small, mostly secreted proteins that chemoattract cells by engaging G protein–coupled receptors (GPCRs) (4, 5) (Table 1). Induction of chemotaxis depends predominantly on coupling to pertussis toxin (PTX)-sensitive $G\alpha i$ proteins, but some chemokine receptors couple to additional G proteins (5–7). Once identified because of their important roles in recruiting innate immune cells and effector T cells to sites of inflammation, chemokines now have a firmly established role in promoting the organization and function of secondary lymphoid tissues (8, 9). The subset of the chemokine family involved in these processes, sometimes referred to as lymphoid or homeostatic chemokines, includes CCL19 (ELC) and CCL21 (SLC) and their shared receptor,

Table 1   Chemokine receptors and their ligands[a]

Receptor	Ligands
CC chemokines	
CCR1	*CCL3 (MIP1α)*, *CCL5 (RANTES)*, *CCL7 (MCP3)*, *CCL8 (MCP2)*, mCCL9 (MRP2), *hCCL13 (MCP4)*, *CCL14 (HCC1)*, *hCCL15 (HCC2)*, *CCL16 (HCC4)*, hCCL23 (MPIF1)
CCR2	CCL2 (MCP1), *CCL7 (MCP3)*, *CCL8 (MCP2)*, mCCL12 (MCP5), *hCCL13 (MCP4)*, *CCL16 (HCC4)*
CCR3	*CCL5 (RANTES)*, *CCL7 (MCP3)*, *CCL8 (MCP2)*, *CCL11 (eotaxin)*, *hCCL13 (MCP4)*, *hCCL15 (HCC2)*, hCCL24 (eotaxin-2), hCCL26 (eotaxin-3), *CCL28 (MEC)*
CCR4	CCL17 (TARC), CCL22 (MDC)
CCR5	*CCL3 (MIP1α)*, CCL4 (MIP1β), *CCL5 (RANTES)*, *CCL8 (MCP2)*, *CCL11 (eotaxin)*, *CCL14 (HCC1)*, *CCL16 (HCC4)*
CCR6	CCL20 (MIP3α, LARC)
CCR7	CCL19 (ELC, MIP3β), CCL21 (SLC, 6Ckine)
CCR8	CCL1 (I309, TCA3)
CCR9	CCL25 (TECK)
CCR10	CCL27 (CTACK), *CCL28 (MEC)*
CXC chemokines	
hCXCR1	*CXCL6 (GCP2)*, *CXCL8 (IL-8)*
CXCR2	CXCL1 (Groα), CXCL2 (Groβ), CXCL3 (Groγ), CXCL5 (ENA78), *CXCL6 (GCP2)*, CXCL7 (NAP2), *CXCL8 (IL-8)*
CXCR3	CXCL9 (MIG), CXCL10 (IP10), CXCL11 (ITAC)
CXCR3b	CXCL4 (PF4), CXCL9 (MIG), CXCL10 (IP10), CXCL11 (ITAC)
CXCR4	CXCL12 (SDF-1)
CXCR5	CXCL13 (BLC, BCA1)
CXCR6	CXCL16–transmembrane chemokine
C chemokines	
XCR1	XCL1 (Lymphotactin), hXCL2 (SCM1b)
CX3C chemokine	
CX3CR1	CX3CL1 (Fractalkine)–transmembrane chemokine

[a]Based on References 4, 5, 128, 191, 192. Chemokines are shown by their standardized nomenclature together with one or more common names in parentheses. Chemokines known to activate more than one receptor are italicized. Some chemokines have antagonistic functions that are not shown (see 5). Chemokines or receptors that are defined only in human or mouse are shown with a corresponding prefix (h or m, respectively). In the case of CXCR2 ligands, the human chemokines are listed; the mouse orthologs do not match individual human ligands and have a different common nomenclature. CXCR3b is a splice variant of CXCR3 (193). CXCL12 has two splice variants (SDF-1α and SDF-1β) that are identical except that SDF-1β has four additional amino acids at the carboxy terminus (194); a third splice variant (SDF-1γ) has been identified in the rat (195). Two CCL21 genes exist in Balb/c mice that encode proteins differing by a single amino acid, termed CCL21-ser and CCL21-leu; in some mouse strains there is an additional copy of the CCL21-leu gene (196, 197). Only a single CCL21 gene has been identified in humans.

CCR7; CXCL13 (BLC) and its receptor CXCR5; and CXCL12 (SDF-1) and its receptor CXCR4 (Table 1).

CHEMOKINES AND LYMPHOID ORGAN ENTRY

Lymphocyte entry to LNs and PPs occurs via high endothelial venules (HEV) and involves a cascade of selectin- (or integrin-) supported rolling, chemokine-mediated integrin activation, and firm integrin-mediated adhesion. The most prominent chemokine functioning on HEV is CCL21, but CXCL12 and CXCL13 also contribute to homeostatic lymphocyte recirculation, and chemokines such as CXCL9 (MIG), CXCL10 (IP10), and CCL2 (MCP1) (Table 1) can be displayed on HEV during inflammation. Current understanding of the events associated with lymphoid organ entry via HEV has been summarized in several excellent reviews (10–12).

Entry to the spleen does not involve HEV; instead, lymphocytes and other blood cells are released into the organ from terminal arterioles that open into the marginal sinus or the red pulp (13, 14). Many of the cells released from these vessels pass via the red pulp into venous sinuses and quickly rejoin circulation. However, in contrast to other blood cell types, a fraction of the lymphocytes rapidly begin to appear within the B and T cell areas of the white-pulp cords (15) (Figure 1). Similar to HEV attachment, $\alpha L \beta 2$ and $\alpha 4$ integrins are involved in lymphocyte migration into white-pulp cords (16), whereas selectins do not appear to be required (17), most likely because the shear forces operating on the cells are substantially lower than within HEV. Deficiency in CXCR5 strongly reduces B lymphocyte accumulation within white-pulp cords, whereas deficiency in CCR7 reduces T cell accumulation in these areas (18, 19). Small numbers of B cells continue to appear within the white pulp of mice deficient in CXCR5 or its ligand, CXCL13, but in animals deficient in both CXCR5 and CCR7, B cell entry is completely blocked (9). Therefore, while lymphocyte entry into the spleen occurs by release from open-ended terminal arterioles, entry to the white-pulp cords is a migration-dependent process that requires the function of integrins and chemokine receptors.

HOMEOSTATIC ORGANIZATION AND ANTIGEN SURVEILLANCE

The B Cell Follicle: CXCR5 and CXCL13

Homing of B cells to lymphoid follicles depends on expression of CXCR5 by B cells and CXCL13 by radiation-resistant follicular stromal cells (20–22). CXCR5 is upregulated during B cell maturation in the bone marrow and is expressed by all mature B cells, including recirculating follicular B cells, marginal zone (MZ) B cells, and peritoneal B1 B cells (23, 24). CXCL13 mRNA is distributed in a striking reticular pattern within follicles, and although CXCL13 protein is distributed more uniformly, the strongest signal is often found in a pattern similar to that of the mRNA-producing cells (25–27) (Figure 1). The CXCL13-expressing stromal cells are likely to be the same cells known from ultrastructural studies as fibroblastic reticular cells, which are involved in ensheathing (and most likely making) the collagen-rich fibers that provide structural support within lymphoid tissues (27). FDC are believed to correspond to a specialized subset of the fibroblastic reticular cells (27). The colocalization of some CXCL13-expressing cells with cells that are positive for FDC markers favors the view that FDC produce CXCL13, although the alternative possibility that FDC are tightly associated with CXCL13-producing stromal cells has not been ruled out. In addition to its expression by stromal cells, CXCL13 can be produced by hematopoietic cells. Expression by macrophages contributes to the CXCR5-dependent accumulation of B1 cells within body cavities (22), and expression by macrophages and DC may contribute to B cell recruitment to sites of inflammation (28–30).

Follicular B cells are highly motile, moving in a "random-walk" through the follicle at ~6 μm/min, a behavior likely to ensure that they efficiently survey the FDC (and each other) for surface-displayed antigen (31). Whether CXCL13 is involved in promoting this motility, either in a chemotactic manner with the B cells moving between local, stromal cell–associated gradients or in a gradient-independent chemokinetic manner, remains to be assessed. Migration toward CXCL13 concentration "peaks" and then movement away into CXCL13 "valleys" would be similar to a process described for axons, whereby the growth cone shows brief periods of movement toward the attractant and then slight movement away during a period of resensitization, followed again by growth toward the attractant (32).

In addition to follicular B cells, the spleen contains a large population of B cells in the splenic MZ, known as MZ B cells (33, 34). This compartment, located at the boundary between the follicles and the red pulp, is separated from the follicles by the marginal sinus, and blood that is released in the marginal sinus filters through this compartment on its way to the red pulp (Figure 1). Correspondingly, MZ B cells play an important role in responses to blood-borne pathogens (33, 34). B cell lodgment in the MZ is independent of CXCR5 and CXCL13 but depends on $\alpha L\beta 2$ and $\alpha 4\beta 1$ integrin-mediated adhesion to ICAM1 and VCAM1, which are integrin-ligands highly expressed in the MZ (35). Consistent with a more adhesive state, MZ B cells in rodents are nonrecirculatory (36). MZ B cell positioning also depends on responsiveness to S1P (37), which is present in high abundance in blood (discussed below). The MZ contains a variety of macrophage populations, and adhesion between MZ B cells and macrophages may contribute to MZ B cell retention (38). Although the factors controlling the positioning of most of these myeloid cells are not well defined, a population of cells located on the inner side of the marginal sinus, identified by their ability to bind the cysteine-rich domain of mannose binding protein, depends on CXCL13 expression for appropriate positioning (39).

The T Zone: CCR7 and Ligands CCL19 and CCL21

T cell and DC migration to lymphoid organ T zones is dependent on CCR7 and its ligands (19, 40). All naive T cells express abundant amounts of CCR7 and exhibit strong chemotactic responses to the two CCR7 ligands, CCL19 and CCL21 (Table 1). T cells migrate within the T zone at an average speed of 12 μm/min, and like B cells in follicles, the movement appears like a random walk (31, 41–43). As with the B cells, whether the movement is indeed random or is directed by local chemoattractant gradients remains an open question. Enumeration of the frequency of naive T cell encounters with a given DC suggests that as many as 5000 T cells can visit a single DC per hour (41, 44). CCL19 and CCL21 are expressed in the T zone by radiation-resistant stromal cells (Figure 1). CCL21 is also made by HEV, whereas CCL19 can be produced by DC (reviewed in 8). The collagen fiber–associated reticular network is even more prominent in the T zone than in follicles, and again the chemokine-producing stromal cells appear to correspond to fibroblastic reticular cells, and chemokine can often be detected in association with the collagen fibers (45–47). Quantitatively, although mRNA of CCL19 and CCL21 is present in similar abundance, CCL21 protein levels are as much as 100-fold higher than those of CCL19 (48). This differential protein abundance may be attributable to the additional C-terminal domain present in CCL21 because its highly basic properties probably favor interactions with proteoglycans and removal of this domain reduces CCL21 activity in vivo (49). Similar differences in protein abundance were also seen when CCL19 and CCL21 were ectopically expressed within the pancreas, providing a possible explanation for the greater efficacy of CCL21 in recruiting cells to an ectopic site (48, 50). It is unclear why two CCR7 ligands are expressed in what is mostly an overlapping pattern in the T zone, but as this property is conserved between mouse and human, it is not likely that the ligands are redundant.

Lymphotoxin-$\alpha 1\beta 2$ and the Regulation of Chemokine Expression

Expression of CXCL13, CCL19, and CCL21 by lymphoid stromal cells is strongly dependent on the cytokine lymphotoxin (LT)-$\alpha 1\beta 2$ signaling via lymphotoxin β-receptor (LTβR) (26, 51–53). Other markers of the stromal cells are also lacking in LT-deficient mice, including MAdCAM1 and FDC markers (54) and the more general follicular stromal marker, BP3, and T-zone stromal marker, gp38 (26, 55). The LTβR is expressed by stromal cells, and the downstream signaling molecules, NF-κB-inducing kinase (NIK), and the NF-κB family members, p52 and relB, are important for normal chemokine expression (52, 56–58). Tumor necrosis factor (TNF) and TNFR1 also regulate expression of splenic CXCL13 and CCL21, although to a weaker extent than LT$\alpha 1\beta 2$/LTβR (26, 51).

B cells provide a major source of LT$\alpha 1\beta 2$ within the spleen, and in mice lacking B cells, splenic CXCL13 and, more surprisingly, CCL21 are poorly induced (21, 55). The importance of B cell–derived LT in splenic chemokine expression is supported by findings in mice in which LT is selectively deleted in B cells using the Cre/LoxP system, although the effects of this deletion were less severe than anticipated from other studies (59). However, as a significant fraction of the lymphotoxin requirement for splenic chemokine induction occurs in a fixed window in neonatal spleen development, it remains important to determine whether CD19-Cre-mediated LTβ gene deletion occurs efficiently in the neonate (55). Naive T cells also make low amounts of LTα1β2, and expression can be augmented by CCR7 ligands and cytokines such as IL-7, but T cells do not seem to be needed for development of chemokine-expressing stromal cells (48, 55). As follicular and T-zone stromal cells both depend on LTα1β2, the basis for differentiation of lymphoid stromal cells into CXCL13-producing versus CCL19- and CCL21-producing cells remains unresolved. In addition to LTα1β2 inducing CXCL13 expression in stromal cells, CXCL13 augments LTα1β2 expression on B cells, generating a positive feedback loop (21). This loop is important for splenic FDC development, and CXCR5- or CXCL13-deficient mice lack FDC except within the GC (21). However, CXCR5 or CXCL13 deficiency causes only a partial loss of LT from B cells, which indicates that additional factors are involved in regulating B cell LTα1β2 expression.

Within LNs, B cells play a much lesser role in regulating chemokine expression than in the spleen; they have no effect on CCL19 or CCL21 levels (55). Instead, the LTα1β2-expressing lymphoid tissue-inducing cell (LTIC) seems likely to play a central role in promoting chemokine upregulation in developing LNs (60, 61). Like B cells, LTICs are CXCR5 positive and CXCL13 responsive, and the failure of most LNs and PPs to develop in CXCR5- or CXCL13-deficient mice is thought to be due to defective recruitment or clustering of these cells (62–64). The role of LTICs in the early steps of LN and PP development has been discussed in detail in recent reviews (61, 65, 66).

BRINGING CELLS TOGETHER FOR THE IMMUNE RESPONSE

Rapid Alterations in Antigen-Presenting Cell Distribution

Antigen enters lymphoid tissues in two forms: as free antigen and associated with antigen-presenting cells. The relative importance of these two routes of entry is likely to vary depending on the type and amount of antigen, as well as the tissue involved. Free antigen arrives in skin-draining LNs within minutes of subcutaneous injection, and much of the material is taken up and degraded by macrophages in the subcapsular sinus and medullary cords (67, 68). Similarly, with antigen arriving in the spleen via the blood, macrophages in the MZ and red pulp are involved in its capture and degradation (33, 69). However, small amounts of material are directed into the lymphoid region of these tissues. As noted above, LNs and spleen contain a network of collagenous fibers that are ensheathed by chemokine-producing stromal cells. These fibers can function as conduits for small antigens, allowing molecules to penetrate within minutes to the DC-rich areas proximal to HEV (45, 70). Evidence that this type of antigen delivery contributes to initiation of adaptive immune responses comes from the findings that DC resident in LNs can acquire antigen within minutes of injection and that T cells can be activated with similar speed (68). The high responsiveness of mature DC to CCL19 and CCL21 and their ability to move into physical contact with chemokine-producing stromal cells are likely to facilitate uptake of antigen from conduits (43, 46, 71).

In addition to containing T-zone DC, spleen and PPs also contain endogenous populations of immature DC located near sites of antigen entry. In the spleen this includes the MZ and the MZ bridging channels (Figure 1). Upon activation, splenic DC migrate rapidly into the T zone, and this requires CCR7 and its ligands (40). One study has also suggested a role for CCR5 in this process in animals infected with *Toxoplasma gondii* (72). Within PPs, a subset of DC that expresses the CCL20 receptor, CCR6, is found in the subepithelial dome region, adjacent to the CCL20 (MIP3α)-expressing follicle-associated epithelium (73) (Table 1). Although some studies have indicated that CCR6 is essential for DC positioning in this compartment, this finding has been debated: Responsiveness to epithelial cell–produced CCL9 (MIP1γ) may be important instead (74–76). Movement of activated DC from the dome region to the T zone is thought to occur in a CCR7-dependent manner (73).

Following exposure to TLR ligands, macrophages migrate quickly from the splenic MZ or LN subcapsular sinus into lymphoid follicles (77–80), possibly ferrying intact antigens for display on FDC. The chemokine requirements for these movements are not yet defined. In the spleen, MZ B cells are also thought to transport antigen into follicles, binding C3-coated antigen via complement receptors 1 and 2 or antibody-coated antigen via FcRs (81, 82). Exposure to TLR signals causes these cells to migrate rapidly into lymphoid follicles, a process that depends on CXCR5 and CXCL13 (35, 81).

The arrival of antigen-bearing DC into LNs from peripheral sites begins several hours after antigen exposure and may not reach its peak for 1–3 days, depending on the type of antigen and DC. Migration of DC from peripheral tissues into lymphatic vessels requires CCR7 and most likely occurs in response to CCL21 that is made by lymphatic endothelium (10, 68, 83). In contrast to CCL21 expression in lymphoid organs, lymphatic CCL21 expression is largely independent of LTα1β2 (53, 84). CCR2 has also been implicated in DC homing to LNs from the skin, although the step that is disrupted is unclear (85, 86). After being transported by lymph to the LN, DC migrate rapidly into the T zone, a process that again involves CCR7 and its ligands (8). However, further cues appear likely to control DC distribution within LNs because CD11b$^+$CD8$^-$ "myeloid" DC are enriched near the T/B boundary, whereas CD11b$^-$CD8$^+$ "lymphoid" DC are distributed throughout the T zone. In addition to the myeloid and lymphoid DC in lymphoid tissues, DC are also present in circulation, including plasmacytoid DC, and these cells may recirculate between secondary lymphoid organs, perhaps using CXCR3 (87–89). DC can also be rapidly recruited from the blood to spleen following pathogen encounter. Injection of *Streptococcus pneumoniae* is associated with rapid appearance of a blood DC subset in the splenic MZ (90). During infection by *Listeria monocytogenes*, a population of TNF- and iNOS-producing DC appears in the spleen in a CCR2-dependent manner (91).

Relocalization of Activated Lymphocytes

Following antigen-receptor engagement, B cells upregulate CCR7 two- to three-fold and exhibit increased responsiveness to the CCR7 ligands, whereas CXCR5 expression and CXCL13 responsiveness remain unchanged (92). This small shift in the balance of chemokine responsiveness appears to be sufficient to cause B cell relocalization from the follicle to the B/T-zone boundary (92) (Figure 2).

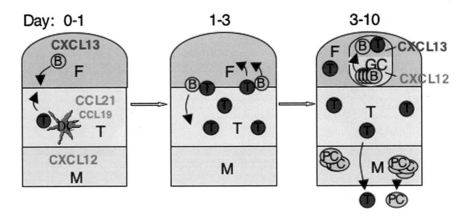

Figure 2   Lymphocyte migration during a T-dependent antibody response. The principal LN compartments, follicle (F), T zone (T), and medulla (M), are color coded according to the predominant chemokine they express, as indicated. Day 0–1: Following antigen encounter, a B cell upregulates CCR7 and moves to the follicle/T-zone boundary in response to CCL21 and CCL19. A CD4 T cell becomes activated after recognizing antigen displayed by a mature T-zone DC, and it upregulates CXCR5 and downregulates CCR7, moving to the follicle/T-zone boundary. Day 1–3: Co-localized antigen-specific B and T cells interact and exchange signals; additional cues (not indicated) are likely to help promote encounters, such as chemokines made by activated B cells. Day 3–10: Activated B cells that become plasmablasts downregulate CXCR5 and CCR7, upregulate CXCR4, and migrate into the CXCL12-rich medulla to become antibody-secreting plasma cells; small numbers of activated B cells retain CXCR5 and localize in the follicle to form a GC. The mature GC contains a CXCL12[+] T-zone proximal dark zone and a CXCL13[+] T-zone distal light zone. Rapidly dividing centroblasts upregulate CXCR4 and lodge in the dark zone in response to CXCL12, whereas centrocytes have reduced CXCR4 and migrate to the light zone at least partly in response to CXCL13. Numerous activated T cells and some plasma cells migrate out of the organ during this phase, although whether chemokines have a role in this exit process is not clear.

Further evidence that it is the balance of chemokine responsiveness that is important rather than the precise level of one chemokine receptor comes from findings with autoantigen-engaged B cells that also locate at the B/T boundary; rather than upregulating CCR7, the cells have reduced amounts of CXCR5 (93, 94). Moreover, treatment of mice with TNF-R agonistic antibodies increases follicular CXCL13 expression and induces movement of autoreactive B cells from the B/T boundary into the follicle (95). Still unclear is how a cell interprets two chemokine signals simultaneously in a manner that causes lodgment at the boundary of the gradients. G protein–coupled receptor kinases and regulator of G protein–signaling molecules can influence the chemokine responsiveness of cells and might therefore contribute to establishment of such balances (96–100).

During initial activation within the T zone, antigen-reactive T cells are observed to swarm around individual antigen-bearing DC and to undergo extensive contacts with these cells (31, 41, 43). Initial encounters between T cells and DC may be promoted by the common attraction of the cells to CCL21/CCL19-producing stromal cells (46). DC also express a variety of chemokines, and there is some evidence for differential chemokine expression by DC, depending on their tissue of origin or the nature of the activating stimulus (89, 101). Although movement of naive T cells toward DC does not appear to involve chemoattraction by the DC, activated and memory T cells may possibly show this behavior (44). For example, some of the DC within skin-draining LNs express CCL22 (MDC) and CCL17 (TARC) (102, 103). As T cells upregulate the CCL17/CCL22 receptor, CCR4, early after activation, this chemokine-receptor system may help ensure that transiently activated T cells move into contact with newly arriving antigen-loaded DC for more persistent interactions (8, 43). Alternatively, differential production of chemokines by DC might favor expansion of distinct T cell subsets. CCR4 expression is associated with skin-homing memory T cells (104). Expression of CCR4 ligands by DC derived from the skin might be a mechanism to promote selective expansion of skin-homing T cells. In this regard, several studies have provided evidence that DC can influence the homing receptor profile of the T cells that they activate (105, 106).

An important function for CD4 T cells is to serve as B cell helpers (Figure 2). Upon activation in the T zone, many CD4 T cells upregulate CXCR5 and undergo a parallel loss of CCL19 and CCL21 responsiveness (107). Downregulation of CCR7 on T cells appears to be sufficient to shift the cells toward the B/T boundary (108). Whether CXCR5 upregulation contributes to their localization at the boundary is not clear, but CXCR5 expression is thought to be essential for their movement into follicles. CXCR5-positive T cells are enriched for cells with potent B-helper activity, presumably indicating that CXCR5 induction occurs together with other gene changes associated with B helper activity, although it is also consistent with the possibility that follicular homing itself promotes T cells to acquire B helper properties (109–112). Antigen engagement induces expression of several chemokines within B cells, and these may act on activated T cells after they reach the B/T boundary, helping to bring the cells into contact (8, 113).

In addition to promoting adaptive immunity, lymphoid organs are involved in helping to achieve the balance between immunity and self-tolerance. $CD4^+CD25^+$ FoxP3-expressing regulatory T cells are important to this process, and these cells can be found in all secondary lymphoid organs (114). Because the suppressive actions of regulatory T cells often depend on cell-cell contact, precisely guided migration is certain to be important to their function. Like naive T cells, most regulatory T cells within lymphoid organs express CCR7 (S. Schwab & J.G. Cyster, unpublished observations). Although only correlative at this time, the delayed but exaggerated immune responses that sometimes occur in CCR7-ligand-deficient paucity of lymph node T cell (plt) mice might reflect disrupted regulatory cell function (115). $CD25^+$ T cells have also been described to express additional receptors, including CCR4 and CCR8, raising the possibility that they interact more efficiently than naive T cells with certain chemokine-producing antigen-presenting cells, a head start that may be important for shutting off responses before they begin (116, 117).

Plasma Cells and Germinal Centers

As activated B cells differentiate into antibody-secreting cells, they markedly downregulate CXCR5 and CCR7 but upregulate CXCR4 (118–120). CXCR4 is critical for normal homing of plasma cells to the red pulp of the spleen and the medullary cords of LNs, the zones of secondary lymphoid organs that express the highest amounts of CXCL12 (118, 121). However, cells lacking CXCR4 are still able to move out of the white pulp cords or the LN cortex, possibly indicating that downregulation of CXCR5 and CCR7 is adequate to lead to the displacement of cells from follicles and T zones. CXCR4 is also required for efficient homing to bone marrow, whereas homing of IgA plasma cells to epithelial tissues appears to involve CCR9 and/or CCR10 (for recent reviews on plasma cell homing, see 121, 122).

Germinal centers normally emerge in the central, CXCL13-rich region of lymphoid follicles (Figure 2), and in mice lacking CXCL13 or CXCR5, GCs are small and mislocalized (20, 21, 123). Like the surrounding lymphoid tissue, germinal centers are organized into compartments; the principal compartments are the T-zone proximal dark zone, made up predominantly of B cell blasts (centroblasts), and the T-zone distal light zone that contains centroblast-derived centrocytes, a dense network of GC FDC and helper T cells. After undergoing somatic mutation, centroblasts move from the dark zone to the light zone where, as centrocytes, they compete to bind antigen and interact with helper T cells (124). Centroblasts have elevated surface levels of CXCR4 compared with centrocytes and follicular B cells, and CXCR4 is required for the development of GC dark and light zones (125). Although CXCL12 is most highly expressed within medullary cords and red pulp, low amounts can also be detected within the GC, with higher abundance in the DZ than in the LZ, and CXCR4 is needed for GC B cells to localize in the dark zone (125). By contrast, CXCL13 is more abundant in the GC light zone, where it is associated with GC FDC. CXCR5 helps guide cells to the light zone and is required for correct positioning of the light zone at the pole of the GC distal to the T zone (125).

Factors Controlling Chemokine Protein Distribution

CXCL12 is notable for the diverse roles it plays, even within a single organ. Present at low amounts within the GC, this chemokine is essential for organization of the cells within this structure, yet it is produced in higher amounts in the adjacent follicular and T-zone compartments and at still higher levels in the nearby medulla (or red pulp) (125). Apparently, these domains of expression can function in isolation despite their proximity, suggesting the existence of mechanisms that tightly limit chemokine spread. Our understanding of the role of chemokine display systems in lymphoid tissues and elsewhere is still rudimentary, although heparan- and chondroitin sulfate–containing proteoglycans are likely to be important (5, 11). Some chemokines may also bind selectively to extracellular matrix proteins, such as collagen or fibronectin (11, 126), and there may be proteins within lymphoid tissues, such as Mac25, that are specialized for chemokine binding and display (127). Chemokine spread may be negatively regulated by the action of proteases, such as dipeptidylpeptidase IV (CD26) and various metalloproteases, that cleave and inactivate many chemokines (5, 128). Whether molecules such as the duffy antigen and D6, nonsignaling chemokine receptors, have roles in limiting chemokine distribution or half-life within lymphoid tissues needs investigation (5). Furthermore, molecules related to the broad-spectrum chemokine antagonists identified within viruses may well exist and act to limit chemokine function, just as negative regulators of morphogens limit theirs (129, 130). A combination of these mechanisms is likely to help ensure that the chemokine-rich lymphoid organ environment maintains well-delineated compartment boundaries.

SPHINGOSINE-1-PHOSPHATE AND LYMPHOID ORGAN EXIT

Lymphocyte Egress from Secondary Lymphoid Organs

Over 40 years ago, the classic experiments of Gowans and coworkers (131) showed that lymphocytes recirculate by traveling from blood to LNs and then into lymph. From these studies it became evident that lymphocytes are continually exiting LNs and PPs into efferent lymphatic vessels and then returning to circulation via the thoracic duct. Ingenious experiments by Ford and coworkers (132, 133) established that lymphocytes also recirculated from the spleen and that most lymphocytes were part of a large pool of recirculating cells. Ultrastructural analysis of LNs identified structures, termed cortical sinusoids, that contained many lymphocytes and connected to the medullary sinuses. These structures were suggested to be involved in exit (134–136) (Figure 3). Once in medullary sinuses, cells are thought to flow freely into efferent lymph (136). Although PPs do not contain medullary sinuses, the lymphoid regions are encompassed by a network of lymphatic vessels,

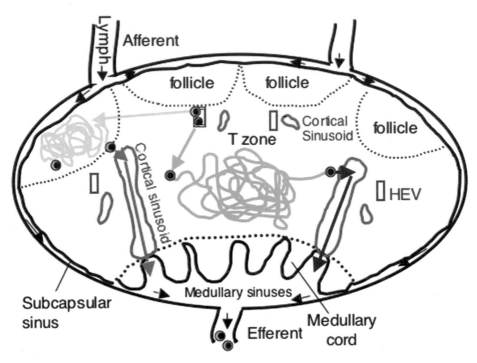

Figure 3   Lymphocyte recirculation through a lymph node. Diagram represents a lymph node cross-section and highlights in color the possible paths taken by a single B cell (*yellow*) or T cell (*blue*). After extensive migration in the follicle or T zone, respectively, the cells travel into the efferent lymphatics. Cortical sinusoids (*brown*), which are lymphatic-related structures present in the outer T zone, connect with the medullary sinuses, and entry into these structures may be the earliest committed step in LN egress. Alternatively, lymphocytes may exit directly into the medullary or subcapsular sinuses.

and cells have been observed migrating into these vessels (137, 138). The exit pathway within spleen has not been well characterized but is likely to involve cells migrating from the white pulp into the red pulp and returning to blood circulation via venous sinuses (139). Early molecular insight into requirements for exit from a lymphoid organ came from the finding that expression of the ADP-ribosylating subunit of PTX in thymocytes blocked their egress from the thymus, implicating the involvement of a Gαi-coupled receptor (140). More recently, studies on a small molecule, FTY720 (2-amino-2-[2-(4-octylphenyl) ethyl] propane-1,3-diol hydrochloride), identified during a screen for immunosuppressant drugs, have proved instructive.

FTY720, a Sequestration-Inducing Drug

Myriocin (ISP-1), the precursor of FTY720, was isolated in a screen for natural products that inhibited the mixed lymphocyte reaction (MLR) (141). Myriocin is a sphingosine-related molecule that binds and inhibits serine palmitoyl-transferase, an enzyme involved in sphingolipid biosynthesis (142). Tests of synthetic myriocin derivatives for an improved ability to prevent skin allograft rejection led to identification of FTY720 (143). FTY720 has protective activity in a variety of animal models of transplant and autoimmune diseases, and clinical trials in renal transplant patients suggest it may have promise as a new type of immunosuppressant (144). The mechanism of FTY720 action in vivo (discussed below) appears to have little or no relationship to the manner of myriocin-mediated MLR inhibition in vitro, demonstrating that serendipity continues to have a role in drug discovery.

Some of the earliest studies with FTY720 showed that it causes rapid loss of lymphocytes from the blood (lymphopenia), reducing numbers by 10- to 100-fold within a few hours (145, 146). The effect is lymphocyte selective, and circulating NK and myeloid cell numbers are not affected (145, 147, 148). In contrast to the effect in blood, lymphocyte numbers in LNs and PPs are slightly increased after 6 to 24 h of treatment (146, 149). Homing into lymphoid organs appears necessary for the effect of FTY720 treatment as L-selectin-low memory T cells and CCR7-deficient T and B cells are less efficiently cleared from the blood (150, 151). A thoracic duct cannulation study in rats demonstrated that naive lymphocytes also disappear from the lymph of FTY720-treated animals (146). Because the only pathway for naive lymphocytes to enter lymph is by exit from lymphoid organs, these data provided some of the first evidence that FTY720 acts by inhibiting lymphoid organ egress. FTY720 treatment also causes accumulation of late-stage CD4 and CD8 single positive cells in the thymus, and intrathymic FITC labeling experiments confirmed that this accumulation is due to a block in thymic egress (147, 152). Furthermore, FTY720 inhibits egress of activated T lymphocytes from LNs that are draining a site of immunization (153). The egress-blocking activity of FTY720 most likely explains many of its immunosuppressive effects, blocking effector cells from reaching transplanted tissue or sites that would normally be targeted by autoreactive cells.

FTY720 is Phosphorylated by Sphingosine Kinase

Myriocin inhibits serine palmitoyl-transferase, but FTY720 has no effect on this enzyme (143). Insight into the mechanism of FTY720 action came with the discovery that it is a substrate for kinases that phosphorylate sphingosine, and within one hour of injection most of the drug exists in the phosphorylated state (149, 154). Two sphingosine kinases have been characterized in mammals, SphK1 and SphK2, and in vitro SphK2 is the more active enzyme in mediating FTY720 phosphorylation (155, 156). The structural similarity of FTY720-phosphate (FTY720-P) to sphingosine-1-phosphate (S1P) led to experiments to test the activity of the drug on S1P receptors, and it was found to engage four of the five known S1P receptors (149, 154). These findings provided the first indication that S1P receptors might be involved in lymphocyte recirculation.

S1P Receptors and Lymphocyte Egress

The first S1P receptor was identified during experiments to define the ligand for endothelial differentiation gene-1 (Edg-1) (157). Cells expressing this 7-transmembrane receptor formed cell-cell aggregates in the presence of serum, and fractionation of the serum revealed that the activity was due to S1P (157). Four additional S1P receptors were subsequently identified: $S1P_2$ (Edg-5), $S1P_3$ (Edg-3), $S1P_4$ (Edg-6), and $S1P_5$ (Edg-8) (158). A related set of receptors (LPA-1, -2, and -3 formerly known as Edg-2, -4, and -7, respectively) bind another serum lysophospholipid, lysophosphatidic acid (LPA) (159). Although originally identified as endothelial differentiation genes, S1P receptors are expressed by many cell types (158). Naive T and B lymphocytes express high amounts of $S1P_1$ and lesser amounts of $S1P_2$, $S1P_3$, and $S1P_4$ (37, 160). Within the thymus, $S1P_1$ mRNA is poorly expressed in immature CD4- and CD8-double-positive cells, but it becomes upregulated as the cells mature to the CD4- and CD8-single-positive stage and is highest on the most mature, L-selectin-high single-positive thymocytes (161, 162).

Although some of the initial findings with FTY720 suggested it may block lymphocyte egress via effects on endothelial cells (149), the finding that one of its target receptors, $S1P_1$, was present at high levels in mature thymocytes and peripheral T cells led to experiments to test whether this receptor was required within lymphocytes during egress. $S1P_1$ deficiency in mice causes embryonic lethality at ∼e13.5 owing to defective blood vessel development, precluding a direct analysis of its role in lymphoid cells (163). However, analysis of $S1P_1$-deficient fetal liver chimeras, or mice carrying LoxP-flanked $S1P_1$ alleles and thymically expresssed Cre recombinase, revealed that $S1P_1$ is essential within T cells for egress from the thymus (161, 162). This intrinsic requirement of $S1P_1$, a Gαi-coupled receptor, within T cells for thymic egress is in agreement with the finding that egress is PTX sensitive (140, 158). When $S1P_1$-deficient thymocytes are transferred intravenously into wild-type recipients, the T cells are able to enter secondary lymphoid organs but they are unable to exit, as measured by their lack of appearance in efferent lymph (161) (Figure 4A). $S1P_1$-deficient B cells are able to exit from the bone marrow of fetal liver chimeras and enter secondary lymphoid organs, but like the T cells, they are very poor in exiting from secondary lymphoid organs (161). Therefore, a common mechanism of egress appears to operate for lymphocytes exiting from thymus and secondary lymphoid organs that depends on $S1P_1$ expression by the lymphocyte. The key role of $S1P_1$ in egress is also indicated by the lack of effect of $S1P_2$ or $S1P_3$ deficiency on egress and the ability of small molecules that selectively bind $S1P_1$ to cause lymphocyte sequestration (159, 164, 165).

Mechanism of FTY720-Induced Lymphocyte Sequestration

In vitro, FTY720-P acts as an agonist on $S1P_1$, $S1P_3$, $S1P_4$, and $S1P_5$, leading to increases in intracellular calcium levels and GTPγS membrane-binding, ERK

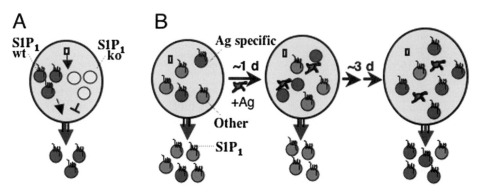

Figure 4 $S1P_1$ is required in lymphocytes for egress and is transiently down-modulated on activated lymphocytes. (*A*) Wild-type lymphocytes (*dark blue*) are able to enter and exit secondary lymphoid organs, whereas $S1P_1$-deficient lymphocytes (*yellow*) are able to enter but are unable to exit. (*B*) During an immune response, induced, for example, by an antigen carried into a lymphoid tissue by a DC (*purple*), antigen-specific T lymphocytes (*red*) downregulate $S1P_1$ and become selectively retained within the antigen-bearing lymphoid organ, whereas lymphocytes of other specificities (*green*) maintain $S1P_1$ expression and continue to recirculate. After 2–3 days of activation and several rounds of cell division, antigen-specific cells re-express $S1P_1$ and again begin leaving the organ and appearing in circulation. In addition to increasing the precursor frequency within the responding lymphoid tissue, transient retention of cells during activation is likely to be important in ensuring that the developing effector cells are correctly programmed in terms of homing receptor and cytokine gene-expression profile before entering circulation.

and AKT phosphorylation, and inhibition of forskolin-induced cAMP in receptor-bearing cells (149, 154, 166). How, then, can FTY720 treatment phenocopy the effect of $S1P_1$ deficiency and block egress? It appears that prolonged exposure to FTY720 causes $S1P_1$ downregulation and inactivation (160, 161). T cells taken from mice treated with FTY720 exhibit a loss of S1P chemotactic responsiveness, and when cells expressing epitope-tagged $S1P_1$ are exposed to FTY720 or the phosphorylated form of the drug, a marked downregulation of the receptor occurs over a period of a few hours, with evidence that the receptor is undergoing degradation (160, 161, 167). Earlier studies had demonstrated that $S1P_1$ is rapidly downregulated following exposure to S1P (168). Therefore, the loss of $S1P_1$ following drug treatment might best be explained by FTY720-P functioning as an $S1P_1$ agonist that cannot be readily dissociated or inactivated following receptor internalization, causing the receptor to be directed to a catabolic pathway. However, further experiments are needed to address this possibility fully. FTY720 also has effects on endothelial cells, such as increasing tight-junction formation and reducing vascular permeability (144, 166). Although these effects might contribute to the therapeutic properties of the drug (169), they are not required for its effect on egress. FTY720's effects on the heart, such as induction of bradycardia, appear to be mediated by $S1P_3$ (164, 165).

S1P Production, Regulation, and Activity

The requirement of $S1P_1$ for thymocyte egress and T and B lymphocyte recirculation indicates that its natural ligand, S1P, is involved in promoting egress. This involvement is supported by the demonstration that infusion of high amounts of S1P causes transient sequestration of lymphocytes, possibly by downregulating $S1P_1$ or disrupting endogenous S1P gradients (149). Although the function of S1P in egress has only recently been defined, the study of S1P production within cells has a long history, and S1P has a large array of physiological roles, including effects on cell migration, adhesion, proliferation, and survival (156, 158, 170). S1P is produced through SphK-mediated phosphorylation of sphingosine, a lipid that can be generated de novo or by breakdown of membrane sphingolipids such as sphingomyelin (Figure 5). Although some extracellular SphK activity has been detected, most of the kinase is intracellular, and the mechanisms controlling S1P release from cells are poorly understood (156, 170). As well as generating extracellular S1P, SphK is important within cells for regulating amounts of sphingosine and of the sphingosine precursor, ceramide, both of which are toxic for many cell types (156, 170). After sphingosine is phosphorylated, it becomes a substrate for S1P

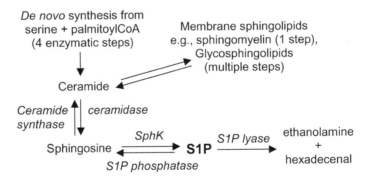

Figure 5   Sphingosine-1-phosphate (S1P) biosynthesis and degradation. Key enzymes (*italicized*) involved in the formation and degradation of S1P are shown. Sphingosine kinase (SphK) is an important point of regulation of S1P synthesis, as it is controlled at the transcriptional level and by phosphorylation, Ca^{2+}/calmodulin binding, and regulated membrane association (156, 172). Sphingolipid biosynthesis occurs predominantly in the Golgi apparatus, whereas degradation occurs in lysosomes. However, the pool of SphK involved in generating extracellular S1P may be separate from the pool involved in sphingolipid metabolism, and it is possibly localized to the plasma membrane. In addition to the pathways indicated, sphingosine can also be obtained in the diet.

lyase, which irreversibly cleaves S1P at the C2-C3 bond to release ethanolamine and hexadecenal (156, 170). S1P levels are also negatively regulated by the actions of S1P phosphatases (SPP1 and SPP2) and possibly by the more general specificity lipid phosphate phophastases (LPPs) (156, 170). SphK, S1P-phosphatase, and S1P lyase enzymes are present in organisms as diverse as yeast and mammals, and appropriate regulation of levels of intracellular S1P, sphingosine, and ceramide is important during yeast responses to stress. In mammalian cells, in addition to being an intermediate in sphingolipid metabolism, S1P can mediate intracellular signaling events, although separating these effects from the extracellular actions of S1P on S1P receptors has been difficult (156, 170).

S1P is present at 100–300 nM in plasma (171, 172) and is also found at high amounts in ovarian ascites (171) and in lymph (M. Matloubian & J.G. Cyster, unpublished observations). Because it is relatively insoluble in aqueous solution, most of the plasma S1P is bound to carriers such as albumin (173). Platelets, which are unique in lacking S1P lyase, contain large amounts of S1P in microvesicles that can be released upon activation, with the local increases in S1P possibly having a role in wound healing (159, 171). Some platelet S1P discharge occurs in the absence of activation, and platelets are considered to be a source of basal plasma S1P. Blood mononuclear cells, neutrophils, and erythrocytes can also efficiently phosphorylate exogenously added sphingosine and discharge S1P into the medium, which suggests a general contribution of hematopoietic cells in maintaining plasma S1P levels (174). This suggestion is also supported by the finding that FTY720 uptake, phosphorylation, and release is more efficient in lymphoid tissues compared with heart, liver, and kidney, despite abundant SphK2 in the latter organs (154). Endothelial cells, by contrast, produce little S1P from exogenous sphingosine and are inefficient in discharging S1P, properties that might help restrict the movement of S1P from circulation into tissues (175).

S1P and Egress Control

One model for the mechanism of S1P action in lymphocyte egress posits that an increasing S1P concentration gradient exists between the interior of the lymphoid tissue and the adjacent blood or lymph, and the lymphocyte response to S1P via $S1P_1$ overcomes the action of retention signals, such as lymphoid chemokines, and promotes egress. Consistent with this model, high concentrations of S1P reduce in vitro responses of activated lymphocytes to lymphoid chemokines (176, 177). Moreover, retention of MZ B cells within the MZ involves $S1P_1$ signals counteracting CXCL13-mediated recruitment, although it is not known whether this effect is directly at the level of CXCR5 or involves changes in molecules that affect responsiveness to other directional cues (37). $S1P_1$ can activate a variety of intracellular pathways in various cell types, including Akt, Erk, Rac, and possibly NF-κB (158). Further characterization of $S1P_1$ signaling in lymphocytes will be important in elucidating the mechanisms regulating thymic egress and lymphocyte recirculation.

In addition to effects on egress, FTY720 treatment and $S1P_1$ deficiency affect surface expression of the activation marker, CD69, albeit with opposite effect; FTY720 causes downregulation and $S1P_1$ deficiency causes constitutive expression (152, 161). $S1P_1$ was also identified as a negative regulator of CD69 expression in a screen for molecules that could prevent phorbol ester-mediated CD69 upregulation in Jurkat cells (178). The differing effects of FTY720 and $S1P_1$ deficiency on this marker, compared with their similar effects on egress, are not yet explained but might indicate that CD69 downregulation occurs because of acute effects of FTY720 signaling prior to $S1P_1$ inactivation. Alternatively, FTY720 may not fully inactivate S1P1 but instead act as a partial agonist, inducing signals that regulate CD69 but that are not adequate to promote egress. AMD3100, a small molecule that inhibits CXCR4 responses to CXCL12, has partial agonist activity (179). The relationship between $S1P_1$, CD69, and egress is intriguing in that transgenic overexpression of CD69 in thymocytes inhibits egress (180, 181). However, the opposing effects of FTY720 and $S1P_1$ deficiency on CD69 expression, the lack of CD69 expression by recirculating lymphocytes, and the lack of effect of CD69 deficiency on egress (182) argue against the conclusion that CD69 is the point of egress control by $S1P_1$.

Retention of Antigen-Specific Cells

Soon after the discovery that lymphocytes recirculate, antigen was shown to cause a transient retention of antigen-reactive cells within lymphoid organs (183, 184) (Figure 4B). This process increases the accumulation of antigen-specific cells in lymphoid organs during an immune response and may help ensure that the cells receive adequate developmental programming before they exit. Correlative evidence suggests that retention occurs because of downregulation of $S1P_1$ within the antigen-activated cells. In vitro, down-modulation of $S1P_1$ mRNA occurs following anti-CD3 and anti-CD28 stimulation of T cells (185). In vivo, antigen-activated T cells downregulate $S1P_1$ mRNA more than 50-fold within one day of activation and they lose S1P chemotactic responsiveness (161). However, after three days, a time when effector cells begin to appear in circulation, $S1P_1$ mRNA abundance is increased and the cells regain S1P responsiveness (161). $S1P_1$ downregulation during lymphocyte activation may also serve to remove negative regulatory effects of $S1P_1$ signaling (178).

Lymphoid Organ Shutdown

In addition to selective retention of antigen-reactive cells, lymphoid organs can undergo a more generalized block or "shutdown" in lymphocyte egress early during the immune response, a process that helps increase precursor frequency in the lymphoid organ (153, 186). Mediators of this nonantigen-selective process include TNF, IFNα/β, and possibly activated DC (187–190). As TNF can induce increased SphK activity (156), one mechanism for shutdown might involve a local overproduction of S1P that disrupts S1P gradients or causes downregulation of lymphocyte $S1P_1$.

CONCLUSION AND FUTURE PERSPECTIVES

Two types of GPCR ligand are now understood to play essential roles in lymphocyte recirculation through lymphoid organs. Proteinaceous ligands (chemokines) are necessary during entry and homing to subcompartments, whereas a lipid (S1P) is required during egress. One key distinction between these systems is that chemokines act as local messengers within the tissue whereas S1P detection appears to serve as a plasma- and lymph-sensing mechanism. Many fundamental questions remain regarding chemokines, S1P, and the regulation of cell migration during adaptive immunity. Much is still to be learned about the transcriptional regulation of chemokine expression within lymphoid tissues. Although $LT\alpha 1\beta 2$-mediated induction of NF-κB molecules is involved, these requirements are common for CCL19, CCL21, and CXCL13, and they fail to explain how follicular and T-zone chemokines are differentially expressed. Also important is defining to what extent lymphoid chemokines function in vivo as chemoattractants. Most data are consistent with the notion that chemokines attract cells that have reached the boundary of a lymphoid compartment, but what about within the compartment, where expression appears more uniform? Do chemokines promote cell motility through local variations in concentration or through chemokinetic effects? Or do they merely function to retain cells within their respective compartments?

The understanding of how S1P functions in lymphocyte egress is only at a beginning. Still unresolved is how $S1P_1$ signaling in lymphocytes promotes egress. This process might involve $S1P_1$ overcoming the retention function of lymphoid chemokines or other molecules, but it could also reflect a chemoattractant role for S1P at the point of egress, helping cells to reverse-transmigrate into lymph or blood. Because S1P is present in abundance in the blood, it is anticipated that $S1P_1$ will be rapidly downregulated on circulating lymphocytes. This downregulation could help ensure a delay in the ability of lymphocytes to exit lymphoid organs immediately following entry and thereby allow the cells to be attracted into the lymphoid tissue parenchyma in response to lymphoid chemokines. Egress of lymphocytes and other cell types from bone marrow appears to be unaffected by FTY720 treatment or $S1P_1$ deficiency, a distinction that is critical to the utility of FTY720 as an immunosuppressant. Although more rigorous analysis is required to test for possible effects on hematopoietic stem cell homing, new questions arise about the requirements for bone marrow egress.

The sophisticated understanding of lymphocyte recirculation control that is emerging should provide new opportunities for developing immunoregulatory agents. Lymphoid chemokine antagonists might have value in the treatment of chronic inflammatory diseases, such as rheumatoid arthritis, because these chemokines are often induced at sites of chronic inflammation. Agents under development to block $LT\alpha 1\beta 2$ function might prove effective in this context. The roles of CXCL12 in the adaptive immune system are diverse, pointing to a variety of potential therapeutic uses for CXCR4 antagonists but also highlighting the need to consider side effects of such therapies. The strong T cell–recruiting activity of CCL21 points to the merit of focusing on this chemokine in antitumor therapies.

Identification of $S1P_1$-specific antagonists is likely to lead to molecules with more selective immunosuppressant activity than FTY720, and improved understanding of the unique features of the lymphocyte egress pathway may lead to identification of further points for therapeutic intervention.

APPENDIX

Abbreviations used: CD26, dipeptidylpeptidase IV; DC, dendritic cells; FDC, follicular dendritic cells; GC, germinal center; GPCRs, G protein–coupled receptors; HEV, high endothelial venules; LNs, lymph nodes; LPA, lysophosphatidic acid; LPPs, lipid phosphate phophastases; LT, cytokine lymphotoxin; LTIC, lymphoid tissue inducing cell; LTβR, lymphotoxin β-receptor; MLR, mixed lymphocyte reaction; MZ, marginal zone; NIK, NF-κB-inducing kinase; PPs, Peyer's patches; PTX, pertussis toxin; S1P, sphingosine-1-phosphate; SphK, sphingosine kinase; TLR, Toll-like receptor; TNF, tumor necrosis factor.

ACKNOWLEDGMENTS/DISCLOSURE STATEMENT

The author thanks Chris Allen, Guy Cinamon, Charles Lo, Takaharu Okada, and Susan Schwab for comments on the manuscript, Charles Lo for help with figures, and all members of his laboratory for contributions that have influenced the writing of this review. The author declares that he has no competing financial interests.

The *Annual Review of Immunology* is online at
http://immunol.annualreviews.org

LITERATURE CITED

1. McMaster PD, Hudack SS. 1935. The formation of agglutinins within lymph nodes. *J. Exp. Med.* 61:783–805
2. Lakkis FG, Arakelov A, Konieczny BT, Inoue Y. 2000. Immunologic 'ignorance' of vascularized organ transplants in the absence of secondary lymphoid tissue. *Nat. Med.* 6:686–88
3. Rennert PD, Hochman PS, Flavell RA, Chaplin DD, Jayaraman S, et al. 2001. Essential role of lymph nodes in contact hypersensitivity revealed in lymphotoxin-α-deficient mice. *J. Exp. Med.* 193:1227–38
4. Zlotnik A, Yoshie O. 2000. Chemokines: a new classification system and their role in immunity. *Immunity* 12:121–27
5. Rot A, von Andrian UH. 2004. Chemokines in innate and adaptive host defense: basic chemokinese grammar for immune cells. *Annu. Rev. Immunol.* 22:891–928
6. Thelen M. 2001. Dancing to the tune of chemokines. *Nat. Immunol.* 2:129–34
7. Tian Y, New DC, Yung LY, Allen RA, Slocombe PM, et al. 2004. Differential chemokine activation of CC chemokine receptor 1-regulated pathways: ligand selective activation of Gα14-coupled pathways. *Eur. J. Immunol.* 34:785–95
8. Cyster JG. 1999. Chemokines and cell migration in secondary lymphoid organs. *Science* 286:2098–102
9. Muller G, Hopken UE, Lipp M. 2003. The impact of CCR7 and CXCR5 on lymphoid

organ development and systemic immunity. *Immunol. Rev.* 195:117–35

10. von Andrian UH, Mempel TR. 2003. Homing and cellular traffic in lymph nodes. *Nat. Rev. Immunol.* 3:867–78

11. Miyasaka M, Tanaka T. 2004. Lymphocyte trafficking across high endothelial venules: dogmas and enigmas. *Nat. Rev. Immunol.* 4:360–70

12. Rosen SD. 2004. Ligands for L-selectin: homing, inflammation, and beyond. *Annu. Rev. Immunol.* 22:129–56

13. Brelinska R, Pilgrim C. 1982. The significance of the subcompartments of the marginal zone for directing lymphocyte traffic within the splenic pulp of the rat. *Cell Tissue Res.* 226:155–65

14. van Ewijk W, Nieuwenhuis P. 1985. Compartments, domains and migration pathways of lymphoid cells in the splenic pulp. *Experientia* 41:199–208

15. Nieuwenhuis P, Ford WL. 1976. Comparative migration of B- and T-lymphocytes in the rat spleen and lymph nodes. *Cell Immunol.* 23:254–67

16. Lo CG, Lu TT, Cyster JG. 2003. Integrin-dependence of lymphocyte entry into the splenic white pulp. *J. Exp. Med.* 197:353–61

17. Nolte MA, Hamann A, Kraal G, Mebius RE. 2002. The strict regulation of lymphocyte migration to splenic white pulp does not involve common homing receptors. *Immunology* 106:299–307

18. Förster R, Mattis AE, Kremmer E, Wolf E, Brem G, Lipp M. 1996. A putative chemokine receptor, BLR1, directs B cell migration to defined lymphoid organs and specific anatomic compartments of the spleen. *Cell* 87:1037–47

19. Förster R, Schubel A, Breitfeld D, Kremmer E, Renner-Muller I, et al. 1999. CCR7 coordinates the primary immune response by establishing functional microenvironments in secondary lymphoid organs. *Cell* 99:23–33

20. Förster R, Mattis AE, Kremmer E, Wolf E, Brem G, Lipp M. 1996. A putative chemokine receptor, BLR1, directs B cell migration to defined lymphoid organs and specific anatomic compartments of the spleen. *Cell* 87:1037–47

21. Ansel KM, Ngo VN, Hyman PL, Luther SA, Förster R, et al. 2000. A chemokine driven positive feedback loop organizes lymphoid follicles. *Nature* 406:309–14

22. Ansel KM, Harris RB, Cyster JG. 2002. CXCL13 is required for b1 cell homing, natural antibody production, and body cavity immunity. *Immunity* 16:67–76

23. Cyster JG, Ngo VN, Ekland EH, Gunn MD, Sedgwick JD, Ansel KM. 1999. Chemokines and B-cell homing to follicles. *Curr. Top. Microbiol Immunol.* 246:87–92

24. Bowman EP, Campbell JJ, Soler D, Dong Z, Manlongat N, et al. 2000. Developmental switches in chemokine response profiles during B cell differentiation and maturation. *J. Exp. Med.* 191:1303–18

25. Gunn MD, Ngo VN, Ansel KM, Ekland EH, Cyster JG, Williams LT. 1998. A B-cell-homing chemokine made in lymphoid follicles activates Burkitt's lymphoma receptor-1. *Nature* 391:799–803

26. Ngo VN, Korner H, Gunn MD, Schmidt KN, Riminton DS, et al. 1999. Lymphotoxin α/β and tumor necrosis factor are required for stromal cell expression of homing chemokines in B and T cell areas of the spleen. *J. Exp. Med.* 189:403–12

27. Cyster JG, Ansel KM, Reif K, Ekland EH, Hyman PL, et al. 2000. Follicular stromal cells and lymphocyte homing to follicles. *Immunol. Rev.* 176:181–93

28. Ishikawa S, Sato T, Abe M, Nagai S, Onai N, et al. 2001. Aberrant high expression of B lymphocyte chemokine (BLC/CXCL13) by CD11b[+]CD11c[+] dendritic cells in murine lupus and preferential chemotaxis of B1 cells towards BLC. *J. Exp. Med.* 193:1393–402

29. Vissers JL, Hartgers FC, Lindhout E, Figdor CG, Adema GJ. 2001. BLC (CXCL13) is expressed by different

dendritic cell subsets in vitro and in vivo. *Eur. J. Immunol.* 31:1544–49

30. Ito T, Ishikawa S, Sato T, Akadegawa K, Yurino H, et al. 2004. Defective B1 cell homing to the peritoneal cavity and preferential recruitment of B1 cells in the target organs in a murine model for systemic lupus erythematosus. *J. Immunol.* 172:3628–34

31. Miller MJ, Wei SH, Parker I, Cahalan MD. 2002. Two-photon imaging of lymphocyte motility and antigen response in intact lymph node. *Science* 296:1869–73

32. Ming GL, Wong ST, Henley J, Yuan XB, Song HJ, et al. 2002. Adaptation in the chemotactic guidance of nerve growth cones. *Nature* 417:411–18

33. Kraal G. 1992. Cells in the marginal zone of the spleen. *Int. Rev. Cytol.* 132:31–73

34. Martin F, Kearney JF. 2002. Marginal-zone B cells. *Nat. Rev. Immunol.* 2:323–35

35. Lu TT, Cyster JG. 2002. Integrin-mediated long-term B cell retention in the splenic marginal zone. *Science* 297:409–12

36. MacLennan ICM, Gray D, Kumararatne DS, Bazin H. 1982. The lymphocytes of splenic marginal zones: a distinct B-cell lineage. *Immunol. Today* 3:305–7

37. Cinamon G, Matloubian M, Lesneski MJ, Xu Y, Low C, et al. 2004. Sphingosine 1-phosphate receptor 1 promotes B cell localization in the splenic marginal zone. *Nat. Immunol.* 5:713–20

38. Karlsson MC, Guinamard R, Bolland S, Sankala M, Steinman RM, Ravetch JV. 2003. Macrophages control the retention and trafficking of B lymphocytes in the splenic marginal zone. *J. Exp. Med.* 198:333–40

39. Yu P, Wang Y, Chin RK, Martinez-Pomares L, Gordon S, et al. 2002. B cells control the migration of a subset of dendritic cells into B cell follicles via CXC chemokine ligand 13 in a lymphotoxin-dependent fashion. *J. Immunol.* 168:5117–23

40. Gunn MD, Kyuwa S, Tam C, Kakiuchi T, Matsuzawa A, et al. 1999. Mice lacking expression of secondary lymphoid organ chemokine have defects in lymphocyte homing and dendritic cell localization. *J. Exp. Med.* 189:451–60

41. Bousso P, Robey E. 2003. Dynamics of CD8[+] T cell priming by dendritic cells in intact lymph nodes. *Nat. Immunol.* 5:579–85

42. Miller MJ, Wei SH, Cahalan MD, Parker I. 2003. Autonomous T cell trafficking examined in vivo with intravital two-photon microscopy. *Proc. Natl. Acad. Sci. USA* 100:2604–9

43. Mempel TR, Henrickson SE, Von Andrian UH. 2004. T-cell priming by dendritic cells in lymph nodes occurs in three distinct phases. *Nature* 427:154–59

44. Miller MJ, Hejazi AS, Wei SH, Cahalan MD, Parker I. 2004. T cell repertoire scanning is promoted by dynamic dendritic cell behavior and random T cell motility in the lymph node. *Proc. Natl. Acad. Sci. USA* 101:998–1003

45. Gretz JE, Anderson AO, Shaw S. 1997. Cords, channels, corridors and conduits: critical architectural elements facilitating cell interactions in the lymph node cortex. *Immunol. Rev.* 156:11–24

46. Luther SA, Tang HL, Hyman PL, Farr AG, Cyster JG. 2000. Coexpression of the chemokines ELC and SLC by T zone stromal cells and deletion of the ELC gene in the plt/plt mouse. *Proc. Natl. Acad. Sci. USA* 97:12694–99

47. Nolte MA, Belien JA, Schadee-Eestermans I, Jansen W, Unger WW, et al. 2003. A conduit system distributes chemokines and small blood-borne molecules through the splenic white pulp. *J. Exp. Med.* 198:505–12

48. Luther SA, Bidgol A, Hargreaves DC, Schmidt A, Xu Y, et al. 2002. Differing activities of homeostatic chemokines CCL19, CCL21, and CXCL12 in lymphocyte and dendritic cell recruitment and lymphoid neogenesis. *J. Immunol.* 169:424–33

49. Stein JV, Rot A, Luo Y, Narasimhaswamy M, Nakano H, et al. 2000. The CC chemokine thymus-derived chemotactic agent 4 (TCA-4, secondary lymphoid tissue chemokine, 6Ckine, exodus-2) triggers lymphocyte function-associated antigen 1-mediated arrest of rolling T lymphocytes in peripheral lymph node high endothelial venules. *J. Exp. Med.* 191:61–76

50. Chen SC, Vassileva G, Kinsley D, Holzmann S, Manfra D, et al. 2002. Ectopic expression of the murine chemokines CCL21a and CCL21b induces the formation of lymph node-like structures in pancreas, but not skin, of transgenic mice. *J. Immunol.* 168:1001–8

51. Kuprash DV, Alimzhanov MB, Tumanov AV, Grivennikov SI, Shakhov AN, et al. 2002. Redundancy in tumor necrosis factor (TNF) and lymphotoxin (LT) signaling in vivo: mice with inactivation of the entire TNF/LT locus versus single-knockout mice. *Mol. Cell. Biol.* 22:8626–34

52. Dejardin E, Droin NM, Delhase M, Haas E, Cao Y, et al. 2002. The lymphotoxin-β receptor induces different patterns of gene expression via two NF-κB pathways. *Immunity* 17:525–35

53. Lo JC, Chin RK, Lee Y, Kang HS, Wang Y, et al. 2003. Differential regulation of CCL21 in lymphoid/nonlymphoid tissues for effectively attracting T cells to peripheral tissues. *J. Clin. Invest.* 112:1495–505

54. Fu Y-X, Chaplin DD. 1999. Development and maturation of secondary lymphoid tissues. *Annu. Rev. Immunol.* 17:399–433

55. Ngo VN, Cornall RJ, Cyster JG. 2001. Splenic T zone development is B cell dependent. *J. Exp. Med.* 194:1649–60

56. Fagarasan S, Shinkura R, Kamata T, Nogaki F, Ikuta K, et al. 2000. Alymphoplasia (aly)-type nuclear factor κB-inducing kinase (NIK) causes defects in secondary lymphoid tissue chemokine receptor signaling and homing of peritoneal cells to the gut-associated lymphatic tissue system. *J. Exp. Med.* 191:1477–86

57. Weih F, Caamano J. 2003. Regulation of secondary lymphoid organ development by the nuclear factor-κB signal transduction pathway. *Immunol. Rev.* 195:91–105

58. Gommerman JL, Browning JL. 2003. Lymphotoxin/light, lymphoid microenvironments and autoimmune disease. *Nat. Rev. Immunol.* 3:642–55

59. Tumanov A, Kuprash D, Lagarkova M, Grivennikov S, Abe K, et al. 2002. Distinct role of surface lymphotoxin expressed by B cells in the organization of secondary lymphoid tissues. *Immunity* 17:239–50

60. Ansel KM, Cyster JG. 2001. Chemokines in lymphopoiesis and lymphoid organ development. *Curr. Opin. Immunol.* 13:172–79

61. Mebius RE. 2003. Organogenesis of lymphoid tissues. *Nat. Rev. Immunol.* 3:292–303

62. Mebius RE, Rennert P, Weissman IL. 1997. Developing lymph nodes collect CD4$^+$CD3$^-$LTβ^+ cells that can differentiate to APC, NK cells, and follicular cells but not T or B cells. *Immunity* 7:493–504

63. Honda K, Nakano H, Yoshida H, Nishikawa S, Rennert P, et al. 2001. Molecular basis for hematopoietic/mesenchymal interaction during initiation of Peyer's patch organogenesis. *J. Exp. Med.* 193:621–30

64. Luther SA, Ansel KM, Cyster JG. 2003. Overlapping Roles of CXCL13, interleukin 7 receptor α, and CCR7 ligands in lymph node development. *J. Exp. Med.* 197:1191–98

65. Eberl G, Littman DR. 2003. The role of the nuclear hormone receptor RORγt in the development of lymph nodes and Peyer's patches. *Immunol. Rev.* 195:81–90

66. Nishikawa S, Honda K, Vieira P, Yoshida H. 2003. Organogenesis of peripheral lymphoid organs. *Immunol. Rev.* 195:72–80

67. Nossal GJ, Abbot A, Mitchell J, Lummus Z. 1968. Antigens in immunity. XV. Ultrastructural features of antigen capture

in primary and secondary lymphoid follicles. *J. Exp. Med.* 127:277–90

68. Itano AA, Jenkins MK. 2003. Antigen presentation to naive CD4 T cells in the lymph node. *Nat. Immunol.* 4:733–39

69. Humphrey JH, Grennan D. 1981. Different macrophage populations distinguished by means of fluorescent polysaccharides. Recognition and properties of marginal-zone macrophages. *Eur. J. Immunol.* 11:221–28

70. Gretz JE, Norbury CC, Anderson AO, Proudfoot AE, Shaw S. 2000. Lymph-borne chemokines and other low molecular weight molecules reach high endothelial venules via specialized conduits while a functional barrier limits access to the lymphocyte microenvironments in lymph node cortex. *J. Exp. Med.* 192:1425–40

71. Kellermann SA, Hudak S, Oldham ER, Liu YJ, McEvoy LM. 1999. The CC chemokine receptor-7 ligands 6Ckine and macrophage inflammatory protein-3β are potent chemoattractants for in vitro- and in vivo-derived dendritic cells. *J. Immunol.* 162:3859–64

72. Aliberti J, Reis e Sousa C, Schito M, Hieny S, Wells T, et al. 2000. CCR5 provides a signal for microbial induced production of IL-12 by CD8α^+ dendritic cells. *Nat. Immunol.* 1:83–87

73. Iwasaki A, Kelsall BL. 2000. Localization of distinct Peyer's patch dendritic cell subsets and their recruitment by chemokines macrophage inflammatory protein (MIP)-3α, MIP-3β, and secondary lymphoid organ chemokine. *J. Exp. Med.* 191:1381–94

74. Cook DN, Prosser DM, Forster R, Zhang J, Kuklin NA, et al. 2000. CCR6 mediates dendritic cell localization, lymphocyte homeostasis, and immune responses in mucosal tissue. *Immunity* 12:495–503

75. Varona R, Villares R, Carramolino L, Goya I, Zaballos A, et al. 2001. CCR6-deficient mice have impaired leukocyte homeostasis and altered contact hypersensitivity and delayed-type hypersensitivity responses. *J. Clin. Invest.* 107:R37–45

76. Zhao X, Sato A, Dela Cruz CS, Linehan M, Luegering A, et al. 2003. CCL9 is secreted by the follicle-associated epithelium and recruits dome region Peyer's patch CD11b$^+$ dendritic cells. *J. Immunol.* 171:2797–803

77. Szakal AK, Holmes KL, Tew JG. 1983. Transport of immune complexes from the subcapsular sinus to lymph node follicles on the surface of nonphagocytic cells, including cells with dendritic morphology. *J. Immunol.* 131:1714–27

78. Groeneveld PH, Erich T, Kraal G. 1986. The differential effects of bacterial lipopolysaccharide (LPS) on splenic non-lymphoid cells demonstrated by monoclonal antibodies. *Immunology* 58:285–90

79. Martinez-Pomares L, Kosco-Vilbois M, Darley E, Tree P, Herren S, et al. 1996. Fc chimeric protein containing the cysteine-rich domain of the murine mannose receptor binds to macrophages from splenic marginal zone and lymph node subcapsular sinus and to germinal centers. *J. Exp. Med.* 184:1927–37

80. Berney C, Herren S, Power CA, Gordon S, Martinez-Pomares L, Kosco-Vilbois MH. 1999. A member of the dendritic cell family that enters B cell follicles and stimulates primary antibody responses identified by a mannose receptor fusion protein. *J. Exp. Med.* 190:851–60

81. Gray D, Kumararatne DS, Lortan J, Khan M, MacLennan IC. 1984. Relation of intra-splenic migration of marginal zone B cells to antigen localization on follicular dendritic cells. *Immunology* 52:659–69

82. Oldfield S, Lortan JE, Hyatt MA, MacLennan IC. 1988. Marginal zone B cells and the localisation of antigen on follicular dendritic cells. *Adv. Exp. Med. Biol.* 237:99–104

83. Cyster JG. 1999. Chemokines and the homing of dendritic cells to the T cell

areas of lymphoid organs. *J. Exp. Med.* 189:447–50

84. Luther SA, Lopez T, Bai W, Hanahan D, Cyster JG. 2000. BLC expression in pancreatic islets causes B cell recruitment and lymphotoxin-dependent lymphoid neogenesis. *Immunity* 12:471–81

85. Sato N, Ahuja SK, Quinones M, Kostecki V, Reddick RL, et al. 2000. CC chemokine receptor (CCR)2 is required for Langerhans cell migration and localization of T helper cell type 1 (Th1)-inducing dendritic cells. Absence of CCR2 shifts the *Leishmania major*-resistant phenotype to a susceptible state dominated by Th2 cytokines, B cell outgrowth, and sustained neutrophilic inflammation. *J. Exp. Med.* 192:205–18

86. Peters W, Dupuis M, Charo IF. 2000. A mechanism for the impaired IFN-γ production in C-C chemokine receptor 2 (CCR2) knockout mice: role of CCR2 in linking the innate and adaptive immune responses. *J. Immunol.* 165:7072–77

87. Penna G, Sozzani S, Adorini L. 2001. Cutting edge: selective usage of chemokine receptors by plasmacytoid dendritic cells. *J. Immunol.* 167:1862–66

88. Krug A, Uppaluri R, Facchetti F, Dorner BG, Sheehan KC, et al. 2002. IFN-producing cells respond to CXCR3 ligands in the presence of CXCL12 and secrete inflammatory chemokines upon activation. *J. Immunol.* 169:6079–83

89. Shortman K, Liu YJ. 2002. Mouse and human dendritic cell subtypes. *Nat. Rev. Immunol.* 2:151–61

90. Balazs M, Martin F, Zhou T, Kearney J. 2002. Blood dendritic cells interact with splenic marginal zone B cells to initiate T-independent immune responses. *Immunity* 17:341–52

91. Serbina NV, Salazar-Mather TP, Biron CA, Kuziel WA, Pamer EG. 2003. TNF/iNOS-producing dendritic cells mediate innate immune defense against bacterial infection. *Immunity* 19:59–70

92. Reif K, Ekland EH, Ohl L, Nakano H,

Lipp M, et al. 2002. Balanced responsiveness to chemoattractants from adjacent zones determines B-cell position. *Nature* 416:94–99

93. Seo SJ, Fields ML, Buckler JL, Reed AJ, Mandik-Nayak L, et al. 2002. The impact of T helper and T regulatory cells on the regulation of anti-double-stranded DNA B cells. *Immunity* 16:535–46

94. Ekland EH, Forster R, Lipp M, Cyster JG. 2004. Requirements for follicular exclusion and competitive elimination of autoantigen binding B cells. *J. Immunol.* 172:4700–8

95. Mandik-Nayak L, Huang G, Sheehan KC, Erikson J, Chaplin DD. 2001. Signaling through TNF receptor p55 in TNF-α-deficient mice alters the CXCL13/CCL19/CCL21 ratio in the spleen and induces maturation and migration of anergic B cells into the B cell follicle. *J. Immunol.* 167:1920–28

96. Bowman EP, Campbell JJ, Druey KM, Scheschonka A, Kehrl JH, Butcher EC. 1998. Regulation of chemotactic and proadhesive responses to chemoattractant receptors by RGS (regulator of G-protein signaling) family members. *J. Biol. Chem.* 273:28040–48

97. Reif K, Cyster JG. 2000. RGS molecule expression in murine B lymphocytes and ability to down-regulate chemotaxis to lymphoid chemokines. *J. Immunol.* 164:4720–29

98. Shi GX, Harrison K, Wilson GL, Moratz C, Kehrl JH. 2002. RGS13 regulates germinal center B lymphocytes responsiveness to CXC chemokine ligand (CXCL)12 and CXCL13. *J. Immunol.* 169:2507–15

99. Kavelaars A, Vroon A, Raatgever RP, Fong AM, Premont RT, et al. 2003. Increased acute inflammation, leukotriene B4-induced chemotaxis, and signaling in mice deficient for G protein-coupled receptor kinase 6. *J. Immunol.* 171:6128–34

100. Fong AM, Premont RT, Richardson RM, Yu YR, Lefkowitz RJ, Patel DD. 2002. Defective lymphocyte chemotaxis

in β-arrestin2- and GRK6-deficient mice. *Proc. Natl. Acad. Sci. USA* 99:7478–83

101. Sallusto F, Palermo B, Lenig D, Miettinen M, Matikainen S, et al. 1999. Distinct patterns and kinetics of chemokine production regulate dendritic cell function. *Eur. J. Immunol.* 29:1617–25

102. Tang HL, Cyster JG. 1999. Chemokine upregulation and activated T cell attraction by maturing dendritic cells. *Science* 284:819–22

103. Alferink J, Lieberam I, Reindl W, Behrens A, Weiss S, et al. 2003. Compartmentalized production of CCL17 in vivo: strong inducibility in peripheral dendritic cells contrasts selective absence from the spleen. *J. Exp. Med.* 197:585–99

104. Reiss Y, Proudfoot AE, Power CA, Campbell JJ, Butcher EC. 2001. CC chemokine receptor (CCR)4 and the CCR10 ligand cutaneous T cell-attracting chemokine (CTACK) in lymphocyte trafficking to inflamed skin. *J. Exp. Med.* 194:1541–47

105. Mora JR, Bono MR, Manjunath N, Weninger W, Cavanagh LL, et al. 2003. Selective imprinting of gut-homing T cells by Peyer's patch dendritic cells. *Nature* 424:88–93

106. Stagg AJ, Hart AL, Knight SC, Kamm MA. 2003. The dendritic cell: its role in intestinal inflammation and relationship with gut bacteria. *Gut* 52:1522–29

107. Ansel KM, McHeyzer-Williams LJ, Ngo VN, McHeyzer-Williams MG, Cyster JG. 1999. In vivo activated CD4 T cells upregulate CXC chemokine receptor 5 and reprogram their response to lymphoid chemokines. *J. Exp. Med.* 190:1123–34

108. Randolph DA, Huang G, Carruthers CJ, Bromley LE, Chaplin DD. 1999. The role of CCR7 in TH1 and TH2 cell localization and delivery of B cell help in vivo. *Science* 286:2159–62

109. Schaerli P, Willimann K, Lang AB, Lipp M, Loetscher P, Moser B. 2000. CXC chemokine receptor 5 expression defines follicular homing T cells with B cell helper function. *J. Exp. Med.* 192:1553–62

110. Breitfeld D, Ohl L, Kremmer E, Ellwart J, Sallusto F, et al. 2000. Follicular B helper T cells express CXC chemokine receptor 5, localize to B cell follicles, and support immunoglobulin production. *J. Exp. Med.* 192:1545–52

111. Kim CH, Rott LS, Clark-Lewis I, Campbell DJ, Wu L, Butcher EC. 2001. Subspecialization of CXCR5$^+$ T cells: B helper activity is focused in a germinal center-localized subset of CXCR5$^+$ T cells. *J. Exp. Med.* 193:1373–81

112. Campbell DJ, Kim CH, Butcher EC. 2001. Separable effector T cell populations specialized for B cell help or tissue inflammation. *Nat. Immunol.* 2:876–81

113. Bystry RS, Aluvihare V, Welch KA, Kallikourdis M, Betz AG. 2001. B cells and professional APCs recruit regulatory T cells via CCL4. *Nat. Immunol.* 2:1126–32

114. Gavin M, Rudensky A. 2003. Control of immune homeostasis by naturally arising regulatory CD4$^+$ T cells. *Curr. Opin. Immunol.* 15:690–96

115. Mori S, Nakano H, Aritomi K, Wang CR, Gunn MD, Kakiuchi T. 2001. Mice lacking expression of the chemokines CCL21-ser and CCL19 (plt mice) demonstrate delayed but enhanced T cell immune responses. *J. Exp. Med.* 193:207–18

116. Iellem A, Mariani M, Lang R, Recalde H, Panina-Bordignon P, et al. 2001. Unique chemotactic response profile and specific expression of chemokine receptors CCR4 and CCR8 by CD4$^+$CD25$^+$ regulatory T cells. *J. Exp. Med.* 194:847–53

117. Annunziato F, Cosmi L, Liotta F, Lazzeri E, Manetti R, et al. 2002. Phenotype, localization, and mechanism of suppression of CD4$^+$CD25$^+$ human thymocytes. *J. Exp. Med.* 196:379–87

118. Hargreaves DC, Hyman PL, Lu TT, Ngo VN, Bidgol A, et al. 2001. A coordinated change in chemokine responsiveness

guides plasma cell movements. *J. Exp. Med.* 194:45–56

119. Wehrli N, Legler DF, Finke D, Toellner K-M, Loetscher P, et al. 2001. Changing responsiveness to chemokines allows medullary plasmablasts to leave lymph nodes. *Eur. J. Immunol.* 31:609–16

120. Hauser AE, Debes GF, Arce S, Cassese G, Hamann A, et al. 2002. Chemotactic responsiveness toward ligands for CXCR3 and CXCR4 is regulated on plasma blasts during the time course of a memory immune response. *J. Immunol.* 169:1277–82

121. Cyster JG. 2003. Homing of antibody secreting cells. *Immunol. Rev.* 194:48–60

122. Kunkel EJ, Butcher EC. 2003. Plasmacell homing. *Nat. Rev. Immunol.* 3:822–29

123. Voigt I, Camacho SA, de Boer BA, Lipp M, Förster R, Berek C. 2000. CXCR5-deficient mice develop functional germinal centers in the splenic T cell zone. *Eur. J. Immunol.* 30:560–67

124. MacLennan ICM. 1994. Germinal centers. *Annu. Rev. Immunol.* 12:117–39

125. Allen CDC, Ansel KM, Low C, Lesley R, Tamamura H, Fujii N, Cyster JG. 2004. Germinal center dark and light zone organization is mediated by CXCR4. *Nat. Immunol.* In press

126. Pelletier AJ, van der Laan LJ, Hildbrand P, Siani MA, Thompson DA, et al. 2000. Presentation of chemokine SDF-1α by fibronectin mediates directed migration of T cells. *Blood* 96:2682–90

127. Nagakubo D, Murai T, Tanaka T, Usui T, Matsumoto M, et al. 2003. A high endothelial venule secretory protein, mac25/angiomodulin, interacts with multiple high endothelial venule-associated molecules including chemokines. *J. Immunol.* 171:553–61

128. Moser B, Wolf M, Walz A, Loetscher P. 2004. Chemokines: multiple levels of leukocyte migration control. *Trends Immunol.* 25:75–84

129. Alexander JM, Nelson CA, van Berkel V, Lau EK, Studts JM, et al. 2002. Structural basis of chemokine sequestration by a herpesvirus decoy receptor. *Cell* 111:343–56

130. Freeman M, Gurdon JB. 2002. Regulatory principles of developmental signaling. *Annu. Rev. Cell Dev. Biol.* 18:515–39

131. Gowans JL, Knight EJ. 1964. The route of re-circulation of lymphocytes in the rat. *Proc. R. Soc. London Ser. B* 159:257–82

132. Ford WL. 1968. The mechanism of lymphopenia produced by chronic irradiation of the rat spleen. *Br. J. Exp. Pathol.* 49:502–10

133. Ford WL. 1969. The immunological and migratory properties of the lymphocytes recirculating through the rat spleen. *Br. J. Exp. Pathol.* 50:257–69

134. Soderstrom N, Stenstrom A. 1969. Outflow paths of cells from the lymph node parenchyma to the efferent lymphatics—observations in thin section histology. *Scand. J. Haematol.* 6:186–96

135. Kelly RH. 1975. Functional anatomy of lymph nodes. I. The paracortical cords. *Int. Arch. Allergy Appl. Immunol.* 48:836–49

136. Belisle C, Sainte-Marie G. 1981. Tridimensional study of the deep cortex of the rat lymph node. III. Morphology of the deep cortex units. *Anat. Rec.* 199:213–26

137. Tsuzuki Y, Miura S, Suematsu M, Kurose I, Shigematsu T, et al. 1996. alpha 4 integrin plays a critical role in early stages of T lymphocyte migration in Peyer's patches of rats. *Int. Immunol.* 8:287–95

138. Azzali G. 2003. Structure, lymphatic vascularization and lymphocyte migration in mucosa-associated lymphoid tissue. *Immunol. Rev.* 195:178–89

139. Bowdler AJ, ed. 1990. *The Spleen. Structure, Function and Clinical Significance.* London: Chapman & Hall Med. 515 pp.

140. Chaffin KE, Perlmutter RM. 1991. A pertussis toxin sensitive process controls thymocyte emigration. *Eur. J. Immunol.* 21:2565–73

141. Fujita T, Inoue K, Yamamoto S, Ikumoto

T, Sasaki S, et al. 1994. Fungal metabolites. Part 11. A potent immunosuppressive activity found in *Isaria sinclairii* metabolite. *J. Antibiot.* 47:208–15

142. Miyake Y, Kozutsumi Y, Nakamura S, Fujita T, Kawasaki T. 1995. Serine palmitoyltransferase is the primary target of a sphingosine-like immunosuppressant, ISP-1/myriocin. *Biochem. Biophys. Res. Commun.* 211:396–403

143. Fujita T, Hirose R, Yoneta M, Sasaki S, Inoue K, et al. 1996. Potent immunosuppressants, 2-alkyl-2-aminopropane-1,3-diols. *J. Med. Chem.* 39:4451–59

144. Brinkmann V, Cyster JG, Hla T. 2004. FTY720: Sphingosine 1-phosphate receptor-1 in the control of lymphocyte egress and endothelial barrier function. *Am. J. Transplant.* 4:1019–25

145. Suzuki S, Enosawa S, Kakefuda T, Shinomiya T, Amari M, et al. 1996. A novel immunosuppressant, FTY720, with a unique mechanism of action, induces long-term graft acceptance in rat and dog allotransplantation. *Transplantation* 61:200–5

146. Chiba K, Yanagawa Y, Masubuchi Y, Kataoka H, Kawaguchi T, et al. 1998. FTY720, a novel immunosuppressant, induces sequestration of circulating mature lymphocytes by acceleration of lymphocyte homing in rats. I. FTY720 selectively decreases the number of circulating mature lymphocytes by acceleration of lymphocyte homing. *J. Immunol.* 160:5037–44

147. Yagi H, Kamba R, Chiba K, Soga H, Yaguchi K, et al. 2000. Immunosuppressant FTY720 inhibits thymocyte emigration. *Eur. J. Immunol.* 30:1435–44

148. Budde K, Schmouder RL, Nashan B, Brunkhorst R, Lücker PW, et al. 2003. Pharmacodynamics of single doses of the novel immunosuppressant FTY720 in stable renal transplant patients. *Am. J. Transplant.* 3:846–54

149. Mandala S, Hajdu R, Bergstrom J, Quackenbush E, Xie J, et al. 2002. Alteration of lymphocyte trafficking by sphingosine-1-phosphate receptor agonists. *Science* 296:346–49

150. Henning G, Ohl L, Junt T, Reiterer P, Brinkmann V, et al. 2001. CC chemokine receptor 7-dependent and -independent pathways for lymphocyte homing: modulation by FTY720. *J. Exp. Med.* 194:1875–81

151. Bohler T, Waiser J, Schuetz M, Neumayer HH, Budde K. 2004. FTY720 exerts differential effects on CD4$^+$ and CD8$^+$ T-lymphocyte subpopulations expressing chemokine and adhesion receptors. *Nephrol. Dial. Transplant.* 19:702–13

152. Rosen H, Alfonso C, Surh CD, McHeyzer-Williams MG. 2003. Rapid induction of medullary thymocyte phenotypic maturation and egress inhibition by nanomolar sphingosine 1-phosphate receptor agonist. *Proc. Natl. Acad. Sci. USA* 100:10907–12

153. Xie JH, Nomura N, Koprak SL, Quackenbush EJ, Forrest MJ, Rosen H. 2003. Sphingosine-1-phosphate receptor agonism impairs the efficiency of the local immune response by altering trafficking of naive and antigen-activated CD4$^+$ T cells. *J. Immunol.* 170:3662–70

154. Brinkmann V, Davis MD, Heise CE, Albert R, Cottens S, et al. 2002. The immune modulator FTY720 targets sphingosine 1-phosphate receptors. *J. Biol. Chem.* 277:21453–57

155. Paugh SW, Payne SG, Barbour SE, Milstien S, Spiegel S. 2003. The immunosuppressant FTY720 is phosphorylated by sphingosine kinase type 2. *FEBS Lett.* 554:189–93

156. Spiegel S, Milstien S. 2003. Sphingosine-1-phosphate: an enigmatic signalling lipid. *Nat. Rev. Mol. Cell Biol.* 4:397–407

157. Lee MJ, Van Brocklyn JR, Thangada S, Liu CH, Hand AR, et al. 1998. Sphingosine-1-phosphate as a ligand for the G protein-coupled receptor EDG-1. *Science* 279:1552–55

158. Hla T. 2003. Signaling and biological actions of sphingosine 1-phosphate. *Pharmacol. Res.* 47:401–7

159. Ishii I, Fukushima N, Ye X, Chun J. 2004. Lysophospholipid receptors: signaling and biology. *Annu. Rev. Biochem.* 73:321–54

160. Graler MH, Goetzl EJ. 2004. The immunosuppressant FTY720 down-regulates sphingosine 1-phosphate G protein-coupled receptors. *FASEB J.* 18: 551–53

161. Matloubian M, Lo CG, Cinamon G, Lesneski MJ, Xu Y, et al. 2004. Lymphocyte egress from thymus and peripheral lymphoid organs is dependent on S1P receptor 1. *Nature* 427:355–60

162. Allende ML, Dreier JL, Mandala S, Proia RL. 2004. Expression of the sphingosine-1-phosphate receptor, S1P$_1$, on T-cells controls thymic emigration. *J. Biol. Chem.* 279:15396–401

163. Liu Y, Wada R, Yamashita T, Mi Y, Deng CX, et al. 2000. Edg-1, the G protein-coupled receptor for sphingosine-1-phosphate, is essential for vascular maturation. *J. Clin. Invest.* 106:951–61

164. Forrest M, Sun SY, Hajdu R, Bergstrom J, Card D, et al. 2004. Immune cell regulation and cardiovascular effects of sphingosine 1-phosphate receptor agonists in rodents are mediated via distinct receptor sub-types. *J. Pharmacol. Exp. Ther.* 309:758–68

165. Sanna MG, Liao J, Jo E, Alfonso C, Ahn MY, et al. 2004. Sphingosine 1-phosphate (S1P) receptor subtypes S1P$_1$ and S1P$_3$, respectively, regulate lymphocyte recirculation and heart rate. *J. Biol. Chem.* 279:13839–48

166. Sanchez T, Estrada-Hernandez T, Paik JH, Wu MT, Venkataraman K, et al. 2003. Phosphorylation and action of the immunomodulator FTY720 inhibits vascular endothelial cell growth factor-induced vascular permeability. *J. Biol. Chem.* 278:47281–90

167. Hale JJ, Neway W, Mills SG, Hajdu R, Ann Keohane C, et al. 2004. Potent S1P receptor agonists replicate the pharmacologic actions of the novel immune modulator FTY720. *Bioorg. Med. Chem. Lett.* 14:3351–55

168. Liu CH, Thangada S, Lee MJ, Van Brocklyn JR, Spiegel S, Hla T. 1999. Ligand-induced trafficking of the sphingosine-1-phosphate receptor EDG-1. *Mol. Biol. Cell* 10:1179–90

169. Peng X, Hassoun PM, Sammani S, McVerry BJ, Burne MJ, et al. 2004. Protective effects of sphingosine 1-phosphate in murine endotoxin-induced inflammatory lung injury. *Am. J. Respir. Crit. Care Med.* 169:1245–51

170. Mandala SM. 2001. Sphingosine-1-phosphate phosphatases. *Prostaglandins Other Lipid Mediat.* 64:143–56

171. Yatomi Y, Ozaki Y, Ohmori T, Igarashi Y. 2001. Sphingosine 1-phosphate: synthesis and release. *Prostaglandins Other Lipid Mediat.* 64:107–22

172. Pyne S, Pyne NJ. 2000. Sphingosine 1-phosphate signalling in mammalian cells. *Biochem. J.* 349:385–402

173. Murata N, Sato K, Kon J, Tomura H, Yanagita M, et al. 2000. Interaction of sphingosine 1-phosphate with plasma components, including lipoproteins, regulates the lipid receptor-mediated actions. *Biochem. J.* 352(Pt. 3):809–15

174. Yang L, Yatomi Y, Miura Y, Satoh K, Ozaki Y. 1999. Metabolism and functional effects of sphingolipids in blood cells. *Br. J. Haematol.* 107:282–93

175. Hisano N, Yatomi Y, Satoh K, Akimoto S, Mitsumata M, et al. 1999. Induction and suppression of endothelial cell apoptosis by sphingolipids: a possible in vitro model for cell-cell interactions between platelets and endothelial cells. *Blood* 93:4293–99

176. Graeler M, Shankar G, Goetzl EJ. 2002. Cutting edge: suppression of T cell chemotaxis by sphingosine 1-phosphate. *J. Immunol.* 169:4084–87

177. Dorsam G, Graeler MH, Seroogy C, Kong

Y, Voice JK, Goetzl EJ. 2003. Transduction of multiple effects of sphingosine 1-phosphate (S1P) on T cell functions by the S1P1 G protein-coupled receptor. *J. Immunol.* 171:3500–7

178. Chu P, Pardo J, Zhao H, Li CC, Pali E, et al. 2003. Systematic identification of regulatory proteins critical for T-cell activation. *J. Biol.* 2:21.1–21.16. doi:10.1186/1475-4924-2-21

179. Zhang WB, Navenot JM, Haribabu B, Tamamura H, Hiramatu K, et al. 2002. A point mutation that confers constitutive activity to CXCR4 reveals that T140 is an inverse agonist and that AMD3100 and ALX40-4C are weak partial agonists. *J. Biol. Chem.* 277:24515–21

180. Nakayama T, Kasprowicz DJ, Yamashita M, Schubert LA, Gillard G, et al. 2002. The generation of mature, single-positive thymocytes in vivo is dysregulated by CD69 blockade or overexpression. *J. Immunol.* 168:87–94

181. Feng C, Woodside KJ, Vance BA, El-Khoury D, Canelles M, et al. 2002. A potential role for CD69 in thymocyte emigration. *Int. Immunol.* 14:535–44

182. Lauzurica P, Sancho D, Torres M, Albella B, Marazuela M, et al. 2000. Phenotypic and functional characteristics of hematopoietic cell lineages in CD69-deficient mice. *Blood* 95:2312–20

183. Sprent J, Miller JFAP, Mitchell GF. 1971. Antigen-induced selective recruitment of circulating lymphocytes. *Cell. Immunol.* 2:171–81

184. Rowley DA, Gowans JL, Atkins RC, Ford WL, Smith ME. 1972. The specific selection of recirculating lymphocytes by antigen in normal and preimmunized rats. *J. Exp. Med.* 136:499–513

185. Graeler M, Goetzl EJ. 2002. Activation-regulated expression and chemotactic function of sphingosine 1-phosphate receptors in mouse splenic T cells. *FASEB J.* 16:1874–78

186. Hall JG, Morris B. 1965. The immediate effect of antigens on the cell output of a lymph node. *Br. J. Exp. Pathol.* 46:450–54

187. Mann EA, Markovic SN, Murasko DM. 1989. Inhibition of lymphocyte recirculation by murine interferon: effects of various interferon preparations and timing of administration. *J. Interferon Res.* 9:35–51

188. Young AJ, Seabrook TJ, Marston WL, Dudler L, Hay JB. 2000. A role for lymphatic endothelium in the sequestration of recirculating $\gamma\delta$ T cells in TNF-α-stimulated lymph nodes. *Eur. J. Immunol.* 30:327–34

189. Martín-Fontecha A, Sebastiani S, Hopken UE, Uguccioni M, Lipp M, et al. 2003. Regulation of dendritic cell migration to the draining lymph node: impact on T lymphocyte traffic and priming. *J. Exp. Med.* 198:615–21

190. McLachlan JB, Hart JP, Pizzo SV, Shelburne CP, Staats HF, et al. 2003. Mast cell-derived tumor necrosis factor induces hypertrophy of draining lymph nodes during infection. *Nat. Immunol.* 4:1199–205

191. Rollins BJ. 1997. Chemokines. *Blood* 90:909–28

192. Youn B-S, Kwon BS. 2000. MIP-1g/MRP-2. In *Cytokine Reference*, ed. JJ Oppenheim, M Feldman, pp. 1237–43. New York: Academic

193. Lasagni L, Francalanci M, Annunziato F, Lazzeri E, Giannini S, et al. 2003. An alternatively spliced variant of CXCR3 mediates the inhibition of endothelial cell growth induced by IP-10, Mig, and I-TAC, and acts as functional receptor for platelet factor 4. *J. Exp. Med.* 197:1537–49

194. Shirozu M, Nakano T, Inazawa J, Tashiro K, Tada H, et al. 1995. Structure and chromosomal localization of the human stromal cell-derived factor 1 (SDF1) gene. *Genomics* 28:495–500

195. Gleichmann M, Gillen C, Czardybon M, Bosse F, Greiner-Petter R, et al. 2000. Cloning and characterization of SDF-1γ, a novel SDF-1 chemokine transcript with developmentally regulated expression in

the nervous system. *Eur. J. Neurosci.* 12: 1857–66

196. Vassileva G, Soto H, Zlotnik A, Nakano H, Kakiuchi T, et al. 1999. The reduced expression of 6Ckine in the *plt* mouse results from the deletion of one of two 6Ckine genes. *J. Exp. Med.* 190:1183–88

197. Nakano H, Gunn MD. 2001. Gene duplications at the chemokine locus on mouse chromosome 4: multiple strain-specific haplotypes and the deletion of secondary lymphoid-organ chemokine and EBI-1 ligand chemokine genes in the *plt* mutation. *J. Immunol.* 166:361–69

Annu. Rev. Immunol. 2005. 23:161–96
doi: 10.1146/annurev.immunol.23.021704.115728
First published online as a Review in Advance on October 20, 2004

MARGINAL ZONE B CELLS

Shiv Pillai, Annaiah Cariappa, and Stewart T. Moran

*Center for Cancer Research, Massachusetts General Hospital and Harvard Medical
School, Boston, Massachusetts 02129; email: pillai@helix.mgh.harvard.edu,
cariappa@helix.mgh.harvard.edu, stmoran@fas.harvard.edu*

Key Words follicular B cells, transitional B cells, B cell receptor, Notch2

■ **Abstract** Our views regarding the origins and functions of splenic marginal zone
B cells have changed considerably over the past few years. Perspectives regarding
the development and function of these cells vary considerably between investigators
studying human and rodent immunology. Marginal zone B cells are now recognized to
constitute a distinct naive B lymphoid lineage. Considerable progress has been made
regarding the mechanisms involved in marginal zone B cell development in the mouse.
Many of the molecular events that participate in the retention of this lineage of B cells
in the marginal zone have been identified. Here, we discuss the functions of these cells
in both innate and adaptive immunity. We also attempt to reconcile differing view-
points regarding the generation and function of marginal zone B cells in rodents and
primates.

INTRODUCTION

In 1901, Weidenreich (1) described a distinguishable concentric collection of cells
surrounding splenic follicles, which he called the Knötchenrand-zone or "the zone
around the small knot." This splenic structure separates the white pulp from the
red pulp and was designated the marginal zone by MacNeal in 1929 (2). The
marginal zone is primarily made up of marginal zone (MZ) B cells, specialized
macrophages, and reticular cells.

In rodents, marginal zone B cells are now recognized as a distinct naive B lineage, separate from mature follicular (FO) B cells and B-1 cells. A small proportion
of memory B cells may also populate the marginal zone in rodents, whereas in
humans most MZ B cells are thought to represent a memory population. The differences between human and rodent MZ B cells are discussed later in the review,
but these populations may be much more similar than is generally recognized. MZ
B cells have long been considered critical determinants of host defense directed
against encapsulated blood-borne bacterial pathogens. These responses were originally believed to be primarily directed against T-independent multivalent antigens.
There is, however, a growing appreciation of a broader role for MZ B cells in both
T-independent and T-dependent immune responses.

In this review, we initially consider some anatomical features of the spleen to place MZ B cells in context. We describe some of the general biological properties that distinguish MZ B cells from B cells that reside in follicles, and we discuss current models for the generation of MZ B cells, based primarily on the study of these cells in rodents. We review the mechanisms involved in the entry of B lymphocytes into the marginal zone and their subsequent retention in this area. We discuss the participation of MZ B cells in host defense and, in the final sections of this review, we consider the biology of human MZ B cells and their relevance to disease.

An extensive overview of the marginal zone of the spleen was provided in a review by Kraal (3), published more than a decade ago. We also refer the interested reader to reviews on MZ B cells published during the past decade (4–6), and to reviews that more broadly deal with the origins of MZ B cells in the context of peripheral B cell development (5, 7–10).

LOCATION, LOCATION, LOCATION: SPLENIC MICROARCHITECTURE SETS THE STAGE

The unique location of MZ B cells permits them to respond very rapidly to blood-borne pathogens. In this section, we briefly consider some unique aspects of splenic microarchitecture in the context of the marginal zone and discuss some of the signaling events that are required for the generation and maintenance of this structure. The term marginal zone is often loosely used, especially in the human literature, to describe anatomical structures outside the spleen. This term should be reserved for a distinguishable and functional facet of splenic microarchitecture.

The Microvasculature of the Spleen in Mice

Most of the blood that flows through the spleen exits the circulation through a structure called the marginal sinus, flows through the marginal zone, and traverses venous sinuses in the spleen before returning to the circulation. Cells in the marginal zone are constantly exposed to large amounts of blood and to any antigens that have access to the systemic circulation.

The splenic artery enters the spleen in the region of the hilum and branches into a number of central or penicillar arterioles that terminate as end arterioles in the red pulp. Central arterioles branch into numerous small follicular arterioles in the white pulp, which direct systemic blood flow into the marginal sinus. This anastomosing, leaky, fenestrated, arteriolar sinus is best defined anatomically in rodents, where it separates the marginal zone from the white pulp (11–13). Some issues that relate to splenic microarchitecture in primates are discussed below. Proximal to their termination in the red pulp, central arterioles are surrounded concentrically by the periarteriolar lymphoid sheath (the T cell zone), B cell follicles, and the marginal zone (Figure 1). Arterial blood encounters decreased resistance when it enters the wider spaces of the marginal sinus. Most naive recirculating lymphocytes that flow into this area are readily drawn in along chemokine gradients into the white pulp.

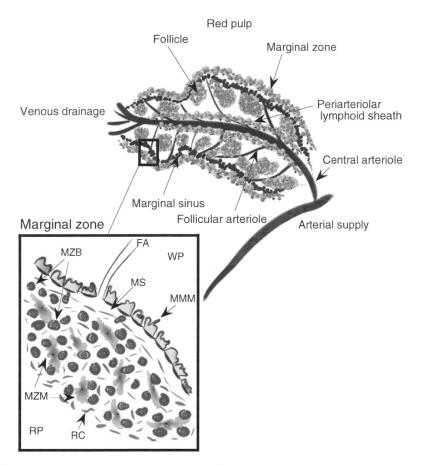

Figure 1 Microvasculature of the spleen. Central arterioles are surrounded concentrically by the periarteriolar lymphoid sheath (or T cell zone) and by the B cell follicles. These arterioles branch into follicular arterioles, which feed into the marginal sinus. The marginal zone lies between the sinus and the red pulp of the spleen. Inset shows the marginal zone area in cross-section. FA, follicular arteriole; RC, reticular cell; RP, red pulp; MS, marginal sinus; MMM, marginal metallophilic macrophage; MZB, marginal zone B cell; MZM, marginal zone macrophage; WP, white pulp.

The majority of the lymphocytes that pass through the marginal sinus are en route to the white pulp or the red pulp and presumably do not possess the appropriate adhesive properties that permit retention in the marginal zone. Apart from splenic follicular precursor B cells that have received cues to differentiate into MZ B cells (discussed below), some circulating memory cells also possess the ability to be retained in the marginal zone (14). These latter cells likely constitute a very small proportion of the B cells in the marginal zone in rodents. Lymphoid cells that do reside in the vicinity of the marginal sinus are particularly well positioned to respond rapidly to blood-borne pathogens.

In humans, the periarteriolar lymphoid sheath has few T cells, and conventional histological studies suggest that follicles are not separated from the marginal zone by a definable sinus (15, 16). The existence of a marginal sinus in primates remains controversial, but corrosion casting studies suggest that large amounts of blood are released into sinuses in or adjacent to the marginal zone in all rodents and primates studied (13). The white pulp in humans is surrounded by inner and outer layers of the marginal zone (these layers are separated in turn by a specialized intervening layer of fibroblasts) and a defined perifollicular zone can be identified outside the marginal zone, separating the latter from the red pulp. This perifollicular zone contains a few sheathed capillaries as well as more numerous blood-filled spaces that lack a defined endothelium. It is presumed that in humans, lymphocytes exit the circulation in the perifollicular zone and enter the white pulp. Although there are differences in splenic architecture and organization in mice and humans, in both species arterial contents enter functionally equivalent areas of decreased resistance, thus facilitating lymphocyte egress. Blood-borne pathogens can be assumed to obtain access readily to the cells of the marginal zone in all species.

Signals Required for the Generation and Maintenance of Splenic Microarchitecture

Signaling mediated by TNF family cytokines, most notably by membrane-bound lymphotoxin (LT) $\alpha\beta 2$, is required for the generation of proper secondary lymphoid organs and for the creation of the microarchitecture of the marginal zone (17–19). In general, LT$\alpha\beta 2$ on the surface of a bone marrow–derived cell induces signaling via the LTβR on stromal cells, resulting in enhanced secretion of homing chemokines and the increased expression of adhesion molecules. LTβR signaling requires NF-κB interacting kinase (NIK), the IκB kinase α (IKKα) activating kinase, that is defective in the naturally occurring *Aly* mutant (20, 21). The LTβR/NIK/IKKα pathway can contribute to the processing of NF-κB2 p100 to p52 (22, 23). Chimeric mice in which cells of hematopoietic origin lack LTα as well as mice in which LTβR signaling is blocked, have very few of the specialized macrophages known to exist in the marginal zone. They express very low levels of homing chemokines for naive B and T lymphocytes, and also have a marked absence of MZ B cells (24, 25). A number of possible mechanisms may link defective LTβR signaling in stromal cells to the absence of MZ B cells. This issue is considered again in the section on MZ B cell retention and migration.

CELLS THAT INHABIT THE MARGINAL ZONE AND THE PHENOTYPIC DEFINITION OF MZ B CELLS

Apart from the cells that are the topic of this review, the marginal zone contains at least two specialized macrophage populations, as well as stromal cells. The stromal cells are often called reticular cells and may include one or more specialized fibroblast populations. Reticular fibers have been described that appear to originate from the sheath of the central arterioles and serve as presumed conduits for the passage of lymphocytes from the white pulp to the red pulp and vice versa. These marginal zone bridging channels, best seen in rodents, are most prominent at the sites where central arterioles enter the white pulp, and where terminal arterioles penetrate the red pulp. A large splenic dendritic cell (DC) population, called marginal DCs, has been observed in the bridging channels, but the function of these DCs is not known (26, 27). Specialized blood-derived $CD11c^{lo}$ DCs may contribute to the differentiation of MZ B cells into plasma cells, but these DCs do not normally inhabit the marginal zone (28). They are discussed later in the review in the context of the activation of MZ B cells by blood-borne particulate antigens.

In rodents, the inner face of the marginal sinus is lined by marginal metallophilic macrophages (MMMs) that can be identified by the MOMA-1 antibody (29). This layer of macrophages is strictly part of the white pulp but is often considered the innermost marker of the marginal zone. MMMs express sialic acid–binding lectins (Siglecs) and contain nonspecific esterases. Kraal (3) postulated that these cells contribute to the detoxification of lipopolysaccharide (LPS). The marginal zone itself contains a network of reticular cells that secrete extracellular matrix components and provide the architectural framework for this region. A distinct population of marginal zone macrophages (MZMs), which can be identified by the ER-TR9 and MARCO (macrophage receptor with collagenous structure) antibodies (30, 31), is interspersed in the marginal zone with what was initially recognized as a specialized population of intermediate-sized lymphocytes. ER-TR9 recognizes the C-type lectin SIGN-RI, and MARCO belongs to the scavenger receptor family. MZMs might participate in the capture of carbohydrate antigens and their presentation to MZ B cells (32) and may also be involved in the retention of lymphocytes in the marginal zone (33). Starting in the mid-1970s, lymphoid cells in the marginal zone were shown to be B lymphocytes on the basis of immunohistochemical staining with antibodies that recognize Igs, Fc receptors, and C3 receptors. They were also considered to be B lymphocytes because they were present in the spleen in the absence of the thymus but could be depleted by anti-IgM treatment (34–38).

Although MZ B cells are defined primarily on the basis of their anatomical localization, the surface expression of a number of markers can also be used to characterize these cells. In rodents the only secondary lymphoid organ in which cells bearing surface markers characteristic of MZ B cells are normally found is the spleen. Unlike follicular B cells that express high levels of IgD and CD23, with either high or low levels of IgM, MZ B cells express high levels of IgM and very low levels of IgD and CD23 (36, 39–41). They also express higher levels of CD21 (complement receptor type II), CD1d (an MHC class Ib protein linked to the presentation of lipid antigens), CD38 (an ADP-ribosyl cyclase), CD9 (a scavenger receptor family protein), and CD25 (the α chain of the IL-2 receptor) than those on follicular B cells (39, 40, 42). The $\beta 2$ integrin, LFA-1, and the $\alpha 4 \beta 1$ integrin are also expressed at higher levels on MZ B cells than on follicular B cells (43). MZ B cells also express higher levels of B7 proteins than do follicular B cells and overall are described as having an "activated" phenotype (40).

MZ B Cells are Sessile and Apparently Long-Lived Cells

Whereas follicular B cells are freely recirculating lymphocytes, MZ B cells are not part of the recirculating pool in rodents. This difference was recognized when it was demonstrated that cannulation and draining of the thoracic duct leads to the depletion of follicular B cells but not of MZ B cells (36). In studies in which one half of the spleen was selectively irradiated, follicular B cells were depleted from the nonirradiated half, whereas the MZ B cells in the nonirradiated portion were not affected (36). In rodents, the absence of cells with an MZ B cell phenotype in tissues other than the spleen underscores the fact that these cells are sessile.

In studies on B cell homeostasis, Rag-2 was knocked in and conditionally deleted at specific times after birth (44). These studies revealed that MZ B cells might represent extremely long-lived cells, apparently surviving as long as the host. It is formally possible that MZ B cells have very long life spans, and that these cells are virtually immortal. A more credible inference, however, is that the spleen might contain a self-renewing progenitor of MZ B cells. Such a notion is consistent with earlier studies indicating that MZ B cells are more sensitive to radiation than follicular B cells, and that exposure to cyclophosphamide leads to the selective depletion of MZ B cells (45). MZ B cell levels are therefore likely to be homeostatically maintained either by self-renewing MZ B cells themselves, or by cycling precursors. Evidence for the possible existence of the latter type of precursor is discussed below.

Temporal Issues That Relate to Marginal Zone Maturation and MZ B Cell Development

The temporally regulated maturation of the microarchitecture of the marginal zone and the development of MZ B cells appear to go hand in hand. Proper development of the marginal zone and of the MZ B cell compartment is delayed until about the age of two years in humans and until 3–4 weeks after birth in rodents (5, 46). Apart from the delayed maturation of MZ B cells, MMMs and MZMs in the spleen are sparse and disorganized early in life. The precise cellular and molecular basis for the delay in MZ B cell maturation remains unclear, but this delay may have a clinical correlation in the inability of infants under the age of two years to mount effective immune responses to selected polysaccharide antigens (47, 48).

PERIPHERAL B CELL POPULATIONS IN THE SPLEEN: THE CELLULAR PATHWAY TO MZ B CELL DEVELOPMENT

During peripheral B cell development, immature B cells migrate from the bone marrow to the spleen, where B cells mature further. To dissect both the cellular and molecular pathways involved in MZ B cell development, one must identify all the splenic precursors of mature FO and MZ B cells.

Peripheral B cells are classified in a number of ways. Important studies have long established that recently generated B cells that express follicular markers, such as high levels of CD23 and IgD, also express high levels of CD24/HSA and are positive for the AA4.1 marker (49–51). CD24 and AA4.1 in this context should be considered as markers that identify recent bone marrow emigrants. These observations helped conceptualize the view that intermediate transitional stages of B cell development do exist. One caveat to be considered with this generally useful view is that many clones of one subset of T2 transitional cells may no longer express CD24 and AA4.1 and may persist as relatively long-lived cells that reside in follicles in all secondary lymphoid organs.

The term T2 "transitional B cell" remains useful to characterize B cells that are $CD23^{hi}IgM^{hi}IgD^{hi}$, but one must recognize, as described below, that there are at least two functionally and developmentally distinct types of T2 cells (9, 10). Another issue to keep in mind is that functionally mature cells that were generated fairly recently may also transiently express markers that characterize recent emigrants from the bone marrow. $IgD^{hi}IgM^{lo}$ FO cells that have recently matured (and therefore express high levels of AA4.1) are sometimes called T3 cells (51). We base most of our understanding of peripheral B cell populations on the analysis of engineered mutants, including B cell antigen receptor (BCR)-knockin mice, and we attempt to reconcile various approaches to peripheral B cell classification. We present a tentative, temporally ordered, cellular pathway for FO and MZ B cell development based on this information in Figure 2.

Newly Formed B Cells

Cells that have recently emerged from the bone marrow and have yet to acquire follicular markers such as IgD and CD23, but that express very low levels of CD21 and invariably express high levels of CD24 and AA4.1, are called T1 or newly formed (NF) B cells. These cells do not require BAFF (B cell–activating factor of the TNF family) for their survival (52–54), but like all B cells they depend on signals from the BCR for survival (55, 56). These cells, after emerging from the marginal sinus, mature and are drawn into follicles following a CXCL13 gradient (57, 58), initially become transitional follicular B cells, and eventually give rise to at least two lineages of B cells, mature FO B cells and MZ B cells. Transitional follicular B cells can be subdivided into two distinct categories.

One Type of T2 Transitional B Cell Population May Persist in All Secondary Lymphoid Organs

All naive B cell populations in the spleen, after the NF/T1 stage, depend on both BAFF and the BCR for survival. One population of T2 transitional cells consists of recirculating $IgM^{hi}IgD^{hi}CD21^{int}$ B cells that exist in primary follicles in all secondary lymphoid organs. This population of cells is not lost in mice with mutations in the Btk (Bruton's tyrosine kinase) pathway or in BCR-knockin mice

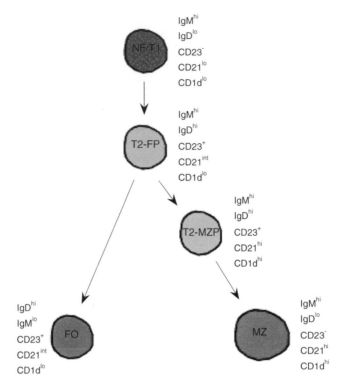

Figure 2 Surface markers that distinguish peripheral B cell populations in the murine spleen. NF (newly formed)/T1 (transitional stage 1) B cells are believed to differentiate into T2-FP (transitional stage 2-follicular precursors), which may either differentiate into mature FO B cells or sequentially into T2-MZP (transitional stage 2-MZ B cell precursors) or MZ (marginal zone) B cells.

that lack FO B cells. In addition, these cells are preserved in other mutant mice, including Aiolos$^{-/-}$ (59) and conditional Notch2$^{-/-}$ mice (60), that retain FO B cells but lack MZ B cells as well as the T2-MZP cells discussed below. These cells are therefore generated and preserved in mice that lack the differentiation signals required to generate mature FO B cells as well as in mice that cannot differentiate into MZ B cells.

Since these IgM^{hi}IgD^{hi}CD21^{int} cells appear to contain precursors of FO cells, and also correspond to the first CD23 expressing B cells described by Allman et al. (51) as T2 cells, we refer to them as T2-FP cells (for transitional type 2 follicular precursors). They can be distinguished from T2-MZP cells (discussed below). T2-FP cells that persist in all B cell follicles presumably represent clones that were neither eliminated by self-tolerance mechanisms nor possess the BCR specificity to mature further into either FO or MZ B cells.

A Second Type of T2 Transitional Cell is a Cycling Precursor of MZ B Cells Restricted to the Spleen in Rodents

A T2 population, that we recognize to be distinct from the population considered in the previous section, was demonstrated by Loder et al. (61) to be cycling cells only seen in the spleen and not in bone marrow, blood, or lymph nodes. These cells were (perhaps erroneously) assumed to be precursors of mature FO B cells. This very same population of $IgM^{hi}IgD^{hi}CD21^{hi}CD1d^{hi}$ and $CD23^{hi}$ cells is lost in Aiolos null mice (59) and in conditional $Notch2^{-/-}$ mice (60), but is preserved in the absence of Btk signals. On the basis of their absence in mice that only lack MZ B cells, we have referred to these missing cells as T2-MZPs for (presumed) MZ B cell precursors (9, 10). These cells are clearly not required precursors of FO B cells because they are missing in Aiolos null mice in which FO B cells are plentiful. Others have since supported our view that these cells are precursors of MZ B cells (60).

Mature FO B Cells are the Only Follicular B Cell Population that is Lost When Btk Signaling is Defective

A distinguishable population of $IgD^{hi}IgM^{lo}CD21^{int}$ B cells is lost in mice that have defects in the Btk pathway (62–72), and we refer to these cells, and these cells alone, as *mature* follicular or FO B cells. FO B cells are the most mature follicular B cell subpopulation.

The term follicular B cell is generally used fairly broadly, but FO cells as defined above should be considered as a distinct and highly differentiated population. It is worth emphasizing that there are at least three distinct categories of $IgD^{hi}CD23^{hi}$ B cells in splenic follicles: FO cells, T2-FP cells, and T2-MZP cells (9, 10). Follicles in lymph nodes contain only two $IgD^{hi}CD23^{hi}$ B cell populations, FO and T2-FP B cells.

MZ B CELL DEVELOPMENT: THE BCR SIGNAL-STRENGTH MODEL AND THE "PRODUCTION BOTTLENECK" MODEL

There appear to be two major driving forces for normal MZ B cell development in replete animals. The primary determinant is the specificity of the BCR, which allows a developing B cell to choose between an FO or an MZ B cell fate. The second major driving force is Notch signaling. B cells selected to mature into the MZ B cell lineage can only do so if they receive additional signals from Notch2 and NF-κB1.

In the following sections, we discuss factors that regulate the commitment of B cells to the MZ B lineage. We discuss a signal-strength model in the context of an FO versus MZ B lymphoid cell-fate decision, and we also consider an alternative, but certainly not mutually exclusive, model that addresses MZ B cell development in the context of the monitoring of bone marrow B cell production. This latter model is referred to as the "production bottleneck" model In a subsequent section, we consider genes that primarily appear to control the retention of B cells in the marginal zone or their migration to this location. Some of these genes may also be required for MZ B cell survival.

Because the signal-strength model suggests that B cell differentiation is driven by self-antigens, it is initially worth considering why the loss of B cells during development has historically been tied to arguments regarding antigen-driven positive selection versus antigen-independent constitutive signaling via the BCR.

Cell Loss During B Cell Development and the Issue of Constitutive BCR Signaling. Does Positive Selection Occur Prior to Lineage Commitment?

Cell loss and repertoire attenuation during early lymphoid ontogeny may be ascribed to both negative and positive selection events. In humans, it has been estimated that about 60%–70% of the primary repertoire is strongly autoreactive and these cells are tolerized and lost either in the bone marrow or as transitional B cells in the periphery (73). In transgenic and knockin models, murine B cells that are strongly autoreactive are negatively selected by receptor editing, deletion, or anergy. However, the proportion of newly generated murine B cells that need to be tolerized is not known. Others (49, 50, 74) have suggested that considerable B cell loss occurs during maturation and that only around 10%–30% of recently generated B cells mature in the periphery. These data suggest, but do not prove, that the survival of peripheral B cells during maturation may be linked to a positive selection event. In the absence of information regarding the proportion of murine B cells that are tolerized during development, we cannot be sure whether the predicted cell losses during peripheral B cell development reflect tolerance or the lack of positive selection.

Most B cell loss during peripheral development is believed to occur at the transitional T2 stage (presumably the T2-FP stage) at which cells first express CD23, inhabit follicles, and acquire the ability to recirculate (51, 75). BAFF is essential for the survival of these transitional cells, as discussed below, and indeed overexpression of BAFF contributes to the survival of many autoreactive clones that would normally have been lost at the T2 (T2-FP in our nomenclature) stage or beyond (76, 77). One could argue, therefore, albeit without certainty, that cell loss during development may be accounted for more by negative selection than by positive selection events.

Positive selection requires that different clones of developing B cells are triggered in a different manner via their BCRs because of differences in receptor affinity for self-antigens. Rajewsky and colleagues (55, 56) have established from conditional deletion experiments that the BCR is absolutely required for the survival of all B cells, including recently generated B lymphocytes. The rapidity with which all B lineage cells are lost in the absence of BCR signals is striking. As has been discussed previously (78, 79), it remains unclear whether BCR-mediated early B cell survival depends on constitutive ligand-independent signaling via the BCR or whether self-antigens drive the BCR-mediated survival of B cells. If the BCR were only to signal in a constitutive ligand-independent fashion, this would further suggest that positive selection is not relevant during the early maturation of peripheral B cells. However, we consider it likely that the BCR does provide baseline constitutive survival signals in all B cells that are not negatively selected, and that self-antigens also play an important role in subsequently mediating lineage commitment events during peripheral B cell maturation. We entertain the possibility that most B cell loss during development is actually linked to negative selection and that positive selection, initiated in follicles at the T2-FP stage, exists primarily to initiate peripheral B cell lineage commitment.

THE BCR SIGNAL-STRENGTH MODEL FOR LINEAGE COMMITMENT IN PERIPHERAL B CELLS

In essence, the signal-strength model that we have proposed (9, 10, 59) encompasses the following steps:

1. A T2-FP cell that receives survival signals via BAFF and constitutive Btk-independent baseline signals via the BCR makes one of two decisions:

2a. If its BCR reacts fairly well with a self-antigen, this B cell is induced to differentiate in a Btk-pathway-dependent manner into an FO B cell.

    OR

2b. If its BCR reacts poorly or not at all with a cognate self-antigen, it continues to survive because of BAFF and constitutive BCR signaling, but in the absence of stronger BCR stimulation it is receptive to inductive signals that drive it to an MZ B cell fate.

The initial impetus for proposing such a model came from studies on Aiolos$^{-/-}$/ Xid double mutant mice (59). Aiolos is a zinc-finger protein of the Ikaros family, expressed primarily in B cells, which may participate in the repression of poorly defined target genes at the level of heterochromatin (80). In the absence of Aiolos, BCR signal strength is enhanced, FO B cell numbers are greater than in wild-type mice, but MZ B cells as well as T2-MZP cells are lost (59, 80). In mice that lack both Aiolos and functional Btk, MZ B cells and T2-MZP cells persist. These data suggest that Aiolos and Btk are in epistasis and that Aiolos is a negative regulator of the Btk pathway (59). In the absence of Aiolos, enhanced Btk signals not only mediate one of the predictable functions of Btk, which is to facilitate FO B cell development, but these "strong" signals also lead to a complete loss of the MZ B cell compartment, a phenotype that would not have previously been predicted to be linked to enhanced BCR signaling. We hypothesized that a cell-fate decision occurs in the spleen, wherein a follicular precursor, possibly a T2-FP cell, has to choose between an FO B cell fate or an MZ B cell fate (Figure 3). Relatively strong

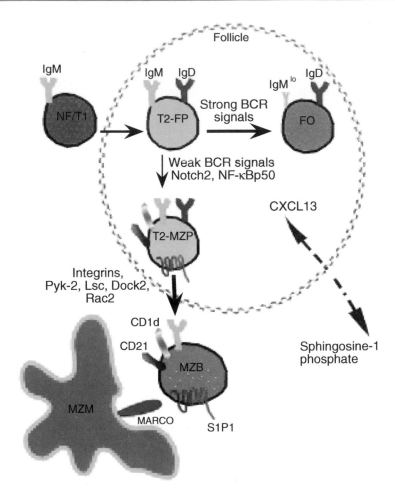

Figure 3 Integration of BCR signal strength and signaling via Notch2 and NF-κB1 at the FO versus MZ B lymphocyte cell-fate transition. S1P$_1$ refers to a sphingosine-1 phosphate receptor. See text for details.

BCR signals mediated through the Btk pathway commit peripheral B cells to an FO B cell fate. Weak signals delivered by the BCR appear to be permissive for MZ B cell development and are incompatible with FO B cell development.

A number of additional pieces of evidence lend support for such a signal-strength hypothesis. Some of these are listed below:

1. In the absence of CD21/CR2, a known positive regulator of BCR signaling, MZ B cells are overrepresented compared with wild-type controls (59).

2. Mice lacking CD22, a negative regulator of BCR signaling, are deficient in MZ B cells (81).

3. Mice in which BCR signaling is impaired because of the presence of a knocked-in light chain mutation, also have increased numbers of MZ B cells (82).

4. Mice in which the tyrosine residues in the Igα ITAM (immunoreceptor tyrosine activation motif) have been modified to phenylalanines exhibit enhanced Ca^{2+} signaling downstream of the BCR and the loss only of MZ B cells (83).

5. The strongest data in support of the signal-strength hypothesis have been obtained from BCR-knockin studies. In replete animals, specific knockin B cell clones exclusively give rise to MZ B cells, traverse the FP and MZP compartments, and are excluded from the FO B cell compartment. Other specific BCRs commit developing B cells exclusively to the FO compartment and are excluded from the MZ B cell compartment (10; A. Cariappa & S. Pillai, unpublished observations). These data strongly suggest that BCR specificity is the primary determining factor that drives a developing B cell to differentiate into an FO B cell or an MZ B cell.

6. The signal-strength model predicts that enhanced Btk signals cause a loss of MZ B cells and an increase in the number of FO B cells. As a corollary, we might therefore predict that defects in the Btk signaling pathway should lead to defects in FO B cell development but should not compromise MZ B cell development. Indeed, all the following result in the loss of FO B cells with the clear preservation of MZ B cells: (*a*) mutations in CD45, a positive regulator of Src family kinases and therefore of Btk activation (66); (*b*) a mutation in BCAP (67); (*c*) an adaptor in B cells for the p85α regulatory subunit of PI3 kinase; (*d*) mutations in p85α (68, 69); (*e*) mutations in Btk itself (59, 62–64, 84); (*f*) a mutation in BLNK (70, 71); (*g*) an adaptor that links Btk to PLCγ2; and (*h*) a mutation in PLCγ2 (72). These data have led to a broadening of the signal-strength model as discussed elsewhere (9, 10), suggesting that "weak" BCR signals suffice for MZ B cell development, "intermediate" BCR signals are required for FO B cell development, and "strong" BCR signals drive B-1 B cell development. The role of self-antigens in the positive selection of B-1 B cells has been clearly demonstrated (85), but a number of other issues, including the stem cell of origin, impinge upon B-1 B cell development. The ontogeny of this lineage is not considered further in this review.

Some data that appear not to agree fully with the signal-strength model should also be taken into account:

1. Although CD19 and CD21 are part of the same complex, in contrast to the phenotype of $CD21^{-/-}$ mice, $CD19^{-/-}$ mice do exhibit a defect in MZ B cell development (86). However, because CD19 may be functionally linked to integrin signaling in conjunction with its associated tetraspanin CD81,

it is possible that the requirement for CD19 during MZ B cell development is not linked to its role in BCR signaling. Integrin signaling, as discussed below, may be critical for the retention or maintenance of MZ B cells.

2. Mice in which the Ebstein-Barr virus LMP2A gene has been integrated into the IgH locus produce either B-1 cells or both MZ and FO B cells, depending on the strength of the promoter used to drive LMP2A expression. LMP2A is thought to act as a surrogate BCR in this model, and therefore it was interpreted that signal strength (as measured by the level of LMP2A expression) might influence B cell development (87). However, the concomitant generation of both FO and MZ B cells in mice in which a weaker promoter drives LMP2A expression may not fully fit the case being made for an FO versus MZ B cell transition. One could argue that the weaker promoter does not fire in an absolutely monomorphic manner, and therefore two "strengths" of signal may sometimes be interpreted in different B cell clones in the same mouse. It is perhaps easier to explain how two self-structures possessing differing affinities for a single BCR might cause a single clone of B cells to differentiate into two different lineages.

3. We have made a case for MZ B cell development being Btk-independent (and this has indeed been verified in many studies). However, there is one case in which the development or survival of MZ B cells bearing a single specific transgene-derived idiotype appeared to be compromised in the absence of Btk signals (86). The Btk dependence of this clone is manifest only when it is in competition with other MZ B cell clones. Btk is now known to be required for the homeostatic proliferation of B cells (88), a phenomenon that is discussed later in this review. It is not surprising that a clone lacking Btk may have fared poorly when it was transferred to a lymphopenic recipient. Although Btk may not be required for "normal" MZ B cell development, its function during MZ B cell activation remains unclear. Xid mice do have a defect in T-independent type 2 responses (88a). This may reflect the absence of B-1 cells as well as a possible defect in MZ B cell activation. The function of Btk in MZ B cells has not so far been examined in replete mice.

Overall, the weight of the evidence, particularly data from mice with knockin BCRs, supports the view that the FO versus MZ B lymphocyte cell-fate decision is driven primarily by differences in BCR signal strength.

What is the Nature of the "Weak" BCR Signal and the "Intermediate" BCR Signal During Peripheral B Cell Development?

What exactly do weak, intermediate, and strong BCR signals mean in biochemical terms? Differences in antigen affinity might be interpreted according to the duration of signaling, the variety of signaling pathways transduced, the amplitude of signaling, or combinations of all three.

The intermediate-strength signal required for BCR-mediated FO B cell maturation is clearly linked to the Btk pathway. Investigators have argued that the Bcl-2 family protein Bcl-XL is induced downstream of the BCR in a Btk-dependent manner (89). Another possible target gene of this or some other intermediate-strength BCR pathway may be the anti-apoptotic Bcl-2 protein. Bcl-2 transgenic animals have virtually no MZ B cells, whereas Bcl-2 null mice present with a marked increase in MZ B cells (90). Bcl-2 may preferentially foster the survival of transitional cells committed to an FO B cell fate at the expense of MZ B cells. Other explanations must be considered for this totally unexpected phenomenon. For poorly understood reasons, Bcl-2 transgenic animals present with enhanced BCR signal strength (90). This Bcl-2 phenotype may be explained by the signal-strength hypothesis as well.

Signaling via the Btk pathway is not required for the survival of NF B cells, transitional B cells, or MZ B cells. Btk-independent BCR signals that contribute to the survival of NF B cells and that may not be sufficient to induce FO B cell development may contribute to the weak signal. The weak signal may represent either constitutive ligand-independent BCR signaling, or it may represent BCR signaling that is driven by self-antigens but is below a signaling threshold required for Btk activation. A number of engineered mouse mutations that compromise MZ B cell development involve genes that might be linked to BCR activation:

1. One potential contributor to the "weak" BCR pathway may be PI3Kp110δ (91–93), which can be activated downstream of the BCR and in whose absence MZ B cells fail to develop.

2. The Btk-independent activation of specific NF-κB dimers downstream of the BCR may also contribute to the weak signal. NF-κB1/p50 is required in a cell-autonomous manner for the generation of MZ B cells (94). The loss of either p65/RelA or c-Rel leads to a less severe but detectable reduction in MZ B cell numbers (94). RelB can contribute to MZ microarchitecture by being part of p52/RelB complexes in stromal cells downstream of the LTβ receptor, but RelB is also required for MZ B cell development in a cell-autonomous manner (95). It is possible, therefore, that p50/RelB heterodimers are required downstream of weak signals delivered by the BCR for MZ B cell development and survival.

3. Activation of NF-κB downstream of the BCR may be mediated by the caspase-recruitment domain 11 (CARD11)/mucosa-associated lymphoid tissue 1 (MALT1)/Bcl-10 complex (96–101). This complex may be activated downstream of the activation of PKCs and may facilitate the lysine-63 ubiquitination of NF-κB essential modifier (NEMO), thus contributing to the activation of the IKK complex (102). These three molecules are necessary for the activation of NF-κB following BCR stimulation, as well as for the development of MZ B cells. Defects in FO B cell development

in mice that lack CARD11, MALT1, or Bcl-10 are minimal. Intriguingly, as is discussed briefly below, both MALT1 and Bcl-10 are activated by translocations in marginal zone–type MALT lymphomas in humans.

4. Another nuclear protein that is required for B cell activation downstream of the BCR is the BOB.1/OBF.1/OCA-B transcriptional coactivator, which binds to and transcriptionally enhances the activity of the Oct-1 and Oct-2 transcription factors. Numerous B cell defects are observed in the absence of BOB.1, including a defect in MZ B cell development (90, 103). B cell migration may also be abnormal in the absence of BOB.1, and it is therefore unclear as to whether BOB.1 represents a component of the weak Btk-independent BCR signal that is required for MZ B cell development, or if it is required for MZ B cell development in a BCR-independent manner.

Notch2 Signaling is Required for MZ B Cell Development

Notch was first described phenotypically in 1917 in *Drosophila* by Morgan (104), and it has since been shown to be instrumental in a host of cell-fate decisions in many organisms. In mice, four Notch genes are expressed differentially in different tissues and cell types and encode closely related integral membrane cell surface receptors (105). These receptors can each interact with one or more of five known ligands. These Notch ligands, Delta-like1, -3, and -4 and Jagged1 and -2, are all integral membrane proteins that are expressed on the surface of a variety of cell types (105). Upon interaction with a ligand, the intracellular portion of the Notch protein is liberated through a proteolytic event, allowing it to translocate to the nucleus, where it forms a ternary complex with RBP-Jκ/CBF1 (the vertebrate homolog of Suppressor of Hairless) and Mastermind, a transcriptional coactivator, to mediate gene transcription (106).

The first indication that the Notch pathway may be required for MZ B cell development was obtained from a B cell–specific conditional knockout of RBP-Jκ, which resulted in a peripheral B cell phenotype similar to that observed in Aiolos null mice—MZ B cells were lost while FO B cell numbers were enhanced (107). A broadly similar phenotype was observed in mice deficient for NF-κB1 (see above). These data suggested that B cells that receive relatively weak signals via the BCR do not spontaneously differentiate in a "default" manner into MZ B cells. Signaling through the Notch pathway and NF-κB are clearly required to generate MZ B cells.

Interestingly, conditional knockout studies have revealed that Delta-like1 (108, in a non-cell-autonomous manner) and Notch2 (60, in a cell-autonomous manner) are both required specifically for MZ B cell development. Mice with one inactivated Notch2 allele are viable and also have a marked reduction in MZ B cells (109). It is likely that Delta-like1 is expressed on some follicular stromal cell, possibly found only in splenic follicles and not in other secondary lymphoid organs, and represents a specific and critical ligand for Notch2. In keeping with a recognized role for Notch signaling in the generation and/or maintenance of MZ B cells, mice harboring a mutation in MINT (Msx2-interacting nuclear target), a negative regulator of Notch signaling, present with an increase in the number of MZ B cells and a decrease in the number of FO B cells (110). In Aiolos$^{-/-}$ mice, and in conditional RBP-J$\kappa^{-/-}$ mice, MZ B cells are lost and FO B cells increase, whereas in conditional Notch2$^{-/-}$ mice MZ B cells are lost and FO B cell numbers are within the normal range. Whether the increase in FO B cell numbers in some mutants, but not in others, represents an interpretable difference is unclear.

There are three Mastermind-like (MAML) proteins in mice (106). Mastermind forms a ternary complex with intracellular Notch and RBP-Jκ and links these proteins to coactivator complexes to facilitate transcription (106). Retroviral transduction of hematopoietic stem cells with a truncated form of MAML1 that only retains the N-terminal intracellular Notch-binding domain (a dominant interfering form of Mastermind) results in an inhibition of MZ B cell development, further underscoring the importance of the Notch pathway in MZ B cell development (111).

The Contribution of BAFF to MZ B Cell Development

The TNF family ligand BAFF/Blys is an essential survival factor for transitional B cells, as revealed by both BAFF inactivation (52–54) and BAFF overexpression studies (112, 113). The BAFF receptor (BAFF-R) is not expressed on NF/T1 cells but is expressed on all other splenic B cell populations (75). Although MZ B cells are markedly reduced in numbers in BAFF$^{-/-}$ mice, this may well be explained by the diminished survival of all follicular precursors of MZ B cells. BAFF transgenic mice present with increased numbers of MZ B cells, presumably because the transitional B cell pool is enhanced and autoreactive transitional and MZ B cells are protected from elimination (77). Until it becomes technically possible to conditionally delete genes in T2-MZP or MZ B cells, it will not be possible to ascertain whether BAFF drives MZ B cell development beyond its role in transitional B cell survival and niche expansion.

The FO Versus MZ B Cell Transition: Integrating BCR Signal Strength and Notch Signals

Our studies suggest the existence of an FO versus MZ B lymphocyte cell-fate decision. Because many mutant mice exist that lack FO B cells but preserve T2-FP, T2-MZP, and MZ B cells, we believe that T2-FP B cells, which also represent a recirculating follicular B cell population, may be the last common precursor of FO and MZ B cells. Although the possibility remains that FO B cells may give rise to T2-MZP and MZ B cells in certain circumstances (such as in conditions of B cell depletion, see below), clearly FO B cells are not a required precursor for either T2-MZP or MZ B cells. T2-FP cells are, however, always present when mutant or knockin mice fail to generate FO cells but exclusively generate T2-MZP and MZ B cells.

Our view is that the initial commitment event to the MZ B lineage is BCR driven, and in a temporal and hierarchical sense, the BCR has precedence over

Notch2. When a specific BCR commits a B cell clone to an FO fate, this clone ignores the presence of Notch2 and its ligand. Clearly, some mechanism must exist whereby relatively strong BCR signaling renders transitional cells in the follicle impervious to the presence of Delta-like1-dependent triggering of Notch2. Conversely, relatively weak BCR signaling may enhance the expression of one or more components of the Notch2 signaling pathway in B cells. The molecular basis for this putative imperviousness to Notch signaling in FO B lymphocyte–committed clones, or for the possible enhanced responsiveness to Notch ligands in MZ B cell–committed lymphoid clones, remains to be elucidated.

It seems likely that the driving signal for FO B cell development may be delivered through the BCR at the T2-FP stage (because MZ B cells can develop from T2-FP cells in the absence of NF B cells) by self-antigens of a relatively high affinity. A striking difference between T2-FP B cells and the preceding NF/T1 cells is the presence of high levels of IgD on T2-FP B cells. These cells may acquire the ability to respond and initiate lineage commitment events in response to self-antigens more readily than NF/T1 cells because they express higher levels of the BCR overall, and higher levels of IgD. IgD has a long cysteine-free hinge region, which facilitates higher "functional affinity" interactions with antigens having a low epitope density (114).

B cell clones that receive only weak signals because their BCRs do not recognize self-antigen with sufficient affinity are presumably receptive to inductive signals delivered by Delta-like1 on a yet-to-be-defined cell, probably of myeloid origin, that resides in the follicular area. Notch signals, weak and Btk-independent BCR signals, possibly BAFF signals, and signals from other presently unidentified cell surface receptors, may contribute either cooperatively or in parallel pathways to the development of MZ B cells.

Teleological Reasons for the Positive Selection of B Cells

Most teleological reasoning does not rise to the level of providing testable hypotheses, but any immunological model would lack soul in the absence of an attempt made in this direction. The positive selection of T cells may well be viewed as a trophic event mediated by self-MHC molecules. The BCR-dependent survival of peripheral B cells mediated either in a tonic/constitutive ligand-independent manner, or driven by self-antigen, may also represent a trophic event initiated possibly to test if a complete receptor has been generated. Constitutive signaling, as discussed above, would ubiquitously provide trophic signals and therefore not mediate true selection.

A second equally compelling reason that would apply only to positive selection mediated by self-antigens (and not to tonic signaling events) is the ability of this process to initiate the generation of lineages from newly produced B cells, which appear homogeneous but differ individually only according to their BCR specificities.

The least satisfying teleological reason is the one that would need to be applied to the following question: Why is weak BCR signaling apparently linked to the specific generation of MZ B cells? One could argue that B cells that react very poorly with self-structures, and that would therefore receive very weak BCR signals from self-antigens, may well represent clones that are worth preserving to deal with pathogen-derived structures with very little resemblance to self. Rather than allow such clones to wither away, Notch ligands and other signals may be designed to "rescue" such B cells and preserve them as part of the innate immune repertoire.

MZ B CELL GENERATION IN THE CONTEXT OF MONITORING BONE MARROW B CELL PRODUCTION: THE "PRODUCTION BOTTLENECK" MODEL

Another model for MZ B cell generation also approaches the issue of MZ B cell generation from broad underpinnings. This "production bottleneck" model has been developed in some depth in a separate review (5), and we discuss some of its aspects here. We believe that the production bottleneck and signal-strength models reflect distinct phenomena, but these models may be brought together in the context of immunodeficiency and homeostatic proliferation.

In essence, the production bottleneck model suggests that in situations of reduced bone marrow B cell production, there is a tendency for enhanced MZ B cell production. This production is driven by what the authors describe may be "an ill-defined compensatory drive" to maintain a diverse repertoire of natural IgM, and expansion of the MZ B cell compartment as well as of peritoneal B-1 cell populations may be a means to this end.

One of the examples cited in support of the bottleneck model is the transfer of limiting numbers of B cells into immunodeficient recipients in bone marrow transplant situations. Large numbers of the transferred cells differentiate rapidly into MZ B cells and plasma cells. Systematic studies on B cells transferred into immunodeficient mice have been performed in the context of examining homeostatic proliferation (88, 115, 116). In these studies, the transferred cells rapidly differentiate into "activated" B cells that phenotypically resemble what we would call T2-MZP cells and MZ B cells. Evidence has been previously provided for the generation of MZ B cells from follicular B cell populations in lymphopenic animals. Rats treated with a single dose of doxorubuicin are depleted of all B cells except recirculating follicular B cells (which probably correspond to FO and T2-FP cells) (117). During recovery, MZ B cells are generated in these rats at a time when NF cells are not seen. These data probably reflect the phenomenon of homeostatic B cell proliferation.

Very little is known about the cellular or molecular pathways involved in the homeostatic proliferation of B cells. One factor that appears to be required for the homeostatic proliferation of B cells is Btk (88). The requirement for Btk strongly suggests that normal MZ B cell development, which is Btk-independent, and the Btk-dependent homeostatic B cell proliferation of B cells, which can contribute to MZ B cell generation, are distinct phenomena. In experiments alluded to earlier, the survival of a specific clone of MZ B cells transferred into partly lymphopenic recipient mice was found to be Btk-dependent (86). We believe that this study, and indeed all studies involving the transfer of B cells into lymphopenic hosts, represent variations to the theme of homeostatic proliferation.

One approach that may partly unify the signal strength and the production bottleneck models is to suggest that there may be a common, final molecular pathway for MZ B cell development, at a point subsequent to the differential requirement for Btk. This common final pathway probably involves the conversion of a T2 FP cell (or even an FO cell that has retained some plasticity) into a cycling T2-MZP cell. A cycling T2-MZP cell may then differentiate into an MZ B cell. It is unclear whether Notch2 is required among other yet-to-be-defined signals.

During normal B cell development in replete mice, the stage is most likely set by BCR specificity, as described in the signal-strength model, and differentiation proceeds from T2-FP to T2-MZP to MZ B cells. In situations of immunodeficiency, the exact humoral mediators involved in homeostatic proliferation and differentiation are not known, but factors such as BAFF (or other unknown factors) might increase the transitional T2 and MZ B cell niche sizes and facilitate MZ B cell expansion. Differentiation may proceed along the same common final pathway, which is probably initiated from T2-FP cells. In the presence of appropriate humoral factors, it is formally possible that differentiation may be initiated from FO B cells as well. The role of BCR specificity in situations of homeostatic proliferation is unclear and should be explored.

MECHANISMS INVOLVED IN B LYMPHOCYTE ENTRY AND RETENTION IN THE MARGINAL ZONE

There is a well-developed paradigm that invokes the sequential role of selectins, chemokines, and integrins in the entry of lymphocytes into lymph nodes across the endothelium of high endothelial venules (HEVs). Lymphocytes are induced to roll by the interaction between selectin ligands on HEVs and selectins on naive lymphocytes. Locally available chemokines then activate integrins, and this results in tight binding of these proteins to integrin ligands on the endothelium. Shear forces that impinge upon lymphocytes emerging in the arteriolar marginal sinus of the spleen are not likely to be as significant as in HEVs, and selectins and selectin ligands may therefore not be relevant in splenic lymphocyte entry. A role for integrins in lymphocyte entry into the white pulp of the spleen has been established. Interactions between the integrins LFA-1 and $\alpha 4\beta 1$ on lymphocytes with their respective ligands, ICAM-1 and VCAM-1, expressed on a splenic radioresistant cell, may mediate an adhesion event that is involved in lymphocyte entry into the spleen (118). This adhesion event probably depends on a yet-to-be-defined chemokine or other $G\alpha i$-protein-coupled receptor because entry can be significantly impaired by exposure to pertussis toxin (118).

Once B cells move from the marginal zone area to the white pulp cords, they may be drawn into the follicles along a CXCL13 gradient. CXCL13 interacts with the CXCR5 chemokine receptor on B cells (57, 58) and thus mediates the proper generation of B cell follicles. For an MZ B cell to evade the powerful draw mediated by CXCR5 signaling, it is induced to move away from this gradient at least in part by signals mediated by $S1P_1$ and $S1P_3$, which are receptors for the lysophospholipid sphingosine-1 phosphate (119). This lysophospholipid is found in fairly abundant concentrations in the blood. $S1P_1$ and $S1P_3$ are expressed at higher levels on MZ B cells than on follicular B cells. Exposure of mice to FTY720, a competitive inhibitor of S1P receptor function, causes the mislocalization of MZ B cells into follicles. In mice that have a genetic defect in $S1P_1$, MZ B cells migrate aberrantly into follicles following a CXCL13 gradient. In mice lacking $S1P_1$ as well as CXCL13, MZ B cells are not mislocalized. $S1P_1$ signaling appears to directly counter the opposing CXCL13-dependent force of attraction that simultaneously draws MZ B cells toward follicles (119).

Of all the known mutants that affect MZ B cells, $S1P_1$-deficiency represents the only genetic model in which MZ B cells are actually generated but remain in the follicle rather than in the marginal zone where they belong. $S1P_1$ signals in a $G\alpha i$-dependent manner. Investigators have previously shown that pertussis toxin displaces MZ B cells from the marginal zone, and this could possibly be explained by the inactivation of $S1P_1$ signaling, although inhibition of CXCL13 should probably have also occurred simultaneously. Mice that lack one member of the $G\alpha i$ family, $G\alpha i2$, have a marked deficiency of MZ B cells, but the molecular and cellular basis of this defect remains poorly understood (120).

Activation of MZ B cells either by antigen or by LPS causes them to migrate initially into follicles. It is presumed that these migration events may facilitate the interaction of MZ B cells with T cells at the T-B interface or possibly, as has been speculated, help draw antigen into follicles (119). This migration, along a CXCL13 gradient, is presumably made possible by the ability of LPS and antigen to induce the downregulation of $S1P_1$ expression.

What are the mechanisms by which MZ B cells are retained in the marginal zone? MZMs may play an important role in retaining MZ B cells in the marginal zone (3, 33). The close interactions that are observed between MZMs and MZ B cells support such a notion. Depletion of the SH2-containing inositol-5 phosphatase (SHIP) in myeloid cells results in the relocation of MZMs to the red pulp and the loss of MZ B cells. The scavenger receptor MARCO on MZMs may bind to a ligand on MZ B cells, but the biochemical basis and relevance of this interaction remains to be established (33).

Another distinct mechanism that has been suggested for the retention of MZ B cells in the marginal zone is the interaction of integrins on B cells with integrin ligands that are induced in the marginal zone in stromal cells by signaling via the LTβR (43). The integrins of relevance in this process are LFA-1, which interacts specifically with ICAM-1 in the marginal zone, and the $\alpha4\beta1$ integrin, which associates primarily with VCAM-1 and fibronectin during this process. Both these integrins are expressed at higher levels on MZ B cells than on follicular B cells. LPS- and antigen-mediated displacement of MZ B cells from the marginal zone to the follicles may be mediated in part by $S1P_1$ downregulation and may also depend on the downregulation of integrin adhesiveness (43).

Integrin signaling has also been indirectly linked to the localization and retention of MZ B cells because many mutants that potentially impinge upon integrin signaling present with MZ B cell deficits. Pyk-2 is a tyrosine kinase that is involved in signaling downstream of integrins (but may also participate in chemokine signaling) and is necessary for the development of MZ B cells (121). Lsc/p115RhoGEF, a specific guanine nucleotide exchange factor for Rho, is also necessary for MZ B cell development (122), and Rho signaling has also been linked to integrin activation. Similarly, the CDM protein DOCK2 (which resembles the *Caenorhabditis elegans* CED-5 and *Drosophila* myoblast city adaptor proteins) is relevant for lymphocyte chemotaxis and for MZ B cell development (123), and may also be biochemically linked to integrin signaling (124). Mice lacking the Rac2 Rho family GTPase have a marked defect in $\alpha 4 \beta 1$ integrin signaling and also lack MZ B cells (125).

An intriguing feature of the above set of mutations is that in all these mutant mice (other than in the $S1P_1$ mutant described earlier) MZ B cells are not mislocalized to the follicles—they are lost altogether. Apparent defects in integrin signaling do not altogether prevent entry of B cells into the spleen, although integrins are believed to be required for the entry of all B cells into the white pulp. One may argue that white pulp entry depends only on an adhesive event, whereas retention in the marginal zone requires signaling as well. These mutations, if they do primarily reflect defects in integrin signaling, may also reveal a role for these signals in the maintenance of MZ B cells.

MZ B CELLS AND HOST DEFENSE

MZ B cells are ideally located to respond to blood-borne pathogens. Along with B-1 B cells, they have been described as cells that are endowed with "natural memory" and that provide a bridge between innate and adaptive immune responses (8). These two types of B cells are believed to be the source of most natural antibodies. Although for many decades MZ B cells were viewed as being key players primarily in responses to polysaccharide antigens, in recent years we have witnessed a growing understanding of the role that these cells play in rapid responses to blood-borne pathogens, and in their ability to participate both in T-independent as well as in T-dependent immune responses. Despite the fact that these cells do not recirculate and may have a restricted repertoire, there are few limits to the range of protective responses that may be obtained from the activation of MZ B cells.

Responses to T-Independent Antigens

MZ B cells have long been functionally linked to immune responses to T-independent type 2 (TI-2) multivalent antigens because of an established requirement for the spleen in these responses (126–129). In humans, splenectomy results in increased susceptibility to encapsulated bacteria (that have polysaccharide capsules) such as *Streptococcus pneumoniae*, *Neisseria meningitides*, or *Hemophilus influenzae* (130, 131). Before the age of two years, humans are unable to mount effective immune responses to encapsulated bacteria because the marginal zone is immature and poorly organized (132, 133). Although these data do not directly implicate MZ B cells in TI-2 responses, more direct evidence was obtained from Pyk-2-deficient mice (121), which lack MZ B cells. These mice have a fairly striking defect in TI-2 responses to artificial multivalent antigens. Mice that lack NF-κB1 have a defect in MZ B cell development (94), and these mice are defective in their ability to handle a number of gram-negative bacteria (134). Mice with an engineered defect in RBP-Jκ (107) lack MZ B cells and are susceptible to blood-borne *Staphylococcus aureus*, but, somewhat surprisingly, do not present with any defects in their responses to artificial TI-2 antigens.

The high levels of CD21 on MZ B cells assist these cells in efficiently capturing complement coated polysaccharides (121). Studies with particulate bacterial antigens have revealed that in the first three days following exposure to blood-borne bacteria, massive waves of plasmablasts are generated by antigen-specific MZ B cells and B-1 cells (135). MZ B cells are intrinsically capable of very rapidly maturing into plasmablasts. This may be due, in part, to the ability of MZ B cells to respond more strongly than follicular B cells, both via the BCR as well as through Toll-like receptors. Resting levels of Blimp-1 are elevated in MZ B cells, suggesting that MZ B cells are poised to rapidly differentiate, in a matter of hours rather than days, into IgM-secreting plasmablasts (135). Activated MZ B cells and plasmablasts are found most prominently in the bridging channels and at the T-B interface, and they presumably mature into plasma cells in the red pulp.

Although the "first" signal for B cell activation is provided by the BCR, the "second" signal for T-independent MZ B cell activation is probably induced by ligands for Toll-like receptors. However, eventual differentiation of an MZ B cell into a plasma cell appears to depend on signals provided by specialized blood-borne DCs.

Blood Dendritic Cells Provide Additional Signals for MZ B Cell Activation and Plasma Cell Differentiation

Blood-borne pathogens that arrive in the marginal zone via the circulation do so in part after being captured by CD11c^{lo} DCs in the circulation (28). DCs, which are generally CD11c^{hi}, are involved in the activation of T cells and contribute to immune responses to protein antigens. DCs also participate in anticarbohydrate responses mediated in the context of whole bacteria (136).

Unique, immature, CD11c^{lo} DCs are activated and rapidly leave the blood after encountering blood-borne bacteria to interact with MZ B cells in the bridging channels of the spleen and at the border between T and B cell areas (28). These cells appear to have enhanced migratory and phagocytic properties compared with other types of activated DCs. The mechanism by which these DCs present multivalent antigens to MZ B cells is unclear. It is possible that lectins on these cells associate with whole bacteria or fragments thereof, thus making these available as antigenic ligands for the BCR. A major function of activated DCs in these TI-2 responses appears to be to provide additional signals to MZ B cells by way of BAFF family ligands. The importance of BAFF interactions with BAFF-R in transitional B cell survival was stressed in a previous section. There are two BAFF family ligands, BAFF and a proliferation-inducing ligand (APRIL), and three receptors, BAFF-R, BCMA, and TACI (reviewed in 137). Blood DCs that have been exposed to *Streptococcus pneumoniae* express enhanced levels of BAFF and APRIL, and TACI-Ig fusion proteins can block the differentiation in vivo of MZ B cells into plasmablasts. Additional signals for MZ B cell differentiation are likely delivered by DCs via the interactions of BAFF or APRIL with BCMA because BCMA appears to be specifically required for the generation or survival of plasma cells (138).

MZ B Cells are Involved in T-Dependent Immune Responses

MZ B cells are endowed with many features that suggest that they are ideally suited for the presentation of protein antigens and for the activation of helper T cells. MZ B cells that are specific for protein antigens may present peptides from these antigens to $CD4^+$ T cells. Although follicular B cells are generally viewed as being unable to activate naive helper T cells in vivo, MZ B cells, in contrast, may in many ways resemble activated DCs. MZ B cells, as noted before, express higher levels of class II antigens and B7 proteins than follicular B cells. MZ B cells are also far more potent activators of naive $CD4^+$ T cells both in vitro and in vivo than follicular B cells, although in the model employed these were primarily of a transitional nature (139).

MZ B cells may be involved in extrafollicular B cell responses to protein (and polysaccharide) antigens (140). These responses occur in the red pulp or the T cell zone–red pulp interface, do not involve germinal center formation, and may be accompanied by class switching and somatic hypermutation (141). These types of responses are considered again in the section below on human MZ B cells. In addition to these extrafollicular B cell responses, it is now clear, from cell transfer studies, that MZ B cells are fully capable of initiating germinal center formation and undergoing somatic hypermutation (142) in responses to artificial antigens. In the case of blood-borne particulate antigens, antibody responses to some protein epitopes are probably initiated by MZ B cells. For some antigens, MZ B cells may be the major source of somatically mutated postgerminal center B cells.

HUMAN MZ B CELLS

Many of the differences in perceptions regarding MZ B cells among immunologists depend on the species being studied. Human MZ B cells share many of the markers and properties of murine MZ B cells. They reside in the splenic marginal zone (among other sites), and are typically $IgM^{hi}IgD^{lo}CD21^{hi}CD23^-$ cells (4). Mice possess only a single CD1 gene, the Cd1d gene, and this is expressed at high levels in murine MZ B cells. Human MZ B cells express high levels of CD1c (143), a distinct isoform. It is likely, though as yet unproven, that human and murine MZ B cells collaborate with NKT cells in responses to lipid antigens. Human MZ B cells, like their rodent counterparts, are considered to represent a first line of defense against blood-borne pathogens, particularly encapsulated bacteria.

In fairly striking contrast to murine MZ B cells, human MZ B cells recirculate freely, are found in many anatomical sites other than the spleen, and appear to be identical to somatically mutated, circulating, IgM^+ memory cells.

About 40% of all circulating human B cells are memory cells, and these cells express CD27, a TNFR family member (144). Another useful marker for human memory B cells is a receptor tyrosine phosphatase called CD148 (145). About half of all human circulating memory cells are isotype-switched cells that are assumed to be postgerminal center memory cells. Most of the remaining human circulating memory cells are called IgM^+ memory cells, the majority of which express both IgM and IgD (IgM^+IgD^+ memory cells). A small number of IgM^+ memory cells have an IgM^+IgD^- phenotype and are referred to as IgM-only memory cells. A very small population of IgD^+IgM^- memory cells (IgD-only memory cells) exists as well. $IgM^+IgD^+CD27^+$ memory cells in the peripheral blood differ from recirculating $IgM^+IgD^+CD27^-$ naive B cells in that the $CD27^+$ population harbors somatic mutations and the $CD27^-$ population does not (144).

Circulating IgM^+ memory cells are lost in individuals with congenital asplenia as well as in patients who have had their spleens removed (143, 146). The absence of these cells has led one group of investigators to suggest that circulating IgM^+ memory B cells are the human analogs of murine B-1a cells, which are also lost when mice are subjected to splenectomy (146). However, because others have shown that human splenic MZ B cells are identical to circulating IgM^+ memory B cells using a number of criteria, including microarray comparisons of gene expression and repertoire modulation after immunization (143), it appears more logical to consider these cells as the developmental and functional human analogs of both murine MZ B cells and B-1a cells.

The somatic mutations observed in human splenic MZ B cells and circulating IgM^+ memory B cells are similar in extent and appear to reflect extrafollicular somatic mutations. In fact, studies on patients with the X-linked hyper-IgM syndrome, harboring mutations in CD40L, suggest that the somatic mutations seen in these human IgM^+ B cells may occur in the absence of significant T-B collaboration, which is somewhat surprising but well documented (143, 147). Intriguingly, somatic mutations in splenic MZ B cells do not appear to require exposure to external antigens because mutations are observed even in very young infants. However, it is unclear if the splenectomized children were previous recipients of the plethora of neonatal immunizations that most children in the developed world receive. MZ B cells in humans may start out as naive nonmutated B cells, as in rodents, but then rapidly diversify further by somatic mutation, either by a poorly understood spontaneous process or, more likely, in response to environmental antigens. These cells carrying somatic mutations continue to reside in the marginal zone, but may also be located in other secondary lymphoid organs.

Are the differences between human and rodent MZ B cells significant? Functionally, in terms of responses to blood-borne pathogens, it is unlikely that there are major differences in these populations. Very little is understood as to why, in rodents, the spleen is the only site of MZ B cell localization, or why exactly the spleen is required for MZ B cell generation in both mice and men. It may be that cycling precursors can only be generated in the spleen, perhaps because specific cell-associated ligands are only available in this organ. There is no intrinsic disadvantage for primates to have evolved the ability to have these immunologically versatile cells reach other sites. Indeed, during the homeostatic proliferation phenomenon in mice, B cells that resemble MZ B cells appear to inhabit all secondary lymphoid organs (115). Immunized rats acquire somatic mutations in their MZ B cells, and these mutations appear to be of the more limited extrafollicular variety, whereas unimmunized rats lack such mutations (117). Somatic mutation in human MZ B cells could be a unique and spontaneous "antigen-independent" diversification mechanism. Alternatively, somatic mutations in human MZ B cells may be of iatrogenic origin in a world where children are provided an accelerated viewing of the antigenic universe.

MZ B CELLS AND DISEASE

Human MZ B cells/IgM$^+$ memory cells are believed to be exquisitely sensitive to triggering by CpG DNA of microbial origin, whereupon they proliferate and differentiate into plasmablasts throughout life, producing antibacterial and other natural antibodies. The antigen-independent polyclonal activation and differentiation of this subset of B cells is considered responsible for "long-term serological memory" (148). Not surprisingly, postsplenectomy infections are associated with an extraordinarily high mortality.

Whether MZ B cells are linked to the pathogenesis of autoimmune disorders in any mechanistic way is unclear. Indeed, the few engineered autoreactive clones that do accumulate in the marginal zone in certain models tend to be of low self-reactivity. Certain autoantibody expressing clones, including class-switched clones, have also been observed to home to the marginal zone (149). The significance of these findings remains unclear. Infiltrates of MZ B cells (essentially IgM$^+$ memory cells) may be of relevance in autoimmune thyroiditis in humans (150), and in Sjogren's syndrome the characteristic lymphoid infiltrate in salivary glands is made up of MZ B cells/IgM$^+$ memory cells (151, 152). There is, however, no reason to believe that MZ B cells are more relevant than other subsets of B cells in the pathogenesis of autoimmune disorders. The extranodal expansion of reactive MZ B cells in certain autoimmune states (including Sjogren's syndrome), as well as in infections, appears to participate in the genesis of certain human lymphomas that are believed to be of MZ B cell origin.

The proclivity for nonspecific mitogens to induce MZ B cell proliferation may also provide a mechanistic link between MZ B cells and many human lymphomas (148). Pathological expansions of MZ B cells range from a condition termed "benign polyclonal B lymphocytosis" of unknown origin (153) to a diverse group of malignancies that are described as marginal zone lymphomas. These are categorized by their site of origin into splenic marginal zone lymphomas, nodal marginal zone lymphomas, and extranodal MALT lymphomas. Splenic marginal zone lymphomas are rare and may sometimes actually be located in the mantle zone (153). Marginal zone lymphomas have also been described in the murine spleen (154). Nodal marginal zone lymphomas are also relatively uncommon and develop in lymph nodes. MALT lymphomas occur at numerous extranodal sites and represent a relatively common type of lymphoid malignancy. These tumors histologically recapitulate the structure of Peyer's patches (155). Reactive B cells are surrounded by a margin of transformed MZ B cells in these tumors. The reactive cells are sometimes of autoimmune origin, or develop in response to infections. In low-grade MALT lymphomas of the gastric mucosa, these tumors are commonly generated as a part of a T cell–dependent immune response to *Helicobacter pylori* antigens. A large proportion of gastric MALT lymphomas cease to grow when *H. pylori* is eradicated. Two translocations are of importance in the genesis of MALT lymphomas that persist after *H. pylori* eradication. The most common cytogenetic abnormality in MALT lymphomas is the t(11;18)(q21;q21) translocation that generates a fusion protein between the N-terminus of cIAP2 and the MALT1 protein. A more rare t(1;14)(p22;q32) translocation contributes to the activation of Bcl-10. As noted earlier, Bcl-10, MALT1, and CARD11 work together to activate NF-κB. The constitutive activation of NF-κB may be required for the survival of many marginal zone lymphomas of the MALT variety.

It remains to be seen whether the growing understanding of the molecular players and pathways that contribute to murine MZ B cell development and survival is relevant to the development and survival of human MZ B cells. A more complete understanding of these mechanisms may find application in specific clinical disorders ranging from Sjogren's syndrome to MALT lymphomas.

FUTURE DIRECTIONS

There are a number of exciting directions that research on MZ B cells is likely to take in the coming years. Many questions remain to be answered regarding the development and function of MZ B cells. How exactly does self-antigen set the stage to select between an FO fate and an MZ B cell fate? What are the signaling events downstream of the BCR that contribute to different peripheral B cell fates? What are the specific targets of Notch2 signaling that yield MZ B cells during development? How do the BCR and Notch2 talk to one another in terms of lineage commitment? What other genes and pathways are involved in MZ B cell maintenance? Are there specific chemokines that are relevant to the migration of MZ B cells and their precursors? Are T2-MZP cells self-renewing progenitors of MZ B cells? What are the molecular and cellular pathways involved in homeostatic proliferation of B cells? How do human MZ B cells develop? Do MZ B cells respond to lipid antigens? Do these cells collaborate with NK T cells? The list is endless, but time flies when you are having fun.

ACKNOWLEDGMENTS

We thank other members of the laboratory for reading this review and for helpful discussions, and Brian Pittner for discussions on IgD. This work was supported by grants AI 33507, AI57486, CA102793, and AI54917 from the NIH.

The *Annual Review of Immunology* is online at
http://immunol.annualreviews.org

LITERATURE CITED

1. Weidenreich F. 1901. Das Gefasssystem der menschlichen Milz. *Arch. Mikrosk. Anat.* 58:247–376
2. MacNeal WJ. 1929. The circulation of blood through the spleen pulp. *Arch. Pathol.* 7:215–27
3. Kraal G. 1992. Cells in the marginal zone of the spleen. *Int. Rev. Cytol.* 132:31–74
4. Spencer J, Perry ME, Dunn-Walters DK. 1998. Human marginal-zone B cells. *Immunol. Today* 19:421–26
5. Martin F, Kearney JF. 2002. Marginal-zone B cells. *Nat. Rev. Immunol.* 2:323–35
6. Zandvoort A, Timens W. 2002. The dual function of the splenic marginal zone: essential for initiation of anti-TI-2 responses but also vital in the general first-line defense against blood-borne antigens. *Clin. Exp. Immunol.* 130:4–11
7. Hardy RR, Hayakawa K. 2001. B cell development pathways. *Annu. Rev. Immunol.* 19:595–621
8. Martin F, Kearney JF. 2000. B-cell subsets and the mature preimmune repertoire. Marginal zone and B1 B cells as part of a "natural immune memory.? *Immunol. Rev.* 175:70–79
9. Cariappa A, Pillai S. 2002. Antigen-dependent B-cell development. *Curr. Opin. Immunol.* 14:241–49
10. Pillai S, Cariappa A, Moran ST. 2004. Positive selection and lineage commitment during peripheral B-lymphocyte development. *Immunol. Rev.* 197:206–18
11. Snook T. 1964. Studies on the perifollicular region of the rat's spleen. *Anat. Rec.* 148:149–59
12. Yamamoto K, Kobayashi T, Murakami T. 1982. Arterial terminals in the rat spleen as demonstrated by scanning electron microscopy of vascular casts. *Scan. Electron Microsc.* 1982:455–58
13. Schmidt EE, MacDonald IC, Groom AC. 1993. Comparative aspects of splenic microcirculatory pathways in mammals: the region bordering the white pulp. *Scan. Microsc.* 7:613–28
14. Liu YJ, Oldfield S, MacLennan IC. 1988. Memory B cells in T cell-dependent antibody responses colonize the splenic marginal zones. *Eur. J. Immunol.* 18:355–62
15. Steiniger B, Barth P, Hellinger A. 2001. The perifollicular and marginal zones of the human splenic white pulp: Do fibroblasts guide lymphocyte immigration? *Am. J. Pathol.* 159:501–12
16. Steiniger B, Ruttinger L, Barth PJ. 2003. The three-dimensional structure of human splenic white pulp compartments. *J. Histochem. Cytochem.* 51:655–64

17. Mebius RE, van Tuijl S, Weissman IL, Randall TD. 1998. Transfer of primitive stem/progenitor bone marrow cells from LT $\alpha^{-/-}$ donors to wild-type hosts: implications for the generation of architectural events in lymphoid B cell domains. *J. Immunol.* 161:3836–43

18. Fu YX, Chaplin DD. 1999. Development and maturation of secondary lymphoid tissues. *Annu. Rev. Immunol.* 17:399–433

19. Ettinger R, Munson SH, Chao CC, Vadeboncoeur M, Toma J, McDevitt HO. 2001. A critical role for lymphotoxin-β receptor in the development of diabetes in nonobese diabetic mice. *J. Exp. Med.* 193:1333–40

20. Shinkura R, Kitada K, Matsuda F, Tashiro K, Ikuta K, et al. 1999. Alymphoplasia is caused by a point mutation in the mouse gene encoding NF-κB-inducing kinase. *Nat. Genet.* 22:74–77

21. Yin L, Wu L, Wesche H, Arthur CD, White JM, et al. 2001. Defective lymphotoxin-β receptor-induced NF-κB transcriptional activity in NIK-deficient mice. *Science* 291:2162–65

22. Senftleben U, Cao Y, Xiao G, Greten FR, Krahn G, et al. 2001. Activation by IKKα of a second, evolutionary conserved, NF-κB signaling pathway. *Science* 293:1495–99

23. Matsushima A, Kaisho T, Rennert PD, Nakano H, Kurosawa K, et al. 2001. Essential role of nuclear factor (NF)-κB-inducing kinase and inhibitor of κB (IκB) kinase α in NF-κB activation through lymphotoxin β receptor, but not through tumor necrosis factor receptor I. *J. Exp. Med.* 193:631–36

24. Banks TA, Rouse BT, Kerley MK, Blair PJ, Godfrey VL, et al. 1995. Lymphotoxin-α-deficient mice. Effects on secondary lymphoid organ development and humoral immune responsiveness. *J. Immunol.* 155:1685–93

25. De Togni P, Goellner J, Ruddle NH, Streeter PR, Fick A, et al. 1994. Abnormal development of peripheral lymphoid organs in mice deficient in lymphotoxin. *Science* 264:703–7

26. Metlay JP, Witmer-Pack MD, Agger R, Crowley MT, Lawless D, Steinman RM. 1990. The distinct leukocyte integrins of mouse spleen dendritic cells as identified with new hamster monoclonal antibodies. *J. Exp. Med.* 171:1753–71

27. Leenen PJ, Radosevic K, Voerman JS, Salomon B, van Rooijen N, et al. 1998. Heterogeneity of mouse spleen dendritic cells: in vivo phagocytic activity, expression of macrophage markers, and subpopulation turnover. *J. Immunol.* 160:2166–73

28. Balazs M, Martin F, Zhou T, Kearney J. 2002. Blood dendritic cells interact with splenic marginal zone B cells to initiate T-independent immune responses. *Immunity* 17:341–52

29. Kraal G, Janse M. 1986. Marginal metallophilic cells of the mouse spleen identified by a monoclonal antibody. *Immunology* 58:665–69

30. Dijkstra CD, Van Vliet E, Dopp EA, van der Lelij AA, Kraal G. 1985. Marginal zone macrophages identified by a monoclonal antibody: characterization of immuno- and enzyme-histochemical properties and functional capacities. *Immunology* 55:23–30

31. Elomaa O, Kangas M, Sahlberg C, Tuukkanen J, Sormunen R, et al. 1995. Cloning of a novel bacteria-binding receptor structurally related to scavenger receptors and expressed in a subset of macrophages. *Cell* 80:603–9

32. Humphrey JH, Grennan D. 1981. Different macrophage populations distinguished by means of fluorescent polysaccharides. Recognition and properties of marginal-zone macrophages. *Eur. J. Immunol.* 11:221–28

33. Karlsson MC, Guinamard R, Bolland S, Sankala M, Steinman RM, Ravetch JV. 2003. Macrophages control the retention and trafficking of B lymphocytes in

the splenic marginal zone. *J. Exp. Med.* 198:333–40

34. Goldschneider I, McGregor DD. 1973. Anatomical distribution of T and B lymphocytes in the rat. Development of lymphocyte-specific antisera. *J. Exp. Med.* 138:1443–65

35. MacLennan IC. 1982. Lymphocytes of splenic marginal zons: a distinct B-cell lineage. *Immunol. Today* 3:305–7

36. Gray D, MacLennan IC, Bazin H, Khan M. 1982. Migrant mu+ delta+ and static mu+ delta- B lymphocyte subsets. *Eur. J. Immunol.* 12:564–69

37. Gray D, McConnell I, Kumararatne DS, MacLennan IC, Humphrey JH, Bazin H. 1984. Marginal zone B cells express CR1 and CR2 receptors. *Eur. J. Immunol.* 14: 47–52

38. Takahashi K, Kozono Y, Waldschmidt TJ, Berthiaume D, Quigg RJ, et al. 1997. Mouse complement receptors type 1 (CR1;CD35) and type 2 (CR2;CD21): expression on normal B cell subpopulations and decreased levels during the development of autoimmunity in MRL/lpr mice. *J. Immunol.* 159:1557–69

39. Oliver AM, Martin F, Gartland GL, Carter RH, Kearney JF. 1997. Marginal zone B cells exhibit unique activation, proliferative and immunoglobulin secretory responses. *Eur. J. Immunol.* 27:2366–74

40. Oliver AM, Martin F, Kearney JF. 1999. IgM^{high}CD21^{high} lymphocytes enriched in the splenic marginal zone generate effector cells more rapidly than the bulk of follicular B cells. *J. Immunol.* 162:7198–207

41. Waldschmidt TJ, Kroese FG, Tygrett LT, Conrad DH, Lynch RG. 1991. The expression of B cell surface receptors. III. The murine low-affinity IgE Fc receptor is not expressed on Ly 1 or 'Ly 1-like' B cells. *Int. Immunol.* 3:305–15

42. Hsu SM. 1985. Phenotypic expression of B lymphocytes. III. Marginal zone B cells in the spleen are characterized by the expression of Tac and alkaline phosphatase. *J. Immunol.* 135:123–30

43. Lu TT, Cyster JG. 2002. Integrin-mediated long-term B cell retention in the splenic marginal zone. *Science* 297:409–12

44. Hao Z, Rajewsky K. 2001. Homeostasis of peripheral B cells in the absence of B cell influx from the bone marrow. *J. Exp. Med.* 194:1151–64

45. Kumararatne DS, Gagnon RF, Smart Y. 1980. Selective loss of large lymphocytes from the marginal zone of the white pulp in rat spleens following a single dose of cyclophosphamide. A study using quantitative histological methods. *Immunology* 40:123–31

46. Lortan J, Gray D, Kumararatne DS, Platteau B, Bazin H, MacLennan IC. 1985. Regulation of the size of the recirculating B cell pool of adult rats. *Adv. Exp. Med. Biol.* 186:593–601

47. Timens W, Boes A, Rozeboom-Uiterwijk T, Poppema S. 1989. Immaturity of the human splenic marginal zone in infancy. Possible contribution to the deficient infant immune response. *J. Immunol.* 143:3200–6

48. Kruschinski C, Zidan M, Debertin AS, von Horsten S, Pabst R. 2004. Age-dependent development of the splenic marginal zone in human infants is associated with different causes of death. *Hum. Pathol.* 35:113–21

49. Allman DM, Ferguson SE, Cancro MP. 1992. Peripheral B cell maturation. I. Immature peripheral B cells in adults are heat-stable antigen^{hi} and exhibit unique signaling characteristics. *J. Immunol.* 149:2533–40

50. Allman DM, Ferguson SE, Lentz VM, Cancro MP. 1993. Peripheral B cell maturation. II. Heat-stable antigen^{hi} splenic B cells are an immature developmental intermediate in the production of long-lived marrow-derived B cells. *J. Immunol.* 151:4431–44

51. Allman D, Lindsley RC, DeMuth W, Rudd K, Shinton SA, Hardy RR. 2001. Resolution of three nonproliferative

immature splenic B cell subsets reveals multiple selection points during peripheral B cell maturation. *J. Immunol.* 167:6834–40

52. Schiemann B, Gommerman JL, Vora K, Cachero TG, Shulga-Morskaya S, et al. 2001. An essential role for BAFF in the normal development of B cells through a BCMA-independent pathway. *Science* 293:2111–14

53. Thompson JS, Bixler SA, Qian F, Vora K, Scott ML, et al. 2001. BAFF-R, a newly identified TNF receptor that specifically interacts with BAFF. *Science* 293:2108–11

54. Schneider P, Takatsuka H, Wilson A, Mackay F, Tardivel A, et al. 2001. Maturation of marginal zone and follicular B cells requires B cell activating factor of the tumor necrosis factor family and is independent of B cell maturation antigen. *J. Exp. Med.* 194:1691–97

55. Lam KP, Kuhn R, Rajewsky K. 1997. In vivo ablation of surface immunoglobulin on mature B cells by inducible gene targeting results in rapid cell death. *Cell* 90:1073–83

56. Kraus M, Alimzhanov MB, Rajewsky N, Rajewsky K. 2004. Survival of resting mature B lymphocytes depends on BCR signaling via the Igα/β heterodimer. *Cell* 117:787–800

57. Forster R, Mattis AE, Kremmer E, Wolf E, Brem G, Lipp M. 1996. A putative chemokine receptor, BLR1, directs B cell migration to defined lymphoid organs and specific anatomic compartments of the spleen. *Cell* 87:1037–47

58. Reif K, Ekland EH, Ohl L, Nakano H, Lipp M, et al. 2002. Balanced responsiveness to chemoattractants from adjacent zones determines B-cell position. *Nature* 416:94–99

59. Cariappa A, Tang M, Parng C, Nebelitskiy E, Carroll M, et al. 2001. The follicular versus marginal zone B lymphocyte cell fate decision is regulated by Aiolos, Btk, and CD21. *Immunity* 14:603–15

60. Saito T, Chiba S, Ichikawa M, Kunisato A, Asai T, et al. 2003. Notch2 is preferentially expressed in mature B cells and indispensable for marginal zone B lineage development. *Immunity* 18:675–85

61. Loder F, Mutschler B, Ray RJ, Paige CJ, Sideras P, et al. 1999. B cell development in the spleen takes place in discrete steps and is determined by the quality of B cell receptor-derived signals. *J. Exp. Med.* 190:75–89

62. Hardy RR, Hayakawa K, Parks DR, Herzenberg LA. 1983. Demonstration of B-cell maturation in X-linked immunodeficient mice by simultaneous three-colour immunofluorescence. *Nature* 306:270–72

63. Khan WN, Alt FW, Gerstein RM, Malynn BA, Larsson I, et al. 1995. Defective B cell development and function in Btk-deficient mice. *Immunity* 3:283–99

64. Kerner JD, Appleby MW, Mohr RN, Chien S, Rawlings DJ, et al. 1995. Impaired expansion of mouse B cell progenitors lacking Btk. *Immunity* 3:301–12

65. Cariappa A, Kim TJ, Pillai S. 1999. Accelerated emigration of B lymphocytes in the Xid mouse. *J. Immunol.* 162:4417–23

66. Byth KF, Conroy LA, Howlett S, Smith AJ, May J, et al. 1996. CD45-null transgenic mice reveal a positive regulatory role for CD45 in early thymocyte development, in the selection of CD4$^+$CD8$^+$ thymocytes, and B cell maturation. *J. Exp. Med.* 183:1707–18

67. Yamazaki T, Takeda K, Gotoh K, Takeshima H, Akira S, Kurosaki T. 2002. Essential immunoregulatory role for BCAP in B cell development and function. *J. Exp. Med.* 195:535–45

68. Fruman DA, Snapper SB, Yballe CM, Davidson L, Yu JY, et al. 1999. Impaired B cell development and proliferation in absence of phosphoinositide 3-kinase p85α. *Science* 283:393–97

69. Suzuki H, Terauchi Y, Fujiwara M, Aizawa S, Yazaki Y, et al. 1999. Xid-like

immunodeficiency in mice with disruption of the p85α subunit of phosphoinositide 3-kinase. *Science* 283:390–92

70. Jumaa H, Wollscheid B, Mitterer M, Wienands J, Reth M, Nielsen PJ. 1999. Abnormal development and function of B lymphocytes in mice deficient for the signaling adaptor protein SLP-65. *Immunity* 11:547–54

71. Pappu R, Cheng AM, Li B, Gong Q, Chiu C, et al. 1999. Requirement for B cell linker protein (BLNK) in B cell development. *Science* 286:1949–54

72. Wang D, Feng J, Wen R, Marine JC, Sangster MY, et al. 2000. Phospholipase Cγ2 is essential in the functions of B cell and several Fc receptors. *Immunity* 13:25–35

73. Wardemann H, Yurasov S, Schaefer A, Young JW, Meffre E, Nussenzweig MC. 2003. Predominant autoantibody production by early human B cell precursors. *Science* 301:1374–77

74. Rolink AG, Andersson J, Melchers F. 1998. Characterization of immature B cells by a novel monoclonal antibody, by turnover and by mitogen reactivity. *Eur. J. Immunol.* 28:3738–48

75. Hsu BL, Harless SM, Lindsley RC, Hilbert DM, Cancro MP. 2002. Cutting edge: BLyS enables survival of transitional and mature B cells through distinct mediators. *J. Immunol.* 168:5993–96

76. Lesley R, Xu Y, Kalled SL, Hess DM, Schwab SR, et al. 2004. Reduced competitiveness of autoantigen-engaged B cells due to increased dependence on BAFF. *Immunity* 20:441–53

77. Thien M, Phan TG, Gardam S, Amesbury M, Basten A, et al. 2004. Excess BAFF rescues self-reactive B cells from peripheral deletion and allows them to enter forbidden follicular and marginal zone niches. *Immunity* 20:785–98

78. Neuberger MS. 1997. Antigen receptor signaling gives lymphocytes a long life. *Cell* 90:971–73

79. Pillai S. 1999. The chosen few? Positive selection and the generation of naive B lymphocytes. *Immunity* 10:493–502

80. Wang JH, Avitahl N, Cariappa A, Friedrich C, Ikeda T, et al. 1998. Aiolos regulates B cell activation and maturation to effector state. *Immunity* 9:543–53

81. Samardzic T, Marinkovic D, Danzer CP, Gerlach J, Nitschke L, Wirth T. 2002. Reduction of marginal zone B cells in CD22-deficient mice. *Eur. J. Immunol.* 32:561–67

82. Sun T, Clark MR, Storb U. 2002. A point mutation in the constant region of Ig lambda1 prevents normal B cell development due to defective BCR signaling. *Immunity* 16:245–55

83. Kraus M, Pao LI, Reichlin A, Hu Y, Canono B, et al. 2001. Interference with immunoglobulin (Ig)α immunoreceptor tyrosine-based activation motif (ITAM) phosphorylation modulates or blocks B cell development, depending on the availability of an Igβ cytoplasmic tail. *J. Exp. Med.* 194:455–69

84. Hendriks RW, de Bruijn MF, Maas A, Dingjan GM, Karis A, Grosveld F. 1996. Inactivation of Btk by insertion of lacZ reveals defects in B cell development only past the pre-B cell stage. *EMBO. J.* 15:4862–72

85. Hayakawa K, Asano M, Shinton SA, Gui M, Allman D, et al. 1999. Positive selection of natural autoreactive B cells. *Science* 285:113–16

86. Martin F, Kearney JF. 2000. Positive selection from newly formed to marginal zone B cells depends on the rate of clonal production, CD19, and *btk. Immunity* 12:39–49

87. Casola S, Otipoby KL, Alimzhanov M, Humme S, Uyttersprot N, et al. 2004. B cell receptor signal strength determines B cell fate. *Nat. Immunol.* 5:317–27

88. Cabatingan MS, Schmidt MR, Sen R, Woodland RT. 2002. Naive B lymphocytes undergo homeostatic proliferation in response to B cell deficit. *J. Immunol.* 169:6795–805

88a. Scher I, Sternberg AD, Berning AK, Paul WE. 1975. X-linked B-lymphocyte immune defect in CBA/N mice. II. Studies of the mechanisms underlying the immune defect. *J. Exp. Med.* 142:637–50

89. Anderson JS, Teutsch M, Dong Z, Wortis HH. 1996. An essential role for Bruton's [corrected] tyrosine kinase in the regulation of B-cell apoptosis. *Proc. Natl. Acad. Sci. USA* 93:10966–71

90. Brunner C, Marinkovic D, Klein J, Samardzic T, Nitschke L, Wirth T. 2003. B cell-specific transgenic expression of Bcl2 rescues early B lymphopoiesis but not B cell responses in BOB.1/OBF.1-deficient mice. *J. Exp. Med.* 197:1205–11

91. Okkenhaug K, Bilancio A, Farjot G, Priddle H, Sancho S, et al. 2002. Impaired B and T cell antigen receptor signaling in p110δ PI 3-kinase mutant mice. *Science* 297:1031–34

92. Clayton E, Bardi G, Bell SE, Chantry D, Downes CP, et al. 2002. A crucial role for the p110δ subunit of phosphatidylinositol 3-kinase in B cell development and activation. *J. Exp. Med.* 196:753–63

93. Jou ST, Carpino N, Takahashi Y, Piekorz R, Chao JR, et al. 2002. Essential, nonredundant role for the phosphoinositide 3-kinase p110δ in signaling by the B-cell receptor complex. *Mol. Cell. Biol.* 22:8580–91

94. Cariappa A, Liou HC, Horwitz BH, Pillai S. 2000. Nuclear factor κB is required for the development of marginal zone B lymphocytes. *J. Exp. Med.* 192:1175–82

95. Weih DS, Yilmaz ZB, Weih F. 2001. Essential role of RelB in germinal center and marginal zone formation and proper expression of homing chemokines. *J. Immunol.* 167:1909–19

96. Xue L, Morris SW, Orihuela C, Tuomanen E, Cui X, et al. 2003. Defective development and function of Bcl10-deficient follicular, marginal zone and B1 B cells. *Nat. Immunol.* 4:857–65

97. Ruefli-Brasse AA, French DM, Dixit VM. 2003. Regulation of NF-κB-dependent lymphocyte activation and development by paracaspase. *Science* 302:1581–84

98. Ruland J, Duncan GS, Wakeham A, Mak TW. 2003. Differential requirement for Malt1 in T and B cell antigen receptor signaling. *Immunity* 19:749–58

99. Egawa T, Albrecht B, Favier B, Sunshine MJ, Mirchandani K, et al. 2003. Requirement for CARMA1 in antigen receptor-induced NF-κB activation and lymphocyte proliferation. *Curr. Biol.* 13:1252–58

100. Hara H, Wada T, Bakal C, Kozieradzki I, Suzuki S, et al. 2003. The MAGUK family protein CARD11 is essential for lymphocyte activation. *Immunity* 18:763–75

101. Jun JE, Wilson LE, Vinuesa CG, Lesage S, Blery M, et al. 2003. Identifying the MAGUK protein Carma-1 as a central regulator of humoral immune responses and atopy by genome-wide mouse mutagenesis. *Immunity* 18:751–62

102. Zhou H, Wertz I, O' Rourke K, Ultsch M, Seshagiri S, et al. 2004. Bcl10 activates the NF-κB pathway through ubiquitination of NEMO. *Nature* 427:167–71

103. Samardzic T, Marinkovic D, Nielsen PJ, Nitschke L, Wirth T. 2002. BOB.1/OBF.1 deficiency affects marginal-zone B-cell compartment. *Mol. Cell. Biol.* 22:8320–31

104. Morgan TH. 1917. The theory of the gene. *Am. Nat.* 51:513–44

105. Radtke F, Wilson A, Mancini SJ, MacDonald HR. 2004. Notch regulation of lymphocyte development and function. *Nat. Immunol.* 5:247–53

106. Wu L, Sun T, Kobayashi K, Gao P, Griffin JD. 2002. Identification of a family of mastermind-like transcriptional coactivators for mammalian notch receptors. *Mol. Cell. Biol.* 22:7688–700

107. Tanigaki K, Han H, Yamamoto N, Tashiro K, Ikegawa M, et al. 2002. Notch-RBP-J signaling is involved in cell fate determination of marginal zone B cells. *Nat. Immunol.* 3:443–50

108. Hozumi K, Negishi N, Suzuki D, Abe N, Sotomaru Y, et al. 2004. Delta-like 1 is

necessary for the generation of marginal zone B cells but not T cells in vivo. *Nat. Immunol.* 5:638–44

109. Witt CM, Won WJ, Hurez V, Klug CA. 2003. Notch2 haploinsufficiency results in diminished B1 B cells and a severe reduction in marginal zone B cells. *J. Immunol.* 171:2783–88

110. Kuroda K, Han H, Tani S, Tanigaki K, Tun T, et al. 2003. Regulation of marginal zone B cell development by MINT, a suppressor of Notch/RBP-J signaling pathway. *Immunity* 18:301–12

111. Maillard I, Weng AP, Carpenter AC, Rodriguez CG, Sai H, et al. 2004. Mastermind critically regulates Notch-mediated lymphoid cell fate decisions. *Blood* 104:1696–702

112. Mackay F, Woodcock SA, Lawton P, Ambrose C, Baetscher M, et al. 1999. Mice transgenic for BAFF develop lymphocytic disorders along with autoimmune manifestations. *J. Exp. Med.* 190:1697–710

113. Khare SD, Sarosi I, Xia XZ, McCabe S, Miner K, et al. 2000. Severe B cell hyperplasia and autoimmune disease in TALL-1 transgenic mice. *Proc. Natl. Acad. Sci. USA* 97:3370–75

114. Loset GA, Roux KH, Zhu P, Michaelsen TE, Sandlie I. 2004. Differential segmental flexibility and reach dictate the antigen binding mode of chimeric IgD and IgM: implications for the function of the B cell receptor. *J. Immunol.* 172:2925–34

115. Agenes F, Freitas AA. 1999. Transfer of small resting B cells into immunodeficient hosts results in the selection of a self-renewing activated B cell population. *J. Exp. Med.* 189:319–30

116. Agenes F, Rosado MM, Freitas AA. 2000. Considerations on B cell homeostasis. *Curr. Top. Microbiol. Immunol.* 252:68–75

117. Dammers PM, de Boer NK, Deenen GJ, Nieuwenhuis P, Kroese FG. 1999. The origin of marginal zone B cells in the rat. *Eur. J. Immunol.* 29:1522–31

118. Lo CG, Lu TT, Cyster JG. 2003. Integrin-dependence of lymphocyte entry into the splenic white pulp. *J. Exp. Med.* 197:353–61

119. Cinamon G, Matloubian M, Lesneski MJ, Xu Y, Low C, et al. 2004. Sphingosine 1-phosphate receptor 1 promotes B cell localization in the splenic marginal zone. *Nat. Immunol.* 5:713–20

120. Dalwadi H, Wei B, Schrage M, Su TT, Rawlings DJ, Braun J. 2003. B cell developmental requirement for the *Gαi2* gene. *J. Immunol.* 170:1707–15

121. Guinamard R, Okigaki M, Schlessinger J, Ravetch JV. 2000. Absence of marginal zone B cells in Pyk-2-deficient mice defines their role in the humoral response. *Nat. Immunol.* 1:31–36

122. Girkontaite I, Missy K, Sakk V, Harenberg A, Tedford K, et al. 2001. Lsc is required for marginal zone B cells, regulation of lymphocyte motility and immune responses. *Nat. Immunol.* 2:855–62

123. Fukui Y, Hashimoto O, Sanui T, Oono T, Koga H, et al. 2001. Haematopoietic cell-specific CDM family protein DOCK2 is essential for lymphocyte migration. *Nature* 412:826–31

124. Sanui T, Inayoshi A, Noda M, Iwata E, Stein JV, et al. 2003. DOCK2 regulates Rac activation and cytoskeletal reorganization through interaction with ELMO1. *Blood* 102:2948–50

125. Croker BA, Tarlinton DM, Cluse LA, Tuxen AJ, Light A, et al. 2002. The Rac2 guanosine triphosphatase regulates B lymphocyte antigen receptor responses and chemotaxis and is required for establishment of B-1a and marginal zone B lymphocytes. *J. Immunol.* 168:3376–86

126. Coil JA, Dickerman JD, Boulton E. 1978. Increased susceptibility of splenectomized mice to infection after exposure to an aerosolized suspension of type III *Streptococcus pneumoniae. Infect. Immun.* 21:412–16

127. Amlot PL, Grennan D, Humphrey JH. 1985. Splenic dependence of the antibody

response to thymus-independent (TI-2) antigens. *Eur. J. Immunol.* 15:508–12

128. Harms G, Hardonk MJ, Timens W. 1996. In vitro complement-dependent binding and in vivo kinetics of pneumococcal polysaccharide TI-2 antigens in the rat spleen marginal zone and follicle. *Infect. Immun.* 64:4220–25

129. Mond JJ, Lees A, Snapper CM. 1995. T cell-independent antigens type 2. *Annu. Rev. Immunol.* 13:655–92

130. Likhite VV. 1976. Immunological impairment and susceptibility to infection after splenectomy. *JAMA* 236:1376–77

131. Holdsworth RJ, Irving AD, Cuschieri A. 1991. Postsplenectomy sepsis and its mortality rate: actual versus perceived risks. *Br. J. Surg.* 78:1031–38

132. Cowan MJ, Ammann AJ, Wara DW, Howie VM, Schultz L, et al. 1978. Pneumococcal polysaccharide immunization in infants and children. *Pediatrics* 62:721–27

133. Totapally BR, Walsh WT. 1998. Pneumococcal bacteremia in childhood: a 6-year experience in a community hospital. *Chest* 113:1207–14

134. Sha WC, Liou HC, Tuomanen EI, Baltimore D. 1995. Targeted disruption of the p50 subunit of NF-κB leads to multifocal defects in immune responses. *Cell* 80:321–30

135. Martin F, Oliver AM, Kearney JF. 2001. Marginal zone and B1 B cells unite in the early response against T-independent blood-borne particulate antigens. *Immunity* 14:617–29

136. Colino J, Shen Y, Snapper CM. 2002. Dendritic cells pulsed with intact *Streptococcus pneumoniae* elicit both protein- and polysaccharide-specific immunoglobulin isotype responses in vivo through distinct mechanisms. *J. Exp. Med.* 195:1–13

137. Mackay F, Ambrose C. 2003. The TNF family members BAFF and APRIL: the growing complexity. *Cytokine Growth Factor Rev.* 14:311–24

138. O' Connor BP, Raman VS, Erickson LD, Cook WJ, Weaver LK, et al. 2004. BCMA is essential for the survival of long-lived bone marrow plasma cells. *J. Exp. Med.* 199:91–98

139. Attanavanich K, Kearney JF. 2004. Marginal zone, but not follicular B cells, are potent activators of naive CD4 T cells. *J. Immunol.* 172:803–11

140. MacLennan IC, Toellner KM, Cunningham AF, Serre K, Sze DM, et al. 2003. Extrafollicular antibody responses. *Immunol. Rev.* 194:8–18

141. William J, Euler C, Christensen S, Shlomchik MJ. 2002. Evolution of autoantibody responses via somatic hypermutation outside of germinal centers. *Science* 297:2066–70

142. Song H, Cerny J. 2003. Functional heterogeneity of marginal zone B cells revealed by their ability to generate both early antibody-forming cells and germinal centers with hypermutation and memory in response to a T-dependent antigen. *J. Exp. Med.* 198:1923–35

143. Weller S, Braun MC, Tan BK, Rosenwald A, Cordier C, et al. 2004. Human blood IgM "memory" B cells are circulating splenic marginal zone B cells harboring a pre-diversified immunoglobulin repertoire. *Blood.* 104:3647–54

144. Klein U, Rajewsky K, Kuppers R. 1998. Human immunoglobulin (Ig)M$^+$IgD$^+$ peripheral blood B cells expressing the CD27 cell surface antigen carry somatically mutated variable region genes: CD27 as a general marker for somatically mutated (memory) B cells. *J. Exp. Med.* 188:1679–89

145. Tangye SG, Liu YJ, Aversa G, Phillips JH, de Vries JE. 1998. Identification of functional human splenic memory B cells by expression of CD148 and CD27. *J. Exp. Med.* 188:1691–703

146. Kruetzmann S, Rosado MM, Weber H, Germing U, Tournilhac O, et al. 2003. Human immunoglobulin M memory B cells controlling *Streptococcus pneumoniae*

infections are generated in the spleen. *J. Exp. Med.* 197:939–45

147. Weller S, Faili A, Garcia C, Braun MC, Le Deist FF, et al. 2001. CD40-CD40L independent Ig gene hypermutation suggests a second B cell diversification pathway in humans. *Proc. Natl. Acad. Sci. USA* 98:1166–70

148. Bernasconi NL, Traggiai E, Lanzavecchia A. 2002. Maintenance of serological memory by polyclonal activation of human memory B cells. *Science* 298:2199–202

149. Li Y, Li H, Weigert M. 2002. Autoreactive B cells in the marginal zone that express dual receptors. *J. Exp. Med.* 195:181–88

150. Segundo C, Rodriguez C, Garcia-Poley A, Aguilar M, Gavilan I, et al. 2001. Thyroid-infiltrating B lymphocytes in Graves' disease are related to marginal zone and memory B cell compartments. *Thyroid* 11:525–30

151. Groom J, Kalled SL, Cutler AH, Olson C, Woodcock SA, et al. 2002. Association of BAFF/BLyS overexpression and altered B cell differentiation with Sjogren's syndrome. *J. Clin. Invest.* 109:59–68

152. Harris NL. 1999. Lymphoid proliferations of the salivary glands. *Am. J. Clin. Pathol.* 111:S94–103

153. Salcedo I, Campos-Caro A, Sampalo A, Reales E, Brieva JA. 2002. Persistent polyclonal B lymphocytosis: an expansion of cells showing IgVH gene mutations and phenotypic features of normal lymphocytes from the CD27$^+$ marginal zone B-cell compartment. *Br. J. Haematol.* 116:662–66

154. Fredrickson TN, Lennert K, Chattopadhyay SK, Morse HC 3rd, Hartley JW. 1999. Splenic marginal zone lymphomas of mice. *Am. J. Pathol.* 154:805–12

155. Cavalli F, Isaacson PG, Gascoyne RD, Zucca E. 2001. MALT lymphomas. *Hematology (Am. Soc. Hematol Educ. Program)* 2001:241–58

156. Quong MW, Martensson A, Langerak AW, Rivera RR, Nemazee D, Murre C. 2004. Receptor editing and marginal zone B cell development are regulated by the helix-loop-helix protein, E2A. *J. Exp. Med.* 199:1101–12

157. Becker-Herman S, Lantner F, Shachar I. 2002. Id2 negatively regulates B cell differentiation in the spleen. *J. Immunol.* 168:5507–13

NOTE ADDED IN PROOF

The Id-family of proteins dimerize with E proteins and antagonize their activity in a dominant negative manner. Interestingly, E2A$^{+/-}$ mice have increased numbers of marginal zone B cells, whereas Id2- and Id3-deficient mice have increased numbers of mature follicular B cells, suggesting that these transcription factors not only play a role in early B cell development but also in splenic B cell differentiation (156, 157).

Annu. Rev. Immunol. 2005. 23:197–223
doi: 10.1146/annurev.immunol.23.021704.115653

HOW NEUTROPHILS KILL MICROBES

Anthony W. Segal

*Center for Molecular Medicine, University College London, London WC1E 6JJ,
United Kingdom; email: t.segal@ucl.ac.uk*

Key Words   bacteria, protease, free radical, microbicidal, ion channel, enzyme

■ **Abstract**   Neutrophils provide the first line of defense of the innate immune system by phagocytosing, killing, and digesting bacteria and fungi. Killing was previously believed to be accomplished by oxygen free radicals and other reactive oxygen species generated by the NADPH oxidase, and by oxidized halides produced by myeloperoxidase. We now know this is incorrect. The oxidase pumps electrons into the phagocytic vacuole, thereby inducing a charge across the membrane that must be compensated. The movement of compensating ions produces conditions in the vacuole conducive to microbial killing and digestion by enzymes released into the vacuole from the cytoplasmic granules.

INTRODUCTION

Neutrophils are highly motile phagocytic cells that constitute the first line of defense of the innate immune system. They were first discovered by Elie Metchnikoff when he inserted rose thorns into starfish larvae and found that wandering mesodermal cells accumulated at the puncture site. He showed these cells to be phagocytic and described the larger cells as macrophagocytes, or macrophages, and the smaller as microphagocytes, now known as granulocytes, of which by far the most numerous are the neutrophils.

The ability of these cells to engulf and degrade bacteria was logically assumed to indicate a killing function. A microbicidal function was ascribed to the contents of their abundant cytoplasmic granules that were discharged into the phagocytic vacuole containing the microbe (1) (Figure 1). Attention was then directed toward the characterization of the granules by electron microscopy, fractionation, and biochemical analysis. Several of the purified granule proteins were shown to kill microbes.

Parallel with studies into microbicidal activity of the granule contents, investigations were undertaken into the metabolism of phagocytosing neutrophils. The neutrophils demonstrated a significant "extra respiration of phagocytosis," which was non-mitochondrial and was associated with a dramatic increase in turnover of the hexose monophosphate (HMP) shunt and the production of large amounts

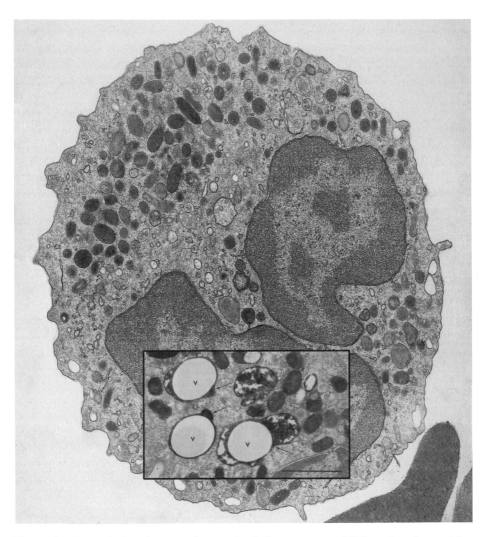

Figure 1   Transmission electron micrograph of a human neutrophil. Inset is an image taken from a neutrophil 20 s after the phagocytosis of latex particles opsonized with IgG (V, vacuole). The section was stained for myeloperoxidase (MPO) to reveal the electron-dense product in the azurophil granules, some of which can be seen degranulating into the phagocytic vacuole (arrows). Bar = 1 μm. (Figure from 17.)

of H_2O_2 (2). These metabolic changes were shown to be essential for microbial killing.

In the late 1960s and early 1970s, a number of related discoveries cast a very different perspective on the killing process. Chronic granulomatous disease (CGD), a profound immunodeficiency to bacterial and fungal infections, was associated with failure of these metabolic changes (3). In addition, myeloperoxidase (MPO)-mediated halogenation, which is microbicidal in the test tube, was also defective in these patients (4).

Soon after its discovery in 1969, superoxide dismutase was used to show that activated neutrophils generate superoxide (5) and that this process is lacking in CGD. This important development provided a direct link between free radical chemistry and biology. At the time, most free radical chemistry was conducted by radiation biologists in test tubes, and its application to biology was purely theoretical. This new discovery was thought to prove that the production of free radical reactions in a biological process was toxic enough to kill organic structures as tough as bacteria and fungal spores. Soon these observations were extrapolated to implicate free radical reactions in a host of pathological processes involving neutrophil infiltration and tissue damage.

During the past few years, the pendulum has swung firmly back to implicating a major primary role for the granule proteins in the killing process (6), with a less direct but still facilitating and activating role for the respiratory burst through the NADPH oxidase. This review concentrates on the elucidation of these recent developments in our understanding of the relationship between the oxidase and granule enzyme activation. Because of the breadth of the subject and space limitations, references are made to authoritative reviews where available.

LIMITATIONS TO UNDERSTANDING KILLING SYSTEMS

Neutrophils are essential for resistance to bacterial and fungal infections. Severe neutropaenia invariably leads to infection by a wide range of organisms (7), most of which are not normally pathogenic, even in CGD. This, coupled with the fact that most CGD patients are able to kill most invading microbes most of the time (8), indicates that killing systems of the neutrophil are highly efficient and multilayered. Investigators once considered oxygen-dependent mechanisms essential for killing invading microbes, but such microbes can in fact be killed by other systems (9). In general, research has concentrated on determining those mechanisms involved in killing the most resistant organisms. The advent of gene-targeting technology allows researchers to determine the roles of the different antimicrobial molecules and their functional interrelationships with various microbes. Additionally, most studies have examined the killing of microbes within the phagocytic vacuole. We do not know whether neutrophils are capable of killing organisms extracellularly in vivo, nor the mechanisms involved if they are.

We have derived the bulk of our detailed information from the study of infection in CGD and the role of the oxidase in microbial killing. Because CGD patients can remain free of infection for many years (8), these methods are imprecise because they only measure some components of the lethal systems. Nonetheless, oxygen-dependent, intravacuolar killing provides a clearly defined set of processes, the examination of which has advanced knowledge of important physiological mechanisms.

THE NADPH OXIDASE

The NADPH oxidase plays a pivotal role in microbial killing because its dysfunction causes CGD, characterized by a profound predisposition to bacterial and fungal infection (8, 10), and killing is compromised under anaerobic conditions (11).

Detailed reviews of the biochemistry and bioenergetics of this system have recently been undertaken (12, 13), to which I refer readers. A schematic representation of the oxidase is shown in Figure 2.

The Electron Transport Chain Through the Membrane

Flavocytochrome b$_{558}$ is the core component of the NADPH oxidase. It is distributed between the plasma membrane and the membrane of the specific granules, and it is incorporated into the wall of the phagocytic vacuole, where it forms a conduit for electrons to be pumped from NADPH in the cytosol onto oxygen in the vacuole.

Flavocytochrome b$_{558}$ is a heterodimer composed of one molecule of p22^{phox} (α-subunit, the product of the *CYBA* gene) and one molecule of gp91^{phox} (β-subunit, *CYBB* gene).

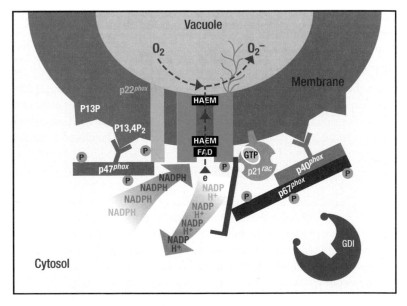

Figure 2   Schematic representation of the NADPH oxidase. Flavocytochrome b$_{558}$ is a heterodimer of gp91^{phox}, which contains the haem- and flavin-binding sites, and p22^{phox}. Electron transport is activated by phosphorylation and translocation to the vacuolar membrane of p47^{phox} and p67^{phox}. p21^{rac}, in the GTP-bound form, is also required (12).

gp91^{phox}

gp91^{phox} contains the entire electron transporting machinery of the flavocytochrome b. It is composed of two major, and very different, domains.

C-TERMINUS: NADPH AND FAD BINDING   The hydrophilic C-terminal (282–570) portion of gp91^{phox} contains the FAD- and NADPH-binding sites. These have distant, but recognizable homology to the large family of ferredoxin-NADP reductase (FNR) proteins, of which cytochrome P450 reductase, nitric oxide (NO) synthase, and yeast ferric reductase are members. This homology has allowed the construction of a model with the depiction of the FAD- and NADPH-binding sites.

N-TERMINUS: HAEM COORDINATION   The hydrophobic N-terminal half of gp91^{phox} contains six membrane-spanning α helices. Helices III and V each contain two histidine residues appropriately positioned (101:209 and 115:222) to coordinate two haem prosthetic groups perpendicular to the plane of the membrane. These histidine residues are completely conserved among all the NADPH OXIDASE (NOX) family members. Site-directed mutagenesis studies support the proposal that these histidine residues form the axial ligands to the haem groups. The predicted placing of the haem groups (one toward the inner face and one toward the outer face) is consistent with their function to transport electrons from the NADPH (via FAD) on the inside (cytosol) across the membrane to the interior of the phagocytic vacuole where molecular O_2 is reduced to form O_2^-. Biological membranes are ~ 25 Å thick, and thus at least two redox centers are required to span them to allow electrons to transfer at kinetically significant rates. The haem groups are nonequivalent and have different redox potentials.

The second (120–167) and third (224–257) external loops of gp91^{phox} contain the N-linked glycosylation sites (asparagines 132, 149, and 240).

p22^{phox} p22^{phox} is a 194 amino acid (~ 21 kDa) protein with a hydrophobic, membrane-spanning N-terminus (1–132). It provides high-affinity binding sites for the cytosolic NADPH oxidase subunits. p47^{phox} binds to a proline-rich domain (151–160) in the cytoplasmic hydrophilic C-terminus and confers stability on gp91^{phox}.

The Activating Proteins in the Cytosol

For electron transport to occur through the flavocytochrome, it must interact with a number of cytosolic proteins that translocate to the membrane of the phagocytic vacuole. This activation depends on a change in the conformation of the flavocytochrome, possibly by displacing the small helix that is predicted in the molecular model to occupy the NADPH-binding site in the inactive state (14) or through the facilitation of electron transfer between the flavin and haem.

Because of their interaction with each other, with lipids, and with phox proteins in the membranes, these cytosolic phox proteins have relatively large numbers of specific interaction domains. Targeting these molecules specifically to that region of the plasma membrane that makes up the wall of the vacuole requires specific local changes, which might include the accumulation of phosphatidylinositol phosphates (PIPs) at this site. Only a small proportion of these cytosolic proteins translocate to the membranes, and these appear to be phosphorylated, as does the flavocytochrome.

$p67^{phox}$ $p67^{phox}$ (NOXA2 from NOX Activator) is a 59,735-Da protein (526 amino acids) with a pI of 6.12. Protein-protein interaction domains include two SH3 domains, two proline-rich regions flanking the central SH3 domain, an N-terminal TPR (tetratricopeptide repeat), and a PB1 domain C-terminal to the central SH3 domain. The TPR domains are thought to bind rac. PB1 domains are known to interact with octicosapeptide motifs, and $p67^{phox}$ binds to $p40^{phox}$ through this domain. $p67^{phox}$ attaches directly to flavocytochrome b_{558}, and at high concentration, in combination with rac or in the form of a $p67^{phox/rac}$ chimera, $p67^{phox}$ is sufficient to induce electron transport.

$p47^{phox}$ $p47^{phox}$ (NOXO2 from NOX Organizer) is a basic protein (pI = 9.6) of molecular weight 44,681 Da (390 amino acids) that is heavily phosphorylated during neutrophil activation. It contains a number of well-defined motifs, including a PX domain (involved in phosphoinositide binding), two SH3 domains (involved in protein-protein interactions), and at least one proline-rich motif (the reciprocal target for SH3 domain interactions). It appears to be an adaptor molecule forming a bridge between $p22^{phox}$ and $p67^{phox}$, and it also binds to cytoplasmic regions of $gp91^{phox}$, thereby stabilizing the attachment of $p67^{phox}$ to flavocytochrome b_{558}. It might also directly influence the function of flavocytochrome b_{558}. The N-terminal regions of $p40^{phox}$ and $p47^{phox}$ contain homologous stretches of 120–130 amino acids that form a structure called the phox homology, or PX domain, which binds to PIPs and directs these proteins to this activated membrane (reviewed in 15).

The two SH3 domains face each other to form a groove in which its C-terminal polybasic region fits. Investigators have suggested that this polybasic region is phosphorylated upon activation, releasing it from its auto-inhibitory role and making the groove accessible to bind the proline-rich tail in the C-terminal portion of $p22^{phox}$.

$p40^{phox}$ $p40^{phox}$ was discovered when it copurified with $p67^{phox}$, to which it is tightly bound. It is a protein of 39,039 Da (339 amino acids), strongly homologous with $p47^{phox}$, with an N-terminal PX domain, followed by an SH3 domain. Toward the C-terminus, there is an octicosapeptide repeat (also known as a PC domain) that seems to be involved in the binding of $p40^{phox}$ to $p67^{phox}$. The protein probably functions as a shuttle partner, transporting $p67^{phox}$, which does not contain a PX domain, to the membrane of the phagocytic vacuole by binding to PIPs.

p21rac   After the discovery of p47^{phox} and p67^{phox}, it became clear that they were not sufficient to reconstitute the active oxidase when combined with membranes. A third protein, a guanosine 5'-triphosphatase (GTP)-dependent factor, was shown to be rac1 or rac2 and was purified from cytosol. The causes of the separation of rac from its complex with guanine nucleotide dissociation inhibitors (GDI) in the cytosol are not known. Rac translocates to the membrane independently from p67^{phox} and p47^{phox}. Its guanosine diphosphate (GDP) is probably exchanged for GTP on the membrane through the action of P-Rex1, a 185-kDa guanine nucleotide exchange factor (GEF) that is activated by phosphatidylinositol-3,4,5-trisphosphate and by the $\beta\gamma$ subunits of heterotrimeric G proteins.

Molecular Genetics of CGD

Defects in any one of four genes give rise to the known forms of CGD. *CYBB* (coding for gp91^{phox}, NOX2) is located on the X chromosome and accounts for about 65% of cases, almost exclusively in males (except in rare female carriers in whom there is extreme lyonization). The other three genes are all autosomal, with defects in *NCF1* (p47^{phox} or NOXO2 protein), *NCF2* (p67^{phox} or NOXA2), and *CYBA* (p22^{phox}), causing approximately 25%, 5%, and 5% of cases, respectively. No instances of CGD have been identified in which a lesion of p40^{phox} is causal.

A small subgroup of CGD patients have what is known as "variant" CGD (16). In these cases there is partial loss of a protein or its function. Often as much as 10%, and up to 30% (H. Malech, personal communication), of normal oxidase activity can be measured.

PRODUCTS OF THE OXIDASE AND THEIR IMPLICATION IN MICROBIAL KILLING

Initiation of NADPH oxidase activity coincides with degranulation, with a lag phase of approximately 20 s (17). It occurs after closure of the vacuole and is limited to the plasma membrane comprising the vacuolar membrane (18). Thus, superoxide cannot be detected on the exterior of a phagocytosing cell (19, 20) unless engulfment is "frustrated" by an overwhelming excess of particles and vacuolar closure becomes impossible.

Because activity of the NADPH oxidase is essential for efficient microbial killing, investigators have focused attention on the products of the oxidase themselves as the lethal agents.

Oxygen radicals and their reaction products, collectively referred to as reactive oxygen species (ROS), are produced as a consequence of NADPH oxidase activity, which pumps superoxide (O_2^-) into the phagocytic vacuole. Because ROS can react with organic molecules, an enormous body of literature has developed that causally links ROS to the death of the microbe.

O_2^- and H_2O_2

The superoxide anion radical has been recognized in chemical systems for many years. Proof of its existence in biology followed the discovery of the enzymatic function of superoxide dismutase, which accelerates the dismutation of $2O_2^- \rightarrow O_2 + O_2^{2-}$ (21). Investigators (5) soon showed that neutrophils produce large amounts of O_2^-, estimated between approximately 1 (22) and 4 (6) M/l in the vacuole. The steady state concentration has been estimated to be in the μM range (22) because dismutation to H_2O_2 (2) is very rapid (23, pp. 60–61) under the prevailing conditions.

Experiments were performed that appeared to demonstrate the killing of microbes by O_2^- generated by xanthine oxidase (24, 25). It is not clear what, if any, ROS other than O_2^- and H_2O_2 (2) are produced in significant quantities in the vacuole.

$HO^\bullet$

O_2^- and H_2O_2 can combine to generate the highly reactive hydroxyl radical ($HO^\bullet$) via the Haber-Weiss reaction. This requires a metal such as iron in the Fenton reaction: $Fe^{2+} + H_2O_2 \rightarrow Fe^{3+} + HO^- + HO^\bullet$. $HO^\bullet$ has been measured in a broken cell preparation (26) and has been implicated as a microbicidal agent (27). These radicals are probably not found in intact cells (28) because lactoferrin, which is unsaturated in neutrophil granules (29, 30), inhibits the generation of $HO^\bullet$ (31) and other free radical reactions (29) by binding free copper and iron. The reaction between HOCl and O_2^- could produce $HO^\bullet$ but does not appear to do so (32).

Cobalt-based radicals could be produced by the Co in cyanocobalamin (33), but a binding protein, transcobalamin 2, present in specific granules, might be there to prevent this from occurring.

Ozone

It has recently been suggested that ozone generated by an antibody-based catalysis is involved in the killing of bacteria within neutrophils (34, 35). Doubt has been subsequently raised, however, on the specificity of the indicator used for ozone, which can apparently also detect O_2^- (36).

Myeloperoxidase-Mediated Halogenation

Myeloperoxidase (MPO) is a di-haem protein composed of two identical heterodimers. Each heterodimer is formed from the post-translational modification of a single polypeptide precursor. The two symmetric halves are linked by disulphide bonds between the two heavy chains. The covalently bound haem has a unique structure and exhibits unusual spectral properties that are responsible for its green color (37). MPO constitutes about 5% of the total neutrophil protein and is present in the cytoplasmic granules at very high concentrations. It makes up about 25% of the granule protein, and this achieves concentrations of about 100 mg/ml (1 mM) in the vacuole.

Investigators thought that this enzyme catalyzes the H_2O_2-dependent oxidation of halides that can react with and kill microbes. Experiments with the MPO-H_2O_2-halide system demonstrated that this enzyme can kill bacteria in the test tube (22, 38–41), and MPO-mediated halogenation has been accepted as an important antimicrobial mechanism for several decades.

A few patients were discovered whose neutrophils lacked MPO and who were also thought to be immunodeficient (42). Recently MPO knockout mice have also shown an undue susceptibility to bacterial and fungal infections (43–45).

Nitric Oxide

Although evidence suggests that neutrophils can induce the synthesis of nitric oxide (NO) synthase during sepsis (46), little evidence implicates the involvement of NO in microbial killing. Even in mice, in the neutrophils of which NO synthase is expressed at much higher levels than in humans, knocking out this molecule has little effect on the killing of microbes for which neutrophils are normally responsible. In contrast, these mice are profoundly susceptible to intracellular organisms such as *S. enterica* and *M. tuberculosis* (47), which classically proliferate within macrophages.

CYTOPLASMIC GRANULES AND THEIR CONTENTS

Researchers have known for almost a century that neutrophils phagocytose and kill microbes. Alexander Fleming discovered and named lysozyme, which he termed "a remarkable bacteriolytic element found in tissues and secretions," including leukocytes (48). He showed that it lysed about two thirds of the bacteria he mixed with it. Researchers subsequently showed that phagocytosis was associated with discharge of the cytoplasmic granules into the vacuole (1) (Figure 1). Attention then focused on microbicidal components within these granules. The first microbicidal granule extract was called phagocytin (49), which was later shown to be composed of an array of cationic antibacterial proteins (50).

Substantial reviews have recently covered this subject (51, 52). Different subsets of granules have been characterized by electron microscopy (53), by various staining techniques, by cell fractionation (54), and by their different functions. There are two predominant types of granules, the azurophil and the specific. They are produced in the promyelocytic and myelocytic stages, and their contents depend on the proteins that are being synthesized at that time as well as on the presence of appropriate signaling peptides (51, 52). The granules also differ in their primary functions, as discussed below.

Azurophil (or Primary) Granules

The azurophils largely contain proteins and peptides directed toward microbial killing and digestion, whereas the specific granules replenish membrane components and help to limit free radical reactions. Azurophil (or primary) granules are the first to be produced. They contain MPO and three predominant neutral proteinases: cathepsin G, elastase, and proteinase 3. Bactericidal/permeability-increasing protein (BPI) was first purified as a factor that permeabilized and killed *E. coli* (55, 56). It has lipopolysaccharide-binding and neutralizing activities (57) and appears to be attached to the granule membrane. Defensins are peptides with molecular weights of 3000–4000 Da, and each contains six disulphide-linked cysteines (58). They exhibit antibacterial activity, but this is inhibited by physiological concentrations of salt. About one third of the total lysozyme (54) is found in these granules.

These granules contain an abundant matrix composed of strongly negatively charged sulphated proteoglycans (59). This matrix strongly binds almost all the peptides and proteins other than lysozyme, which are strongly cationic. This sequestration together with the acidic pH at which the granule interior is maintained (60) keeps these enzymes in a quiescent, inactivated state.

Specific (or Secondary) Granules

Specific granules contain unsaturated (61) lactoferrin, which binds and sequesters iron and copper; transcobalamin II, which binds cyanocobalamin; about two thirds of the lysozyme (54); neutrophil gelatinase-associated lipocalin (62); and a number of membrane proteins also present in the plasma membrane, including flavocytochrome b_{558} of the NADPH oxidase (63).

Gelatinase (or Tertiary) Granules

Some granules contain gelatinase in the absence of lactoferrin, although most of the lactoferrin-containing specific granules also contain gelatinase (64). The designation of granules as "gelatinase granule" refers to granules that contain gelatinase but not lactoferrin; they may represent one end of the spectrum of a single type of granule with the same contents but in differing proportions.

Lysosomes

Lysosomes contain acid hydrolases. The activity of these enzymes appears to fractionate with the azurophil granules. They are, however, released into the phagocytic vacuole much later than the azurophil contents and therefore must be in a distinct compartment (17).

Secretory Vesicles

These endocytic vesicles contain serum albumin (65) and are probably the empty vesicular structures described previously (66). They provide a valuable reservoir of membrane components. Their reassociation with the plasma membrane replenishes that which is consumed during phagocytosis, as well as its component proteins such as complement receptor (67) and flavocytochrome b_{558}.

CONDITIONS IN THE PHAGOCYTIC VACUOLE

One must clearly understand the conditions in the phagocytic vacuole when attempting to define killing mechanisms. A heavily opsonized particle is taken up into the phagocytic vacuole within 20 s (17, 68), and killing is almost immediate (68). The apparent delay in many assays results from a low collision frequency between neutrophils and microbes, which is due to low densities of both, coupled with slow mixing (69) and suboptimal opsonization.

To determine the concentration of the vacuolar contents, one must know the volume of the space between the surface of the organism and the membrane of the phagocytic vacuole. It is certainly very small (17) (Figure 1), and possibly negligible, as has been shown in macrophages (70).

The human neutrophil has numerous granules, the contents of which are released into the vacuole and squeezed onto the surface of the organism in very high concentrations, almost like attaching a limpet mine to a target (17). Researchers have estimated that the granule protein makes up about 40% of the vacuolar volume (22), achieving protein concentrations of about 500 mg/ml (6). It was initially thought that the specific granules degranulated first, followed by the azurophils. These studies were conducted on rabbit neutrophils, and alkaline phosphatase, which we now know to be a marker for membranes, was used as the marker for the specific granules (71). In fact, both of these granule types fuse with the phagocytic vacuole with roughly similar kinetics approximately 20 s after particle uptake (17). The acid hydrolases only enter the vacuole after about 5 min, when the pH has started to fall to levels appropriate for the optimal activity of these enzymes.

Investigators had initially reported that the pH in the vacuole fell to about 6 after 3 min and to 4 after 6 min (72). However, subsequent studies have shown that the NADPH oxidase elevates the pH to about 7.8–8.0 in the first 3 min after phagocytosis, after which it gradually falls to about 7.0 after 10–15 min (68, 73, 74). The NADPH oxidase consumes 0.2 fmols of O_2 when a particle the size of a bacterium is engulfed. This equates to massive amounts of O_2^-, on the order of 1–4 Mols/l, that are injected into the vacuole.

NEUTRAL PROTEASES ARE ESSENTIAL FOR BACTERIAL AND FUNGAL KILLING

Although the proposal that ROS are toxic to ingested microbes was attractive, it was never adequately tested under the conditions pertaining to the phagocytic vacuole. The opportunity was provided by the development of gene targeting. This technique allowed the production of a mouse model that lacks the major neutrophil proteases: neutrophil elastase (NE) (6, 75), cathepsin G (6), or both enzymes (6, 76, 77) (Figure 3).

NE-deficient mice were excessively susceptible to infection with Gram-negative (*K. pneumoniae* and *E. coli*) (75) but not Gram-positive (*S. aureus*) bacteria. NE

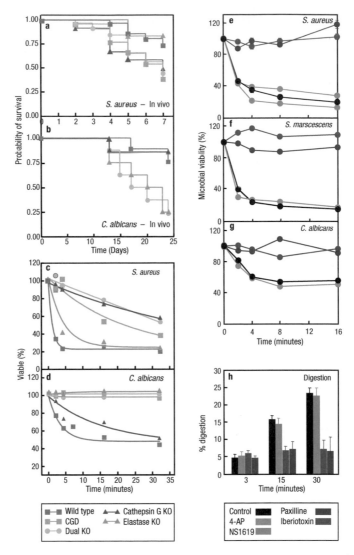

Figure 3 The neutral proteases elastase and cathepsin G as well as K^+ flux are required for microbial killing and digestion by neutrophils. Cathepsin G, neutrophil elastase (NE), and $p47^{phox}$ (CGD) knockout mice are susceptible to *S. aureus* (a) and *C. albicans* (b) in vivo, and their neutrophils kill these organisms poorly in the test tube (c) and (d) (adapted from 6). Inhibition of the BK_{Ca} K^+ channel with specific inhibitors paxilline (PAX) and iberiotoxin (IBTX) prevents killing of *S. aureus* (e), *S. marscescens* (f), and *C. albicans* (g) by neutrophils, whereas the opener NS1619 and nonspecific inhibitor 4-aminopyridine were without effect. The BK_{Ca} K^+ channel blockers also inhibited digestion of radiolabeled, killed *S. aureus* (h) (adapted from 74). Neither the loss of the proteases nor blockage of the BK_{Ca} channel affected phagocytosis, oxidase activity, or iodination.

was also necessary for protection against *C. albicans* (6). Both enzymes were required to kill *A. fumigatus*. The loss of cathepsin G alone was found by others (77) to be without effect on the killing of various of bacteria. The loss of both NE and cathepsin G conferred as profound a defect of bacterial killing as was observed with the CGD mouse model (6).

In these studies on protease-deficient mice, microbial killing was abolished despite a completely normal respiratory burst and normal levels of iodination. This established that ROS and metabolites of the action of MPO generated in the vacuole are not sufficient to kill these bacteria and fungi.

Thus, it was clear that the combination of NADPH oxidase activity and neutral protease enzymes are require for microbial killing to take place. This raises the question of the connection between these two processes.

THE RELATIONSHIP BETWEEN THE NADPH OXIDASE AND KILLING BY GRANULE CONTENTS

Activity of the NADPH Oxidase Alters the Appearance of the Contents of the Phagocytic Vacuole

The activity of the NADPH oxidase alters the appearance of the contents of phagocytic vacuoles in electron micrographs of neutrophils examined soon after they had phagocytosed bacteria (6). In normal cells, the contents of the vacuole had a diffuse, almost ground-glass appearance, with very few intact aggregates of granule contents. By contrast, in CGD cells there was little dispersion, with obvious clumping of the granular contents. This abnormal appearance was also apparent in vacuoles from a patient with variant CGD with 10% of the normal oxidase activity.

These obvious structural differences, coupled with the massive amounts of O_2^- injected into the vacuole and the fact that 10% of this amount of O_2^- in variant CGD (amounting to some 100–400 mMols/l) was insufficient, suggested to researchers that the oxidase was exerting some physico-chemical influence on the granule contents rather than simply producing ROS or substrate for MPO. Segal and colleagues (6) therefore turned their attention to electron transport across the membrane and its consequences for the movement of other ions.

Charge Compensation Across the Vacuolar Wall

The oxidase is electrogenic, transferring electrons, unaccompanied by protons, across the vacuolar membrane (78–81). The vacuolar volume is about 0.2 μm^3, with a membrane surface area of about 1.65 μm^2. In each vacuole, 0.8–2.0 fmols of O_2^- are produced, and thus about 5–10 $\times$ 10^8 electrons pass across each μ^2 of membrane. The charge on one electron is 1.6 $\times$ 10^{-19} coulombs, so 3–7 $\times$ 10^8 charges in one square micron would produce from 4.6 $\times$ 10^{-3} to 1.2 $\times$ 10^{-2} coulombs/cm^2. With the capacitance of the membrane at approximately 1 microfarad/cm^2 (82), this charge would depolarize the membrane potential by 4,600–11,700 volts!

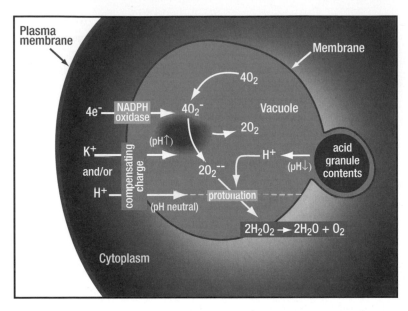

Figure 4   Activity of the NADPH oxidase depolarizes the membrane. The nature of the compensating charge governs the changes in vacuolar pH and tonicity. Electrons are transported across the vacuolar membrane to form O_2^-, which dismutates to O_2^{2-}. O_2^- and O_2^{2-} become protonated to form HO_2 and H_2O_2, thereby consuming protons and elevating the pH in the vacuole despite the entry of acidic granule contents. This process can only occur if part of the charge is compensated by ions other than protons, which in part occurs through the passage of K^+ ions (6, 74).

Depolarization of the membrane to +190 mV shuts down NADPH oxidase activity completely (83). Thus, for significant oxidase activity to occur, the charge must be compensated.

The changes in the vacuolar pH, which is elevated from that of the extracellular medium to 7.8–8.0 (68) despite the release into the vacuole of 500 mg/ml of acidic granule protein contents (6), hold the key to understanding the nature of the compensating ions (Figure 4). These granule contents are maintained at pH 5.0 in the granule by a proton pump (60) and have strong buffering powers. About 400 μmol potassium hydroxide is required per gram of granule protein to elevate the pH from 5.0 to 8.0 (6).

The vacuole becomes alkaline despite the entry of acidic granule contents, indicating that the O_2^- and O_2^{2-} are consuming protons in the vacuole. This would not happen if each electron passing across the membrane was accompanied by a proton, demonstrating that compensating charges cannot be solely in the form of H^+ from the cytoplasm.

The major cation in the cytoplasm is K^+, which accumulates in the vacuole at concentrations of up to about 600 mM as a consequence of oxidase activity

(6). Transport of K^+ ions is markedly diminished when the pH rises above 8.0, indicating that the K^+ channel provides an important self-regulating mechanism for elevating the vacuolar pH while also ensuring that it does not go too high.

K^+ flux only accounts for about 6% of the compensating charge (6). The putative proton channel discussed below does not appear to compensate for all the rest of the charge because its inhibition with Zn^{2+} and Cd^{2+} fails to block the NADPH oxidase (74). Therefore, some other major ion flux must also be involved. As is described below, this is accomplished by the flux of chloride ions through a glycine-gated, strychnine-sensitive channel.

The K^+ Enters the Phagocytic Vacuole Through BK_{Ca} Channels

K^+ enters the vacuole through the large conductance Ca^{2+}-activated K^+ channel (74). Iberiotoxin (IBTX) and paxilline (PAX), both highly selective and potent inhibitors of this channel (84, 85), prevent the alkalinization of the vacuole, confirming the importance of the influx of K^+ into the vacuole on alkalinization of this compartment. The IC_{50} values for this effect were in the region of 10 nM for IBTX and PAX, consistent with their IC_{50} for channel block. In addition, the BK_{Ca} channel opener, NS1619 (86), significantly augmented the rise in pH to supranormal levels. A variety of blockers and openers of other K^+ channels were without effect.

[86]Rb^+ release from activated neutrophils after stimulation with phorbol myristate acctate (PMA) was also induced by NS1619 and even further enhanced by the combination of this opener and PMA. PMA-induced and NS1619-induced efflux were both completely abrogated by IBTX and PAX. The same was found to apply to eosinophils.

BK_{Ca} channels are classically opened by the combination of membrane depolarization and elevated cytosolic Ca^{2+} (87). The same holds true for this channel in neutrophils and eosinophils. Neither depolarizing the membrane nor elevating the cytosolic Ca^{2+} was sufficient to fully open the K^+ channel, whereas the combination of the two caused as much channel opening as did stimulation with PMA. Although PMA stimulation is well known to depolarize the neutrophil plasma membrane (88), it is generally thought not to elevate cytosolic Ca^{2+}. One mechanism by which this might occur is through a drop in pH just beneath the plasma membrane as a consequence of charge separation induced by the oxidase. Corresponding elevations in Ca^{2+} and falls in pH were seen just beneath the plasma membrane in activated cells (74).

Charge Compensation by Protons

Protons remain in the cytoplasm as a result of charge separation, which occurs when the electrons are transported from NADPH across the wall of the phagocytic vacuole. Additional protons are produced in the cytosol by the HMP shunt, which generates NADPH (89), as well as during the production of energy by glycolysis. This proton generation by an active oxidase, estimated to be about 150 mMols/l (90), causes an initial slight fall in cytosolic pH that rapidly returns to normal.

Three mechanisms appear to be associated with the extrusion of these protons, which are extruded in roughly equimolar quantities with the O_2^- that is generated (91, 92). The predominant one is a Na^+/H^+ antiport (93, 94). Its inhibition by the removal of extracellular Na^+ or blockage with amiloride causes acidification of the cytosol upon stimulation of the cells. In addition, both Zn^{2+} and Cd^{2+}-sensitive proton channels (95, 96) and vacuolar (V)-type H^+ pumps, inhibited by bafilomycins (90), are also present.

Investigators generally agree that the charge induced by electron translocation (I_e) through the NADPH oxidase is compensated by proton efflux (78, 83, 97), although the identity of the proposed channel is currently highly contentious. One school of thought holds that protons pass through voltage-gated proton channels that are distinct from any NADPH oxidase component (98). The opposing view is that they pass through flavocytochrome b_{558} of the oxidase, gp91^{phox}, itself (99–101).

One of the hallmarks of the assumption that I_e is largely compensated by proton fluxes is that both Zn^{2+} and Cd^{2+}, known proton channel blockers (98, 102, 103), were also thought to inhibit O_2^- production (83, 97). The discrepancy between the low μM concentrations of these cations that block proton channels and the mM concentrations needed to inhibit cytochrome c reduction was recently explained by the voltage dependence of I_e. Zn^{2+} and Cd^{2+} shift the threshold voltage for activating voltage-gated proton channels into the steeply voltage-dependent region of I_e, thereby attenuating O_2^- production (83).

However, Zn^{2+} and Cd^{2+} inhibition of voltage-gated proton channels do not inhibit the NADPH oxidase: They have no effect on PMA-induced oxygen consumption, the true measure of oxidase activity. Zn^{2+} and Cd^{2+} interfere with the reduction of cytochrome c by accelerating the dismutation of O^{2-} to H_2O_2 (74). In a system in which xanthine-xanthine oxidase generated O_2^-, 3 mM concentrations of these elements induced the dismutation of O_2^- to H_2O_2 at a rate indistinguishable from that catalyzed by superoxide dismutase (1 μg/ml). Zn^{2+}, at concentrations three orders of magnitude greater than those causing almost complete blockage to proton channels, was also without effect on the currents measured in electrophysiological studies performed on neutrophils, eosinophils, or on PMA-induced ^{86}Rb efflux from these cells (74). This does not mean that H^+ movement through proton channels does not compensate some of the charge, but only that the justification hitherto provided is incorrect.

Charge Compensation by Cl⁻

We showed that K^+ accounts for only about 5%–10% of the compensation of the total electron transport, and, contrary to the description in a recent critique of our work (104), we never claimed that it was the only compensating ion. More recently, we (J. Ahluwalia, G. Gabella, S. Pope, A. Warley, A. Segal, unpublished) have discovered that that Cl^-, passing through strychnine-sensitive, glycine-activated homomeric channels, compensates about 90% of the charge. These channels were characterized by patch clamping whole cells and isolated phagocytic vacuoles, and by Western blotting. The removal of Cl^- or the blockage of this channel abolished both the respiratory burst and microbial killing. High concentrations of Cl^- and glycine required for the optimal function of these channels are contained within the cytoplasmic granules, which empty into the vacuole. NADPH oxidase activity was lost when the granules were removed and regained when Cl^- was reintroduced into the vacuole. Lysozyme, cathepsin G, and elastase were inactivated by hypertonic Cl^-, the removal of which would be important for their function. These Cl^- fluxes provide a direct couple between the extent of degranulation and oxidase activity required to activate the released enzymes.

The Movement of K^+ into the Vacuole Activates NE and Cathepsin G

The contents of the cytoplasmic azurophil granules are not freely in solution. They are almost exclusively highly cationic proteins that are strongly bound to the highly negatively charged proteoglycans heparin and chondroitin sulphate (59), in which state they are inactive. They are activated in the vacuole both by the elevation in pH described above and by the hypertonic K^+. The latter breaks the charged interaction between the enzymes and the matrix, releasing them in a soluble form (6) (Figure 5). For these hypertonic conditions to develop, water must be prevented from entering the vacuole in response to the osmotic attraction of the salts. This is achieved by encasing the vacuole in a meshwork of cytoskeletal proteins, including paxillin and vinculin.

The importance of the accumulation of K^+ in the vacuole was shown when this was diminished either with the K^+ ionophore valinomycin (6), or by blocking the BK_{Ca} channel with the specific inhibitors IBTX or PAX (74). In both cases, microbial killing and digestion was almost completely prevented (Figure 3) despite the generation of normal quantities of ROS and normal levels of iodination.

Why Was the Importance of Granule Contents in the Killing Process so Overshadowed by ROS and MPO-Mediated Halogenation?

The theory that microbes are killed within the phagocytic vacuole by ROS had fertile ground on which to develop. The lack of production of O_2^- and H_2O_2 in anaerobic cells and in CGD with impaired killing under these conditions supported this theory (3, 11), as did the concept of toxicity engendered in the name "reactive oxygen species." Although experiments were performed in support of these ideas, the conditions under which they were performed in no way reflected the conditions pertaining in the vacuole. They were often done at the wrong pH, and never in the presence of the enormously high concentrations of protein that occur naturally.

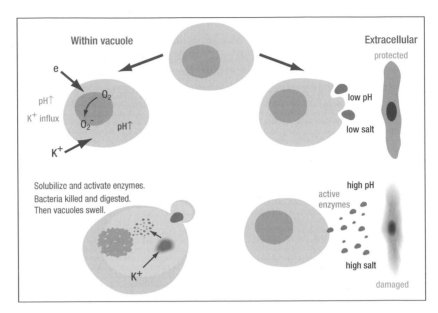

Figure 5   Schematic representation of interaction between NADPH oxidase and granule proteases. Electron transport through flavocytochrome b_{558} consumes protons in the vacuole, elevating pH to a level optimal for neutral proteases, which are also activated by K^+ driven into the vacuole to compensate the charge across the membrane. The hypertonic K^+ solubilizes the cationic granule proteases and peptides by displacing them from the anionic sulphated proteoglycan granule matrix. The requirement for an alkaline, hypertonic environment restricts the toxicity of these proteins to the vacuolar compartment, thereby limiting damage to normal tissues.

O_2^-

Initial studies claimed that killing occurred by O_2^- generated by the reaction of xanthine with xanthine oxidase, but in fact in those experiments the microbes were killed in the absence of the substrate xanthine, and killing was not inhibited by superoxide dismutase (24). In a similar experiment, no killing of bacteria by O_2^- was observed after 15 min (25).

H_2O_2

H_2O_2, which is used as a topical antiseptic (105), is produced by neutrophils and has been thought of as capable of killing microbes within them (106, 107). Supportive evidence was provided by the finding that catalase-negative organisms rarely infect patients with CGD (108). The explanation was that these bacteria generated enough H_2O_2 to catalyze their own MPO-mediated halogenation within the vacuole of the neutrophil (109, 110). In vitro mutagenesis was used to generate strains of *S. aureus* containing varying levels of catalase, and their virulence in mice was found to be inversely proportional to their catalase content (111). Recently, however, doubts have been cast on this theory. Catalase-deficient *A. nidulans* (112) and *S. aureus* (113) are as virulent as the catalase-positive varieties in mouse models of CGD, and the bacteria could never come near to producing the relatively enormous quantities of H_2O_2 generated even by cells from patients with variant CGD.

When glucose oxidase was administered to CGD cells in liposomes, it appeared to correct the killing defect (114, 115). However, no explanation was provided as to how glucose would gain access to the vacuole in adequate amounts to generate sufficient quantities of H_2O_2, and the killing of bacteria in the extracellular medium was not excluded.

MPO

Experiments that demonstrated that the MPO-H_2O_2-halide system can kill bacteria in the test tube (22, 38–41) were conducted under nonphysiological conditions, with relatively low concentrations of MPO (50 μg/ml rather than 100 mgs/ml), at low pH (5.0 rather than 7.8–8.0), and, most important of all, in the absence of the high levels of proteins (approximately 500 mgs/ml) found in the vacuole. When bacteria were exposed to 100 mM H_2O_2 or 1 mM HOCl in the presence of 25 mg/ml granule proteins (technically much more manageable than the experimentally determined 500 mg/ml), killing was almost abolished (116).

Neutrophils clearly iodinate and chlorinate proteins when bacteria are phagocytosed, and this halogenation is dependent on an active NADPH oxidase and MPO (118). However, it is largely the proteins of the neutrophil granule rather than the microbial proteins that are iodinated (116, 119) and chlorinated (120), a highly inefficient system if its primary purpose is to halogenate bacterial proteins. Further indications as to the inefficiency of the proposed system come from the amounts of H_2O_2 generated. It seems highly unlikely that substrate would need to be provided at molar concentrations and that the 100 mM H_2O_2 produced by patients with variant CGD would be insufficient when it is effective at 50 μM in the test tube (38).

A few patients were discovered whose neutrophils lacked MPO who were also thought to be immunodeficient (42), and an MPO knockout mouse was shown to be susceptible to yeast but not bacterial infection (45). However, the advent of automated differential leukocyte counting machines, in which the identification of neutrophils depended on a peroxidase stain, revealed that about 1 in 2000 of the general population are MPO-deficient without any undue predisposition to infection (121). The neutrophils of birds also lack MPO (122).

One possible function of MPO is to protect the digestive enzymes from oxidative denaturation (123) by removing H_2O_2 from the phagocytic vacuole. MPO has catalase activity (124), but this only functions efficiently if the compound II that accumulates is reduced back to the native enzyme. This reduction can be achieved by the high concentrations of O_2^- in the vacuole with which MPO forms an adduct to produce compound III (125). The impaired microbial killing observed in the MPO knockout mouse (126) could result from oxidative inactivation of antimicrobial proteins by the H_2O_2 that accumulates under these conditions (106).

MPO may also have dual functions, one as a catalase under the conditions pertaining in the vacuole, but another in a microbicidal capacity outside the cell where enzyme and substrate is much more dilute, and the pH, which is generally low at sites of infection and inflammation, is more conducive to halogenation reactions.

CONCLUDING REMARKS AND PERSPECTIVES

The complexity of the NADPH oxidase and its associated ion fluxes might seem excessive for the apparently simple purpose of activating enzymes within the phagosome. These enzymes, however, have the potential to be highly destructive to normal tissues, and yet organs housing the most exuberant inflammation and neutrophil infiltration can undergo resolution and return completely to normal a week or two later. Some of the neutrophil are removed by apoptosis, but many also necrose with the resultant release of their granules. The requirement of the combination of hypertonicity and alkalinity, neither of which occurs naturally in inflammatory foci, for the activation of these enzymes severely limits the toxicity of granules released into the tissues (Figure 5).

The demonstration that ROS and MPO-mediated halogenation are not the primary killing systems they were long believed to be has reopened many questions relating to mechanisms of innate immunity in the neutrophil. The roles of the different granule constituents in the killing and digestion of specific organisms is of interest, as are the consequences of the interaction of ROS with these granule contents on their biophysical, biochemical, and hence antimicrobial properties.

A number of problems still need to be resolved to clarify the mechanisms involved in charge compensation across the vacuolar membrane. These include the relationship between the channels conducting these charges and electron transport through flavocytochrome b_{558} and the mechanisms responsible for activating, regulating, and integrating the fluxes of these different ions.

ACKNOWLEDGMENTS

I thank the Wellcome Trust and CGD Research Trust for support, and Jatinder Ahluwalia, Simon Pope, and Daniel Marks for reading the manuscript. I apologize to all investigators whose work has not been cited owing to space restrictions.

The *Annual Review of Immunology* is online at
http://immunol.annualreviews.org

LITERATURE CITED

1. Cohn ZA, Hirsch JG. 1960. The influence of phagocytosis on the intracellular distribution of granule-associated components of polymorphonuclear leucocytes. *J. Exp. Med.* 112:1015–22

2. Iyer GYN, Islam DMF, Quastel JH. 1961. Biochemical aspects of phagocytosis. *Nature* 192:535–41

3. Holmes B, Page AR, Good RA. 1967. Studies of the metabolic activity of

leukocytes from patients with a genetic abnormality of phagocyte function. *J. Clin. Invest.* 46:1422–32

4. Klebanoff SJ, White LR. 1969. Iodination defect in the leukocytes of a patient with chronic granulomatous disease of childhood. *N. Engl. J. Med.* 280:460–66

5. Babior BM, Kipnes RS, Curnutte JT. 1973. Biological defence mechanisms: the production by leukocytes of superoxide, a potential bactericidal agent. *J. Clin. Invest.* 52:741–44

6. Reeves EP, Lu H, Jacobs HL, Messina CG, Bolsover S, et al. 2002. Killing activity of neutrophils is mediated through activation of proteases by K$^+$ flux. *Nature* 416:291–97

7. Vento S, Cainelli F. 2003. Infections in patients with cancer undergoing chemotherapy: aetiology, prevention, and treatment. *Lancet Oncol.* 4:595–604

8. Winkelstein JA, Marino MC, Johnston RBJ, Boyle J, Curnutte J, et al. 2000. Chronic granulomatous disease. Report on a national registry of 368 patients. *Medicine (Baltimore)* 79:155–69

9. Segal AW, Harper AM, Garcia RC, Merzbach D. 1982. The action of cells from patients with chronic granulomatous disease on *Staphylococcus aureus. J. Med. Microbiol.* 15:441–49

10. Thrasher AJ, Keep NH, Wientjes F, Segal AW. 1994. Chronic granulomatous disease. *Biochim. Biophys. Acta* 1227:1–24

11. Mandell GL. 1974. Bactericidal activity of aerobic and anaerobic polymorphonuclear neutrophils. *Infect. Immun.* 9:337–41

12. Cross AR, Segal AW. 2004. The NADPH oxidase of professional phagocytes— prototype of the NOX electron transport chain systems. *Biochem. Biophysica Acta—Bioenergetics* 1657:1–22

13. Vignais PV. 2002. The superoxide-generating NADPH oxidase: structural aspects and activation mechanism. *Cell. Mol. Life Sci.* 59:1428–59

14. Taylor WR, Jones DT, Segal AW. 1993. A structural model for the nucleotide binding domains of the flavocytochrome b$_{-245}$ β-chain. *Protein Sci.* 2:1675–85

15. Wientjes FB, Segal AW. 2003. PX domain takes shape. *Curr. Opin. Hematol.* 10:2–7

16. Lew PD, Southwick FS, Stossel TP, Whitin JC, Simons E, Cohen HJ. 1981. A variant of chronic granulomatous disease: deficient oxidative metabolism due to a low-affinity NADPH oxidase. *N. Engl. J. Med.* 305:1329–33

17. Segal AW, Dorling J, Coade S. 1980. Kinetics of fusion of the cytoplasmic granules with phagocytic vacuoles in human polymorphonuclear leukocytes. Biochemical and morphological studies. *J. Cell Biol.* 85:42–59

18. Briggs RT, Robinson JM, Karnovsky ML, Karnovsky MJ. 1986. Superoxide production by polymorphonuclear leukocytes. A cytochemical approach. *Histochemistry* 84:371–78

19. Segal AW, Meshulam T. 1979. Production of superoxide by neutrophils: a reappraisal. *FEBS Lett.* 100:27–32

20. Thomas MJ, Hedrick CC, Smith S, Pang J, Jerome WG, et al. 1992. Superoxide generation by the human polymorphonuclear leukocyte in response to latex beads. *J. Leukoc. Biol.* 51:591–96

21. McCord JM, Fridovich I. 1969. Superoxide dismutase. An enzymic function for erythrocuprein (hemocuprein). *J. Biol. Chem.* 244:6049–55

22. Hampton MB, Kettle AJ, Winterbourn CC. 1998. Inside the neutrophil phagosome: oxidants, myeloperoxidase, and bacterial killing. *Blood* 92:3007–17

23. Halliwell B, Gutteridge JMC. 1999. *Free Radicals in Biology and Medicine.* New York: Oxford Univ. Press

24. Babior BM, Curnutte JT, Kipnes RS. 1975. Biological defense mechanisms. Evidence for the participation of superoxide in bacterial killing by xanthine oxidase. *J. Lab. Clin. Med.* 85:235–44

25. Rosen H, Klebanoff SJ. 1979. Bactericidal activity of a superoxide

anion-generating system. A model for the polymorphonuclear leukocyte. *J. Exp. Med.* 149:27–39

26. Ambruso DR, Johnston RB Jr. 1981. Lactoferrin enhances hydroxyl radical production by human neutrophils, neutrophil particulate fractions, and an enzymatic generating system. *J. Clin. Invest.* 67:352–60

27. Rosen H. 1980. Role of hydroxyl radical in polymorphonuclear leukocyte-mediated bactericidal activity. *Agents Actions Suppl.* 7:180–84

28. Cohen MS, Britigan BE, Pou S, Rosen GM. 1991. Application of spin trapping to human phagocytic cells: insight into conditions for formation and limitation of hydroxyl radical. *Free Radic. Res. Commun.* 12–13(Pt. 1):17–25

29. Gutteridge JM, Paterson SK, Segal AW, Halliwell B. 1981. Inhibition of lipid peroxidation by the iron-binding protein lactoferrin. *Biochem. J.* 199:259–61

30. Winterbourn CC. 1983. Lactoferrin-catalysed hydroxyl radical production. Additional requirement for a chelating agent. *Biochem. J.* 210:15–19

31. Britigan BE, Hassett DJ, Rosen GM, Hamill DR, Cohen MS. 1989. Neutrophil degranulation inhibits potential hydroxyl-radical formation. Relative impact of myeloperoxidase and lactoferrin release on hydroxyl-radical production by iron-supplemented neutrophils assessed by spin-trapping techniques. *Biochem. J.* 264:447–55

32. Rosen GM, Pou S, Ramos CL, Cohen MS, Britigan BE. 1995. Free radicals and phagocytic cells. *FASEB J.* 9:200–9

33. Banerjee R, Ragsdale SW. 2003. The many faces of vitamin B12: catalysis by cobalamin-dependent enzymes. *Annu. Rev. Biochem.* 72:209–47

34. Wentworth P Jr , McDunn JE, Wentworth AD, Takeuchi C, Nieva J, et al. 2002. Evidence for antibody-catalyzed ozone formation in bacterial killing and inflammation. *Science* 298:2195–99

35. Babior BM, Takeuchi C, Ruedi J, Gutierrez A, Wentworth P Jr . 2003. Investigating antibody-catalyzed ozone generation by human neutrophils. *Proc. Natl. Acad. Sci. USA* 100:3031–34

36. Kettle AJ, Clark BM, Winterbourn CC. 2004. Superoxide converts indigo carmine to isatin sulfonic acid: implications for the hypothesis that neutrophils produce ozone. *J. Biol. Chem.* 279:18521–25

37. Fiedler TJ, Davey CA, Fenna RE. 2000. X-ray crystal structure and characterization of halide-binding sites of human myeloperoxidase at 1.8 Å resolution. *J. Biol. Chem.* 275:11964–71

38. Klebanoff SJ. 1968. Myeloperoxidase-halide-hydrogen peroxide antibacterial system. *J. Bacteriol.* 95:2131–38

39. Klebanoff SJ. 1975. Antimicrobial mechanisms in neutrophilic polymorphonuclear leukocytes. *Semin. Hematol.* 12:117–42

40. Klebanoff SJ. 1967. Iodination of bacteria: a bactericidal mechanism. *J. Exp. Med.* 126:1063–78

41. Hampton MB, Kettle AJ, Winterbourn CC. 1996. Involvement of superoxide and myeloperoxidase in oxygen-dependent killing of *Staphylococcus aureus* by neutrophils. *Infect. Immun.* 64:3512–17

42. Lehrer RI, Hanifin J, Cline MJ. 1969. Defective bactericidal activity in myeloperoxidase-deficient human neutrophils. *Nature* 223:78–79

43. Aratani Y, Kura F, Watanabe H, Akagawa H, Takano Y, et al. 2000. Differential host susceptibility to pulmonary infections with bacteria and fungi in mice deficient in myeloperoxidase. *J. Infect. Dis.* 182:1276–79

44. Gaut JP, Yeh GC, Tran HD, Byun J, Henderson JP, et al. 2001. Neutrophils employ the myeloperoxidase system to generate antimicrobial brominating and chlorinating oxidants during sepsis. *Proc. Natl. Acad. Sci. USA* 98:11961–66

45. Aratani Y, Koyama H, Nyui S, Suzuki K, Kura F, Maeda N. 1999. Severe

impairment in early host defense against *Candida albicans* in mice deficient in myeloperoxidase. *Infect. Immun.* 67: 1828–36

46. Wheeler MA, Smith SD, Garcia-Cardena G, Nathan CF, Weiss RM, Sessa WC. 1997. Bacterial infection induces nitric oxide synthase in human neutrophils. *J. Clin. Invest.* 99:110–16

47. Chakravortty D, Hensel M. 2003. Inducible nitric oxide synthase and control of intracellular bacterial pathogens. *Microbes. Infect.* 5:621–27

48. Fleming A. 1922. On a remarkable bacteriolytic element found in tissues and secretions. *Proc. R. Soc. London* 93:306-317

49. Hirsch JG. 1956. Phagocytin: a bactericidal substance from polymorphonuclear leucocytes. *J. Exp. Med.* 103:589–611

50. Zeya HI, Spitznagel JK. 1968. Arginine-rich proteins of polymorphonuclear leukocyte lysosomes. Antimicrobial specificity and biochemical heterogeneity. *J. Exp. Med.* 127:927–41

51. Borregaard N, Cowland JB. 1997. Granules of the human neutrophilic polymorphonuclear leukocyte. *Blood* 89:3503–21

52. Gullberg U, Bengtsson N, Bulow E, Garwicz D, Lindmark A, Olsson I. 1999. Processing and targeting of granule proteins in human neutrophils. *J. Immunol. Methods* 232:201–10

53. Bainton DF. 1993. Neutrophilic leukocyte granules: from structure to function. *Adv. Exp. Med. Biol.* 336:17–33

54. Baggiolini M, Hirsch JG, De Duve C. 1969. Resolution of granules from rabbit heterophil leukocytes into distinct populations by zonal sedimentation. *J. Cell Biol.* 40:529–41

55. Weiss J, Franson RC, Beckerdite S, Schmeidler K, Elsbach P. 1975. Partial characterization and purification of a rabbit granulocyte factor that increases permeability of *Escherichia coli*. *J. Clin. Invest.* 55:33–42

56. Weiss J, Elsbach P, Olsson I, Odeberg H. 1978. Purification and characterization of a potent bactericidal and membrane active protein from the granules of human polymorphonuclear leukocytes. *J. Biol. Chem.* 253:2664–72

57. Ooi CE, Weiss J, Doerfler ME, Elsbach P. 1991. Endotoxin-neutralizing properties of the 25 kD N-terminal fragment and a newly isolated 30 kD C-terminal fragment of the 55–60 kD bactericidal/permeability-increasing protein of human neutrophils. *J. Exp. Med.* 174:649–55

58. Ganz T. 2003. Defensins: antimicrobial peptides of innate immunity. *Nat. Rev. Immunol.* 3:710–20

59. Kolset SO, Gallagher JT. 1990. Proteoglycans in haemopoietic cells. *Biochim. Biophys. Acta* 1032:191–211

60. Styrt B, Klempner MS. 1982. Internal pH of human neutrophil lysosomes. *FEBS Lett.* 149:113–16

61. Bullen JJ, Armstrong JA. 1979. The role of lactoferrin in the bactericidal function of polymorphonuclear leucocytes. *Immunology* 36:781–91

62. Bundgaard JR, Sengelov H, Borregaard N, Kjeldsen L. 1994. Molecular cloning and expression of a cDNA encoding NGAL: a lipocalin expressed in human neutrophils. *Biochem. Biophys. Res. Commun.* 202:1468–75

63. Segal AW, Jones OT. 1979. The subcellular distribution and some properties of the cytochrome b component of the microbicidal oxidase system of human neutrophils. *Biochem. J.* 182:181–88

64. Hibbs MS, Bainton DF. 1989. Human neutrophil gelatinase is a component of specific granules. *J. Clin. Invest* 84:1395–402

65. Borregaard N, Kjeldsen L, Rygaard K, Bastholm L, Nielsen MH, et al. 1992. Stimulus-dependent secretion of plasma proteins from human neutrophils. *J. Clin. Invest.* 90:86–96

66. Baggiolini M, Hirsch JG, De Duve C.

1970. Further biochemical and morphological studies of granule fractions from rabbit heterophil leukocytes. *J. Cell Biol.* 45:586–97

67. Sengelov H, Kjeldsen L, Kroeze W, Berger M, Borregaard N. 1994. Secretory vesicles are the intracellular reservoir of complement receptor 1 in human neutrophils. *J. Immunol.* 153:804–10

68. Segal AW, Geisow M, Garcia R, Harper A, Miller R. 1981. The respiratory burst of phagocytic cells is associated with a rise in vacuolar pH. *Nature* 290:406–9

69. Holmes B, Quie PG, Windhorst DB, Good RA. 1966. Fatal granulomatous disease of childhood. An inborn abnormality of phagocytic function. *Lancet* 1:1225–28

70. Wright SD, Silverstein SC. 1984. Phagocytosing macrophages exclude proteins from the zones of contact with opsonized targets. *Nature* 309:359–61

71. Bainton DF. 1973. Sequential degranulation of the two types of polymorphonuclear leukocyte granules during phagocytosis of microorganisms. *J. Cell Biol.* 58:249–64

72. Jensen MS, Bainton DF. 1973. Temporal changes in pH within the phagocytic vacuole of the polymorphonuclear neutrophilic leukocyte. *J. Cell Biol.* 56:379–88

73. Cech P, Lehrer RI. 1984. Phagolysosomal pH of human neutrophils. *Blood* 63:88–95

74. Ahluwalia J, Tinker A, Clapp LH, Duchen MR, Abramov AY, et al. 2004. The large-conductance Ca^{2+}-activated K^+ channel is essential for innate immunity. *Nature* 427:853–58

75. Belaaouaj A, McCarthy R, Baumann M, Gao Z, Ley TJ, et al. 1998. Mice lacking neutrophil elastase reveal impaired host defense against Gram negative bacterial sepsis. *Nat. Med.* 4:615–18

76. Tkalcevic J, Novelli M, Phylactides M, Iredale JP, Segal AW, Roes J. 2000. Impaired immunity and enhanced resistance to endotoxin in the absence of neutrophil elastase and cathepsin G. *Immunity* 12:201–10

77. MacIvor DM, Shapiro SD, Pham CT, Belaaouaj A, Abraham SN, Ley TJ. 1999. Normal neutrophil function in cathepsin G-deficient mice. *Blood* 94:4282–93

78. Henderson LM, Chappell JB, Jones OT. 1987. The superoxide-generating NADPH oxidase of human neutrophils is electrogenic and associated with an H^+ channel. *Biochem. J.* 246:325–29

79. Kapus A, Szaszi K, Ligeti E. 1992. Phorbol 12-myristate 13-acetate activates an electrogenic H^+-conducting pathway in the membrane of neutrophils. *Biochem. J.* 281:697–701

80. DeCoursey TE, Cherny VV. 1993. Potential, pH, and arachidonate gate hydrogen ion currents in human neutrophils. *Biophys. J.* 65:1590–98

81. Schrenzel J, Serrander L, Banfi B, Nusse O, Fouyouzi R, et al. 1998. Electron currents generated by the human phagocyte NADPH oxidase. *Nature* 392:734–37

82. Pauly H, Packer L, Schwan HP. 1960. Electrical properties of mitochondrial membranes. *J. Biophys. Biochem. Cytol.* 7:589–601

83. DeCoursey TE, Morgan D, Cherny VV. 2003. The voltage dependence of NADPH oxidase reveals why phagocytes need proton channels. *Nature* 422:531–34

84. Sanchez M, McManus OB. 1996. Paxilline inhibition of the alpha-subunit of the high-conductance calcium-activated potassium channel. *Neuropharmacology* 35:963–68

85. Galvez A, Gimenez-Gallego G, Reuben JP, Roy-Contancin L, Feigenbaum P, et al. 1990. Purification and characterization of a unique, potent, peptidyl probe for the high conductance calcium-activated potassium channel from venom of the scorpion *Buthus tamulus*. *J. Biol. Chem.* 265:11083–90

86. Lawson K. 2000. Potassium channel openers as potential therapeutic weapons

in ion channel disease. *Kidney Int.* 57: 838–45

87. Kaczorowski GJ, Knaus HG, Leonard RJ, McManus OB, Garcia ML. 1996. High-conductance calcium-activated potassium channels; structure, pharmacology, and function. *J. Bioenerg. Biomembr.* 28:255–67

88. Jankowski A, Grinstein S. 1999. A non-invasive fluorimetric procedure for measurement of membrane potential. Quantification of the NADPH oxidase-induced depolarization in activated neutrophils. *J. Biol. Chem.* 274:26098–104

89. Borregaard N, Schwartz JH, Tauber AI. 1984. Proton secretion by stimulated neutrophils. Significance of hexose monophosphate shunt activity as source of electrons and protons for the respiratory burst. *J. Clin. Invest.* 74:455–59

90. Nanda A, Gukovskaya A, Tseng J, Grinstein S. 1992. Activation of vacuolar-type proton pumps by protein kinase C. Role in neutrophil pH regulation. *J. Biol. Chem.* 267:22740–46

91. Takanaka K, O'Brien PJ. 1988. Proton release associated with respiratory burst of polymorphonuclear leukocytes. *J. Biochem. (Tokyo)* 103:656–60

92. van Zwieten R, Wever R, Hamers MN, Weening RS, Roos D. 1981. Extracellular proton release by stimulated neutrophils. *J. Clin. Invest.* 68:310–13

93. Simchowitz L. 1985. Chemotactic factor-induced activation of Na^+/H^+ exchange in human neutrophils. II. Intracellular pH changes. *J. Biol. Chem.* 260:13248–55

94. Grinstein S, Furuya W. 1986. Cytoplasmic pH regulation in phorbol ester-activated human neutrophils. *Am. J. Physiol.* 251(Pt. 1):C55–65

95. Henderson LM, Chappell JB, Jones OT. 1988. Internal pH changes associated with the activity of NADPH oxidase of human neutrophils. Further evidence for the presence of an H^+ conducting channel. *Biochem. J.* 251:563–67

96. Nanda A, Grinstein S. 1991. Protein kinase C activates an H^+ (equivalent) conductance in the plasma membrane of human neutrophils. *Proc. Natl. Acad. Sci. USA* 88:10816–20

97. Henderson LM, Chappell JB, Jones OT. 1988. Superoxide generation by the electrogenic NADPH oxidase of human neutrophils is limited by the movement of a compensating charge. *Biochem. J.* 255:285–90

98. DeCoursey TE, Morgan D, Cherny VV. 2002. The gp91^{phox} component of NADPH oxidase is not a voltage-gated proton channel. *J. Gen. Physiol.* 120:773–79

99. Henderson LM, Meech RW. 1999. Evidence that the product of the human X-linked CGD gene, gp91-*phox*, is a voltage-gated H^+ pathway. *J. Gen. Physiol.* 114:771–86

100. Maturana A, Arnaudeau S, Ryser S, Banfi B, Hossle JP, et al. 2001. Heme histidine ligands within gp91^{phox} modulate proton conduction by the phagocyte NADPH oxidase. *J. Biol. Chem.* 276:30277–84

101. Nanda A, Romanek R, Curnutte JT, Grinstein S. 1994. Assessment of the contribution of the cytochrome b moiety of the NADPH oxidase to the transmembrane H^+ conductance of leukocytes. *J. Biol. Chem.* 269:27280–85

102. Thomas RC, Meech RW. 1982. Hydrogen ion currents and intracellular pH in depolarized voltage-clamped snail neurones. *Nature* 299:826–28

103. Henderson LM, Chappell JB, Jones OT. 1988. Internal pH changes associated with the activity of NADPH oxidase of human neutrophils. Further evidence for the presence of an H^+ conducting channel. *Biochem. J.* 251:563–67

104. DeCoursey TE. 2004. During the respiratory burst, do phagocytes need proton channels or potassium channels, or both? *Sci. STKE* 2004:E21

105. Miyasaki KT, Genco RJ, Wilson ME.

1986. Antimicrobial properties of hydrogen peroxide and sodium bicarbonate individually and in combination against selected oral, gram-negative, facultative bacteria. *J. Dent. Res.* 65:1142–48

106. Locksley RM, Wilson CB, Klebanoff SJ. 1983. Increased respiratory burst in myeloperoxidase-deficient monocytes. *Blood* 62:902–9

107. Clifford DP, Repine JE. 1982. Hydrogen peroxide mediated killing of bacteria. *Mol. Cell Biochem.* 49:143–49

108. Gallin JI, Buescher ES, Seligmann BE, Nath J, Gaither T, Katz P. 1983. NIH conference. Recent advances in chronic granulomatous disease. *Ann. Intern. Med.* 99:657–74

109. Holmes B, Good RA. 1972. Laboratory models of chronic granulomatous disease. *J. Reticuloendothel. Soc.* 12:216–37

110. Pitt J, Bernheimer HP. 1974. Role of peroxide in phagocytic killing of pneumococci. *Infect. Immun.* 9:48–52

111. Mandell GL. 1975. Catalase, superoxide dismutase, and virulence of *Staphylococcus aureus*. In vitro and in vivo studies with emphasis on staphylococcal-leukocyte interaction. *J. Clin. Invest.* 55: 561–66

112. Chang YC. 1998. Virulence of catalase-deficient *Aspergillus nidulans* in $p47^{phox-/-}$ mice. Implications for fungal pathogenicity and host defense in chronic granulomatous disease. *J. Clin. Invest.* 101:1843–50

113. Messina CG, Reeves EP, Roes J, Segal AW. 2002. Catalase negative *Staphylococcus aureus* retain virulence in mouse model of chronic granulomatous disease. *FEBS Lett.* 518:107–10

114. Ismail G, Boxer LA, Baehner RL. 1979. Utilization of liposomes for correction of the metabolic and bactericidal deficiencies in chronic granulomatous disease. *Pediatr. Res.* 13:769–73

115. Gerber CE, Bruchelt G, Falk UB, Kimpfler A, Hauschild O, et al. 2001. Reconstitution of bactericidal activity in chronic granulomatous disease cells by glucose-oxidase-containing liposomes. *Blood* 98:3097–105

116. Reeves EP, Nagl M, Godovac-Zimmermann J, Segal AW. 2003. Reassessment of the microbicidal activity of reactive oxygen species and hypochlorous acid with reference to the phagocytic vacuole of the neutrophil granulocyte. *J. Med. Microbiol.* 52:643–51

117. Deleted in proof

118. Klebanoff SJ, Clark RA. 1977. Iodination by human polymorphonuclear leukocytes: a re-evaluation. *J. Lab. Clin. Med.* 89:675–86

119. Segal AW, Garcia RC, Harper AM, Banga JP. 1983. Iodination by stimulated human neutrophils. Studies on its stoichiometry, subcellular localization and relevance to microbial killing. *Biochem. J.* 210:215–25

120. Chapman AL, Hampton MB, Senthilmohan R, Winterbourn CC, Kettle AJ. 2002. Chlorination of bacterial and neutrophil proteins during phagocytosis and killing of *Staphylococcus aureus*. *J. Biol. Chem.* 277:9757–62

121. Nauseef WM. 1988. Myeloperoxidase deficiency. *Hematol. Oncol. Clin. N. Am.* 2:135–58

122. Penniall R, Spitznagel JK. 1975. Chicken neutrophils: oxidative metabolism in phagocytic cells devoid of myeloperoxidase. *Proc. Natl. Acad. Sci. USA* 72:5012–15

123. Kobayashi M, Tanaka T, Usui T. 1982. Inactivation of lysosomal enzymes by the respiratory burst of polymorphonuclear leukocytes. Possible involvement of myeloperoxidase-H_2O_2-halide system. *J. Lab. Clin. Med.* 100:896–907

124. Kettle AJ, Winterbourn CC. 2001. A kinetic analysis of the catalase activity of myeloperoxidase. *Biochemistry* 40: 10204–12

125. Winterbourn CC, Garcia RC, Segal AW. 1985. Production of the superoxide

adduct of myeloperoxidase (compound III) by stimulated human neutrophils and its reactivity with hydrogen peroxide and chloride. *Biochem. J.* 228:583–92

126. Aratani Y, Kura F, Watanabe H, Akagawa H, Takano Y, et al. 2002. Critical role of myeloperoxidase and nicotinamide adenine dinucleotide phosphate-oxidase in high-burden systemic infection of mice with *Candida albicans. J. Infect. Dis.* 185:1833–37

Annu. Rev. Immunol. 2005. 23:225–74
doi: 10.1146/annurev.immunol.23.021704.115526
Copyright © 2005 by Annual Reviews. All rights reserved
First published online as a Review in Advance on November 11, 2004

NK Cell Recognition

Lewis L. Lanier

*Department of Microbiology and Immunology and the Cancer Research Institute,
University of California, San Francisco School of Medicine, San Francisco,
California 94143-0414; email: lanier@itsa.ucsf.edu*

Key Words   innate immunity, immune receptors, signal transduction

■ **Abstract**   The integrated processing of signals transduced by activating and inhibitory cell surface receptors regulates NK cell effector functions. Here, I review
the structure, function, and ligand specificity of the receptors responsible for NK cell
recognition.

INTRODUCTION

Natural killer (NK) cells distinguish between normal healthy cells and abnormal cells by using a sophisticated repertoire of cell surface receptors that control
their activation, proliferation, and effector functions.[1] Germline genes that do not
require somatic recombination encode these receptors; thus, NK cells represent
an arm of the innate immune system. Although they lack the ability to generate
antigen-specific receptors by somatic cell genetic alterations, NK cells in many
aspects are more closely related to T cells, with which they share a common
bipotential progenitor, than to other populations of leukocytes of the innate immune system (reviewed in 1, 2). In particular, NK cells share a common killing
mechanism with CD8[+] cytotoxic T lymphocytes (CTL) (i.e., using perforin and
granzymes). Like CTL and CD4[+] Th1 cells, NK cells secrete interferon-γ (IFN-
γ). Despite a similar pattern of cytokine production to CTL and CD4[+] Th1 cells,
an important distinction is that NK cells are unable to produce IL-2. While the
term "NK receptor" has been used to describe molecules that were first discovered on NK cells, the majority of these NK receptors are expressed on at least a
subset of T lymphocytes, in particular on $\gamma\delta$TCR[+] T cells and on activated CD8[+]
T cells.

Emerging evidence suggests that NK cells, previously considered an ancient
immune effector cell type, have more likely coevolved with T cells, given that
both of these lymphocytes are focused on recognition of conventional and nonconventional major histocompatibility complex (MHC) molecules. In this regard,

---

[1]See Appendix for a full list of abbreviations used.

NK cells distinguish themselves from phagocytes (macrophages and granulocytes) that rely solely on conserved pattern-recognition receptors, for example, the toll-like receptors. Functional MHC molecules are present in cartilaginous fish, but not in more primitive species. Similarly, NK cells, as they are currently defined, also have not been identified in species lower than fish. Thus, based on their lineage relationships, receptor repertoire, and effector functions, NK cells appear to be a transitional cell type bridging the innate and adaptive immune systems.

Understanding NK cell recognition is more complex than for B cells and T cells, where the antigen receptors dominate the differentiation, activation, and effector function of these lymphocytes. Rather than being regulated by any one receptor, NK cells appear to work by the integration of numerous signals from receptors that would be designated "adhesion molecules" or "costimulatory receptors" on T cells. Further, the activation of NK cells is stringently controlled by inhibitory receptors that presumably function as a fail-safe to avoid inadvertent stimulation, which may result in harm to normal healthy cells in the host.

NK cell recognition involves the initial binding to potential target cells, interactions between activating and inhibitory receptors with ligands available on the target, and the integration of signals transmitted by these receptors, which determines whether the NK cell detaches and moves on or stays and responds. NK cells respond by reorganizing and releasing cytotoxic granules and by transcribing and secreting cytokines. Recent studies have demonstrated reorientation of the relevant receptors into an "NK synapse" during NK cell encounters with potential target cells (3–7), as observed previously in the interaction between T cells and antigen-presenting cells. NK cells differ from naive T cells in that mature NK cells are poised as effector cells for an immediate response. These "ready-to-go" cells express granzymes and perforin, and their lytic response can be triggered within minutes, without requiring transcription, translation, or cell proliferation. Recent studies by Locksley and colleagues (8) have shown that NK cells constitutively express prestored transcripts for IFN-γ that are immediately available to initiate cytokine synthesis upon activation. Even at their earliest stages of development, IFN-γ transcripts are present in the NK cell progenitors in the mouse bone marrow (8). Thus, there is no equivalent in the NK cell lineage that corresponds to a "naive" T cell, which must undergo proliferation, chromatin remodeling of cytokine genes, and de novo transcription and translation of granzymes and perforin before it becomes a competent effector cell. In this regard, the phenotype of a "resting" NK cell is more similar to an effector CD8$^+$ T cell with respect to expression of cell surface receptors and effector molecules. Indeed, many NK receptors are expressed on CD8$^+$ T cells (and some CD4$^+$ T cells) only after their conversion to effector or memory cells (reviewed in 9). The ready-to-go state of NK cells and the fact that NK cell receptors are invariant and constitutively present on a large proportion of cells within the population make these cells well suited for early defense.

THE "MISSING-SELF HYPOTHESIS" REVISITED

Initially, NK cells were described as non-MHC-restricted in their recognition process because of their ability to kill target cells that either lacked MHC or expressed various allogeneic MHC molecules. However, Karre and colleagues (10) noted that rather than ignore MHC, NK cells appear to be actively inhibited from responding when they encounter certain tumor cells that express MHC class I. Subsequently, the ability of NK cells to recognize and eliminate normal host hematopoietic cells that lack MHC class I was substantiated by demonstrating NK cell–dependent rejection of bone marrow cells from β2-microglobulin-deficient syngeneic mice (11, 12). According to the "missing-self" hypothesis (13), NK cells were proposed to provide immune surveillance for cells that had downregulated MHC class I, an event that frequently accompanies cellular transformation or infection with certain viruses. Until recently, a common misconception has been that NK cells attack any cell lacking MHC molecules because the potential target cell cannot engage an inhibitory NK cell receptor for MHC class I. This notion is counterintuitive given documentation of the events involving cell-cell binding, Ca^{2+} mobilization, and synapse formation when NK cells encounter susceptible target cells that lack MHC class I. A contemporary modification of the missing-self hypothesis might state, "NK cells patrol for abnormal cells that lack MHC class I or overexpress ligands for activating NK cell receptors" (Figure 1). In essence, the inhibitory MHC class I receptors on NK cells serve as a rheostat, regulating and dampening signals transduced through activating receptors. When NK cells and potential target cells meet, the information is interpreted by an analog, not a binary process. Experimental evidence suggests that the MHC class I inhibitory receptors may serve only to dampen, rather than completely terminate, NK cell effector function and that the amount of MHC class I on the surface of the target is proportional to the degree of inhibition. In experimental models, when multiple activating NK cell receptors are engaged simultaneously (14) or when a sufficiently potent activating NK receptor is stimulated (15, 16), NK cells are capable of effectively eliminating cells even if their inhibitory receptors for MHC class I are ligated.

A corollary of the missing-self hypothesis is that failure of NK cells to respond to a potential target can be due either to active inhibition mediated by the inhibitory receptors or alternatively, to the absence of sufficient activation signals to initiate a response (Figure 1). An example of the latter situation may be represented by encounters between human erythrocytes and circulating peripheral blood NK cells. Although human red blood cells do not express MHC class I, NK cells do not attack them; therefore, erythrocytes may lack ligands capable of engaging the activating NK cell receptors. An alternative explanation for the inability of NK cells to harm normal tissues with low (e.g., neural tissues) or no (e.g., erythrocytes) MHC class I is the possibility that this target cell protection is mediated by inhibitory receptors recognizing non-MHC ligands. As precedence, macrophages express the SIRPα inhibitory receptor that inhibits their phagocytosis of erythrocytes expressing its ligand CD47 (17). Recent studies have demonstrated that an inhibitory NK receptor

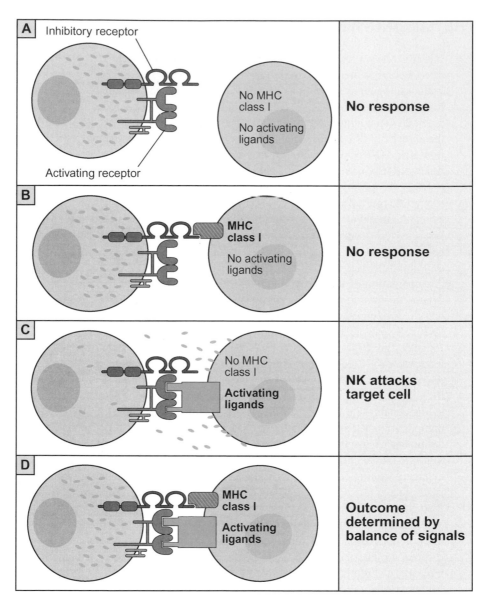

Figure 1 "Missing-self" revisited. Graphic depiction of encounters between NK cells and potential targets and possible outcomes. In some circumstances, inhibitory receptors recognizing ligands other than MHC class I proteins may suppress NK cell responses. When interacting with target cells expressing ligands for both inhibitory and activating receptors, the outcome is determined by the summation of the strength of signals. The amount of activating and inhibitory receptors on the NK cells and the amount of ligands on the target cell, as well as the qualitative differences in the signals transduced, determine the extent of the NK cell response.

of the mouse NKR-P1 (Klrb1) family (NKR-P1d) recognizes mouse Clr-b (also known as Ocil), a cell-surface glycoprotein broadly expressed on many cell types (except erythrocytes) (18, 19). In addition, other inhibitory receptors on NK cells, e.g., LAIR-1 (20, 21), MAFA (Klrg1) (22, 23), gp49B1 (24–27), CD66a (28, 29), Siglec7 (30, 31), many with undefined ligands, might conceivably participate in the modulation of NK cell responses against cells lacking or expressing low levels of MHC class I. Whereas the role of the inhibitory NK cell receptors for MHC class I has been clearly established, the physiological significance of these other inhibitory receptors, especially in protecting MHC class I–deficient cells, awaits in vivo confirmation.

NK RECEPTOR SIGNAL TRANSDUCTION: GENERAL PARADIGMS

Signaling by many inhibitory and activating NK receptors is mediated by conserved sequences within the cytoplasmic domains of these receptors or their associated adapter proteins. All of the well-defined inhibitory NK cell receptors possess in their cytoplasmic domains one or more copies of the consensus sequence Ile/Val/Leu/Ser-x-Tyr-x-x-Leu/Val, where x denotes any amino acid. Referred to as an immunoreceptor tyrosine-based inhibitory motif (ITIM), it was first described in FcγRIIb, an Fc receptor for IgG expressed on B cells that is responsible for suppressing signaling through surface immunoglobulin (32). ITIMs are found in all inhibitory NK receptors, as well as in many other receptors expressed on hematopoietic cells (reviewed in 33). Upon ligand binding, the tyrosine residue in the ITIM is phosphorylated, likely by a Src family kinase, and phosphatases are recruited through their SH2-domains. As detailed below, there is evidence for the recruitment of the tyrosine-specific phosphatases SHP (SH2-containing protein-tyrosine phosphatase)-1 and SHP-2, or the phospholipid-specific phosphatase SHIP (SH2-containing inositol polyphosphate 5-phosphatase), depending on the particular receptor analyzed. These phosphatases work at a membrane proximal location, dampening or preventing NK cell effector functions, i.e., cytotoxicity and cytokine production. SHIP functions to degrade phosphatidylinositol-3,4,5-trisphosphate (PI-3,4,5-P$_3$) to phosphatidylinositol-3, 4-bisphosphate (PI-3,4-P$_2$), thereby preventing sustained Ca^{2+}-dependent signaling. In NK cells, depending on the particular activating and inhibitory receptors engaged, recruitment and activation of SHP-1 and SHP-2 by the inhibitory receptors results in decreased phosphorylation of numerous intracellular signaling proteins, including FcεRIγ, ZAP70, Syk, PLCγ1, PLCγ2, Shc, LAT, SLP76, and Vav-1 (34–38). It is uncertain whether these signaling proteins serve as direct substrates of the phosphatases or are prevented from being phosphorylated by indirect mechanisms resulting from SHP-1 or SHP-2 activity.

Several activating NK receptors share a common signaling pathway with the T cell and B cell antigen receptors, using adapter proteins containing an immunoreceptor tyrosine-based activation motif (ITAM). The ITAM is defined by the prototype sequence, Asp/Glu-x-x-Tyr-x-x-Leu/Ile x_{6-8} Tyr xx Leu/Ile, where x denotes any amino acid with 6 to 8 amino acids between the two Tyr xx Leu/Ile elements (39). NK cells express three ITAM-containing adapter proteins: FcεRIγ (40), CD3ζ (41), and DAP12 (42) [also called KARAP (43)]. Indeed, the first activating NK receptor identified (44, 45), and the best characterized, is CD16, the low-affinity Fc receptor for IgG that is responsible for antibody-dependent cellular cytotoxicity (ADCC) (reviewed in 46, 47). Human CD16 can associate with FcεRIγ (40) and/or CD3ζ (48), whereas mouse CD16 only pairs with FcεRIγ (49). As discussed in detail below, these ITAM-bearing adapter proteins can associate with several NK cell receptors, in addition to CD16, thereby providing signaling function. Upon tyrosine phosphorylation of the ITAM, the tyrosine kinases Syk and ZAP70 (both of which are expressed in NK cells) are recruited via their SH2 domains and stimulate downstream events, causing a Ca^{2+} influx, degranulation, and transcription of cytokine and chemokine genes. Surprisingly, Syk and ZAP70 are not required for NK cell development, and many effector functions are intact in mice that are genetically deficient in both of these kinases (50, 51). A similar phenotype (i.e., the presence of mature NK cells with certain effector functions maintained) is observed in "triple knockout" mice lacking FcεRIγ, CD3ζ, and DAP12 (K. Ogasawara & L.L. Lanier, unpublished observation). Together, these findings imply that, unlike B and T lymphocytes, a single signaling pathway does not dominate the differentiation and effector functions mediated by NK cells.

In this review, I provide an overview of the structure, signal transduction, and biological function of the activating and inhibitory NK receptors, with particular emphasis on those receptors with defined physiological ligands. I discuss the different classes of NK receptors defined by their ligand specificity, i.e., receptors for MHC class I, receptors for MHC class I–related ligands, and receptors for host-encoded non-MHC ligands. By this presentation, I hope to highlight features common to each family and unique to certain molecules and ligands.

RECOGNITION OF MHC CLASS I LIGANDS

NK receptors recognizing "classical" and "nonclassical" class I molecules encoded by genes within the MHC have been identified, including the rodent Ly49 receptors, human killer cell immunoglobulin-like receptors (KIR), and conserved CD94/NKG2 receptor family. By contrast, there is no credible evidence that NK cells recognize MHC class II molecules based on the analysis of class II–deficient mice and in vitro functional studies using human or mouse target cells expressing MHC class II. Thus, NK cells apparently specialize in immune surveillance focused on monitoring cells for aberrant expression of MHC class I molecules.

Ly49 Receptors

A molecular explanation for the missing-self hypothesis was provided first by the demonstration by Yokoyama and colleagues (52) that the subset of NK cells expressing the Ly49A receptor were preferentially unable to kill certain tumor cells expressing H-2D^d. *Ly49A* is the prototypic member of a small gene family that encodes type II transmembrane-anchored glycoproteins expressed on subsets of NK cells and memory T cells. The number of *Ly49* genes varies in different mouse strains, and there is evidence for extensive allelic polymorphism (53). The *Ly49* genes are best characterized in the C57BL/6 and 129/J mouse strains (54, 55), where 14 genes have been identified in a cluster within the NK complex on mouse chromosome 6 (56). Most of these genes encode inhibitory receptors with ITIMs in their cytoplasmic domains, whereas others (e.g., *Ly49D* and *Ly49H* in C57BL/6 mice) are activating receptors that lack ITIMs and associate noncovalently with the ITAM-bearing DAP12 adapter molecule (57). A positively charged arginine in the transmembrane domain of the activating Ly49 receptors permits interaction with the negatively charged aspartic acid residue in the transmembrane of DAP12; in the absence of DAP12, the activating Ly49 receptors are not stably expressed on the cell surface (57). In DAP12-deficient mice, the activating Ly49 receptors are only poorly expressed on the cell surface and they are nonfunctional (58), indicating that other signaling adapter molecules cannot substitute for DAP12. Salient and remarkable features of the Ly49 receptors include the following: (*a*) Each NK cell within the population transcribes on average from one to four *Ly49* genes, as determined by RT-PCR analysis of single NK cells in the fetal and adult NK cell population (59); (*b*) *Ly49* genes can be expressed in a monoallelic fashion (60, 61) by a unique stochastic mechanism of gene regulation (62); (*c*) both the frequency of cells expressing a particular Ly49 receptor and the amount of Ly49 on the cell surface is subtly influenced by expression of H-2 in the host (reviewed in 63, 64); (*d*) Ly49 glycoproteins are members of the C-type lectin-like receptor family comprised of a single lectin-like extracellular domain and are expressed as disulfide-bonded homodimers (heterodimers of Ly49 proteins encoded by different genes have not been detected); and (*e*) expression of *Ly49* genes is stably maintained within the clonal progeny of a mature NK cell (reviewed in 63, 64).

The *Ly49* gene family appears to have evolved by gene duplication and gene conversion. The genomic organization of the *Ly49* genes, with the domains for the ligand-binding extracellular, transmembrane, and cytoplasmic segments encoded by independent exons, provides an ideal arrangement for receptor diversification. By "shuffling the deck" of *Ly49* exons during meiosis, exons encoding the extracellular domain of an inhibitory receptor could be placed in proximity to exons for the transmembrane and cytoplasmic domains of an activating receptor. Such an event likely occurred to generate an inhibitory receptor in C57L mice that has an extracellular domain quite similar to the activating Ly49D receptor and the transmembrane and cytoplasmic domain (containing an ITIM) of the inhibitory Ly49A receptor in C57BL/6 mice (65). The expression of Ly49 glycoproteins as homodimers, rather than heterodimers, may be an important feature, to prevent association between the inhibitory and activating isoforms.

Structures of inhibitory Ly49 and H-2 complexes and mutational analysis of the receptor and ligand have provided detailed insights into NK cell recognition

(66, 67; reviewed in 68). The homodimeric Ly49A receptor binds to H-2D^d at two distinct sites, one of which involves the α1 and α2 domains of MHC class I, whereas the second interaction site spans the α1, α2, α3 domains and β2-microglobulin (66, 69). Heterogeneity may exist in Ly49 receptors with regard to ligand binding in that complexes of Ly49C and H-2K^b differ from the binding observed between Ly49A and H-2D^d (67). Ly49 binding to MHC class I requires the presence of a bound peptide within the H-2 groove, but no consensus has emerged on the biological relevance of this. Studies of the Ly49A receptor indicate that any peptide would suffice (70, 71), whereas some degree of peptide selectivity has been reported for Ly49C and Ly49I (72, 73). Despite the fact that the Ly49 proteins have evolved from the C-type lectin family, ligand specificity appears principally dependent on protein-protein binding, although carbohydrate recognition could conceivably play a minor role in the interaction. Determining the precise ligand specificity of the Ly49 receptors is complicated by the following factors: (*a*) Binding assays using tetrameric H-2 complexes are biased by the inclusion of only a single peptide in the H-2 groove; (*b*) cell-cell binding assays using Ly49 and H-2 transfected cells may be inadequate to detect low-affinity interactions that are nonetheless biologically relevant; (*c*) Ly49 receptors appear to cross-react broadly with different H-2 alleles, and only the highest-affinity interactions may be revealed by conventional binding assays using soluble recombinant proteins or transfectants; and (*d*) interactions that occur on the surface of an NK cell in *cis* between Ly49 receptors and their own H-2 molecules may not be revealed using the receptors and ligands in solution (74).

While the inhibitory Ly49 receptors presumably function to prevent auto-aggression by NK cells, a biological rationale for the DAP12-associated activating Ly49 receptors with specificity for H-2 has remained an enigma. In C57BL/6 mice, Ly49D has been shown by using in vitro cytotoxicity assays to recognize H-2D^d, and has been implicated in the rejection of H-2D^d bone marrow allografts in C57BL/6 recipients (75–78). However, direct interactions between Ly49D and H-2 have not been documented by using either H-2D^d tetramers (72) or Ly49D reporter cell assays (79), implying either that the affinity of Ly49D for H-2D^d is lower than the inhibitory Ly49 receptors for this ligand or that coreceptors or costimulatory molecules on the NK cell may be necessary to trigger a functional response against H-2D^d-bearing target cells. Nonetheless, ligation of the DAP12-associated Ly49D receptor has been shown to potently activate cytotoxicity, as well as initiate transcription of numerous cytokines and chemokines (80). The activating Ly49P and Ly49W receptors in NOD mice also have been shown to recognize H-2D^d ligands (81, 82), but their biological role has not been investigated.

Thus, although the relevance of the activating receptors reactive with H-2 has been documented in allogeneic bone marrow transplantation, their importance in physiological immune responses is still unclear. In a H-2$^{b/d}$ heterozygous host, the subset of NK cells expressing Ly49D may attack host cells that have lost H-2^b but retained H-2^d due to transformation or viral infection. In this scenario, these cells would appear allogeneic and elicit a response in the subset of NK cells expressing

Ly49D that lack an inhibitory receptor able to recognize H-2^b. Ly49D$^+$ NK cells in mice expressing H-2D^d are apparently not depleted or rendered stably unresponsive, but rather these cells are regulated by the presence of inhibitory receptors for self MHC class I (75). Further studies suggest that the suppressive action of the inhibitory Ly49 receptors on these Ly49D$^+$ NK cells can be overcome in the presence of IL-12 or IL-18, thereby permitting NK cell activation even in the presence of H-2 ligands for their inhibitory receptors (83). Thus, during inflammation when IL-12 or IL-18 are abundant, local NK cells may indeed become autoreactive in order to augment the immune response by the production of IFN-γ and the secretion of chemokines to attract other immune cells. Although detrimental if systemic or sustained, a localized, transient autoreaction by NK cells at a site of infection may be valuable in the earliest stages of an immune response.

It is possible that the physiological high-affinity ligands of the activating Ly49 receptors are not host self-proteins, and that the interactions with H-2 represent weak, biologically unimportant cross reactivity. This notion is supported by studies of the DAP12-associated Ly49H receptor, which is responsible for the resistance of C57BL/6 mice to infection with mouse cytomegalovirus (MCMV) (84–87). Whereas Ly49H does not bind to any known H-2 molecule, it binds with high affinity to the m157 viral glycoprotein that is encoded by MCMV and is expressed on the cell surface of MCMV-infected cells (88, 89). An *m157*-deletion mutant of MCMV has severely decreased virulence in C57BL/6 mice, confirming that m157 is a virulence factor (90). Expression of a *Ly49H* transgene confers resistance to MCMV infection in BALB/c mice (which do not express an endogenous *Ly49H* gene and are a MCMV-susceptible mouse strain) (86). Passage of MCMV in C57BL/6 mice or RAG1$^{-/-}$ mice on the C57BL/6 background results in loss-of-function mutations in the *m157* gene (91, 92), demonstrating immune selection of MCMV, a double-stranded DNA herpesvirus, due to NK cell–mediated immunity. Given the rapid elimination of *m157* in MCMV-resistant C57BL/6 mice, why did this viral gene evolve? This is likely explained by the finding that the m157 protein has structural homology to MHC class I and in certain MCMV-susceptible mouse strains, the m157 glycoprotein binds to inhibitory Ly49 receptors, such as Ly49I in 129/J mice (88). Presumably, at some time in the past, MCMV captured a host *H-2* gene that would bind inhibitory Ly49 receptors, like Ly49I, and evolved m157 to function as a virulence factor by suppressing NK cell–mediated immunity. Because the *Ly49* genes are rapidly evolving, the inhibitory Ly49I-related gene may have been transformed by gene conversion from an inhibitory into an activating Ly49H-related receptor in mice related to the C57BL/6 strain. Further, whereas the inhibitory Ly49I-like receptors retained the ability to bind both host H-2 and viral m157 glycoproteins, the activating Ly49H receptor may have evolved to bind m157 with high affinity, but lost reactivity with H-2 to prevent autoimmunity. This hypothesis, although impossible to formally prove, would be supported if other pathogen-encoded ligands can be found for the families of NK cell receptors that have activating and inhibitory isoforms. Rat CMV has a structural homolog of m157, so a search for rat Ly49 receptors functionally corresponding to Ly49H and

Ly49I is warranted. The conversion of an inhibitory human KIR into an activating KIR is also suggested by comparing the sequences of the highly related KIR2DL2 and KIR2DS2 proteins. Whereas two ITIMs are present in the cytoplasmic domain of KIR2DL2, a stop codon in the cytoplasmic domain of the activating *KIR2S2* gene results in premature termination of the protein, thus leaving the ITIM as an ancestral relic in the 3' untranslated region (93).

A search for human *Ly49* genes on chromosome 12p12.3-p13.2, the region syntenic to mouse chromosome 6, has revealed the existence of a single pseudogene that is poorly transcribed (94, 95). Similarly, a single nonfunctional *Ly49* gene is present in our closest ancestors (chimpanzee and gorilla), but a single intact *Ly49* gene has been identified in baboon, orangutan, cow, pig, dog, and cat, and an ITIM is present in the cytoplasmic domain of the nonprimate species, but not in the putative baboon or orangutan Ly49 protein (96–98). Southern blot analysis of horse genomic DNA suggests the existence of multiple *Ly49* genes (97), and at least six full-length cDNAs encoding five potential inhibitory receptors and one activating receptor have been identified (99). Thus, in rodents and horses Ly49 may function as the predominant NK receptors for MHC class I, whereas other species may have devised a different solution to mediate this function.

Killer Cell Immunoglobulin-Like Receptors

Humans do not have *Ly49* genes, but as a remarkable example of convergent evolution, an NK receptor system with all of the same general features has arisen to provide the same function in primates. The human *KIR* gene family contains 15 genes and 2 pseudogenes that are closely linked on chromosome 19q13.4. The number of *KIR* genes in the genome of any given individual varies within the population. Two common haplotypes, designated A and B, have been defined based on the number of genes present, and allelic polymorphism at each of the loci has been identified (100). However, further studies indicate the existence of at least 37 haplotypes, based on gene content, as the KIR genotype of more individuals has been evaluated (reviewed in 101; also see http://www.ncbi.nlm.nih.gov:80/books/bv.fcgi?call=bv. View..ShowTOC&rid=mono_003.TOC&depth=2). A database serving as a central depository for KIR sequences can be accessed at http://www.ebi.ac.uk:80/ipd/kir/index.html. A minimal A haplotype may have as few as five intact genes (but more typically seven genes), whereas B haplotypes may contain up to ten intact genes. Only three common "framework" genes are shared by all haplotypes (*KIR3DL3*, *KIR2DL4*, and *KIR3DL2*), and the allelic variants of some *KIR* genes are unable to generate functional receptors that can be stably expressed on the cell surface (102–105).

An analysis of the region of the chromosome containing the human *KIR* genes (106) and a comparison of *KIR* genes in humans and higher primates (98, 107, 108) indicates that these genes are rapidly evolving. Their close proximity in the genome and the high degree of nucleic acid identity between these genes facilitates KIR diversification by readily permitting asymmetric recombination (106,

109, 110). As a consequence, discriminating between alleles and loci becomes difficult and represents a technical challenge for laboratories performing KIR typing to study the potential role of these molecules in disease resistance or susceptibility. In addition to primates, *KIR*-like genes have been identified in cow (111) and horse (99). Two mouse genes similar to human *KIR3DL* have been found on the mouse X-chromosome, and these are transcribed in mouse NK cells and thymocytes, although the function of these proteins has not been established (112, 113).

The human *KIR* genes are expressed by subsets of NK cells (114, 115), $\gamma \delta$TCR$^+$ T cells, and memory/effector $\alpha \beta$TCR$^+$ T cells (usually CD8$^+$ T cells and some CD4$^+$ T cells, but not thymocytes or naive T cells) (116, 117). Once a given *KIR* gene is expressed in a T cell clone or NK cell, it is stably maintained in the progeny of these cells (118, 119). This pattern of expression appears to be regulated by methylation of the silent *KIR* loci, which can also result in monoallelic expression of KIR in NK cell clones (120, 121). T cell clones possessing an identically rearranged TCRα and TCRβ chain can stably express different *KIR* genes in their clonal progeny, indicating that the *KIR* genes are activated after the TcR rearrangements have occurred in the T cell clone (122–124).

Unlike the Ly49 proteins that are C-type lectins in structure, KIR evolved from the Ig superfamily, and these receptors are type I transmembrane glycoproteins with two Ig-like domains (designated KIR2D) or three Ig-like domains (designated KIR3D) in the extracellular region (125–127) (Table 1). The Ig-like domains have been designated D0, D1, and D2, with the D0 domain being the most N-terminal in KIR3D proteins, followed by the D1 and D2 domains. A short stalk region separates the Ig-like domains from the transmembrane segment, and the cytoplasmic domains are variable in length; some receptors possess long (L) cytoplasmic domains with one or two ITIM sequences, and other receptors have short (S) cytoplasmic domains without ITIM. KIR with short cytoplasmic domains (KIR2DS and KIR3DS) have a Lys residue, centrally located within their transmembrane region that is required for association with the DAP12 adapter protein. The inhibitory and activating receptors within the KIR family are encoded by separate genes and are not generated by alternative splicing of a single gene. However, in the case of one KIR3D gene, some alleles encode inhibitory receptors, e.g., KIR3DL1, whereas other alleles of this same gene encode putative activating receptors, e.g., KIR3DS1.

Despite their structural differences, the KIR and Ly49 receptor families share many common features: (*a*) Both are small gene families (10–15 closely linked genes) that arose by gene duplication and have diversified by gene conversion; (*b*) both demonstrate substantial genetic polymorphism and can be expressed in a mono-allelic fashion; (*c*) both are expressed on subsets of NK cells and memory T cells by a stochastic process, with the receptor repertoire in the individual being shaped by subtle influences of the host MHC class I haplotype; (*d*) both families contain genes that encode inhibitory receptors with ITIMs in their cytoplasmic domains and activating receptors that associate with the ITAM-bearing DAP12

TABLE 1 Human NK receptors (and their signaling adapters) for MHC class I

Gene	Other Names	CD	Function	Signaling	Ligand
TYROBP	DAP12, KARAP		Activation	Syk, ZAP70	N/A
HCST	DAP10, KAP10		Activation	p85 PI3K	N/A
FCE1G	FcεRIγ		Activation	Syk, ZAP70	N/A
LILRB1	ILT2/LIR1	CD85j	Inhibition	ITIM	HLA-A,B,C,E,F,G, CMV UL18
KIR3DL3		CD158z	Inhibition	ITIM	?
KIR2DL3		CD158b2	Inhibition	ITIM	HLA-C S77/N80
KIR2DL2		CD158b1	Inhibition	ITIM	HLA-C S77/N80
KIR2DL1		CD158a	Inhibition	ITIM	HLA-C N77/K80
KIR2DL4		CD158d	Inhibition/ Activation?	FcεRIγ/ITIM?	HLA-G?
KIR3DL1		CD158e1	Inhibition	ITIM	HLA-Bw4
KIR3DS1		CD158e2	Activation	DAP12[a]	?
KIR2DL5A		CD158f	Inhibition	ITIM	?
KIR2DL5B			Inhibition	ITIM	?
KIR2DS3			Activation	DAP12	?
KIR2DS5		CD158g	Activation	DAP12	?
KIR2DS1		CD158h	Activation	DAP12	HLA-C, weakly
KIR2DS2		CD158j	Activation	DAP12	?
KIR2DS4		CD158i	Activation	DAP12	HLA-C, weakly
KIR3DL2		CD158k	Inhibition	ITIM	HLA-A?
KLRD1/ KLRC1		CD94/ NKG2A	Inhibition	ITIM	HLA-E
KLRD1/ KLRC2		CD94/ NKG2C	Activation	DAP12	HLA-E
KLRC3		NKG2E	?	?	?
KLRC4		NKG2F	?	?	?

[a]Based on sequence similarities, KIR2DS1, KIR2DS3, KIR2DS5, and KIR3DS1 probably associate with DAP12; however, this has formally been shown only with KIR2DS2 and KIR2DS4. The KIR2DL and KIR3DL all express ITIM and are assumed to transmit inhibitory signals. NKG2B is a splice variant of the *NKG2A* (*KLRC1*) gene and NKG2H is a splice variant of the *NKG2E* (*KLRC3*) gene.

adapter protein; and (*e*) both recognize polymorphic determinants on MHC class I ligands.

KIR recognize HLA-A, HLA-B, and HLA-C proteins (Table 1; Figure 2). Members of the KIR2D subfamily recognize a polymorphism in HLA-C proteins at positions 77 and 80 on the α1 domain of the HLA-C heavy chain (128). All known alleles of HLA-C have either Ser at position 77 and Asn at position 80 or Asn at position 77 and Lys at position 80, and these are recognized by different isoforms of KIR2DL. KIR3DL1 has been shown to react with HLA-B and certain HLA-A proteins that possess the Bw4 serological epitope, defined by residues 77–83 in the α1 domain (129, 130). KIR3DL2 has been shown to recognize certain HLA-A ligands; however, the precise specificity of this receptor has not been defined (131–133). An intact HLA class I trimer, composed of heavy chain, β2-microglobulin, and peptide, is required for KIR recognition. KIR can discriminate between different peptides presented by HLA-A, -B, or -C. Residues at positions 7 and 8 in the peptide have been implicated as the most important (133–139). Although KIR recognition is clearly both peptide dependent and peptide selective, these receptors do not distinguish self from nonself peptides; thus, the biological relevance is not obvious. Co-crystals of KIR2DL1 with HLA-Cw4 and KIR2DL2 with HLA-Cw3 (140) have defined these interactions in exquisite molecular detail (reviewed in 68).

Although the specificity of the inhibitory KIR have been extensively characterized, very little is known about the ligands for the KIR2DS and KIR3DS molecules. The similarity between several pairs of the activating and inhibitory KIR suggests they arose by gene duplication. However, in all cases studied, the activating KIR either does not bind HLA class I, or binds with an affinity much weaker than that of the paired inhibitory KIR. For example, whereas KIR2DL1 and KIR2DS1 differ by only 7 amino acids in their extracellular domain, KIR2DL1 binds to HLA-C*0401 much more strongly than KIR2DS1 (141). Similarly, KIR2DL2 and KIR2DL3 bind to HLA-C*0304, but KIR2DS2, whose extracellular domain differs from KIR2DL2 and KIR2DL3 by only 3 or 4 amino acids, respectively, failed to bind any HLA class I molecule examined. Conversion of a tyrosine at position 45 in KIR2DS2 to a phenylalanine, which is present in KIR2DL2 and KIR2DL3, enabled the mutant KIR2DS2 to bind HLA-C (141, 142). KIR2DS4 also binds only weakly to HLA-Cw4 and does not bind to HLA-Cw6, unlike KIR2DL1, which binds both of these HLA-C proteins (143). Thus, it appears that as a class the activating KIR, like the activating Ly49 receptors in mice, demonstrate low or no binding to HLA class I molecules. This feature may well have been selected for during the evolution of these receptors to minimize the risk of autoimmunity.

KIR2DL4 is the most distinct gene in the KIR family. The *KIR2DL4* promoter differs substantially from all other *KIR* genes, and both alleles are expressed in essentially all activated NK cells (121, 144, 145). Additionally, unlike other KIR, KIR2DL4 is constitutively expressed only on the surface of the CD56[bright] subset of peripheral blood NK cells (104, 146). On the CD56[dim] subset, KIR2DL4 expression is induced when NK cells are stimulated to proliferate in culture. The

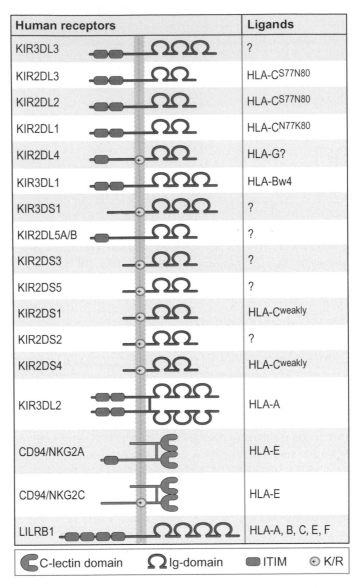

Figure 2   Graphic depiction of human NK cell receptors for MHC class I. Inhibitory KIR (i.e., KIR2DL and KIR3DL), LILRB1, and CD94/NKG2A contain ITIMs in their cytoplasmic domains. CD94/NKG2C and the KIR molecules lacking ITIMs and having a charged residue in their transmembrane domains (i.e., KIR2DS and KIR3DS) likely pair with the DAP12 signaling adapter. KIR2DL4 is an exception; it possesses an ITIM in its cytoplasmic domain and is associated with the FcεRIγ signaling adapter. MHC class I ligands for the receptors, if known, are shown.

KIR2DL4 protein is also unique in that unlike other KIR2D molecules, which have the D1 and D2 Ig-like domains in their extracellular region, KIR2DL4 is composed of D0 and D2 Ig-like domains (D0 is the first Ig-like domain of the KIR3D subfamily) (147). Other structural features of KIR2DL4 are also remarkable. The KIR2DL4 transmembrane region has an Arg residue, rather than the Lys residue found in the other activating KIR, and it is more membrane proximal, near the extracellular region. Unlike other activating KIR, KIR2DL4 associates with the FcεRIγ adapter protein, but not with DAP12 (146; L.L. Lanier & D. Rosen, unpublished observation) and has a functional ITIM in its cytoplasmic domain (148, 149). Despite the presence of an ITIM, cross-linking KIR2DL4 with mAb induces the production of IFN-γ in resting NK cells and triggers cytotoxicity and IFN-γ production in IL-2-activated NK cells (104, 150, 151). *KIR2DL4* is polymorphic (152), and one allele (designated 9A) that is prevalent in the human population is transcribed only at low levels and encodes a protein that is not stably expressed on the cell surface (104, 151). Some studies suggest that HLA-G may serve as a ligand for KIR2DL4 (153–155); however, this has not been validated in other experimental systems (156, 157).

Binding of inhibitory KIR to their MHC class I ligands on potential target cells results in suppression of cytotoxicity and cytokine secretion by KIR-bearing NK cells and T cells. As mentioned above, recruitment of SHP-1 to the tyrosine-phosphorylated ITIM in the KIR has been implicated as the predominant mechanism of inhibition of effector cell function (158–161). The activating KIR, which lack ITIM in their cytoplasmic domains, signal by association with the ITAM-bearing DAP12 adapter protein (42, 43). Because of the conserved Lys residue in the transmembrane of the KIR2DS and KIR3DS proteins, it is assumed that all of these receptors associate with DAP12; however, this has been demonstrated directly only with KIR2DS2. Whereas all NK cells express DAP12, this adapter protein is found only in a minor subset of T cells. A unique population of $CD4^+$ $CD28^-$ T cells from patients with rheumatoid arthritis has been shown to express an activating KIR molecule in the absence of DAP12 (162). Cross-linking KIR2DS2 on these T cells causes phosphorylation of JNK (c-Jun-NH_2-terminal protein kinase), but not activation of ERK 1/2 (extracellular signal-regulated kinase). Snyder and colleagues (162) have speculated that KIR2DS2 may contribute to the T cell–mediated autoimmune disease.

There is emerging evidence implicating KIR in human autoimmune disorders. In addition to studies documenting activating KIR-bearing $CD4^+$ T cells in patients with rheumatoid arthritis (162, 163), epidemiological data have shown that individuals possessing a *KIR2DS2* gene and certain *HLA-C* alleles are more predisposed to rheumatoid arthritis with vascular complications than are healthy individuals or arthritis patients without vascular complications (164). Similarly, individuals possessing genes encoding the activating KIR2DS1 or KIR2DS receptors are at greater risk for psoriatic arthritis, but only if these individuals lack HLA-C alleles that can bind to their inhibitory KIR2DL receptors (109). A similar correlation has been observed in patients with scleroderma (165), and KIR2DS1 has been linked to risk for psoriasis vulgaris (166). Collectively, these studies provide hints that expression of activating KIR, in the absence of an inhibitory receptor for self MHC class I, may contribute to autoimmune disorders. This may be of particular significance if activating KIR are expressed in effector T cells, where they may synergize with the signals transduced by TcR that may otherwise be insufficient for an autoantigen alone to elicit an autoimmune response. Additionally, activating KIR enhancement of TcR signaling in CD4$^+$ T cells has previously been documented in vitro (167).

KIR, albeit perhaps detrimental in autoimmunity, may be beneficial in immune responses to tumors or viral pathogens. HIV-infected individuals homozygous for HLA-Bw4 progress more slowly to AIDS and live longer than individuals with other HLA haplotypes (168). Further studies indicated that the protective effect was more pronounced in the subset of individuals expressing an HLA-Bw4 allele with Ile at position 80 and when the individual possessed a *KIR3DS1* gene. No ligand has yet been identified for KIR3DS1, and given the small genome of HIV, it is unlikely that HIV directly encodes a protein recognized by KIR3DS1, as is the case with Ly49H recognition of the m157 MCMV glycoprotein. Nonetheless, an HIV-derived peptide or perhaps a host protein induced by HIV infection might conceivably be presented by HLA-Bw4 to NK or T cells expressing an activating KIR3DS1. Lack of antibodies against KIR3DS1 has hampered progress in testing these hypotheses. An understanding of KIR recognition may be useful clinically in the context of hematopoietic stem cell transplantation for the treatment of cancer (reviewed in 169). Velardi and colleagues (170) observed that deliberate mismatch of HLA-C between donor and recipient may be beneficial in eliciting a graft-versus-leukemia effect in the treatment of acute myeloid leukemia (AML). Presumably, donor-derived NK cells that lack an inhibitory KIR for the allogeneic HLA-C molecules expressed on the host leukemia cells are able to respond to and eliminate residual disease. Although a retrospective analysis of HLA-C disparity in AML patients who experience relapse after stem cell transplantation has not provided conclusive evidence to support this hypothesis (171–173), the KIR haplotype of the donors was not evaluated in these prior studies, and the conditioning regimens in the different patient populations were different. Unlike allogeneic T cells that can cause severe graft-versus-host disease in the recipient, allogeneic NK cells may have a better capacity to discriminate tumor cells from normal healthy tissues.

CB94/NKG2 Receptors

The *CD94* and *NKG2* family of genes are present in the genomes of human (174, 175), rat (176, 177), and mouse (178–180) and encode receptors that recognize nonconventional MHC class Ib ligands (human HLA-E and mouse Qa1^b) (Figure 2; Table 1). These genes are located within the NK complex on human chromosome 12p12.3-p13.2 and on the syntenic region of mouse chromosome 6 (Figure 3). In mouse and human, a single *CD94* gene is closely genetically linked to four NKG2 family genes in human (*NKG2A*, *-C*, *-E*, and *-F*) (174) and three genes in

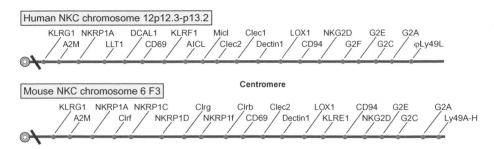

Figure 3   The human and mouse NK complex. Graphic depiction (not to scale) of the genes within the NK complex on human chromosome 12p12.3-p13.2 and mouse chromosome 6. The assignment of gene order for certain mouse genes is provisional.

mouse (*NKG2A, -C, -E*) (178, 179). Unlike the *Ly49* and *KIR* genes, the *CD94* and *NKG2* genes have limited polymorphism, and the minor allelic variants have not been shown to affect the function of these receptors (181). An ancestor of the mammalian CD94/NKG2 genes has been identified in teleostean fish (182) and in tunicates (183), suggesting that this receptor system may be involved in primordial self-nonself discrimination.

CD94 and *NKG2* encode type II transmembrane proteins of the C-type lectin-like family. CD94 can be expressed on the cell surface as a disulfide-linked homodimer or as a disulfide-linked heterodimer with NKG2A or NKG2C (179, 184, 185). NKG2A has an ITIM in its cytoplasmic domain and CD94/NKG2A heterodimers function as inhibitory receptors (37, 186–188). Conversely, CD94/NKG2C heterodimers serve as activating receptors and require association with the DAP12 adapter protein for stable expression on the cell surface and for signaling (189). The Lys residue in the transmembrane region of NKG2C associates with the Asp residue in the transmembrane segment of DAP12 and is required to generate a stable receptor complex (189). Although the extracellular domain of human NKG2E is very similar to NKG2C and has a Lys residue in its transmembrane region, we have been unable to demonstrate that human NKG2E associates with DAP12 (L.L. Lanier, unpublished observation). Human NKG2F has a cytoplasmic domain and transmembrane segment containing a charged residue but lacks an extracellular region due to a premature stop codon that disrupts the lectin-like domain (190). In mouse, CD94/NKG2C and CD94/NKG2E both appear to pair with DAP12 (179). Although CD94 homodimers can be expressed on the cell surface, they do not bind HLA-E or Qa1[b] (179, 184), and it is unlikely that they transmit signals because CD94 lacks a cytoplasmic domain.

CD94/NKG2 receptors are expressed on most NK cells and $\gamma\delta$TCR[+] T cells and on a subset of effector/memory CD8[+] $\alpha\beta$TCR[+] T cells (191, 192). Within the NK cell population in human peripheral blood, CD94/NKG2A and CD94/NKG2C receptors are expressed on overlapping subsets of NK cells, apparently in a stochastic fashion in that the frequency of double positive cells (i.e., CD94/NKG2A[+],

CD94/NKG2C$^+$) is, as expected, essentially the percentage calculated by multiplying the percentages of NK cells expressing each receptor (L.L. Lanier, unpublished observation). Expression of CD94/NKG2 receptors appears earlier in NK cell ontogeny than Ly49 in mice (193, 194) or KIR in humans (195, 196). Unlike the KIR and Ly49 receptors that are stably maintained once expressed, CD94/NKG2 receptors on NK cells and T cells are modulated by cytokines in the environment. IL-15 (197), TGF-β (198), and IL-12 (199) have been shown to induce CD94/NKG2 on human T cells in vitro. Expression of the inhibitory CD94/NKG2A receptor can also be regulated by TcR activation and reciprocally CD94/NKG2A can negatively regulate TcR-dependent signaling (200).

Human CD94/NKG2A and CD94/NKG2C bind HLA-E (201–203), and the mouse receptors bind Qa1^b (179). Unlike Ly49 and KIR, the CD94/NKG2 receptors do not demonstrate extensive polymorphism, perhaps because their ligands also demonstrate very little allelic variation. An intriguing feature of HLA-E and Qa1^b is that the most abundant peptides bound in the groove of these class Ib molecules are derived from the leader segments of other MHC class I proteins (202, 204–206), although peptides other than class I leader segments are also able to bind HLA-E and Qa1^b (207, 208). Of note, the leader peptides of HLA-E and Qa1^b do not bind to their own antigen-binding pockets; therefore, expression of HLA-E and Qa1^b on the cell surface is dependent upon availability of leader peptides provided by HLA-A, -B, -C, -G, or H-2, respectively. Therefore, CD94/NKG2 receptors are able to monitor the status of the classical and certain nonconventional MHC class I proteins (e.g., HLA-G) in a cell by using HLA-E and Qa1^b as surrogates.

Why then do the inhibitory CD94/NKG2A and activating CD94/NKG2C receptors both seemingly bind the same ligand? As with the KIR and Ly49 receptors, the inhibitory CD94/NKG2A receptor appears to bind ligand with a higher affinity than the activating CD94/NKG2C receptor (209). In addition, evidence suggests that the peptides bound to HLA-E or Qa1^b can differentially affect recognition by the inhibitory and activating receptors (209–211). A biological consequence of this is suggested by the studies of Michaelsson and colleagues (212), who have shown that peptides derived from heat shock protein 60 (hsp60) bind to HLA-E; however, these HLA-E molecules containing hsp60 peptides are not able to bind the inhibitory CD94/NKG2A receptor. Thus, HLA-E on "stressed" cells may fail to bind to the inhibitory CD94/NKG2A receptors, thereby permitting NK cells to eliminate these abnormal cells. It is tempting to speculate that certain peptides, perhaps from pathogens, may bind to HLA-E or Qa1^b and preferentially engage the activating CD94/NKG2C receptors. Although this has not yet been found, a human cytomegalovirus (HCMV) gene encodes a protein, UL40, with a leader segment that is permissive for binding HLA-E (213–216). Whereas classical MHC class I molecules are downregulated during HCMV infection, the UL40 leader peptide may substitute for MHC class I, thereby maintaining cell surface expression of HLA-E on the infected cells. UL40 may function as a virulence factor by evading NK cell recognition by this mechanism.

CD94/NKG2A receptors have also been implicated in an immune response against polyoma virus (217). Although CTL are generated in susceptible strains of mice infected with polyoma virus, these CTL express CD94/NKG2A receptors that suppress their lytic activity against virus-infected cells. CD94/NKG2A receptors are also rapidly induced on antigen-specific $CD8^+$ T cells after infection of mice with lymphocytic choriomeningitis virus (LCMV) or *Listeria monocytogenes* (218); however, the CD94/NKG2A receptor did not affect the antiviral function of LCMV-specific CTL (219). Of the other inhibitory NK receptors detected on activated $CD8^+$ T cells in human and mouse, CD94/NKG2A is the most prevalent and is induced both by TcR signaling and cytokines. It has been proposed that inhibitory NK receptors on T cells may increase the signaling threshold so that CTL will preferentially kill target cells expressing high-affinity ligands for their TcR, thereby limiting damage to uninfected cells that may express low-affinity self-antigens (116). Additionally, inhibitory NK receptors on T cells might diminish TcR signaling to prevent T cell activation–induced cell death, resulting in prolonged survival of the effector T cells and the generation of memory (220, 221).

LILR

The human *LILR* family of genes (also known as LIR, ILT, and CD85) is located on human chromosome 19q13.4 just centromeric of the *KIR* genes. Of the 13 *LILR* genes, two, *LILRB1* (ILT2/LIR1) and *LILRB2* (ILT4/LIR2), encode inhibitory receptors that bind MHC class I (222, 223); however, LILRB2 is not expressed on NK cells. LILRB1, a cell surface glycoprotein with four Ig-like domains in the extracellular region and four ITIMs in its cytoplasmic domain (Figure 2; Table 1), is variably expressed on peripheral blood NK cells (ranging from undetectable to ~75% of NK cells) and a subset of T cells, but is highly and uniformly expressed on B cells and monocytes (222, 223). In contrast to other NK receptors for MHC class I, LILRB1 binds with low affinity to a conserved region in the $\alpha3$ domain of essentially all HLA class I glycoproteins, including HLA-A, -B, -C, -E, -F, and -G (224, 225). UL18, a glycoprotein encoded by HCMV that has structural homology to MHC class I (226), binds to LILRB1 with a 1000-fold higher affinity than to HLA class I ligands (222, 224). Thus, UL18 may serve as a decoy ligand to engage the inhibitory LILRB1 receptors on leukocytes during viral infection, thus suppressing antiviral responses. Whereas LILRB1 receptors on NK cells can suppress their activation upon encountering HLA class I–bearing targets (227), in general the KIR and CD94/NKG2 receptors appear to play a more dominant role. Given that LILRB1 is highly expressed on B cells and monocytes, perhaps this receptor has a more significant role in the regulation of these leukocytes that lack KIR and CD94/NKG2 receptor systems. The mouse orthologs of the human LILR family, the mouse *PIR* genes (228, 229), encode receptors able to bind H-2, but these do not appear to be expressed on mouse NK cells (230, 231).

RECOGNITION OF MHC CLASS I–RELATED LIGANDS

NKG2D Receptor

The NKG2D receptor recognizes cell surface glycoproteins structurally related to MHC class I, but most of these ligands are not encoded by genes in the MHC complex and do not function as peptide-binding structures for the presentation of antigens to T cells (Figure 4) (reviewed in 232). The *NKG2D* gene is in the NK complex on human chromosome 12p12.3-p13.2, and the mouse gene is at a syntenic location on chromosome 6. Unlike the KIR and Ly49 family of receptors, NKG2D is encoded by a single gene that demonstrates essentially no polymorphism in mice (233) or humans (174, 181) and it is an activating receptor. The name NKG2D is a misnomer because the *NKG2D* gene has very little homology to the *NKG2A, NKG2C, NKG2E,* and *NKG2F* genes, which are highly related to each other and likely evolved by gene duplication. The original NKG2D cDNA represented a rare and unusually spliced transcript that contained a small fragment of NKG2A in the 5′ untranslated region, which was not subsequently found in the most abundant full-length transcripts (174).

NKG2D is a type II transmembrane-anchored glycoprotein expressed as a disulfide-linked homodimer on the surface of all mouse and human NK cells and most $\gamma\delta$TCR$^+$ T cells (234, 235). NKG2D does not form dimers with CD94 (236). All human CD8$^+$ T cells, including naive T cells in cord blood, constitutively express NKG2D (234), whereas in mice expression of NKG2D on mouse CD8$^+$ T cells requires activation (235). The expression of NKG2D on T cells and NK

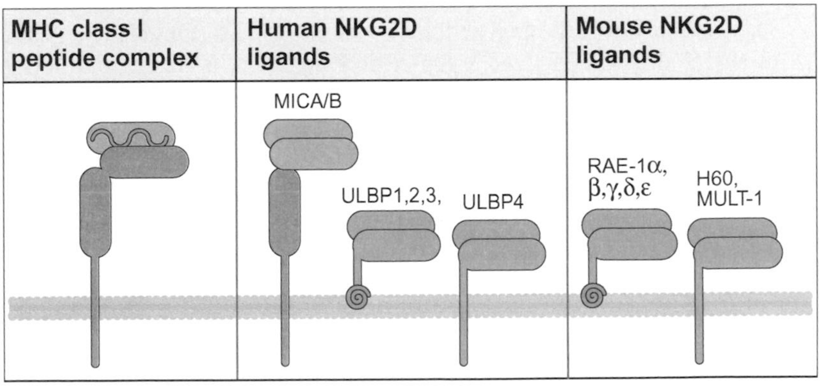

Figure 4   NKG2D ligands. Graphic depiction of the structures of the ligands for human and mouse NKG2D, compared with a conventional MHC class I protein. ULBP1, -2, -3, and -4 are the human orthologs of the mouse RAE-1/H60/MULT1 molecules. Human ULBP1, -2, -3 and mouse RAE-1 proteins are attached to the cell membrane by a phosphatidylinositol glycan anchor, whereas human MICA, MICB, and ULBP4 and mouse H60 and MULT1 have a membrane-spanning transmembrane domain.

cells can be increased by culture in IL-15 or TNF-α (237, 238), but is significantly downregulated in the presence of TGF-β (239, 240).

The adapter proteins associated with NKG2D are also different in human and mouse. In mouse, two isoforms of NKG2D that are generated by alternative splicing have been described. These NKG2D proteins differ in the presence or absence of 13 amino acids at the N terminus in the cytoplasmic domain (241). The longer protein (NKG2D-L) exclusively associates with the DAP10 adapter protein, whereas the short isoform (NKG2D-S) is promiscuous and can pair with either DAP12 or DAP10 (241, 242). By contrast, humans express only an NKG2D-L protein, which exclusively uses DAP10 for signaling (236, 243–245). This difference in mouse and human NKG2D has been localized to the transmembrane region; the human NKG2D transmembrane segment is able to associate only with DAP10 and not DAP12, whereas the mouse NKG2D transmembrane region binds both DAP10 and DAP12 (246). The 13 amino acids at the N terminus of mouse NKG2D-L apparently prevent association with DAP12 (246). Differential use of DAP10 and DAP12 by NKG2D has functional consequences in that the ITAM-containing DAP12 adapter activates the Syk and ZAP70 tyrosine kinases in NK cells (42), whereas DAP10 has a Tyr-x-x-Met (where x denotes any amino acid) in its cytoplasmic domain that upon phosphorylation binds to the p85 subunit of phosphatidylinositol-3 kinase (PI3K) (236). Mouse CD8$^+$ T cells usually express DAP10, but not DAP12, so that NKG2D signaling in mouse T cells exclusively uses the DAP10 pathway (241, 242). Expression of NKG2D on the cell surface requires coassociation with DAP10; without an adapter protein, NKG2D is retained in the cytoplasm and degraded (236, 243, 246).

Stimulation of NK cells through NKG2D triggers cell-mediated cytotoxicity and in some cases induces secretion of cytokines and chemokines. Given that the cytoplasmic domain of human DAP10 comprises only 21 amino acids and contains known motifs only for binding PI3K and Grb2, it is remarkable that NKG2D signaling initiates such potent activation. Stimulation of human peripheral blood NK cells with soluble recombinant NKG2D ligands causes activation of the PI3K and Akt signaling pathways, as expected, but also results in the phosphorylation of JAK2 (Janus kinase 2), STAT5, ERK1/2 and MEK1/2 (phospho-mitogen-activated protein kinase 1/2) (238). Furthermore, cross-linking of NKG2D on human NK cells with an anti-NKG2D mAb activates Vav1, Rho family GTPases, and PLC-γ2 (245). NKG2D signaling in human NK cells does not involve the activation of Syk or ZAP70 tyrosine kinases. Similarly, NKG2D-dependent cytolytic activity is largely intact in mice that are genetically deficient in DAP12 or both Syk and ZAP70 (51).

NKG2D binds to a family of ligands with structural homology to MHC class I (reviewed in 247). Human ligands are MICA, MICB, ULBP1, ULBP2, ULBP3, and ULBP4 (234, 248, 249), and the mouse ligands are RAE-1α, RAE-1β, RAE-1γ, RAE-1δ, RAE-1ε, H60, and MULT1 (15, 250–252). MICA and MICB are encoded by genes within the human MHC, linked to HLA-B (253), but the other mouse and human NKG2D ligands are not. The *RAE-1*, *H60*, and *MULT1* genes are linked on mouse chromosome 10. The RAE-1 proteins are highly related (>85% identity); however, the H60 and MULT1 proteins show less than 25% homology with the RAE-1 proteins or to each other. The human *ULBP* genes (also called *Raet1*) are orthologs of the mouse *RAE-1* genes and are found in a cluster of 10 related genes or pseudogenes on the opposite end of the human chromosome 6 relative to the MHC complex (254). A comparison of the ULBP and MIC proteins indicates that they share less than 20% homology with each other or with any of the mouse ligands. The human ULBP1, -2, -3, and mouse RAE-1 glycoproteins are anchored to the membrane by phosphatidylinositol-glycan, whereas human ULBP4, MICA, MICB, and mouse H60 and MULT1 are likely anchored by transmembrane-spanning segments. All ligands have $\alpha 1$ and $\alpha 2$ domains forming an MHC class I–like fold; however, none is likely to have open peptide-binding grooves, based on the crystal structures of the proteins that have been solved (255–258). MICA and MICB, unlike ULBP or the mouse NKG2D ligands, have an $\alpha 3$ domain, but unlike HLA class I proteins, they do not bind $\beta 2$-microglobulin (259). Given the low homology between the MIC and ULBP proteins in humans and the RAE-1 and H60 and MULT1 proteins in mice, it is remarkable that all bind with relative high affinity to NKG2D. Analysis of the structure of NKG2D-ULBP3, NKG2D-MICA, and NKG2D-RAE-1β complexes indicates that the receptor and ligand interfaces are remarkably similar, despite their use of completely different residues for binding (255, 256, 258).

The *MIC* genes are very polymorphic, with 54 alleles of *MICA* and 18 alleles of *MICB* (http://mhc-x.u-strasbg.fr/human.htm), and there is also evidence for limited polymorphism in the *ULBP* genes. Although not examined comprehensively, allelic variants of MICA proteins can bind with different affinities to NKG2D (260, 261). The mouse *RAE-1* genes are also polymorphic, and in analyzing different mouse strains, it is difficult to distinguish between genes and alleles in the absence of genomic sequences. Little is known about the transcriptional regulation of the genes encoding the NKG2D ligands. Spies and colleagues (262) have identified a heat shock response element in the *MIC* genes and shown induction of MIC transcripts in stressed cells. In mice, the *RAE-1* genes were initially discovered because they were induced by retinoic acid treatment of a teratocarcinoma cell line, and they are abundantly expressed in embryonic mice, but silent in adult mice (263, 264). *RAE-1* transcription is induced in mouse macrophages in response to Toll-like receptor signaling (265) and by viral infection (266). Further studies are necessary to understand why so many human and mouse genes have been devoted to producing ligands for a single invariant receptor (i.e., NKG2D) and what is driving the polymorphism of these genes.

NKG2D has been implicated in immunity against viruses and tumors. The seminal experiment defining the missing-self hypothesis was the ability of NK cells in C57BL/6 mice to reject the H-2 class I–deficient variant (RMA/S) of the MHC class I–bearing RMA lymphoma (10). RMA cells lack expression of NKG2D ligands and are resistant to NK cell–mediated cytotoxicity in vivo and in vitro. However, when RMA cells were transfected with RAE-1 or H60 they were rendered susceptible to lysis by NK cells in vitro and were rejected in vivo (15, 16, 250). With certain immunogenic tumors, expression of NKG2D ligands can augment the generation of $CD8^+$ CTL and perhaps also induce a $CD4^+$ T helper response (15, 267). The mechanism whereby RAE-1-bearing tumors induce a T helper response has not been defined, but it is probably not by direct recognition of RAE-1 on the tumors because mouse $CD4^+$ T cells do not express NKG2D even when stimulated through their TcR.

The importance of NKG2D in antiviral immunity is best exemplified by the study of immunity to mouse and human CMV. Using a soluble recombinant UL16 protein encoded by HCMV, Cosman and colleagues (248, 249) cloned the ULBP-1 cDNA and by sequence homology identified the ULBP2, -3, and -4 molecules. UL16 binds ULBP1, ULBP2, and MICB, but not MICA, ULBP3, or ULBP4. UL16 has a lower affinity than NKG2D, and rather than compete for ligand binding UL16 intersects the NKG2D ligands intracellularly and prevents their expression on the surface of the infected cell, thereby diminishing susceptibility of the infected cells to NKG2D-dependent NK cell effector functions (268–271). UL16 associates with ULBP1, -2, or MICB in the endoplasmic reticulum or cis-Golgi compartments and prevents maturation and transport of the proteins to the cell surface (268, 270). Expression of MICA (which is resistant to downregulation by UL16) on target cells has been shown to costimulate proliferation and cytokine production by HCMV-specific CTL clones, indicating that NKG2D on $CD8^+$ T cells may play a role in adaptive immunity (272). Similarly, the MCMV genome encodes viral proteins that prevent expression of the mouse NKG2D ligands on the surface of infected cells (266, 273, 274). The MCMV m152 viral protein, which previously has been shown to block expression of H-2 class I glycoproteins on the surface of infected cells (275), also causes intracellular retention of the RAE-1 proteins, but does not affect H60 or MULT1 expression (266). Deletion of the *m152* gene causes moderate attenuation of viral replication in BALB/c mice, and this can be restored by administration of a blocking anti-NKG2D mAb (266). Another MCMV viral protein, m155, selectively targets H60 for intracellular degradation but does not prevent RAE-1 or MULT1 expression (274). Growth of an *m155*-deficient MCMV is severely attenuated in scid mice (276); however, viral replication of the *m155*-deficient MCMV was equivalent to wild-type virus when BALB/c mice were treated with a neutralizing anti-NKG2D mAb or if NK cells were depleted by antiasialo-GM1 sera (274). Thus, both human and mouse CMV prevent NKG2D-dependent immunity, indicating the importance of this immune receptor.

Like CMV, tumors have found means to escape NKG2D-mediated immune surveillance. While both mouse and human tumors frequently express NKG2D ligands (250, 277, 278), some tumors secrete or release these ligands, which then serve as decoys to subvert NK cell and T cell immune responses (279–281). Soluble MIC proteins have been detected in the sera of cancer patients, and in these individuals the levels of NKG2D on their T cells are significantly decreased (279, 280). TGF-β1, which is frequently produced by tumors, also downregulates expression of NKG2D on lymphocytes (239). Perhaps treatment with IL-15, which is able to elevate NKG2D on T cells and NK cells, may serve as a useful therapy to overcome these tumor-evasion mechanisms.

Although NKG2D-mediated responses are beneficial in immune responses against tumors and pathogens, evidence is emerging that this system may also be deleterious by contributing to autoimmunity. In humans, MICA has been detected on synoviocytes in the joints of patients with rheumatoid arthritis, accompanied by the presence of an unusual subset of CD4$^+$ T cells that lack CD28 but express NKG2D (282). NKG2D has also been implicated in the development of autoimmune diabetes in NOD mice (283). RAE-1 was detected on the surface of islet cells in the pancreas of NOD mice, and treating NOD mice with a neutralizing, nondepleting anti-NKG2D mAb completely prevented disease. Anti-NKG2D mAb treatment was shown to inhibit the expansion of NKG2D-bearing autoreactive CD8$^+$ T cells in NOD mice (283). However, NK cells also participate in the onset of diabetes in NOD mice, and disease can be eliminated by depleting NK cells, suggesting that an NK cell–mediated NKG2D-dependent process may also be involved (284). Collectively, these studies suggest NKG2D as an attractive target for therapeutic intervention in autoimmune diseases.

RECOGNITION OF HOST-ENCODED NON-MHC LIGANDS

NK cells have evolved several receptor systems to sense MHC class I or MHC class I–like molecules that regulate their responses. However, they possess additional mechanisms that regulate their behavior upon encountering potential targets that lack expression of MHC or MHC-related proteins. For example, the mouse RMA/S T cell lymphoma, mouse B16 melanoma cells, and the human 721.221 B lymphoblastoid cell line are sensitive to NK cell–mediated cytotoxicity, yet none of these transformed cell lines express MHC class I or ligands for NKG2D. In addition, the observation that mice deficient in Syk and ZAP70 retain the ability to kill RMA/S implies the existence of non-ITAM-based activation pathways in NK cells (50, 51). Unlike the ITAM-dependent NK receptors, which upon engagement can directly trigger cytotoxicity and cytokine production, it is unclear whether some of the other NK receptors may serve as "costimulatory" receptors, augmenting the signaling from other unidentified receptors, rather than independently initiating a response. Alternatively, it can be argued that a certain threshold of signaling is required to overcome the action of the inhibitory NK receptors and that this can be achieved by the simultaneous engagement of several costimulatory receptors that individually are unable to initiate effector functions. This latter mechanism represents a fail-safe system, whereby a potential target cell would be required not only to display diminished levels of ligands for inhibitory NK receptors, but also to overexpress the ligands for multiple costimulatory NK receptors. Such a system, with checks and balances, would minimize the chance of accidental attack against normal, healthy cells. Here, I present a summary of the NK receptors for

TABLE 2   Human NK receptors for host-encoded non-MHC ligands

Gene	Species	Other names	CD	Function	Signaling	Ligand
	Mouse	NKR-P1A		Activation?	FcεRIγ	?
	Mouse	NKR-P1C		Activation	FcεRIγ	?
	Mouse	NKR-P1D		Inhibition	ITIM	Clr-b
	Mouse	NKR-P1F		Activation	FcεRIγ	Clr-g
KLRB1	Human	NKR-P1A	CD161	?	?	?
KLRK1	Mouse	NKG2D[a]		Activation	DAP10, DAP12	RAE-1 $\alpha,\beta,\gamma,\delta,\varepsilon$; H60; MULT1
KLRK1	Human	NKG2D		Activation	DAP10	MICA/B; ULBP1,2,3,4
CD244	Mouse	2B4	CD244	Inhibition	?	CD48
CD244	Human	2B4	CD244	Activation	SAP	CD48
CD226	Human	DNAM-1	CD226	Activation	?	CD112, CD155
CD96	Human		CD96	Activation	?	CD155
PILRb	Mouse	PILR1β		Activation	DAP12	PILR-L

[a]A splice variant of mouse NKG2D, NKG2D-S associates with DAP12 or DAP10 adapter protein, whereas the mouse NKG2D-L splice variant and all human NKG2D proteins associate only with DAP10.

which host-encoded non-MHC ligands have been defined that activate or inhibit NK cell responses (Table 2).

NKR-P1 Receptors

NK1.1 is the prototype antigen defining mouse NK cells in C57BL/6 mice (285). In mouse, NK1.1 is a polymorphic antigen encoded by a member of the *NKR-P1* gene family, which is located in the NK complex on mouse chromosome 6 (286–288). In C57BL/6 mice, four genes, *NKR-P1A*, *NKR-P1C*, *NKR-P1D*, and *NKR-P1F*, encode type II membrane glycoproteins of the C-type lectin-like family. Orthologs of the mouse *NKR-P1* genes were first discovered in the rat (289). In contrast to rodents that have several *NKR-P1* genes, only a single, nonpolymorphic *NKR-P1* gene exists in the human genome (290). The PK136 mAb (291) commonly used to detect NK cells and NK1.1$^+$ T cells reacts with the *NKR-P1C* gene product in C57BL/6 mice, but binds to other polymorphic NKR-P1 family members in other mouse strains (292). The cytoplasmic domain of mouse NKR-P1D contains an ITIM, indicating inhibitory function, whereas the NKR-P1A, -C, and -F lack ITIM and have a charged residue in the transmembrane domains and are presumably activating receptors. Arase and colleagues (293, 294) have demonstrated that mouse NKR-P1C associates with the ITAM-containing FcεRIγ adapter, and cross-linking with anti-NK1.1 mAb induces NK cell–mediated cytotoxicity and cytokine production. Presumably, NKR-P1A and NKR-P1F also pair with FcεRIγ and behave in a similar fashion, although this has not been demonstrated owing to lack of antibodies against these receptors. The cytoplasmic domain of human NKR-P1A does not contain ITIM sequences, and the transmembrane region lacks charged amino acids, so how human NKR-P1A signals (if indeed it does) is not known (290).

NKR-P1C is expressed by all NK cells in C57BL/6 mice and is present on a heterogeneous subset of T cells (including $CD4^-8^-$, $CD4^+$, and $CD8^+$ T cells) commonly referred to as NKT cells, some of which recognize CD1d antigens (295; reviewed in 296). Expression of human NKR-P1A (also called CD161) is remarkably different; it is present on only a subset of peripheral blood NK cells and is much more abundantly expressed on T cells than is mouse NK1.1. In adult humans, NKR-P1A is on about 25% of peripheral T cells, including $CD4^+$ and $CD8^+$ T cells (mostly with an effector/memory phenotype) and $\gamma\delta TCR^+$ T cells (290). It is also found on a subset of $CD3^+$ cells in the fetal thymus and liver (290).

The function of mouse NKR-P1C is still unknown, but protein ligands for two other family members, NKR-P1D and NKR-P1F, have been identified (18, 19). The ligands for these receptors are themselves type II membrane glycoproteins of the C-type lectin family encoded by genes within the mouse NK complex. The inhibitory NKR-P1D receptor, which is expressed on most NK cells in C57BL/6 mice (19), recognizes Clr-b (297), a cell surface glycoprotein present on essentially all hematopoietic cells, including T cells, B cells, NK cells, myeloid cells, and thymocytes (18). RMA/S cells transfected with Clr-b yielded cells that were more resistant than parental RMA/S cells to NK cell–mediated lysis in vitro, and this protection was reversed in the presence of anti-NKR-P1D mAb (19). It is interesting to note that another name for Clr-b is osteoclast inhibitory lectin (298, 299), particularly in light of studies showing a defect in osteoclast function in mice lacking FcεRIγ (300, 301). Whether osteoclasts express NKR-P1D has not been evaluated.

NKR-P1F binds to Clr-g, another C-type lectin encoded by a gene in the mouse NK complex (297). Whereas Clr-b is transcribed in a broad range of cells and tissues [consistent with results using the anti-Clr-b mAb (18)], Clr-g appears to be transcribed preferentially in activated NK cells, which also express its receptor, NKR-P1F (297).

Like the contraction of the human *NKR-P1* gene family, only a single gene exists with homology to the mouse *Clr* genes. Based on chromosomal location and structure, the human *LLT1* gene likely represents the human ortholog of mouse *Clr* (302). Human NK cells transcribe *LLT1*, and an anti-LLT1 mAb has been reported to induce IFN-γ in NK cells (303). Anti-NKR-P1A mAbs have been shown either to induce or inhibit NK cell–mediated redirected cytotoxicity against Fc receptor–bearing targets or to have no effect (175). In addition, anti-NKR-P1A mAb have been reported to costimulate CD1d-specific human T cell proliferation (304), to suppress *trans*-endothelial cell migration of $CD4^+$ T cells (305), and to induce proliferation of immature thymocytes (306). How these signaling events occur and why variable results were obtained in different NK or T cell population remain a mystery, given the existence of only a single, nonpolymorphic human *NKR-P1A* gene with no known signaling motifs. This topic requires future attention.

2B4 Receptor

2B4 (also called CD244) and its ligand CD48 (307, 308) are members of the CD2 family of Ig-related proteins encoded by a cluster of related genes on human chromosome 1q22 and mouse chromosome 1. Human and mouse 2B4 were discovered by screening for mAbs that would activate human and mouse NK cells, respectively (309, 310), and were recognized as being related when the genes encoding these receptors were cloned (311–315). 2B4 is present on all human and mouse NK cells, most $\gamma\delta$TCR$^+$ T cells, and CD8$^+$ T cells (typically the subset with an effector/memory phenotype) (309, 310, 316, 317), and in humans 2B4 is also present on monocytes and basophils (315).

2B4 has two Ig-like domains in the extracellular region and its cytoplasmic tail contains four Thr-x-Tyr-x-x-Leu/Ile motifs. This motif defines a family of receptors using a common signaling pathway; the prototype member is SLAM (CD150) (reviewed in 318) and includes the NTB-A (319) and CRACC (320) receptors also expressed by NK cells and able to activate their lytic activity. Upon phosphorylation of the tyrosine in the Thr-x-Tyr-x-x-Leu/Ile motif, probably by the Src family kinase Fyn, 2B4 binds to the SHP-1 and SHP-2 tyrosine phosphatases as well as to the SAP (also called SH2D1A) intracellular adapter protein. However, there are conflicting reports regarding association between 2B4 and SHP-1 or SHP-2, depending on whether the experiments were conducted in NK cells or by transfection into other host cells (313, 321–324). 2B4 signaling involves LAT and Vav1 activation (325–327). The function of 2B4 may be different in human and mouse NK cells. F(ab')$_2$ fragments of anti-mouse 2B4 can augment the NK cell–mediated cytolysis of certain tumors (309), and NK cells from *2B4*-deficient mice demonstrate enhanced responses against target cells expressing CD48 (328). Therefore, in mice 2B4 apparently functions as an inhibitory NK cell receptor. By contrast, in mature human NK cells 2B4 behaves as an activating receptor. Whether 2B4 is capable of independently triggering effector cell functions or rather serves as a costimulatory receptor is unresolved (310, 314, 315, 329).

The strongest evidence supporting an activating role in human NK cells comes from the demonstration that transfection of CD48 into certain NK-resistant target cells renders them susceptible to NK cell–mediated cytotoxicity and triggers the production of IFN-γ by the human NK cells and this can be blocked by anti-CD48 mAb and anti-human 2B4 mAb (330, 331; T. Sun & L.L. Lanier, unpublished observations). However, even in humans the story is more complicated. In patients with a loss-of-function mutation in the X-linked *SAP* gene, NK cells are no longer able to be activated through the 2B4 receptor (321, 322, 331, 332); however, in one case 2B4 in a *SAP*-deficient individual appeared to mediate inhibitory function (321). Furthermore, immature human NK cells generated in vitro from CD34$^+$ progenitors express 2B4 receptors that mediate inhibitory function, presumably because these immature NK cells lack SAP (333). The molecular basis for these discordant findings in mice and humans has not been established. Moreover, another adapter protein with structural homology to SAP, called EAT2 (reviewed in 318), has been identified, and it has not been established whether SAP and EAT2 are differentially expressed in human and mouse NK cells. 2B4 may be a multifunctional receptor in both humans and mice, causing different functional outcomes depending on the stage of NK cell differentiation and activation.

DNAM-1 Receptor

DNAM-1 receptor (also called CD226) is a member of the Ig superfamily, encoded by a gene on human chromosome 18q22.3, that is expressed by human NK cells, T cells, a subset of B cells, monocytes, and platelets (334–336). CD112 (also known as polio virus receptor, PVR) and CD155 (also called nectin-2) have been identified as ligands for DNAM-1 (337, 338). Interactions between DNAM-1 on NK cells and CD112 and CD155 on tumor cells augments NK cell–mediated cytotoxicity and cytokine production, and these ligands are frequently overexpressed on human tumor cells (337–339; A. Shibuya, personal communication). In NK cells, DNAM-1 can be detected in a complex containing LFA-1 (CD11a/CD18), and ligation of LFA-1 causes Fyn-dependent phosphorylation of tyrosine residues in the cytoplasmic domain of DNAM-1 that are necessary for DNAM-1-dependent NK cell functions (340, 341). Migration of monocytes through the intercellular endothelial cell junctions involves DNAM-1 on monocytes and CD155 on vascular endothelial cells (342), suggesting the possibility of a similar role in NK cell trafficking. NK cells express CD96 (also called Tactile), which only shows ~20% homology with DNAM-1 and has been shown to also recognize CD155 and promote NK cell adhesion and activation (343). Although CD112 and CD155 are broadly distributed on many tissues throughout the body, these cells may be normally spared from NK cell–mediated attack if these cells express HLA class I ligands for the inhibitory KIR or CD94/NKG2A receptors. These studies suggest that DNAM-1 and CD96 may regulate both NK cell migration and cellular activation.

PILR Receptor

The activating PILRβ receptor was cloned from a mouse NK cell cDNA library using a screening strategy designed to find receptors able to associate with the DAP12 signaling adapter (344). PILRβ is a type I glycoprotein that has a Lys residue in its transmembrane region that permits association with DAP12. Prior studies using a yeast two-hybrid screening technique to isolate proteins interacting with SHP-1 led to the discovery of human PILRα, an inhibitory receptor with an ITIM in its cytoplasmic domain (345). Of note, the cytoplasmic domain of mouse and human PILRα also has a Thr-x-Tyr-x-x-Leu/Ile motif, similar to that found in 2B4; however, it has not been determined whether this can associate with SHP-2 or SAP (or EAT2). Database searches for human and mouse receptors also revealed the existence of the pair of genes encoding the inhibitory PILRα (also called FDF03) and activating PILRβ (also called FDFACT) receptors in both humans (on chromosome 7q22.7) and mice (chromosome 5) (346). A ligand, designated PILR-L, that binds both mouse PILRα and PILRβ has been identified; it is a small transmembrane-anchored cell surface protein with homology to the CD99 gene family (344). In mice, the DAP12-associated mouse PILRβ receptor is present on NK cells, as well as on dendritic cells. Activated mouse NK cells are able to kill PILR-L-bearing target cells, and dendritic cells exposed to cells with PILR-L secrete TNF-α and nitric oxide (344). Human PILRα and PILRβ are predominantly expressed in the myeloid lineage, including monocytes, dendritic cells, macrophages, and granulocytes; however, unlike in mice, PILRβ has not been detected on human NK cells (346). PILRβ is the most recently described of the NK receptors with defined ligands. The physiological role of this molecule in NK cell–dependent (and dendritic cell–mediated) immune responses is still far from being understood.

CONCLUSIONS

Our understanding of NK cell recognition and signaling, and their role in immune responses has advanced considerably since NK cells were referred to as "null cells" because they presumably lacked any cell surface antigens and were deemed nonspecific. Despite extensive progress in elucidating the role of NK cells in innate immunity, many aspects of NK cell biology are unexplained and unexplored. Given the breadth of the NK cell field, I have limited this review to focus on the NK recognition structures for which physiological cellular ligands have been identified. Indeed, many of the most intriguing and specific NK receptors are still poorly understood with respect to ligand specificity and signaling properties. For example, the natural cytotoxicity receptors (reviewed in 347), encompassing NKp30 (348) [also called 1C7 (349)], NKp44 (350, 351), and NKp46 (352), represent an important family of orphan receptors that will undoubtedly be implicated in the antitumor and antiviral functions of NK cells once their physiological ligands are uncovered. Moreover, future studies defining the molecules used by NK cells to communicate with dendritic cells, macrophages, and T cells during immune responses against pathogens and tumors and in autoimmunity promise to reveal the importance of NK cells in the immune system.

APPENDIX

Abbreviations used: AML, acute myeloid leukemia; CTL, cytotoxic T lymphocytes; ERK1/2, extracellar signal-regulated kinases 1/2; HCMV, human cytomegalovirus; hsp60, heat shock protein 60; IFN-γ, interferon-γ; ITAM, immunoreceptor tyrosine-based activation motif; ITIM, immunoreceptor tyrosine-based inhibitory motif; JAK2, Janus kinase 2; KIR, human killer cell immunoglobulin-like receptors; MCMV, mouse cytomegalovirus; MEK1/2, phospho-mitogen-activated protein kinase 1/2; MHC, major histocompatibility complex; NK, natural killer; PI-3, phosphatidylinositol-3; PVR, polio virus receptor; SHIP, SH2-containing inositol polyphosphate 5-phosphatase; SHP, SH2-containing protein-tyrosine phosphatase.

ACKNOWLEDGMENTS

L.L.L. is an American Cancer Society Research Professor and is funded by National Institutes of Health grants CA89294, CA89189, CA095137, and AI52127. Thanks to David Rosen, Melissa Lodoen, Koetsu Ogasawara, Jessica Hamerman, Will Carr, Stuart Tangye, Hilary Warren, Hisashi Arase, Bill Seaman, and Akira Shibuya for helpful discussions.

**The *Annual Review of Immunology* is online at
http://immunol.annualreviews.org**

LITERATURE CITED

1. Spits H, Blom B, Jaleco AC, Weijer K, Verschuren MC, et al. 1998. Early stages in the development of human T, natural killer and thymic dendritic cells. *Immunol. Rev.* 165:75–86

2. Colucci F, Caligiuri MA, Di Santo JP. 2003. What does it take to make a natural killer? *Nat. Rev. Immunol.* 3:413–25

3. Davis DM, Chiu I, Fassett M, Cohen GB, Mandelboim O, Strominger JL. 1999. The human natural killer cell immune synapse. *Proc. Natl. Acad. Sci. USA* 96:15062–67

4. Lou Z, Jevremovic D, Billadeau DD, Leibson PJ. 2000. A balance between positive and negative signals in cytotoxic lymphocytes regulates the polarization of lipid rafts during the development of cell-mediated killing. *J. Exp. Med.* 19:347–54

5. Vyas YM, Mehta KM, Morgan M, Maniar H, Butros L, et al. 2001. Spatial organization of signal transduction molecules in the NK cell immune synapses during MHC class I-regulated noncytolytic and cytolytic interactions. *J. Immunol.* 167:4358–67

6. Vyas YM, Maniar H, Dupont B. 2002. Cutting edge: Differential segregation of the SRC homology 2-containing protein tyrosine phosphatase-1 within the early NK cell immune synapse distinguishes noncytolytic from cytolytic interactions. *J. Immunol.* 168:3150–54

7. Orange JS, Harris KE, Andzelm MM, Valter MM, Geha RS, Strominger JL. 2003. The mature activating natural killer cell immunologic synapse is formed in distinct stages. *Proc. Natl. Acad. Sci. USA* 100:14151–56

8. Stetson DB, Mohrs M, Reinhardt RL, Baron JL, Wang ZE, et al. 2003. Constitutive cytokine mRNAs mark natural killer (NK) and NK T cells poised for rapid effector function. *J. Exp. Med.* 198:1069–76

9. Vivier E, Anfossi N. 2004. Inhibitory NK-cell receptors on T cells: witness of the past, actors of the future. *Nat. Rev. Immunol.* 4:190–98

10. Karre K, Ljunggren HG, Piontek G, Kiessling R. 1986. Selective rejection of H-2-deficient lymphoma variants suggests alternative immune defense strategy. *Nature* 319:675–78

11. Hoglund P, Ohlen C, Carbone E, Franksson L, Ljunggren H-G, et al.

1991. Recognition of β_2-microglobulin-negative (β_2m-) T-cell blasts by natural killer cells from normal but not from β_2m-mice: nonresponsiveness controlled by β_2m-bone marrow in chimeric mice. *Proc. Natl. Acad. Sci. USA* 88:10332–36

12. Bix M, Liao N-S, Zijlstra M, Loring J, Jaenisch R, Raulet D. 1991. Rejection of class I MHC-deficient haemopoietic cells by irradiated MHC-matched mice. *Nature* 349:329–31

13. Ljunggren H-G, Karre K. 1990. In search of the 'missing self': MHC molecules and NK cell recognition. *Immunol. Today* 11:237–44

14. Lanier LL, Corliss B, Phillips JH. 1997. Arousal and inhibition of human NK cells. *Immunol. Rev.* 155:145–54

15. Diefenbach A, Jensen ER, Jamieson AM, Raulet DH. 2001. Rae1 and H60 ligands of the NKG2D receptor stimulate tumour immunity. *Nature* 413:165–71

16. Cerwenka A, Baron JL, Lanier LL. 2001. Ectopic expression of retinoic acid early inducible-1 gene (RAE-1) permits natural killer cell-mediated rejection of a MHC class I-bearing tumor in vivo. *Proc. Natl. Acad. Sci. USA* 98:11521–26

17. Oldenborg PA, Zheleznyak A, Fang YF, Lagenaur CF, Gresham HD, Lindberg FP. 2000. Role of CD47 as a marker of self on red blood cells. *Science* 288:2051–54

18. Carlyle JR, Jamieson AM, Gasser S, Clingan CS, Arase H, Raulet DH. 2004. Missing self-recognition of Ocil/Clr-b by inhibitory NKR-P1 natural killer cell receptors. *Proc. Natl. Acad. Sci. USA* 101:3527–32

19. Iizuka K, Naidenko OV, Plougastel BF, Fremont DH, Yokoyama WM. 2003. Genetically linked C-type lectin-related ligands for the NKRP1 family of natural killer cell receptors. *Nat. Immunol.* 4:801–7

20. Meyaard L, Adema GJ, Chang C, Woollatt E, Sutherland GR, et al. 1997. LAIR-1, a novel inhibitory receptor expressed on human mononuclear leukocytes. *Immunity* 7:283–90

21. Poggi A, Tomasello E, Revello V, Nanni L, Costa P, Moretta L. 1997. p40 molecule regulates NK cell activation mediated by NK receptors for HLA class I antigens and TCR-mediated triggering of T lymphocytes. *Int. Immunol.* 9:1271–79

22. Butcher S, Arney KL, Cook GP. 1998. MAFA-L, an ITIM-containing receptor encoded by the human NK cell gene complex and expressed by basophils and NK cells. *Eur. J. Immunol.* 28:3755–62

23. Hanke T, Corral L, Vance RE, Raulet DH. 1998. 2F1 antigen, the mouse homolog of the rat "mast cell function-associated antigen", is a lectin-like type II transmembrane receptor expressed by natural killer cells. *Eur. J. Immunol.* 28:4409–17

24. Rojo S, Burshtyn DN, Long EO, Wagtmann N. 1997. Type I transmembrane receptor with inhibitory function in mouse mast cells and NK cells. *J. Immunol.* 158:9–12

25. Wang LL, Mehta IK, LeBlanc PA, Yokoyama WM. 1997. Mouse natural killer cells express gp49B1, a structural homologue of human killer inhibitory receptors. *J. Immunol.* 158:13–17

26. Castells MC, Klickstein LB, Hassani K, Cumplido JA, Lacouture ME, et al. 2001. gp49B1-α(v)β3 interaction inhibits antigen-induced mast cell activation. *Nat. Immunol.* 2:436–42

27. Gu X, Laouar A, Wan J, Daheshia M, Lieberman J, et al. 2003. The gp49B1 inhibitory receptor regulates the IFN-γ responses of T cells and NK cells. *J. Immunol.* 170:4095–101

28. Moller MJ, Kammerer R, Grunert F, von Kliest S. 1996. Biliary glycoprotein (BGP) expression on T cells and on a natural killer cell subpopulation. *Int. J. Cancer* 65:740–45

29. Markel G, Lieberman N, Katz G, Arnon TI, Lotem M, et al. 2002. CD66a interactions between human melanoma and NK cells: a novel class I MHC-independent

inhibitory mechanism of cytotoxicity. *J. Immunol.* 168:2803–10

30. Nicoll G, Ni J, Liu D, Klenerman P, Munday J, et al. 1999. Identification and characterization of a novel siglec, siglec-7, expressed by human natural killer cells and monocytes. *J. Biol. Chem.* 274:34089–95

31. Nicoll G, Avril T, Lock K, Furukawa K, Bovin N, Crocker PR. 2003. Ganglioside GD3 expression on target cells can modulate NK cell cytotoxicity via siglec-7-dependent and -independent mechanisms. *Eur. J. Immunol.* 33:1642–48

32. Muta T, Kurosaki T, Misulovin Z, Sanchez M, Nussenzweig MC, Ravetch RV. 1994. A 13-amino acid motif in the cytoplasmic domain of FcγRIIB modulates B-cell receptor signalling. *Nature* 368:70–73

33. Ravetch JV, Lanier LL. 2000. Immune inhibitory receptors. *Science* 290:84–89

34. Valiante NM, Phillips JH, Lanier LL, Parham P. 1996. Killer cell inhibitory receptor recognition of human leukocyte antigen (HLA) class I blocks formation of a pp36/PLC-γ signaling complex in human natural killer (NK) cells. *J. Exp. Med.* 184:2243–50

35. Binstadt BA, Brumbaugh KM, Dick CJ, Scharenberg AM, Williams BL, et al. 1996. Sequential involvement of Lck and SHP-1 with MHC-recognizing receptors on NK cells inhibits FcR-initiated tyrosine kinase activation. *Immunity* 5:629–38

36. Binstadt BA, Billadeau DD, Jevremovic D, Williams BL, Fang N, et al. 1998. SLP-76 is a direct substrate of SHP-1 recruited to killer cell inhibitory receptors. *J. Biol. Chem.* 273:27518–23

37. Palmieri G, Tullio V, Zingoni A, Piccoli M, Frati L, et al. 1999. CD94/NKG2-A inhibitory complex blocks CD16-triggered syk and extracellular regulated kinase activation, leading to cytotoxic function of human NK cells. *J. Immunol.* 162:7181–88

38. Stebbins CC, Watzl C, Billadeau DD, Leibson PJ, Burshtyn DN, Long EO. 2003. Vav1 dephosphorylation by the tyrosine phosphatase SHP-1 as a mechanism for inhibition of cellular cytotoxicity. *Mol. Cell Biol.* 23:6291–99

39. Reth M. 1989. Antigen receptor tail clue. *Nature* 338:383–84

40. Hibbs ML, Selvaraj P, Carpen O, Springer TA, Kuster H, et al. 1989. Mechanisms for regulating expression of membrane isoforms of FcγRIII (CD16). *Science* 246:1608–11

41. Anderson P, Caligiuri M, Ritz J, Schlossman SF. 1989. CD3-negative natural killer cells express ζ TCR as part of a novel molecular complex. *Nature* 341:159–62

42. Lanier LL, Corliss BC, Wu J, Leong C, Phillips JH. 1998. Immunoreceptor DAP12 bearing a tyrosine-based activation motif is involved in activating NK cells. *Nature* 391:703–7

43. Olcese L, Cambiaggi A, Semenzato G, Bottino C, Moretta A, Vivier E. 1997. Human killer cell activatory receptors for MHC class I molecules are included in a multimeric complex expressed by Natural Killer cells. *J. Immunol.* 158:5083–86

44. Perussia B, Starr S, Abraham S, Fanning V, Trinchieri G. 1983. Human natural killer cells analyzed by B73.1, a monoclonal antibody blocking Fc receptor functions. I. Characterization of the lymphocyte subset reactive with B73.1. *J. Immunol.* 130:2133–41

45. Lanier LL, Le AM, Phillips JH, Warner NL, Babcock GF. 1983. Subpopulations of human natural killer cells defined by expression of the Leu-7 (HNK-1) and Leu-11 (NK-15) antigens. *J. Immunol.* 131:1789–96

46. Lanier LL. 1998. NK cell receptors. *Annu. Rev. Immunol.* 16:359–93

47. Ravetch JV, Bolland S. 2001. IgG Fc receptors. *Annu. Rev. Immunol.* 19:275–90

48. Lanier LL, Yu G, Phillips JH. 1989. Co-association of CD3ζ with a receptor (CD16) for IgG Fc on human natural killer cells. *Nature* 342:803–5

49. Kurosaki T, Gander I, Ravetch JV. 1991.

A subunit common to an IgG Fc receptor and the T-cell receptor mediates assembly through different interactions. *Proc. Natl. Acad. Sci. USA* 88:3837–41

50. Colucci F, Schweighoffer E, Tomasello E, Turner M, Ortaldo JR, et al. 2002. Natural cytotoxicity uncoupled from the Syk and ZAP-70 intracellular kinases. *Nat. Immunol.* 3:288–94

51. Zompi S, Hamerman JA, Ogasawara K, Schweighoffer E, Tybulewicz VL, et al. 2003. NKG2D triggers cytotoxicity in mouse NK cells lacking DAP12 or Syk family kinases. *Nat. Immunol.* 4:565–72

52. Karlhofer FM, Ribuado RK, Yokoyama WM. 1992. MHC class I alloantigen specificity of Ly-49+ IL-2-activated natural killer cells. *Nature* 358:66–70

53. Mehta IK, Wang J, Roland J, Margulies DH, Yokoyama WM. 2001. Ly49A allelic variation and MHC class I specificity. *Immunogenetics* 53:572–83

54. Wilhelm BT, Gagnier L, Mager DL. 2002. Sequence analysis of the ly49 cluster in C57BL/6 mice: a rapidly evolving multigene family in the immune system. *Genomics* 80:646–61

55. Makrigiannis AP, Pau AT, Saleh A, Winkler-Pickett R, Ortaldo JR, Anderson SK. 2001. Class I MHC-binding characteristics of the 129/J Ly49 repertoire. *J. Immunol.* 166:5034–43

56. Yokoyama WM, Plougastel BF. 2003. Immune functions encoded by the natural killer gene complex. *Nat. Rev. Immunol.* 3:304–16

57. Smith KM, Wu J, Bakker ABH, Phillips JH, Lanier LL. 1998. Cutting Edge: Ly49D and Ly49H associate with mouse DAP12 and form activating receptors. *J. Immunol.* 161:7–10

58. Bakker ABH, Hoek RM, Cerwenka A, Blom B, Lucian L, et al. 2000. DAP12-deficient mice fail to develop autoimmunity due to impaired antigen priming. *Immunity* 13:345–53

59. Kubota A, Kubota S, Lohwasser S, Mager DL, Takei F. 1999. Diversity of NK cell receptor repertoire in adult and neonatal mice. *J. Immunol.* 163:212–16

60. Held W, Roland J, Raulet DH. 1995. Allelic exclusion of Ly49-family genes encoding class I MHC-specific receptors on NK cells. *Nature* 376:355–58

61. Held W, Raulet DH. 1997. Expression of the Ly49A gene in murine natural killer cell clones is predominantly but not exclusively mono-allelic. *Eur. J. Immunol.* 27:2876–84

62. Saleh A, Davies GE, Pascal V, Wright PW, Hodge DL, et al. 2004. Identification of probabilistic transcriptional switches in the Ly49 gene cluster: a novel eukaryotic mechanism for selective gene activation. *Immunity* 21:1–20

63. Raulet DH, Vance RE, McMahon CW. 2001. Regulation of the natural killer cell receptor repertoire. *Annu. Rev. Immunol.* 19:291–330

64. Veinotte LL, Wilhelm BT, Mager DL, Takei F. 2003. Acquisition of MHC-specific receptors on murine natural killer cells. *Crit. Rev. Immunol.* 23:251–66

65. Mehta IK, Smith HR, Wang J, Margulies DH, Yokoyama WM. 2001. A "chimeric" C57L-derived Ly49 inhibitory receptor resembling the Ly49d activation receptor. *Cell. Immunol.* 209:29–41

66. Tormo J, Natarajan K, Margulies DH, Mariuzza RA. 1999. Crystal structure of a lectin-like natural killer cell receptor bound to its MHC class I ligand. *Nature* 402:623–31

67. Dam J, Guan R, Natarajan K, Dimasi N, Chlewicki LK, et al. 2003. Variable MHC class I engagement by Ly49 natural killer cell receptors demonstrated by the crystal structure of Ly49C bound to H-2K(b). *Nat. Immunol.* 4:1213–22

68. Natarajan K, Dimasi N, Wang J, Mariuzza RA, Margulies DH. 2002. Structure and function of natural killer cell receptors: multiple molecular solutions to self, nonself discrimination. *Annu. Rev. Immunol.* 20:853–85

69. Wang J, Whitman MC, Natarajan K,

Tormo J, Mariuzza RA, Margulies DH. 2002. Binding of the natural killer cell inhibitory receptor Ly49A to its major histocompatibility complex class I ligand. Crucial contacts include both H-2Dd and β 2-microglobulin. *J. Biol. Chem.* 277: 1433–42

70. Orihuela M, Margulies DH, Yokoyama WM. 1996. The NK cell receptor Ly-49A recognizes a peptide-induced conformational determinant on its MHC class I ligand. *Proc. Natl. Acad. Sci. USA* 93: 11792–97

71. Correa I, Raulet DH. 1995. Binding of diverse peptides to MHC class I molecules inhibits target cell lysis by activated natural killer cells. *Immunity* 2:61–71

72. Hanke T, Takizawa H, McMahon CW, Busch DH, Pamer EG, et al. 1999. Direct assessment of MHC class I binding by seven Ly49 inhibitory NK cell receptors. *Immunity* 11:67–77

73. Michaelsson J, Achour A, Salcedo M, Kase-Sjostrom A, Sundback J, et al. 2000. Visualization of inhibitory Ly49 receptor specificity with soluble major histocompatibility complex class I tetramers. *Eur. J. Immunol.* 30:300–7

74. Doucey MA, Scarpellino L, Zimmer J, Guillaume P, Luescher IF, et al. 2004. Cis association of Ly49A with MHC class I restricts natural killer cell inhibition. *Nat. Immunol.* 5:328–36

75. George TC, Ortaldo JR, Lemieux S, Kumar V, Bennett M. 1999. Tolerance and alloreactivity of the Ly49D subset of murine NK cells. *J. Immunol.* 163:1859–67

76. George TC, Mason LH, Ortaldo JR, Kumar V, Bennett M. 1999. Positive recognition of MHC class I molecules by the Ly49D receptor of murine NK cells. *J. Immunol.* 162:2035–43

77. Nakamura MC, Linnemeyer PA, Niemi EC, Mason LH, Ortaldo JR, et al. 1999. Mouse Ly-49D recognizes H-2Dd and activates natural killer cell cytotoxicity. *J. Exp. Med.* 189:493–500

78. Mason LH, Willette-Brown J, Mason AT, McVicar D, Ortaldo JR. 2000. Interaction of Ly-49D$^+$NK cells with H-2Dd Target cells leads to Dap-12 phosphorylation and IFN-γ secretion. *J. Immunol.* 164:603–11

79. Furukawa H, Iizuka K, Poursine-Laurent J, Shastri N, Yokoyama WM. 2002. A ligand for the murine NK activation receptor Ly-49D: activation of tolerized NK cells from β_2-microglobulin-deficient mice. *J. Immunol.* 169:126–36

80. Ortaldo JR, Bere EW, Hodge D, Young HA. 2001. Activating ly-49 NK receptors: central role in cytokine and chemokine production. *J. Immunol.* 166:4994–99

81. Silver ET, Gong D, Hazes B, Kane KP. 2001. Ly-49W, an activating receptor of nonobese diabetic mice with close homology to the inhibitory receptor Ly-49G, recognizes H-2D(k) and H-2D(d). *J. Immunol.* 166:2333–41

82. Silver ET, Gong DE, Chang CS, Amrani A, Santamaria P, Kane KP. 2000. Ly-49P activates NK-mediated lysis by recognizing H-2Dd. *J. Immunol.* 165:1771–81

83. Ortaldo JR, Young HA. 2003. Expression of IFN-γ upon triggering of activating Ly49D NK receptors in vitro and in vivo: costimulation with IL-12 or IL-18 overrides inhibitory receptors. *J. Immunol.* 170:1763–69

84. Brown MG, Dokun AO, Heusel JW, Smith HR, Beckman DL, et al. 2001. Vital involvement of a natural killer cell activation receptor in resistance to viral infection. *Science* 292:934–37

85. Daniels KA, Devora G, Lai WC, O'Donnell CL, Bennett M, Welsh RM. 2001. Murine cytomegalovirus is regulated by a discrete subset of natural killer cells reactive with monoclonal antibody to Ly49H. *J. Exp. Med.* 194:29–44

86. Lee SH, Zafer A, de Repentigny Y, Kothary R, Tremblay ML, et al. 2003. Transgenic expression of the activating natural killer receptor Ly49H confers resistance to cytomegalovirus in genetically susceptible mice. *J. Exp. Med.* 197:515–26

87. Sjolin H, Tomasello E, Mousavi-Jazi M, Bartolazzi A, Karre K, et al. 2002. Pivotal role of KARAP/DAP12 adaptor molecule in the natural killer cell-mediated resistance to murine cytomegalovirus infection. *J. Exp. Med.* 195:825–34

88. Arase H, Mocarski ES, Campbell AE, Hill AB, Lanier LL. 2002. Direct recognition of cytomegalovirus by activating and inhibitory NK cell receptors. *Science* 296:1323–26

89. Smith HR, Heusel JW, Mehta IK, Kim S, Dorner BG, et al. 2002. Recognition of a virus-encoded ligand by a natural killer cell activation receptor. *Proc. Natl. Acad. Sci. USA* 99:8826–31

90. Bubi I, Wagner M, Krmpoti A, Saulig T, Kim S, et al. 2004. Gain of virulence caused by loss of a gene in murine cytomegalovirus. *J. Virol.* 78:7536–44

91. Voigt V, Forbes CA, Tonkin JN, Degli-Esposti MA, Smith HR, et al. 2003. Murine cytomegalovirus m157 mutation and variation leads to immune evasion of natural killer cells. *Proc. Natl. Acad. Sci. USA* 100:13483–88

92. French AR, Pingel JT, Wagner M, Bubic I, Yang L, et al. 2004. Escape of mutant double-stranded DNA virus from innate immune control. *Immunity* 20:747–56

93. Arase H, Lanier LL. 2004. Specific recognition of virus-infected cells by paired NK receptors. *Rev. Med. Virol.* 14:83–93

94. Westgaard IH, Berg SF, Orstavik S, Fossum S, Dissen E. 1998. Identification of a human member of the Ly-49 multigene family. *Eur. J. Immunol.* 28:1839–46

95. Barten R, Trowsdale J. 1999. The human Ly-49L gene. *Immunogenetics* 49:731–34

96. Mager DL, McQueen KL, Wee V, Freeman JD. 2001. Evolution of natural killer cell receptors. Coexistence of functional Ly49 and KIR genes in baboons. *Curr. Biol.* 11:626–30

97. Gagnier L, Wilhelm BT, Mager DL. 2003. Ly49 genes in non-rodent mammals. *Immunogenetics* 55:109–15

98. Guethlein LA, Flodin LR, Adams EJ, Parham P. 2002. NK cell receptors of the orangutan (*Pongo pygmaeus*): a pivotal species for tracking the coevolution of killer cell Ig-like receptors with MHC-C. *J. Immunol.* 169:220–29

99. Takahashi T, Yawata M, Raudsepp T, Lear TL, Chowdhary BP, et al. 2004. Natural killer cell receptors in the horse: evidence for the existence of multiple transcribed LY49 genes. *Eur. J. Immunol.* 34:773–84

100. Uhrberg M, Valiante NM, Shum BP, Shilling HG, Lienert-Weidenbach K, et al. 1997. Human diversity in killer cell inhibitory receptor (KIR) genes. *Immunity* 7:753–63

101. Vilches C, Parham P. 2002. KIR: Diverse, rapidly evolving receptors of innate and adaptive immunity. *Annu. Rev. Immunol.* 20:217–51

102. Maxwell LD, Wallace A, Middleton D, Curran MD. 2002. A common KIR2DS4 deletion variant in the human that predicts a soluble KIR molecule analogous to the KIR1D molecule observed in the rhesus monkey. *Tissue Antigens* 60:254–58

103. Hsu KC, Liu XR, Selvakumar A, Mickelson E, O'Reilly RJ, Dupont B. 2002. Killer Ig-like receptor haplotype analysis by gene content: evidence for genomic diversity with a minimum of six basic framework haplotypes, each with multiple subsets. *J. Immunol.* 169:5118–29

104. Goodridge JP, Witt CS, Christiansen FT, Warren HS. 2003. KIR2DL4 (CD158d) genotype influences expression and function in NK cells. *J. Immunol.* 171:1768–74

105. Pando MJ, Gardiner CM, Gleimer M, McQueen KL, Parham P. 2003. The protein made from a common allele of KIR3DL1 (3DL1*004) is poorly expressed at cell surfaces due to substitution at positions 86 in Ig domain 0 and 182 in Ig domain 1. *J. Immunol.* 171:6640–49

106. Wilson MJ, Torkar M, Haude A, Milne S, Jones T, et al. 2000. Plasticity in the organization and sequences of human KIR/ILT gene families. *Proc. Natl. Acad. Sci. USA* 97:4778–83

107. Khakoo SI, Rajalingam R, Shum BP, Weidenbach K, Flodin L, et al. 2000. Rapid evolution of NK cell receptor systems demonstrated by comparison of chimpanzees and humans. *Immunity* 12:687–98

108. Rajalingam R, Parham P, Abi-Rached L. 2004. Domain shuffling has been the main mechanism forming new hominoid killer cell Ig-like receptors. *J. Immunol.* 172:356–69

109. Martin MP, Nelson G, Lee JH, Pellett F, Gao X, et al. 2002. Cutting edge: susceptibility to psoriatic arthritis: influence of activating killer Ig-like receptor genes in the absence of specific HLA-C alleles. *J. Immunol.* 169:2818–22

110. Martin AM, Kulski JK, Gaudieri S, Witt CS, Freitas EM, et al. 2004. Comparative genomic analysis, diversity and evolution of two KIR haplotypes A and B. *Gene* 335:121–31

111. Storset AK, Slettedal IO, Williams JL, Law A, Dissen E. 2003. Natural killer cell receptors in cattle: A bovine killer cell immunoglobulin-like receptor multigene family contains members with divergent signaling motifs. *Eur. J. Immunol.* 33:980–90

112. Hoelsbrekken SE, Nylenna O, Saether PC, Slettedal IO, Ryan JC, et al. 2003. Cutting edge: molecular cloning of a killer cell Ig-like receptor in the mouse and rat. *J. Immunol.* 170:2259–63

113. Welch AY, Kasahara M, Spain LM. 2003. Identification of the mouse killer immunoglobulin-like receptor-like (Kirl) gene family mapping to chromosome X. *Immunogenetics* 54:782–90

114. Moretta A, Bottino C, Pende D, Tripodi G, Tambussi G, et al. 1990. Identification of four subsets of human CD3-CD16⁺ natural killer (NK) cells by the expression of clonally distributed functional surface molecules: correlation between subset assignment of NK clones and ability to mediate specific alloantigen recognition. *J. Exp. Med.* 172:1589–98

115. Litwin V, Gumperz J, Parham P, Phillips JH, Lanier LL. 1994. NKB1: An NK cell receptor involved in the recognition of polymorphic HLA-B molecules. *J. Exp. Med.* 180:537–43

116. Phillips JH, Gumperz JE, Parham P, Lanier LL. 1995. Superantigen-dependent, cell-mediated cytotoxicity inhibited by MHC class I receptors on T lymphocytes. *Science* 268:403–5

117. Ferrini S, Cambiaggi A, Meazza R, Sforzini S, Marciano S, et al. 1994. T cell clones expressing the natural killer cell-related p58 receptor molecule display heterogeneity in phenotypic properties and p58 function. *Eur. J. Immunol.* 24:2294–98

118. Gumperz JE, Valiante NM, Parham P, Lanier LL, Tyan D. 1996. Heterogeneous phenotypes of expression of the NKB1 natural killer cell class I receptor among individuals of different HLA types appear genetically regulated, but not linked to MHC haplotype. *J. Exp. Med.* 183:1817–27

119. Shilling HG, Young N, Guethlein LA, Cheng NW, Gardiner CM, et al. 2002. Genetic control of human NK cell repertoire. *J. Immunol.* 169:239–47

120. Santourlidis S, Trompeter HI, Weinhold S, Eisermann B, Meyer KL, et al. 2002. Crucial role of DNA methylation in determination of clonally distributed killer cell Ig-like receptor expression patterns in NK cells. *J. Immunol.* 169:4253–61

121. Chan HW, Kurago ZB, Stewart CA, Wilson MJ, Martin MP, et al. 2003. DNA methylation maintains allele-specific KIR gene expression in human natural killer cells. *J. Exp. Med.* 197:245–55

122. Uhrberg M, Valiante NM, Young NT, Lanier LL, Phillips JH, Parham P. 2001. The repertoire of killer cell Ig-like receptor and CD94:NKG2A receptors in T cells: clones sharing identical $\alpha\beta$ TCR rearrangement express highly diverse killer cell Ig-like receptor patterns. *J. Immunol.* 166:3923–32

123. Vely F, Peyrat MA, Couedel C, Morcet JF, Halary F, et al. 2001. Regulation of inhibitory and activating killer-cell Ig-like receptor expression occurs in T cells after termination of TCR rearrangements. *J. Immunol.* 166:2487–94

124. Snyder MR, Muegge LO, Offord C, O'Fallon WM, Bajzer Z, et al. 2002. Formation of the killer Ig-like receptor repertoire on CD4$^+$CD28(null) T cells. *J. Immunol.* 168:3839–46

125. Colonna M, Samaridis J. 1995. Cloning of Ig-superfamily members associated with HLA-C and HLA-B recognition by human NK cells. *Science* 268:405–8

126. Wagtmann N, Biassoni R, Cantoni C, Verdiani S, Malnati MS, et al. 1995. Molecular clones of the p58 natural killer cell receptor reveal Ig-related molecules with diversity in both the extra- and intracellular domains. *Immunity* 2:439–49

127. D'Andrea A, Chang C, Franz-Bacon K, McClanahan T, Phillips JH, Lanier LL. 1995. Cutting edge: molecular cloning of NKB1: a natural killer cell receptor for HLA-B allotypes. *J. Immunol.* 155:2306–10

128. Colonna M, Spies T, Strominger JL, Ciccone E, Moretta A, et al. 1992. Alloantigen recognition by two human natural killer cell clones is associated with HLA-C or a closely linked gene. *Proc. Natl. Acad. Sci. USA* 89:7983–85

129. Gumperz JE, Litwin V, Phillips JH, Lanier LL, Parham P. 1995. The Bw4 public epitope of HLA-B molecules confers reactivity with NK cell clones that express NKB1, a putative HLA receptor. *J. Exp. Med.* 181:1133–44

130. Gumperz JE, Barber LD, Valiante NM, Percival L, Phillips JH, et al. 1997. Conserved and variable residues within the Bw4 motif of HLA-B make separable contributions to recognition by the NKB1 killer cell-inhibitory receptor. *J. Immunol.* 158:5237–41

131. Dohring C, Scheidegger D, Samaridis J, Cella M, Colonna M. 1996. A human killer inhibitory receptor specific for HLA-A. *J. Immunol.* 156:3098–101

132. Pende D, Biassoni R, Cantoni C, Verdiani S, Falco M, et al. 1996. The natural killer cell receptor specific for HLA-A allotypes: a novel member of the p58/p70 family of inhibitory receptors that is characterized by three immunoglobulin-like domains and is expressed as a 140-kD disulphide-linked dimer. *J. Exp. Med.* 184:505–18

133. Hansasuta P, Dong T, Thananchai H, Weekes M, Willberg C, et al. 2004. Recognition of HLA-A3 and HLA-A11 by KIR3DL2 is peptide-specific. *Eur. J. Immunol.* 34:1673–79

134. Malnati MS, Peruzzi M, Parker KC, Biddison WE, Ciccone E, et al. 1995. Peptide specificity in the recognition of MHC class I by natural killer cell clones. *Science* 267:1016–18

135. Peruzzi M, Wagtmann N, Long EO. 1996. A p70 killer cell inhibitory receptor specific for several HLA-B allotypes discriminates among peptides bound to HLA-B*2705. *J. Exp. Med.* 184:1585–90

136. Peruzzi M, Parker KC, Long EO, Malnati MS. 1996. Peptide sequence requirements for the recognition of HLA-B*2705 by specific natural killer cells. *J. Immunol.* 157:3350–56

137. Gavioli R, Zhang Q-J, Masucci MG. 1996. HLA-A11-mediated protection from NK cell-mediated lysis: role of HLA-A11-presented peptides. *Hum. Immunol.* 49:1–12

138. Rajagopalan S, Long EO. 1997. The direct binding of a p58 killer cell inhibitory receptor to human histocompatibility leukocyte antigen (HLA)-Cw4 exhibits peptide specificity. *J. Exp. Med.* 185:1523–28

139. Zappacosta F, Borrego F, Brooks AG, Parker KC, Coligan JE. 1997. Peptides isolated from HLA-CW*0304 confer different degrees of protection from natural killer cell-mediated lysis. *Proc. Natl. Acad. Sci. USA* 94:6313–18

140. Boyington JC, Motyka SA, Schuck P,

Brooks AG, Sun PD. 2000. Crystal structure of an NK cell immunoglobulin-like receptor in complex with its class I MHC ligand. *Nature* 405:537–43

141. Winter CC, Gumperz JE, Parham P, Long EO, Wagtmann N. 1998. Direct binding and functional transfer of NK cell inhibitory receptors reveal novel patterns of HLA-C allotype recognition. *J. Immunol.* 161:571–77

142. Vales-Gomez M, Reyburn HT, Erskine RA, Strominger J. 1998. Differential binding to HLA-C of p50-activating and p58-inhibitory natural killer cell receptors. *Proc. Natl. Acad. Sci. USA* 95: 14326–31

143. Katz G, Markel G, Mizrahi S, Arnon TI, Mandelboim O. 2001. Recognition of HLA-Cw4 but not HLA-Cw6 by the NK cell receptor killer cell Ig-like receptor two-domain short tail number 4. *J. Immunol.* 166:7260–67

144. Valiante NM, Uhrberg M, Shilling HG, Lienert-Weidenbach K, Arnett KL, et al. 1997. Functionally and structurally distinct NK cell receptor repertoires in the peripheral blood of two human donors. *Immunity* 7:739–51

145. Stewart CA, Van Bergen J, Trowsdale J. 2003. Different and divergent regulation of the KIR2DL4 and KIR3DL1 promoters. *J. Immunol.* 170:6073–81

146. Kikuchi-Maki A, Catina TL, Campbell KS. 2004. Structure-function analysis of KIR2DL4: an activating NK cell receptor exhibiting limited expression in humans. *Int. Nat. Killer Cell Works., 20th,* Abstr. No. B051

147. Selvakumar A, Steffens U, Dupont B. 1996. NK cell receptor gene of the KIR family with two Ig domains but highest homology to KIR receptors with three Ig domains. *Tissue Antigens* 48:285–95

148. Faure M, Long EO. 2002. KIR2DL4 (CD158d), an NK cell-activating receptor with inhibitory potential. *J. Immunol.* 168:6208–14

149. Yusa S, Catina TL, Campbell KS. 2002.

SHP-1- and phosphotyrosine-independent inhibitory signaling by a killer cell Ig-like receptor cytoplasmic domain in human NK cells. *J. Immunol.* 168:5047–57

150. Rajagopalan S, Fu J, Long EO. 2001. Cutting edge: induction of IFN-γ production but not cytotoxicity by the killer cell Ig-like receptor KIR2dl4 (CD158d) in resting NK cells. *J. Immunol.* 167:1877–81

151. Kikuchi-Maki A, Yusa S, Catina TL, Campbell KS. 2003. KIR2DL4 is an IL-2-regulated NK cell receptor that exhibits limited expression in humans but triggers strong IFN-γ production. *J. Immunol.* 171:3415–25

152. Witt CS, Whiteway JM, Warren HS, Barden A, Rogers M, et al. 2002. Alleles of the KIR2DL4 receptor and their lack of association with pre-eclampsia. *Eur. J. Immunol.* 32:18–29

153. Rajagopalan S, Long EO. 1999. An HLA-G-specific receptor expressed on all natural killer cells. *J. Exp. Med.* 189:1093–110

154. Cantoni C, Verdiani S, Falco M, Pessino A, Conte R, et al. 1998. p49, a putative HLA class I-specific inhibitory NK receptor belonging to the immunoglobulin superfamily. *Eur. J. Immunol.* 28:1980–90

155. Ponte M, Cantoni C, Biassoni R, Tradori-Cappai A, Bentivoglio G, et al. 1999. Inhibitory receptors sensing HLA-G1 molecules in pregnancy: Decidua-associated natural killer cells express LIR-1 and CD94/NKG2A and acquire p49, a novel HLA-G1-specific receptor. *Proc. Natl. Acad. Sci. USA* 96:5674–79

156. Boyson JE, Erskine R, Whitman MC, Chiu M, Lau JM, et al. 2002. Disulfide bond-mediated dimerization of HLA-G on the cell surface. *Proc. Natl. Acad. Sci. USA* 99:16180–85

157. Allan DS, Colonna M, Lanier LL, Churakova TD, Abrams JA, et al. 1999. Tetrameric complexes of HLA-G bind to peripheral blood myelomonocytic cells. *J. Exp. Med.* 189:1149

158. Campbell KS, Dessing M, Lopez-Botet M, Cella M, Colonna M. 1996.

Tyrosine phosphorylation of a human killer inhibitory receptor recruits protein tyrosine phosphatase 1C. *J. Exp. Med.* 184:93–100

159. Burshtyn DN, Scharenberg AM, Wagtmann N, Rajagopalan S, Berrada K, et al. 1996. Recruitment of tyrosine phosphatase HCP by the killer cell inhibitory receptor. *Immunity* 4:77–85

160. Fry A, Lanier LL, Weiss A. 1996. Phosphotyrosines in the KIR motif of NKB1 are required for negative signaling and for association with PTP1C. *J. Exp. Med.* 184:295–300

161. Olcese L, Lang P, Vely F, Cambiaggi A, Marguet D, et al. 1996. Human and mouse killer-cell inhibitory receptors recruit PTP1C and PTP1D protein tyrosine phosphatases. *J. Immunol.* 156:4531–34

162. Snyder MR, Lucas M, Vivier E, Weyand CM, Goronzy JJ. 2003. Selective activation of the c-Jun NH(2)-terminal protein kinase signaling pathway by stimulatory KIR in the absence of KARAP/DAP12 in CD4+T Cells. *J. Exp. Med.* 197:437–49

163. Namekawa T, Snyder MR, Yen JH, Goehring BE, Leibson PJ, et al. 2000. Killer cell activating receptors function as costimulatory molecules on CD4+ CD28null T cells clonally expanded in rheumatoid arthritis. *J. Immunol.* 165:1138–45

164. Yen JH, Moore BE, Nakajima T, Scholl D, Schaid DJ, et al. 2001. Major histocompatibility complex class I-recognizing receptors are disease risk genes in rheumatoid arthritis. *J. Exp. Med.* 193:1159–68

165. Momot T, Koch S, Hunzelmann N, Krieg T, Ulbricht K, et al. 2004. Association of killer cell immunoglobulin-like receptors with scleroderma. *Arthritis Rheum.* 50:1561–65

166. Suzuki Y, Hamamoto Y, Ogasawara Y, Ishikawa K, Yoshikawa Y, et al. 2004. Genetic polymorphisms of killer cell immunoglobulin-like receptors are associated with susceptibility to psoriasis vulgaris. *J. Invest. Dermatol.* 122:1133–36

167. Mandelboim O, Davis DM, Reyburn HT, Vales-Gomez M, Sheu EG, et al. 1996. Enhancement of class II-restricted T cell responses by costimulatory NK receptors for class I MHC proteins. *Science* 274:2097–100

168. Flores-Villanueva PO, Yunis EJ, Delgado JC, Vittinghoff E, Buchbinder S, et al. 2001. Control of HIV-1 viremia and protection from AIDS are associated with HLA-Bw4 homozygosity. *Proc. Natl. Acad. Sci. USA* 98:5140–45

169. Parham P, McQueen KL. 2003. Alloreactive killer cells: hindrance and help for haematopoietic transplants. *Nat. Rev. Immunol.* 3:108–22

170. Ruggeri L, Capanni M, Urbani E, Perruccio K, Shlomchik WD, et al. 2002. Effectiveness of donor natural killer cell alloreactivity in mismatched hematopoietic transplants. *Science* 295:2097–100

171. Bishara A, De Santis D, Witt CC, Brautbar C, Christiansen FT, et al. 2004. The beneficial role of inhibitory KIR genes of HLA class I NK epitopes in haploidentically mismatched stem cell allografts may be masked by residual donor-alloreactive T cells causing GVHD. *Tissue Antigens* 63:204–11

172. Davies SM, Ruggieri L, DeFor T, Wagner JE, Weisdorf DJ, et al. 2002. Evaluation of KIR ligand incompatibility in mismatched unrelated donor hematopoietic transplants. Killer immunoglobulin-like receptor. *Blood* 100:3825–27

173. Giebel S, Locatelli F, Lamparelli T, Velardi A, Davies S, et al. 2003. Survival advantage with KIR ligand incompatibility in hematopoietic stem cell transplantation from unrelated donors. *Blood* 102:814–19

174. Houchins JP, Yabe T, McSherry C, Bach FH. 1991. DNA sequence analysis of NKG2, a family of related cDNA clones encoding type II integral membrane proteins on human natural killer cells. *J. Exp. Med.* 173:1017–20

175. Chang C, Rodriguez A, Carretero M, Lopez-Botet M, Phillips JH, Lanier LL.

1995. Molecular characterization of human CD94: a type II membrane glycoprotein related to the C-type lectin superfamily. *Eur. J. Immunol.* 25:2433–37

176. Dissen E, Ber SF, Westgaard IH, Fossum S. 1997. Molecular characterization of a gene in the rat homologous to human CD94. *Eur. J. Immunol.* 27:2080–86

177. Berg SF, Dissen E, Westgaard IH, Fossum S. 1998. Two genes in the rat homologous to human NKG2. *Eur. J. Immunol.* 28:444 50

178. Lohwasser S, Hande P, Mager DL, Takei F. 1999. Cloning of murine NKG2A, B and C: second family of C-type lectin receptors on murine NK cells. *Eur. J. Immunol.* 29:755–61

179. Vance RE, Jamieson AM, Raulet DH. 1999. Recognition of the class Ib molecule Qa-1b by putative activating receptors CD94/NKG2C and CD94/NKG2E on mouse natural killer cells. *J. Exp. Med.* 190:1801–12

180. Vance RE, Kraft JR, Altman JD, Jensen PE, Raulet DH. 1998. Mouse CD94/NKG2A is a natural killer cell receptor for the nonclassical major histocompatibility complex (MHC) class I molecule Qa-1(b). *J. Exp. Med.* 188: 1841–48

181. Shum BP, Flodin LR, Muir DG, Rajalingam R, Khakoo SI, et al. 2002. Conservation and variation in human and common chimpanzee CD94 and NKG2 genes. *J. Immunol.* 168:240–52

182. Sato A, Mayer WE, Overath P, Klein J. 2003. Genes encoding putative natural killer cell C-type lectin receptors in teleostean fishes. *Proc. Natl. Acad. Sci. USA* 100:7779–84

183. Khalturin K, Becker M, Rinkevich B, Bosch TC. 2003. Urochordates and the origin of natural killer cells: identification of a CD94/NKR-P1-related receptor in blood cells of Botryllus. *Proc. Natl. Acad. Sci. USA* 100:622–27

184. Lazetic S, Chang C, Houchins JP, Lanier LL, Phillips JH. 1996. Cutting edge: human NK cell receptors involved in MHC class I recognition are disulfide-linked heterodimers of CD94 and NKG2 subunits. *J. Immunol.* 157:4741–45

185. Brooks AG, Posch PE, Scorzelli CJ, Borrego F, Coligan JE. 1997. NKG2A complexed with CD94 defines a novel inhibitory NK cell receptor. *J. Exp. Med.* 185:795–800

186. Houchins JP, Lanier LL, Niemi E, Phillips JH, Ryan JC. 1997. Natural killer cell cytolytic activity is inhibited by NKG2-A and activated by NKG2-C. *J. Immunol.* 158:3603–9

187. Carretero M, Cantoni C, Bellon T, Bottino C, Biassoni R, et al. 1997. The CD94 and NKG2-A C type lectins covalently assemble to form a natural killer cell inhibitory receptor for HLA class I molecules. *Eur. J. Immunol.* 27:563–75

188. Le Drean E, Vely F, Olcese L, Cambiaggi A, Guia S, et al. 1998. Inhibition of antigen-induced T cell response and antibody-induced NK cell cytotoxicity by NKG2A: association of NKG2A with SHP-1 and SHP-2 protein-tyrosine phosphatase. *Eur. J. Immunol.* 28:264–76

189. Lanier LL, Corliss B, Wu J, Phillips JH. 1998. Association of DAP12 with activating CD94/NKG2C NK cell receptors. *Immunity* 8:693–701

190. Plougastel B, Trowsdale J. 1997. Cloning of NKG2-F, a new member of the NKG2 family of human natural killer cell receptor genes. *Eur. J. Immunol.* 27:2835–39

191. Aramburu J, Balboa MA, Ramirez A, Silva A, Acevedo A, et al. 1990. A novel functional cell surface dimer (Kp43) expressed by natural killer cells and T cell receptor-γ/δ^+T lymphocytes. I. Inhibition of the IL-2 dependent proliferation by anti-Kp43 monoclonal antibody. *J. Immunol.* 144:3238–47

192. Toyama-Sorimachi N, Taguchi Y, Yagita H, Kitamura F, Kawasaki A, et al. 2001. Mouse CD94 participates in Qa-1-mediated self recognition by NK cells and

delivers inhibitory signals independent of Ly-49. *J. Immunol.* 166:3771–79

193. Sivakumar PV, Gunturi A, Salcedo M, Schatzle JD, Lai WC, et al. 1999. Expression of functional CD94/NKG2A inhibitory receptors on fetal NK1.1⁺Ly-49-cells: a possible mechanism of tolerance during NK cell development. *J. Immunol.* 162:6976–80

194. Kim S, Iizuka K, Kang HS, Dokun A, French AR, et al. 2002. In vivo developmental stages in murine natural killer cell maturation. *Nat. Immunol.* 3:523–28

195. Mingari MC, Vitale C, Cantoni C, Bellomo R, Ponte M, et al. 1997. Interleukin-15-induced maturation of human natural killer cells from early thymic precursors: selective expression of CD94/NKG2A as the only HLA class I-specific inhibitory receptor. *Eur. J. Immunol.* 27:1374–80

196. Miller JS, McCullar V. 2001. Human natural killer cells with polyclonal lectin and immunoglobulin-like receptors develop from single hematopoietic stem cells with preferential expression of NKG2A and KIR2DL2/L3/S2. *Blood* 98:705–13

197. Mingari MC, Ponte M, Bertone S, Schiavetti F, Vitale C, et al. 1998. HLA class I-specific inhibitory receptors in human T lymphocytes: interleukin-15-induced expression of CD94/NKG2A in superantigen- or alloantigen-activated CD8⁺T cells. *Proc. Natl. Acad. Sci. USA* 95:1172–77

198. Bertone S, Schiavetti F, Bellomo R, Vitale C, Ponte M, Moretta L, Mingari MC. 1999. Transforming growth factor-β-induced expression of CD94/NKG2A inhibitory receptors in human T lymphocytes. *Eur. J. Immunol* 29:23–29

199. Derre L, Corvaisier M, Pandolfino MC, Diez E, Jotereau F, Gervois N. 2002. Expression of CD94/NKG2-A on human T lymphocytes is induced by IL-12: implications for adoptive immunotherapy. *J. Immunol.* 168:4864–70

200. Jabri B, Selby JM, Negulescu H, Lee L, Roberts AI, et al. 2002. TCR specificity dictates CD94/NKG2A expression by human CTL. *Immunity* 17:487–99

201. Braud VM, Allan DSJ, O'Callaghan CA, Soderstrom K, D'Andrea A, et al. 1998. HLA-E binds to natural killer cell receptors CD94/NKG2A, B, and C. *Nature* 391:795–98

202. Borrego F, Ulbrecht M, Weiss EH, Coligan JE, Brooks AG. 1998. Recognition of human histocompatibility leukocyte antigen (HLA)-E complexed with HLA class I signal sequence-derived peptides by CD94/NKG2 confers protection from natural killer cell-mediated lysis. *J. Exp. Med.* 187:813–18

203. Lee N, Llano M, Carretero M, Ishitani A, Navarro F, et al. 1998. HLA-E is a major ligand for the NK inhibitory receptor CD94/NKG2A. *Proc. Natl. Acad. Sci. USA* 95:5199–204

204. Aldrich CJ, DeCloux A, Woods AS, Cotter RJ, Soloski MJ, Forman J. 1994. Identification of a TAP-dependent leader peptide recognized by alloreactive T cells specific for a class Ib antigen. *Cell* 79: 649–58

205. Braud V, Jones EY, McMichael A. 1997. The human major histocompatibility complex class Ib molecule HLA-E binds signal sequence-derived peptides with primary anchor residues at positions 2 and 9. *Eur. J. Immunol.* 27:1164–69

206. Lee N, Goodlett DR, Ishitani A, Marquardt H, Geraghty DE. 1998. HLA-E surface expression depends on binding of TAP-dependent peptides derived from certain HLA class I signal sequences. *J. Immunol.* 160:4951–60

207. Davies A, Kalb S, Liang B, Aldrich CJ, Lemonnier FA, et al. 2003. A peptide from heat shock protein 60 is the dominant peptide bound to Qa-1 in the absence of the MHC class Ia leader sequence peptide Qdm. *J. Immunol.* 170:5027–33

208. Miller JD, Weber DA, Ibegbu C, Pohl J, Altman JD, Jensen PE. 2003. Analysis of HLA-E peptide-binding specificity and contact residues in bound peptide

required for recognition by CD94/NKG2. *J. Immunol.* 171:1369–75

209. Valés-Gómez M, Reyburn HT, Erskine RA, Lopez-Botet M, Strominger JL. 1999. Kinetics and peptide dependency of the binding of the inhibitory NK receptor CD94/NKG2-A and the activating receptor CD94/NKG2-C to HLA-E. *EMBO J.* 18:4250–60

210. Llano M, Lee N, Navarro F, Garcia P, Albar JP, et al. 1998. HLA-E-bound peptides influence recognition by inhibitory and triggering CD94/NKG2 receptors: preferential response to an HLA-G-derived nonamer. *Eur. J. Immunol.* 28:2854–63

211. Kraft JR, Vance RE, Pohl J, Martin AM, Raulet DH, Jensen PE. 2000. Analysis of Qa-1(b) peptide binding specificity and the capacity of CD94/NKG2A to discriminate between Qa-1-peptide complexes. *J. Exp. Med.* 192:613–24

212. Michaelsson J, Teixeira De Matos C, Achour A, Lanier LL, Karre K, Soderstrom K. 2002. A signal peptide derived from hsp60 binds HLA-E and interferes with CD94/NKG2A recognition. *J. Exp. Med.* 196:1403–14

213. Tomasec P, Braud VM, Rickards C, Powell MB, McSharry BP, et al. 2000. Surface expression of HLA-E-, an inhibitor of natural killer cells, enhanced by human cytomegalovirus gpUL40. *Science* 287:1031–33

214. Ulbrecht M, Martinozzi S, Grzeschik M, Hengel H, Ellwart JW, et al. 2000. Cutting edge: the human cytomegalovirus UL40 gene product contains a ligand for HLA-E and prevents NK cell-mediated lysis. *J. Immunol.* 164:5019–22

215. Cerboni C, Mousavi-Jazi M, Wakiguchi H, Carbone E, Karre K, Soderstrom K. 2001. Synergistic effect of IFN-γ and human cytomegalovirus protein UL40 in the HLA-E-dependent protection from NK cell-mediated cytotoxicity. *Eur. J. Immunol.* 31:2926–35

216. Wang EC, McSharry B, Retiere C, Tomasec P, Williams S, et al. 2002. UL40-mediated NK evasion during productive infection with human cytomegalovirus. *Proc. Natl. Acad. Sci. USA* 99:7570–75

217. Moser JM, Gibbs J, Jensen PE, Lukacher AE. 2002. CD94-NKG2A receptors regulate antiviral CD8[+]T cell responses. *Nat. Immunol.* 3:189–95

218. McMahon CW, Zajac AJ, Jamieson AM, Corral L, Hammer GE, et al. 2002. Viral and bacterial infections induce expression of multiple NK cell receptors in responding CD8[+] T cells. *J. Immunol.* 169:1444–52

219. Miller JD, Peters M, Oran AE, Beresford GW, Harrington L, et al. 2002. CD94/NKG2 Expression does not inhibit cytotoxic function of lymphocytic choriomeningitis virus-specific CD8[+] T cells. *J. Immunol.* 169:693–701

220. Ugolini S, Arpin C, Anfossi N, Walzer T, Cambiaggi A, et al. 2001. Involvement of inhibitory NKRs in the survival of a subset of memory-phenotype CD8[+] T cells. *Nat. Immunol.* 2:430–35

221. Gunturi A, Berg RE, Forman J. 2003. Preferential survival of CD8 T and NK cells expressing high levels of CD94. *J. Immunol.* 170:1737–45

222. Cosman D, Fanger N, Borges L, Kibin M, Chin W, et al. 1997. A novel immunoglobulin superfamily receptor for cellular and viral MHC class I molecules. *Immunity* 7:273–82

223. Colonna M, Navarro F, Bellon T, Llano M, Garcia P, et al. 1997. A common inhibitory receptor for major histocompatibility complex class I molecules on human lymphoid and myelomonocytic cells. *J. Exp. Med.* 186:1809–18

224. Chapman TL, Heikeman AP, Bjorkman PJ. 1999. The inhibitory receptor LIR-1 uses a common binding interaction to recognize class I MHC molecules and the viral homolog UL18. *Immunity* 11:603–13

225. Lepin EJ, Bastin JM, Allan DS, Roncador G, Braud VM, et al. 2000. Functional characterization of HLA-F and binding of

HLA-F tetramers to ILT2 and ILT4 receptors. *Eur. J. Immunol.* 30:3552–61

226. Beck S, Barrell BG. 1988. Human cytomegalovirus encodes a glycoprotein homologous to MHC class-I antigens. *Nature* 331:269–72

227. Navarro F, Llano M, Bellon T, Colonna M, Geraghty DE, Lopez-Botet M. 1999. The ILT2(LIR1) and CD94/NKG2A NK cell receptors respectively recognize HLA-G1 and HLA-E molecules co-expressed on target cells. *Eur. J. Immunol.* 29:277–83

228. Kubagawa H, Burrows PD, Cooper MD. 1997. A novel pair of immunoglobulin-like receptors expressed by B cells and myeloid cells. *Proc. Natl. Acad. Sci. USA* 94:5261–66

229. Hayami K, Fukuta D, Nishikawa Y, Yamashita Y, Inui M, et al. 1997. Molecular cloning of a novel murine cell-surface glycoprotein homologous to killer cell inhibitory receptors. *J. Biol. Chem.* 272:7320–27

230. Kubagawa H, Chen CC, Le Hong Ho L, Shimada TS, Gartland L, et al. 1999. Biochemical nature and cellular distribution of the paired immunoglobulin-like receptors, PIR-A and PIR-B. *J. Exp. Med.* 189:309–18

231. Nakamura A, Kobayashi E, Takai T. 2004. Exacerbated graft-versus-host disease in Pirb$^{-/-}$ mice. *Nat. Immunol.* 5:623–29

232. Raulet DH. 2003. Roles of the NKG2D immunoreceptor and its ligands. *Nat. Rev. Immunol.* 3:781–90

233. Ho EL, Carayannopoulos LN, Poursine-Laurent J, Kinder J, Plougastel B, et al. 2002. Costimulation of multiple NK cell activation receptors by NKG2D. *J. Immunol.* 169:3667–75

234. Bauer S, Groh V, Wu J, Steinle A, Phillips JH, et al. 1999. Activation of natural killer cells and T cells by NKG2D, a receptor for stress-inducible MICA. *Science* 285:727–30

235. Jamieson AM, Diefenbach A, McMahon CW, Xiong N, Carlyle JR, Raulet DH.

2002. The role of the NKG2D immunoreceptor in immune cell activation and natural killing. *Immunity* 17:19–29

236. Wu J, Song Y, Bakker ABH, Bauer S, Groh V, et al. 1999. An activating receptor complex on natural killer and T cells formed by NKG2D and DAP10. *Science* 285:730–32

237. Roberts AI, Lee L, Schwarz E, Groh V, Spies T, et al. 2001. Cutting edge: NKG2D receptors induced by IL-15 costimulate CD28-negative effector CTL in the tissue microenvironment. *J. Immunol.* 167:5527–30

238. Sutherland CL, Chalupny NJ, Schooley K, VandenBos T, Kubin M, Cosman D. 2002. UL16-binding proteins, novel MHC class I-related proteins, bind to NKG2D and activate multiple signaling pathways in primary NK cells. *J. Immunol.* 168:671–79

239. Castriconi R, Cantoni C, Della Chiesa M, Vitale M, Marcenaro E, et al. 2003. Transforming growth factor β 1 inhibits expression of NKp30 and NKG2D receptors: consequences for the NK-mediated killing of dendritic cells. *Proc. Natl. Acad. Sci. USA* 100:4120–25

240. Lee JC, Lee KM, Kim DW, Heo DS. 2004. Elevated TGF-β1 secretion and down-modulation of NKG2D underlies impaired NK cytotoxicity in cancer patients. *J. Immunol.* 172:7335–40

241. Diefenbach A, Tomasello E, Lucas M, Jamieson AM, Hsia JK, et al. 2002. Selective associations with signaling proteins determine stimulatory versus costimulatory activity of NKG2D. *Nat. Immunol.* 3:1142–49

242. Gilfillan S, Ho EL, Cella M, Yokoyama WM, Colonna M. 2002. NKG2D recruits two distinct adapters to trigger NK cell activation and costimulation. *Nat. Immunol.* 3:1150–55

243. Wu J, Cherwinski H, Spies T, Phillips JH, Lanier LL. 2000. DAP10 and DAP12 form distinct, but functionally cooperative, receptor complexes in natural killer cells. *J. Exp. Med.* 192:1059–68

244. Andre P, Castriconi R, Espeli M, Anfossi N, Juarez T, et al. 2004. Comparative analysis of human NK cell activation induced by NKG2D and natural cytotoxicity receptors. *Eur. J. Immunol.* 34:961–71

245. Billadeau DD, Upshaw JL, Schoon RA, Dick CJ, Leibson PJ. 2003. NKG2D-DAP10 triggers human NK cell-mediated killing via a Syk-independent regulatory pathway. *Nat. Immunol.* 4:557–64

246. Rosen DB, Araki M, Hamerman JA, Chen T, Yamamura T, Lanier LL. 2004. A structural basis for the association of DAP12 with mouse, but not human, NKG2D. *J. Immunol.* 173:2470–78

247. Radaev S, Sun PD. 2003. Structure and function of natural killer cell surface receptors. *Annu. Rev. Biophys. Biomol. Struct.* 32:93–114

248. Cosman D, Mullberg J, Sutherland CL, Chin W, Armitage R, et al. 2001. ULBPs, novel MHC class I-related molecules, bind to CMV glycoprotein UL16 and stimulate NK cytotoxicity through the NKG2D receptor. *Immunity* 14:123–33

249. Jan Chalupny N, Sutherland CL, Lawrence WA, Rein-Weston A, Cosman D. 2003. ULBP4 is a novel ligand for human NKG2D. *Biochem. Biophys. Res. Commun.* 305:129–35

250. Cerwenka A, Bakker AB, McClanahan T, Wagner J, Wu J, et al. 2000. Retinoic acid early inducible genes define a ligand family for the activating NKG2D receptor in mice. *Immunity* 12:721–27

251. Carayannopoulos LN, Naidenko OV, Fremont DH, Yokoyama WM. 2002. Cutting edge: murine UL16-binding protein-like transcript 1: a newly described transcript encoding a high-affinity ligand for murine NKG2D. *J. Immunol.* 169:4079–83

252. Diefenbach A, Hsia JK, Hsiung MY, Raulet DH. 2003. A novel ligand for the NKG2D receptor activates NK cells and macrophages and induces tumor immunity. *Eur. J. Immunol.* 33:381–91

253. Bahram S, Bresnahan M, Geraghty DE, Spies T. 1994. A second lineage of mammalian major histocompatibility complex class I genes. *Proc. Natl. Acad. Sci. USA* 91:6259–63

254. Radosavljevic M, Cuillerier B, Wilson MJ, Clement O, Wicker S, et al. 2002. A cluster of ten novel MHC class I related genes on human chromosome 6q24.2-q25.3. *Genomics* 79:114–23

255. Li P, Morris DL, Willcox BE, Steinle A, Spies T, Strong RK. 2001. Complex structure of the activating immunoreceptor NKG2D and its MHC class I-like ligand MICA. *Nat. Immunol.* 2:443–51

256. Li P, McDermott G, Strong RK. 2002. Crystal structures of RAE-1β and its complex with the activating immunoreceptor NKG2D. *Immunity* 16:77–86

257. Holmes MA, Li P, Petersdorf EW, Strong RK. 2002. Structural studies of allelic diversity of the MHC class I homolog MIC-B, a stress-inducible ligand for the activating immunoreceptor NKG2D. *J. Immunol.* 169:1395–400

258. Radaev S, Rostro B, Brooks AG, Colonna M, Sun PD. 2001. Conformational plasticity revealed by the cocrystal structure of NKG2D and its class I MHC-like ligand ULBP3. *Immunity* 15:1039–49

259. Li P, Willie ST, Bauer S, Morris DL, Spies T, Strong RK. 1999. Crystal structure of the MHC class I homolog MIC-A, a $\gamma\delta$ T cell ligand. *Immunity* 10:577–84

260. Li Z, Groh V, Strong RK, Spies T. 2000. A single amino acid substitution causes loss of expression of a MICA allele. *Immunogenetics* 51:246–48

261. Steinle A, Li P, Morris DL, Groh V, Lanier LL, Strong RK, Spies T. 2001. Interactions of human NKG2D with its ligands MICA, MICB, and homologs of the mouse RAE-1 protein family. *Immunogenetics* 53:279–87

262. Groh V, Bahram S, Bauer S, Herman A, Beauchamp M, Spies T. 1996. Cell stress-regulated human major histocompatibility complex class I gene expressed in gastrointestinal epithelium. *Proc. Natl. Acad. Sci. USA* 93:12445–50

263. Nomura M, Zou Z, Joh T, Takihara Y, Matsuda Y, Shimada K. 1996. Genomic structures and characterization of Rae1 family members encoding GPI-anchored cell surface proteins and expressed predominantly in embryonic mouse brain. *J. Biochem.* 120:987–95

264. Zou Z, Nomura M, Takihara Y, Yasunaga T, Shimada K. 1996. Isolation and characterization of retinoic acid-inducible cDNA clones in F9 cells: a novel cDNA family encodes cell surface proteins sharing partial homology with MHC class I molecules. *J. Biochem.* 119:319–28

265. Hamerman JA, Ogasawara K, Lanier LL. 2004. Cutting edge: Toll-like receptor signaling in macrophages induces ligands for the NKG2D receptor. *J. Immunol.* 172:2001–5

266. Lodoen M, Ogasawara K, Hamerman JA, Arase H, Houchins JP, et al. 2003. NKG2D-mediated natural killer cell protection against cytomegalovirus is impaired by viral gp40 modulation of retinoic acid early inducible 1 gene molecules. *J. Exp. Med.* 197:1245–53

267. Westwood JA, Kelly JM, Tanner JE, Kershaw MH, Smyth MJ, Hayakawa Y. 2004. Cutting Edge: novel priming of tumor-specific immunity by NKG2D-triggered NK cell-mediated tumor rejection and Th1-independent CD4$^+$T cell pathway. *J. Immunol.* 172:757–61

268. Wu J, Chalupny NJ, Manley TJ, Riddell SR, Cosman D, Spies T. 2003. Intracellular retention of the MHC class I-related chain B ligand of NKG2D by the human cytomegalovirus UL16 glycoprotein. *J. Immunol.* 170:4196–200

269. Welte SA, Sinzger C, Lutz SZ, Singh-Jasuja H, Sampaio KL, et al. 2003. Selective intracellular retention of virally induced NKG2D ligands by the human cytomegalovirus UL16 glycoprotein. *Eur. J. Immunol.* 33:194–203

270. Dunn C, Chalupny NJ, Sutherland CL, Dosch S, Sivakumar PV, et al. 2003. Human cytomegalovirus glycoprotein UL16 causes intracellular sequestration of NKG2D ligands, protecting against natural killer cell cytotoxicity. *J. Exp. Med.* 197:1427–39

271. Rolle A, Mousavi-Jazi M, Eriksson M, Odeberg J, Soderberg-Naucler C, et al. 2003. Effects of human cytomegalovirus infection on ligands for the activating NKG2D receptor of NK cells: up-regulation of UL16-binding protein (ULBP)1 and ULBP2 is counteracted by the viral UL16 protein. *J. Immunol.* 171:902–8

272. Groh V, Rhinehart R, Randolph-Habecker J, Topp MS, Riddell SR, Spies T. 2001. Costimulation of CD8$\alpha\beta$ T cells by NKG2D via engagement by MIC induced on virus-infected cells. *Nat. Immunol.* 2:255–60

273. Krmpotic A, Busch DH, Bubic I, Gebhardt F, Hengel H, et al. 2002. MCMV glycoprotein gp40 confers virus resistance to CD8$^+$ T cells and NK cells in vivo. *Nat. Immunol.* 3:529–35

274. Lodoen M, Abenes G, Umamoto S, Houchins JP, Li F, Lanier LL. 2004. The cytomegalovirus m155 gene product subverts NK cell antiviral protection by disruption of H60-NKG2D interactions. *J. Exp. Med.* 200:1075–81

275. Ziegler H, Thale R, Lucin P, Muranyi W, Flohr T, et al. 1997. A mouse cytomegalovirus glycoprotein retains MHC class I complexes in the ERGIC/cis-Golgi compartments. *Immunity* 6:57–66

276. Abenes G, Chan K, Lee M, Haghjoo E, Zhu J, et al. 2004. Murine cytomegalovirus with a transposon insertional mutation at open reading frame m155 is deficient in growth and virulence in mice. *J. Virol.* 78:6891–99

277. Groh V, Rhinehart R, Secrist H, Bauer S, Grabstein KH, Spies T. 1999. Broad tumor-associated expression and recognition by tumor-derived $\gamma\delta$ T cells of MICA and MICB. *Proc. Natl. Acad. Sci. USA* 96:6879–84

278. Diefenbach A, Jamieson AM, Liu SD,

Shastri N, Raulet DH. 2000. Ligands for the murine NKG2D receptor: expression by tumor cells and activation of NK cells and macrophages. *Nat. Immunol.* 1:119–26

279. Groh V, Wu J, Yee C, Spies T. 2002. Tumour-derived soluble MIC ligands impair expression of NKG2D and T-cell activation. *Nature* 419:734–38

280. Doubrovina ES, Doubrovin MM, Vider E, Sisson RB, O'Reilly RJ, et al. 2003. Evasion from NK cell immunity by MHC class I chain-related molecules expressing colon adenocarcinoma. *J. Immunol.* 171:6891–99

281. Salih HR, Rammensee HG, Steinle A. 2002. Cutting edge: down-regulation of MICA on human tumors by proteolytic shedding. *J. Immunol.* 169:4098–102

282. Groh V, Bruhl A, El-Gabalawy H, Nelson JL, Spies T. 2003. Stimulation of T cell autoreactivity by anomalous expression of NKG2D and its MIC ligands in rheumatoid arthritis. *Proc. Natl. Acad. Sci. USA* 100:9452–57

283. Ogasawara K, Hamerman JA, Ehrlich LR, Bour-Jordan H, Santamaria P, et al. 2004. NKG2D blockade prevents autoimmune diabetes in NOD mice. *Immunity* 20:757–67

284. Poirot L, Benoist C, Mathis D. 2004. Natural killer cells distinguish innocuous and destructive forms of pancreatic islet autoimmunity. *Proc. Natl. Acad. Sci. USA* 101:8102–7

285. Glimcher L, Shen FW, Cantor H. 1977. Identification of a cell-surface antigen selectively expressed on the natural killer cell. *J. Exp. Med.* 145:1–9

286. Yokoyama WM, Ryan JC, Hunter JJ, Smith HRC, Stark M, Seaman WE. 1991. cDNA cloning of mouse NKR-P1 and genetic linkage with Ly-49: identification of a natural killer cell gene complex on mouse chromosome 6. *J. Immunol.* 147:3229–36

287. Giorda R, Weisberg EP, Ip TK, Trucco M. 1992. Genomic structure and strain-specific expression of the natural killer cell receptor NKR-P1. *J. Immunol.* 149: 1957–63

288. Ryan JC, Turck J, Niemi EC, Yokoyama WM, Seaman WE. 1992. Molecular cloning of the NK1.1 antigen, a member of the NKR-P1 family of natural killer cell activation molecules. *J. Immunol.* 149:1631–35

289. Giorda R, Rudert WA, Vavassori C, Chambers WH, Hiserodt JC, Trucco M. 1990. NKR-P1, a signal transduction molecule on natural killer cells. *Science* 249:1298–300

290. Lanier LL, Chang C, Phillips JH. 1994. Human NKR-P1A: a disulfide linked homodimer of the C-type lectin superfamily expressed by a subset of NK and T lymphocytes. *J. Immunol.* 153:2417–28

291. Koo GC, Peppard JR. 1984. Establishment of monoclonal anti-NK1.1 antibody. *Hybridoma* 3:301

292. Carlyle JR, Martin A, Mehra A, Attisano L, Tsui FW, Zuniga-Pflucker JC. 1999. Mouse NKR-P1B, a novel NK1.1 antigen with inhibitory function. *J. Immunol.* 162:5917–23

293. Arase H, Arase N, Saito T. 1996. Interferon γ production by natural killer (NK) cells and NK1.1$^+$ T cells upon NKR-P1 cross-linking. *J. Exp. Med.* 183:2391–96

294. Arase N, Arase H, Park SY, Ohno H, Ra C, Saito T. 1997. Association with FcRg is essential for activation signal through NKR-P1 (CD161) in natural killer (NK) cells and NK1.1$^+$T cells. *J. Exp. Med.* 186:1957–63

295. Bendelac A, Lantz O, Quimby ME, Yewdell JW, Bennink JR, Brutkiewicz RR. 1995. CD1 recognition by mouse NK1$^+$T lymphocytes. *Science* 268:863–65

296. Godfrey DI, Hammond KJ, Poulton LD, Smyth MJ, Baxter AG. 2000. NKT cells: facts, functions and fallacies. *Immunol. Today* 21:573–83

297. Plougastel B, Dubbelde C, Yokoyama

WM. 2001. Cloning of Clr, a new family of lectin-like genes localized between mouse Nkrp1a and Cd69. *Immunogenetics* 53:209–14

298. Zhou H, Kartsogiannis V, Hu YS, Elliott J, Quinn JM, et al. 2001. A novel osteoblast-derived C-type lectin that inhibits osteoclast formation. *J. Biol. Chem.* 276:14916–23

299. Hu YS, Zhou H, Myers D, Quinn JM, Atkins GJ, et al. 2004. Isolation of a human homolog of osteoclast inhibitory lectin that inhibits the formation and function of osteoclasts. *J. Bone Miner. Res.* 19:89–99

300. Mocsai A, Humphrey MB, Van Ziffle JA, Hu Y, Burghardt A, et al. 2004. The immunomodulatory adapter proteins DAP12 and Fc receptor γ-chain (FcRγ) regulate development of functional osteoclasts through the Syk tyrosine kinase. *Proc. Natl. Acad. Sci. USA* 101:6158–63

301. Koga T, Inui M, Inoue K, Kim S, Suematsu A, et al. 2004. Costimulatory signals mediated by the ITAM motif cooperate with RANKL for bone homeostasis. *Nature* 428:758–63

302. Boles KS, Barten R, Kumaresan PR, Trowsdale J, Mathew PA. 1999. Cloning of a new lectin-like receptor expressed on human NK cells. *Immunogenetics* 50:1–7

303. Mathew PA, Chuang SS, Vaidya SV, Kumaresan PR, Boles KS, Pham HT. 2004. The LLT1 receptor induces IFN-γ production by human natural killer cells. *Mol. Immunol.* 40:1157–63

304. Exley M, Porcelli S, Furman M, Garcia J, Balk S. 1998. CD161 (NKR-P1A) costimulation of CD1d-dependent activation of human T cells expressing invariant Vα24JαQ T cell receptor α chains. *J. Exp. Med.* 188:867–76

305. Poggi A, Costa P, Zocchi MR, Moretta L. 1997. NKRP1A molecule is involved in transendothelial migration of CD4+human T lymphocytes. *Immunol Lett* 57:121–23

306. Poggi A, Costa P, Morelli L, Cantoni C, Pella N, et al. 1996. Expression of human NKRP1A by CD34+immature thymocytes: NKRP1A-mediated regulation of proliferation and cytolytic activity. *Eur. J. Immunol.* 26:12660–72

307. Brown MH, Boles K, Anton van der Merwe P, Kumar V, Mathew PA, Barclay NA. 1998. 2B4, the natural killer and T cell immunoglobulin superfamily surface protein, is a ligand for CD48. *J. Exp. Med.* 188:2083–90

308. Latchman Y, McKay PF, Reiser H. 1998. Identification of the 2B4 molecule as a counter-receptor for CD48. *J. Immunol.* 161:5809–12

309. Garni-Wagner BA, Purohit A, Mathew PA, Bennett M, Kumar K. 1993. A novel function-associated molecule related to non-MHC-restricted cytotoxicity mediated by activated natural killer cells and T cells. *J. Immunol.* 151:60–70

310. Valiante NM, Trinchieri G. 1993. Identification of a novel signal transduction surface molecule on human cytotoxic lymphocytes. *J. Exp. Med.* 178:1397–406

311. Mathew PA, Garni-Wagner BA, Land K, Takashima A, Stoneman E, et al. 1993. Cloning and characterization of the 2B4 gene encoding a molecule associated with non-MHC-restricted killing mediated by activated natural killer cells and T cells. *J. Immunol.* 151:5328–37

312. Boles KS, Nakajima H, Colonna M, Chuang SS, Stepp SE, et al. 1999. Molecular characterization of a novel human natural killer cell receptor homologous to mouse 2B4. *Tissue Antigens* 54:27–34

313. Tangye SG, Lazetic S, Woollatt E, Sutherland GR, Lanier LL, Phillips JH. 1999. Cutting Edge: human 2B4, an activating NK cell receptor, recruits the protein tyrosine phosphatase SHP-2 and the adaptor signaling protein SAP. *J. Immunol.* 162:6981–85

314. Kubin MZ, Parshley DL, Din W, Waugh JY, Davis-Smith T, et al. 1999. Molecular cloning and biological characterization of NK cell activation-inducing ligand,

a counterstructure for CD48. *Eur. J. Immunol.* 29:3466–77

315. Nakajima H, Cella M, Langen H, Friedlein A, Colonna M. 1999. Activating interactions in human NK cell recognition: the role of 2B4-CD48. *Eur. J. Immunol.* 29:1676–83

316. Speiser DE, Colonna M, Ayyoub M, Cella M, Pittet MJ, et al. 2001. The activatory receptor 2B4 is expressed in vivo by human CD8$^+$ effector $\alpha\beta$ T cells. *J. Immunol.* 167:6165–70

317. Peritt D, Sesok-Pizzini DA, Schretzenmair R, Macgregor RR, Valiante NM, et al. 1999. C1.7 antigen expression on CD8$^+$ T cells is activation dependent: increased proportion of C1.7$^+$CD8$^+$ T cells in HIV-1-infected patients with progressing disease. *J. Immunol.* 162:7563–68

318. Engel P, Eck MJ, Terhorst C. 2003. The SAP and SLAM families in immune responses and X-linked lymphoproliferative disease. *Nat. Rev. Immunol.* 3:813–21

319. Bottino C, Falco M, Parolini S, Marcenaro E, Augugliaro R, et al. 2001. Ntb-a, a novel sh2d1a-associated surface molecule contributing to the inability of natural killer cells to kill Epstein-Barr virus-infected B cells in x-linked lymphoproliferative disease. *J. Exp. Med.* 194:235–46

320. Bouchon A, Cella M, Grierson HL, Cohen JI, Colonna M. 2001. Cutting edge: activation of NK cell-mediated cytotoxicity by a SAP-independent receptor of the CD2 family. *J. Immunol.* 167:5517–21

321. Parolini S, Bottino C, Falco M, Augugliaro R, Giliani S, et al. 2000. X-linked lymphoproliferative disease. 2B4 molecules displaying inhibitory rather than activating function are responsible for the inability of natural killer cells to kill Epstein-Barr virus-infected cells. *J. Exp. Med.* 192:337–46

322. Nakajima H, Cella M, Bouchon A, Grierson HL, Lewis J, et al. 2000. Patients with X-linked lymphoproliferative disease have a defect in 2B4 receptor-mediated NK cell cytotoxicity. *Eur. J. Immunol.* 30:3309–18

323. Schatzle JD, Sheu S, Stepp SE, Mathew PA, Bennett M, Kumar V. 1999. Characterization of inhibitory and stimulatory forms of the murine natural killer cell receptor 2B4. *Proc. Natl. Acad. Sci. USA* 96:3870–75

324. Chen R, Relouzat F, Roncagalli R, Aoukaty A, Tan R, et al. 2004. Molecular dissection of 2B4 signaling: implications for signal transduction by SLAM-related receptors. *Mol. Cell Biol.* 24:5144–56

325. Bottino C, Augugliaro R, Castriconi R, Nanni M, Biassoni R, et al. 2000. Analysis of the molecular mechanism involved in 2B4-mediated NK cell activation: evidence that human 2B4 is physically and functionally associated with the linker for activation of T cells. *Eur. J. Immunol.* 30:3718–22

326. Riteau B, Barber DF, Long EO. 2003. Vav1 phosphorylation is induced by β2 integrin engagement on natural killer cells upstream of actin cytoskeleton and lipid raft reorganization. *J. Exp. Med.* 198:469–74

327. Klem J, Verrett PC, Kumar V, Schatzle JD. 2002. 2B4 is constitutively associated with linker for the activation of T cells in glycolipid-enriched microdomains: properties required for 2B4 lytic function. *J. Immunol.* 169:55–62

328. Lee KM, McNerney ME, Stepp SE, Mathew PA, Schatzle JD, et al. 2004. 2B4 Acts as a non-major histocompatibility complex binding inhibitory receptor on mouse natural killer cells. *J. Exp. Med.* 199:1245–54

329. Sivori S, Parolini S, Falco M, Marcenaro E, Biassoni R, et al. 2000. 2B4 functions as a co-receptor in human NK cell activation. *Eur. J. Immunol.* 30:787–93

330. Tangye SG, Phillips JH, Lanier LL. 2000. The CD2-subset of the Ig superfamily of cell surface molecules: receptor-ligand pairs expressed by NK cells and other immune cells. *Semin. Immunol.* 12:149–57

331. Tangye SG, Phillips JH, Lanier LL, Nichols KE. 2000. Cutting Edge: functional requirement for SAP in 2B4-mediated activation of human natural killer cells as revealed by the X-linked lymphoproliferative syndrome. *J. Immunol.* 165:2932–36

332. Benoit L, Wang X, Pabst HF, Dutz J, Tan R. 2000. Defective NK cell activation in X-linked lymphoproliferative disease. *J. Immunol.* 165:3549–53

333. Sivori S, Falco M, Marcenaro E, Parolini S, Biassoni R, et al. 2002. Early expression of triggering receptors and regulatory role of 2B4 in human natural killer cell precursors undergoing in vitro differentiation. *Proc. Natl. Acad. Sci. USA* 99:4526–31

334. Burns GF, Triglia T, Werkmeister JA, Begley CG, Boyd AW. 1985. TLiSA1, a human T lineage-specific activation antigen involved in the differentiation of cytotoxic T lymphocytes and anomalous killer cells from their precursors. *J. Exp. Med.* 161:1063–78

335. Scott JL, Dunn SM, Hillam AJ, Walton S, Berndt MC, et al. 1989. Characterization of a novel membrane glycoprotein involved in platelet activation. *J. Biol. Chem.* 264:13475–82

336. Shibuya A, Campbell D, Hannum C, Yssel H, Franz-Bacon K, et al. 1996. DNAM-1, a novel adhesion molecule involved in the cytolytic function of T lymphocytes. *Immunity* 4:573–81

337. Bottino C, Castriconi R, Pende D, Rivera P, Nanni M, et al. 2003. Identification of PVR (CD155) and Nectin-2 (CD112) as cell surface ligands for the human DNAM-1 (CD226) activating molecule. *J. Exp. Med.* 198:557–67

338. Tahara-Hanaoka S, Shibuya K, Onoda Y, Zhang H, Yamazaki S, et al. 2004. Functional characterization of DNAM-1 (CD226) interaction with its ligands PVR (CD155) and nectin-2 (PRR-2/CD112). *Int. Immunol.* 16:533–38

339. Masson D, Jarry A, Baury B, Blanchardie P, Laboisse C, et al. 2001. Overexpression of the CD155 gene in human colorectal carcinoma. *Gut* 49:236–40

340. Shibuya K, Lanier LL, Phillips JH, Ochs HD, Shimizu K, et al. 1999. Physical and functional association of LFA-1 with DNAM-1 adhesion molecule. *Immunity* 11:615–23

341. Shibuya K, Shirakawa J, Kameyama T, Honda S, Tahara-Hanaoka S, et al. 2003. CD226 (DNAM-1) is involved in lymphocyte function-associated antigen 1 costimulatory signal for naive T cell differentiation and proliferation. *J. Exp. Med.* 198:1829–39

342. Reymond N, Imbert AM, Devilard E, Fabre S, Chabannon C, et al. 2004. DNAM-1 and PVR regulate monocyte migration through endothelial junctions. *J. Exp. Med.* 199:1331–41

343. Fuchs A, Cella M, Giurisato E, Shaw AS, Colonna M. 2004. Cutting edge: CD96 (tactile) promotes NK cell-target cell adhesion by interacting with the poliovirus receptor (CD155). *J. Immunol.* 172:3994–98

344. Shiratori I, Ogasawara K, Saito T, Lanier LL, Arase H. 2004. Activation of natural killer cells and dendritic cells upon recognition of a novel CD99-like ligand by paired immunoglobulin-like Type 2 receptor. *J. Exp. Med.* 199:525–33

345. Mousseau DD, Banville D, L'Abbe D, Bouchard P, Shen S-H. 2000. PILRα, a novel immunoreceptor tyrosine-based inhibitory motif-bearing protein, recruits SHP-1 upon tyrosine phosphorylation and is paired with the truncated counterpart PILRβ. *J. Biol. Chem.* 275:4467–74

346. Fournier N, Chalus L, Durand I, Garcia E, Pin JJ, et al. 2000. FDF03, a novel inhibitory receptor of the immunoglobulin superfamily, is expressed by human dendritic and myeloid cells. *J. Immunol.* 165:1197–209

347. Moretta A, Bottino C, Vitale M, Pende D, Cantoni C, et al. 2001. Activating receptors and coreceptors involved in

human natural killer cell-mediated cytolysis. *Annu. Rev. Immunol.* 19:197–223

348. Pende D, Parolini S, Pessino A, Sivori S, Augugliaro R, et al. 1999. Identification and molecular characterization of NKP30, a novel triggering receptor involved in natural cytotoxicity mediated by human natural killer cells. *J. Exp. Med.* 190:1505–16

349. Nalabolu SR, Shukla H, Nallur G, Parimoo S, Weissman SM. 1996. Genes in a 220-kb region spanning the TNF cluster in human MHC. *Genomics* 31:215–22

350. Vitale M, Bottino C, Sivori S, Sanseverino L, Castriconi R, et al. 1998. NKp44, a novel triggering surface molecule specifically expressed by activated natural killer cells, is involved in non-major histocompatibility complex-restricted tumor cell lysis. *J. Exp. Med.* 187:2065–72

351. Cantoni C, Bottino C, Vitale M, Pessino A, Augugliaro R, et al. 1999. NKp44, a triggering receptor involved in tumor cell lysis by activated human natural killer cells, is a novel member of the immunoglobulin superfamily. *J. Exp. Med.* 189:787–96

352. Pessino A, Sivori S, Bottino C, Malaspina A, Morelli L, et al. 1998. Molecular cloning of NKp46: a novel member of the immunoglobulin superfamily involved in triggering of natural cytotoxicity. *J. Exp. Med.* 188:953–60

Annu. Rev. Immunol. 2005. 23:275–306
doi: 10.1146/annurev.immunol.23.021704.115633
First published online as a Review in Advance on November 11, 2004

IPC: Professional Type 1 Interferon-Producing Cells and Plasmacytoid Dendritic Cell Precursors

Yong-Jun Liu

*Department of Immunology and Center for Cancer Immunology Research,
University of Texas, M.D. Anderson Cancer Center, Houston, Texas 77030;
email: yjliu@mdanderson.org*

Key Words pDC, type 1 interferon, dendritic cells, Toll-like receptor

■ **Abstract** Type 1 interferon-(α, β, ω)-producing cells (IPCs), also known as plasmacytoid dendritic cell precursors (pDCs), represent 0.2%–0.8% of peripheral blood mononuclear cells in both humans and mice. IPCs display plasma cell morphology, selectively express Toll-like receptor (TLR)-7 and TLR9, and are specialized in rapidly secreting massive amounts of type 1 interferon following viral stimulation. IPCs can promote the function of natural killer cells, B cells, T cells, and myeloid DCs through type 1 interferons during an antiviral immune response. At a later stage of viral infection, IPCs differentiate into a unique type of mature dendritic cell, which directly regulates the function of T cells and thus links innate and adaptive immune responses. After more than two decades of effort by researchers, IPCs finally claim their place in the hematopoietic chart as the most important cell type in antiviral innate immunity. Understanding IPC biology holds future promise for developing cures for infectious diseases, cancer, and autoimmune diseases.

UNCOVERING THE MYSTERY OF TYPE 1 INTERFERON-PRODUCING CELLS AND PLASMACYTOID DENDRITIC CELLS

From Plasmacytoid T Cells to Plasmacytoid Monocytes

In 1958, pathologists K. Lennert and W. Remmele (1) reported a histological observation of cells with plasma cell morphology in the T cell areas of human reactive lymph nodes. These plasma cells were named "T-associated plasma cells." In 1983, A.C. Feller et al. (2) found that the T-associated plasma cells expressed CD4 (OKT4), a marker for helper/inducer T cells, but that they did not express B cell antigen or immunoglobulin. T-associated plasma cells were renamed "plasmacytoid T cells" and were suggested to be the counterparts of plasma cells of the B cell system that secrete T cell lymphokines instead of immunoglobulins.

The name "plasmacytoid T cells" was later questioned by Dr. F. Facchetti (3), who found that plasmacytoid T cells did not express T cell receptor (TCR)

component CD3, but that they did express MHC class II and some myeloid antigens. He suggested that the plasmacytoid T cells should be renamed "plasmacytoid monocytes" (3).

From Plasmacytoid Monocytes to Plasmacytoid Predendritic Cells

In 1993, we identified two subsets of CD4$^+$CD3$^-$ cells in human tonsils: (a) CD4$^+$CD3$^-$CD11c$^+$ dendritic cells (DCs) within germinal centers, which can activate/coactivate naive T cells and germinal center B cells (4, 5), and (b) CD4$^+$ CD3 CD11c$^-$ cells, localized within the T cell–rich areas around high endothelial venules (HEV), which displayed a lymphoid-plasmacytoid morphology. These CD4$^+$CD3$^-$CD11c$^-$ cells can differentiate into mature DCs when cultured with interleukin (IL)-3 or IL-3 plus CD40L (6).

Two subsequent events were critical for us to make the connection between the CD4$^+$CD3$^-$CD11c$^-$ pre-DCs and the plasmacytoid monocytes. In October 1994, I met Dr. F. Facchetti, an expert on plasmacytoid monocytes, at the European Group for Immunodeficiency Symposium in Spain. After I presented our work on the CD4$^+$CD3$^-$CD11c$^+$ GCDC, Dr. Facchetti asked me if I knew a cell type called plasmacytoid monocytes, which also had a CD4$^+$CD3$^-$ phenotype. Dr. Facchetti kindly sent me a copy of his PhD thesis, entitled "The Plasmacytoid Monocyte," and wrote, "Dear Dr. Liu, the term 'plasmacytoid monocytes' that I suggested for these cells is now accepted by the literature; this, unfortunately, does not say anything on the function of these cells and on what they are capable to secrete. I am afraid that it will be very difficult to isolate plasmacytoid monocytes from lymph nodes and cultivate them." Because the plasmacytoid monocytes described in his thesis were localized in the T cell areas, whereas the CD4$^+$CD3$^-$CD11c$^+$ GCDC were found in B cell follicles, we concluded that the CD4$^+$CD3$^-$CD11c$^+$ GCDC were not plasmacytoid monocytes.

A second key event occurred in 1996. Gerardin Grouard, a PhD student in my laboratory, presented her work on the CD4$^+$CD3$^-$CD11c$^+$ GCDCs at the Les Embiez Conference for the European Network of Immunologists in southern France, where she met Dr. Luis Filgueira of the University of Zurich. Dr. Filgueira kindly offered to perform an electron microscopic (EM) study on the tonsillar DC subsets. When the EM photographs came back, we were astonished by the plasma cell morphology of every CD4$^+$CD3$^-$CD11c$^-$ cell. We immediately realized that the CD4$^+$CD3$^-$CD11c$^-$ pre-DC may be identical to the plasmacytoid monocytes described in Dr. Facchetti's PhD thesis (3), as well as to the DR$^+$CD11c$^-$ blood DCs reported by O'Doherty et al. (7).

After extensive studies on the CD4$^+$CD3$^-$CD11c$^-$ pre-DC, we concluded (5) that (a) we had isolated the plasmacytoid T cell/monocytes; (b) plasmacytoid T cell/monocytes did not express immunoglobulin or TCR; (c) plasmacytoid T cell/monocytes can differentiate into mature DCs when cultured with IL-3 or IL-3 plus CD40L, and therefore should be named plasmacytoid dendritic cell precursors (pDCs); (*d*) pDCs are unrelated to monocytes and may be of lymphoid lineage because they lack many of the myeloid antigens and phagocytic activity; and (*e*) pDCs are similar to the blood DR$^+$CD11c$^-$ immature DC (7). In 1997, Olweus et al. (8) reported that pDCs express a very high level of IL-3Rα (CD123) and may represent myeloid cells.

From Plasmacytoid DC to Natural Type IPCs

We had thus solved one of the mysteries of the plasmacytoid T cells/monocytes and concluded that they represent a unique subset of DC precursors, now called plasmacytoid DCs (pDCs) (6). We were still puzzled, however, by their plasmacytoid morphology.

The connection between pDCs and their function as professional type 1 IPCs was made on April 17, 1998, at Albert Einstein College of Medicine, where I was visiting Drs. Anne Davidson and Betty Diamond and giving a seminar on human B cell and DC subsets. I told the audience that I was puzzled by the plasmacytoid morphology of pDCs and did not have any idea what these cells did. Dr. Fred Siegal told me that pDCs really smelled like a cell type called "the natural interferon-producing cells."

Although all nucleated cells can produce type 1 interferon (IFN) upon infection by an appropriate virus, it became clear in the late 1970s that there is a blood cell type that has the ability to produce more type 1 IFN than other cell types (3). Initial studies suggested that natural killer (NK) cells were the major type 1 IPCs following viral infections, and NK cells activated themselves by type 1 IFNs in an autocrine fashion (9, 10). Subsequent studies using monoclonal antibodies specific for NK cells, B cells, T cells, monocytes, and macrophages concluded, however, that IPCs were not any of these (11, 12). Interestingly, IPCs were found to express MHC class II (13, 14), suggesting that IPCs might represent blood DCs (14). One cell-sorting study suggested that IPCs were conventional DCs, which have the conventional DC morphology and the ability to induce a strong allogeneic mixed lymphocyte reaction (MLR) (15). However, an earlier study showed that an IPC-enriched population was unable to induce MLR (16). The field was obviously frustrated by the inability to purify a homogeneous population of IPCs and to perform a definitive study. This situation was pointed out by Fitzgerald-Bocarsly in 1993 regarding the identity of IPCs: "Although much progress has been made in the past several years regarding their enrichment and characterization, these cells are still identified as much by what they are not (i.e., not T cells, B cells, NK cells, stem cells, or macrophages) as by what they are (i.e., low density, HLA-DR$^+$ cells)" (17). In 1996, Svensson et al. (18) took a more direct approach by analyzing the surface phenotype of intracellular IFN-α^+ blood mononuclear cells after a 5-h stimulation with herpes simplex virus (HSV). Svensson et al. (18) reported for the first time the most comprehensive surface phenotype of IPCs, as CD4$^+$DR$^+$CD45RA$^+$CD11c$^-$CD11b$^-$CD14$^-$CD13$^-$CD33$^-$CD16$^-$CD80$^-$CD86$^-$. The limitation of this study was that the use of HSV to activate the cells, followed by fixation and treatment with detergent for intracellular IFN-α staining, had some effects on the original phenotype of the cells, and most importantly it prevented further study of these cells. For example, the HSV-treated IPCs were found to express CD83 and CD45RO, lack rough endoplasmic reticulum, and have the ability to stimulate proliferation of T cells of HSV-immune donors. These are obviously not the phenotype and properties of freshly isolated IPCs.

Because of the phenotypic similarities between pDCs (6) and IPCs (18), we investigated, in collaboration with Dr. Fred Siegal, whether highly purified viable pDCs (with over 99% purity) were indeed IPCs. We reported our conclusions at the 5th International Symposium on Dendritic Cells in Fundamental and Clinical Immunology in September 1998 (19), as well as in a manuscript published in a June 1999 issue of *Science* (20). We reported the following findings: (*a*) pDCs produced 100–1000 times more type 1 IFN than the other blood cell types following HSV activation and indeed represent IPCs, and (*b*) IPCs rapidly lose the ability to produce large amounts of type 1 IFN following maturation into DCs in culture with IL-3 or HSV. We concluded that pDCs indeed represent IPCs. These findings suggest that, upon recognition of microbial pathogens, IPCs rapidly produce type 1 IFN as effector cells of the innate immune system and subsequently differentiate into DCs to trigger adaptive immune responses.

Human pDC/IPCs were also reported to be isolated from human peripheral blood on the basis of their expression of immunoglobulin-like transcript receptor 3 (ILT3), but not ILT1 (21). Because these ILT3$^+$ILT1$^-$ cells respond to lipopolysaccharide (LPS) by producing large amounts of IL-12p70 (20), and because human pDC/IPCs do not express Toll-like receptor (TLR)-4 and do not respond to LPS (22–24), it is not clear whether these cells represent pDC/IPCs.

Identification of pDC/IPCs in Mice, Rat, Pig, and Monkey

In 2001, three groups identified and isolated mouse pDC/IPCs from lymphoid tissues as CD11c$^+$B220$^+$Gr-1$^+$CD45Rb^{high}CD11b$^-$ cells (25–27). Researchers also recently identified pDC/IPCs from monkey (28), pig (29, 29a), and rat (30).

ISOLATION AND CHARACTERIZATION OF HUMAN pDC/IPCs

Isolation of Human pDC/IPCs

At least three different methods have been developed to isolate pDC/IPCs from human blood and tonsils. These include (*a*) isolation of CD4$^+$CD11c$^-$Lin$^-$ (CD3, CD14, CD16, CD19, CD56) cells by three-color immunofluorescence cell sorting (6); (*b*) isolation of CD123^{high}HLA-DR$^+$Lin$^-$ cells by three-color immunofluorescence cell sorting (8); and (*c*) isolation of BDCA2$^+$ or BDCA4$^+$ cells by immunofluorescence cell sorting or magnetic bead cell sorting (31, 32). We prefer to isolate pDC/IPCs by using the first method (CD4$^+$CD11c$^-$Lin$^-$ cell sorting) because it gives high purity and does not appear to interfere with the function of pDC/IPCs. The second method (CD123^{high}HLA-DR$^+$Lin$^-$ cell sorting) may give rise to basophil contamination. Although BDCA2 is very specific for pDC/IPCs, anti-BDCA2 may inhibit pDC/IPC production of IFN-α. Many laboratories are currently using anti-BDCA4 magnetic bead isolation kits. Because BDCA4 is also expressed on a small fraction of CD11c$^+$ myeloid DCs (mDCs) and T cells (33), the third method does not give pure pDC/IPCs (34).

pDC/IPC Morphology

On Giemsa staining under light microscopy, human pDC/IPCs indeed look like plasma cells. They are slightly smaller than CD14$^+$ monocytes, but bigger than resting lymphocytes (Figure 1A). Whereas a monocyte displays a horseshoe-shaped nucleus (Figure 1B), a pDC/IPC displays an eccentric kidney-shaped nucleus (Figure 1B). And whereas monocytes have many vesicles in the cytoplasm, pDC/IPCs have a basophilic cytoplasm that contains a pale Golgi zone. By scanning

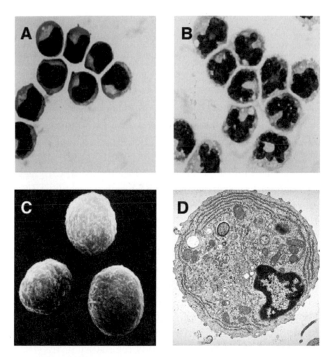

Figure 1   Morphology of pDCs/IPCs. (*A*) Giesma staining of pDCs/IPCs; (*B*) Giemsa staining of monocytes; (*C*) scanning EM of pDCs/IPCs; (*D*) transmission EM of pDCs/IPCs.

EM, pDC/IPCs display a smooth, round, lymphoid morphology and are 8–10 μm in diameter (Figure 1C). By transmission EM, pDC/IPCs display nuclei with marginal heterochromatin and cytoplasm containing well-developed rough endoplasmic reticulum, small Golgi apparatus, and many mitochondria (Figure 1D). Within the isolated mouse pDC/IPC population, only about 20% has plasmacytoid morphology under the EM (26).

Surface Phenotype of pDC/IPCs

Human pDC/IPCs do not express the lineage-specific markers for all the known cell types within the immune system, including surface and cytoplasmic immunoglobulin and CD19 (B cells), TCR and CD3 complexes (T cells), CD14 (monocytes), CD16 and CD56 (NK cells), and CD11c (myeloid DCs). Although pDC/IPCs were named plasmacytoid monocytes because of their expression of MHC class II and myeloid antigen such as CD68, pDC/IPCs do not express most of the antigens expressed on myeloid cells, such as CD11b, CD13, CD14, or CD33. They also do not express nonspecific esterase, and they lack phagocytic activity. These facts together suggest that pDC/IPCs belong to an independent cell lineage within the immune system. A summary of the phenotypic and functional characteristics of human and mouse DC subsets, including pDC/IPCs, is presented in Tables 1 and 2.

pDC/IPC DEVELOPMENT

The developmental path and molecular regulation of pDC/IPC are not fully understood. Today, FLT3L ligand is the only known cytokine that is critical for pDC/IPC development from hematopoietic stem cells (HSCs) in humans and mice (35–38). The ability of FLT3L to promote pDC/IPC development in vivo was confirmed by experiments showing that administration of FLT3L into human volunteers led to an increase in the number of peripheral blood pDC/IPC in humans (39), and that FLT3L-transgenic mice have increased numbers of pDC/IPC, whereas FLT3L-deficient mice have less pDC/IPC (38, 40).

The notion that pDCs are of lymphoid origin had been supported by findings that the gene transcripts of pre-T cell receptor α (pTα), λ5, Spi-B, as well as IgH D-J gene rearrangements could be found in pDCs, but not by mDCs (41, 42). Moreover, overexpression of the dominant-negative transcription factors Id2 or Id3 blocks development of pDC/IPC, T cells, and B cells, but not of myeloid DCs (mDCs) (43). However, more recent studies revealed that FLT3$^+$ cells within either common lymphoid progenitors (CLP) or common myeloid progenitors (CMP) could differentiate into both mDCs and pDCs in cultures and in vivo (44, 45). In addition, studies in mice deficient in IFN regulatory factor (IRF)-8, a critical transcriptional factor for the myeloid cell lineage (46), demonstrated that the generation of pDC/IPCs, CD8α^+ DCs, epidermal DCs, and dermal DCs were all impaired (47). As a result of these seemingly divergent findings, several different hypotheses

TABLE 1   Human peripheral blood DC and DC precursors

Phenotype	pDC/IPC	Monocytes	CD11c$^+$ immature DC
Myeloid marker			
CD11b	−	+	+
CD11c	−	+	+
CD13	−	+	+
CD14	−	+	−
CD33	−	+	+
Lymphoid marker			
Pre-Ta	+	−	−
Ig1-like 14.1	+	−	−
Spi-B	+	−	−
Pattern recognition receptors			
TLR1	+	++	+
TLR2	−	++	+
TLR3	−	−	++
TLR4	−	++	+
TLR5	−	+	+
TLR6	+	+	+
TLR7	++	−	−
TLR8	−	++	++
TLR9	++	−	−
TLR10	+	−	+
Mannose R	−	+/−	+/−
BDCA2	+	−	−
CD1a, b, c, d	−	+/−	+/−
Other differentially expressed antigens			
CD4	++	+	+
CD45RA	+	−	−
CD45RO	−	+	+
IL-3R	+++	+	+
GM-CSFR	+	++	++
Function			
IFN-α/β production	++++	+	+
IL-12 production	−	++	++
Phagocytosis	−	++	++

have been proposed regarding the developmental origin of pDCs, including the existence of a common DC precursor in blood that can give rise to all DC subsets (48), pDCs arising as a branch of the committed lymphoid lineage (6, 42) and lineage conversion (49).

A recent study by Akashi's group (50) shows that although CMP do not express RAG gene products and IgHD-J rearrangement, pDCs derived from CMP express

TABLE 2   Phenotype and function of mouse DC subsets

	CD8a$^+$CD4$^-$	CD8a$^-$CD4$^-$	CD8a$^-$CD4$^+$	IPCs
Phenotype				
CD8	+	−	−	+/−
CD11b	−	+	+	−
CD11c	+	+	+	+
CD4	−	+	+	+/−
B220	−	−	−	+
Ly6c	−	−	−	+
CD45RB	+	+	+	+++
DEC-205	+	+/−	−	−
Function				
IL-12	+++	−	−	+
IFN-γ	++	−	−	−
IFN-α	+	−	−	+++
Cross-priming of CD8 T cells	+	−	−	−

RAG gene products and show IgHD-J rearrangement. This study suggests that pDCs represent a very unique hematopoietic lineage, whose development may be much more flexible than both conventional lymphoid (B, T, NK) and myeloid (monocyte and granulocytes) cells.

LOCALIZATION, MIGRATION, AND LIFE SPAN OF pDC/IPCs

The identification of human pDC/IPCs in fetal liver, thymus, and bone marrow suggests that pDC/IPCs develop from HSCs within these primary lymphoid tissues (35). Transfer of CD34$^+$ hematopoietic progenitor cells into SCID mice leads to generation of human pDC/IPCs in mouse bone marrow and human thymic transplants (51–53). During adult life, pDC/IPCs appear to be produced constantly from bone marrow. Injection of FLT3L or granulocyte colony-stimulating factor (G-CSF) into healthy human volunteers leads to a significant increase in the number of peripheral blood pDC/IPCs (39). G-CSF may promote pDC/IPC immobilization from bone marrow. After leaving the bone marrow, pDC/IPCs appear to migrate into the T cell–rich areas of the secondary lymphoid tissues through HEV in lymph nodes (Figure 2) and mucosa-associated lymphoid tissues, as well as through marginal zones of the spleen under steady-state conditions (6, 21, 32, 54–57). This migration behavior is much like that of B and T lymphocytes. By contrast, monocytes and immature mDCs appear to migrate into nonlymphoid tissues and then migrate into the T cell–rich areas of secondary lymph nodes through afferent lymph upon activation (Figure 2). This unique migration property of pDC/IPCs appears to be associated with their expression of CD62L and

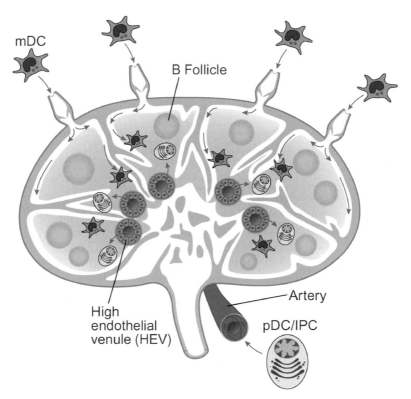

Figure 2   Migration pathways of pDC/IPCs versus myeloid DC (mDC) into a lymph node. pDC/IPC migrate into a lymph node through blood and high endothelial venules (HEV). mDC migrate into a lymph node through afferent lymphatics. Both pDC/IPC and mDC are localized in the T cell–rich areas.

CCR7, which interact sequentially with L-selectin ligands expressed by HEV and chemokines ELC/CCL19 and SLC/CCL21 expressed by HEV and stromal cells within the T cell–rich areas (57, 58). In mice, pDC/IPCs differentiate into a unique subset of CD8$^+$ DCs following viral infection (59, 60). The study of the kinetics of bromodeoxyuridine labeling and adoptive transfer experiments suggests that pDC/IPCs in mice have a relatively long average life span of about two weeks (59).

INNATE IMMUNE RESPONSE BY pDC/IPCs

pDC/IPCs Selectively Express Intracellular TLR7 and TLR9 that Respectively Recognize Single-Stranded RNA and Double-Stranded DNA

The remarkable functional plasticity of DCs at the precursor stage or immature stage has brought into question the existence of different DC subsets or lineages.

Within the immune system, evolutionary force drove the development of multiple subsets of B and T lymphocytes, which rapidly and efficiently respond to common microbial antigens. Unlike conventional B and T cells, B-1 B cells, $\gamma\delta$ T cells, and NKT cells express restricted and distinct antigen receptors, capable of recognizing common antigens derived from bacteria or damaged host cells, a phenomenon called by Klaus Rejewsky (61) "evolutionary immunological memory." We hypothesized that if separate DC lineages/subsets with specialized functions really exist, they might express different sets of Toll-like receptors (TLRs), the ancient microbial pattern recognition receptors highly conserved from *Drosophila* to humans (62–65). We and other investigators demonstrated that, whereas monocytes preferentially expressed TLR1, -2, -4, -5, -6, and -8, pDC/IPCs strongly expressed TLR7 and -9 (Table 1) (22–24, 66). In accordance with these TLR expression profiles, monocytes responded to the known microbial ligands for TLR2 (peptidoglycan, lipoteichoic acid) and TLR4 (LPS) by producing tumor necrosis factor (TNF)-α and IL-6. In contrast, pDC/IPCs produced large amounts of IFN-α in response to DNA virus and CpG oligodeoxynucleotides (CpG ODNs) (TLR9 ligand) or single-stranded viral RNA (TLR7 ligand) (22–24, 66–70). A recent study demonstrated that whereas monocytes and mDCs preferentially express bacteria-recognizing TLR2, -4, -5, and -6 on the cell surface, pDC/IPCs preferentially express virus-recognizing TLR7 and TLR9 within the intracellular endosomal compartments (71, 72) (Figure 3). Interestingly, CD11c$^+$ mDCs were found to express TLR3, suggesting CD11c$^+$ mDCs may play a critical role in recognizing dsRNA viruses. The remarkable differences among monocytes, CD11c$^+$ immature DC, and pDC/IPCs in their TLR repertoire expression and responsiveness to microbial antigens suggests that these myeloid-related DC/DC precursors and pDC/IPCs may have developed through different evolutionary trails to preferentially recognize bacteria and viruses respectively (Figure 3).

pDC/IPCs are Professional Type 1 IPCs

Upon activation with a virus, pDC/IPCs produce a huge amount of type 1 IFN (1–2 U/cell, or 3–10 pg/cell) within 24 h, which is 100 to 1000 times more than that produced by any other blood cell type (20). The type 1 IFN responses from pDC/IPCs have the following features (34, 73):

1. pDC/IPCs do not contain pre-existing mRNA transcripts for type 1 IFNs before viral stimulation.
2. Type 1 IFN mRNA can be detected in pDC/IPCs as early as 4 h following viral stimulation, and the level reaches its peak at 12 h.
3. From 6 to 12 h following viral stimulation, about 50% of total mRNA expressed by pDC/IPCs encodes for type 1 IFNs, including all types of IFN-α, IFN-β, IFN-ω, IFN-λ and IFN-τ (H. Kanzler, W. Cao & Y.-J. Liu, unpublished observation).

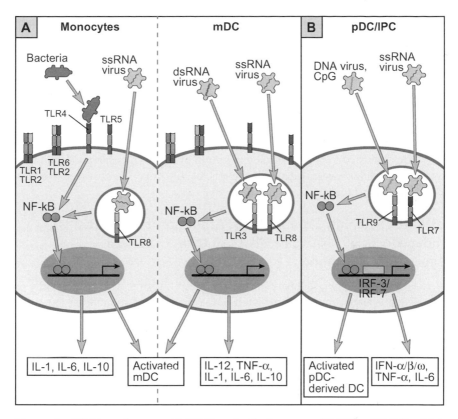

Figure 3 Within endosome, pDC/IPCs selectively express TLR7 and TLR9, which recognize single-stranded RNA and double-stranded DNA viruses, respectively (*right*). Signaling through TLR7 and TLR9 leads to activation of pDCs to secrete large amounts of type 1 IFN and to differentiate into mature DCs. Monocytes preferentially express TLR1, -2, -4, -5, and -6 that recognize different bacterial products. Signaling these TLRs leads to activation of monocytes to secrete TNF-α, IL-1, IL-6, and IL-10, and to differentiate into mature DCs (*left*). Similar to monocytes, mDCs express TLR1, -2, -4, -5, and -6. However, mDC but not monocytes express TLR3, which recognizes double-stranded RNA virus (*middle*). Signaling TLR3 leads to activation of mDCs to produce large amounts of IL-12, IL-1, and IL-6 and a small amount of type 1 IFN.

4. pDC/IPCs produce most IFN-α protein within the first 24 h following viral stimulation.

5. After the first 24 h of viral stimulation, pDC/IPCs make only moderate amounts of IFN-α, and these activated pDC/IPCs become refractory to secondary stimulation with the same virus or different virus (H. Kanzler, W. Cao & Y.-J. Liu, unpublished observation).

6. Human pDC/IPCs produce moderate amounts of TNF-α and IL-6, but not IL-1α, IL-1β, IL-3, IL-10, IL-12, IL-15, IL-18, IFN-γ, lymphotoxin-α, or granulocyte-macrophage colony-stimulating factor (GM-CSF) at protein levels following viral stimulation.

These data suggest that pDC/IPCs are dedicated to producing type 1 IFNs in antiviral innate immunity. The innate immune system has apparently evolved to have different cell types dedicated to fight against each of the three major microbes: bacteria, viruses, and parasites. Although monocyte/macrophages and neutrophils are dedicated to phagocytosis and killing of bacteria, eosinophils, and basophils, mast cells are dedicated to killing parasites. IPCs may have evolved to control viral infection (Figure 4).

pDC/IPCs Rapidly Produce Large Amounts of IFN-α that is Independent of Positive Feedback of IFN-β Through Type 1 IFN Receptors

The molecular mechanisms underlying the ability of pDC/IPCs to rapidly produce such a large amount of type I IFN following viral stimulation are still poorly understood. The molecular regulation of IFN-α production has been extensively studied in fibroblasts, and a positive feedback model was proposed (74). Upon viral infection, transcriptional factor IRF-3 is phosphorylated and translocated into the nucleus, where it activates IFN-β gene transcription. IFN-β secreted by

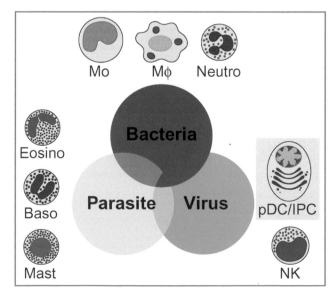

Figure 4   The innate immune system has dedicated cell types to control infections by three major microbes.

the virus-infected cells activates Jak/Stat signaling pathways, leading to formation of both ISGF3 transcriptional complexes, which in turn activates the transcription of IRF-7. The de novo synthesis of IRF-7 strongly activates the transcription of IFN-α and IFN-β genes. The rapid and robust transcription of both IFN-α and IFN-β genes and production of IFN-α and IFN-β proteins by pDC/IPCs following viral stimulation suggests that the regulation of IFN-α production in pDC/IPCs may not be mediated by the positive feedback effect of IFN-β. This hypothesis is supported by the finding that, unlike fibroblasts, pDC/IPCs express high IRF-7 constitutively, which may contribute partly to the extraordinary ability of pDC/IPCs to rapidly produce a huge amount of IFN-α without the autocrine IFN-β feedback mechanism (75–78). This hypothesis was directly tested in a study that used type 1 IFN receptor–deficient mice; fibroblasts derived from these mice produced much less IFN-α than fibroblasts derived from the wild-type mice. However, pDC/IPCs derived from both type 1 IFN receptor–deficient mice and wild-type mice produced similar amounts of IFN-α in response to vesicular stomatitis virus, suggesting that the ability of pDC/IPCs to produce large amounts of IFN-α is independent of the positive feedback regulation through the type 1 IFN receptors (79).

Human pDC/IPCs Have a Limited Ability to Produce IL-12

There have been considerable debates on whether pDC/IPCs can produce large amounts of IL-12, like mDCs. Our previous studies showed that pDC/IPCs (20,000 cells), freshly isolated on the basis of the CD4$^+$CD11c$^-$Lin$^-$ phenotype, produced low to undetectable amounts (less than 10 pg/ml) of IL-12 p70 following activation with HSV or CpG ODN AAC-30 (22). By contrast, Cella et al. (21) showed that pDC/IPCs (10,000 cells) isolated on the basis of the ILT3$^+$ILT1$^-$ phenotype produced high levels of IL-12 p70 in response to LPS (808 pg/ml) and to CD40L (2100 pg/ml). Krug et al. (23) showed that pDC/IPCs (100,000 cells) isolated by magnetic beads on the basis of BDCA4 expression did not produce significant amounts of IL-12 p70 in response to LPS alone, CpG ODN alone, or CD40L alone, but produced high levels of IL-12 p70 (more than 6000 pg/ml) in response to a combination of CD40L and B-type CpG ODN-2006. These two observations challenge the concept that specialized cells are the main producers of either type 1 IFNs or IL-12. The following evidence suggests that the observations by Cella et al. (21) and Krug et al. (23) that human pDC/IPCs produced large amounts of IL-12 p70 following activation were due mainly to mDC in their experiments.

1. The conclusion that human pDC/IPCs isolated on the basis of ILT3$^+$ILT1$^-$ produce large amounts of IL-12 p70 (808 pg/ml) in response to LPS is incorrect (21) because the pDC/IPCs did not express LPS receptor TLR4 (22–24, 66).

2. The finding that human pDC/IPCs isolated on the basis of ILT3$^+$ILT1$^-$ produce large amounts of IL-12 p70 (2100 pg/ml) in response to CD40L alone (21) was not confirmed by other studies (22, 23, 34, 80, 81).

3. Krug et al. (23) used positive magnetic bead selection of BDCA4-expressing cells to purify human pDC/IPCs. First, it is very difficult to achieve high purity of pDC/IPCs (over 99%) by magnetic bead selection. Second, BDCA4, also known as neuropilin-1, is expressed by monocyte-derived DCs, activated CD11c$^+$ mDCs, and a subpopulation of CD3$^+$CD57$^+$ T cells (33). Therefore, human pDC/IPCs isolated by magnetic bead selection of BDCA4$^+$ cells may contain mDCs.

4. We have recently isolated BDCA4$^+$ cells according to the methods described by Krug et al. (23). These cells were activated by CD40L plus A-type CpG ODN-2216, B-type CpG ODN-2006, or C-type CpG ODN-C274. At 6 h, 8 h, and 10 h after stimulation, intracellular expression of IFN-α and IL-12 p70 by activated BDCA4 cells was analyzed by three-color immunofluorescence flow cytometry. We found that cells producing IL-12 p70 were mainly the contaminating CD11c$^+$ mDCs, but not CD11c$^-$ pDC/IPCs. No cells produced both IFN-α and IL-12 p70, thus confirming the result of a recent study by Duramad et al. (82).

A more direct demonstration that mDCs and pDC/IPCs have specialized functions in producing IL-12 versus type 1 IFN, respectively, came from a study using a molecule called R848, which triggers TLR8 on mDCs and TLR7 on pDC/IPCs. This study showed that, whereas mDCs preferentially produced IL-12 in response to R848, pDC/IPCs produced IFN-α (83). This finding further supports the concept that pDC/IPCs are specialized to produce IFN-α, but not IL-12, in response to microbial stimulation.

Findings of recent studies suggest that, unlike human pDC/IPCs, mouse pDC/IPCs have the capacity to produce both IFN-α and IL-12 (25–27). This may indeed represent the species difference between human and mouse pDC/IPC. Mouse and human pDC/IPCs also have some significant differences in surface phenotype, in particular the expression of TLRs (84, 85).

Myeloid DCs are Specialized in Producing IL-12, but not Type 1 IFNs

All nucleated cells, including mDCs, have the capacity to produce type 1 IFNs when stimulated or infected by an appropriate virus through a universal PKR-mediated pathway. The uniqueness of pDC/IPCs is that they are able to produce more type 1 IFN than any other cell types and to dedicate 50% of their transcription to making type 1 IFN mRNAs following viral infection (20, 34). The concept that there is a specialized cell type that is dedicated to producing type 1 IFNs during viral infection was recently questioned by a study in mice showing that CD11c^{high} mDCs produced as much IFN-α as pDC/IPCs when high doses of naked synthetic poly I:C were electroporated into the cells (86). We have reexamined the production of IFN-α by human pDC/IPCs, CD11c$^+$ mDCs, and monocyte-derived DCs isolated from the same donor in response to seven different TLR ligands alone, or in combination with CD40L, and four different viruses (HSV, influenza virus,

Saidai virus, HIV) (T. Ito & Y.-J. Liu, manuscript in preparation). We found that the maximal IFN-α production by pDC/IPCs is at least 70 times more than the maximal IFN-α produced by mDCs in response to any of the just described stimuli. By contrast, the maximal amount of IL-12 p70 produced by mDCs is at least 10 times more than the maximal amounts of IL-12 p70 produced by pDC/IPCs in response to any of these stimuli (34). These data further support the concept that pDC/IPCs are professional IPCs and are evolved to become the key effector cells in antiviral innate immunity. Obviously, pDC/IPCs may not be responsible for the innate immune responses to all types of viruses because pDC/IPCs do not express TLR3 to recognize dsRNA viruses, and some viruses may develop the immunoinvasion mechanisms.

REGULATION OF T CELL–MEDIATED IMMUNE RESPONSES BY pDC/IPCs

pDC/IPC Differentiation to Mature DCs Through Two Pathways

pDC/IPCs express low levels of MHC class II and low to undetectable levels of CD80 and CD86, and pDC/IPCs are incapable of stimulating significant antigen-specific T cell proliferation. In vitro studies suggest that pDC/IPCs have two pathways to differentiate into mature DCs and acquire the capacity to directly talk to T cells: (*a*) the IL-3-dependent pathway, in which human pDC/IPCs express strikingly high levels of IL-3 receptors (8, 80) and differentiate into DCs in culture with IL-3 or IL-3 plus CD40L (6, 8); and (*b*) the IFN-α- and TNF-α-dependent pathway, in which pDC/IPCs express TLR7 and TLR9. Signaling through TLR7 and TLR9 by viruses or by synthetic CpG ODN stimulates pDC/IPCs to produce IFN-α and TNF-α, two cytokines that induce pDC/IPCs to differentiate into DCs (73). Whereas pDC-derived mature DCs induced by IL-3 and CD40L preferentially prime naive CD4$^+$ T cells to produce IL-4, IL-5, and IL-10 (80), pDC-derived mature DCs induced by virus preferentially prime naive CD4$^+$ T cells to produce IFN-γ and IL-10 (73). These studies suggest that, like immature mDCs, pDCs also display functional plasticity in terms of priming different effector T cell responses, depending on the type of maturation signals (Figure 5A). The biological significance of pDC/IPC differentiation into DCs in the presence of IL-3 is unknown. Investigators (73) have proposed that IL-3 may be produced by basophils, eosinophils, and mast cells during parasite infection, and pDC/IPC-derived DCs may play a role triggering antiparasite adaptive T helper 2 (Th2) immune responses. Two recent studies in mice (59, 60) demonstrate that pDC/IPCs indeed differentiate into DCs following viral infection in vivo. These studies indicate that IPCs represent a unique cell lineage within the immune system, which first plays a critical role as effector cells in antimicrobial innate immune responses and subsequently differentiates into professional antigen-presenting cells to initiate adaptive immune responses (84) (Figure 5A).

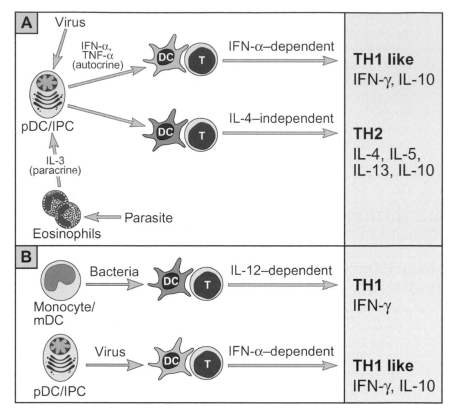

Figure 5 (*A*) Functional plasticity of pDC/IPC-derived DCs. Upon viral infection, pDCs differentiate into DCs mediated by autocrine IFN-α and TNF-α, which prime naive CD4$^+$ T cells to produce IFN-γ and IL-10. Upon parasite infection, pDCs differentiate into DCs mediated by paracrine IL-3 released by mast cells, eosinophils, and basophils, which prime naive CD4$^+$ T cells to produce Th2 cytokines IL-4, -5, -10, and -13. (*B*) Two distinct antigen-presenting cell systems in humans have the capacity to prime naive CD4$^+$ T cells to produce IFN-γ: Bacteria-activated mDC mainly use IL-12, whereas viral-induced pDC-derived DC use type 1 IFN.

pDC-Derived DCs Induce Th1 by IFN-α but not IL-12

pDC/IPCs rapidly produce huge amounts of type 1 IFNs (50,000 to 100,000 pg/ml) within the first 24 h after viral stimulation. Within the following 48 to 72 h, activated pDC/IPCs undergo differentiation into mature DCs, which express high levels of MHC class I and class II and costimulatory molecules CD80 and CD86, and pDC-derived mature DCs produce lower but significant amounts of type 1 IFNs (1000 to 5000 pg/ml). The virus-induced pDC-derived DCs induce human naive CD4$^+$ allogeneic T cells to undergo strong proliferation and differentiation into IFN-γ- and

IL-10-producing cells (73). Interestingly, the ability of virus-induced pDC-derived DCs to induce naive CD4$^+$ T cells to produce IFN-γ is dependent on type 1 IFN, but independent of IL-12 (73). The results of this study suggest that there are two distinct antigen-presenting cell systems in humans that have the capacity to prime naive CD4$^+$ T cells to produce IFN-γ: Bacteria-activated mDCs mainly use IL-12, whereas viral-induced pDC-derived DCs use type 1 IFN (Figure 5B).

pDC-Derived DCs Induce Th2 through OX40L

Previous studies showed that human pDC-derived DCs induced by IL-3 preferentially prime Th2 responses (73, 80, 87). A recent study demonstrated that pDC-derived DCs induced by IL-3 express high levels of surface OX40L, and neutralizing monoclonal antibody to OX40L significantly inhibited the ability of pDC-derived DCs to prime naive CD4$^+$ T cells to produce Th2 cytokines, including IL-4, IL-5, and IL-13 (34).

pDC-Derived DCs and their Ability to Prime Naive
Versus Memory T Cells

It is unclear whether pDC-derived DCs can directly prime naive T cells. Two recent studies in mice suggest that mouse pDC-derived DCs induced by CpG ODN-1826 fail to induce antigen-specific naive T cell responses but that they can induce antigen-specific memory recall responses in vivo (60, 88). During influenza viral infection, however, pDC-derived DCs appear able to prime virus-specific primary and secondary CD4$^+$ and CD8$^+$ T cell immune responses in vitro and in vivo (60, 89). CpG ODN-1826 may be less potent than influenza virus in activating pDCs.

pDC-Derived DCs and Presentation of Endogenous
and Exogenous Antigens

Unlike mDCs, pDCs are poor in phagocytosis and macropinocytosis (6). A recent study demonstrated that pDC-derived DCs induced by CpG ODN were capable of priming CD8$^+$ T cell responses to endogenous antigens or peptides, but not those to exogenous antigens (90). This finding, together with the previous findings that pDCs selectively express intracellular TLR7 and TLR9 and are poor in phagocytosis and pinocytosis, suggests that pDC and pDC-derived DCs may be more specialized in presenting viral antigens and endogenous self-antigens.

pDc/IPC and Cross-Priming

Although pDCs have the capacity to process and present viral antigen after viral infection, their ability to cross-present exogenous antigens appears to be limited. Previous studies demonstrated that the CD8$^+$ DC subset is the major antigen-presenting cell that has the capacity to cross-present exogenous antigens to CD8$^+$ T cells (91, 92). A recent study showed that the ability of mDCs to cross-prime

CD8$^+$ T cells during viral infection depends on type 1 IFN (93). Because pDC/IPCs represent the major producer of type 1 IFNs during viral infection, it is highly likely that pDCs can promote the ability of mDCs to cross-prime CD8$^+$ T cell responses to exogenous antigens.

pDc/IPCs and Regulatory T Cells

Freshly isolated resting pDC/IPCs express low levels of MHC class I, class II, and CD86 and no detectable level of CD80. Although resting pDC/IPCs do not have the capacity to induce strong T cell proliferation, they appear to prime naive CD4$^+$ T cells to differentiate into IL-10-producing Tr1 cells in cultures in both humans (94) and mice (95, 96). In contrast to mDCs, the pDC/IPC's ability to prime T cells to produce IL-10 is maintained even after differentiation into mature activated DCs. IL-3- and CD40-activated pDC-derived DCs prime naive CD4$^+$ T cells to Th2 (producing IL-4, IL-5, and IL-10) (34, 80, 87) and naive CD8$^+$ T cells to CD8$^+$ T suppressor cells (producing IL-10) (81). Virus-induced pDC-derived DCs prime naive T cells to produce IFN-γ and IL-10 (73). These studies suggest that pDC-derived DCs have an intrinsic ability to prime naive T cells to produce IL-10, regardless of their maturation stages and activation signals. In addition, CpG-ODN-induced pDC-derived DCs were shown to induce the generation of CD4$^+$CD25$^+$ Tr cells in vitro (73a). Results of two recent studies suggest that pDC/IPCs may indeed play a critical role in suppressing asthmatic immune responses to inhaled antigens (97), or in suppressing immune responses that mediate *Leishmania major* infection in mice (98). We hypothesize that pDC/IPCs may represent naturally occurring regulatory DCs when directly presenting antigens to T cells, either at a resting stage or at a mature DC stage. pDC/IPCs may trigger productive T cell–mediated immune responses through activation of mDCs (see next section).

pDC/IPCs REGULATE THE FUNCTION OF CONVENTIONAL MYELOID DC BY TYPE 1 IFN

The possible cross-talk between pDCs and mDCs and the ability of pDC/IPCs to induce a productive, adaptive, T cell–mediated immune response through activating mDCs were suggested in three different types of studies. pDC/IPCs in systemic lupus erythematosus (SLE) patients appear to be constantly activated through TLR9 by self-chromatin-antichromatin antibody complexes to produce type 1 IFNs (99–101). Type 1 IFNs within the sera of SLE patients strongly activate monocytes and immature mDCs, which subsequently induce strong Th1-mediated immune responses (102, 103). A recent study (89) showed that human pDC/IPCs could induce a bystander maturation of mDCs in response to HIV infection in vitro by producing type 1 IFN and TNF-α. During immune responses to double-stranded RNA or viral infection in mice, mDCs fail to undergo maturation in the absence of type 1 IFN receptors (104, 105). The exposure to type 1 IFN at immature stages of mDCs lead to their activation and enhanced production of IL-12, IL-15, IL-18, and IL-23 (87, 106–110).

Together, the above studies suggest that during a viral infection, pDC/IPCs are activated to produce large amounts of type 1 IFNs within the first 24 h. These type 1 IFNs not only have immediate antiviral effects but also strongly activate viral-infected monocytes and mDCs to present viral antigens to T cells, which subsequently induce strong T cell–mediated antiviral responses (Figure 6).

After a productive antiviral adaptive immune response is established, pDC/IPCs or pDC-derived DCs appear to have several strategies to contract the effector phase and at the same time enhance the memory phase of an immune response (Figure 7): (*a*) At a late stage of an immune response, pDC-derived DCs may prime naive T cells to produce IL-10 (37, 73, 80); (*b*) type 1 IFN may directly act on mature mDCs to inhibit their ability to produce IL-12 (110, 111); (*c*) type 1 IFN may directly prime both mDCs and T cells to produce IL-10 (112–114); and (*d*) type 1 IFN contributes to the maintenance of memory T cells (115, 116). The ability of type 1 IFN to inhibit IL-12 production by mature DCs and to prime mDCs and T cells to produce IL-10 may offer a partial explanation for the therapeutic window allowing IFN-β to be an effective treatment for multiple sclerosis.

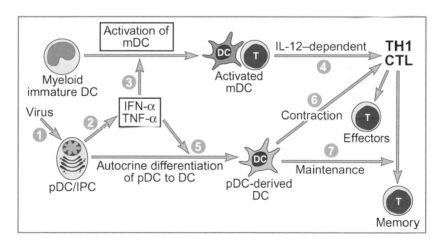

Figure 6 pDC/IPCs regulate the function of mDC. Viral infection (1) induces pDC/IPCs to produce type 1 IFN and TNF-α (2), which then activate monocytes or mDCs (3) to upregulate costimulatory molecules and secrete IL-12; the activated mDCs induce strong Th1 and cytotoxic T lymphocyte responses (4); pDC/IPCs differentiate into mature DCs by autocrine IFN-α and TNF-α (5); pDC-derived DCs prime naive T cells to produce IL-10, which may contribute to the contraction of the effector phase of T cell responses (6); pDC-derived DCs may also enhance the generation and maintenance of memory T cells through type 1 IFN and other mechanisms (7).

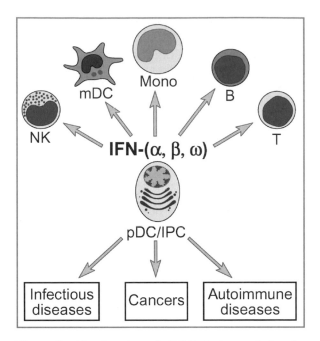

Figure 7 The function of pDC/IPCs in regulating the functions of other immune cells and in the control and pathogenesis of human diseases.

REGULATION OF NK CELL FUNCTION BY pDC/IPCs

Historically, investigators (14, 117, 118) have shown that NK cell activation during viral infection depends on the presence of a population of HLA-DR$^+$ accessory cells (now known as pDC/IPCs). The importance of IPCs in induced NK cell activation was directly demonstrated by using highly purified pDC/IPCs and NK cells (104). Previous studies (119, 120) suggested that CpG ODN directly activates NK cells. However, highly purified NK cells are not activated by CpG (121, 122). This is consistent with the finding that NK cells do not express TLR9 (36, 122). In collaboration with Dr. W. Chen, we have recently demonstrated that NK cells isolated by the most commonly used methods all contain 1%–2% pDC/IPCs (36). When these contaminating pDC/IPCs are depleted by monoclonal antibody BDCA2 or BDCA4 from NK cell preparation, CpG ODN fails to activate NK cells.

REGULATION OF B CELL FUNCTION BY pDC/IPCs

Jego et al. (123) recently showed that, when total peripheral blood mononuclear cells from a donor vaccinated with influenza vaccine were cultured with influenza virus, large amounts of virus-specific polyclonal IgG antibodies were induced. This in vitro virus-specific antibody response could be completely abolished by depleting pDC/IPCs from total blood mononuclear cells. This study further showed that two cytokines secreted by virus-activated pDC/IPCs, IFN-α and IL-6 (73), acted sequentially to drive virus-specific B cells to differentiate into plasma blasts and then mature plasma cells (123).

pDC/IPCs AND HUMAN DISEASES

HIV

The expression of CD4, CXCR4, and CCR5 by human pDC/IPCs suggests that they may be the targets of HIV infection (6, 58). Immunohistochemical staining of tonsils and thymus from HIV-infected individuals reveals the presence of HIV p24$^+$ pDC/IPCs, indicating that pDC/IPCs are productively infected by HIV virus (124, 125). Earlier studies showed that peripheral blood mononuclear cells from patients with AIDS had a decreased ability to produce IFN-α in response to HSV stimulation (126, 127). Recent studies demonstrate that peripheral blood pDC/IPC numbers are decreased in advanced stages of HIV infection (128–131). Loss of circulating pDC/IPCs correlated with a high HIV viral load and the occurrence of opportunistic infections and Kaposi sarcoma (128).

Systemic Lupus Erythematosus (SLE)

A link between IFN-α and human SLE was originally made by two clinical observations: (*a*) the development of SLE during IFN-α therapy in a 23-year-old woman with a metastatic carcinoma (132), and (*b*) the finding in many SLE patients of increased serum levels of type 1 IFNs (133–135). The numbers of circulating pDC/IPCs are decreased in patients with SLE, but large numbers of activated pDC/IPCs infiltrate the skin lesions and actively produce type 1 IFN in these patients (101, 136, 137). pDC/IPCs appear to be activated by immune complexes consisting of antidouble-stranded DNA antibodies and DNA derived from apoptotic cells (138). The high levels of IFN-α in the sera of SLE patients were found to activate mDCs to trigger T cell–mediated autoimmunity (102), as well as to promote differentiation of B cells into antibody-secreting plasma cells (123). Recent studies demonstrate that the expression of type 1 IFN genes and IFN-induced genes represent the most striking molecular signatures of SLE peripheral blood cells (139–142). Type 1 IFNs may represent the most important effector molecules in SLE pathology, as well as targets for treating SLE.

Cancer

Both immature mDCs and pDC/IPCs infiltrate solid tumors (143–145). Tumor-infiltrating immature mDCs appear to be refractory to stimulation by LPS or CD40L and lack the ability to activate T cells (144, 146). These tumor-infiltrating immature mDCs likely present tumor antigens continuously and induce tumor-specific regulatory T cells (147, 148). In breast cancer, high numbers of infiltrating CD123$^+$ pDC/IPCs are correlated with an increased risk of tumor dissemination and relapse (149). In ovarian epithelial cell carcinomas, large numbers of pDC/IPCs were found in ascitic fluids. These pDC/IPCs were incapable of activating T cells and instead induced IL-10-producing regulatory T cells (150). A recent study suggests that pDC/IPCs within the tumor draining lymph nodes may express indoleamine 2,3-dioxygenase (IDO), which may create a local microenvironment that is potently suppressive of host anti-tumor T cell responses (151). These findings suggest that both immature mDCs and pDC/IPCs within the solid tumor are incapable of inducing antitumor immune responses but instead may induce regulatory T cells that inhibit antitumor immunity. In a mouse tumor model, Vicari et al. (144) showed that CpG ODN plus anti-IL-10 neutralizing mAb could activate the tumor-infiltrating DCs to induce robust antitumor cytotoxic T cell responses and tumor rejection in vivo. Because pDC/IPCs are the major cell type expressing TLR9, this study suggests that CpG ODN may activate tumor-infiltrating pDC/IPC to produce type 1 IFN and TNF-α, which then activate tumor-infiltrating immature mDCs to induce antitumor T cell responses. Targeting pDC/IPCs by CpG ODN to activate the adjacent tumor-infiltrating mDCs may represent a promising strategy for developing cancer vaccines.

CONCLUSION

pDC/IPCs represent a separate hematopoietic lineage, which appears to be closer to B lineage than to myeloid lineage. These cells are continuously produced from HSC within the bone marrow and then released into the peripheral blood stream. Unlike myeloid cells that enter the secondary lymphoid nodes from afferent lymphatics, pDC/IPCs enter the lymph nodes through HEV (like the T and B lymphocytes) and then colonize the T cell–rich areas. Under steady state, pDC/IPCs appear to play a critical role in maintaining peripheral immune tolerance. This may be due to the ability of resting pDC/IPCs to prime naive T cells to produce IL-10. Unlike monocytes and mDCs that preferentially express TLR2, -4, -5, and -6, pDC/IPCs express TLR7 and -9 within the endosomal compartment. Upon viral infection, pDC/IPCs rapidly produce large amounts of type 1 IFNs, which not only have direct inhibitory effects on viral replication but also contribute to the activation of NK cells, B cells, T cells, and mDCs, leading to the induction and expansion of an antiviral immune response (Figure 7). The ability of activated pDC/IPCs to activate myeloid immature DC through type 1 IFN appears to be critical for the induction of T cell–mediated antiviral immunity. After producing large amounts of type 1 IFN, pDC/IPCs rapidly differentiate into mature DCs through an autocrine mechanism mediated by type 1 IFNs and TNF-α. At this stage, pDC/IPC-derived DCs may contribute to the contraction of the effector phase of T cell responses and at the same time to the establishment of T cell memory.

Several fascinating questions will challenge us during the next few years, including the following: (*a*) What regulates pDC/IPC development from stem cells, and how and when is pDC/IPC development separated from B cell development? (*b*) What regulates the rapid and massive type I IFN production? (*c*) Are there

IFN-independent pathways by which pDC/IPCs regulate the function of other immune cells? and (*d*) How can we harness pDC/IPC biology to develop immunotherapy for viral infectious diseases, cancer, and autoimmune diseases?

ACKNOWLEDGMENTS

The author thanks the past and present members of the laboratory for their contribution to the discovery and characterization of pDC/IPCs; Drs. X.F. Qin, W. Cao, T. Ito, and Y.H. Wang for their comments on the manuscript; Mrs. Misty Hajek for her invaluable assistance in preparing this manuscript; and Drs. J. Banchereau, F. Siegal, J. Levy, and W. Chen for collaboration. This work is supported by the University of Texas M.D. Anderson Cancer Center and the National Institutes of Health.

The *Annual Review of Immunology* is online at
http://immunol.annualreviews.org

LITERATURE CITED

1. Lennert K, Remmele W. 1958. Karyometric research on lymph node cells in man. I. Germinoblasts, lymphoblasts and lymphocytes. *Acta Haematol.* 19:99–113 (In German)

2. Feller AC, Lennert K, Stein H, Bruhn HD, Wuthe HH. 1983. Immunohistology and aetiology of histiocytic necrotizing lymphadenitis. Report of three instructive cases. *Histopathology* 7:825–39

3. Facchetti F, de Wolf-Peeters C, Mason DY, Pulford K, van den Oord JJ, Desmet VJ. 1988. Plasmacytoid T cells. Immunohistochemical evidence for their monocyte/macrophage origin. *Am. J. Pathol.* 133:15–21

4. Grouard G, Durand I, Filgueira L, Banchereau J, Liu YJ. 1996. Dendritic cells capable of stimulating T cells in germinal centres. *Nature* 384:364–67

5. Dubois B, Barthelemy C, Durand I, Liu YJ, Caux C, Briere F. 1999. Toward a role of dendritic cells in the germinal center reaction: triggering of B cell proliferation and isotype switching. *J. Immunol.* 162:3428–36

6. Grouard G, Rissoan MC, Filgueira L, Durand I, Banchereau J, Liu YJ. 1997. The enigmatic plasmacytoid T cells develop into dendritic cells with interleukin (IL)-3 and CD40-ligand. *J. Exp. Med.* 185:1101–11

7. O'Doherty U, Peng M, Gezelter S, Swiggard WJ, Betjes M, et al. 1994. Human blood contains two subsets of dendritic cells, one immunologically mature and the other immature. *Immunology* 82:487–93

8. Olweus J, BitMansour A, Warnke R, Thompson PA, Carballido J, Picker LJ, et al. 1997. Dendritic cell ontogeny: a human dendritic cell lineage of myeloid origin. *Proc. Natl. Acad. Sci. USA* 94:12551–56

9. Timonen T, Saksela E, Virtanen J, Cantell K. 1980. Natural killer cells are responsible for the interferon production induced in human lymphocytes by tumor cell contact. *Eur. J. Immunol.* 10:422–27

10. Djeu JY, Stocks N, Zoon K, Stanton GJ, Timonen T, Herberman RB. 1982. Positive self regulation of cytotoxicity in human natural killer cells by production of interferon upon exposure to influenza and

herpes viruses. *J. Exp. Med.* 156:1222–34

11. Yamaguchi T, Handa K, Shimizu Y, Abo T, Kumagai K. 1977. Target cells for interferon production in human leukocytes stimulated by Sendai virus. *J. Immunol.* 118:1931–35

12. Peter HH, Dallugge H, Zawatzky R, Euler S, Leibold W, Kirchner H. 1980. Human peripheral null lymphocytes. II. Producers of type-1 interferon upon stimulation with tumor cells, Herpes simplex virus and Corynebacterium parvum. *Eur. J. Immunol.* 10:547–55

13. Abb J, Abb H, Deinhardt F. 1983. Phenotype of human α-interferon producing leucocytes identified by monoclonal antibodies. *Clin. Exp. Immunol.* 52:179–84

14. Perussia B, Fanning V, Trinchieri G. 1985. A leukocyte subset bearing HLA-DR antigens is responsible for in vitro α interferon production in response to viruses. *Nat. Immun. Cell Growth Regul.* 4:120–37

15. Ferbas JJ, Toso JF, Logar AJ, Navratil JS, Rinaldo CR Jr. 1994. CD4$^+$ blood dendritic cells are potent producers of IFN-α in response to in vitro HIV-1 infection. *J. Immunol.* 152:4649–62

16. Chehimi J, Starr SE, Kawashima H, Miller DS, Trinchieri G, et al. 1989. Dendritic cells and IFN-α-producing cells are two functionally distinct non-B, non-monocytic HLA-DR$^+$ cell subsets in human peripheral blood. *Immunology* 68:488–90

17. Fitzgerald-Bocarsly P. 1993. Human natural interferon-α producing cells. *Pharmacol. Ther.* 60:39–62

18. Svensson H, Johannisson A, Nikkila T, Alm GV, Cederblad B. 1996. The cell surface phenotype of human natural interferon-α producing cells as determined by flow cytometry. *Scand. J. Immunol.* 44:164–72

19. Siegal FP, Kadowaki N, Shodell M, Liu YJ. 1998. Evidence for identity of the (natural) interferon (IFN) producing cell (NIPC) and the CD11c- precursor of DC2. *J. Leukoc. Biol.* 2(Suppl.):18

20. Siegal FP, Kadowaki N, Shodell M, Fitzgerald-Bocarsly PA, Shah K, et al. 1999. The nature of the principal type 1 interferon-producing cells in human blood. *Science* 284:1835–37

21. Cella M, Jarrossay D, Facchetti F, Alebardi O, Nakajima H, et al. 1999. Plasmacytoid monocytes migrate to inflamed lymph nodes and produce large amounts of type I interferon. *Nat. Med.* 5:919–23

22. Kadowaki N, Ho S, Antonenko S, Malefyt RW, Kastelein RA, et al. 2001. Subsets of human dendritic cell precursors express different Toll-like receptors and respond to different microbial antigens. *J. Exp. Med.* 194:863–69

23. Krug A, Towarowski A, Britsch S, Rothenfusser S, Hornung V, et al. 2001. Toll-like receptor expression reveals CpG DNA as a unique microbial stimulus for plasmacytoid dendritic cells which synergizes with CD40 ligand to induce high amounts of IL-12. *Eur. J. Immunol.* 31:3026–37

24. Jarrossay D, Napolitani G, Colonna M, Sallusto F, Lanzavecchia A. 2001. Specialization and complementarity in microbial molecule recognition by human myeloid and plasmacytoid dendritic cells. *Eur. J. Immunol.* 31:3388–93

25. Nakano H, Yanagita M, Gunn MD. 2001. CD11c$^+$B220$^+$Gr-1$^+$ cells in mouse lymph nodes and spleen display characteristics of plasmacytoid dendritic cells. *J. Exp. Med.* 194:1171–78

26. Asselin-Paturel C, Boonstra A, Dalod M, Durand I, Yessaad N, et al. 2001. Mouse type I IFN-producing cells are immature APCs with plasmacytoid morphology. *Nat. Immunol.* 2:1144–50

27. Bjorck P. 2001. Isolation and characterization of plasmacytoid dendritic cells from Flt3 ligand and granulocyte-macrophage colony-stimulating factor-treated mice. *Blood* 98:3520–26

28. Coates PT, Barratt-Boyes SM, Zhang L, Donnenberg VS, O'Connell PJ, et al. 2003. Dendritic cell subsets in blood and lymphoid tissue of rhesus monkeys and their mobilization with Flt3 ligand. *Blood* 102:2513–21

29. Guzylack-Piriou L, Balmelli C, McCullough KC, Summerfield A. 2004. Type-A CpG oligonucleotides activate exclusively porcine natural interferon-producing cells to secrete interferon-α, tumour necrosis factor-α and interleukin-12. *Immunology* 112:28–37

29a. Domeika K, Magnusson M, Eloranta ML, Fuxler L, Alm GV, Fossum C. 2004. Characteristics of oligodeoxyribonucleotides that induce interferon (IFN)-α in the pig and the phenotype of the IFN-α producing cells. *Vet. Immunol. Immunopathol.* 101:87–102

30. Hubert FX, Voisine C, Louvet C, Heslan M, Josien R. 2004. Rat plasmacytoid dendritic cells are an abundant subset of MHC class II+ CD4+CD11b⁻OX62⁻ and type 1 IFN-producing cells that exhibit selective expression of Toll-like receptors 7 and 9 and strong responsiveness to CpG. *J. Immunol.* 172:7485–94

31. Dzionek A, Fuchs A, Schmidt P, Cremer S, Zysk M, et al. 2000. BDCA-2, BDCA-3, and BDCA-4: three markers for distinct subsets of dendritic cells in human peripheral blood. *J. Immunol.* 165:6037–46

32. Dzionek A, Sohma Y, Nagafune J, Cella M, Colonna M, et al. 2001. BDCA-2, a novel plasmacytoid dendritic cell-specific type II C-type lectin, mediates antigen capture and is a potent inhibitor of interferon α/β induction. *J. Exp. Med.* 194:1823–34

33. Dzionek A, Inagaki Y, Okawa K, Nagafune J, Rock J, et al. 2002. Plasmacytoid dendritic cells: from specific surface markers to specific cellular functions. *Hum. Immunol.* 63:1133–48

34. Ito T, Amakawa R, Inaba M, Hori T, Ota M, et al. 2004. Plasmacytoid dendritic cells regulate Th cell responses through OX40 ligand and type I IFNs. *J. Immunol.* 172:4253–59

35. Blom B, Ho S, Antonenko S, Liu YJ. 2000. Generation of interferon α-producing predendritic cell (Pre-DC)2 from human CD34+ hematopoietic stem cells. *J. Exp. Med.* 192:1785–96

36. Chen W, Antonenko S, Sederstrom JM, Liang X, Chan AS, et al. 2004. Thrombopoietin cooperates with FLT3-ligand in the generation of plasmacytoid dendritic cell precursors from human hematopoietic progenitors. *Blood* 103:2547–53

37. Gilliet M, Boonstra A, Paturel C, Antonenko S, Xu XL, et al. 2002. The development of murine plasmacytoid dendritic cell precursors is differentially regulated by FLT3-ligand and granulocyte/macrophage colony-stimulating factor. *J. Exp. Med.* 195:953–58

38. Brawand P, Fitzpatrick DR, Greenfield BW, Brasel K, Maliszewski CR, De Smedt T. 2002. Murine plasmacytoid predendritic cells generated from Flt3 ligand-supplemented bone marrow cultures are immature APCs. *J. Immunol.* 169:6711–19

39. Pulendran B, Banchereau J, Burkeholder S, Kraus E, Guinet E, et al. 2000. Flt3-ligand and granulocyte colony-stimulating factor mobilize distinct human dendritic cell subsets in vivo. *J. Immunol.* 165:566–72

40. Manfra DJ, Chen SC, Jensen KK, Fine JS, Wiekowski MT, Lira SA. 2003. Conditional expression of murine Flt3 ligand leads to expansion of multiple dendritic cell subsets in peripheral blood and tissues of transgenic mice. *J. Immunol.* 170:2843–52

41. Rissoan MC, Duhen T, Bridon JM, Bendriss-Vermare N, Peronne C, et al. 2002. Subtractive hybridization reveals the expression of immunoglobulin-like transcript 7, Eph-B1, granzyme B, and 3 novel transcripts in human plasmacytoid dendritic cells. *Blood* 100:3295–303

42. Corcoran L, Ferrero I, Vremec D, Lucas

K, Waithman J, et al. 2003. The lymphoid past of mouse plasmacytoid cells and thymic dendritic cells. *J. Immunol.* 170:4926–32

43. Spits H, Couwenberg F, Bakker AQ, Weijer K, Uittenbogaart CH. 2000. Id2 and Id3 inhibit development of CD34+ stem cells into predendritic cell (pre-DC)2 but not into pre-DC1. Evidence for a lymphoid origin of pre-DC2. *J. Exp. Med.* 192:1775–84

44. Karsunky H, Merad M, Cozzio A, Weissman IL, Manz MG. 2003. Flt3 ligand regulates dendritic cell development from Flt3+ lymphoid and myeloid-committed progenitors to Flt3+ dendritic cells in vivo. *J. Exp. Med.* 198:305–13

45. D'Amico A, Wu L. 2003. The early progenitors of mouse dendritic cells and plasmacytoid predendritic cells are within the bone marrow hemopoietic precursors expressing Flt3. *J. Exp. Med.* 198: 293–303

46. Tamura T, Ozato K. 2002. ICSBP/IRF-8: its regulatory roles in the development of myeloid cells. *J. Interferon Cytokine Res.* 22:145–52

47. Aliberti J, Schulz O, Pennington DJ, Tsujimura H, Reis e Sousa C, et al. 2003. Essential role for ICSBP in the in vivo development of murine CD8α+ dendritic cells. *Blood* 101:305–10

48. del Hoyo GM, Martin P, Vargas HH, Ruiz S, Arias CF, Ardavin C. 2002. Characterization of a common precursor population for dendritic cells. *Nature* 415: 1043–47

49. Comeau MR, Van der Vuurst de Vries AR, Maliszewski CR, Galibert L. 2002. CD123bright plasmacytoid predendritic cells: Progenitors undergoing cell fate conversion? *J. Immunol.* 169:75–83

50. Shigematsu H, Reizis B, Iwasaki H, Mizuno S, Hu D, et al. 2004. Plasmacytoid dendritic cells activate lymphoid-specific genetic programs irrespective of their cellular origin. *Immunity* 21:43–53

51. Palucka AK, Gatlin J, Blanck JP, Melkus MW, Clayton S, et al. 2003. Human dendritic cell subsets in NOD/SCID mice engrafted with CD34+ hematopoietic progenitors. *Blood* 102:3302–10

52. Weijer K, Uittenbogaart CH, Voordouw A, Couwenberg F, Seppen J, et al. 2002. Intrathymic and extrathymic development of human plasmacytoid dendritic cell precursors in vivo. *Blood* 99:2752–59

53. Traggiai E, Chicha L, Mazzucchelli L, Bronz L, Piffaretti JC, et al. 2004. Development of a human adaptive immune system in cord blood cell-transplanted mice. *Science* 304:104–7

54. Penna G, Vulcano M, Sozzani S, Adorini L. 2002. Differential migration behavior and chemokine production by myeloid and plasmacytoid dendritic cells. *Hum. Immunol.* 63:1164–71

55. Blasius A, Vermi W, Krug A, Facchetti F, Cella M, Colonna M. 2004. A cell-surface molecule selectively expressed on murine natural interferon-producing cells that blocks secretion of interferon-α. *Blood* 103:4201–6

56. Asselin-Paturel C, Brizard G, Pin JJ, Briere F, Trinchieri G. 2003. Mouse strain differences in plasmacytoid dendritic cell frequency and function revealed by a novel monoclonal antibody. *J. Immunol.* 171:6466–77

57. Yoneyama H, Matsuno K, Zhang Y, Nishiwaki T, Kitabatake M, et al. 2004. Evidence for recruitment of plasmacytoid dendritic cell precursors to inflamed lymph nodes through high endothelial venules. *Int. Immunol.* 16:915–28

58. Penna G, Sozzani S, Adorini L. 2001. Cutting edge: selective usage of chemokine receptors by plasmacytoid dendritic cells. *J. Immunol.* 167:1862–66

59. O'Keeffe M, Hochrein H, Vremec D, Caminschi I, Miller JL, et al. 2002. Mouse plasmacytoid cells: long-lived cells, heterogeneous in surface phenotype and function, that differentiate into CD8+

dendritic cells only after microbial stimulus. *J. Exp. Med.* 196:1307–19

60. Schlecht G, Garcia S, Escriou N, Freitas AA, Leclerc C, Dadaglio G. 2004. Murine plasmacytoid dendritic cells induce effector/memory CD8$^+$ T cell responses in vivo after viral stimulation. *Blood* 104: 1808–15

61. Rajewsky K. 1989. Evolutionary and somatic immunological memory. In *Progress in Immunology VII*, ed. A Kudo, S Bauer, F Melchers, pp. 397–403. Berlin: Springer-Verlag

62. Janeway CA Jr, Medzhitov R. 2002. Innate immune recognition. *Annu. Rev. Immunol.* 20:197–216

63. Takeda K, Kaisho T, Akira S. 2003. Toll-like receptors. *Annu. Rev. Immunol.* 21:335–76

64. Aderem A, Ulevitch RJ. 2000. Toll-like receptors in the induction of the innate immune response. *Nature* 406:782–87

65. Beutler B. 2000. Endotoxin, Toll-like receptor 4, and the afferent limb of innate immunity. *Curr. Opin. Microbiol.* 3:23–28

66. Bauer S, Kirschning CJ, Hacker H, Redecke V, Hausmann S, et al. 2001. Human TLR9 confers responsiveness to bacterial DNA via species-specific CpG motif recognition. *Proc. Natl. Acad. Sci. USA* 98:9237–42

67. Lund J, Sato A, Akira S, Medzhitov R, Iwasaki A. 2003. Toll-like receptor 9-mediated recognition of herpes simplex virus-2 by plasmacytoid dendritic cells. *J. Exp. Med.* 198:513–20

68. Lund JM, Alexopoulou L, Sato A, Karow M, Adams NC, et al. 2004. Recognition of single-stranded RNA viruses by Toll-like receptor 7. *Proc. Natl. Acad. Sci. USA* 101:5598–603

69. Heil F, Hemmi H, Hochrein H, Ampenberger F, Kirschning C, et al. 2004. Species-specific recognition of single-stranded RNA via Toll-like receptor 7 and 8. *Science* 303:1526–29

70. Diebold SS, Kaisho T, Hemmi H, Akira S, Reis e Sousa C. 2004. Innate antiviral responses by means of TLR7-mediated recognition of single-stranded RNA. *Science* 303:1529–31

71. Latz E, Schoenemeyer A, Visintin A, Fitzgerald KA, Monks BG, et al. 2004. TLR9 signals after translocating from the ER to CpG DNA in the lysosome. *Nat. Immunol.* 5:190–98

72. Ahmad-Nejad P, Hacker H, Rutz M, Bauer S, Vabulas RM, Wagner H. 2002. Bacterial CpG-DNA and lipopolysaccharides activate Toll-like receptors at distinct cellular compartments. *Eur. J. Immunol.* 32:1958–68

73a. Moseman EA, Liang X, Dawson AJ, Panoskaltsis-Mortari A, Krieg AM, et al. 2004. Human plasmacytoid dendritic cells activated by CpG oligodeoxynucleotides induce the generation of CD4$^+$CD25$^+$ regulatory T cells. *J. Immunol.* 173:4433–42

73. Kadowaki N, Antonenko S, Lau JY, Liu YJ. 2000. Natural interferon α/β-producing cells link innate and adaptive immunity. *J. Exp. Med.* 192:219–26

74. Taniguchi T, Takaoka A. 2002. The interferon-α/β system in antiviral responses: a multimodal machinery of gene regulation by the IRF family of transcription factors. *Curr. Opin. Immunol.* 14:111–16

75. Coccia EM, Severa M, Giacomini E, Monneron D, Remoli ME, et al. 2004. Viral infection and Toll-like receptor agonists induce a differential expression of type I and λ interferons in human plasmacytoid and monocyte-derived dendritic cells. *Eur. J. Immunol.* 34:796–805

76. Izaguirre A, Barnes BJ, Amrute S, Yeow WS, Megjugorac N, et al. 2003. Comparative analysis of IRF and IFN-α expression in human plasmacytoid and monocyte-derived dendritic cells. *J. Leukoc. Biol.* 74:1125–38

77. Kerkmann M, Rothenfusser S, Hornung V, Towarowski A, Wagner M, et al. 2003. Activation with CpG-A and CpG-B

oligonucleotides reveals two distinct regulatory pathways of type I IFN synthesis in human plasmacytoid dendritic cells. *J. Immunol.* 170:4465–74

78. Takauji R, Iho S, Takatsuka H, Yamamoto S, Takahashi T, et al. 2002. CpG-DNA-induced IFN-α production involves p38 MAPK-dependent STAT1 phosphorylation in human plasmacytoid dendritic cell precursors. *J. Leukoc. Biol.* 72:1011–19

79. Barchet W, Cella M, Odermatt B, Asselin-Paturel C, Colonna M, Kalinke U. 2002. Virus-induced interferon α production by a dendritic cell subset in the absence of feedback signaling in vivo. *J. Exp. Med.* 195:507–16

80. Rissoan MC, Soumelis V, Kadowaki N, Grouard G, Briere F, et al. 1999. Reciprocal control of T helper cell and dendritic cell differentiation. *Science* 283:1183–86

81. Gilliet M, Liu YJ. 2002. Generation of human CD8 T regulatory cells by CD40 ligand-activated plasmacytoid dendritic cells. *J. Exp. Med.* 195:695–704

82. Duramad O, Fearon KL, Chan JH, Kanzler H, Marshall JD, et al. 2003. IL-10 regulates plasmacytoid dendritic cell response to CpG-containing immunostimulatory sequences. *Blood* 102:4487–92

83. Ito T, Amakawa R, Kaisho T, Hemmi H, Tajima K, et al. 2002. Interferon-α and interleukin-12 are induced differentially by Toll-like receptor 7 ligands in human blood dendritic cell subsets. *J. Exp. Med.* 195:1507–12

84. Shortman K, Liu YJ. 2002. Mouse and human dendritic cell subtypes. *Nat. Rev. Immunol.* 2:151–61

85. Boonstra A, Asselin-Paturel C, Gilliet M, Crain C, Trinchieri G, et al. 2003. Flexibility of mouse classical and plasmacytoid-derived dendritic cells in directing T helper type 1 and 2 cell development: dependency on antigen dose and differential Toll-like receptor ligation. *J. Exp. Med.* 197:101–9

86. Diebold SS, Montoya M, Unger H, Alex-opoulou L, Roy P, et al. 2003. Viral infection switches non-plasmacytoid dendritic cells into high interferon producers. *Nature* 424:324–28

87. Ito T, Amakawa R, Inaba M, Ikehara S, Inaba K, Fukuhara S. 2001. Differential regulation of human blood dendritic cell subsets by IFNs. *J. Immunol.* 166:2961–69

88. Krug A, Veeraswamy R, Pekosz A, Kanagawa O, Unanue ER, et al. 2003. Interferon-producing cells fail to induce proliferation of naive T cells but can promote expansion and T helper 1 differentiation of antigen-experienced unpolarized T cells. *J. Exp. Med.* 197:899–906

89. Fonteneau JF, Larsson M, Beignon AS, McKenna K, Dasilva I, et al. 2004. Human immunodeficiency virus type 1 activates plasmacytoid dendritic cells and concomitantly induces the bystander maturation of myeloid dendritic cells. *J. Virol.* 78:5223–32

90. Salio M, Palmowski MJ, Atzberger A, Hermans IF, Cerundolo V. 2004. CpG-matured murine plasmacytoid dendritic cells are capable of in vivo priming of functional CD8 T cell responses to endogenous but not exogenous antigens. *J. Exp. Med.* 199:567–79

91. den Haan JM, Lehar SM, Bevan MJ. 2000. CD8[+] but not CD8[−] dendritic cells cross-prime cytotoxic T cells in vivo. *J. Exp. Med.* 192:1685–96

92. Belz GT, Vremec D, Febbraio M, Corcoran L, Shortman K, et al. 2002. CD36 is differentially expressed by CD8[+] splenic dendritic cells but is not required for cross-presentation in vivo. *J. Immunol.* 168:6066–70

93. Le Bon A, Etchart N, Rossmann C, Ashton M, Hou S, et al. 2003. Cross-priming of CD8[+] T cells stimulated by virus-induced type I interferon. *Nat. Immunol.* 4:1009–15

94. Kuwana M, Kaburaki J, Wright TM, Kawakami Y, Ikeda Y. 2001. Induction of antigen-specific human CD4[+] T cell

anergy by peripheral blood DC2 precursors. *Eur. J. Immunol.* 31:2547–57

95. Martin P, Del Hoyo GM, Anjuere F, Arias CF, Vargas HH, et al. 2002. Characterization of a new subpopulation of mouse CD8α^+ B220$^+$ dendritic cells endowed with type 1 interferon production capacity and tolerogenic potential. *Blood* 100:383–90

96. Bilsborough J, George TC, Norment A, Viney JL. 2003. Mucosal CD8α^+ DC, with a plasmacytoid phenotype, induce differentiation and support function of T cells with regulatory properties. *Immunology* 108:481–92

97. De Heer HJ, Hammad H, Soullie T, Hijdra D, Vos N, et al. 2004. Essential role of lung plasmacytoid dendritic cells in preventing asthmatic reactions to harmless inhaled antigen. *J. Exp. Med.* 200:89–98

98. Baldwin T, Henri S, Curtis J, O'Keeffe M, Vremec D, et al. 2004. Dendritic cell populations in *Leishmania major*-infected skin and draining lymph nodes. *Infect. Immun.* 72:1991–2001

99. Lovgren T, Eloranta ML, Bave U, Alm GV, Ronnblom L. 2004. Induction of interferon-α production in plasmacytoid dendritic cells by immune complexes containing nucleic acid released by necrotic or late apoptotic cells and lupus IgG. *Arthritis Rheum.* 50:1861–72

100. Ronnblom L, Alm GV. 2002. The natural interferon-α producing cells in systemic lupus erythematosus. *Hum. Immunol.* 63:1181–93

101. Farkas L, Beiske K, Lund-Johansen F, Brandtzaeg P, Jahnsen FL. 2001. Plasmacytoid dendritic cells (natural interferon-α/β-producing cells) accumulate in cutaneous lupus erythematosus lesions. *Am. J. Pathol.* 159:237–43

102. Blanco P, Palucka AK, Gill M, Pascual V, Bancereau J. 2001. Induction of dendritic cell differentiation by IFN-α in systemic lupus erythematosus. *Science* 294:1540–43

103. Palucka AK, Bancereau J, Blanco P, Pascual V. 2002. The interplay of dendritic cell subsets in systemic lupus erythematosus. *Immunol. Cell Biol.* 80:484–88

104. Dalod M, Hamilton T, Salomon R, Salazar-Mather TP, Henry SC, et al. 2003. Dendritic cell responses to early murine cytomegalovirus infection: subset functional specialization and differential regulation by interferon α/β. *J. Exp. Med.* 197:885–98

105. Honda K, Sakaguchi S, Nakajima C, Watanabe A, Yanai H, et al. 2003. Selective contribution of IFN-α/β signaling to the maturation of dendritic cells induced by double-stranded RNA or viral infection. *Proc. Natl. Acad. Sci. USA* 100:10872–77

106. Luft T, Pang KC, Thomas E, Hertzog P, Hart DN, et al. 1998. Type I IFNs enhance the terminal differentiation of dendritic cells. *J. Immunol.* 161:1947–53

107. Paquette RL, Hsu NC, Kiertscher SM, Park AN, Tran L, et al. 1998. Interferon-α and granulocyte-macrophage colony-stimulating factor differentiate peripheral blood monocytes into potent antigen-presenting cells. *J. Leukoc. Biol.* 64:358–67

108. Santodonato L, D'Agostino G, Nisini R, Mariotti S, Monque DM, et al. 2003. Monocyte-derived dendritic cells generated after a short-term culture with IFN-α and granulocyte-macrophage colony-stimulating factor stimulate a potent Epstein-Barr virus-specific CD8$^+$ T cell response. *J. Immunol.* 170:5195–202

109. Santini SM, Lapenta C, Logozzi M, Parlato S, Spada M, et al. 2000. Type I interferon as a powerful adjuvant for monocyte-derived dendritic cell development and activity in vitro and in Hu-PBL-SCID mice. *J. Exp. Med.* 191:1777–88

110. Nagai T, Devergne O, Mueller TF, Perkins DL, van Seventer JM, van Seventer GA. 2003. Timing of IFN-β exposure during human dendritic cell maturation and naive Th cell stimulation has contrasting effects on Th1 subset generation: a role for IFN-β-mediated regulation of IL-12 family

cytokines and IL-18 in naive Th cell differentiation. *J. Immunol.* 171:5233–43

111. Heystek HC, den Drijver B, Kapsenberg ML, van Lier RA, de Jong EC. 2003. Type I IFNs differentially modulate IL-12p70 production by human dendritic cells depending on the maturation status of the cells and counteract IFN-γ-mediated signaling. *Clin. Immunol.* 107:170–77

112. Aman MJ, Tretter T, Eisenbeis I, Bug G, Decker T, et al. 1996. Interferon-α stimulates production of interleukin-10 in activated CD4⁺ T cells and monocytes. *Blood* 87:4731–36

113. Rep MH, Hintzen RQ, Polman CH, van Lier RA. 1996. Recombinant interferon-β blocks proliferation but enhances interleukin-10 secretion by activated human T-cells. *J. Neuroimmunol.* 67:111–18

114. Curreli S, Romerio F, Secchiero P, Zella D. 2002. IFN-α2b increases interleukin-10 expression in primary activated human CD8⁺ T cells. *J. Interferon Cytokine Res.* 22:1167–73

115. Tough DF, Sun S, Zhang X, Sprent J. 1999. Stimulation of naive and memory T cells by cytokines. *Immunol. Rev.* 170:39–47

116. Marrack P, Kappler J, Mitchell T. 1999. Type I interferons keep activated T cells alive. *J. Exp. Med.* 189:521–30

117. Bandyopadhyay S, Perussia B, Trinchieri G, Miller DS, Starr SE. 1986. Requirement for HLA-DR⁺ accessory cells in natural killing of cytomegalovirus-infected fibroblasts. *J. Exp. Med.* 164:180–95

118. Oh SH, Bandyopadhyay S, Miller DS, Starr SE. 1987. Cooperation between CD16(Leu-11b)+ NK cells and HLA-DR⁺ cells in natural killing of herpesvirus-infected fibroblasts. *J. Immunol.* 139:2799–802

119. Yamamoto S, Yamamoto T, Iho S, Tokunaga T. 2000. Activation of NK cell (human and mouse) by immunostimulatory DNA sequence. *Springer Semin. Immunopathol.* 22:35–43

120. Vollmer J, Weeratna R, Payette P, Jurk

M, Schetter C, et al. 2004. Characterization of three CpG oligodeoxynucleotide classes with distinct immunostimulatory activities. *Eur. J. Immunol.* 34:251–62

121. Ballas ZK, Rasmussen WL, Krieg AM. 1996. Induction of NK activity in murine and human cells by CpG motifs in oligodeoxynucleotides and bacterial DNA. *J. Immunol.* 157:1840–45

122. Hornung V, Rothenfusser S, Britsch S, Krug A, Jahrsdorfer B, et al. 2002. Quantitative expression of Toll-like receptor 1–10 mRNA in cellular subsets of human peripheral blood mononuclear cells and sensitivity to CpG oligodeoxynucleotides. *J. Immunol.* 168:4531–37

123. Jego G, Palucka AK, Blanck JP, Chalouni C, Pascual V, Banchereau J. 2003. Plasmacytoid dendritic cells induce plasma cell differentiation through type I interferon and interleukin 6. *Immunity* 19:225–34

124. Fong L, Mengozzi M, Abbey NW, Herndier BG, Engleman EG. 2002. Productive infection of plasmacytoid dendritic cells with human immunodeficiency virus type 1 is triggered by CD40 ligation. *J. Virol.* 76:11033–41

125. Keir ME, Stoddart CA, Linquist-Stepps V, Moreno ME, McCune JM. 2002. IFN-α secretion by type 2 predendritic cells up-regulates MHC class I in the HIV-1-infected thymus. *J. Immunol.* 168:325–31

126. Lopez C, Fitzgerald PA, Siegal FP. 1983. Severe acquired immune deficiency syndrome in male homosexuals: diminished capacity to make interferon-α in vitro associated with severe opportunistic infections. *J. Infect. Dis.* 148:962–66

127. Siegal FP, Lopez C, Fitzgerald PA, Shah K, Baron P, et al. 1986. Opportunistic infections in acquired immune deficiency syndrome result from synergistic defects of both the natural and adaptive components of cellular immunity. *J. Clin. Invest.* 78:115–23

128. Soumelis V, Scott I, Gheyas F, Bouhour D, Cozon G, et al. 2001. Depletion

of circulating natural type 1 interferon-producing cells in HIV-infected AIDS patients. *Blood* 98:906–12

129. Pacanowski J, Kahi S, Baillet M, Lebon P, Deveau C, et al. 2001. Reduced blood CD123$^+$ (lymphoid) and CD11c$^+$ (myeloid) dendritic cell numbers in primary HIV-1 infection. *Blood* 98:3016–21

130. Feldman S, Stein D, Amrute S, Denny T, Garcia Z, et al. 2001. Decreased interferon-α production in HIV-infected patients correlates with numerical and functional deficiencies in circulating type 2 dendritic cell precursors. *Clin. Immunol.* 101:201–10

131. Chehimi J, Campbell DE, Azzoni L, Bacheller D, Papasavvas E, et al. 2002. Persistent decreases in blood plasmacytoid dendritic cell number and function despite effective highly active antiretroviral therapy and increased blood myeloid dendritic cells in HIV-infected individuals. *J. Immunol.* 168:4796–801

132. Ronnblom LE, Alm GV, Oberg KE. 1990. Possible induction of systemic lupus erythematosus by interferon-α treatment in a patient with a malignant carcinoid tumour. *J. Intern. Med.* 227:207–10

133. Preble OT, Black RJ, Friedman RM, Klippel JH, Vilcek J. 1982. Systemic lupus erythematosus: presence in human serum of an unusual acid-labile leukocyte interferon. *Science* 216:429–31

134. Strannegard O, Hermodsson S, Westberg G. 1982. Interferon and natural killer cells in systemic lupus erythematosus. *Clin. Exp. Immunol.* 50:246–52

135. Ytterberg SR, Schnitzer TJ. 1982. Serum interferon levels in patients with systemic lupus erythematosus. *Arthritis Rheum.* 25:401–6

136. Cederblad B, Blomberg S, Vallin H, Perers A, Alm GV, Ronnblom L. 1998. Patients with systemic lupus erythematosus have reduced numbers of circulating natural interferon-α-producing cells. *J. Autoimmun.* 11:465–70

137. Blomberg S, Eloranta ML, Cederblad B, Nordlin K, Alm GV, Ronnblom L. 2001. Presence of cutaneous interferon-α producing cells in patients with systemic lupus erythematosus. *Lupus* 10:484–90

138. Vallin H, Perers A, Alm GV, Ronnblom L. 1999. Anti-double-stranded DNA antibodies and immunostimulatory plasmid DNA in combination mimic the endogenous IFN-α inducer in systemic lupus erythematosus. *J. Immunol.* 163:6306–13

139. Bennett L, Palucka AK, Arce E, Cantrell V, Borvak J, et al. 2003. Interferon and granulopoiesis signatures in systemic lupus erythematosus blood. *J. Exp. Med.* 197:711–23

140. Crow MK, Kirou KA, Wohlgemuth J. 2003. Microarray analysis of interferon-regulated genes in SLE. *Autoimmunity* 36:481–90

141. Baechler EC, Batliwalla FM, Karypis G, Gaffney PM, Ortmann WA, et al. 2003. Interferon-inducible gene expression signature in peripheral blood cells of patients with severe lupus. *Proc. Natl. Acad. Sci. USA* 100:2610–15

142. Han GM, Chen SL, Shen N, Ye S, Bao CD, Gu YY. 2003. Analysis of gene expression profiles in human systemic lupus erythematosus using oligonucleotide microarray. *Genes Immun.* 4:177–86

143. Bell D, Chomarat P, Broyles D, Netto G, Harb GM, et al. 1999. In breast carcinoma tissue, immature dendritic cells reside within the tumor, whereas mature dendritic cells are located in peritumoral areas. *J. Exp. Med.* 190:1417–26

144. Vicari AP, Chiodoni C, Vaure C, Ait-Yahia S, Dercamp C, et al. 2002. Reversal of tumor-induced dendritic cell paralysis by CpG immunostimulatory oligonucleotide and anti-interleukin 10 receptor antibody. *J. Exp. Med.* 196:541–49

145. Vermi W, Bonecchi R, Facchetti F, Bianchi D, Sozzani S, et al. 2003. Recruitment of immature plasmacytoid

dendritic cells (plasmacytoid monocytes) and myeloid dendritic cells in primary cutaneous melanomas. *J. Pathol.* 200: 255–68

146. Chaux P, Favre N, Martin M, Martin F. 1997. Tumor-infiltrating dendritic cells are defective in their antigen-presenting function and inducible B7 expression in rats. *Int. J. Cancer* 72:619–24

147. Mahnke K, Qian Y, Knop J, Enk AH. 2003. Induction of CD4$^+$/CD25$^+$ regulatory T cells by targeting of antigens to immature dendritic cells. *Blood* 101:4862–69

148. Dhodapkar MV, Steinman RM. 2002. Antigen-bearing immature dendritic cells induce peptide-specific CD8$^+$ regulatory T cells in vivo in humans. *Blood* 100:174–77

149. Treilleux I, Lebecque S, Goddard S, Pin JJ, Bremond A, et al. 2002. *Dendritic cell infiltration, chemokine and chemokine receptors expression in primary breast carcinomas: correlation with nodal involvement and outcome.* Presented at Annu. Meet. Am. Soc. Clin. Oncol., 38th, Orlando, Fla. Abstr. 1802

150. Zou W, Machelon V, Coulomb-L'Hermin A, Borvak J, Nome F, et al. 2001. Stromal-derived factor-1 in human tumors recruits and alters the function of plasmacytoid precursor dendritic cells. *Nat. Med.* 7:1339–46

151. Munn DH, Sharma MD, Hou D, Baban B, Lee JR, et al. 2004. Expression of indoleamine 2,3-dioxygenase by plasmacytoid dendritic cells in tumor-draining lymph nodes. *J. Clin. Invest.* 114:280–90

Annu. Rev. Immunol. 2005. 23:307–36
doi: 10.1146/annurev.immunol.23.021704.115843
First published online as a Review in Advance on November 11, 2004

TYPE I INTERFERONS (α/β) IN IMMUNITY AND AUTOIMMUNITY

Argyrios N. Theofilopoulos, Roberto Baccala,
Bruce Beutler, and Dwight H. Kono

*Immunology Department, The Scripps Research Institute, La Jolla, California 92037;
email: argyrio@scripps.edu, rbaccala@scripps.edu, bruce@scripps.edu,
dkono@scripps.edu*

Key Words   plasmacytoid cells, TLR, innate immunity, lupus, IDDM

■ **Abstract**   The significance of type I interferons (IFN-α/β) in biology and medicine renders research on their activities continuously relevant to our understanding of normal and abnormal (auto) immune responses. This relevance is bolstered by discoveries that unambiguously establish IFN-α/β, among the multitude of cytokines, as dominant in defining qualitative and quantitative characteristics of innate and adaptive immune processes. Recent advances elucidating the biology of these key cytokines include better definition of their complex signaling pathways, determination of their importance in modifying the effects of other cytokines, the role of Toll-like receptors in their induction, their major cellular producers, and their broad and diverse impact on both cellular and humoral immune responses. Consequently, the role of IFN-α/β in the pathogenesis of autoimmunity remains at the forefront of scientific inquiry and has begun to illuminate the mechanisms by which these molecules promote or inhibit systemic and organ-specific autoimmune diseases.

INTRODUCTION

The multiple subtypes of α-interferons and the single β-interferon belong to the type I family of interferons (IFNs) and, together with the related but distinct single-member type II IFN (IFN-γ), constitute one of the most important classes of cytokines (1–3).[1] They exert a vast array of biologic functions, the most pronounced being those affecting the immune system. The broad effects of IFN-α/β extend to the development of immunocyte lineages and sublineages, innate immunity, and almost every aspect of cellular and humoral adaptive immune responses. The diverse biological properties of these highly pleiotropic cytokines can be accounted for by the fact that signaling through their receptors leads to modulation in expression of hundreds of genes, as shown by recent microarray data (4–6). New

---

[1]See Appendix for a full list of abbreviations used.

0732-0582/05/0423-0307$14.00

307

molecular tools have helped investigators define the intricate pathways by which these mediators affect many cell biologic processes, creating an ever-expanding body of literature that is sometimes difficult to integrate. Nonetheless, a clear picture of several aspects of their biology has emerged, including signaling processes, priming capacity, cross-talk among themselves and other cytokines, receptors and ligands involved in their production, and their major cellular producers. These discoveries have advanced our understanding of the role of these molecules not only in normal immunologic responses but also in the abnormal processes that provoke autoimmune diseases. This review encompasses selected aspects of the biology of type I IFNs related to these recent advances, with focus on their role in autoimmunity.

TYPE I IFN MEMBERS, RECEPTORS, AND SIGNALING

Type I IFNs belong to the class II family of α-helical cytokines, which includes type II IFN-γ, the newly identified IFN-λs, IL-10, and several IL-10 homologs (IL-19, IL-20, IL-22, IL-24, IL-26) (7–9). The composition, receptors, and signaling pathways of type I IFNs have been reviewed in depth (1, 2), and only a brief description is made here.

Type I IFNs constitute a multi-member cytokine family (IFN-α subtypes, -β, -ε, -κ, -ω, -δ, and -τ). Of these, IFN-δ and IFN-τ are not found in humans, IFN-ε is expressed in the placenta and may play a role in reproduction, and IFN-κ is expressed in keratinocytes. From an immunologic perspective, therefore, IFN-α and IFN-β are the main types of interest. IFN-β is represented by a single member, while both the human and mouse genomes contain more than 20 different *IFN-α* genes, of which 13 encode functional polypeptides. The multiple intronless IFN-α genes were likely generated by repeated gene duplications and recombinations. Although the reason(s) for multiple IFN-α subtypes is not fully understood, evidence suggests that they have distinct functions. Moreover, their expression, and the qualitative and quantitative profiles of in vitro–induced genes, depend on the stimulating agent, cell type, and donor (10).

Recently, two research groups identified a novel class of human type I-like IFNs, termed IFN-λ1, -λ2, and -λ3 (11), or IL-28A, IL-28B, and IL-29 (12), respectively. Although IFN-λs are functionally similar to type I IFNs, their genes have distinct sequence and chromosomal locations and, unlike the IFN-αs, have several introns. Moreover, they do not use the IFN-α receptor (IFNAR), but rather signal through a heterodimeric receptor composed of a specific ligand-binding R1 chain (also termed IL-28R), and a second chain (IL-10R2) that also serves as the R2 subunit for the IL-10, IL-22, and IL-26 receptors (8).

IFN-α and -β share a ubiquitously expressed heterodimeric receptor composed of IFNAR1 and IFNAR2 subunits. Evidence suggests that the IFNAR2 serves as the ligand-binding chain, but both chains are required for signal transduction. In general, various cell types display small numbers of these high-affinity receptors (200 to 6000 per cell; dissociation constant of 10^{-9}–10^{-11}). IFN-α/β binding leads to ligand-induced receptor dimerization, and then to auto- and transphosphorylation of the two receptor-associated Janus protein tyrosine kinases (Tyk2 on IFNAR1 and Jak1 on IFNAR2). Phosphorylation of the Janus kinases results in phosphorylation of the intracellular domain of IFNAR1 and creation of docking sites for STAT2 (preassociated with STAT1 on IFNAR2), which is phosphorylated and serves as a platform for recruitment and phosphorylation of STAT1. The phosphorylated STAT1/STAT2 heterodimers then dissociate from the receptor and translocate into the nucleus through an unknown mechanism, where they associate with the IFN regulatory factor 9 (IRF-9, also referred to as p48) to form the heterotrimeric complex IFN-stimulated gene factor 3 (ISGF3). The ISGF3 then binds to upstream regulatory consensus sequences of IFN-α/β-inducible genes (IFN-stimulated response elements, or ISRE) and initiates transcription. A similar signaling mechanism has been invoked for IFN-λs (11, 12). IFN-α/β activate several other pathways, including formation of STAT1 homodimers that can stimulate transcription of genes containing the IFN-γ-activated sequence (GAS).

Negative regulation of type I IFN signaling is accomplished by various mechanisms, including receptor internalization and degradation, dephosphorylation of Jaks and STATs by several phosphatases, induction of suppressors of cytokine signaling (SOCS), and repression of STAT-mediated gene activation by protein inhibitors of activated STATs (PIAS) (13).

PRIMING AND CROSS-TALK OF TYPE I IFNs WITH OTHER CYTOKINES

IFN-α/β production is initiated at the early stages of the innate immune response and, therefore, it is likely to be the dominant factor in shaping downstream events in the innate and adaptive immune responses. Indeed, it appears that a major role for IFN-α/β is the induction of a priming state through which production and regulation of other mediators, including cytokines, are affected. Therefore, in addressing the role of IFN-α/β in immunity and autoimmunity, it is important to recognize that, in addition to direct action, their effects may be mediated by synergistic or antagonistic interactions with other cytokines.

A relevant finding in this regard is that low constitutive levels of IFN-α/β are prerequisites for enhancement of IFN-α/β production subsequent to viral infection (14, 15). Basal IFN-α/β levels also appear to be required for efficient IFN-γ signaling because responses to IFN-γ are defective in the presence of antibodies to IFN-α/β or in the absence of IFNAR1 (15, 16). Because the defective IFN-γ response by IFNAR1-null cells is associated with impaired dimerization of STAT1, investigators concluded that IFNAR signaling induced by spontaneous subthreshold levels of IFN-α/β (which do not substantially activate downstream signaling events) provides docking sites on tyrosine residues of IFNAR1 for more efficient STAT1 recruitment after stimulation of IFN-γ receptor (IFNGR). Further evidence suggests that this cooperation is mediated by the creation of a receptosome composed of the IFNAR1 chain brought into close proximity with the IFNGR2 chain at caveolar membrane domains. The physical interaction between IFNAR1 and IFNGR2 and the increased STAT1 recruitment leads to at least a tenfold enhancement of otherwise weak IFN-γ signaling.

IFN-α/β signaling also upregulates IFN-γ production by dendritic cells (DCs) and T cells and thereby favors the induction and maintenance of Th1 cells (17–20). Furthermore, IFN-α/β acting in concert with T cell–receptor signaling can induce IFN-γ production by STAT4 activation (21, 22). The converse, i.e., influence of IFN-γ on IFN-α/β, is also true because IFN-γ pretreatment of cells markedly sensitizes them to IFN-α, largely owing to increased synthesis of ISGΓ3 (23, 24). A recent study has shown that enhancement of IFN-α signaling by IFN-γ is caused by increased STAT1 expression and depends on the tyrosine kinase Syk and on adaptor proteins that activate Syk through immunoreceptor tyrosine activation motifs (24a). Thus, type I and II IFNs may reciprocally affect each other's production and signaling, and some of the effects on normal and abnormal (auto) immune responses following blockade of IFN-α/β or IFN-γ signaling may result from modifications in the activity of the other type.

Type I IFNs, acting directly or indirectly, can influence the expression and function of a variety of other cytokines (25). For example, like IFN-γ, basal levels of IFN-α/β can enhance IL-6 signaling by providing docking sites for STAT1 and STAT3 on the phosphorylated IFNAR1, which may be brought into close proximity to the gp130 chain of the IL-6R (26). IFN-α/β also enhance production of the anti-inflammatory transforming growth factor β (TGF-β), IL-1 receptor antagonist, and soluble tumor necrosis factor (TNF) receptors (25). In contrast, IFNs inhibit activation of STAT6 by IL-4 by inducing SOCS-1 expression (27). IFN-α/β negatively regulate IL-12 expression but upregulate expression of the high-affinity IL-12Rβ2 subunit in CD4$^+$ T cells. Under conditions of high concentrations of IFN-α/β, inhibition of IL-12 production may dominate, whereas upregulation of the IL-12Rβ2 may be biologically important under low concentrations (3). IFN-α/β or their inducers can also elicit high IL-15 expression by DCs, thereby causing strong and selective stimulation of memory-phenotype CD8$^+$ T cells (28). Moreover, IL-10 may partially exert its Th2-polarizing and anti-inflammatory activities by reducing IFN-α/β (and IFN-γ) signaling through suppression of STAT1-phosphorylation (29). Conversely, priming with IFN-α (or IFN-γ) confers a proinflammatory gain of function on IL-10 by enhancing IFN-γ-inducible STAT1-dependent genes (30). This finding may explain the suspected pathogenic role of IL-10 in human lupus in which IFN-α levels are increased (31), as well as the inhibition of disease in (NZBxW)F$_1$ mice with anti-IL-10 antibody treatment (32).

Crossregulation of IFN-α/β and TNF-α production has also been reported with reciprocal suppressive effects. Investigators have proposed that the prevalence of one of these two cytokines may affect the type of autoimmune disease an individual develops with, for example, IFN-α/β predominance leading to lupus and TNF-α to rheumatoid arthritis (RA) (33, 34). Support for this concept is, however, inferential because, despite earlier reports on the beneficial role of TNF-α in mouse lupus models, other studies have shown that TNF-α may also exert proinflammatory and tissue-damaging effects in this disease (35, 36). Moreover, this single-cytokine-based paradigm is difficult to reconcile with the broad spectrum of diseases affected by IFN-α/β or TNF-α.

A variety of additional cross-talk between IFN-α/β-engaged Jak-STATs and other pathways, such as the NF-κB, the integrin signaling and the p53 apoptotic pathways, has been detected, as have effects of IFNs on a large set of cytokines and chemokines that might influence immunocyte maturation, homing, effector functions, and apoptosis (25, 37, 38).

PLASMACYTOID CELLS AS THE MAJOR PRODUCERS OF IFN-α/β

Although virtually all cells can produce IFN-α/β in response to viral and bacterial pathogens, plasmacytoid dendritic cells (pDCs), or "natural IFN-producing cells" (NIPCs), are the most potent, producing up to 1000-fold more IFN-α/β (and IFN-λ) than other cell types (39, 40). Immature mouse pDCs have the phenotype $CD11b^- CD8\alpha^- CD11c^{+/-} B220^+ Ly6C^+$ MHC class $II^{+/-}$, whereas the human peripheral blood counterpart has the phenotype $CD4^+ CD123^+ HLADR^+ CD68^+ CD45RA^+ CD11c^-$ (41). pDCs appear to derive from a common precursor for all types of DCs (42) and can develop efficiently from both myeloid- and lymphoid-committed progenitors (42a). Three human pDC surface markers, termed blood DC antigen (BDCA)-2, BDCA-3, and BDCA-4, have recently been identified, but the corresponding antibodies do not cross-react with mouse pDC (43). BDCA-2 is an endocytic type II C-type lectin that can capture and internalize antigen, whereas BDCA-4, identical to neuropilin-1, is apparently important for the interaction between DCs and T cells. In vitro ligation of pDC with anti-BDCA-2 and, less well, with anti-BDCA-4 inhibited IFN-α induction by these cells (43, 44), suggesting their potential therapeutic utility. Recently, a novel rat mAb (120G8) was found to exhibit high specificity for mouse pDC and to retain reactivity with these cells even after their maturation to a conventional DC phenotype (45).

Functionally, immature pDCs exhibit low allostimulatory activity and can even be tolerogenic (46), but activation with viruses, unmethylated CpG-DNA, IL-3, or CD40L and without evident proliferation allows them to become mature DCs expressing high levels of class I and class II MHC, costimulatory CD80 and CD86 molecules, as well as CD8α, thereby resembling conventional DCs (41). The number of pDCs in lymphoid organs is very low, and there is considerable mouse strain variation (45, 47), but mobilization with Flt3L or Flt3L and GM-CSF results in a striking increase of these cells in bone marrow and spleen (48–50).

As indicated, the most distinguishing feature of human and mouse pDCs is their production of large amounts of IFN-α/β in the precursor stage. This production is further enhanced upon stimulation of endosomal Toll-like receptors (TLR) present in these cells, such as TLR7 and TLR9, with ssRNA, hypomethylated CpGs in bacterial DNA, or certain types of autoantigen-autoantibody immune complexes (see below). The reason for the extraordinary production of IFN-α/β by pDCs is unclear, but a high constitutive expression of IRF-7 compared with other types of DC has been suggested (40, 51).

Although the high production of IFN-α/β by pDCs has been emphasized, biologically relevant levels of these cytokines are also produced by conventional myeloid DCs (CD11c^{hi}B220$^-$Ly6C$^-$) (17, 52). Moreover, conventional DCs can be switched to produce the same high amounts of IFN-α/β as pDCs when infected with certain types of DC-tropic dsRNA viruses, or when dsRNA is introduced by in vitro transfection into their cytoplasm to mimic direct viral infection (53). In this case, induction of IFN-α/β does not depend on expression of TLR3 or the adaptor molecule MyD88 (see below), but rather on the cytosolic dsRNA-binding enzyme protein kinase R.

IFN-α/β-ASSOCIATED TRANSCRIPTION FACTORS AND THEIR IMMUNOLOGIC EFFECTS

IFNs induce, and their expression is regulated by, several transcription factors that exert significant effects on the immune system. One class of these factors with a helix-turn-helix DNA-binding motif, collectively termed IFN regulatory factors (IRF), encompasses at least nine members (IRF-1 to IRF-9; see Table 1) (54, 55). Among them, IRF-4, -5, and -7 are primarily expressed in lymphoid cells, whereas others are ubiquitously expressed and are induced or hyperinduced by IFN-α/β.

Gene knockouts of some IRFs have shown that these transcription factors exert profound effects on immune system development and function. *Irf-1* gene-deleted mice show severe defects in NK cells, NK1$^+$ T cells, and intestinal intraepithelial $\gamma\delta^+$ T cells, attributed to the absence of IL-15 (56, 57). These mice also show severe defects in CD8$^+$ thymocyte development and defects in positive and negative selection owing to abnormalities in TCR signaling and induction of genes required for CD8$^+$ lineage commitment (58, 59). Primarily as a consequence of impaired IL-12 production, IRF-1-deficient mice also fail to mount Th1 responses (60, 61), and these mice show disease reduction in several Th1-mediated autoimmunity models, including collagen-induced arthritis (62), experimental encephalomyelitis (62), and diabetes in non-obese diabetic (NOD) mice (63). Deletion of IRF-2 also leads to defective NK cell development and Th1 differentiation, indicating that IRF-1 and IRF-2 do not compensate for one another, but act synergistically in these processes (64). Nonetheless, deletion of IRF-2 leads to upregulation of IFN-α/β-induced genes and an inflammatory skin disease resembling psoriasis (65). Thus, IRF-2 appears to act both as agonist and antagonist of the highly homologous IRF-1 for ISRE-responsive genes.

TABLE 1 Interferon regulatory factor (IRF) genes and autoimmunity

Factor	Induction	Targets	Knockout mice
IRF-1	Type I and II IFNs	Upstream *cis* elements of IFN-α/β genes (activator)	Deficient in iNOS, IL-12, CD8-positive T cells, NK cells, γδ T cells, Th1 responses, protection from autoimmunity
IRF-2	Type I and II IFNs	Upstream *cis* elements of IFN-α/β genes (antagonist for IRF-1, but also activator of some genes)	Defective NK and Th1 cell differentiation; upregulation of IFNα/β and development of an inflammatory skin disease
IRF-3	Viral infection, TLRs	IFN-β and IFN-α	Essential for IFN-β induction; resistance to LPS-induced endotoxin shock
IRF-4	Antigen receptor activation, TLR, mitogen, cytokine or coreceptor stimulation, but not IFNs (B and T cells)	Ig light-chain, CD20, CD23, IL-4, ISRE	Lymphoproliferation, other abnormalities in B and T cell homeostasis, along with reduced humoral responses, serum Ig, and Th differentiation
IRF-5	Viral infection, type I IFN, p53	IFN-α and -β, chemokines, cell cycle regulatory and apoptotic genes	Not done
IRF-6	Unknown	Unknown	Not done
IRF-7	IFN-α, but not IFN-γ, TLR, DNA-damaging agents (UV light), EBV LMP-1	IFN-α and -β	Not done
IRF-8	IFN-γ	ISRE	Absence of pDC in lymphoid organs, reduced CD8α⁺ DCs and lack of response to TLR3 or TLR9, defects in macrophage function, chronic myeloid leukemia–like syndrome
IRF-9	Type I and II IFNs	Forms trimolecular complexes with STAT1:STAT1 or STAT1:STAT2	Not done

IRF-4-deleted mice also exhibit immunologic defects, including splenomegaly, lymphadenopathy, reduced humoral responses and serum Ig levels, compromised Th1 and Th2 differentiation, and other abnormalities in T and B cell homeostasis (66, 67). Finally, deletion of IRF-8 (primarily induced by IFN-γ and marginally by IFN-α/β), also called IFN consensus sequence binding protein (ICSBP), leads to a variety of immunologic defects (54), including absence of pDCs in lymphoid organs, marked reduction and defective activation of CD8α^+DCs, and lack of responses to TLR3 and TLR9 stimuli (68–70).

Another class of IFN-induced transcription factors is that encoded by the *Ifi200* gene family, which in the mouse includes *Ifi202a, Ifi202b, Ifi203, Ifi204*, and *D3*, forming a tight cluster on the distal part of chromosome 1 (71). Although the role of the Ifi200 family of proteins has not been fully elucidated, there is evidence that they act as negative regulators of cell growth and apoptosis. A polymorphism leading to increased expression of the Ifi202 phosphoprotein has been associated with a major lupus-predisposing locus (*Nba-2*) of NZB mice (72).

Overall, IFN-α/β-associated transcription factors seem to regulate expression of many genes whose products are fundamental to the development, regulation, and function of the innate and adaptive immune system.

TOLL-LIKE RECEPTORS, INNATE IMMUNITY, AND AUTOIMMUNITY

High production of type I IFNs is initiated in response to pathogen sensing by the innate immune system. A large body of recent studies has demonstrated that this sensing is mediated by one or more of the 13 mammalian TLR paralogs (73, 74, 74a). Although the exact ligands for some of these receptors remain unidentified, each appears to recognize a limited set of molecules from distinct types of pathogens. For example, dsRNA is the ligand for TLR3, ssRNA for TLR7 (mouse) or TLR8 (human), lipopolysaccharide (LPS) for TLR4, and prokaryotic unmethylated CpG-DNA for TLR9. TLRs on cell surface membranes (TLR1, 2, 4, 5, 6 and perhaps 11) sense proteins or lipids from bacteria, fungi, or protozoa, whereas TLRs on endosomal membranes (TLR3, 7, 8, and 9) detect bacterial and viral nucleic acids. TLR-mediated signals, through engagement of several adaptor molecules and subsequent activation of primary and secondary kinases, the NF-κB pathway, and IRF-3, initiate transcription of hundreds to thousands of genes, including those encoding inflammatory cytokines such as TNF-α and type I IFNs. These cytokines, in turn, modulate gene expression as well.

The Toll-interleukin-1 receptor (TIR) domain-containing cytoplasmic adaptors participating in TLR-mediated signaling include myeloid differentiation factor 88 (MyD88), TIR-containing adaptor protein/MyD88 adaptor-like (TIRAP-Mal), TIR-containing adaptor-inducing IFNβ/TIR-containing adaptor molecule-1 (TRIF/TICAM-1), and TRIF-related adaptor molecule (TRAM). Although most TLRs signal via the MyD88 adaptor, TLR3 signals exclusively through a

MyD88-independent pathway in which TRIF is the adaptor, and TLR4 uses the MyD88 pathway (which in the case of this receptor requires both MyD88 and Mal) as well as an alternative pathway with both TRIF and TRAM as adaptors (75–78a).

MyD88 and/or Mal elicit activation of IL-1 receptor-associated kinase-4 (IRAK-4), a serine kinase that phosphorylates IRAK-1, and recruits TNF receptor-associated factor-6 (TRAF-6), a scaffold protein that causes activation of many other protein kinases, leading to activation of IκB kinase and, ultimately, to nuclear translocation of NF-κB. By contrast, TRIF acts alone (when activated by TLR3) or in conjunction with TRAM (when activated by TLR4) to recruit Tank-binding kinase-1 (TBK1), a protein kinase responsible for phosphorylation of IRF-3, a key transcription factor that leads to type I IFN gene transcription (Figure 1).

Not only TLR3 and TLR4, but also TLR7 and TLR9 can activate expression of the type I IFN genes. Because TLR7 and TLR9 do not use TRIF or TRAM, the

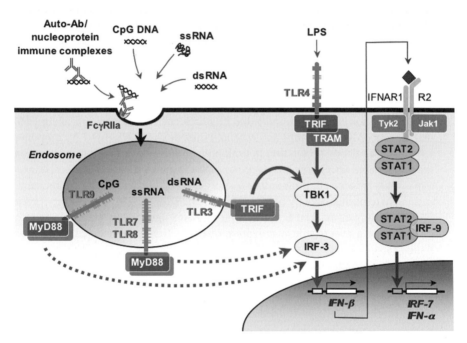

Figure 1 TLRs engaged in IFN-α/β production. Endogenous ligands, such as apoptotic/necrotic material and nucleoproteins complexed with autoantibodies, and exogenous ligands, such as bacterial lipopolysaccharide (LPS), bacterial hypomethylated CpG-DNA, and viral ssRNA or dsRNA, bind to the indicated TLRs on cell surfaces or in endosomal compartments. TLR signaling, involving specific adaptor molecules, recruits the protein kinase TBK1, which phosphorylates IRF-3 and initiates IFN-β transcription. Subsequent signaling through IFNAR leads to IRF-7 and IFN-α expression.

pathway for activation has remained mysterious. Conceivably, other adaptors yet unknown or other members of the IRF family may trigger enhanced IFN-α/β transcription by TLR7 and TLR9. Among the principal effects of TLR signaling and cytokine production is activation of antigen-presenting cells (APCs), upregulation of costimulatory molecules, and the subsequent initiation of a vigorous adaptive immune response.

Although under normal circumstances TLRs do not recognize self, signaling through these receptors may play important secondary and even primary roles in the loss of self-tolerance and induction of autoimmunity. For example, enhanced proliferative responses of rheumatoid factor idiotype-bearing B cells to chromatin-antibody immune complexes resulted from endocytosis of these immune complexes and engagement of TLR9 (79). In another study, DNA with unmethylated CpG motifs efficiently stimulated anti-DNA idiotype-expressing B cells (80). On the basis of these findings, investigators also speculated that self-RNA released by damaged tissues and bound to autoantibodies, when endocytosed, could lead to TLR7- or TLR8-driven DC activation as well as stimulation of self-reactive B cells (81, 82). These findings do not provide a primary explanation for the escape of B cells from self-tolerance, but they do suggest an important secondary mechanism that enhances or sustains production of antideoxyribonucleoprotein autoantibodies in lupus. That this B cell activation mechanism is secondary to the pathogenesis of systemic autoimmunity is supported by the observation that injection of bacterial DNA induces antibodies against mammalian dsDNA only in lupus-predisposed mice containing the corresponding nontolerized B cell precursors, not in normal background mice in which such precursors are anergized or deleted (83). Moreover, although repeated injections of LPS (lipid A component) lead to autoantibody production in both lupus-predisposed and normal mice, only the predisposed mice show histologic manifestations of disease (84). Resistance to CpG DNA-induced autoimmunity by anergic B cells under normal circumstances is thought to be mediated by two distinct mechanisms, an active regulatory process involving antigen-induced B cell receptor (BCR) signaling to the ERK inhibitory pathway and a selective desensitization of BCRs from mitogenic calcineurin signaling (85).

The above findings argue for a secondary role of TLR signaling in enhancing humoral autoimmunity. Engagement of TLRs, however, may still be considered a potential primary trigger for both humoral- and cell-mediated autoimmune diseases. In this case, the postulated mechanism is activation of APC by the induced cytokines (particularly IFNs) leading to upregulation of MHC and costimulatory molecules, which then may facilitate engagement of low-affinity, nontolerant, self-reactive T cells present in the periphery but normally nonengaged and, therefore, quiescent. For instance, B10.S mice transgenic for a T cell receptor specific for the encephalitogenic myelin proteolipid protein peptide are normally resistant to spontaneous experimental allergic encephalomyelitis (EAE) induction owing to a low state of APC activation, but tolerance can be broken and EAE can develop after APC activation by TLR9 or TLR4 engagement (86). Thus, activation of APC via innate immune receptor engagement can break self-tolerance and trigger the development of autoimmunity even in a genetically resistant strain. In this context, infection with certain pathogens has frequently been associated with autoimmune manifestations. Although the mechanism is most often attributed to mimicry between self and foreign epitopes, the alternative possibility that tissue destruction causes availability of previously sequestered self-antigens in regional lymph nodes (87, 88), and/or direct APC activation through TLR signaling and engagement of otherwise quiescent self-reactive T cells, is highly plausible. Figure 2 represents how engagement of TLRs by endogenous or exogenous ligands may lead to systemic or organ-specific autoimmune diseases.

IFN-α/β AND ADAPTIVE IMMUNE RESPONSES

IFN-α/β exert multiple direct and indirect effects on the adaptive immune system that impact almost every cell type and function (3, 52, 89).

IFN-α/β are major inducers of immature DC activation, leading to upregulation of MHC (especially class I MHC), chemokines and chemokine receptors, and costimulatory molecules (CD40, CD80, CD86), which in turn leads to efficient homing in secondary lymphoid organs and CD8$^+$ or CD4$^+$ T cell responses. These effects can be exercised locally or at a distance. IFN-α/β-induced maturation of DCs can also promote cross-priming of CD8$^+$ T cells against virally infected targets (90). IFN-α/β keep activated CD8$^+$ and CD4$^+$ T cells alive and enhance their proliferation by acting either directly (91) or indirectly through induction of IL-15 by APCs (28, 92). Moreover, efficient activation of naive CD8$^+$ T cells appears to be dependent on IFN-α/β-induced IP-10 and CXCR3 (93). Indeed, in vivo proliferation of T cells was reduced in IFNAR1-deficient lupus mice, as was the self-MHC + self-peptide-mediated homeostatic proliferation of such T cells upon transfer into the wild-type lymphopenic syngeneic host (19). IFN-α/β also promote NK cell cytotoxicity, which appears to depend on STAT1 (94) as well as macrophage development, maturation, and iNOS production (54).

IFN-α/β are also known to exert potent antiproliferative and proapoptotic effects on T cells (95), which has made it difficult to explain how clonal expansion of effector T cells occur in the event of an infection when large amounts of IFNs are produced. A potential answer to this enigma is that early in the antiviral response, T cells are under the control of regulatory processes that downregulate the transcriptional response to IFNs, thereby facilitating proliferation of effector cells (96). The antiproliferative and proapoptotic effects of IFN-α/β are associated with a variety of molecular changes, including increases in both cyclin kinase inhibitors and several proapoptotic molecules (Fas/FasL, p53, Bax, Bak), as well as with activation of procaspases 8 and 3 (95).

Although crucial to viral defense, the role of type I IFNs in immunity against bacterial pathogens is less clear. Surprisingly, three recent studies with IFNAR-deficient mice infected with a Gram-positive intracellular bacterium (*Listeria*

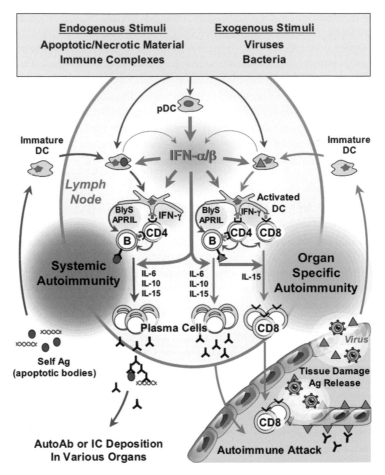

Figure 2 Mechanisms by which IFN-α/β may contribute to the pathogenesis of systemic and organ-specific autoimmune diseases in predisposed backgrounds. Engagement of TLR by endogenous or exogenous stimuli leads to IFN-α/β production primarily by pDCs and, to a lesser extent, DCs. IFN-α/β then induce DC activation, leading to high expression of MHC class I (and secondarily class II by IFN-γ) and costimulatory molecules. Production of BLyS and APRIL is also initiated and, together with T cell help and other cytokines, induces B cell differentiation to plasma cells and autoantibody production. The diverse autoantibodies and/or immune complexes (IC) bind to cell surfaces and tissues and cause systemic autoimmune diseases. Similar mechanisms may also cause organ-specific autoimmune diseases, but tissue damage and availability of previously sequestered self-antigens in regional lymph nodes is required for engagement of nontolerant cytotoxic CD8 T cells. Presentation of the released tissue-specific self-antigens by B cells to helper CD4 T cells may also occur, leading to autoantibody production. In both systemic and organ-specific autoimmune diseases, IFN-α/β may also directly promote survival and proliferation of self-reactive T and B cells.

monocytogenes) provided evidence that the absence of type I IFN signaling rendered the mice more resistant to infection (96a–c). The exact mechanism of this effect is not clear, but presumably signaling by IFNs enhances lymphocyte apoptosis caused by bacterial pore-forming toxins. Whether these findings are applicable to other bacterial infections remains to be determined.

Type I IFNs also exert a variety of effects on the development and function of B cells. Thus, IFN-α/β enhance BCR-dependent mature B2 cell responses and increase survival and resistance to Fas-mediated apoptosis (97). Signaling by IFNAR, acting directly or indirectly through other cytokines/chemokines, is also required for normal development and proliferation of the B1 subset (19), which is thought to be a major producer of autoantibodies. Moreover, type I IFNs, acting indirectly through DC activation, exert strong adjuvant effects by markedly enhancing antibody responses and promoting Ig isotype switching (98).

IFN-α (and IFN-γ) also upregulates expression of the two major B cell survival factors, the B lymphocyte stimulator (BLyS, also known as BAFF, TALL-1, THANK, and zTNF4), and a proliferation-inducing ligand (APRIL) in DCs and monocytes, a finding that might explain the antiapoptotic effect of IFN-α/β on B cells. Furthermore, BLyS and APRIL, in conjunction with other cytokines (IL-10, TGF-β), can induce CD40-independent Ig class-switch recombination from Cμ to Cγ and/or Cα genes in B cells (99). Secretion of class-switched antibodies then follows upon BCR engagement together with IL-15. Moreover, virus-triggered pDCs, acting through IFN-α/β, induce CD40-activated B cells to differentiate initially into plasmablasts, which in the presence of IL-6 differentiate into Ig-secreting plasma cells (100). These findings further demonstrate the ability of IFN-α/β to promote humoral immune responses and point toward another mechanism by which IFN-α/β may induce hypergammaglobulinemia and autoantibody production in lupus-predisposed individuals (101). In further support of the role of B cell trophic factors in systemic autoimmunity, mice transgenic for BLyS (*Tnfsf13b* gene) have vastly increased numbers of mature B cells and develop humoral, cellular, and histologic manifestations resembling lupus or Sjögren's syndrome (102, 103), as do mice lacking the transmembrane activator and calcium modulator ligand interactor (TACI), which apparently acts as an inhibitor of BLyS (104). Similarly, mice with conditional SOCS-1 deficiency in DCs showed high levels of BLyS and APRIL, resulting in B cell expansion and autoantibody production (105). In contrast, lupus-predisposed mice treated with recombinant receptors for BLyS and APRIL (BAFFR or TACI) exhibit reduced disease (106, 107). Humans and mice with systemic autoimmune syndromes have high levels of BLyS in their serum that correlate with autoantibody titers, suggesting that BLyS may be an attractive therapeutic target (108).

As with T cells, IFN-α/β can also exert inhibitory effects on B cell development and survival. Thus, bone marrow and spleen cellularity were shown to be greatly reduced in IFN-α-treated mice, and B-lineage cells were reduced by more than 80%, particularly the CD19$^+$ pro-B cells (109). This effect was attributed to the IFN-α opposing effects on IL-7. However, no defects in B cell development were observed in mice lacking the IFNAR1 chain (19). Moreover, as noted above, IFN-α/β may inhibit apoptosis of mature B cells.

IFN-α/β IN AUTOIMMUNE DISEASES

Given the diverse and potent effects of IFN-α/β in the innate and adaptive immune system, it is not surprising that these cytokines play a pivotal pathogenic role in several autoimmune diseases (Table 2). Among them, evidence linking IFN-α/β with the pathogenesis of lupus and insulin-dependent diabetes mellitus (IDDM) in humans and rodent models is the most convincing.

Systemic Lupus Erythematosus (SLE)

Increased levels of IFN-α in the serum of lupus patients were first noted over 25 years ago (110) and subsequently confirmed in several studies (reviewed in 111). Surprisingly, increases in IFN-α are not associated with consistent increases in IFN-β, perhaps reflecting a degree of independent regulation between these two types of IFN. Although other cytokines are also increased in lupus sera, IFN-α levels best coincide with disease exacerbations (112). IFN-α treatment for a variety of unrelated conditions (viral infections, tumors) also sometimes exacerbates or even induces a wide spectrum of autoimmune manifestations, including lupus (reviewed in 113). Convincing evidence for a role of IFN-α in lupus pathogenesis was provided by the recent finding that sera of lupus patients, particularly during active disease, induced in vitro maturation of normal blood monocytes into efficient antigen-presenting DCs, and the active factor for this effect was IFN-α (114). In addition, recent microarray studies with peripheral blood mononuclear cells of lupus patients showed gene expression "signatures" distinguishable from controls by higher representation of IFN-α- and IFN-γ-inducible transcripts, a characteristic that was a marker of more severe and active disease (5, 6, 115–117). Further independent analysis of the above data suggested that genes preferentially regulated by IFN-α may predominate in early disease samples, while those regulated by IFN-γ may appear at later stages. Therefore, investigators hypothesized that IFN-α plays a role in the proximal events of disease pathogenesis, and IFN-γ contributes to the later chronic inflammation and target organ damage (117). However, a more recent microarray analysis of laser-captured glomeruli from lupus patients shows type I IFN response elements among the four dominant clusters of overexpressed genes, whereas IFN-γ-induced transcripts were less prominent (118). In all the above microarray studies, it was surprising that expression levels for IFN-α/β (or IFN-γ) were normal. This finding might be explained by the severe reduction of pDCs in the peripheral blood of lupus patients, presumably owing to their migration to tissues following acquisition of IFN-α/β-induced chemokine receptors (119).

Why lupus patients have higher levels of IFN-α has not been fully explained, but both exogenous and endogenous inducers may be considered. With regard to

TABLE 2   Type I IFNs and autoimmunity

Disease	Findings related to IFN-α/β	Effects of type I IFN
Systemic lupus erythematosus (SLE)	Increased serum levels of IFN-α IFN-α levels correlate with disease exacerbation Peripheral blood cell IFN gene expression "signatures" IFNAR knockout NZB and B6-*lpr* mice have reduced disease IFNAR knockout MRL-*lpr* mice develop more severe disease	Induction and exacerbation (humans and mice)
Insulin-dependent diabetes mellitus (IDDM)	Increased serum levels and pancreas mRNA expression of IFN-α Transgenic expression of IFN-α in pancreatic β-islet cells causes overt diabetes Diabetes in several rat and mouse models is induced/exacerbated by high dose poly I:C (IFN-α inducer)	Occasionally occurs during IFN-α treatment for unrelated diseases (humans) Decreased incidence and severity of diabetes in NOD and BB rats Low dose poly I:C prevents diabetes in BB rats (possibly by generation of suppressor/regulatory T cells) Oral IFN-α delayed onset of diabetes in NOD and IDDM patients (phase I study)
Multiple sclerosis (MS)/EAE	EAE is exacerbated in IFN-β-deficient mice	Used in the treatment of MS
Rheumatoid arthritis (RA)	IFN-α levels increased in synovial fluid IFN-β treatment can inhibit collagen-induced arthritis in mice and rhesus monkeys	Rarely associated with IFN-α treatment Beneficial in phase I trials
Myasthenia gravis	IFN-α can inhibit EAMG	Rarely occurs following IFN-α treatment
Autoimmune hemolytic anemia	Reduced in NZB mice deficient for IFNAR	Rarely occurs following IFN-α treatment

exogenous inducers, viral and bacterial pathogens obviously may be the culprits but, despite many efforts, investigators have not identified a specific pathogen for this disease. Nevertheless, IFN-α/β production may be a common pathway by which infection by a variety of pathogens or other exogenous type I IFN stimuli induce or exacerbate systemic autoimmunity in susceptible individuals, as often seen in SLE following infection or UV light exposure. As discussed earlier, however, there is also evidence for IFN-α/β endogenous inducers, such as products of apoptotic or necrotic cells combined with lupus serum autoantibodies (119, 120). "Interferogenic" anti-DNA and anti-ribonucleoprotein (anti-RNP) complexes with DNA or RNA, respectively, reportedly can stimulate IFN-α/β production through FcγRIIa binding and internalization (119). This finding is consistent with the recent suggestion that mammalian RNA, which is capable of binding to IFN-α/β-inducing endosomal TLRs, is prevented from activating cells because of compartmentalization away from the endosomes. Thus, only the anti-RNP/RNP complexes, taken up in the endosomes, could result in activation of the relevant TLRs and production of IFN-α/β. Regardless of the exact inducer, a model has been set forth according to which lupus results from an unabated activation of myeloid DCs through IFN-α produced by pDCs (34).

Early evidence of acceleration of disease severity and onset by IFN-α/β or its inducers (dsRNA, poly I:C) in lupus-predisposed New Zealand Black (NZB) mice (121–124) was reinforced by the recent demonstration that lupus disease was significantly reduced in IFNAR1-deficient NZB mice (19). The gene encoding the IFNAR1 on distal chromosome 16 is not within the known NZB susceptibility loci (125). Compared with littermate controls, homozygous IFNAR-deleted mice had significantly reduced autoantibodies, hemolytic anemia, kidney disease, and mortality. These reductions were intermediate in the heterozygous-deleted mice, indicating therapeutic effectiveness for even partial reduction in IFN-α/β signaling. As expected for the potent pleiotropic effects of type I IFNs, receptor-deficient mice had reductions in numbers and proliferation of most immunocyte subsets, and, of course, defects of in vitro maturation and function of DCs in response to exogenous IFN-α. Interestingly, there was no reduction in the high levels of the Ifi202 phosphoprotein, attributed to a mutation in the promoter of the *Ifi202* gene that is associated with a major NZB predisposing locus (72). This finding agrees with previous and recent studies indicating that, in addition to IFN-α/β, other factors, such as IL-6, can also induce Ifi202 expression (71, 126). The data indicate that the adverse effects mediated by the *Nba-2*-associated *Ifi202* allele as well as those by other predisposing loci of the NZB mice are attenuated in the absence of IFN-α/β signaling.

Another interesting finding in IFNAR1-deficient NZB mice was a significant decrease in the frequency of IFN-γ-producing CD4$^+$ and CD8$^+$ T cells. This decrease correlates with reductions in the Th1-mediated IgG2a subclass of anti-DNA autoantibodies, consistent with crossregulation of IFN-γ production and signaling by IFN-α/β, as discussed earlier. Considering that, like IFN-α/β, IFN-γ also adversely affects disease in several murine lupus models (127), one may argue that therapies based on blocking either class of IFNs may reduce the detrimental activities of both. This possibility needs to be directly tested, as it would be important to determine whether blocking IFN-α/β signaling is also effective when applied after the developmental stage and, in particular, after disease manifestations have appeared.

In addition to NZB mice, disease reduction was reported in IFNAR1-deleted B6.Fas^{lpr} mice (128) but, surprisingly, not in similarly deleted MRL-Fas^{lpr} mice (129). No clear reason aside from the differences in disease severity (mild in B6.Fas^{lpr}, severe in MRL-Fas^{lpr}) was given for these opposite responses.

Because IFNs exert potent pleiotropic effects, their role as pathogenic effectors in this disease is likely to be mediated by multiple mechanisms, including enhanced DC maturation and self-Ag presentation; promotion of T and B cell differentiation, proliferation, and survival; disturbances in the balance of anti- and proinflammatory cytokines; and induction of chemokines and receptors that promote homing of inflammatory cells in tissues.

Overall, IFN-α/β signaling appears to be a master switch that activates all or most of the above pathways, leading to pathogenicity in lupus-predisposed backgrounds. It has not been established, however, whether this switch is turned on in lupus because of a primary defect, such as hyperproduction or hyper-responsiveness to stimuli and/or a higher number of IFN-α/β-producing cells, or because of a secondary abnormality, such as a viral or bacterial trigger, or increased levels of apoptotic cells and autoantigen-autoantibody immune complexes.

Insulin-Dependent Diabetes Mellitus (IDDM)

Considerable data supporting a link between IFN-α and IDDM (type 1 diabetes) in humans and rodent models have been reported, with both inducing/enhancing and inhibitory effects (reviewed in 130, 131).

Increased levels of IFN-α in the serum and increased mRNA expression of quite limited (but different among individuals) IFN-α subtype profiles in the pancreas of IDDM patients have been detected (132). Moreover, as with certain other autoimmune diseases, type 1 diabetes occasionally appears during IFN-α treatment of unrelated diseases such as chronic hepatitis or tumors (133, 134). The fact that IDDM is primarily a childhood disease while these rare cases involve IFN-α-treated adults suggests more than chance occurrence. Correlation of Coxsackie B virus infections with increased levels of IFN-α in plasma and blood cells in type 1 diabetes has also been detected (135).

Evidence supporting a central role for type I IFNs in the pathogenesis of IDDM has also been obtained in rodent models. Thus, normal background mice with transgenic expression of IFN-α (136), IFN-β (137), and even IFN-κ (138) in the β cells of the pancreas develop overt diabetes with inflammatory infiltrates, destruction of β cells, and hyperglycemia. IDDM was prevented by treating IFN-α-expressing transgenic mice with a mAb against the IFN-α subtype encoded by the transgene (136). Diabetes was also induced/accelerated with injections of the strong IFN-α/β inducer poly I:C in disease-susceptible BioBreeding (BB) rats (139, 140), the mouse model of streptozotocin-induced diabetes (140), and diabetes induced by a variant of the encephalomyocarditis virus (EMC-D) (141). Injections of poly I:C also promoted diabetes in mice transgenic for islet expression of the costimulatory molecule B7.1 immunized with an insulin self-peptide (142, 143).

In contrast, administration of recombinant IFN-α decreased the incidence and severity of diabetes in both NOD mice (144) and BB rats (145). Continuous administration of poly I:C alone or in combination with rIL-2 in NOD mice also prevented glycosuria, presumably by inducing some type of regulatory T cells (146). Similarly, poly I:C at low doses (0.05–0.1 μg/g body weight) prevented insulitis and diabetes in BB rats (147), in contrast to the previously reported enhancement of disease with 100-fold higher doses (5 μg/g). This differential effect was attributed to generation of suppressor/regulatory T cells at low, but not high, poly I:C doses. Oral administration of IFN-α also significantly delayed the onset of diabetes in NOD mice (148) and, to a lesser degree, in a phase I open trial in humans with recent-onset IDDM (149). Thus, as with TNF-α (150), the effects of IFN-α in IDDM appear dependent on disease stage, i.e., IFN-α may promote initiation of the aberrant autoimmune response at the early stages, but may suppress proliferation and survival of autoreactive T cells at late stages. Alternatively, by promoting T cell survival, IFN-α/β may correct the lymphopenia thought to be a major contributor to autoimmune pathogenesis in NOD mice (151) and systemic autoimmune disease in general (152).

Several mechanisms can be invoked for the induction of IFN-α in IDDM and how IFN-α promotes early disease phases. The first suspect for induction is infection by pancreatotropic viruses, although with the possible exception of enteroviruses no firm association between viral infections and autoimmune diabetes has yet been established (153). Still, a viral etiology cannot be excluded because obstacles exist in tissue availability, and viral traces may have disappeared by the time clinical manifestations become evident. Paradoxically, however, infections with certain viruses can suppress the survival and function of DCs and T cells, with IFN-α/β being a major mediator of this suppression (154). Consequently, lymphocytic choriomeningitis virus (LCMV) infection can abrogate diabetes in both the NOD (155) and the transgenic RIP-LCMV (156) models. Other cytokines (i.e., IFN-β, IFN-γ, and IL-2) produced by epithelial cells, DCs, and other cell types, as well as proinflammatory products of damaged cells, may constitute alternative means for local IFN-α production.

Both immunologic and nonimmunologic effects may contribute to IFN-α-mediated tissue damage (reviewed in 130). The immunologic processes, as outlined earlier, include DC activation, proliferation, and survival of naive and memory T cells, autoantibody production, and Ig class switch. Nonimmunologic effects of relevance to diabetes may include decreased insulin synthesis, suppression of mitochondrial function and ATP levels leading to decreased glucose-stimulated insulin secretion, suppression of cell division, and increased apoptosis.

Other Autoimmune Diseases

Detrimental or beneficial effects of IFN-α/β in several other autoimmune diseases have been reported, primarily in multiple sclerosis (MS) and EAE and, to a lesser extent, in RA, Sjögren's syndrome, myasthenia gravis, autoimmune hemolytic anemia, thyroiditis, uveitis, Behcet's disease, and others. The use of IFN-β, IFN-α, or combinations thereof in treating MS is well known (157). Moreover, mice deficient in IFN-β showed augmented and chronic EAE (158). Despite many studies in humans with MS and the EAE mouse model, the precise mechanisms by which type I IFNs exert their modest beneficial effects in MS remain largely unresolved, although they may be mediated by a combination of antiviral, anti-inflammatory, anti-proliferative, proapoptotic and other immunomodulatory activities.

As with lupus and type 1 diabetes, RA-like manifestations are rare in patients receiving IFN-α therapy for unrelated disorders (159), and IFN-α levels may be increased in synovial fluids of RA patients. On the other hand, IFN-β reportedly inhibited collagen-induced arthritis in mice (160) and rhesus monkeys (161) and had some beneficial effects in RA (162) and Sjögren's syndrome (163).

Myasthenia subsequent to IFN-α treatment has also been reported (164). However, IFN-α treatment inhibited experimental autoimmune myasthenia gravis (EAMG) with both reductions in anti-AChR autoantibody titers and suppression of CD4$^+$ T cell responses to AChR and its immunodominant peptide (165).

Autoimmune hemolytic anemia also sometimes follows treatment with IFN-α for unrelated disorders (166). Moreover, as discussed earlier, hemolytic anemia was significantly reduced in IFNAR1-deficient NZB mice (19).

Thus, although not yet adequately defined, it is evident that IFN-α/β have a major effect on virtually all autoimmune diseases. IFN-α/β are therefore an excellent candidate target for therapeutic intervention. Such intervention, however, must consider the disease-specific effects of IFN-α/β in autoimmunity and their importance in immune surveillance. In the latter, more precise targeting of autoimmune pathways related to IFN-α/β may potentially be obtained by targeting three main areas, the inducers of type I IFNs (TLRs, immune complexes), specific type I IFN family members and subtypes, and finally, IFN-α/β effector pathways, such as IRFs and IFIs.

CONCLUSIONS

Type I IFNs (α/β) are central to a vast array of immunologic functions. Their induction early in the innate immune response provides a priming mechanism that orchestrates many subsequent processes in innate as well as adaptive immune responses. The outcome can be promotion or inhibition of these responses, but the conditions under which one or the other prevails remain to be precisely defined. These cytokines also occupy center stage in the pathogenesis of several systemic and organ-specific autoimmune diseases, where again their effects can be detrimental or beneficial. What renders these molecules destructive when there is a predisposition to autoimmunity? Are there primary defects in the production of, or response to, type I IFNs in autoimmunity, or are the IFNs simply part of the pathway required for any immunologic response? It is essential to determine how a physiologically protective molecule is rendered harmful. Answering these questions is central to devising IFN-related therapies for autoimmune diseases, with the crucial caveat that, because these molecules are essential in normal immunologic processes, such interventions should be carefully designed.

APPENDIX

Abbreviations used: APC, antigen-presenting cell; APRIL, a proliferation-inducing ligand; BB, BioBreeding; BCR, B cell receptor; BDCA, blood DC antigen; DC, dendritic cell; EAE, experimental allergic encephalomyelitis; EAMG, experimental autoimmune myasthenia gravis; EMC-D, encephalomyocarditis virus D variant; GM-CSF, granulocyte macrophage-colony stimulating factor; ICSBP, IFN consensus sequence binding protein; IDDM, insulin-dependent diabetes mellitus; IFN, interferon; IFNAR, IFN alpha receptor; IFNGR, IFN-γ receptor; IRAK-4, IL-1 receptor-associated kinase 4; IRF, IFN regulatory factor; ISGF3, IFN-stimulated gene factor 3; ISRE, IFN-stimulated response elements; LCMV, lymphocytic choriomeningitis virus; LPS, lipopolysaccharide; MS, multiple sclerosis; MyD88, myeloid differentiation factor 88; Mal, MyD88 adaptor-like; NIPC, natural IFN-producing cell; NOD, non-obese diabetic; NZB, New Zealand Black; pDC, plasmacytoid dendritic cell; PIAS, protein inhibitors of activated STATs; RA, rheumatoid arthritis; RNP, ribonucleoprotein; SLE, systemic lupus erythematosus; SOCS, suppressors of cytokine signaling; TACI, transmembrane activator and calcium modulator ligand interactor; TBK1, Tank-binding kinase 1; TGF-β, transforming growth factor β; TICAM, TIR-containing adaptor molecule; TIR, Toll-interleukin-1 receptor; TIRAP, TIR-containing adaptor protein; TLR, Toll-like receptor; TNF, tumor necrosis factor; TRAF-6, TNF receptor-associated factor 6; TRAM, TRIF-related adaptor molecule; TRIF, TIR-containing adaptor inducing IFN.

ACKNOWLEDGMENTS

This is Publication No. 16777-IMM from the Department of Immunology, The Scripps Research Institute, 10550 N. Torrey Pines Rd., La Jolla, CA 92037. The work of the authors discussed herein was supported, in part, by NIH grants AR39555, AR31203, and AR42242. The authors thank M. Kat Occhipinti-Bender for editorial work. Please note that space limitations do not allow citation of many excellent original publications, and we apologize for these omissions.

The *Annual Review of Immunology* is online at
http://immunol.annualreviews.org

LITERATURE CITED

1. Stark GR, Kerr IM, Williams BR, Silverman RH, Schreiber RD. 1998. How cells respond to interferons. *Annu. Rev. Biochem.* 67:227–64

2. Pestka S. 2000. The human interferon α species and receptors. *Biopolymers* 55: 254–87

3. Biron CA. 2001. Interferons α and β as immune regulators—a new look. *Immunity* 14:661–64

4. Der SD, Zhou A, Williams BR, Silverman RH. 1998. Identification of genes differentially regulated by interferon α, β, or γ using oligonucleotide arrays. *Proc. Natl. Acad. Sci. USA* 95:15623–28

5. Baechler EC, Batliwalla FM, Karypis G, Gaffney PM, Ortmann WA, et al. 2003. Interferon-inducible gene expression signature in peripheral blood cells of patients with severe lupus. *Proc. Natl. Acad. Sci. USA* 100:2610–15

6. Bennett L, Palucka AK, Arce E, Cantrell V, Borvak J, et al. 2003. Interferon and granulopoiesis signatures in systemic lupus erythematosus blood. *J. Exp. Med.* 197:711–23

7. Pestka S, Krause CD, Sarkar D, Walter MR, Shi Y, et al. 2004. Interleukin-10 and related cytokines and receptors. *Annu. Rev. Immunol.* 22:929–79

8. Donnelly RP, Sheikh F, Kotenko SV, Dickensheets H. 2004. The expanded family of class II cytokines that share the IL-10 receptor-2 (IL-10R2) chain. *J. Leukoc. Biol.* 76:314–21

9. Kotenko SV, Langer JA. 2004. Full house: 12 receptors for 27 cytokines. *Int. Immunopharmacol.* 4:593–608

10. Schlaak JF, Hilkens CM, Costa-Pereira AP, Strobl B, Aberger F, et al. 2002. Cell-type and donor-specific transcriptional responses to interferon-α. Use of customized gene arrays. *J. Biol. Chem.* 277:49428–37

11. Kotenko SV, Gallagher G, Baurin VV, Lewis-Antes A, Shen M, et al. 2003. IFN-λs mediate antiviral protection through a distinct class II cytokine receptor complex. *Nat. Immunol.* 4:69–77

12. Sheppard P, Kindsvogel W, Xu W, Henderson K, Schlutsmeyer S, et al. 2003. IL-28, IL-29 and their class II cytokine receptor IL-28R. *Nat. Immunol.* 4:63–68

13. Shuai K, Liu B. 2003. Regulation of JAK-STAT signalling in the immune system. *Nat. Rev. Immunol.* 3:900–11

14. Hata N, Sato M, Takaoka A, Asagiri M, Tanaka N, et al. 2001. Constitutive IFN-α/β signal for efficient IFN-α/β gene induction by virus. *Biochem. Biophys. Res. Commun.* 285:518–25

15. Taniguchi T, Takaoka A. 2001. A weak signal for strong responses: interferon-α/β revisited. *Nat. Rev. Mol. Cell Biol.* 2:378–86

16. Takaoka A, Mitani Y, Suemori H, Sato M, Yokochi T, et al. 2000. Cross talk between interferon γ and -α/β signaling components in caveolar membrane domains. *Science* 288:2357–60

17. Montoya M, Schiavoni G, Mattei F, Gresser I, Belardelli F, et al. 2002. Type I interferons produced by dendritic cells promote their phenotypic and functional activation. *Blood* 99:3263–71

18. Brinkmann V, Geiger T, Alkan S, Heusser CH. 1993. Interferon α increases the frequency of interferon γ-producing human CD4$^+$ T cells. *J. Exp. Med.* 178:1655–63

19. Santiago-Raber ML, Baccala R, Haraldsson KM, Choubey D, Stewart TA, et al. 2003. Type-I interferon receptor deficiency reduces lupus-like disease in NZB mice. *J. Exp. Med.* 197:777–88

20. Cousens LP, Peterson R, Hsu S, Dorner A, Altman JD, et al. 1999. Two roads diverged: interferon α/β- and interleukin 12-mediated pathways in promoting T cell interferon γ responses during viral infection. *J. Exp. Med.* 189:1315–28

21. Nguyen KB, Cousens LP, Doughty LA, Pien GC, Durbin JE, et al. 2000. Interferon α/β-mediated inhibition and promotion of interferon γ: STAT1 resolves a paradox. *Nat. Immunol.* 1:70–76

22. Nguyen KB, Watford WT, Salomon R, Hofmann SR, Pien GC, et al. 2002. Critical role for STAT4 activation by type 1 interferons in the interferon-γ response to viral infection. *Science* 297:2063–66

23. Darnell JE Jr, Kerr IM, Stark GR. 1994. Jak-STAT pathways and transcriptional activation in response to IFNs and other extracellular signaling proteins. *Science* 264:1415–21

24. Levy DE, Lew DJ, Decker T, Kessler DS, Darnell JE Jr. 1990. Synergistic interaction between interferon-α and interferon-γ through induced synthesis of one subunit of the transcription factor ISGF3. *EMBO J.* 9:1105–11

24a. Tassiulas I, Hu X, Ho H, Kashyap Y, Paik P, Hu Y, et al. 2004. Amplification of IFN-α-induced STAT1 activation and inflammatory function by Syk and ITAM-containing adaptors. *Nat. Immunol.* 5:1181–89

25. Brassard DL, Grace MJ, Bordens RW. 2002. Interferon-α as an immunotherapeutic protein. *J. Leukoc. Biol.* 71:565–81

26. Mitani Y, Takaoka A, Kim SH, Kato Y, Yokochi T, et al. 2001. Cross talk of the interferon-α/β signalling complex with gp130 for effective interleukin-6 signalling. *Genes Cells* 6:631–40

27. Dickensheets HL, Venkataraman C, Schindler U, Donnelly RP. 1999. Interferons inhibit activation of STAT6 by interleukin 4 in human monocytes by inducing SOCS-1 gene expression. *Proc. Natl. Acad. Sci. USA* 96:10800–5

28. Zhang X, Sun S, Hwang I, Tough DF, Sprent J. 1998. Potent and selective stimulation of memory-phenotype CD8[+] T cells in vivo by IL-15. *Immunity* 8:591–99

29. Ito S, Ansari P, Sakatsume M, Dickensheets H, Vazquez N, et al. 1999. Interleukin-10 inhibits expression of both interferon α- and interferon γ-induced genes by suppressing tyrosine phosphorylation of STAT1. *Blood* 93:1456–63

30. Sharif MN, Tassiulas I, Hu Y, Mecklenbrauker I, Tarakhovsky A, et al. 2004. IFN-α priming results in a gain of proinflammatory function by IL-10: implications for systemic lupus erythematosus pathogenesis. *J. Immunol.* 172:6476–81

31. Llorente L, Richaud-Patin Y. 2003. The role of interleukin-10 in systemic lupus erythematosus. *J. Autoimmun.* 20:287–89

32. Ishida H, Muchamuel T, Sakaguchi S, Andrade S, Menon S, et al. 1994. Continuous administration of anti-interleukin 10 antibodies delays onset of autoimmunity in NZB/W F1 mice. *J. Exp. Med.* 179:305–10

33. Ivashkiv LB. 2003. Type I interferon modulation of cellular responses to cytokines and infectious pathogens: potential role in SLE pathogenesis. *Autoimmunity* 36:473–79

34. Banchereau J, Pascual V, Palucka AK. 2004. Autoimmunity through cytokine-induced dendritic cell activation. *Immunity* 20:539–50

35. Theofilopoulos AN, Lawson BR. 1999. Tumour necrosis factor and other cytokines in murine lupus. *Ann. Rheum. Dis.* 58(Suppl. 1):I49–55

36. Aringer M, Smolen JS. 2003. SLE—Complex cytokine effects in a complex autoimmune disease: tumor necrosis factor in systemic lupus erythematosus. *Arthritis Res. Ther.* 5:172–77

37. O'Shea JJ, Gadina M, Schreiber RD. 2002. Cytokine signaling in 2002: new surprises in the Jak/Stat pathway. *Cell* 109(Suppl):S121–31

38. Takaoka A, Hayakawa S, Yanai H, Stoiber

D, Negishi H, et al. 2003. Integration of interferon-α/β signalling to p53 responses in tumour suppression and antiviral defence. *Nature* 424:516–23

39. Colonna M, Krug A, Cella M. 2002. Interferon-producing cells: on the front line in immune responses against pathogens. *Curr. Opin. Immunol.* 14:373–79

40. Coccia EM, Severa M, Giacomini E, Monneron D, Remoli ME, et al. 2004. Viral infection and Toll-like receptor agonists induce a differential expression of type I and λ interferons in human plasmacytoid and monocyte-derived dendritic cells. *Eur. J. Immunol.* 34:796–805

41. Shortman K, Liu YJ. 2002. Mouse and human dendritic cell subtypes. *Nat. Rev. Immunol.* 2:151–61

42. del Hoyo GM, Martin P, Vargas HH, Ruiz S, Arias CF, et al. 2002. Characterization of a common precursor population for dendritic cells. *Nature* 415:1043–47

42a. Shigematsu H, Reizis B, Iwasaki H, Mizuno S, Hu D, et al. 2004. Plasmacytoid dendritic cells activate lymphoid-specific genetic programs irrespective of their cellular origin. *Immunity* 21:43–53

43. Dzionek A, Inagaki Y, Okawa K, Nagafune J, Röck J, et al. 2002. Plasmacytoid dendritic cells: from specific surface markers to specific cellular functions. *Hum. Immunol.* 63:1133–48

44. Blomberg S, Eloranta ML, Magnusson M, Alm GV, Ronnblom L. 2003. Expression of the markers BDCA-2 and BDCA-4 and production of interferon-α by plasmacytoid dendritic cells in systemic lupus erythematosus. *Arthritis. Rheum.* 48:2524–32

45. Asselin-Paturel C, Brizard G, Pin JJ, Briere F, Trinchieri G. 2003. Mouse strain differences in plasmacytoid dendritic cell frequency and function revealed by a novel monoclonal antibody. *J. Immunol.* 171:6466–77

46. Martin P, del Hoyo GM, Anjuere F, Arias CF, Vargas HH, et al. 2002. Characterization of a new subpopulation of mouse CD8α^+ B220$^+$ dendritic cells endowed with type 1 interferon production capacity and tolerogenic potential. *Blood* 100:383–90

47. Nakano H, Yanagita M, Gunn MD. 2001. CD11c$^+$B220$^+$Gr-1$^+$ cells in mouse lymph nodes and spleen display characteristics of plasmacytoid dendritic cells. *J. Exp. Med.* 194:1171–78

48. Bjorck P. 2001. Isolation and characterization of plasmacytoid dendritic cells from Flt3 ligand and granulocyte-macrophage colony-stimulating factor-treated mice. *Blood* 98:3520–26

49. Gilliet M, Boonstra A, Paturel C, Antonenko S, Xu XL, et al. 2002. The development of murine plasmacytoid dendritic cell precursors is differentially regulated by FLT3-ligand and granulocyte/macrophage colony-stimulating factor. *J. Exp. Med.* 195:953–58

50. D'Amico A, Wu L. 2003. The early progenitors of mouse dendritic cells and plasmacytoid predendritic cells are within the bone marrow hemopoietic precursors expressing Flt3. *J. Exp. Med.* 198:293–303

51. Izaguirre A, Barnes BJ, Amrute S, Yeow WS, Megjugorac N, et al. 2003. Comparative analysis of IRF and IFN-α expression in human plasmacytoid and monocyte-derived dendritic cells. *J. Leukoc. Biol.* 74:1125–38

52. Santini SM, Di Pucchio T, Lapenta C, Parlato S, Logozzi M, et al. 2002. The natural alliance between type I interferon and dendritic cells and its role in linking innate and adaptive immunity. *J. Interferon Cytokine Res.* 22:1071–80

53. Diebold SS, Montoya M, Unger H, Alexopoulou L, Roy P, et al. 2003. Viral infection switches non-plasmacytoid dendritic cells into high interferon producers. *Nature* 424:324–28

54. Taniguchi T, Ogasawara K, Takaoka A, Tanaka N. 2001. IRF family of transcription factors as regulators of host defense. *Annu. Rev. Immunol.* 19:623–55

55. Sato M, Taniguchi T, Tanaka N. 2001. The interferon system and interferon regulatory factor transcription factors—studies from gene knockout mice. *Cytokine Growth Factor Rev.* 12:133–42

56. Ohteki T, Yoshida H, Matsuyama T, Duncan GS, Mak TW, et al. 1998. The transcription factor interferon regulatory factor 1 (IRF-1) is important during the maturation of natural killer 1.1^+ T cell receptor-α/β^+ ($NK1^+$ T) cells, natural killer cells, and intestinal intraepithelial T cells. *J. Exp. Med.* 187:967–72

57. Ogasawara K, Hida S, Azimi N, Tagaya Y, Sato T, et al. 1998. Requirement for IRF-1 in the microenvironment supporting development of natural killer cells. *Nature* 391:700–3

58. Matsuyama T, Kimura T, Kitagawa M, Pfeffer K, Kawakami T, et al. 1993. Targeted disruption of IRF-1 or IRF-2 results in abnormal type I IFN gene induction and aberrant lymphocyte development. *Cell* 75:83–97

59. Penninger JM, Sirard C, Mittrucker HW, Chidgey A, Kozieradzki I, et al. 1997. The interferon regulatory transcription factor IRF-1 controls positive and negative selection of $CD8^+$ thymocytes. *Immunity* 7:243–54

60. Taki S, Sato T, Ogasawara K, Fukuda T, Sato M, et al. 1997. Multistage regulation of Th1-type immune responses by the transcription factor IRF-1. *Immunity* 6:673–79

61. Lohoff M, Ferrick D, Mittrucker HW, Duncan GS, Bischof S, et al. 1997. Interferon regulatory factor-1 is required for a T helper 1 immune response in vivo. *Immunity* 6:681–89

62. Tada Y, Ho A, Matsuyama T, Mak TW. 1997. Reduced incidence and severity of antigen-induced autoimmune diseases in mice lacking interferon regulatory factor-1. *J. Exp. Med.* 185:231–38

63. Nakazawa T, Satoh J, Takahashi K, Sakata Y, Ikehata F, et al. 2001. Complete suppression of insulitis and diabetes in NOD mice lacking interferon regulatory factor-1. *J. Autoimmun.* 17:119–25

64. Lohoff M, Duncan GS, Ferrick D, Mittrucker HW, Bischof S, et al. 2000. Deficiency in the transcription factor interferon regulatory factor (IRF)-2 leads to severely compromised development of natural killer and T helper type 1 cells. *J. Exp. Med.* 192:325–36

65. Hida S, Ogasawara K, Sato K, Abe M, Takayanagi H, et al. 2000. $CD8^+$ T cell-mediated skin disease in mice lacking IRF-2, the transcriptional attenuator of interferon-α/β signaling. *Immunity* 13:643–55

66. Mittrucker HW, Matsuyama T, Grossman A, Kundig TM, Potter J, et al. 1997. Requirement for the transcription factor LSIRF/IRF4 for mature B and T lymphocyte function. *Science* 275:540–43

67. Lohoff M, Mittrucker HW, Prechtl S, Bischof S, Sommer F, et al. 2002. Dysregulated T helper cell differentiation in the absence of interferon regulatory factor 4. *Proc. Natl. Acad. Sci. USA* 99:11808–12

68. Schiavoni G, Mattei F, Sestili P, Borghi P, Venditti M, et al. 2002. ICSBP is essential for the development of mouse type I interferon-producing cells and for the generation and activation of $CD8\alpha^+$ dendritic cells. *J. Exp. Med.* 196:1415–25

69. Tsujimura H, Tamura T, Ozato K. 2003. Cutting edge: IFN consensus sequence binding protein/IFN regulatory factor 8 drives the development of type I IFN-producing plasmacytoid dendritic cells. *J. Immunol.* 170:1131–35

70. Tsujimura H, Tamura T, Kong HJ, Nishiyama A, Ishii KJ, et al. 2004. Toll-like receptor 9 signaling activates NF-κB through IFN regulatory factor-8/IFN consensus sequence binding protein in dendritic cells. *J. Immunol.* 172:6820–27

71. Choubey D, Kotzin BL. 2002. Interferon-inducible p202 in the susceptibility to systemic lupus. *Front. Biosci.* 7:e252–62

72. Rozzo SJ, Allard JD, Choubey D, Vyse TJ, Izui S, et al. 2001. Evidence for an

interferon-inducible gene, Ifi202, in the susceptibility to systemic lupus. *Immunity* 15:435–43

73. Takeda K, Kaisho T, Akira S. 2003. Toll-like receptors. *Annu. Rev. Immunol.* 21: 335–76

74. Beutler B, Hoebe K, Du X, Ulevitch RJ. 2003. How we detect microbes and respond to them: the Toll-like receptors and their transducers. *J. Leukoc. Biol.* 74:479–85

74a. Iwasaki A, Medzhitov R. 2004. Toll-like receptor control of the adaptive immune responses. *Nat. Immunol.* 5:987–95

75. Hoebe K, Du X, Georgel P, Janssen E, Tabeta K, et al. 2003. Identification of Lps2 as a key transducer of MyD88-independent TIR signalling. *Nature* 424: 743–48

76. Yamamoto M, Sato S, Hemmi H, Hoshino K, Kaisho T, et al. 2003. Role of adaptor TRIF in the MyD88-independent toll-like receptor signaling pathway. *Science* 301:640–43

77. Yamamoto M, Sato S, Hemmi H, Uematsu S, Hoshino K, et al. 2003. TRAM is specifically involved in the Toll-like receptor 4-mediated MyD88-independent signaling pathway. *Nat. Immunol.* 4:1144–50

78. Hoebe K, Janssen EM, Kim SO, Alexopoulou L, Flavell RA, et al. 2003. Upregulation of costimulatory molecules induced by lipopolysaccharide and double-stranded RNA occurs by Trif-dependent and Trif-independent pathways. *Nat. Immunol.* 4:1223–29

78a. McGettrick AF, O'Neill LA. 2004. The expanding family of MyD88-like adaptors in Toll-like receptor signal transduction. *Mol. Immunol.* 41:577–82

79. Leadbetter EA, Rifkin IR, Hohlbaum AM, Beaudette BC, Shlomchik MJ, et al. 2002. Chromatin-IgG complexes activate B cells by dual engagement of IgM and Toll-like receptors. *Nature* 416:603–07

80. Viglianti GA, Lau CM, Hanley TM, Miko BA, Shlomchik MJ, et al. 2003. Activation of autoreactive B cells by CpG dsDNA. *Immunity* 19:837–47

81. Heil F, Hemmi H, Hochrein H, Ampenberger F, Kirschning C, et al. 2004. Species-specific recognition of single-stranded RNA via Toll-like receptor 7 and 8. *Science* 303:1526–29

82. O'Neill LA. 2004. After the Toll rush. *Science* 303:1481–82

83. Wloch MK, Alexander AL, Pippen AM, Pisetsky DS, Gilkeson, et al. 1997. Molecular properties of anti-DNA induced in preautoimmune NZB/W mice by immunization with bacterial DNA. *J. Immunol.* 158:4500–6

84. Hang L, Slack JH, Amundson C, Izui S, Theofilopoulos AN, et al. 1983. Induction of murine autoimmune disease by chronic polyclonal B cell activation. *J. Exp. Med.* 157:874–83

85. Rui L, Vinuesa CG, Blasioli J, Goodnow CC. 2003. Resistance to CpG DNA-induced autoimmunity through tolerogenic B cell antigen receptor ERK signaling. *Nat. Immunol.* 4:594–600

86. Waldner H, Collins M, Kuchroo VK. 2004. Activation of antigen-presenting cells by microbial products breaks self tolerance and induces autoimmune disease. *J. Clin. Invest.* 113;990–97

87. Turley S, Poirot L, Hattori M, Benoist C, Mathis D. 2003. Physiological β cell death triggers priming of self-reactive T cells by dendritic cells in a type-1 diabetes model. *J. Exp. Med.* 198:1527–37

88. Horwitz MS, Bradley LM, Harbertson J, Krahl T, Lee J, et al. 1998. Diabetes induced by Coxsackie virus: initiation by bystander damage and not molecular mimicry. *Nat. Med.* 4:781–85

89. Le Bon A, Tough DF. 2002. Links between innate and adaptive immunity via type I interferon. *Curr. Opin. Immunol.* 14:432–36

90. Le Bon A, Etchart N, Rossmann C, Ashton M, Hou S, et al. 2003. Cross-priming of CD8$^+$ T cells stimulated by

virus-induced type I interferon. *Nat. Immunol.* 4:1009–15

91. Marrack P, Kappler J, Mitchell T. 1999. Type I interferons keep activated T cells alive. *J. Exp. Med.* 189:521–30

92. Tough DF, Borrow P, Sprent J. 1996. Induction of bystander T cell proliferation by viruses and type I interferon in vivo. *Science* 272:1947–50

93. Ogasawara K, Hida S, Weng Y, Saiura A, Sato K, et al. 2002. Requirement of the IFN-α/β-induced CXCR3 chemokine signalling for CD8$^+$ T cell activation. *Genes Cells* 7:309–20

94. Lee CK, Rao DT, Gertner R, Gimeno R, Frey AB, et al. 2000. Distinct requirements for IFNs and STAT1 in NK cell function. *J. Immunol.* 165:3571–77

95. Chawla-Sarkar M, Lindner DJ, Liu YF, Williams BR, Sen GC, et al. 2003. Apoptosis and interferons: role of interferon-stimulated genes as mediators of apoptosis. *Apoptosis* 8:237–49

96. Dondi E, Rogge L, Lutfalla G, Uze G, Pellegrini S. 2003. Down-modulation of responses to type I IFN upon T cell activation. *J. Immunol.* 170:749–56

96a. Carrero JA, Calderon B, Unanue ER. 2004. Type I interferon sensitizes lymphocytes to apoptosis and reduces resistance to *Listeria* infection. *J. Exp. Med.* 200:535–40

96b. O'Connell RM, Saha SK, Vaidya SA, Bruhn KW, Miranda GA, et al. 2004. Type I interferon production enhances susceptibility to *Listeria monocytogenes* infection. *J. Exp. Med.* 200:437–45

96c. Auerbuch V, Brockstedt DG, Meyer-Morse N, O'Riordan M, Portnoy DA. 2004. Mice lacking the type I interferon receptor are resistant to *Listeria monocytogenes*. *J. Exp. Med.* 200:527–33

97. Braun D, Caramalho I, Demengeot J. 2002. IFN-α/β enhances BCR-dependent B cell responses. *Int. Immunol.* 14:411–19

98. Le Bon A, Schiavoni G, D'Agostino G, Gresser I, Belardelli F, et al. 2001. Type I

interferons potently enhance humoral immunity and can promote isotype switching by stimulating dendritic cells in vivo. *Immunity* 14:461–70

99. Litinskiy MB, Nardelli B, Hilbert DM, He B, Schaffer A, et al. 2002. DCs induce CD40-independent immunoglobulin class switching through BLyS and APRIL. *Nat. Immunol.* 3:822–29

100. Jego G, Palucka AK, Blanck JP, Chalouni C, Pascual V, et al. 2003. Plasmacytoid dendritic cells induce plasma cell differentiation through type I interferon and interleukin 6. *Immunity* 19:225–34

101. MacLennan I, Vinuesa C. 2002. Dendritic cells, BAFF, and APRIL: innate players in adaptive antibody responses. *Immunity* 17:235–38

102. Khare SD, Sarosi I, Xia XZ, McCabe S, Miner K, et al. 2000. Severe B cell hyperplasia and autoimmune disease in TALL-1 transgenic mice. *Proc. Natl. Acad. Sci. USA* 97:3370–75

103. Mackay F, Woodcock SA, Lawton P, Ambrose C, Baetscher M, et al. 1999. Mice transgenic for BAFF develop lymphocytic disorders along with autoimmune manifestations. *J. Exp. Med.* 190:1697–710

104. Seshasayee D, Valdez P, Yan M, Dixit VM, Tumas D, et al. 2003. Loss of TACI causes fatal lymphoproliferation and autoimmunity, establishing TACI as an inhibitory BLyS receptor. *Immunity* 18:279–88

105. Hanada T, Yoshida H, Kato S, Tanaka K, Masutani K, et al. 2003. Suppressor of cytokine signaling-1 is essential for suppressing dendritic cell activation and systemic autoimmunity. *Immunity* 19:437–50

106. Gross JA, Johnston J, Mudri S, Enselman R, Dillon SR, et al. 2000. TACI and BCMA are receptors for a TNF homologue implicated in B-cell autoimmune disease. *Nature* 404:995–99

107. Liu W, Szalai A, Zhao L, Liu D, Martin F, et al. 2004. Control of spontaneous B

lymphocyte autoimmunity with adeno-virus-encoded soluble TACI. *Arthritis Rheum.* 50:1884–96

108. Stohl W. 2004. A therapeutic role for BLyS antagonists. *Lupus* 13:317–22

109. Lin Q, Dong C, Cooper MD. 1998. Impairment of T and B cell development by treatment with a type I interferon. *J. Exp. Med.* 187:79–87

110. Hooks JJ, Moutsopoulos HM, Geis SA, Stahl NI, Decker JL, et al. 1979. Immune interferon in the circulation of patients with autoimmune disease. *N. Engl. J. Med.* 301:5–8

111. Ronnblom L, Alm GV. 2001. An etiopathogenic role for the type I IFN system in SLE. *Trends Immunol.* 22:427–31

112. Bengtsson AA, Sturfelt G, Truedsson L, Blomberg J, Alm G, et al. 2000. Activation of type I interferon system in systemic lupus erythematosus correlates with disease activity but not with antiretroviral antibodies. *Lupus* 9:664–71

113. Gota C, Calabrese L. 2003. Induction of clinical autoimmune disease by therapeutic interferon-α. *Autoimmunity* 36:511–18

114. Blanco P, Palucka AK, Gill M, Pascual V, Banchereau J. 2001. Induction of dendritic cell differentiation by IFN-α in systemic lupus erythematosus. *Science* 294:1540–43

115. Han GM, Chen SL, Shen N, Ye S, Bao CD, et al. 2003. Analysis of gene expression profiles in human systemic lupus erythematosus using oligonucleotide microarray. *Genes Immun.* 4:177–86

116. Alcorta D, Preston G, Munger W, Sullivan P, Yang JJ, et al. 2002. Microarray studies of gene expression in circulating leukocytes in kidney diseases. *Exp. Nephrol.* 10:139–49

117. Crow MK. 2003. Interferon-α: a new target for therapy in systemic lupus erythematosus? *Arthritis Rheum.* 48:2396–401

118. Peterson KS, Huang JF, Zhu J, D'Agati V, Liu X, et al. 2004. Characterization of heterogeneity in the molecular pathogenesis of lupus nephritis from transcrip-tional profiles of laser-captured glomeruli. *J. Clin. Invest.* 113:1722–33

119. Ronnblom L, Eloranta ML, Alm GV. 2003. Role of natural interferon-α producing cells (plasmacytoid dendritic cells) in autoimmunity. *Autoimmunity* 36:463–72

120. Lovgren T, Eloranta ML, Bave U, Alm GV, Ronnblom L. 2004. Induction of interferon-α production in plasmacytoid dendritic cells by immune complexes containing nucleic acid released by necrotic or late apoptotic cells and lupus IgG. *Arthritis Rheum.* 50:1861–72

121. Heremans H, Billiau A, Colombatti A, Hilgers J, de Somer P. 1978. Interferon treatment of NZB mice: accelerated progression of autoimmune disease. *Infect. Immun.* 21:925–30

122. Adam C, Thoua Y, Ronco P, Verroust P, Tovey M, et al. 1980. The effect of exogenous interferon: acceleration of autoimmune and renal diseases in (NZB/W) F1 mice. *Clin. Exp. Immunol.* 40:373–82

123. Sergiescu D, Cerutti I, Efthymiou E, Kahan A, Chany C. 1979. Adverse effects of interferon treatment on the life span of NZB mice. *Biomedicine* 31:48–51

124. Hasegawa K, Hayashi T. 2003. Synthetic CpG oligodeoxynucleotides accelerate the development of lupus nephritis during preactive phase in NZB x NZWF1 mice. *Lupus* 12:838–45

125. Kono DH, Baccala R, Theofilopoulos AN. 2004. Genes and genetics of murine lupus. In *Systemic Lupus Erythematosus*, ed. RG Lahita, pp. 225–63. San Diego: Elsevier

126. Pramanik R, Jorgensen TN, Xin H, Kotzin BL, Choubey D. 2004. Interleukin-6 induces expression of Ifi202, an interferon-inducible candidate gene for lupus susceptibility. *J. Biol. Chem.* 279:16121–27

127. Theofilopoulos AN, Koundouris S, Kono DH, Lawson BR. 2001. The role of IFN-γ in systemic lupus erythematosus: a challenge to the Th1/Th2 paradigm in autoimmunity. *Arthritis Res.* 3:136–41

128. Braun D, Geraldes P, Demengeot J. 2003. Type I interferon controls the onset and

severity of autoimmune manifestations in lpr mice. *J. Autoimmun.* 20:15–25

129. Hron JD, Peng SL. 2004. Type I IFN protects against murine lupus. *J. Immunol.* 173: 2134–42

130. Stewart TA. 2003. Neutralizing interferon α as a therapeutic approach to autoimmune diseases. *Cytokine Growth Factor Rev.* 14:139–54

131. Devendra D, Eisenbarth GS. 2004. Interferon α—a potential link in the pathogenesis of viral-induced type 1 diabetes and autoimmunity. *Clin. Immunol.* 111:225–33

132. Huang X, Yuang J, Goddard A, Foulis A, James RF, et al. 1995. Interferon expression in the pancreases of patients with type I diabetes. *Diabetes* 44:658–64

133. Fabris P, Floreani A, Tositti G, Vergani D, De Lalla F, et al. 2003. Type 1 diabetes mellitus in patients with chronic hepatitis C before and after interferon therapy. *Aliment. Pharmacol. Ther.* 18:549–58

134. Guerci AP, Guerci B, Levy-Marchal C, Ongagna J, Ziegler O, et al. 1994. Onset of insulin-dependent diabetes mellitus after interferon-α therapy for hairy cell leukaemia. *Lancet* 343:1167–68

135. Chehadeh W, Weill J, Vantyghem MC, Alm G, Lefebvre J, et al. 2000. Increased level of interferon-α in blood of patients with insulin-dependent diabetes mellitus: relationship with coxsackievirus B infection. *J. Infect. Dis.* 181:1929–39

136. Stewart TA, Hultgren B, Huang X, Pitts-Meek S, Hully J, et al. 1993. Induction of type I diabetes by interferon-α in transgenic mice. *Science* 260:1942–46

137. Pelegrin M, Devedjian JC, Costa C, Visa J, Solanes G, et al. 1998. Evidence from transgenic mice that interferon-β may be involved in the onset of diabetes mellitus. *J. Biol. Chem.* 273:12332–40

138. Vassileva G, Chen SC, Zeng M, Abbondanzo S, Jensen K, et al. 2003. Expression of a novel murine type I IFN in the pancreatic islets induces diabetes in mice. *J. Immunol.* 170:5748–55

139. Ewel CH, Sobel DO, Zeligs BJ, Bellanti JA. 1992. Poly I:C accelerates development of diabetes mellitus in diabetes-prone BB rat. *Diabetes* 41:1016–21

140. Huang X, Hultgren B, Dybdal N, Stewart TA. 1994. Islet expression of interferon-α precedes diabetes in both the BB rat and streptozotocin-treated mice. *Immunity* 1:469–78

141. Giron DJ, Agostini HJ, Thomas DC. 1988. Effect of interferons and poly(I):poly(C) on the pathogenesis of the diabetogenic variant of encephalomyocarditis virus in different mouse strains. *J. Interferon. Res.* 8:745–53

142. Moriyama H, Wen L, Abiru N, Liu E, Yu L, et al. 2002. Induction and acceleration of insulitis/diabetes in mice with a viral mimic (polyinosinic-polycytidylic acid) and an insulin self-peptide. *Proc. Natl. Acad. Sci. USA* 99:5539–44

143. Paronen J, Liu E, Moriyama H, Devendra D, Ide A, et al. 2004. Genetic differentiation of poly I:C from B:9–23 peptide induced experimental autoimmune diabetes. *J. Autoimmun.* 22:307–13

144. Sobel DO, Ahvazi B. 1998. Alpha-interferon inhibits the development of diabetes in NOD mice. *Diabetes* 47:1867–72

145. Sobel DO, Creswell K, Yoon JW, Holterman D. 1998. Alpha interferon administration paradoxically inhibits the development of diabetes in BB rats. *Life Sci.* 62:1293–302

146. Serreze DV, Hamaguchi K, Leiter EH. 1989. Immunostimulation circumvents diabetes in NOD/Lt mice. *J. Autoimmun.* 2:759–76

147. Sobel DO, Goyal D, Ahvazi B, Yoon JW, Chung YH, et al. 1998. Low dose poly I:C prevents diabetes in the diabetes prone BB rat. *J. Autoimmun.* 11:343–52

148. Tanaka-Kataoka M, Kunikata T, Takayama S, Iwaki K, Fujii M, et al. 1999. Oral use of interferon-α delays the onset of insulin-dependent diabetes mellitus in nonobese diabetes mice.

J. Interferon Cytokine Res. 19:877–79

149. Brod SA. 2002. Ingested type I interferon: a potential treatment for autoimmunity. *J. Interferon Cytokine Res.* 22:1153–66

150. Yang XD, Tisch R, Singer SM, Cao ZA, Liblau RS, et al. 1994. Effect of tumor necrosis factor α on insulin-dependent diabetes mellitus in NOD mice. I. The early development of autoimmunity and the diabetogenic process. *J. Exp. Med.* 180:995–1004

151. King C, Ilic A, Koelsch K, Sarvetnick N. 2004. Homeostatic expansion of T cells during immune insufficiency generates autoimmunity. *Cell* 117:265–77

152. Theofilopoulos AN, Dummer W, Kono DH. 2001. T cell homeostasis and systemic autoimmunity. *J. Clin. Invest.* 108:335–40

153. Jaeckel E, Manns M, Von Herrath M. 2002. Viruses and diabetes. *Ann. N.Y. Acad. Sci.* 958:7–25

154. Sevilla N, McGavern DB, Teng C, Kunz S, Oldstone MB. 2004. Viral targeting of hematopoietic progenitors and inhibition of DC maturation as a dual strategy for immune subversion. *J. Clin. Invest.* 113:737–45

155. Oldstone MB. 1990. Viruses as therapeutic agents. I. Treatment of nonobese insulin-dependent diabetes mice with virus prevents insulin-dependent diabetes mellitus while maintaining general immune competence. *J. Exp. Med.* 171:2077–89

156. Christen U, Benke D, Wolfe T, Rodrigo E, Rhode A, et al. 2004. Cure of prediabetic mice by viral infections involves lymphocyte recruitment along an IP-10 gradient. *J. Clin. Invest.* 113:74–84

157. Hafler DA. 2004. Multiple sclerosis. *J. Clin. Invest.* 113:788–94

158. Teige I, Treschow A, Teige A, Mattsson R, Navikas V, et al. 2003. IFN-β gene deletion leads to augmented and chronic demyelinating experimental autoimmune encephalomyelitis. *J. Immunol.* 170:4776–84

159. Passos de Souza E, Evangelista Segundo PT, Jose FF, Lemaire D, Santiago M. 2001. Rheumatoid arthritis induced by α-interferon therapy. *Clin. Rheumatol.* 20:297–99

160. Van Holten J, Reedquist K, Sattonet-Roche P, Smeets TJ, Plater-Zyberk C, et al. 2004. Treatment with recombinant interferon-β reduces inflammation and slows cartilage destruction in the collagen-induced arthritis model of rheumatoid arthritis. *Arthritis Res. Ther.* 6:R239–49

161. Tak PP, Hart BA, Kraan MC, Jonker M, Smeets TJ, et al. 1999. The effects of interferon β treatment on arthritis. *Rheumatology* 38:362–69

162. van Holten J, Plater-Zyberk C, Tak PP. 2002. Interferon-β for treatment of rheumatoid arthritis? *Arthritis Res.* 4:346–52

163. Cummins MJ, Papas A, Kammer GM, Fox PC. 2003. Treatment of primary Sjögren's syndrome with low-dose human interferon α administered by the oromucosal route: combined phase III results. *Arthritis Rheum.* 49:585–93

164. Borgia G, Reynaud L, Gentile I, Cerini R, Ciampi R, et al. 2001. Myasthenia gravis during low-dose IFN-α therapy for chronic hepatitis C. *J. Interferon Cytokine Res.* 21:469–70

165. Deng C, Goluszko E, Baron S, Wu B, Christadoss P. 1996. IFN-α therapy is effective in suppressing the clinical experimental myasthenia gravis. *J. Immunol.* 157:5675–82

166. Andriani A, Bibas M, Callea V, De Renzo A, Chiurazzi F, et al. 1996. Autoimmune hemolytic anemia during α interferon treatment in nine patients with hematological diseases. *Haematologica* 81:258–60

167. Kawai T, Sato S, Ishii KJ, Coban C, Hemmi H, et al. 2004. Interferon-α induction through Toll-like receptors involves

a direct interaction of IRF7 with MyD88 and TRAF6. *Nat. Immunol.* 5:1061–68

168. Barchet W, Cella M, Odermatt B, Asselin-Paturel C, Colonna M, Kalinke U. 2002. Virus-induced interferon α production by a dendritic cell subset in the absence of

feedback signaling in vivo. *J. Exp. Med.* 195:507–16

169. Liu Y-J. 2005. IPC: Professional type 1 interferon-producing cells and plasmacytoid dendritic cell precursors. *Annu. Rev. Immunol.* 23:275–306

NOTE ADDED IN PROOF

A very recent study (167) has indicated that signaling through TLR7, TLR8, and TLR9 leads to MyD88 association with IRF-7 and direct induction of IFN-α (i.e., without prior IRF-3 induction and IFN-β signaling through IFNAR; see Figure 1). Earlier studies showed that, unlike fibroblasts, pDCs derived from both IFNAR-deficient mice and wild-type mice produced similar amounts of IFN-α in response to vesicular stomatitis virus (168). The combined findings suggest that production of large amounts of IFN-α by pDC is independent of the positive feedback regulation through the IFNAR, presumably due to high constitutive expression of IRF-7 by these cells (169).

Annu. Rev. Immunol. 2005. 23:337–66
doi: 10.1146/annurev.immunol.23.021704.115756
First published online as a Review in Advance on November 12, 2004

Pentraxins at the Crossroads Between Innate Immunity, Inflammation, Matrix Deposition, and Female Fertility

Cecilia Garlanda,[1*] Barbara Bottazzi,[1*] Antonio Bastone,[1] and Alberto Mantovani[1,2]

[1]Istituto di Ricerche Farmacologiche Mario Negri, 20157 Milan, Italy; [2]Institute of General Pathology, Faculty of Medicine, University of Milan, Italy; email: garlanda@marionegri.it; bottazzib@marionegri.it; bastone@marionegri.it; mantovani@marionegri.it

Key Words inflammatory response, immune response, extracellular matrix, fertility, neurodegeneration

■ **Abstract** C reactive protein, the first innate immunity receptor identified, and serum amyloid P component are classic short pentraxins produced in the liver. Long pentraxins, including the prototype PTX3, are expressed in a variety of tissues. Some long pentraxins are expressed in the brain and some are involved in neuronal plasticity and degeneration. PTX3 is produced by a variety of cells and tissues, most notably dendritic cells and macrophages, in response to Toll-like receptor (TLR) engagement and inflammatory cytokines. PTX3 acts as a functional ancestor of antibodies, recognizing microbes, activating complement, and facilitating pathogen recognition by phagocytes, hence playing a nonredundant role in resistance against selected pathogens. In addition, PTX3 is essential in female fertility because it acts as a nodal point for the assembly of the cumulus oophorus hyaluronan-rich extracellular matrix. Thus, the prototypic long pentraxin PTX3 is a multifunctional soluble pattern recognition receptor at the crossroads between innate immunity, inflammation, matrix deposition, and female fertility.

The serum obtained from human beings and monkeys during the acute phase of diverse infections contains a protein which is precipitable by the C polysaccharide of pneumococcus (8).

---

*Cecilia Garlanda and Barbara Bottazzi have equally contributed to the Pentraxin Project and to this review.

0732-0582/05/0423-0337$14.00

INTRODUCTION

Innate immunity is a first line of resistance against pathogens, and it plays a key role in the activation and orientation of adaptive immunity and in the maintenance of tissue integrity and repair. Recognition of pathogens and damaged tissues is mediated by pattern recognition receptors (PRRs) (1). Innate defense mechanisms consist of a cellular and a humoral arm. Cellular PRRs belong to different functional and structural groups, which include the Toll-like receptors (TLR), scavenger receptors, lectin receptors, and G protein–coupled receptors for formyl peptides (2). The humoral arm of innate immunity is also diverse; it includes collectins (mannose-binding lectin, surfactant protein A and D, C1q), ficolins, and pentraxins.

Pentraxins are a superfamily of evolutionarily conserved proteins characterized by a structural motif, the pentraxin domain (3–6). C reactive protein (CRP), which together with serum amyloid P (SAP) component constitutes the short pentraxin arm of the superfamily, was the first PRR to be identified, as vividly illustrated by the words of Abernethy & Avery, above (7, 8). CRP was originally described and named for its ability to bind in a Ca-dependent manner the C-polysaccharide of *Streptococcus pneumoniae*.

PTX3 (9, 10) and subsequently identified long pentraxins (11–18) were identified in the 1990s as cytokine-inducible genes or molecules expressed in specific tissues (e.g., neurons, spermatozoa). Short and long pentraxins are conserved in evolution from arachnids and insects to humans. Their conservation is testimony to their role in complex organisms. Structural analysis and gene-modified mice have provided a new level of understanding of the role of pentraxins in immunity and homeostasis.

In this review, we summarize current understanding of the structure and function of pentraxins. Our focus is primarily on the more recently discovered long pentraxin family and its prototypic member PTX3, but we also discuss recent progress on the structure and functions of the classic short pentraxins CRP and SAP. Current research suggests that pentraxins are an essential component of the humoral arm of innate immunity, activated following pathogen recognition by cellular PRR. Moreover, pentraxins are multifunctional proteins at the crossroads between immunity and inflammation, extracellular matrix construction, and female fertility.

THE PENTRAXIN SUPERFAMILY

Members

Pentraxins are characterized by the presence in their carboxy-terminal of a 200 amino acid pentraxin domain, with an 8 amino acid–long conserved pentraxin signature (HxCxS/TWxS, where x is any amino acid) (Figure 1A). The first pentraxin described was CRP, identified in human serum during the 1930s as the prototypic acute phase response protein (7) produced by the liver in inflammatory or infectious conditions. Human SAP was subsequently identified as a relative of CRP for the amino acid sequence homology (51%) and for the similar appearance in electron microscopy (annular disc-like structure with pentameric symmetry) (3, 4, 19). CRP and SAP orthologs in different mammal species share substantial sequence homology, with notable differences including serum basal levels and changes during the acute phase response, CRP and SAP being the main acute phase reactants in human and mouse, respectively. In the arthropod *Limulus polyphemus*, different forms of CRP and SAP were identified as abundant constituents of the hemolymph (20–22) involved in recognizing and destroying pathogens.

During the early 1990s, a new pentraxin domain–containing secreted protein was identified as an IL-1-inducible gene in endothelial cells (PTX3) or as a TNF-stimulated gene (TSG-14) in fibroblasts (9, 10). The main structural property of the long pentraxin PTX3 that differentiated it from CRP and SAP was the presence of a 174 amino acid–long amino-terminal domain, not present in CRP and SAP, coupled to the pentraxin domain (Figure 1*A*).

The long pentraxins sharing the same general organization identified after PTX3 include guinea pig apexin (14, 23), neuronal pentraxin (NP) 1 or NPTX1 (11, 13), NP2 (also called Narp or NPTX2) (12, 16), and neuronal pentraxin receptor (NPR), a transmembrane molecule (17, 18) (see below). The amino acid sequence identity among members of this subfamily is relatively high in the carboxy-pentraxin domain and ranges from 28% between human PTX3 (hPTX3) and hNP1 to 68% between hNP1 and hNP2. By contrast, in the amino-terminal domain a low level of similarity is found (about 10% for PTX3 versus NP1). However, identity in the amino-terminal domain among the neuronal pentraxins is higher and ranges between 28% and 38%, suggesting the existence of subclasses of molecules among the long pentraxins. The homology between NP1 and PTX3 or between NP2 and PTX3 at the N-terminal level is restricted to the extreme N-terminus; this characteristic and the longer size of NP1 and NP2 suggest the presence of a third domain localized between the N-terminal and the pentraxin domains (24). Ortholog molecules have been found so far for PTX3, NP1, NP2, and NPR not only in human, mouse, and rat, but also in lower vertebrates such as zebrafish and pufferfish (Y. Martinez, unpublished results) (Figure 1*B*). The ortholog of apexin has not been clearly defined. We recently identified a new evolutionarily conserved member of the long pentraxin family, PTX4 (Y. Martinez, unpublished results). Long pentraxins have been identified in *Xenopus laevis* (XL-PXN1) (15) and in insects. In *Drosophila melanogaster*, Swiss cheese protein is a long (1425 amino acids) pentraxin that, when mutated, is responsible for age-dependent neurodegeneration (25).

Phylogeny

The pentraxin domain is highly conserved in mammals, in lower vertebrates (*Xenopus laevis, Danio rerio*, the zebrafish, *Takifugu rubripes*, the pufferfish), and in arthropods (the arachnids *Limulus polyphemus* and *Tachypleus tridentatus*, the horseshoe crabs, and the insect *Drosophila melanogaster*). Phylogenetic tree analysis allows the identification of five main groups of molecules (Figure 1*B*).

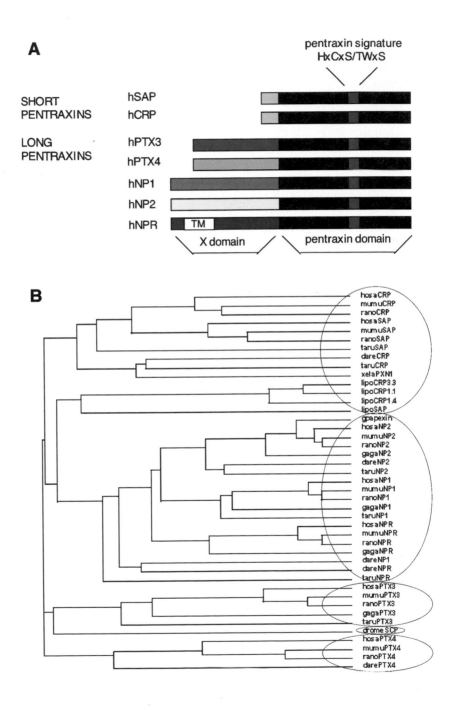

The first group of molecules includes the short pentraxins that diverged from the common ancestor of all pentraxins. The duplication event that gave rise to CRP and SAP may have occurred very early in evolution, as both can be found in chordates as well as in arthropods (20). Interestingly, XL-PXN1 *Xenopus laevis*, which is a long pentraxin, clusters with the short pentraxins, possibly because of the low level of homology between its N-terminal domain and that of the other long pentraxins. The second group includes the neuronal pentraxins that cluster as a subclass of long pentraxins found in mammals as well as in lower vertebrates. On the basis of branch length, NPR is the oldest group that diverged from a common ancestor of neuronal pentraxins; subsequently NP2 and finally NP1 appeared. Apexin clusters with the neuronal pentraxins and in particular with NP2. The third group includes only PTX3, whose sequence has been identified in mammals as well as in birds (*Gallus gallus*) and in the most ancient vertebrate *Takifugu rubripes*. PTX3 originated very early in the pentraxin evolution, directly from the common ancestor of the whole family. The fourth group includes PTX4 and its orthologs, found in mammals as well as in the zebrafish. Like PTX3, PTX4 originated directly from the common ancestors of the pentraxins very early in the evolution of pentraxins, at the divergence of vertebrates. The last group is represented by *Drosophila melanogaster* Swiss cheese protein, a long pentraxin involved in glia-neuron interaction (25). Swiss cheese protein originated from the common ancestor of pentraxins, and interestingly it localizes in the phylogenetic tree close to PTX3. The lack of relationship among the five groups of long pentraxins identified in this analysis suggests that they originated independently by fusion events between the gene encoding the ancestral pentraxin domain and other unrelated sequences.

SHORT PENTRAXINS

Short pentraxins are 25-kDa proteins characterized by a common structural organization in five (six in *Limulus polyphemus*) or ten identical subunits arranged in a pentameric radial symmetry. Human CRP and SAP are the prototypic short pentraxins: they share approximately 51% amino acid sequence identity and are thought to have originated from a single gene duplication (26).

Figure 1   The pentraxin superfamily. (*A*) Human short and long pentraxins. TM: transmembrane domain. (*B*) Phylogeny of pentraxins. The dendogram was organized by the neighbor-joining (NJ) algorithm with molecular evolutionary genetics analysis (MEGA) version 2.1. Circles identify related molecules. Abbreviations are as follows: hosa, *Homo sapiens* (human); mumu, *Mus musculus* (house mouse); rano, *Rattus norvegicus* (norway rat); gaga, *Gallus gallus* (domestic fowl); xela, *Xenopus laevis* (african clawed frog); dare, *Danio rerio* (zebrafish); taru, *Takifugu rubripes* (pufferfish); drome, *Drosophila melanogaster* (fruit fly); gp, *Cavia porcellus* (guinea pig); lipo, *Limulus polyphemus* (horshoe crab).

Structure

Human CRP is composed of five identical nonglycosilated protomers. The amino acids sequence includes two cysteines in position 36 and 97 conserved in all the members of the pentraxin family and involved in intrachain disulfide bonds. Each CRP protomer has a characteristic lectin fold composed of two-layered ß sheets with flattened jellyroll topology; five protomers are noncovalently associated to form a pentamer with a total molecular weight of 115,135 Da (27).

The human CRP gene is located on chromosome 1q23 and is organized in two exons, the first exon coding for the leader peptide and the first two amino acids of the mature protein and the second exon coding for the remaining 204 amino acids. The promoter region of human CRP comprises two acute phase response elements, each containing a binding site for the liver-specific transcription factor HNF1 (28), and two C/EBP (CCAAT/enhancer binding protein β) binding sites, both necessary and sufficient for IL-6-induced transcription (29, 30). STAT3 has also been found to participate in transducing the effects of IL-6 on CRP expression (31). In addition, a nonconsensus κB site overlapping the proximal C/EBP binding site has been identified (32). Binding of Rel P50 to the κB site in response to IL-1 enhances and stabilizes binding of C/EBP to the CRP promoter (33) and amplifies CRP expression.

CRP levels in plasma of healthy adults are barely detectable (≤ 3 mg/l) but increase as much as 1000-fold following an acute phase stimulus as a result of accelerated rates of transcription in the liver (4). Circulating CRP is produced only by hepatocytes (4), mainly in response to the proinflammatory cytokine IL-6. IL-1 may also contribute as an additional signal acting synergistically with IL-6 in the induction of CRP mRNA (34). Other cells, such as lymphocytes and monocyte/macrophages, are able to synthesize CRP, but apparently these cells do not contribute to CRP plasma levels.

SAP is a highly conserved plasma glycoprotein composed of 5 or 10 identical subunits noncovalently associated in pentameric rings interacting face to face (35). SAP is a normal component of basement membranes (36) and is the main acute phase protein in mice, whereas in human serum it is constitutively present at 30 to 50 μg/ml. The human gene maps to chromosome 1 in close physical and genetic linkage with the CRP gene and shares with CRP the same organization in two exons, the first one coding for the signal peptide and the second for the mature protein. The mature SAP protomer is 204 amino acids long and has a molecular mass of 25,462 Da; in the presence of physiological levels of calcium, human SAP is a pentamer with a molecular mass of 127,310 Da, although at pH 8.0 in the absence of calcium, SAP consists of pentameric and decameric forms (37–39). Unlike CRP, each SAP protomer is glycosilated with a single N-linked biantennary oligosaccharide at Asn[32] (38).

According to the three-dimensional structure derived by X-ray diffraction (35), human SAP has a tertiary fold, which resembles that of legume lectins as Concanavalin A. SAP protomers have a flattened ß-jelly roll topology with a single long elix folded on the top of the ß-sheet. The five subunits are arranged in a ring around a hole and are held together by hydrogen bonds and salt bridges. The decamer is stabilized by ionic interactions between the two pentamers. Each SAP subunit can bind two calcium ions, and residues involved in calcium binding are conserved in all SAPs.

Ligands

The physiological functions attributed to CRP and SAP involve Ca^{2+}-dependent ligand binding (Table 1). The first ligand described for CRP was the C-polysaccharide of *Streptococcus pneumoniae*: This interaction is due to a direct binding

TABLE 1   Differential ligand recognition by PTX3 and short pentraxins

	PTX3	CRP	SAP
Membrane moieties:			
PC	−	+	−
PE	−	−	+
Galactomannan[a]	+	NT	NT
LPS	−	−	+
OmpA	+	NT	NT
Complement components:			
C1q	+	+	+
C4b-binding protein	−	−	l
Cytokines—Growth factors:			
FGF2	+	+/−	NT
IL-1; other growth factors, cytokines and chemokines	−	NT	NT
Matrix proteins:			
TSG6	+	NT	NT
Laminin	−	+	+
Type IV collagen	−	−	+
Fibronectin	−	+	+
Chondroitin sulfate	−	NT	+
Hyaluronic acid	−	NT	NT
Microbes:			
Aspergillus fumigatus	+	+	NT
Pseudomonas aeruginosa	+	NT	NT
Salmonella typhimurium	+	−	+
Paracoccidioides brasiliensis	+	NT	NT
Zymosan	+	+	+
Miscellaneous:			
Apoptotic cells	+	+	+
Histones	+	+	+
Heparin	−	−	+
MoβDG[b]	−	−	+

[a] based on competition data.
[b] 4,6-O-(1-carboxyethylidene)-β-D-galactopyranoside.

of CRP to phosphorylcholine (PC), a major constituent of C-type capsule polysac-charides. Moreover, CRP binds various pathogens, including fungi, yeasts, and bacteria (40). CRP has additional calcium-dependent binding specificity for chro-matin, histones, and small nuclear ribonucleoprotein U1, as well as glycans and phospholipids (4). In the absence of calcium, CRP binds polycations such as poly-L-lysine, poly-L-arginine, and myelin basic protein.

SAP is a calcium-dependent lectin originally characterized for its binding to agarose and in particular for the agarose component 4,6-cyclin pyruvate acetal of β-D-galactose (41). Like CRP, SAP binds various bacteria, such as *Streptococcus pyogenes* and *Neisseria meningitidis* (42, 43). Moreover, binding to influenza virus (44) and to lipopolysaccharide (LPS) has also been reported (42, 45). Other ligands for SAP include: carbohydrate determinants such as heparin, 6-phosphorylated mannose, and 3-sulfated saccharides (46); matrix components such as laminin, type IV collagen, fibronectin, and proteoglycans; and C4b-binding protein and all forms of amyloid fibrils. In addition, SAP is the major DNA- and chromatin-binding protein in plasma (47, 48).

CRP and SAP, aggregated or attached to most of their ligands, can bind to C1q, the recognition subunit of the classical complement pathway (49), interacting to a specific region of its collagen-like domain and activating the classical comple-ment cascade (50, 51). Complement activation by short pentraxins may be one of the mechanisms leading to the removal of cellular debris. Consistent with this hypothesis, both CRP and SAP bind in a calcium-dependent way apoptotic cells enhancing phagocytosis by macrophages (52, 53).

The observation of enhanced phagocytosis of apoptotic cells opsonized with SAP and CRP in the absence of complement suggests the existence of specific receptors for pentraxins on phagocytic cells. A specific and saturable binding to all three classes of Fcγ receptors has been demonstrated for both CRP and SAP (54, 55), and the interaction with Fcγ seems able to mediate phagocytosis of apoptotic cells as well as zymosan (56, 57). However, some scientists have questioned the interpretation of these data, suggesting instead that binding of CRP to Fcγ receptors is not demonstrable when F(ab')2 anti-CRP antibodies are used and that binding may be influenced by CRP contamination with traces of IgG (58, 59).

Functions

Although much is known about the biochemical characteristics of short pentraxins and their use as markers in different pathological situations, the actual function of these molecules remains, to some extent, elusive. An important contribution to the understanding of the in vivo role of CRP and SAP comes from the generation of genetically modified mice. Here, a stumbling block in understanding the biology of short pentraxins is represented by the different regulation of CRP and SAP in mouse and human.

Several reports concerning CRP transgenic (CRPtg) mice have been published in recent years, although no data are available on CRP knockout animals. Early observations showed that administration of human CRP increases survival of mice infected with *Streptococcus pneumoniae* and this effect is likely mediated by the strong reaction of CRP toward the PC moiety present on the cell wall of these bacteria. According to these data, CRPtg mice infected with *Streptococcus pneumoniae* (60) are resistant to infections, showing longer survival time and lower mortality than non-tg littermates. Similarly, CRP administration protects against *Haemophilus influenzae*, a pathogen expressing PC (61, 62). Finally, CRPtg animals are resistant to infections with the Gram-negative pathogen *Salmonella enterica* (63), even in the absence of CRP binding.

The effects of CRP are not limited to protection against pathogens: CRPtg mice are also protected in a model of experimental allergic encephalomyelitis (64), and administration of human CRP offers a transient protection against systemic lupus erythematosus (SLE) in SLE-prone mice (NZB/NZW) (65). The protective effect may be mediated by CRP binding to nuclear antigens relevant for SLE, such as chromatin, histones, and small nuclear ribonucleoprotein U1, as well as by binding and opsonization of apoptotic cells. Recent research shows that development of disease is delayed and survival is increased in NZB/NZW mice carrying the human CRP transgene (66); this protection is associated with the ability of CRP to limit renal damage by preventing deposition of immune complexes.

Conflicting reports concern a possible protective role of CRP toward bacterial LPS. Mice expressing the rabbit CRP gene are resistant to the lethal effect of LPS (67); similarly, human CRP administration is protective in some experimental models (42, 68), although protection of mice against LPS lethality by passive administration of CRP is not a general phenomenon (69). Such conflicting reports may reflect an inherent variability of models in which CRPs from different species and purity were used, associated to differences in the animal strains and to heterogeneity of LPS preparations.

The availability of *sap* knockout ($sap^{-/-}$) mice (70) helped to advance understanding of the biological role of this protein. Surprisingly, SAP plays a dual role in bacterial infections, exhibiting a host defense function against pathogens to which it does not bind. When SAP binds to bacteria, a strong antiopsonic effect is observed, resulting in enhanced virulence of the infectious agent (42).

SAP is a universal constituent of the amyloid deposits that are characteristic of systemic amyloidosis, Alzheimer's disease, and prion diseases. SAP binds to amyloid fibrils (71) and stabilizes the deposits, participating in the pathogenesis of the disease. The role of SAP in amyloidogenesis has been investigated in vivo in $sap^{-/-}$ animals: in these mice, the appearance of amyloid deposits is delayed and their quantity is reduced (70). Pharmacologic targeting of SAP may represent an innovative therapeutic strategy (72). Furthermore, $sap^{-/-}$ mice spontaneously develop antinuclear autoimmunity and severe glomerulonephritis (73), a phenotype resembling human SLE. These results strongly support a role for SAP in the protection against chromatin-induced autoimmunity.

THE PROTOTYPIC LONG PENTRAXIN PTX3

Gene and Protein Organization

The human PTX3 gene, localized on human chromosome 3 band q25, is organized in three exons separated by two introns. The first two exons code for the leader peptide and the N-terminal domain of the protein, respectively, and the third exon encodes the pentraxin domain, matching exactly the other members of the pentraxin family (9).

The PTX3 protein is 381 amino acids long, including a signal peptide of 17 amino acids. The mature secreted protein has a predicted molecular weight of 40,165 Da and consists of a C-terminal 203 amino acids pentraxin-like domain coupled with an N-terminal portion of 178 amino acids unrelated to other known proteins. Scientists have observed a significant alignment between PTX3 C-terminal domain and classical short pentraxins, with 57% of conserved amino acids and 17% of identical amino acids. Analysis of human PTX3 sequence indicates the presence of an N-linked glycosilation site in the C-terminal domain at Asn^{220} that accounts for the higher molecular weight observed in SDS-PAGE under reducing conditions (45 kDa versus the predicted 40 kDa). The C-terminal domain contains a canonical pentraxin signature and two cysteines at amino acid positions 210 and 271 of PTX3 conserved in all members of the pentraxin family.

Gel electrophoresis under native conditions demonstrates that PTX3 protomers are assembled to form multimers predominantly of 440 kDa apparent molecular mass, corresponding to decamers; moreover, gel filtration reveals higher forms eluting in a region corresponding to an apparent molecular mass of 900 kDa, which suggests that two decamers of PTX3 may associate to form an eicosamer (74). In contrast to CRP and SAP pentamers, the decameric form of PTX3 (Figure 2) depends on interchain disulfide bonds, as demonstrated by SDS-PAGE in the absence of reducing agents. A similar model was proposed for NP1 and Narp (75).

Human and murine PTX3, localized in the synthenic region of chromosome 3 (q24–28), are highly conserved: Both proteins are 381 amino acids long and share 82% of identical amino acids and 92% of conserved amino acids. According to modelling, the PTX3 pentraxin domain well accommodates on the tertiary fold of SAP, with almost all the ß-strands and the α-helical segments conserved (76).

Gene Regulation and Production

The human PTX3 proximal promoter contains Pu1, AP-1, NF-κB, Sp1, and NF-IL-6 sites. The NF-κB proximal site in the mouse and human promoter is essential for induction by IL-1 and TNF (77, 78). No induction of the human promoter was observed with IL-6 (77). Therefore, analysis so far of the PTX3 proximal promoter accounts for induction by TLR agonists, IL-1, and TNF, but not for recently discovered costimuli (e.g., IL-10; see below).

A variety of cell types can produce PTX3 in vitro upon exposure to primary inflammatory signals (Figure 2). These include endothelial cells, smooth muscle

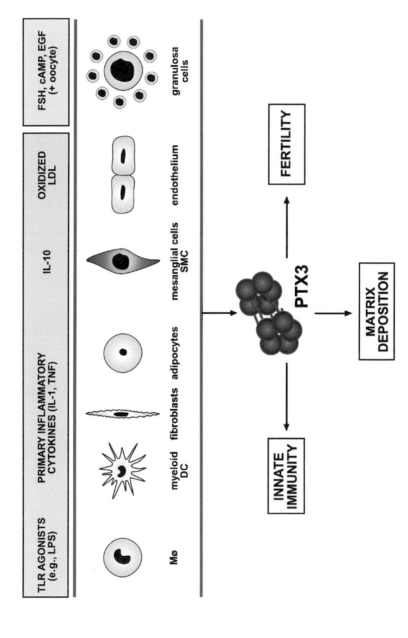

Figure 2   Cellular sources and inducers of the long pentraxin PTX3.

cells (SMCs), adipocytes, fibroblasts, mononuclear phagocytes, and dendritic cells (DCs) (9, 10, 76, 79–84). We recently reassessed the relative capacity of different cell types to produce PTX3 and found that DCs produce the highest amounts (79). PTX3 production is induced by primary inflammatory signals, such as IL-1, TNF, and microbial moieties (e.g., LPS, lipoarabinomannans) (9, 85). Specifically, agonists for different members of the TLR family stimulate PTX3 production. IL-6 is generally a poor inducer of PTX3 (80). However, PTX3 was found to be expressed in Castleman's disease, propelled by IL-6 (86), and it is induced in Kaposi's sarcoma cells by viral IL-6 encoded by human herpesvirus-8 (87).

IFN-γ and IL-10 have divergent effects on PTX3 production. IFN-γ inhibits PTX3 expression and production in different cellular contexts (24, 82, 88). IL-4 and IL-13 do not affect PTX3 production, whereas, surprisingly, IL-10 was found by transcriptional profiling to induce PTX3 expression in DCs and monocytes and to costimulate PTX3 production with LPS (89; A. Doni, unpublished data). PTX3 is therefore part of the genetic program expressed by M2 mononuclear phagocytes and IL-10-treated DCs. Given its role in matrix organization, PTX3 expression in these cells is likely to be related to the orchestration of matrix deposition, tissue repair, and remodeling (90).

DCs are major producers of PTX3 on a per-cell basis (79). Interestingly, production of PTX3 is restricted to myeloid DCs, whereas IFN-producing plasmacytoid DCs are unable to produce PTX3 in response to appropriate agonists, possibly because of autocrine inhibition by IFN. PTX3 production by DCs and neighboring macrophages is likely to facilitate pathogen recognition and activation of an appropriate adaptive immune response (see below).

Vascular endothelial cells and SMCs produce copious amounts of PTX3 in response to inflammatory signals, including oxydized low density lipoproteins (ox-LDL) (9, 84) (Figure 2). PTX3-producing macrophages, endothelial cells, and SMCs have been identified in human atherosclerotic lesions (91). These results have provided a basis for testing the potential of PTX3 as a novel diagnostic tool in vascular disorders.

In vivo injection of LPS in mice induces PTX3 expression and high blood levels (76, 92). A variety of tissues express PTX3, with two aspects emerging. First, expression is most prominent in the heart and skeletal muscle. Second, in contrast to SAP, PTX3 is expressed at low levels in the liver. Unlike neuronal long pentraxins, PTX3 is not constitutively expressed in the central nervous system (CNS). Following exposure to inflammatory signals (LPS, IL-1, TNF), infectious agents (*Candida albicans, Cryptococcus neoformans*), autoimmune reactions (experimental allergic encephalomyelitis), or limbic seizures, PTX3 is expressed and produced in the CNS (81, 93, 94).

Northern blot analysis revealed that *ptx3* mRNA was expressed in the mouse ovary during the preovulatory period, showing close temporal correlation to matrix deposition by cumulus cells. In situ analysis revealed that *ptx3* mRNA expression was confined to cumulus cells and to a few granulosa cells lining the follicle antrum of preovulatory follicles. Western blot and immunofluorescence analysis indicated that PTX3 was associated with the extracellular matrix of wild-type cumuli. In the cumulus oophorus, expression of PTX3 is orchestrated by hormonal ovulatory stimuli (follicle-stimulating hormone or human chorionic gonadotropin), by oocyte-derived soluble factors, and in particular a member of the transforming growth factor β (TGFβ) family, growth differentiation factor-9 (GDF-9) (95, 96) (see below).

In addition PTX3 has been identified in a variety of gene expression or proteomic profiling efforts ranging from astrocyte secreted proteins to space flown fibroblasts (e.g., 97, 98).

Ligands

The first described and best characterized ligand of PTX3 is the complement component C1q (74, 99) (Table 1). Unlike classical pentraxins, PTX3 interacts with C1q in a calcium-independent manner, without a previous aggregation of the protein. Interaction of PTX3 with plastic-immobilized C1q induces activation of the classical complement pathway, as demonstrated by an increased deposition of C3 and C4. In contrast, fluid-phase PTX3 binding to C1q inhibits complement activation via competitive blocking of relevant interaction sites (99).

Like CRP and SAP, PTX3 binds to apoptotic cells, inhibiting their recognition by DCs (100). Binding occurs late in the apoptotic process and, unlike classic short pentraxins, PTX3 binding is calcium-independent. In addition, preincubation of apoptotic cells with PTX3 enhances C1q binding and C3 deposition on the cell surface, suggesting a role for PTX3 in the complement-mediated clearance of apoptotic cells (99).

PTX3 also binds selected pathogens, including conidia of *Aspergillus fumigatus*, *Pseudomonas aeruginosa*, *Salmonella typhimurium*, *Paracoccidioides brasiliensis*, zymosan, but not *Escherichia coli*, *Burkholderia cepacia*, *Listeria monocytogenes*, or *Candida albicans* (101, 102).

The microbial moieties recognized by PTX3 have not been completely defined (Table 1). As expected on the basis of structural analysis (74, 76), PTX3 does not bind LPS; moreover, it does not bind classical short pentraxin ligands [PC, phosphoethanolamine (PE) and high pyruvate agarose]. Binding of PTX3 to *A. fumigatus* is competed by galactomannan (101). Mannan recognition is consistent with binding to zymosan (102). We recently identified outer membrane protein A (OmpA) as a bacterial moiety specifically bound by PTX3 (P. Jeannin & B. Bottazzi, unpublished observation). Matrix components (fibronectin, type IV collagen) are recognized by SAP but not by PTX3. In contrast, PTX3 binds the matrix component TNFα-induced protein 6 (TNFAIP6 or TSG-6) (96), a multifunctional protein usually associated with inflammation (103, 104). By binding to TSG-6, PTX3 acts as a nodal point for the assembly of hyaluronic acid (HA)-rich extracellular matrix, which is essential for female fertility (96).

PTX3 binds fibroblast growth factor 2 (FGF2) but not other members of the FGF family or cytokines and chemokines (Table 1). The angiogenic activity of FGF2 in vitro and in vivo is blocked by PTX3 (105).

Role in Innate Immunity

The investigation of $ptx3^{-/-}$ mice, generated by homologous recombination, has been invaluable to understanding the in vivo function of PTX3 (96, 101). *Ptx3*-deficient mice are viable and display a normal life span in a conventional mouse facility. The only apparent abnormality is a severe deficiency in female fertility (see below).

As discussed above, PTX3 binds conidia of the opportunistic fungus *A. fumigatus* as well as selected Gram-positive and Gram-negative bacteria. Upon binding to *A. fumigatus* conidia, recombinant PTX3 facilitated the internalization and the killing of conidia, as well as the production of monocyte chemotactic protein-1 (MCP-1, also known as CCL-2) by mononuclear phagocytes. Conidia rapidly induced PTX3 production in vitro in murine and human mononuclear phagocytes and DCs (Figure 3). PTX3 plasma levels were increased in mice infected with *A. fumigatus* and in neutropenic patients with hematologic malignancies and *A. fumigatus* systemic infection (101).

$Ptx3^{-/-}$ mice were extremely susceptible to invasive pulmonary aspergillosis (IPA) in terms of mortality, lung and brain colonization, and lung inflammatory response. The specificity of the role played by PTX3 in the susceptibility to IPA is demonstrated by the complete protective effect of $ptx3^{-/-}$ mice treatment with recombinant PTX3. The therapeutic potential of PTX3 in IPA is also suggested by its protective effect in a murine IPA model of allogeneic, T cell–depleted bone marrow transplantation (106).

In $ptx3^{-/-}$ mice, the defective recognition of *A. fumigatus* conidia by the host, and in particular by phagocytes and DCs, was associated with the lack of development of appropriate and protective T helper cell type 1 (Th1) antifungal responses and with an unbalanced cytokine profile skewed toward a Th2 response. In this context, the role played by PTX3 in regulating the development of detrimental Th2 responses involved in allergic brochopulmonary aspergillosis needs to be further investigated.

In models of bacterial infections, such as *P. aeruginosa* lung infection (a pathogen recognized by PTX3), $ptx3^{-/-}$ mice showed a partial increase in mortality and lung colonization. In contrast, susceptibility to *L. monocytogenes* and to intra-abdominal sepsis caused by caecal ligation and puncture were not affected by PTX3 deficiency (101; C. Garlanda, unpublished results). These results suggest that PTX3 deficiency does not cause a generalized impairment of host resistance to microbial pathogens and that PTX3 is involved in recognition and resistance against specific microorganisms.

These results demonstrate that PTX3 acts as a soluble PRR with an essential role in resistance against selected pathogens, in particular *A. fumigatus* (Figure 3). The regulated expression of this molecule in macrophages and DCs suggests that PTX3, unlike the short pentraxins made in the liver, represents a mechanism of amplification of innate resistance against pathogens mainly acting locally at the site of infection and inflammation.

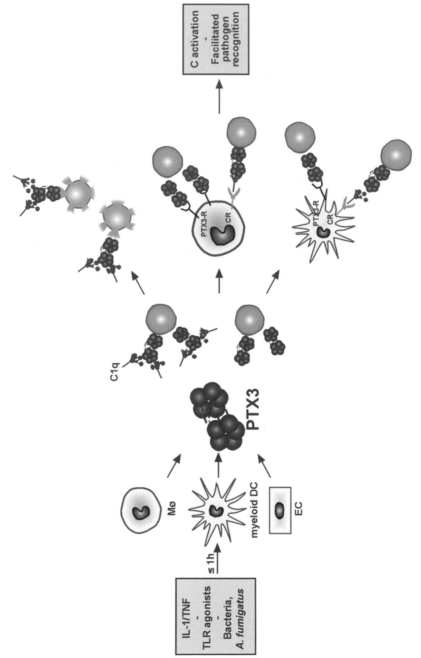

Figure 3 Role of the long pentraxin PTX3 in antimicrobial resistance. PTX3-R, putative PTX3 receptor(s).

Role in Inflammation

PTX3 blood levels are low (about 25 ng/ml in mice, <2 ng/ml in humans) in normal conditions but increase rapidly (peak at 6–8 h) and dramatically (200–800 ng/ml) during endotoxic shock, sepsis, and other inflammatory conditions (107, 108).

The in vivo role of PTX3 in inflammatory conditions has been investigated using PTX3 transgenic mice overexpressing the murine gene under the control of its own promoter (109) and in $ptx3^{-/-}$ mice generated by homologous recombination (101; C. Garlanda, unpublished results). PTX3 transgenic mice showed increased resistance to LPS toxicity and to cecal ligation and puncture (109). Transgenic mice showed higher levels of IL-10, and macrophages were primed for increased nitric oxide production in response to IFN-γ and TNF (109).

In sharp contrast to the data on transgenic mice, $ptx3^{-/-}$ mice showed normal susceptibility to LPS toxicity (in terms of mortality, cytokine levels, and PMN recruitment in the lungs) and normal susceptibility to cecal ligation and puncture (101; C. Garlanda, unpublished). Moreover, PTX3 per se failed to affect cytokine production in vivo and in macrophages in vitro (C. Garlanda & B. Bottazzi, unpublished observation). The reason for the divergence of results obtained in PTX3 transgenic and deficient mice is not clear.

PTX3-overexpressing mice showed exacerbated inflammatory response following intestinal ischemia reperfusion injury (110). In a model of skeletal muscle ischemia and reperfusion injury, we observed PTX3 transcript induction, but we failed to find differences between wild-type and PTX3-deficient mice in tissue damage, assessed as polymorphonuclear cell infiltration (myeloperoxidase activity) and Creatine Kinase activity in the injured muscle (R. Latini, unpublished results).

PTX3 is expressed in the CNS under a variety of inflammatory conditions (81, see above), including kainate-induced seizures (93). PTX3 is induced in glial cells following seizure-induced cytokine (IL-1) production, which amplifies damage. The susceptibility to kainate-induced seizures in $ptx3^{-/-}$ mice was similar to that observed in their wild-type littermates, but $ptx3^{-/-}$ mice had more widespread and severe neuronal damage. These results suggest that PTX3 confers resistance to neurodegeneration, because its absence from the brain tissue is associated with an increased number of degenerating neurons. In analogy with findings on apoptotic cells (100), PTX3 may bind to dying neurons and rescue them from otherwise irreversible damage. Alternatively, it may interact with neuronal pentraxins and modulate their function (see below).

PTX3 in Extracellular Matrix Architecture and Female Fertility

$Ptx3^{-/-}$ mice generated by homologous recombination displayed a severe defect in female fertility (95, 101). The infertility or severe subfertility of $ptx3$-deficient mice was tracked to an abnormal cumulus oophorus, characterized by an unstable extracellular matrix in which cumulus cells were uniformly dispersed instead of radiating out from a central oocyte (96).

As discussed above, *ptx3* mRNA was expressed in the mouse ovary by cumulus cells during the preovulatory period, and the protein was associated with the extracellular matrix of the cumuli, where it plays a role in assembling the HA-enriched matrix of the cumulus. A crucial step of cumulus matrix assembly is the transfer and covalent linkage of the heavy chains of serum inter α trypsin inhibitor (IαI) protein to HA or to the HA-binding glycoprotein TSG-6. Consistently, mice deficient in the light chain of IαI, bikunin, (111), or in TSG-6 (112) are infertile because of instability of the cumulus matrix and lack of oocyte fertilization, like $ptx3^{-/-}$ mice. Binding experiments performed to investigate a possible interaction between PTX3 and TSG-6, which is synthesized by cumulus cells in parallel with PTX3 (95), revealed that PTX3 binds to full-length human TSG-6 or to Link_TSG-6 (i.e., its HA-binding domain) at a site distinct from its HA-binding surface (96). Competition studies suggest that each protomer in a PTX3 10/20-mer can bind an individual TSG-6 molecule and, therefore, may form a multi-molecular complex that acts as a "node" for cross-linking HA chains in the cumulus matrix, therefore serving as an additional way of cross-linking the matrix.

Furthermore, cytofluorimetric and immunofluorescence analysis and sperm migration/entrapment assays indicated that spermatozoa bound soluble and immobilized PTX3, suggesting that PTX3 embedded in the matrix of the cumulus could also direct guidance and entrapment of spermatozoa, thus facilitating the fertilization process (96).

PTX3 is expressed in the human periovulatory cumulus oophorus and is conserved between mouse and human. Therefore, it is likely that PTX3 may play the same role in human female fertility and that PTX3 deficiency might be a cause of unexplained infertility in women despite a normal ovulation.

Several lines of evidence point to analogies between the process of ovulation and inflammation (113, 114) and indicate that prostaglandins and cytokines play a central role in mediating the hormone regulation of cumulus matrix component synthesis. In addition to a hormonal ovulatory stimulus, oocyte soluble factors, and in particular GDF-9, a member of the TGFβ family (95, 115), are required for eliciting hyaluronan synthesis, cumulus expansion, and temporally and anatomically restricted PTX3 expression during the periovulatory period (116, 117). The synthesis of PTX3 during both ovulation and inflammation adds a further element linking these fundamental processes (Figure 4).

PTX3 is assembled predominantly as a large multimer complex consisting of two decamers (74). PTX3/TSG-6 complexes might thus serve as anchoring sites for multiple HA molecules, thereby substantially strengthening and stabilizing the HA network. In both physiological and pathological conditions, HA-protein interaction is crucial for the formation and stability of extracellular matrix in several tissues (118, 119). The finding that the long pentraxin PTX3 is a component of the extracellular matrix of the cumulus oophorus, essential for HA organization, raises the probability of a similar localization and function of this molecule in certain

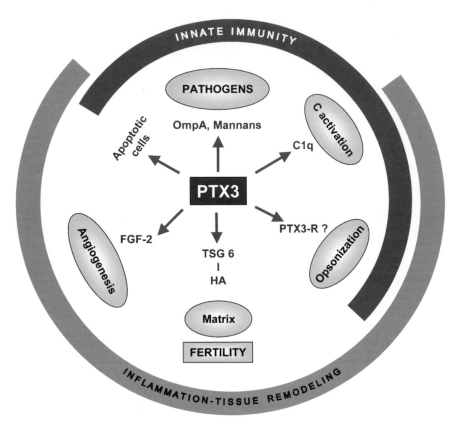

Figure 4   PTX3 ligands and function in innate immunity, inflammation, and tissue remodeling.

HA-enriched inflammatory tissues, such as in rheumatoid arthritis, where TSG-6 is also expressed (103, 120).

Human Pathology

The relationship to a classic diagnostic (CRP), now experiencing a renaissance in cardiovascular disorders (4, 121), and the data obtained from studies of gene-modified mice have given impetus to efforts aimed at assessing the usefulness of PTX3 in diverse human pathological conditions. The hypothesis driving many previous and ongoing efforts is that PTX3, unlike CRP (made in the liver and induced primarily by IL-6), may represent a rapid marker for primary local activation of innate immunity and inflammation (Figure 5). Indeed, in all clinical studies conducted so far, the correlation between levels of PTX3 and CRP was loose or nonsignificant (107, 108). A second general characteristic emerging from studies of blood levels in murine and human pathology is the rapidity of PTX3 increase,

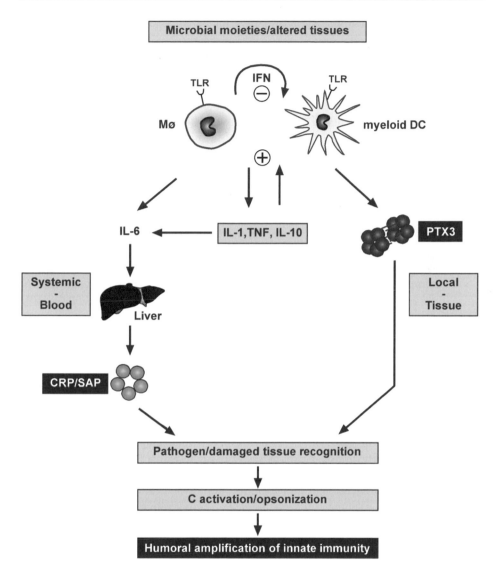

Figure 5   Pentraxins in humoral innate immunity. Inducibility of CRP or SAP is species dependent (see text).

compared to CRP, consistent with its original identification as an immediate early gene (108).

Increased levels of PTX3 have been observed in diverse infectious disorders, including sepsis, *A. fumigatus* infections, tuberculosis, and dengue (101, 107; G. Peri, unpublished data). In some of these disorders, PTX3 levels correlated with disease activity or severity.

Pentraxins, including SAP and PTX3, bind apoptotic cells and release nuclear components, regulate their clearance, and gate the activation of autoimmunity (100). Increased levels of PTX3 have been observed in a restricted set of autoimmune disorders (e.g., in the blood in small vessel vasculitis and in the synovial fluid in rheumatoid arthritis), but not in others (e.g., SLE, Crohn's disease) (122, 123; G. Peri & A. Doni, unpublished results). In small vessel vasculitis, PTX3 levels correlate with clinical activity of the disease and represent a candidate marker for monitoring the disease (122).

Inflammation is a critical component of ischemic heart disorders, and CRP has emerged as a valuable diagnostic tool (for a critical appraisal, see 4). The high levels of expression in the heart during inflammatory reactions, the production by vascular cells in response to inflammatory signals (9) and oxLDL (84), and the occurrence in atherosclerotic lesions (91) prompted studies on PTX3 levels in acute myocardial infarction (108, 124). In a recent study with a cohort of 748 patients, PTX3, measured along with established markers including CRP, emerged as the only independent predictor of mortality (124). It remains to be elucidated whether this impressive correlation with outcome actually reflects a role in the pathogenesis of damage, for instance by amplifying the complement and coagulation cascades (125, 126).

Results in gene-targeted mice have revealed a nonredundant function of PTX3 in female fertility (95, 96). PTX3 is produced and present in the human cumulus oophorus, and it was recently suggested that cumulus PTX3 transcript levels correlate with oocyte quality (127).

PTX3 is a humoral effector molecule of innate immunity; it binds selected pathogens, activates complement, facilitates cellular recognition and disposal, and acts as a matrix component. The molecular partner of PTX3 in the matrix identified so far (Figures 4 and 5), TSG-6, is a candidate chondroprotective agent in rheumatoid arthritis (103). Current research suggests that PTX3 may well fulfill a similar function.

PTX3 synergizes with conventional antifungal agents in the treatment of *A. fumigatus* infections (106). This recent finding reinforces the hypothesis of PTX3 as a candidate new agent for the treatment or profylaxis of *A. fumigatus* infections in immunocompromised patients.

OTHER LONG PENTRAXINS

Researchers have identified a set of long pentraxins in neuronal tissues (Figure 1). NP1 (or NPTXI) was originally identified as a protein binding taipoxin, the presynaptic-acting snake venom neurotoxin (11). NP2 (or NPTXII) was cloned by low stringency hybridization (12) or as Narp, an early gene induced by physiologic synaptic activity (16). Unlike NP1, NP2/Narp is expressed in a wide range of non-nervous tissues, prominently in the testis (12). NP2 has homology with apexin, a guinea pig long pentraxin identified in the acrosome of spermatozoa (14, 23).

Recent analysis suggests that apexin is not the guinea pig ortholog of NP2 (Y. Martinez, unpublished data). NPR is an integral membrane pentraxin, coexpressed in the brain with NP1, that binds NP1 and taipoxin (17, 18).

Various functions have been attributed to neuronal pentraxins. On the basis of its binding to taipoxin, NP1 was postulated to have a role in synaptic uptake. NP1 is induced during low K^+-induced apoptotic death of cerebellar granule cells (128) and during hypoxic-ischemic injury of the neonatal brain (129). NP1 antisense nucleotides protect neuronal cells against death induced by hypoxia or by the glutamate analog AMPA (α-amino-3-hydroxy-5-methyl-4 isoxazole-propionic acid) (129).

Narp, which binds agar (16), and NP1 form heterocomplexes in the brain via covalent links involving cysteines in the N-terminal, nonpentraxin domain, as PTX3 does. The pentraxin domains associate with AMPA-type gutamate receptors. NP1 and Narp together have superadditive synaptogenic activity. These two neuronal pentraxins, and possibly NPR, would contribute to activity-dependent (Narp) and -independent (NP1) synaptogenesis and to synaptic plasticity (75). NP1-deficient mice have been generated but show no apparent phenotype (75). This negative finding may reflect redundancy of neuronal pentraxins.

PTX3 is expressed by neuronal cells and astrocytes following exposure to infectious agents, inflammatory cytokines, stroke, experimental autoimmune encephalomyelitis, and limbic seizures (81, 93, 94). In limbic seizures, gene-targeted mice revealed a protective role for PTX3 in seizure-induced neurodegeneration (93). It remains to be established whether PTX3 can form heterocomplexes with neuronal pentraxins and regulate their function.

Scientists have identified pentraxin-like domains in diverse molecules expressed in peripheral tissues. For instance, vascular inducible G protein–coupled receptor (GPCR, VIGR) is induced by LPS or thrombin in endothelial cells and consists of an N-terminal pentraxin-like domain on top of an adhesin-type GPCR (130). Similarly, the ectodomain of very large GPCR1 (VLGR-1) contains a pentraxin domain. Interestingly, VLGR-1 is expressed in the developing brain (131). The function of these and other pentraxin-like domain-containing molecules is at present unknown.

OVERVIEW AND PERSPECTIVE

Pentraxins are evolutionary conserved humoral PRRs. Strong evidence, including evidence from studies of gene-modified mice, suggests that at least some of these molecules play a nonredundant role in innate resistance against microbes. Available information suggests that the short pentraxins CRP and SAP and the long pentraxin PTX3 have different ligand specificity (Table 1). Thus, pentraxins provide the innate immune system with a repertoire of diverse receptors with distinct specificity.

In terms of regulation of production, members of the pentraxin family can be distinguished as inducible (or inflammatory) and constitutive (or homeostatic).

Constitutive versus inducible production may vary in different species, as discussed above for CRP and SAP in humans versus rodents. Copious amounts of the short pentraxins CRP and SAP are made in the liver as the end result of the pathogen recognition–cytokine cascade (Figure 5). In contrast, long pentraxins are generally expressed at extrahepatic sites, and the prototypic molecule PTX3 is directly induced by TLR engagement and primary inflammatory cytokines. Therefore, liver-derived short pentraxins and tissue-expressed long pentraxins (PTX3) are likely to fulfill complementary functions, acting primarily at a systemic and local tissue level, respectively (Figure 5).

The regulation of production and effector functions of at least some members of the pentraxin superfamily (e.g., CRP or PTX3) are strongly reminescent of antibodies. Their production is induced by recognition via TLR of microbial nonself or altered self (oxLDL), directly (PTX3) or indirectly (short pentraxins) (Figure 5). Short pentraxins and PTX3 recognize microbial structures or altered self (apoptotic cells), activate complement, and facilitate recognition and disposal by macrophages, thus acting as a humoral amplification loop of innate immunity. Therefore, inducible pentraxins act as bona fide functional proto-antibodies.

Innate resistance to pathogens is one of the many facets of pentraxins. PTX3 is divergently regulated by IFN-γ and IL-10 and is essential for activation of a polarized type 1 response to *A. fumigatus* (89, 101). Pentraxins bind apoptotic cells, nucleosomes, and nuclear components, and SAP-deficient mice are prone to develop autoimmunity (73). Therefore, as for other innate immunity receptors, pentraxins can contribute to the orientation of adaptive immunity and to the vetoing of autoimmunity.

Members of the pentraxin family are involved in neuronal function (NP1, NP2, NPR), regulation of neurodegeneration (NP1, PTX3, SAP), construction of extracellular matrices (PTX3, SAP), and female fertility (PTX3). The latter two related functions, rather than immunity, most likely underlie the high conservation in mammals of PTX3. Therefore, pentraxins are soluble multifunctional PRRs at the crossroads between innate and adaptative immunity, inflammation, matrix deposition, and female fertility. It will be important to assess whether, in analogy to CRP and SAP, the newly discovered long pentraxins can contribute to clinical medicine as diagnostic or therapeutic agents.

ACKNOWLEDGMENTS

This work was supported by Associazione Italiana per la Ricerca sul Cancro (AIRC), Ministero Istruzione Università e Ricerca (MIUR), CNR, European Commission. We wish to thank people who, over the years, were part of the Pentraxin Project in our department (in particular Giuseppe Peri, Andrea Doni, and Annunciata Vecchi) and external collaborators (in particular Luigina Romani, Roberto Latini, Antonia Salustri, and Giovanni Salvatori) for invaluable help, suggestions, and illuminating discussions. We thank Yeny Martinez for preparing Figure 1*B*.

The *Annual Review of Immunology* is online at
http://immunol.annualreviews.org

LITERATURE CITED

1. Medzhitov R. 2001. Toll-like receptors and innate immunity. *Nat. Rev. Immunol.* 1:135–45

2. Gordon S. 2002. Pattern recognition receptors: doubling up for the innate immune response. *Cell* 111:927–30

3. Szalai AJ, Agrawal A, Greenhough TJ, Volanakis JE. 1999. C-reactive protein: structural biology and host defense function. *Clin. Chem. Lab. Med.* 37:265–70

4. Pepys MB, Hirschfield GM. 2003. C-reactive protein: a critical update. *J. Clin. Invest.* 111:1805–12

5. Pepys MB, Baltz ML. 1983. Acute phase proteins with special reference to C-reactive protein and related proteins (pentaxins) and serum amyloid A protein. *Adv. Immunol.* 34:141–212

6. Mantovani A, Garlanda C, Bottazzi B. 2003. Pentraxin 3, a non-redundant soluble pattern recognition receptor involved in innate immunity. *Vaccine* 21(Suppl. 2):S43–47

7. Tillet WS, Francis T Jr. 1930. Serological reactions in pneumonia with a non protein somatic fraction of pneumococcus. *J. Exp. Med.* 52:561–85

8. Abernethy TJ, Avery OT. 1941. The occurence during acute infections of a protein not normally present in the blood. I. Distribution of the reactive protein in patients' sera and the effect of calcium on the flocculation reaction with C. polysaccharide of pneumococcus. *J. Exp. Med.* 73:173–82

9. Breviario F, d'Aniello EM, Golay J, Peri G, Bottazzi B, et al. 1992. Interleukin-1-inducible genes in endothelial cells. Cloning of a new gene related to C-reactive protein and serum amyloid P component. *J. Biol. Chem.* 267:22190–97

10. Lee GW, Lee TH, Vilcek J. 1993. TSG-14, a tumor necrosis factor- and IL-1-inducible protein, is a novel member of the pentaxin family of acute phase proteins. *J. Immunol.* 150:1804–12

11. Schlimgen AK, Helms JA, Vogel H, Perin MS. 1995. Neuronal pentraxin, a secreted protein with homology to acute phase proteins of the immune system. *Neuron* 14:519–26

12. Hsu YC, Perin MS. 1995. Human neuronal pentraxin II (NPTX2): conservation, genomic structure, and chromosomal localization. *Genomics* 28:220–27

13. Omeis IA, Hsu YC, Perin MS. 1996. Mouse and human neuronal pentraxin 1 (NPTX1): conservation, genomic structure, and chromosomal localization. *Genomics* 36:543–45

14. Noland TD, Friday BB, Maulit MT, Gerton GL. 1994. The sperm acrosomal matrix contains a novel member of the pentaxin family of calcium-dependent binding proteins. *J. Biol. Chem.* 269:32607–14

15. Seery LT, Schoenberg DR, Barbaux S, Sharp PM, Whitehead AS. 1993. Identification of a novel member of the pentraxin family in *Xenopus laevis*. *Proc. R. Soc. London Ser. B* 253:263–70

16. Tsui CC, Copeland NG, Gilbert DJ, Jenkins NA, Barnes C, Worley PF. 1996. Narp, a novel member of the pentraxin family, promotes neurite outgrowth and is dynamically regulated by neuronal activity. *J. Neurosci.* 16:2463–78

17. Dodds DC, Omeis IA, Cushman SJ, Helms JA, Perin MS. 1997. Neuronal pentraxin receptor, a novel putative integral membrane pentraxin that interacts with neuronal pentraxin 1 and 2 and taipoxin-associated calcium-binding protein 49. *J. Biol. Chem.* 272:21488–94

18. Kirkpatrick LL, Matzuk MM, Dodds DC, Perin MS. 2000. Biochemical interactions of the neuronal pentraxins. Neuronal pentraxin (NP) receptor binds to taipoxin and taipoxin-associated calcium-binding protein 49 via NP1 and NP2. *J. Biol. Chem.* 275:17786–92

19. Gewurz H, Zhang XH, Lint TF. 1995. Structure and function of the pentraxins. *Curr. Opin. Immunol.* 7:54–64

20. Shrive AK, Metcalfe AM, Cartwright JR, Greenhough TJ. 1999. C-reactive protein and SAP-like pentraxin are both present in *Limulus polyphemus* haemolymph: crystal structure of *Limulus* SAP. *J. Mol. Biol.* 290:997–1008

21. Armstrong PB, Swarnakar S, Srimal S, Misquith S, Hahn EA, et al. 1996. A cytolytic function for a sialic acid-binding lectin that is a member of the pentraxin family of proteins. *J. Biol. Chem.* 271:14717–21

22. Liu TY, Robey FA, Wang CM. 1982. Structural studies on C-reactive protein. *Ann. NY Acad. Sci.* 389:151–62

23. Reid MS, Blobel CP. 1994. Apexin, an acrosomal pentaxin. *J. Biol. Chem.* 269: 32615–20

24. Goodman AR, Cardozo T, Abagyan R, Altmeyer A, Wisniewski HG, Vilcek J. 1996. Long pentraxins: an emerging group of proteins with diverse functions. *Cytokine Growth Factor Rev.* 7:191–202

25. Kretzschmar D, Hasan G, Sharma S, Heisenberg M, Benzer S. 1997. The swiss cheese mutant causes glial hyperwrapping and brain degeneration in *Drosophila*. *J. Neurosci.* 17:7425–32

26. Rubio N, Sharp PM, Rits M, Zahedi K, Whitehead AS. 1993. Structure, expression, and evolution of guinea pig serum amyloid P component and C-reactive protein. *J. Biochem.* 113:277–84

27. Shrive AK, Cheetham GM, Holden D, Myles DA, Turnell WG, et al. 1996. Three dimensional structure of human C-reactive protein. *Nat. Struct. Biol.* 3:346–54

28. Toniatti C, Demartis A, Monaci P, Nicosia A, Ciliberto G. 1990. Synergistic transactivation of the human C-reactive protein promoter by transcription factor HNF-1 binding at two distinct sites. *EMBO J.* 9:4467–75

29. Li SP, Goldman ND. 1996. Regulation of human C-reactive protein gene expression by two synergistic IL-6 responsive elements. *Biochemistry* 35:9060–68

30. Ramji DP, Vitelli A, Tronche F, Cortese R, Ciliberto G. 1993. The two C/EBP isoforms, IL-6DBP/NF-IL6 and C/EBP δ/NF-IL6 β, are induced by IL-6 to promote acute phase gene transcription via different mechanisms. *Nucleic Acids Res.* 21:289–94

31. Zhang D, Sun M, Samols D, Kushner I. 1996. STAT3 participates in transcriptional activation of the C-reactive protein gene by interleukin-6. *J. Biol. Chem.* 271:9503–9

32. Cha-Molstad H, Agrawal A, Zhang D, Samols D, Kushner I. 2000. The Rel family member P50 mediates cytokine-induced C-reactive protein expression by a novel mechanism. *J. Immunol.* 165: 4592–97

33. Agrawal A, Cha-Molstad H, Samols D, Kushner I. 2001. Transactivation of C-reactive protein by IL-6 requires synergistic interaction of CCAAT/enhancer binding protein β (C/EBP β) and Rel p50. *J. Immunol.* 166:2378–84

34. Zhang D, Jiang SL, Rzewnicki D, Samols D, Kushner I. 1995. The effect of interleukin-1 on C-reactive protein expression in Hep3B cells is exerted at the transcriptional level. *Biochem. J.* 310(Part 1):143–48

35. Emsley J, White HE, O'Hara BP, Oliva G, Srinivasan N, et al. 1994. Structure of pentameric human serum amyloid P component. *Nature* 367:338–45

36. Zahedi K. 1997. Characterization of the binding of serum amyloid P to laminin. *J. Biol. Chem.* 272:2143–48

37. Aquilina JA, Robinson CV. 2003.

Investigating interactions of the pentraxins serum amyloid P component and C-reactive protein by mass spectrometry. *Biochem. J.* 375:323–28

38. Pepys MB, Rademacher TW, Amatayakul-Chantler S, Williams P, Noble GE, et al. 1994. Human serum amyloid P component is an invariant constituent of amyloid deposits and has a uniquely homogeneous glycostructure. *Proc. Natl. Acad. Sci. USA* 91:5602–6

39. Hutchinson WL, Hohenester E, Pepys MB. 2000. Human serum amyloid P component is a single uncomplexed pentamer in whole serum. *Mol. Med.* 6:482–93

40. Szalai AJ. 2002. The antimicrobial activity of C-reactive protein. *Microbes Infect.* 4:201–5

41. Hind CR, Collins PM, Renn D, Cook RB, Caspi D, et al. 1984. Binding specificity of serum amyloid P component for the pyruvate acetal of galactose. *J. Exp. Med.* 159:1058–69

42. Noursadeghi M, Bickerstaff MC, Gallimore JR, Herbert J, Cohen J, Pepys MB. 2000. Role of serum amyloid P component in bacterial infection: protection of the host or protection of the pathogen. *Proc. Natl. Acad. Sci. USA* 97:14584–89

43. Hind CR, Collins PM, Baltz ML, Pepys MB. 1985. Human serum amyloid P component, a circulating lectin with specificity for the cyclic 4,6-pyruvate acetal of galactose. Interactions with various bacteria. *Biochem. J.* 225:107–11

44. Andersen O, Vilsgaard Ravn K, Juul Sorensen I, Jonson G, Holm Nielsen E, Svehag SE. 1997. Serum amyloid P component binds to influenza A virus haemagglutinin and inhibits the virus infection in vitro. *Scand. J. Immunol.* 46:331–37

45. de Haas CJ, van der Tol ME, Van Kessel KP, Verhoef J, Van Strijp JA. 1998. A synthetic lipopolysaccharide-binding peptide based on amino acids 27–39 of serum amyloid P component inhibits lipopolysaccharide-induced responses in human blood. *J. Immunol.* 161:3607–15

46. Loveless RW, Floyd-O'Sullivan G, Raynes JG, Yuen CT, Feizi T. 1992. Human serum amyloid P is a multispecific adhesive protein whose ligands include 6-phosphorylated mannose and the 3-sulphated saccharides galactose, N-acetylgalactosamine and glucuronic acid. *EMBO J.* 11:813–19

47. Pepys MB, Butler PJ. 1987. Serum amyloid P component is the major calcium-dependent specific DNA binding protein of the serum. *Biochem. Biophys. Res. Commun.* 148:308–13

48. Butler PJ, Tennent GA, Pepys MB. 1990. Pentraxin-chromatin interactions: serum amyloid P component specifically displaces H1-type histones and solubilizes native long chromatin. *J. Exp. Med.* 172:13–18

49. Nauta AJ, Daha MR, van Kooten C, Roos A. 2003. Recognition and clearance of apoptotic cells: a role for complement and pentraxins. *Trends Immunol.* 24:148–54

50. Jiang H, Robey FA, Gewurz H. 1992. Localization of sites through which C-reactive protein binds and activates complement to residues 14–26 and 76–92 of the human C1q A chain. *J. Exp. Med.* 175:1373–79

51. Ying SC, Gewurz AT, Jiang H, Gewurz H. 1993. Human serum amyloid P component oligomers bind and activate the classical complement pathway via residues 14–26 and 76–92 of the A chain collagen-like region of C1q. *J. Immunol.* 150:169–76

52. Gershov D, Kim S, Brot N, Elkon KB. 2000. C-Reactive protein binds to apoptotic cells, protects the cells from assembly of the terminal complement components, and sustains an antiinflammatory innate immune response: implications for systemic autoimmunity. *J. Exp. Med.* 192:1353–64

53. Familian A, Zwart B, Huisman HG, Rensink I, Roem D, et al. 2001. Chromatin-independent binding of serum

amyloid P component to apoptotic cells. *J. Immunol.* 167:647–54

54. Bharadwaj D, Stein MP, Volzer M, Mold C, Du Clos TW. 1999. The major receptor for C-reactive protein on leukocytes is Fcγ receptor II. *J. Exp. Med.* 190:585–90

55. Bharadwaj D, Mold C, Markham E, Du Clos TW. 2001. Serum amyloid P component binds to Fcγ receptors and opsonizes particles for phagocytosis. *J. Immunol.* 166:6735–41

56. Mold C, Baca R, Du Clos TW. 2002. Serum amyloid P component and C-reactive protein opsonize apoptotic cells for phagocytosis through Fcγ receptors. *J. Autoimmun.* 19:147–54

57. Mold C, Gresham HD, Du Clos TW. 2001. Serum amyloid P component and C-reactive protein mediate phagocytosis through murine FcγRs. *J. Immunol.* 166:1200–5

58. Hundt M, Zielinska-Skowronek M, Schmidt RE. 2001. Lack of specific receptors for C-reactive protein on white blood cells. *Eur. J. Immunol.* 31:3475–83

59. Saeland E, van Royen A, Hendriksen K, Vile-Weekhout H, Rijkers GT, et al. 2001. Human C-reactive protein does not bind to FcγRIIa on phagocytic cells. *J. Clin. Invest.* 107:641–43

60. Szalai AJ, Briles DE, Volanakis JE. 1995. Human C-reactive protein is protective against fatal *Streptococcus pneumoniae* infection in transgenic mice. *J. Immunol.* 155:2557–63

61. Weiser JN, Pan N, McGowan KL, Musher D, Martin A, Richards J. 1998. Phosphorylcholine on the lipopolysaccharide of *Haemophilus influenzae* contributes to persistence in the respiratory tract and sensitivity to serum killing mediated by C-reactive protein. *J. Exp. Med.* 187:631–40

62. Lysenko E, Richards JC, Cox AD, Stewart A, Martin A, et al. 2000. The position of phosphorylcholine on the lipopolysaccharide of *Haemophilus influenzae* af-

fects binding and sensitivity to C-reactive protein-mediated killing. *Mol. Microbiol.* 35:234–45

63. Szalai AJ, VanCott JL, McGhee JR, Volanakis JE, Benjamin WH Jr. 2000. Human C-reactive protein is protective against fatal *Salmonella enterica* serovar typhimurium infection in transgenic mice. *Infect. Immun.* 68:5652–56

64. Szalai AJ, Nataf S, Hu XZ, Barnum SR. 2002. Experimental allergic encephalomyelitis is inhibited in transgenic mice expressing human C-reactive protein. *J. Immunol.* 168:5792–97

65. Du Clos TW, Zlock LT, Hicks PS, Mold C. 1994. Decreased autoantibody levels and enhanced survival of (NZB × NZW) F1 mice treated with C-reactive protein. *Clin. Immunol. Immunopathol.* 70:22–27

66. Szalai AJ, Weaver CT, McCrory MA, van Ginkel FW, Reiman RM, et al. 2003. Delayed lupus onset in (NZB × NZW)F1 mice expressing a human C-reactive protein transgene. *Arthritis Rheum.* 48:1602–11

67. Xia D, Samols D. 1997. Transgenic mice expressing rabbit C-reactive protein are resistant to endotoxemia. *Proc. Natl. Acad. Sci. USA* 94:2575–80

68. Mold C, Rodriguez W, Rodic-Polic B, Du Clos TW. 2002. C-reactive protein mediates protection from lipopolysaccharide through interactions with FcγR. *J. Immunol.* 169:7019–25

69. Hirschfield GM, Herbert J, Kahan MC, Pepys MB. 2003. Human C-reactive protein does not protect against acute lipopolysaccharide challenge in mice. *J. Immunol.* 171:6046–51

70. Botto M, Hawkins PN, Bickerstaff MC, Herbert J, Bygrave AE, et al. 1997. Amyloid deposition is delayed in mice with targeted deletion of the serum amyloid P component gene. *Nat. Med.* 3:855–59

71. Tennent GA, Lovat LB, Pepys MB. 1995. Serum amyloid P component prevents proteolysis of the amyloid fibrils

of Alzheimer disease and systemic amyloidosis. *Proc. Natl. Acad. Sci. USA* 92: 4299–303

72. Pepys MB, Herbert J, Hutchinson WL, Tennent GA, Lachmann HJ, et al. 2002. Targeted pharmacological depletion of serum amyloid P component for treatment of human amyloidosis. *Nature* 417:254–59

73. Bickerstaff MC, Botto M, Hutchinson WL, Herbert J, Tennent GA, et al. 1999. Serum amyloid P component controls chromatin degradation and prevents antinuclear autoimmunity. *Nat. Med.* 5:694–97

74. Bottazzi B, Vouret-Craviari V, Bastone A, De Gioia L, Matteucci C, et al. 1997. Multimer formation and ligand recognition by the long pentraxin PTX3. Similarities and differences with the short pentraxins C-reactive protein and serum amyloid P component. *J. Biol. Chem.* 272:32817–23

75. Xu DS, Hopf C, Reddy R, Cho RW, Guo LP, et al. 2003. Narp and NP1 form heterocomplexes that function in developmental and activity-dependent synaptic plasticity. *Neuron* 39:513–28

76. Introna M, Alles VV, Castellano M, Picardi G, De Gioia L, et al. 1996. Cloning of mouse ptx3, a new member of the pentraxin gene family expressed at extrahepatic sites. *Blood* 87:1862–72

77. Basile A, Sica A, d'Aniello E, Breviario F, Garrido G, et al. 1997. Characterization of the promoter for the human long pentraxin PTX3. Role of NF-κB in tumor necrosis factor-α and interleukin-1β regulation. *J. Biol. Chem.* 272:8172–78

78. Altmeyer A, Klampfer L, Goodman AR, Vilcek J. 1995. Promoter structure and transcriptional activation of the murine TSG-14 gene encoding a tumor necrosis factor/interleukin-1-inducible pentraxin protein. *J. Biol. Chem.* 270:25584–90

79. Doni A, Peri G, Chieppa M, Allavena P, Pasqualini F, et al. 2003. Production of the soluble pattern recognition receptor PTX3 by myeloid, but not plasmacytoid, dendritic cells. *Eur. J. Immunol.* 33:2886–93

80. Alles VV, Bottazzi B, Peri G, Golay J, Introna M, Mantovani A. 1994. Inducible expression of PTX3, a new member of the pentraxin family, in human mononuclear phagocytes. *Blood* 84:3483–93

81. Polentarutti N, Bottazzi B, Di Santo E, Blasi E, Agnello D, et al. 2000. Inducible expression of the long pentraxin PTX3 in the central nervous system. *J. Neuroimmunol.* 106:87–94

82. Goodman AR, Levy DE, Reis LF, Vilcek J. 2000. Differential regulation of TSG-14 expression in murine fibroblasts and peritoneal macrophages. *J. Leukoc. Biol.* 67:387–95

83. Abderrahim-Ferkoune A, Bezy O, Chiellini C, Maffei M, Grimaldi P, et al. 2003. Characterization of the long pentraxin PTX3 as a TNF α-induced secreted protein of adipose cells. *J. Lipid Res.* 44:994–1000

84. Klouche M, Peri G, Knabbe C, Eckstein HH, Schmid FX, et al. 2004. Modified atherogenic lipoproteins induce expression of pentraxin-3 by human vascular smooth muscle cells. *Atherosclerosis* 175:221–28

85. Vouret-Craviari V, Matteucci C, Peri G, Poli G, Introna M, Mantovani A. 1997. Expression of a long pentraxin, PTX3, by monocytes exposed to the mycobacterial cell wall component lipoarabinomannan. *Infect. Immun.* 65:1345–50

86. Malaguarnera L, Pilastro MR, Vicari L, Di Marco R, Malaguarnera M, Messina A. 2000. PTX3 gene expression in Castleman's disease. *Eur. J. Haematol.* 64:132–34

87. Klouche M, Brockmeyer N, Knabbe C, Rose-John S. 2002. Human herpesvirus 8-derived viral IL-6 induces PTX3 expression in Kaposi's sarcoma cells. *AIDS* 16:F9–18

88. Polentarutti N, Picardi G, Basile A, Cenzuales S, Rivolta A, et al. 1998. Interferon-γ inhibits expression of the long pentraxin PTX3 in human monocytes. *Eur. J. Immunol.* 28:496–501

89. Perrier P, Martinez FO, Locati M, Bianchi G, Nebuloni M, et al. 2004. Distinct transcriptional programs activated by interleukin-10 with or without lipopolysaccharide in dendritic cells: induction of the B cell-activating chemokine, CXC chemokine ligand 13. *J. Immunol.* 172:7031–42

90. Mantovani A, Sozzani S, Locati M, Allavena P, Sica A. 2002. Macrophage polarization: tumor-associated macrophages as a paradigm for polarized M2 mononuclear phagocytes. *Trends Immunol.* 23:549–55

91. Rolph MS, Zimmer S, Bottazzi B, Garlanda C, Mantovani A, Hansson GK. 2002. Production of the long pentraxin PTX3 in advanced atherosclerotic plaques. *Arterioscler. Thromb. Vasc. Biol.* 22:E10–18

92. Lee GW, Goodman AR, Lee TH, Vilcek J. 1994. Relationship of TSG-14 protein to the pentraxin family of major acute phase proteins. *J. Immunol.* 153:3700–7

93. Ravizza T, Moneta D, Bottazzi B, Peri G, Garlanda C, et al. 2001. Dynamic induction of the long pentraxin PTX3 in the CNS after limbic seizures: evidence for a protective role in seizure-induced neurodegeneration. *Neuroscience* 105:43–53

94. Agnello D, Carvelli L, Muzio V, Villa P, Bottazzi B, et al. 2000. Increased peripheral benzodiazepine binding sites and pentraxin 3 expression in the spinal cord during EAE: relation to inflammatory cytokines and modulation by dexamethasone and rolipram. *J. Neuroimmunol.* 109:105–11

95. Varani S, Elvin JA, Yan CN, DeMayo J, DeMayo FJ, et al. 2002. Knockout of pentraxin 3, a downstream target of growth differentiation factor-9, causes female subfertility. *Mol. Endocrinol.* 16:1154–67

96. Salustri A, Garlanda C, Hirsch E, De Acetis M, Maccagno A, et al. 2004. PTX3 plays a key role in the organization of the cumulus oophorus extracellular matrix and in in vivo fertilization. *Development* 131:1577–86

97. Lafon-Cazal M, Adjali O, Galeotti N, Poncet J, Jouin P, et al. 2003. Proteomic analysis of astrocytic secretion in the mouse. Comparison with the cerebrospinal fluid proteome. *J. Biol. Chem.* 278:24438–48

98. Semov A, Semova N, Lacelle C, Marcotte R, Petroulakis E, et al. 2002. Alterations in TNF- and IL-related gene expression in space-flown WI38 human fibroblasts. *FASEB J.* 16:899–901

99. Nauta AJ, Bottazzi B, Mantovani A, Salvatori G, Kishore U, et al. 2003. Biochemical and functional characterization of the interaction between pentraxin 3 and C1q. *Eur. J. Immunol.* 33:465–73

100. Rovere P, Peri G, Fazzini F, Bottazzi B, Doni A, et al. 2000. The long pentraxin PTX3 binds to apoptotic cells and regulates their clearance by antigen-presenting dendritic cells. *Blood* 96:4300–6

101. Garlanda C, Hirsch E, Bozza S, Salustri A, De Acetis M, et al. 2002. Non-redundant role of the long pentraxin PTX3 in antifungal innate immune response. *Nature* 420:182–86

102. Diniz SN, Nomizo R, Cisalpino PS, Teixeira MM, Brown GD, et al. 2004. PTX3 function as an opsonin for the dectin-1-dependent internalization of zymosan by macrophages. *J. Leukoc. Biol.* 75:649–56

103. Milner CM, Day AJ. 2003. TSG-6: a multifunctional protein associated with inflammation. *J. Cell Sci.* 116:1863–73

104. Wisniewski HG, Vilcek J. 2004. Cytokine-induced gene expression at the crossroads of innate immunity, inflammation and fertility: TSG-6 and PTX3/TSG-14. *Cytokine Growth Factor Rev.* 15:129–46

105. Rusnati M, Camozzi M, Moroni E, Bottazzi B, Peri G, et al. 2004. Selective recognition of fibroblast growth factor-2 by the long pentraxin PTX3 inhibits angiogenesis. *Blood* 104:92–99

106. Gaziano R, Bozza S, Bellocchio S, Perruccio K, Montagnoli C, et al. 2004. Combination therapy with pentraxin 3 and antifungals in experimental aspergillosis. *Antimicrob. Agents Chemother.* 48:4414–21

107. Muller B, Peri G, Doni A, Torri V, Landmann R, et al. 2001. Circulating levels of the long pentraxin PTX3 correlate with severity of infection in critically ill patients. *Crit. Care Med.* 29:1404–7

108. Peri G, Introna M, Corradi D, Iacuitti G, Signorini S, et al. 2000. PTX3, a prototypic long pentraxin, is an early indicator of acute myocardial infarction in man. *Circulation* 102:636–41

109. Dias AA, Goodman AR, Dos Santos JL, Gomes RN, Altmeyer A, et al. 2001. TSG-14 transgenic mice have improved survival to endotoxemia and to CLP-induced sepsis. *J. Leukoc. Biol.* 69:928–36

110. Souza DG, Soares AC, Pinho V, Torloni H, Reis LF, et al. 2002. Increased mortality and inflammation in tumor necrosis factor-stimulated gene-14 transgenic mice after ischemia and reperfusion injury. *Am. J. Pathol.* 160:1755–65

111. Zhuo L, Yoneda M, Zhao M, Yingsung W, Yoshida N, et al. 2001. Defect in SHAP-hyaluronan complex causes severe female infertility. A study by inactivation of the bikunin gene in mice. *J. Biol. Chem.* 276:7693–96

112. Fulop C, Szanto S, Mukhopadhyay D, Bardos T, Kamath RV, et al. 2003. Impaired cumulus mucification and female sterility in tumor necrosis factor-induced protein-6 deficient mice. *Development* 130:2253–61

113. Richards JS, Russell DL, Ochsner S, Espey LL. 2002. Ovulation: new dimensions and new regulators of the inflammatory-like response. *Annu. Rev. Physiol.* 64:69–92

114. Espey LL. 1994. Current status of the hypothesis that mammalian ovulation is comparable to an inflammatory reaction. *Biol. Reprod.* 50:233–38

115. Elvin JA, Clark AT, Wang P, Wolfman NM, Matzuk MM. 1999. Paracrine actions of growth differentiation factor-9 in the mammalian ovary. *Mol. Endocrinol.* 13:1035–48

116. Salustri A, Yanagishita M, Hascall VC. 1990. Mouse oocytes regulate hyaluronic acid synthesis and mucification by FSH-stimulated cumulus cells. *Dev. Biol.* 138:26–32

117. Buccione R, Vanderhyden BC, Caron PJ, Eppig JJ. 1990. FSH-induced expansion of the mouse cumulus oophorus in vitro is dependent upon a specific factor(s) secreted by the oocyte. *Dev. Biol.* 138:16–25

118. Day AJ, Prestwich GD. 2002. Hyaluronan-binding proteins: tying up the giant. *J. Biol. Chem.* 277:4585–88

119. Tammi MI, Day AJ, Turley EA. 2002. Hyaluronan and homeostasis: a balancing act. *J. Biol. Chem.* 277:4581–84

120. Wisniewski HG, Vilcek J. 2004. Cytokine-induced gene expression at the crossroads of innate immunity, inflammation and fertility: TSG-6 and PTX3/TSG-14. *Cytokine Growth Factor Rev.* 15:129–46

121. Hirschfield GM, Pepys MB. 2003. C-reactive protein and cardiovascular disease: new insights from an old molecule. *Q. J. Med.* 96:793–807

122. Fazzini F, Peri G, Doni A, Dell'Antonio G, Dal Cin E, et al. 2001. PTX3 in small-vessel vasculitides: an independent indicator of disease activity produced at sites of inflammation. *Arthritis Rheum.* 44:2841–50

123. Luchetti MM, Piccinini G, Mantovani A, Peri G, Matteucci C, et al. 2000. Expression and production of the long pentraxin PTX3 in rheumatoid arthritis (RA). *Clin. Exp. Immunol.* 119:196–202

124. Latini R, Maggioni AP, Peri G, Gonzini L, Lucci D, et al. 2004. Prognostic significance of the long pentraxin PTX3 in acute myocardial infarction. *Circulation* 110:2349–54

125. Napoleone E, Di Santo A, Peri G, Mantovani A, de Gaetano G, et al. 2004. The long

pentraxin PTX3 up-regulates tissue factor in activated monocytes: another link between inflammation and clotting activation. *J. Leukoc. Biol.* 76:203–9

126. Napoleone E, Di Santo A, Bastone A, Peri G, Mantovani A, et al. 2002. Long pentraxin PTX3 upregulates tissue factor expression in human endothelial cells: a novel link between vascular inflammation and clotting activation. *Arterioscler. Thromb. Vasc. Biol.* 22:782–87

127. Zhang XQJ, Moyse J, Jarari N, Confino E, Kazer R. 2003. Pentraxin-3 gene expression in cumulus cells may be a molecular marker for egg quality. *Fertil. Steril.* 80(Suppl. 3):S81

128. DeGregorio-Rocasolano N, Gasull T, Trullas R. 2001. Overexpression of neuronal pentraxin 1 is involved in neuronal death evoked by low K^+ in cerebellar granule cells. *J. Biol. Chem.* 276:796–803

129. Hossain MA, Russell JC, O'Brien R, Laterra J. 2004. Neuronal pentraxin 1: a novel mediator of hypoxic-ischemic injury in neonatal brain. *J. Neurosci.* 24:4187–96

130. Stehlik C, Kroismayr R, Dorfleutner A, Binder BR, Lipp J. 2004. VIGR—a novel inducible adhesion family G-protein coupled receptor in endothelial cells. *FEBS Lett.* 569:149–55

131. McMillan DR, Kayes-Wandover KM, Richardson JA, White PC. 2002. Very large G protein-coupled receptor-1, the largest known cell surface protein, is highly expressed in the developing central nervous system. *J. Biol. Chem.* 277:785–92

Annu. Rev. Immunol. 2005. 23:367–86
doi: 10.1146/annurev.immunol.23.021704.115723
First published online as a Review in Advance on November 19, 2004

Maintenance of Serum Antibody Levels

Rudolf A. Manz,[1] Anja E. Hauser,[1] Falk Hiepe,[1,2] and Andreas Radbruch[1,2]

[1]Deutsches Rheumaforschungszentrum, [2]Charité-Universitätsmedizin Berlin,
10117 Berlin, Germany; email: manz@drfz.de, anja.hauser@yale.edu,
falk.hiepe@charite.de, radbruch@drfz.de

Key Words humoral immunity, immunological memory, autoantibodies, plasma cells, plasma blasts

■ **Abstract** In vertebrates, serum antibodies are an essential component of innate and adaptive immunity and immunological memory. They also can contribute significantly to immunopathology. Their composition is the result of tightly regulated differentiation of B lymphocytes into antibody-secreting plasma blasts and plasma cells. The survival of antibody-secreting cells determines their contribution to the immune response in which they were generated and to long-lasting immunity, as provided by stable serum antibody levels. Short-lived plasma blasts and/or plasma cells secrete antibodies for a reactive immune response. Short-lived plasma blasts can become long-lived plasma cells, probably by competition with preexisting plasma cells for occupation of a limited number of survival niches in the body, in a process not yet fully understood. Limitation of the number of long-lived plasma cells allows the immune system to maintain a stable humoral immunological memory over long periods, to react to new pathogenic challenges, and to adapt the humoral memory in response to these antigens.

INTRODUCTION

More than a century ago, Behring & Kitasato (1) discovered that a component of serum, later termed antibodies, can transfer specific immunity to other animals. Since then, antibodies have been extensively characterized in molecular detail. The genes encoding them and their exclusive use in B lymphocytes have revealed the most astounding mechanisms to generate more than a million different antibodies with different specificities and different functions (classes), to increase the affinity of antibodies by somatic hypermutation, and to ensure that each B lymphocyte expresses only antibodies of one specificity, by exclusion of alleles from expression (2). It has become clear that antibodies are involved in innate and adaptive immunity, contribute to immunopathology, and can be critically involved in the pathogenesis of autoimmune diseases. B lymphocytes use them in their membrane-bound form as antigen receptors, triggering their activation and

0732-0582/05/0423-0367$14.00

enabling them to present the antigen efficiently to T helper lymphocytes. Activation of B lymphocytes can result in their differentiation into antibody-secreting cells (ASCs), plasma blasts and plasma cells. Despite their relevance for the understanding of immunity, little is known about these cells, which have often been regarded as short-lived endstages of B cell differentiation, and of limited relevance. This view has been challenged recently. Here, we review the current concepts on the biology of ASCs with respect to their contribution to the maintenance of serum antibody levels, humoral immunity, and humoral memory.

Serum antibodies are derived from different types of ASCs, reflecting the dual role of B lymphocytes in both innate and adaptive immunity. ASCs of the B1 lineage express antibodies binding with low affinities to multiple antigens, often microbial structures shared by a variety of pathogens. These antibodies are usually of the IgM, IgA, or IgG3 subclass. Prenatal induction of antibody secretion by B1-derived ASCs, producing "natural antibodies," also contributes to this "innate" component of serum antibody levels, which probably is maintained throughout life (3, 4). The production of natural antibodies can be regarded as a first line of defense against pathogens, and it also might be involved in the regulation of the respective immune responses (5, 6). In response to antigen, ASCs also develop from B2 lymphocytes, in a specific humoral immune reaction that peaks at about 1 to 2 weeks after antigenic insult. Secondary encounter with antigen results in the secretion of antibodies of increased affinity to the antigen, an increased peak of specific serum antibody titer, and persistent levels of antibodies in the serum. Following vaccination or infection, persistent levels of specific antibodies are detectable in human serum for decades. They are protective, in that they neutralize or eliminate the pathogen and its toxic products upon reinfection (7, 8). In mice, too, humoral memory for specific pathogens is persistent (9). Owing to transfer of maternal antibodies via milk and placenta (6, 10), protective antibodies of adaptive immune responses of the mother are present already at birth, i.e., before the developing immune system has encountered the respective pathogens.

After the discovery of antibodies, another 60 years passed before the cells secreting the antibodies were identified by A. Fagraeus in rabbit spleen as "plasma cells," long known for their prominent cytoplasm and well-developed endoplasmatic reticulum (as reviewed in 11). In spleen and other secondary lymphoid organs, ASCs develop from B lymphocytes, either from B1 cells of the marginal zones, in immune responses against components of microbial cell membranes, or from follicular B2 cells, which can differentiate either into ASCs or into memory B cells. The development and biology of B memory cells is described in detail in this volume by McHeyzer-Williams (11a). Plasma cell differentiation is accompanied by a switch from expression of the membrane-bound form of the antibodies to expression of the secreted form, and by an enormous increase in production of antibody molecules per cell. Plasma cells can synthesize and secrete several thousand antibody molecules per second (12, 13). Thus, the antibody levels in serum and other body fluids can be maintained by a relatively small population of ASCs, which make up only about 0.1% to 1.0% of the cells of secondary lymphoid organs and the bone marrow (14–16). In contrast, the half-life of antibody molecules in serum is less than 3 weeks (17, 18). Maintenance of specific serum antibody levels requires continuous secretion of antibodies and thus persistence of ASCs.

ANTIBODY ISOTYPES IN SERUM

Sera of immune competent donors mainly contain antibodies of the IgG, IgA, and IgM classes (19). IgD and IgE are present in serum at only low concentrations, together making up less than 1% of total serum immunoglobulin. Maternal and B1 cell–derived antibodies, generated by various mechanisms, as discussed below, provide high concentrations of immunoglobulins in serum at birth (Figure 1). When maternal antibodies decay, antibody levels provided by ASCs of the newborn rise slowly during infancy and childhood to concentrations which thereafter remain remarkably stable during adulthood (19), with only small variations until old age. Serum antibody levels of individuals older than 95 years can show an increase in IgA, IgG1, and IgG3 (20), leaving it unclear whether this is cause or consequence of reaching old age.

Serum levels vary considerably for antibodies of the different classes (19). Making up about 85% of total serum antibody levels in humans, antibodies of the IgG subclasses are most abundant. This is partly due to their rather long half-life. IgG can shuttle between serum and endothelium surfaces, where it is bound by FcRn, protecting it from degradation (21). IgA is estimated to have the highest rate of biosynthesis, with up to 66 mg/kg of body weight daily, compared with 34 mg of IgG and 7.9 mg of IgM (22, 23). In serum, however, monomeric IgA accounts for 7%–15% of the serum antibody. Most IgA is secreted as a dimer within mucosal fluids (24). Roughly 5% of serum antibody is IgM, mainly pentameric (25, 26).

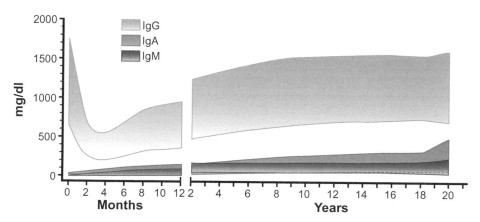

Figure 1   Antibody titers in serum. Levels of IgG, IgA, and IgM increase slowly until adulthood and remain stable thereafter (19).

Owing to its low rate of synthesis of 0.4 mg/kg per day and its high susceptibility to degradation (27), IgD is rare among serum antibodies, contributing only 0.3%. With an average concentration of less than 0.0003 mg/ml in nonatopic adults, the concentration of IgE is the lowest of all serum antibody classes, accounting for 0.02% of total serum antibody. This low level is due to the very low synthesis rate of 0.0016 mg/kg per day, as well as to the short half-life of IgE in serum of 2.5 days (28).

PRENATAL AND NEONATAL SERUM ANTIBODIES

In the serum of newborns, before they have contacted any pathogens, antibodies are already present. IgG levels in fetal serum are comparable to IgG levels of the mother (19). A fraction of these antibodies is produced by ASCs, which developed from B1 lymphocytes (29). The antibodies produced by these cells are often polyreactive and bind with low affinities to multiple antigens (30), including microbial surfaces, thus providing protection against many common environmental pathogens. However, because these "innate" antibodies do not bind with high affinities (30), their protective capacities are limited.

In primates, newborns also have "adaptive" antibodies, transferred to them from their mothers through the placenta. Owing to the structure of this organ in primates, maternal blood makes direct contact with the fetal trophoblast, allowing selective transfer of IgG to the fetus (31). All mammalian newborns are provided with maternal antibodies by transfer of immunoglobulins via milk (32). In humans and primates, the principle antibody class contained within the colostrum is IgA; in most domestic animals it is IgG. The low proteolytic activity in the gastrointestinal tract of newborns and colostral trypsin inhibitors prevent the degradation of immunoglobulins through the first days of life (33).

For the transfer of antibodies both via milk and via the placenta, the major histocompatibility complex class I–related molecule FcRn (34) plays an important role. FcRn-cDNA and -protein have been isolated from human syncytiotrophoblast (35–37), and FcRn colocalizes with IgG in endosomes of syncytiotrophoblast cells (38). Endothelial cells pinocytose IgG and probably transfer it to the fetal circulation. Carnivores have an endotheliochorial placenta where the fetal chorionic epithelium is in contact with the endothelium of the maternal capillaries. In these species, only 5%–10% of the IgG in the mother's serum is passed to the serum of the offspring through the placenta. The syndesmochorial placenta of ruminants (chorionic epithelium in contact with uterine tissues) and epitheliochorial placenta of horses and pigs (chorionic epithelium in contact with intact uterine epithelium) do not allow the passage of antibodies. Newborns of these animals take up antibodies with colostrum only (39). In rodents as well, the transfer of IgG from milk is quantitatively much more important than that via the placenta (40, 41). Independent of the route of transfer, however, newborns are already equipped with maternal adaptive serum antibodies, representing the humoral memory of the mother, and their own innate serum antibodies, both at concentrations similar to those of adults.

PRODUCTION OF SERUM ANTIBODIES

Histologically, cells with prominent endoplasmic reticulum and large cytoplasm had been termed "plasma cells," before researchers knew their function. In 1948, A. Fagraeus reported that the presence of "plasma cells" in rabbit spleen was strictly correlated to antibody production following immunization. In 1955, Coons and collaborators demonstrated, by immunofluorescence, the presence of antibodies inside plasma cells. In 1959, G. Nossal finally provided the evidence that these cells were indeed secreting the antibodies they expressed (reviewed in 11). Today, ASCs would be distinguished as "plasma blasts," the early stages of differentiation from an activated B cell and still proliferating, and "plasma cells," the endstage of differentiation and no longer proliferating. Plasma cells can be short-lived or long-lived, as discussed below.

SITES OF ANTIBODY SECRETION

Mucosal Immune Responses

After immunization via the gut-associated lymphoid tissue, ASCs are generated in intestinal and nonintestinal mucosal tissue (42). Most of the antibodies secreted here are of the IgA isotype. Most IgA dimerizes because the IgA-secreting cells also express the joining chain protein required for and mediating dimerization. Dimeric IgA is transcytosed by epithelial cells and transported to their extracorporal surface, where it serves as a component of mucus and an important first line of defense against pathogens of the environment (43). The majority of ASCs induced by immunization with rotavirus, a typical intestinal pathogen, is found in Peyer's patches and intestinal lamina propria, whereas fewer ASCs are located in spleen and bone marrow (44).

A fraction of mucosal IgA plasma cells are descendants of B1 cells, induced to undergo class switch and plasma cell differentiation locally (45). Others are derived from B2 cells, activated with help from T cells in Peyer's patches (46). In response to activation, these ASCs leave the intestine via the draining mesenteric lymph nodes, begin to secrete antibodies while circulating through spleen, and finally relocate to the lamina propria of the gut (47).

Homing of activated B cells and ASCs to the various mucosal sites is a complex process, controlled by chemoattraction, adhesion receptors, and other signaling receptors. CCL28, the ligand of CCR10, is expressed in different mucosal sites and tissues (48). Almost all IgA-secreting cells migrate toward CCL28 (42, 49, 50). This attraction probably allows IgA-secreting cells to spread IgA-mediated protection all over the mucosa. Selective attraction of a fraction of IgA plasma cells to the small intestine is mediated by CCR9 (42). In the mucosa, expression of CCL25, the ligand of CCR9, is restricted to the crypt epithelium (51) and endothelial cells (52) of the small intestine. CCR9-deficient mice have reduced numbers of plasma cells in their small intestine and a low IgA response to oral antigens

(53). The homing of ASCs from mucosal immune responses to mucosal tissue is further mediated by their expression of mucosa-specific adhesion molecules. In contrast to ASCs induced by systemic immunization, those induced by mucosal immunization mainly express $\alpha 4\beta 7$-integrin (54).

Systemic Immune Responses

Antigen entering the body via skin or blood induces an antibody response in secondary lymphoid tissues such as lymph nodes and spleen (55). Antibody-secreting cells appear after about three days, and are present for a few more days (56). These cells are a mixture of plasma blasts and plasma cells and are located in the vicinity of CD11c[high] dendritic cells (DCs) in the extrafollicular foci of the spleen and medullary cord of lymph nodes. ASCs not associated with these CD11c[high] DCs most likely undergo apoptosis (57).

In immune responses that depend on the help of T lymphocytes for the activation and differentiation of the B lymphocytes, ASCs can migrate from lymph nodes and spleen to the bone marrow (58–60). Here, antigen-specific plasma cells can be detected for many years after immunization (9, 61–63). Bone marrow plasma cells are selected for the production of antibodies with high affinity (64). Antibodies secreted by bone marrow plasma cells can be of higher affinity than those expressed by memory B cells binding to the same antigen (65).

ASCs translocate from secondary lymphoid tissue to bone marrow via the bloodstream and lymphatics. In sheep, 60 h after secondary immunization a sharp increase in numbers of lymphoblasts is detectable in the efferent lymph of lymph nodes draining the site of immunization (66). In human blood, the number of antigen-specific ASCs increases transiently after immunization, with a peak at 6 days after immunization (67). In guinea pig, an influx of mononuclear cells from blood into the bone marrow has been observed during the first 3 days after intravascular administration of antigen (68).

Only recently has the molecular basis for migration of ASCs from secondary lymphoid organs to bone marrow begun to emerge. ASCs express several adhesion molecules, which could be involved in homing and selective survival in particular tissues, although so far tissue-specificity has not been demonstrated for any of the adhesion molecules. Among these adhesion molecules are VLA-4, VLA-5, CD9, CD44, and CD138 (syndecan-1) (14, 69, 70). However, chemokine receptors CXCR3 and CXCR4 are involved in the regulation of migration of ASCs from systemic immune responses (60, 71). Unlike B cells, which are attracted by CXCL13, CCL19, and CCL21 (72), ASCs from murine spleen are attracted by CXCL12, the ligand for CXCR4 (73). CXCL12 (SDF-1α) is expressed in the red pulp of spleen, the medullary cords of lymph nodes, and bone marrow stroma. However, only plasma blasts respond to CXCL12 by migration, whereas plasma cells do not (60). Plasma cells also express CXCR4, and they respond to CXCL12 by improved survival (74). Compared with wild-type cells, CXCR4-deficient ASCs are localized differently in spleen and are about threefold reduced in numbers in bone marrow (73). Thus, CXCR4 is probably one, but not the only, receptor of ASCs controlling their homing into the bone marrow. IgA-secreting cells from mucosal lymphoid tissues can migrate toward CXCL12, too (42, 49), suggesting that these cells may have the choice of homing to mucosal tissue or bone marrow. Investigators have yet to elucidate whether persistent antibody responses of mucosal immune responses are maintained by ASCs of mucosal tissues or of bone marrow.

Another chemokine receptor expressed by ASCs is CXCR3 (60, 75). CXCL9, CXCL10, and CXCL11, the ligands for CXCR3, are expressed by cells of inflamed tissues and also by a subset of high endothelial venule cells, which surround the B cell follicles in the draining lymph nodes (76). ASCs can readily be detected in chronically inflamed tissue (77, 78). After immunization of NZB/W mice, antigen-specific ASCs migrate not only to the bone marrow, but in similar numbers also to the chronically inflamed kidneys (75, 77). Although the contribution of these plasma cells to the maintenance of serum antibody levels is less clear, they provide high local antibody concentrations in the inflamed tissue. In protective immune responses, this may help to combat the immunizing pathogen at the reactive site. In autoimmunity and allergy, local antibody secretion may contribute to pathogenesis of the inflamed organs.

ANTIBODY-SECRETING CELLS OF THE B1 LINEAGE

A fraction of serum antibodies is usually referred to as "natural" antibodies, mainly IgM, IgA, and IgG3 (3, 79, 80) (Table 1). In mice, these antibodies are secreted by cells of the B1 lineage, distinct from cells of the B2 lineage by their early appearance during fetal development, tissue distribution, phenotye, and capacity of self-renewal (81, 82). The original definition of "natural" antibody invoked the idea that such antibodies are present before the immune system sees the respective antigens. This is a controversial definition because of the antibodies' polyreactivity, which makes it difficult to determine whether the cells secreting "natural" antibodies are generated in response to antigen, addressing the B cell's antigen-receptor (surface antibody), or in response to "mitogenic" signals addressing the B cell's pattern recognition receptors for pathogen-associated molecular patterns (PAMP) (e.g., receptors for lipopolysaccarides, demethylated bacterial DNA, etc.) (83).

TABLE 1 B1 and B2 cell contributions to protective antibody titers

	B1 cells	**B2 cells**
Stimulation by	Microbial antigens; autoantigens	Antigen (possible contribution of polyclonal activation by microbial agents)
T dependence	Mainly T-independent	T-independent and T-dependent
Dominant antibody classes	IgM; IgA	IgG
ASC	Short-lived	Short-lived and long-lived

In adult mice, cells of the B1 lineage account for only a few percent of all B lymphocytes, but they contribute at least 50% of the serum IgM. The features of natural antibodies and the B1 lineage cells that secrete them, have already been described and reviewed (see 29, 84, 85). In brief, at least two mechanisms are discussed that could drive B1 lymphocytes into differentiation into ASCs, stimulation by microbial antigens and/or mitogens of the gut flora and stimulation by autoantigens. Stimulation of B1 cells in mucosal tissue by microbial antigens of the gut enhances the production of natural antibody titers (83, 86, 87). The comparison of serum antibodies of preimmune mice living in normal versus germ-free environments suggests that cells secreting natural antibodies specific for bacterial antigens are generated in response to stimulation with bacteria (87a). Independent of T cell help, stimulation of B1 lymphocytes by antigens or "mitogens" from the gut flora leads to the production of IgA by B1 lineage ASCs at mucosal sites (88). These antibodies do not contribute significantly to serum antibody, but rather to mucosal antibody levels.

The activation of B1 lymphocytes by autoantigens and their differentiation into ASCs has been demonstrated recently for mice expressing a transgene for hen egg lysozyme (HEL) somatically, and a transgenic HEL-specific antibody in their B cells (89). Intracellular but not membrane-bound or secreted HEL induced the activation and proliferation of B1 cells in the peritoneal cavity. HEL-specific IgM-secreting cells were found in the red pulp cords of the spleen, but not in the bone marrow or lymph nodes. HEL-specific IgM was readily detectable in the sera in amounts matching the fraction of natural antibodies binding to intracellular self-antigens in wild-type mice. Such autoreactive antibodies are present in the sera of most individuals, regardless of whether they suffer from autoimmune disorders. Although definitive evidence is still lacking that the HEL-specific ASCs in their double transgenic mice belong to the B1 lineage, the experiment of Ferry and colleagues (89) shows that natural autoantibodies can be generated by intracellular autoantigens. This is in line with the presence of natural antibodies in human cord blood (86, 90) and in germ-free mice (87) and their polyreactive specificities, including autoantigens, e.g., phosphatidylcholine.

In view of the continuous activation of B1 cells by bacterial antigens, mitogens and autoantigens, and the constant levels of serum antibody levels attributed to this chronic stimulation, it seems that ASCs of the B1 lineage are short-lived and constantly replaced by newly formed plasma blasts and plasma cells, although the lifetime and terminal differentiation of these cells is still poorly characterized.

AQUIRED HUMORAL IMMUNITY

After infection or intentional immunization, antigen-specific antibodies of high affinity can be detected in blood for long periods, up to the lifetime of the individual. The levels of these serum antibodies are maintained even in the apparent absence of the antigen. This "humoral" memory can effectively protect against reinfection (7). Both mucosal and systemic infections can induce long-lasting humoral immunity, but antibodies induced by systemic infection persist even longer and in human serum are present for several decades after their original induction (91).

The induction phase of an immune response against protein antigens lasts a few days, while large numbers of antigen-specific antibody-secreting plasma blasts are generated in secondary lymphoid tissues (56, 92). After migration to the bone marrow and terminal differentiation into plasma cells, these ASCs maintain the levels of specific serum antibodies, as discussed below. The induction phase can be extended in case of persisting antigen, and specific antibody levels in serum may be maintained by the long-lasting immune response itself, while it lasts (93). Extended formation of specific plasma blasts could result from the continuous activation of memory B cells by antigen, trapped on follicular DCs, or constantly generated de novo from proliferating pathogen, as long as it is not eliminated (93, 94). The relative contribution of these mechanisms to the maintenance of serum-antibody levels is not yet entirely clear. In the absence of chronic immune reactions, however, maintenance of humoral memory and most of the serum antibodies not secreted by B1 lineage cells is probably provided by long-lived plasma cells of the bone marrow (95, 96). Researchers have known for some time that bone marrow is the principal site of persistent antibody production in an established humoral memory response (58, 63).

LONG-LIVED PLASMA CELLS

In a secondary immune response of mice to ovalbumin, 60 days after immunization the formation of proliferating plasma blasts and plasma cells stops, as has been shown by labeling proliferating cells with Bromo-deoxy-uridine. Accordingly, in an immune response to phycoerythrin, the specific memory B cells largely cease to proliferate after several weeks (97).

In the immune response to ovalbumin, a population of long-lived, nonproliferating, antigen-specific plasma cells persists in bone marrow and maintains the levels of specific serum antibodies. These plasma cells can be transferred and will continue to secrete antibodies even in antigen-free recipients (92, 96). In this particular study (96), however, after the initial 6 weeks of analysis, the numbers of specific, long-lived plasma cells in the bone marrow did not change detectably until analysis was terminated, i.e., for another 14 weeks, indicating that in an established memory phase, long-lived plasma cells of the bone marrow have a half-life exceeding that of the individual. The half-life of long-lived bone marrow plasma cells formed in response to lymphocytic choriomeningitis virus has been estimated to be around 5 months (95). This may underestimate the true half-life because in those experiments the mice were treated with gamma irradiation or mitomycin C, probably affecting the survival of plasma cells. The survival of plasma cells in the bone marrow is not an intrinsic property of the plasma cell. Rather, plasma cell survival seems to depend on the ability of the plasma cell to respond to a combination of signals provided by its environment (74, 98). Survival niches providing such signals are apparently scattered throughout the bone marrow (99). Their number seems to be limited because the frequencies of plasma cells in bone marrow are constant at about 0.5% throughout life and in different species (14, 15, 58). This constant frequency implies that newly generated plasma blasts, when migrating to the bone marrow, have to compete with established plasma cells for their survival niches. Competition for the limited number of plasma cell survival niches in the bone marrow offers an intriguing explanation for the regulation of serum antibody levels provided by plasma cells of the B2 lineage (75, 100). The concept would be even more attractive if survival niches for ASCs in bone marrow were shared or overlapped with niches for other lymphocytes (101) and hematopoietic stem cells (102, 103), generating additional levels of regulation.

Although the exact combination of signals making up a plasma cell survival niche in bone marrow is still not known, several signals have been identified that prolong survival of bone marrow plasma cells ex vivo. Stromal cells of bone marrow provide such signals (74, 98, 104) and protect plasma cells from apoptosis (105, 106). The signals identified so far include direct adhesive interactions between bone marrow reticular stromal cells and plasma cells, as well as the cytokines IL-6, SDF-1α (CXCL12), and TNF-α. Although the interruption of CXCR4/CXCL12 signaling in CXCR4-deficient mice leads to a threefold reduction of bone marrow plasma cells (73), an effect hard to attribute to impaired migration of plasma blasts versus impaired survival of plasma cells, IL-6-deficient mice have normal numbers of bone marrow plasma cells, showing that in vivo this signal is redundant (74). VLA-4 may be an important molecular link between stromal cells and plasma cells (98).

Another survival signal for plasma cells might be Blys/BAFF. Blys-deficient mice have reduced levels of serum antibodies (107, 108). Plasma cells express B cell maturation antigen (BCMA), a receptor for Blys. Blys and APRIL, another ligand of BCMA, prolong survival of ASCs in vitro, in particular in the presence of IL-6 (109). Blocking Blys in vivo reduces plasma cell numbers in bone marrow by 65% and increases apoptosis of plasma blasts in spleen about fourfold. Thus, it remains to be demonstrated whether BCMA signaling is required for the establishment of plasma blasts in the bone marrow or for the continued survival of plasma cells there.

PLASMA CELL TURNOVER

For mice, researchers have shown that long-lived plasma cells can maintain specific serum antibody levels for the lifetime of the animals (95, 96). For humans, researchers still debate whether long-lived plasma cells can survive for a lifetime or whether they have a defined half-life, which requires their constant replacement, although at a low rate (Figure 2). Recently it has been proposed that, in the absence of antigen, polyclonal activation of memory B cells in response to cytokine signals

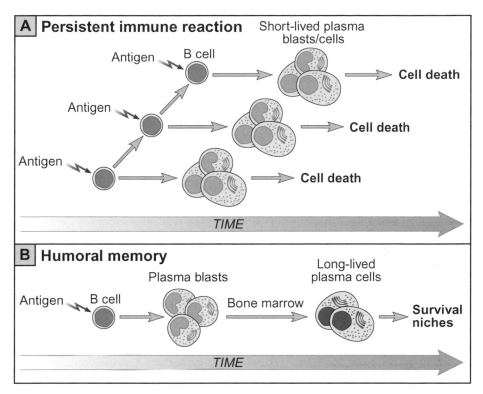

Figure 2   Mechanisms leading to maintenance of specific antibody titers following immunization. Prolonged antigenic stimulation can lead to the continuous activation of B cells and formation of short-lived plasma blasts and plasma cells during persistent immune reactions, e.g., during chronic infections. Long-lived plasma cells maintain specific humoral antibody memory in the absence of persistent antigenic stimulation. It has been proposed that chronic but low-level polyclonal activation of memory B cells generates plasma cells that substitute for old plasma cells within longer periods.

and pathogen-pattern signals in the course of immune reactions generates plasma blasts representing the repertoire of the memory B cells and replaces old plasma cells (110). Indeed, after intentional immunization with one antigen, ASCs specific for recall antigens appeared in the blood at very low frequencies. The actual contribution of this phenomenon to the maintenance of serum antibody levels remains to be demonstrated. An alternative explanation for the appearance of such cells is that they are long-lived plasma cells of the bone marrow, dislocated from their niches by the newly formed plasma blasts specific for the immunizing antigen (75, 100).

The concept of competition between newly generated plasma blasts and old plasma cells for bone marrow survival niches implies that the maintenance of humoral memory for a specific antigen is regulated by the frequency and strength of subsequent immune responses, i.e., the memory for more recent antigens is established at the expense of the memory for "old" antigens not encountered anymore. Memory for old antigens could be refreshed when such antigens are encountered again and levels of specific antibodies in serum have dropped below protective concentrations. Activation of memory B cells representing the reactive memory would then generate plasma blasts again, which could migrate to the bone marrow and enhance the levels of specific antibodies in serum.

SERUM ANTIBODIES IN IMMUNOPATHOLOGY

The immune system has evolved to provide specific protection to pathogens and, as is evident from immunodeficiencies, is indispensable for the successful survival of vertebrates. If successful, however, immune reactions bear the risk of developing into chronic immunopathology and autoreactivity. Antibodies play a pivotal role in this pathology. Antibodies specific for self-antigens are a common feature of systemic and organ-specific autoimmune diseases (111, 112). Autoantibodies can contribute to the pathogenesis of autoimmune diseases either directly, by classic effector mechanisms, or through extensive formation of immune complexes with autoantigens, creating a deposition problem (5). In chronic autoimmune processes, the levels of serum antibodies increase considerably (hypergammaglobulinemia) as a consequence of chronic activation of autoreactive B cells and their differentiation into ASCs (113–115).

The role of autoantibodies in the pathogenesis of autoimmune diseases can be easily depicted for systemic lupus erythematosus (SLE). Antibodies binding to double-stranded DNA (dsDNA) characterize human and murine forms of SLE, and their levels in serum are an excellent correlate of disease activity. These autoantibodies can cause severe manifestations of disease, such as nephritis and vascular injury (116). During flares of SLE, serum levels of autoantibodies directed against dsDNA, nucleosomes, or SmD1 increase (116–118). In SLE patients with sustained disease activity despite rigorous immunosuppressive treatment, pathogenic anti-dsDNA autoantibodies persist in serum (119, 120). Also, in patients suffering from other autoimmune disorders, autoantibodies to particular autoantigens remain present in serum following immunosuppression (121–125). The persistence of autoantibodies in serum upon immunosuppression is a clear hint that such autoantibodies are secreted by long-lived plasma cells, refractory to immunosuppression and feedback signals from antigen-antibody complexes. The existence of long-lived, nonproliferating autoreactive plasma cells has been demonstrated directly in the murine NZB/W model of SLE (126). In these mice, both long-lived autoreactive plasma cells and short-lived, constantly de novo generated plasma blasts and plasma cells contribute to autoantibody levels, with a ratio of 1:3, as evidenced for dsDNA-specific ASCs. Accordingly, immunosuppression of autoimmune patients by selective depletion of B lymphocytes, but not plasma cells, with anti-CD20 antibodies (Rituximab) does not lead to complete disappearance of autoantibodies (127–129). In sera of rheumatoid arthritis patients improving clinically upon Rituximab treatment, the levels of IgM-, IgA-, and IgG-rheumatoid factor, i.e., autoantibodies to immunoglobulin and autoantibodies to citrullinated peptides, dropped significantly (130). This drop was not observed or was less significant in patients not responding to the treatment with an improved clinical outcome. Interestingly, the serum levels of antibodies to microbial antigens, e.g., pneumococcal capsular polysaccharide, and the levels of tetanus-specific antibodies did not change significantly upon treatment (129, 130). The resistance of protective old serum antibodies to Rituximab demonstrates that these antibody levels are maintained by long-lived plasma cells, which do not express CD20 (70). Autoantibodies, in turn, can be secreted by either long-lived plasma cells or short-lived plasma blasts/plasma cells, which can be visualized in peripheral blood during flares of the disease (131, 132), the generation of which is interrupted by anti-CD20. Whether autoASCs can become long-lived plasma cells may depend on the timing and mode of their generation, as well as whether they belong to the B1 or B2 lineage.

CONCLUDING REMARKS

Blood is an organ of life and defense. Secreted antibodies of blood provide specific protection against pathogens the individual has encountered in the past. The regulation of antibody concentrations in the blood is apparently based on simple principles. Secreted antibodies decay with constant rates independent of their specificity. They are also synthesized at constant rates, by ASCs. The antibody levels in serum can thus be regulated by regulating the numbers of cells synthesizing them. Antibody-secreting plasma blasts are generated in high numbers during immune reactions, but their average lifespan is short. To maintain humoral memory, i.e., stable levels of specific antibodies in serum over long time periods in the apparent absence of antigen, ASCs can be recruited to a pool of long-lived plasma cells. Survival of the plasma cells is dependent on defined signals provided in a limited number of survival niches in the body, most prominently in the bone marrow. Thus, competition between newly generated plasma blasts and old plasma cells for occupancy of survival niches makes humoral memory flexible to add new specificities, allows its regeneration from memory B cells, and keeps the serum antibody levels constant. "Blood is a very special juice," as the German poet J.W. Goethe has said.

ACKNOWLEDGMENTS

We gratefully acknowledge the assistance of Christine Raulfs and graphics support of Luise Fehlig. Without the continuous discussion in the DRFZ B cell club, the concepts discussed here would not have been developed. This work was supported by the Deutsche Forschungsgemeinschaft through grants SFB421, SFB618,

KFO 105, and MA 2273 and RI 1056/2–1 and the European Commission through framework 5 Project MEMOVAX.

The *Annual Review of Immunology* is online at
http://immunol.annualreviews.org

LITERATURE CITED

1. Behring E, Kitasato S. 1890. Ueber das Zustandekommen der Diphtherie-Immunität und der Tetanus-Immunität bei Thieren. *Dtsch. Med. Wochenschr.* 16(49): 1113–14
2. Rajewsky K. 1996. Clonal selection and learning in the antibody system. *Nature* 381:751–58
3. Boyden SV. 1966. Natural antibodies and the immune response. *Adv. Immunol.* 5:1–28
4. Michael JG. 1969. Natural antibodies. *Curr. Top. Microbiol. Immunol.* 48:43–62
5. Martin F, Chan AC. 2004. Pathogenic roles of B cells in human autoimmunity; insights from the clinic. *Immunity* 20: 517–27
6. Ochsenbein AF, Fehr T, Lutz C, Suter M, Brombacher F, et al. 1999. Control of early viral and bacterial distribution and disease by natural antibodies. *Science* 286:2156–59
7. Ahmed R, Gray D. 1996. Immunological memory and protective immunity: understanding their relation. *Science* 272:54–60
8. Hammarlund E, Lewis MW, Hansen SG, Strelow LI, Nelson JA, et al. 2003. Duration of antiviral immunity after smallpox vaccination. *Nat. Med.* 9:1131–37
9. Slifka MK, Matloubian M, Ahmed R. 1995. Bone marrow is a major site of long-term antibody production after acute viral infection. *J. Virol.* 69:1895–902
10. Simister NE, Story CM. 1997. Human placental Fc receptors and the transmission of antibodies from mother to fetus. *J. Reprod. Immunol.* 37:1–23
11. Nossal GJ. 2002. One cell, one anti-

body: prelude and aftermath. *Immunol. Rev.* 185:15–23
11a. McHeyzer-Williams M, McHeyzer-Williams L. 2004. Antigen-specific memory B cell development. *Annu. Rev. Immunol.* 23:487–513
12. Helmreich E, Kern M, Eisen HN. 1961. The secretion of antibody by isolated lymph node cells. *J. Biol. Chem.* 236:464–73
13. Hibi T, Dosch HM. 1986. Limiting dilution analysis of the B cell compartment in human bone marrow. *Eur. J. Immunol.* 16:139–45
14. Arce S, Luger E, Muehlinghaus G, Cassese G, Hauser A, et al. 2004. CD38 low IgG-secreting cells are precursors of various CD38 high-expressing plasma cell populations. *J. Leukoc. Biol.* 75:1022–28
15. Brieva JA, Roldan E, De la Sen ML, Rodriguez C. 1991. Human in vivo-induced spontaneous IgG-secreting cells from tonsil, blood and bone marrow exhibit different phenotype and functional level of maturation. *Immunology* 72:580–83
16. Haaijman JJ, Schuit HR, Hijmans W. 1977. Immunoglobulin-containing cells in different lymphoid organs of the CBA mouse during its life-span. *Immunology* 32:427–34
17. Vieira P, Rajewsky K. 1988. The half-lives of serum immunoglobulins in adult mice. *Eur. J. Immunol.* 18:313–36
18. Talbot PJ, Buchmeier MJ. 1987. Catabolism of homologous murine monoclonal hybridoma IgG antibodies in mice. *Immunology* 60:485–89
19. Bienvenu J, Whicher J, Chir B, Aguzzi F. 1996. Immunoglobulins. In *Serum

Proteins in Clinical Medicine, ed. RF Ritchie, O Navolotskaia, pp. 1–16. Scarborough, ME: Found. Blood Res.

20. Radl J, Sepers JM, Skvaril F, Morell A, Hijmans W. 1975. Immunoglobulin patterns in humans over 95 years of age. *Clin. Exp. Immunol.* 22:84–90

21. Ghetie V, Ward ES. 2000. Multiple roles for the major histocompatibility complex class I- related receptor FcRn. *Annu. Rev. Immunol.* 18:739–66

22. Rifai A, Fadden K, Morrison SL, Chintalacharuvu KR. 2000. The N-glycans determine the differential blood clearance and hepatic uptake of human immunoglobulin (Ig)A1 and IgA2 isotypes. *J. Exp. Med.* 191:2171–82

23. Mestecky J, McGhee JR. 1987. Immunoglobulin A (IgA): molecular and cellular interactions involved in IgA biosynthesis and immune response. *Adv. Immunol.* 40:153–245

24. Kerr MA. 1990. The structure and function of human IgA. *Biochem. J.* 271:285–96

25. Metzger H. 1970. Structure and function of gamma M macroglobulins. *Adv. Immunol.* 12:57–116

26. Parkhouse RM, Askonas BA, Dourmashkin RR. 1970. Electron microscopic studies of mouse immunoglobulin M; structure and reconstitution following reduction. *Immunology* 18:575–84

27. Spiegelberg HL. 1977. The structure and biology of human IgD. *Immunol. Rev.* 37: 3–24

28. Waldmann TA. 1969. Disorders of immunoglobulin metabolism. *N. Engl. J. Med.* 281:1170–77

29. Herzenberg LA, Stall AM, Lalor PA, Sidman C, Moore WA, Parks DR. 1986. The Ly-1 B cell lineage. *Immunol. Rev.* 93:81–102

30. Casali P, Schettino EW. 1996. Structure and function of natural antibodies. *Curr. Top. Microbiol. Immunol.* 210:167–79

31. Sheldrake RF, Husband AJ, Watson DL, Cripps AW. 1984. Selective transport of serum-derived IgA into mucosal secretions. *J. Immunol.* 132:363–68

32. Lilius EM, Marnila P. 2001. The role of colostral antibodies in prevention of microbial infections. *Curr. Opin. Infect. Dis.* 14:295–300

33. Telemo E, Westrom BR, Ekstrom G, Karlsson BW. 1987. Intestinal macromolecular transmission in the young rat: influence of protease inhibitors during development. *Biol. Neonate* 52:141–48

34. Simister NE, Mostov KE. 1989. An Fc receptor structurally related to MHC class I antigens. *Nature* 337:184–87

35. Story CM, Mikulska JE, Simister NE. 1994. A major histocompatibility complex class I-like Fc receptor cloned from human placenta: possible role in transfer of immunoglobulin G from mother to fetus. *J. Exp. Med.* 180:2377–81

36. Simister NE, Story CM, Chen HL, Hunt JS. 1996. An IgG-transporting Fc receptor expressed in the syncytiotrophoblast of human placenta. *Eur. J. Immunol.* 26: 1527–31

37. Leach JL, Sedmak DD, Osborne JM, Rahill B, Lairmore MD, Anderson CL. 1996. Isolation from human placenta of the IgG transporter, FcRn, and localization to the syncytiotrophoblast: implications for maternal-fetal antibody transport. *J. Immunol.* 157:3317–22

38. Kristoffersen EK, Matre R. 1996. Colocalization of the neonatal Fc gamma receptor and IgG in human placental term syncytiotrophoblasts. *Eur. J. Immunol.* 26:1668–71

39. Tizard I. 2001. The protective properties of milk and colostrum in non-human species. *Adv. Nutr. Res.* 10:139–66

40. Roberts DM, Guenthert M, Rodewald R. 1990. Isolation and characterization of the Fc receptor from the fetal yolk sac of the rat. *J. Cell Biol.* 111:1867–76

41. Ghetie V, Hubbard JG, Kim JK, Tsen MF, Lee Y, Ward ES. 1996. Abnormally short serum half-lives of IgG in beta

2-microglobulin-deficient mice. *Eur. J. Immunol.* 26:690–96

42. Lazarus NH, Kunkel EJ, Johnston B, Wilson E, Youngman KR, Butcher EC. 2003. A common mucosal chemokine (mucosae-associated epithelial chemokine/CCL28) selectively attracts IgA plasmablasts. *J. Immunol.* 170:3799–805

43. Kato H, Kato R, Fujihashi K, McGhee JR. 2001. Role of mucosal antibodies in viral infections. *Curr. Top. Microbiol. Immunol.* 260:201–28

44. Youngman KR, Franco MA, Kuklin NA, Rott LS, Butcher EC, Greenberg HB. 2002. Correlation of tissue distribution, developmental phenotype, and intestinal homing receptor expression of antigen-specific B cells during the murine anti-rotavirus immune response. *J. Immunol.* 168:2173–81

45. Fagarasan S, Kinoshita K, Muramatsu M, Ikuta K, Honjo T. 2001. In situ class switching and differentiation to IgA-producing cells in the gut lamina propria. *Nature* 413:639–43

46. Bowman EP, Kuklin NA, Youngman KR, Lazarus NH, Kunkel EJ, et al. 2002. The intestinal chemokine thymus-expressed chemokine (CCL25) attracts IgA antibody-secreting cells. *J. Exp. Med.* 195:269–75

47. Lamm ME, Phillips-Quagliata JM. 2002. Origin and homing of intestinal IgA antibody-secreting cells. *J. Exp. Med.* 195:F5–8

48. Pan JL, Kunkel EJ, Gosslar U, Lazarus N, Langdon P, et al. 2000. A novel chemokine ligand for CCR10 and CCR3 expressed by epithelial cells in mucosal tissues. *J. Immunol.* 165:2943–49

49. Kunkel EJ, Kim CH, Lazarus NH, Vierra MA, Soler D, et al. 2003. CCR10 expression is a common feature of circulating and mucosal epithelial tissue IgA Ab-secreting cells. *J. Clin. Invest.* 111:1001–10

50. Hieshima K, Ohtani H, Shibano M, Izawa D, Nakayama T, et al. 2003. CCL28

has dual roles in mucosal immunity as a chemokine with broad-spectrum antimicrobial activity. *J. Immunol.* 170:1452–61

51. Kunkel EJ, Campbell JJ, Haraldsen G, Pan JL, Boisvert J, et al. 2000. Lymphocyte CC chemokine receptor 9 and epithelial thymus-expressed chemokine (TECK) expression distinguish the small intestinal immune compartment: epithelial expression of tissue-specific chemokines as an organizing principle in regional immunity. *J. Exp. Med.* 192:761–67

52. Papadakis KA, Prehn J, Nelson V, Cheng L, Binder SW, et al. 2000. The role of thymus-expressed chemokine and its receptor CCR9 on lymphocytes in the regional specialization of the mucosal immune system. *J. Immunol.* 165:5069–76

53. Pabst O, Ohl L, Wendland M, Wurbel MA, Kremmer E, et al. 2004. Chemokine receptor CCR9 contributes to the localization of plasma cells to the small intestine. *J. Exp. Med.* 199:411–16

54. Quiding-Jarbrink M, Nordstrom I, Granstrom G, Kilander A, Jertborn M, et al. 1997. Differential expression of tissue-specific adhesion molecules on human circulating antibody-forming cells after systemic, enteric, and nasal immunizations. A molecular basis for the compartmentalization of effector B cell responses. *J. Clin. Invest.* 99:1281–86

55. Liu YJ, Zhang J, Lane PJ, Chan EY, MacLennan IC. 1991. Sites of specific B cell activation in primary and secondary responses to T cell-dependent and T cell-independent antigens. *Eur. J. Immunol.* 21:2951–62

56. Smith KG, Hewitson TD, Nossal GJ, Tarlinton DM. 1996. The phenotype and fate of the antibody-forming cells of the splenic foci. *Eur. J. Immunol.* 26:444–48

57. de Vinuesa CG, Gulbranson-Judge A, Khan M, O'Leary P, Cascalho M, et al. 1999. Dendritic cells associated with plasmablast survival. *Eur. J. Immunol.* 29:3712–21

58. McMillan R, Longmire RL, Yelenosky

R, Lang JE, Heath V, Craddock CG. 1972. Immunoglobulin synthesis by human lymphoid tissues: normal bone marrow as a major site of IgG production. *J. Immunol.* 109:1386–94

59. Benner R, van Oudenaren A. 1975. Antibody formation in mouse bone marrow. IV. The influence of splenectomy on the bone marrow plaque-forming cell response to sheep red blood cells. *Cell Immunol.* 19:167–82

60. Hauser AE, Debes GF, Arce S, Cassese G, Hamann A, et al. 2002. Chemotactic responsiveness toward ligands for CXCR3 and CXCR4 is regulated on plasma blasts during the time course of a memory immune response. *J. Immunol.* 169:1277–82

61. Dilosa RM, Maeda K, Masuda A, Szakal AK, Tew JG. 1991. Germinal center B cells and antibody production in the bone marrow. *J. Immunol.* 146:4071–77

62. Benner R, Hijmans W, Haaijman JJ. 1981. The bone marrow: the major source of serum immunoglobulins, but still a neglected site of antibody formation. *Clin. Exp. Immunol.* 46:1–8

63. Tew JG, DiLosa RM, Burton GF, Kosco MH, Kupp LI, et al. 1992. Germinal centers and antibody production in bone marrow. *Immunol. Rev.* 126:99–112

64. Takahashi Y, Dutta PR, Cerasoli DM, Kelsoe G. 1998. In situ studies of the primary immune response to (4-hydroxy-3-nitrophenyl)acetyl. V. Affinity maturation develops in two stages of clonal selection. *J. Exp. Med.* 187:885–95

65. Smith KG, Light A, Nossal GJ, Tarlinton DM. 1997. The extent of affinity maturation differs between the memory and antibody-forming cell compartments in the primary immune response. *EMBO J.* 16:2996–3006

66. Hay JB, Murphy MJ, Morris B, Bessis MC. 1972. Quantitative studies on the proliferation and differentiation of antibody-forming cells in lymph. *Am. J. Pathol.* 66:1–24

67. Cupps TR, Goldsmith PK, Volkman DJ, Gerin JL, Purcell RH, Fauci AS. 1984. Activation of human peripheral blood B cells following immunization with hepatitis B surface antigen vaccine. *Cell Immunol.* 86:145–54

68. Koch G, Osmond DG, Julius MH, Benner R. 1981. The mechanism of thymus-dependent antibody formation in bone marrow. *J. Immunol.* 126:1447–51

69. Ridley RC, Xiao H, Hata H, Woodliff J, Epstein J, Sanderson RD. 1993. Expression of syndecan regulates human myeloma plasma cell adhesion to type I collagen. *Blood* 81:767–74

70. Medina F, Segundo C, Campos-Caro A, Gonzalez-Garcia I, Brieva JA. 2002. The heterogeneity shown by human plasma cells from tonsil, blood, and bone marrow reveals graded stages of increasing maturity, but local profiles of adhesion molecule expression. *Blood* 99:2154–61

71. Wehrli N, Legler DF, Finke D, Toellner KM, Loetscher P, et al. 2001. Changing responsiveness to chemokines allows medullary plasmablasts to leave lymph nodes. *Eur. J. Immunol.* 31:609–16

72. Reif K, Ekland EH, Ohl L, Nakano H, Lipp M, et al. 2002. Balanced responsiveness to chemoattractants from adjacent zones determines B-cell position. *Nature* 416:94–99

73. Hargreaves DC, Hyman PL, Lu TT, Ngo VN, Bidgol A, et al. 2001. A coordinated change in chemokine responsiveness guides plasma cell movements. *J. Exp. Med.* 194:45–56

74. Cassese G, Arce S, Hauser AE, Lehnert K, Moewes B, et al. 2003. Plasma cell survival is mediated by synergistic effects of cytokines and adhesion-dependent signals. *J. Immunol.* 171:1684–90

75. Manz RA, Arce S, Cassese G, Hauser AE, Hiepe F, Radbruch A. 2002. Humoral immunity and long-lived plasma cells. *Curr. Opin. Immunol.* 14:517–21

76. Janatpour MJ, Hudak S, Sathe M, Sedgwick JD, McEvoy LM. 2001. Tumor necrosis factor-dependent segmental

control of MIG expression by high endothelial venules in inflamed lymph nodes regulates monocyte recruitment. *J. Exp. Med.* 194:1375–84

77. Cassese G, Lindenau S, de Boer B, Arce S, Hauser A, et al. 2001. Inflamed kidneys of NZB/W mice are a major site for the homeostasis of plasma cells. *Eur. J. Immunol.* 31:2726–32

78. Mallison SM 3rd, Szakal AK, Ranney RR, Tew JG. 1988. Antibody synthesis specific for nonoral antigens in inflamed gingiva. *Infect. Immun.* 56:823–30

79. Hook WA, Toussaint AJ, Simonton LA, Muschel LH. 1966. Appearance of natural antibodies in young rabbits. *Nature* 210:543–44

80. Cohen IR, Norins LC. 1966. Natural human antibodies to gram-negative bacteria: immunoglobulins G, A, and M. *Science* 152:1257–59

81. Kantor AB. 1991. The development and repertoire of B-1 cells (CD5 B cells). *Immunol. Today* 12:389–91

82. Kasaian MT, Ikematsu H, Casali P. 1992. Identification and analysis of a novel human surface CD5$^-$ B lymphocyte subset producing natural antibodies. *J. Immunol.* 148:2690–702

83. Jiang HQ, Thurnheer MC, Zuercher AW, Boiko NV, Bos NA, Cebra JJ. 2004. Interactions of commensal gut microbes with subsets of B- and T-cells in the murine host. *Vaccine* 22:805–11

84. Kantor AB, Herzenberg LA. 1993. Origin of murine B cell lineages. *Annu. Rev. Immunol.* 11:501–38

85. Hardy RR, Carmack CE, Li YS, Hayakawa K. 1994. Distinctive developmental origins and specificities of murine CD5$^+$ B cells. *Immunol. Rev.* 137:91–118

86. Tlaskalova-Hogenova H, Mandel L, Stepankova R, Bartova J, Barot R, et al. 1992. Autoimmunity: from physiology to pathology. Natural antibodies, mucosal immunity and development of B cell repertoire. *Folia Biol.* 38:202–15

87. Coutinho A, Kazatchkine MD, Avrameas S. 1995. Natural autoantibodies. *Curr. Opin. Immunol.* 7:812–18

87a. Bos NA, Kimura H, Meeuwsen CG, De Visser H, Hazenberg MP, et al. 1989. Serum immunoglobulin levels and naturally occurring antibodies against carbohydrate antigens in germ-free BALB/c mice fed chemically defined ultrafiltered diet. *Eur. J. Immunol.* 19:2335–39

88. Macpherson AJ, Gatto D, Sainsbury E, Harriman GR, Hengartner H, Zinkernagel RM. 2000. A primitive T cell-independent mechanism of intestinal mucosal IgA responses to commensal bacteria. *Science* 288:2222–26

89. Ferry H, Jones M, Vaux DJ, Roberts IS, Cornall R. 2003. The cellular location of self-antigen determines the positive and negative selection of autoreactive B cells. *J. Exp. Med.* 198:1415–25

90. Mouthon L, Nobrega A, Nicolas N, Kaveri SV, Barreau C, et al. 1995. Invariance and restriction toward a limited set of self-antigens characterize neonatal IgM antibody repertoires and prevail in autoreactive repertoires of healthy adults. *Proc. Natl. Acad. Sci. USA* 92:3839–43

91. Slifka MK, Ahmed R. 1996. Long-term humoral immunity against viruses: revisiting the issue of plasma cell longevity. *Trends Microbiol.* 4:394–400

92. Manz RA, Lohning M, Cassese G, Thiel A, Radbruch A. 1998. Survival of long-lived plasma cells is independent of antigen. *Int. Immunol.* 10:1703–11

93. Tew JG, Phipps RP, Mandel TE. 1980. The maintenance and regulation of the humoral immune response: persisting antigen and the role of follicular antigen-binding dendritic cells as accessory cells. *Immunol. Rev.* 53:175–201

94. Bachmann MF, Odermatt B, Hengartner H, Zinkernagel RM. 1996. Induction of long-lived germinal centers associated with persisting antigen after viral infection. *J. Exp. Med.* 183:2259–69

95. Slifka MK, Antia R, Whitmire JK, Ahmed R. 1998. Humoral immunity due to

long-lived plasma cells. *Immunity* 8:363–72

96. Manz RA, Thiel A, Radbruch A. 1997. Lifetime of plasma cells in the bone marrow. *Nature* 388:133–34

97. Schittek B, Rajewsky K. 1990. Maintenance of B-cell memory by long-lived cells generated from proliferating precursors. *Nature* 346:749–51

98. Wols HAM, Underhill GH, Kansas GS, Witte PL. 2002. The role of bone marrow-derived stromal cells in the maintenance of plasma cell longevity. *J. Immunol.* 169:4213–21

99. Tokoyoda K, Egawa T, Sugiyama T, Choi BI, Nagasawa T. 2004. Cellular niches controlling B lymphocyte behavior within bone marrow during development. *Immunity* 20:707–18

100. Manz RA, Radbruch A. 2002. Plasma cells for a lifetime? *Eur. J. Immunol.* 32:923–27

101. Freitas AA, Rocha B. 2000. Population biology of lymphocytes: the flight for survival. *Annu. Rev. Immunol.* 18:83–111

102. Zhang JW, Niu C, Ye L, Huang HY, He X, et al. 2003. Identification of the haematopoietic stem cell niche and control of the niche size. *Nature* 425:836–41

103. Calvi LM, Adams GB, Weibrecht KW, Weber JM, Olson DP, et al. 2003. Osteoblastic cells regulate the hacmatopoietic stem cell niche. *Nature* 425:841–46

104. Roldan E, Brieva JA. 1991. Terminal differentiation of human bone marrow cells capable of spontaneous and high-rate immunoglobulin secretion: role of bone marrow stromal cells and interleukin 6. *Eur. J. Immunol.* 21:2671–77

105. Merville P, Dechanet J, Desmouliere A, Durand I, de Bouteiller O, et al. 1996. Bcl-2+ tonsillar plasma cells are rescued from apoptosis by bone marrow fibroblasts. *J. Exp. Med.* 183:227–36

106. Kawano MM, Mihara K, Huang N, Tsujimoto T, Kuramoto A. 1995. Differentiation of early plasma cells on bone marrow stromal cells requires interleukin-6 for escaping from apoptosis. *Blood* 85:487–94

107. Gross JA, Dillon SR, Mudri S, Johnston J, Littau A, et al. 2001. TACI-Ig neutralizes molecules critical for B cell development and autoimmune disease: impaired B cell maturation in mice lacking BLyS. *Immunity* 15:289–302

108. Schiemann B, Gommerman JL, Vora K, Cachero TG, Shulga-Morskaya S, et al. 2001. An essential role for BAFF in the normal development of B cells through a BCMA-independent pathway. *Science* 293:2111–14

109. O'Connor BP, Raman VS, Erickson LD, Cook WJ, Weaver LK, et al. 2004. BCMA is essential for the survival of long-lived bone marrow plasma cells. *J. Exp. Med.* 199:91–98

110. Bernasconi NL, Traggiai E, Lanzavecchia A. 2002. Maintenance of serological memory by polyclonal activation of human memory B cells. *Science* 298:2199–202

111. Martin F, Kearney JF. 2000. B-cell subsets and the mature preimmune repertoire. Marginal zone and B1 B cells as part of a "natural immune memory." *Immunol. Rev.* 175:70–79

112. Davidson A, Diamond B. 2001. Autoimmune diseases. *N. Engl. J. Med.* 345:340–50

113. Cheema GS, Roschke V, Hilbert DM, Stohl W. 2001. Elevated serum B lymphocyte stimulator levels in patients with systemic immune-based rheumatic diseases. *Arthritis Rheum.* 44:1313–19

114. Groom J, Kalled SL, Cutler AH, Olson C, Woodcock SA, et al. 2002. Association of BAFF/BLyS overexpression and altered B cell differentiation with Sjögren's syndrome. *J. Clin. Invest.* 109:59–68

115. Zhang J, Roschke V, Baker KP, Wang Z, Alarcon GS, et al. 2001. Cutting edge: a role for B lymphocyte stimulator in systemic lupus erythematosus. *J. Immunol.* 166:6–10

116. Hahn BH. 1998. Antibodies to DNA. *N. Engl. J. Med.* 338:1359–68

117. Riemekasten G, Marell J, Trebeljahr G, Klein R, Hausdorf G, et al. 1998. A novel epitope on the C-terminus of SmD1 is recognized by the majority of sera from patients with systemic lupus erythematosus. *J. Clin. Invest.* 102:754–63

118. Bruns A, Blass S, Hausdorf G, Burmester GR, Hiepe F. 2000. Nucleosomes are major T and B cell autoantigens in systemic lupus erythematosus. *Arthritis Rheum.* 43:2307–15

119. Rosen O, Thiel A, Massenkeil G, Hiepe F, Haupl T, et al. 2000. Autologous stem-cell transplantation in refractory autoimmune diseases after in vivo immunoablation and ex vivo depletion of mononuclear cells. *Arthritis Res.* 2:327–36

120. Traynor AE, Schroeder J, Rosa RM, Cheng D, Stefka J, et al. 2000. Treatment of severe systemic lupus erythematosus with high-dose chemotherapy and haemopoietic stem-cell transplantation: a phase I study. *Lancet* 356: 701–7

121. Izumi N, Fuse I, Furukawa T, Uesugi Y, Tsuchiyama J, et al. 2003. Long-term production of pre-existing alloantibodies to E and c after allogenic BMT in a patient with aplastic anemia resulting in delayed hemolytic anemia. *Transfusion* 43:241–45

122. Wahren M, Tengner P, Gunnarsson I, Lundberg I, Hedfors E, et al. 1998. Ro/SS-A and La/SS-B antibody level variation in patients with Sjögren's syndrome and systemic lupus erythematosus. *J. Autoimmun.* 11:29–38

123. Westman KW, Bygren PG, Ericsson UB, Hoier-Madsen M, Wieslander J, Erfurth EM. 1998. Persistent high prevalence of thyroid antibodies after immunosuppressive therapy in subjects with glomerulonephritis. A prospective three-year follow-up study. *Am. J. Nephrol.* 18:274–79

124. De Block CE, De Leeuw IH, Rooman RP, Winnock F, Du Caju MV, Van Gaal LF. 2000. Gastric parietal cell antibodies are associated with glutamic acid decarboxylase-65 antibodies and the HLA DQA1*0501-DQB1*0301 haplotype in type 1 diabetes mellitus. *Diabet. Med.* 17: 618–22

125. Decochez K, Tits J, Coolens JL, Van Gaal L, Krzentowski G, et al. 2000. High frequency of persisting or increasing islet-specific autoantibody levels after diagnosis of type 1 diabetes presenting before 40 years of age. *Diabetes Care* 23:838–44

126. Hoyer BF, Moser K, Hauser AE, Peddinghaus A, Voigt C, et al. 2004. Short-lived plasmablasts and long-lived plasma cells contribute to chronic humoral autoimmunity in NZB/W mice. *J. Exp. Med.* 199:1577–84

127. Leandro MJ, Edwards JC, Cambridge G, Ehrenstein MR, Isenberg DA. 2002. An open study of B lymphocyte depletion in systemic lupus erythematosus. *Arthritis Rheum.* 46:2673–77

128. Silverman GJ, Weisman S. 2003. Rituximab therapy and autoimmune disorders: prospects for anti-B cell therapy. *Arthritis Rheum.* 48:1484–92

129. Edwards JC, Szczepanski L, Szechinski J, Filipowicz-Sosnowska A, Emery P, et al. 2004. Efficacy of B-cell-targeted therapy with rituximab in patients with rheumatoid arthritis. *N. Engl. J. Med.* 350:2572–81

130. Cambridge G, Leandro MJ, Edwards JC, Ehrenstein MR, Salden M, et al. 2003. Serologic changes following B lymphocyte depletion therapy for rheumatoid arthritis. *Arthritis Rheum.* 48:2146–54

131. Jacobi AM, Odendahl M, Reiter K, Bruns A, Burmester GR, et al. 2003. Correlation between circulating CD27[high] plasma cells and disease activity in patients with systemic lupus erythematosus. *Arthritis Rheum.* 48:1332–42

132. Odendahl M, Jacobi A, Hansen A, Feist E, Hiepe F, et al. 2000. Disturbed peripheral B lymphocyte homeostasis in systemic lupus erythematosus. *J. Immunol.* 165:5970–79

Annu. Rev. Immunol. 2005. 23:387–414
doi: 10.1146/annurev.immunol.23.021704.115616
Copyright © 2005 by Annual Reviews. All rights reserved
First published online as a Review in Advance on November 19, 2004

CATERPILLER: A Novel Gene Family Important in Immunity, Cell Death, and Diseases

Jenny P-Y. Ting and Beckley K. Davis

*Department of Microbiology and Immunology, Lineberger Comprehensive Cancer Center,
University of North Carolina, Chapel Hill, North Carolina 27599;
email: jenny_ting@med.unc.edu; antigen@med.unc.edu*

Key Words   innate immunity, NOD, NALP, plant *R* genes

■ **Abstract**   The newly discovered CATERPILLER (CLR) gene family encodes proteins with a variable but limited number of N-terminal domains, followed by a nucleotide-binding domain (NBD) and leucine-rich repeats (LRR). The N-terminal domain consists of transactivation, CARD, Pyrin, or BIR domains, with a minority containing undefined domains. These proteins are remarkably similar in structure to the TIR-NBD-LRR and CC-NBD-LRR disease resistance (R) proteins that mediate immune responses in plants. The NBD-LRR architecture is conserved in plants and vertebrates, but only remnants are found in worms and flies. The CLRs regulate inflammatory and apoptotic responses, and some act as sensors that detect pathogen products. Several CLR genes have been genetically linked to susceptibility to immunologic disorders. We describe prominent family members, including CIITA, CARD4/NOD1, NOD2/CARD15, CIAS1, CARD7/NALP1, and NAIP, in more detail. We also discuss implied roles of these proteins in diversifying immune detection and in providing a check-and-balance during inflammation.

INTRODUCTION

A major challenge faced by the immune system is the recognition of an enormous array of antigens that are not only divergent in their composition but that also undergo constant changes. To survive, each species develops a system of immune diversity that responds properly to these antigens. Immunoglobulin (Ig) and T cell receptor (TCR) are at the forefront of immune recognition and diversity in adaptive immunity of vertebrates. Of equal importance is the innate immune system. This arm of immunity is conserved in nearly all taxa and is clearly more ancient than the adaptive immune system. The Toll receptors, first discovered in *Drosophila*, have been evolutionarily preserved from fly to human, and in human are known as Toll-like receptors (TLR) (1, 2). TLRs are pattern recognition receptors that recognize different pathogen-associated molecular patterns (PAMPs) rather than pathogen-specific determinants, thus allowing the immune system to recognize invariant pathogenic and/or synthetic products. To date there are at least 11 TLRs,

0732-0582/05/0423-0387$14.00

and they recognize pathogen products singly or in combination with other TLRs, thus diversifying their recognition potential. Another major challenge faced by the immune system is the ability to limit damage during inflammation and immune responses to pathogens. This regulation is achieved by immune tolerance and by the presence of negative regulatory mechanisms to repress both adaptive and innate immune response. Dysregulation of the immune system can lead to autoimmunity, autoinflammation, and/or immunodeficiency. These challenges of the immune system are met by many families of proteins that participate in both innate and adaptive immunity. This review describes a new family of immune regulatory genes, which we first christened the CATERPILLER (CLR) family (3). Subsequently, these proteins have also been called NOD (4). The pyrin-containing subgroup of this family has also received different designations, including NALP, PAN, and PYPAF (5–8).[1] CLR family members provide important arsenals for immune response in animals, but they also have counterparts in plants and are likely to rival TLRs in their fundamental importance for the function of ancient immune systems. This review addresses the recent advances in CLR evolution, biology, and function in immunity and human diseases.

The CATERPILLER Family

CLR genes encode cytoplasmic proteins with a tripartite domain architecture that shares structural similarities with a subclass of plant disease resistance (*R*) genes (Figure 1 and Table 1). The N-terminus is composed of an effector domain, typically a Pyrin, CARD, transactivation, or BIR domain. A minority contains an undefined N-terminal domain that predicts a similar fold (our unpublished observation) to that found in Pyrin, CARD, and death effector domain (9). The known effector domains are thought to regulate homotypic/heterotypic interactions (9–14). A large nucleotide-binding domain (NACHT, NB-ARC, or NOD) that immediately follows the effector domain might function to regulate self-oligomerization and other regulatory functions (15, 16). The C-terminus is composed of a series of leucine-rich repeats (LRR) that are variable in composition and number. The LRR regions have been implicated in autoregulation, ligand binding, and protein-protein interactions (15, 17–20). This overall domain organization in CLR proteins suggests that these proteins exist as higher order complexes, as is seen with CIITA (class II transactivator), CIAS1 (cold-induced autoinflammatory syndrome), and CARD7/NALP1 (12, 21–23). These proteins are primary candidates to expand the diversity of recognition and sensor molecules for immune detection, to modulate signals elicited by pathogens, to downregulate an ongoing inflammatory response, and/or to induce apoptosis.

Although the founding member of this family, CIITA, was discovered more than a decade ago (24), most members of this family are newly discovered. Among the members, a remarkable number are genetically associated with susceptibility to

---

[1]See Appendix for a full list of abbreviations used.

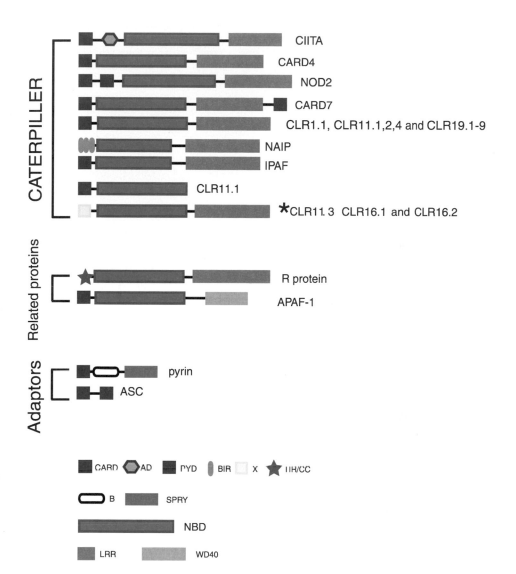

Figure 1   Domain structure of the CLR family and associated proteins. Apaf-1 and R proteins are shown as related proteins. PYD, pyrin domain; CARD, caspase-recruitment domain; AD, activation domain; BIR, baculovirus IAP repeat; X, uncharacterized and unrelated; TIR/CC, Toll-IL-1 receptor or coiled-coil domain; FIIND, domain with function to find; NBD, nucleotide-binding domain; LRR, leucine-rich repeat; WD40, WD40 repeat region; B, zinc finger-B box; SPRY, Spla and Ryanodine receptor. An asterisk designates three unrelated proteins that share little homology. These proteins contain unrelated N-termini and variable C-termini LRRs.

TABLE 1   CATERPILLERs in the human genome

CLR name	Synonym[a]	N-terminus[b]	Location	Isoform[c]
CLR1.1	CIAS1[d], PYPAF1, NALP3	PYD	Chr.1q44	Yes
CLR2.1	CARD12[d], IPAF, CLAN	CARD	Chr.2p22	Yes
CLR5.1	NAIP[d], Birc1	BIRx3	Chr.5q13.2	Yes
CLR7.1	CARD4[d], NOD1	CARD	Chr.7p14	Yes
CLR11.1[d]	NALP10, NOD8, PAN5, PYNOD	PYD	Chr.11p15.4	NP[e,f]
CLR11.2[d]	NALP14, NOD5, PAN8	PYD	Chr.11p15.4	Yes
CLR11.3[d]	NOD9	X	Chr.11q23	Yes
CLR11.4	PYPAF5[d], NALP6, PAN3	PYD	Chr.11p15.5	Yes
CLR16.1[d]	NOD27, PAN14	X	Chr.16q13	Yes
CLR16.2[d]	NOD3	X	Chr.16p13.3	NP
CLR16.3	NOD2[d], CARD15	CARDx2	Chr.16q12	Yes
CLR17.1	CARD7[d], NALP1, DEFCAP, NAC	PYD	Chr.17p13.1	Yes
CLR19.1[d]	NALP9, NOD6, PAN12	PYD	Chr.19q13.42	NP
CLR19.2[d]	NALP8, NOD16, PAN4	PYD	Chr.19q13.43	NP
CLR19.3	PYPAF7[d], monarch-1, NALP12, PAN6	PYD	Chr.19q13.42	Yes
CLR19.4	PYPAF3[d], NALP7, NOD12, PAN7	PYD	Chr.19q13.42	Yes
CLR19.5	PYPAF4[d], PAN2, NALP4	PYD	Chr.19q13.42	Yes
CLR19.6	PYPAF6[d], NALP11, NOD17, PAN10	PYD	Chr.19q13.42	NP
CLR19.7[d]	NALP13, NOD14, PAN13	PYD	Chr.19q13.43	Yes
CLR19.8	MATER[d], PYPAF8, NALP5, PAN11	PYD	Chr.19q13.43	NP
CLR19.9	NBS1[d], PYPAF2, NALP2, PAN1	PYD	Chr.19q13.42	Yes
CIITA	CIITA[d]	CARD/AD	Chr.16p13.13	Yes
CLRpseudoX.1	NOD24		Chr.Xp11.1	
CLRpseudoX.2	NOD13		Chr.Xq23	
CLRpseudo12.1	NOD25		Chr.12q24.32	

[a]Synonym nomenclature represents the chronology of publication.
[b]N-terminal domains: PYD, pyrin domain; CARD, caspase-recruitment domain; BIR, baculovirus IAP repeat domain; X, undefined and unrelated; AD, activation domain.
[c]Based on published reports, public database entries and our unpublished observations.
[d]First publication.
[e]NP, none published in available databases.
[f]An uncharacterized mRNA species from reference (156).

immune disorders in humans. The expression of these proteins ranges from those with more restricted expression in immune cells to those with a broad pattern of expression (25), suggesting that as a family they may function in a variety of tissues and serve both immune and nonimmune functions.

Plant Disease Resistance Genes

A brief description of the *R* genes in plants is warranted as they are likely to provide invaluable clues for the new *CLR* gene family. Disease resistance in plants relies heavily on large families of highly polymorphic R proteins that are composed of different structural domains. A complete discussion of *R* genes is beyond the scope of this review and the readers can refer to several excellent reviews (26, 27); however, much can be gleaned from the analysis of *R* genes. The R proteins are highly polymorphic but structurally conserved; some contain a NBD called NB-ARC that is closely homologous to the NACHT domain, followed by LRRs. The N-terminal domain of plant R proteins is variable, with either TIR or CC domains. Nonetheless, several R proteins have no recognizable N-terminal domains (26). The only known function of these proteins is in plant disease resistance, and they are believed to constitute the major immune defense network. R proteins are crucial for the immune defense against bacteria, virus, fungi, nematodes, insects, oomycetes, and even synthetic products such as insecticides (27). As a reflection of their importance, they are estimated to comprise >1% of the *Arabidopsis* and *Oryza* genomes, and to date more than 125 and 600 *R* genes have been found in these genomes, respectively (28, 29).

R proteins mediate the recognition of pathogen-derived molecules, which are encoded by pathogen *avr* (avirulence) genes. The avirulence designation arises from the observation that R proteins can neutralize pathogens that express specific Avr proteins, rendering the pathogen avirulent. In this scenario, the Avr protein elicits a protective defense response in the host genotypes that expresses the appropriate *R* gene product, leading to a hypersensitive response (HR). The HR includes programmed cell death of the infected cells, causing a necrotic lesion and the release of antimicrobial products that contribute to the inhibition of pathogen spread (26, 30). In contrast, *avr* genes provide a selective advantage to pathogens that infect a host genotype lacking the appropriate *R* gene, leading to pathogen spread, thus explaining the evolutionary preservation of *avr* genes in the pathogen (31, 32).

The most straightforward hypothesis for R protein and Avr interaction is direct receptor-ligand type interaction. However, investigators have demonstrated very few such interactions. The few examples of an R protein that interacts directly with its respective Avr product include Pto from tomato (a non-NBD-LRR R protein) and Pi-ta from rice (33). Even among these interactions, in vivo evidence in plants is lacking, and a more complex picture has emerged. For example, the interaction of Pi-ta and Avr-Pi-ta is detected in a yeast two-hybrid system using the LRR domain as bait, but the full-length Pi-ta protein fails to interact with the Avr protein in a yeast two-hybrid screen (34). The lack of direct interactions has led to several hypotheses evoking indirect interactions in protein complexes, additional cofactors or receptors, or R protein–mediated modification and detection of proteins that interact with Avr or vice versa. One of the most prominent hypotheses that arose from the formation of a protein complex but that does not require direct interaction of R with cognate Avr is the "guard hypothesis." In this hypothesis, the R protein acts as a guard and interacts with a host protein that is directly targeted by the Avr product in its function as a virulence factor. This minimally tripartite interaction causes the generation of an HR, whereas in the absence of the R protein, pathogen virulence occurs. Indeed, evidence exists that R proteins from *Arabadopsis* interact with proteins other than their corresponding Avr proteins. For example, the RIN4 protein is found to interact with RPM1 and RPS2 (40, 41). Also, RPS5 appears to indirectly recognize AvrPphB, possibly via a cleavage product of the AvrPphB and PBS-1 protein complex (36). The "guard hypothesis" is further exemplified by the observation that resistance to the Avr-Pto product from *Pseudomonas syringae* requires two tomato host gene products, the Pto serine threonine kinase atypical R protein and the non-Avr-Pto binding NBD-LRR protein Prf (37–39). Intriguingly, the vertebrate CARD4/NOD1 and NOD2/CARD15 are thought to sense intracellular bacterial products and facilitate the cellular response (42–45) in a function parallel to the R proteins.

Evolution of the CATERPILLER Family: Plants and Mammals

A comparison of sequences from across kingdom boundaries demonstrates that CLR and R proteins form distinct clades or groups, but they are clearly related (Figure 2). Phylogenetic analysis demonstrates that the R proteins as a whole are related to the CLR family as a whole, but whether they appear to be cryptically orthologous or homologous is not known.

Further comparisons of related sequences reveal ~85 vertebrate CLR orthologs and related proteins in mice, rats, humans, and two teleost fish species (Figure 2). The mammalian CLR proteins (represented by human, rat, and mouse sequences) typically form a single clade (Figure 2). However, we were unable to assign murine (both mouse and rat) orthologs for CLR19.6, CLR19.2, and CLR19.7, indicating differences in the composition of the CLR family across species. Nonetheless, these genes are present and highly conserved (~95%) in the genome of *Pan troglodytes* (chimp). CLR19.4 and CLR19.9 appear to be paralogous in humans, with a single mouse sequence equally related to both. CLR genes are also found in murine rodents, but are absent in humans. Otherwise, human, mouse, and rat CLR orthologs have similar domain architecture and are located in syntenic regions within their respective genomes (J. Harton, unpublished observation).

Database searches of *Brachydanio rerio* and *Takifugu rubripes* reveal at least four orthologous CLR proteins in teleost fish: CARD4/NOD1, NOD2/CARD15 (46), CLR16.2, and CLR11.3. A single sequence from *Brachydanio* groups near the CIITA clade. The dearth of CLR genes in teleost fish might reflect different

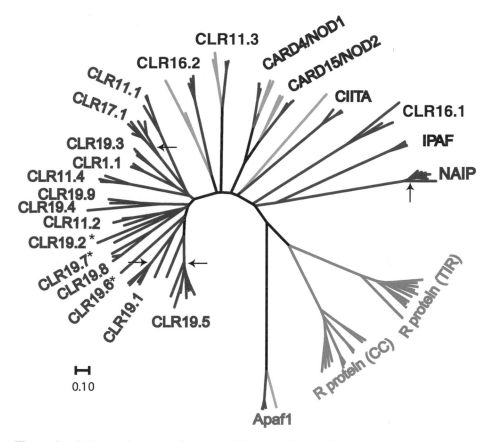

Figure 2   CLR proteins are a diverse multigene family that is related to the plant R proteins. Full-length proteins were aligned, using Clustal X, and used to construct dendrograms by the neighbor-joining method using MEGA2 software. Apaf-1 is shown as a related sequence. Known proteins and putative orthologs from human, mouse, rat, and teleost fish are shown. Each branch represents a sequence. (Text color code: *green*, plant R proteins; *purple*, NAIPs; *blue*, CARD-containing CLRs; *black*, unrelated N-termini CLRs; *red*, Pyrin-containing CLRs. Line color code: *green*, plant; *brown*, mammalian; *light blue*, teleost fish lineages. Arrows represent murine-specific duplications; asterisks represent human-specific CLRs.)

evolutionary histories (owing to putative genome-wide or segmental duplications) or different immunological strategies between mammals and fish (47, 48).

Repeated database searches of *Drosophila* and *Caenorhabditis* genomes yielded sequences showing weak similarities with known CLR, but these sequences did not conform to the tripartite domain architecture used to define CLR proteins (3). Both *Drosophila* and *Caenorhabditis* contain the individual domains necessary for some CLR proteins, such as the NACHT and LRR domains. N-terminal effector domains are less common and less well conserved. There are examples of invertebrate CARD domains in *Drosophila* (Dronc and DARK) and *Caenorhabditis* (CED-3 and CED-4) genomes. The Pyrin domain appears to be vertebrate-specific. Nonetheless, there is a paucity of Pyrin-containing proteins in teleost fish. *Caspy/Caspy2* and *zASC* are the only known fish genes to encode a Pyrin domain (14, 49). These results suggest that the vertebrate CLR family arose at or near the teleost lineage, coincident with the emergence of the adaptive immune system, possibly to co-opt different mechanisms to integrate the newly emerged adaptive immune system.

The patchwork appearance of CLR genes during evolution might reflect the dynamic nature of the different genomes and the selective pressures maintained on each population. Genome-wide duplications are quite rare in vertebrate genomes, however; plants undergo more frequent duplication events (50, 51). This strategy might account for the lack of orthology seen between the *R* genes and the *CLR* genes owing to a birth and death process during gene evolution (52). Gene duplication is thought to aid in driving diversity. By relaxing the selective pressures on the paralogs, a duplicated gene is able to drift into pseudogeny (nonfunctionalization) or acquire a new function (neo-functionalization) or a complementary function (subfunctionalization) (52).

Prominent Members of the Human CATERPILLER Family

The role of CLR proteins in vertebrate physiology is less understood than the role of R proteins in host-parasite interactions in plants; however, several members have been well studied and are likely to shed light on the rest of the CLR family. These are exemplified by CIITA, CARD4/NOD1, NOD2/CARD15, CIAS1, NAIP, and CARD7/NALP1. As some genes and proteins have several names, they are ordered here according to publication date.

CIITA, THE CLASS II TRANSACTIVATOR   The *MHC2TA* gene that codes for the CIITA protein was identified by complementation cloning of the RJ2.2.5 cell line, an in vitro–selected MHC class II negative cell line (53). Mutations of *MHC2TA* were found to be the genetic defect associated with bare lymphocyte syndrome type II (BLS) (24), a disorder caused by reduced or absent MHC class II gene expression (readers are referred to more extensive reviews of CIITA in References 54–57). The CIITA protein does not bind DNA, but instead serves as a scaffold or interaction interface for DNA-binding transcription factors that recognize the MHC class II promoter, which include NF-Y, RFX, and CREB. In addition, CIITA also coordinates the recruitment of histone modifying enzymes and contains a histone acetylase domain within its own N-terminus (58). CIITA is a potent transcriptional activator that is specific in its induction of genes important for the function of antigen-presenting cells, including MHC class II, HLA-DM, Ii, MHC class I, and plexin-A1 (59–62). The latter is a modulator of actin polarization that is important for dendritic cell (DC) function. The potency of CIITA is demonstrated by the near abrogation of MHC class II upon its removal in mice and the near-absence of MHC class II expression in most patients lacking functional CIITA (63, 64).

CIITA is a founding member of the family of NTPases called the NACHT (65). The NACHT domain, which was also used to define the NTPases of the CLR family, consists of seven signature motifs, including the ATP/GTPase-specific P-loop, Mg^{2+}-binding site (the Walker A and B motifs), and five additional motifs. The NACHT domain is unique in that motif VII contains a conserved array of polar, aromatic, and hydrophobic residues that is not seen in any other NTPase family (65). Structure-function analyses of CIITA have revealed the presence of both conventional domains expected of transcription activators, as well as unorthodox motifs. The N-terminal acidic domain (residues 1–125) is required for transactivation function (66, 67). This domain also contains a CARD-like region that lacks CARD activity (68). The mid-section of the protein consists of the NACHT domain (residues 337–702), which was later confirmed to possess weak GTP-binding activity (69, 70). This domain is involved in protein oligomerization and is important in nuclear import and export (15, 71–73). Researchers have suggested that the multimerization of CIITA might be similar to the induced proximity of Apaf-1 that enhances interactions with other proteins in the complex (15). CIITA also contains a C-terminal LRR that affects nuclear translocation and self-association (15, 18).

CARD4/NOD1   The protein christened caspase recruitment domain 4 (CARD4), or nucleotide-binding oligomerization domain 1 (NOD1) protein, was reported in 1999 by two groups on the basis of a search of the genomic database for homologs of the nematode CED-4 protein and its mammalian homolog, Apaf-1 (10, 74). Apaf-1 is a pivotal intermediary in apoptosis that interacts with cytosolic cytochrome C through the C-terminal tryptophan-aspartic acid repeat domain called WD40 (75). In the presence of ATP/dATP, this interaction leads to the unfolding of its N-terminal CARD domain and oligomerization (76, 77). The uncovered CARD domain undergoes homophilic interaction with the CARD domain of procaspase-9, resulting in caspase activation and eventually cell death (76, 77). Whereas Apaf-1 contains WD40 repeats that regulate Apaf-1 activation, CARD4/NOD1 contains LRRs (Figure 1).

The initial discovery showed that the introduction of overexpressed CARD4/NOD1 activated NF-κB and caspase-9, the latter leading to enhanced apoptosis. CARD4/NOD1 interacts with the CARD-containing serine-threonine kinase called Rip2/RICK/CARDIAK (10). Cells from Rip2$^{-/-}$ mice are deficient in NF-κB activation by CARD4/NOD1 and NOD2/CARD15 proteins (78, 79). During bacterial infection, the activation of NF-κB and c-Jun N-terminal kinase (JNK) by invasive *Shigella flexneri* is accompanied by CARD4/NOD1 oligomerization, which leads to the recruitment of Rip2 and the IKK complex (80).

Initially, researchers thought that CARD4/NOD1 mediates LPS-induced NF-κB and caspase-1 activation (81, 82); however, these results were obtained with commercial LPS preparations (43). Two seminal reports found that CARD4/NOD1 detects a proteoglycan contaminant present in commercial LPS that consists of a diaminopimelate-containing *N*-acetylglucosamine-*N*-acetylmuramic acid (Glc-NAc-MurNAc) tripeptide motif found in Gram-negative bacteria (42, 43). Diaminopimelic acid (DAP) is unique to Gram-negative proteoglycans, whereas Gram-positive bacteria have a lysine residue at the third peptide position that does not appear to activate CARD4/NOD1. However, some controversy remains because the two research groups reported opposite findings with extracts derived from the Gram-positive *Bacillus subtilis*. The minimal inducing moiety is composed of D-Glu-DAP or D-Gln-DAP devoid of the sugar component (42). Bone marrow–derived macrophages from CARD4/NOD1$^{-/-}$ mice show a defective response to D-glu-DAP (42). Likewise, epithelial cells transfected with dominant-negative CARD4/NOD1 inhibit bacteria-induced NF-κB activation (80). Importantly, there is no evidence for the direct binding or recognition of proteoglycans by CARD4/NOD1 because the experiments relied on ectopic and overexpression of CARD4/NOD1 and NF-κB activation by the inducing DAP-containing molecule. Based on plant R protein analysis, it is possible that an indirect rather than a direct mode of interaction occurs. As CARD4/NOD1 is expressed broadly in multiple tissues, it is hypothesized to serve an important and broad bacterial sensing function in multiple tissues.

NOD2/CARD15   NOD2/CARD15 is another member of the CARD-containing subfamily of CLRs. It shares many common properties with CARD4/NOD1, yet also has important distinguishing features. The N-terminus of NOD2/CARD15 contains two CARD domains instead of one (83) (Figure 1). Its expression is more restricted and is limited to monocytes, epithelial cells (83, 84), and Paneth cells in the intestine (85, 86). Expression of *NOD2/CARD15* in intestinal cells is of particular interest because this gene has been identified as the first susceptibility gene for Crohn's disease (CD) (87, 88), an intestinal inflammatory disorder, as well as a susceptibility locus for Blau syndrome (BS) (89). Overexpressed NOD2/CARD15 also induces NF-κB activation in response to commercial LPS, and activation requires the kinase IKKγ. As does CARD4/NOD1, NOD2/CARD15 interacts with Rip2/RICK via a homophilic CARD-CARD interaction, and this correlates with NF-κB activation (83). As evidence of its intracellular bacterial sensing role, the presence of NOD2/CARD15 is necessary for NF-κB activation by a contaminant in LPS, the proteoglycan muramyl dipeptide (44, 45, 90). Because muramyl dipeptide is the common moiety of proteoglycans derived from both Gram-positive and Gram-negative bacteria, investigators have proposed that NOD2/CARD15 has a broad role in the sensing of both types of bacteria in restricted cell types like macrophages or Paneth cells.

CIAS/CRYOPYRIN/PYPAF1/NALP3/CLR1.1   Hoffman et al. (91) identified *CIAS1* as a gene that segregated in family members affected with the familial cold urticaria (FCU) syndrome and Muckle-Wells syndrome (MWS), and the protein encoded by this gene is called cryopyrin. Soon after, another group reported the same gene and called it *PYPAF1* (92). Finally, a separate report (93) verified mutations of the gene in patients with inherited and periodic MWS and called the gene *NALP3*. Further analysis indicates that mutations in *CIAS1* are also found in the neonatal-onset multi-system inflammatory disease (NOMID), also known as chronic infantile neurologic cutaneous articular (CINCA) syndrome (94).

CIAS1 has a highly restricted expression pattern. It is not found in a large panel of tissues and transformed cell lines, but it is found primarily in peripheral blood leukocytes and most prominently in monocytes, although some expression is found in granulocytes, mouse mast cells, and T cells (92, 95). Molecular and functional studies have provided clues to the function of cryopyrin; nonetheless, a conflicting picture has also arisen, probably because many of these studies relied on overexpression systems using less physiologically relevant cell types. Manji et al. (92) first used a yeast two-hybrid system to show that cryopyrin interacts with the apoptosis-associated speck-like protein containing a CARD (ASC) protein, a Pyrin-CARD-containing protein, likely through a homophilic pyrin-pyrin interaction. In this report, cryopyrin does not activate a NF-κB reporter gene per se, but significantly activates NF-κB when combined with a low level of ASC. Although interaction between the two proteins could not be demonstrated by coimmunoprecipitation in transfected cells or as recombinant proteins, the proteins colocalize to punctuate structures in the cytoplasm of cells (92, 96). The synergistic effect of cryopyrin with ASC on NF-κB and procaspase-1 activation has been supported by other work using an overexpression system (97). However, we and others have found that CIAS1 alone can reduce NF-κB activation, or reduce procaspase-1-mediated processing of pro-IL-1β to mature IL-1β (98, 99). This inhibitory function of CIAS1 is dependent on the presence of both NBD and LRR domains and is not mediated by either alone, or by the pyrin domain (99). These conflicting data indicate that CIAS1 is inhibitory or inert with regard to NF-κB and IL-1β production when expressed alone, but it may vary with the concentrations used (98, 100), which points to the importance of future experiments that rely on knockdown, knockout, and/or knockin strategies.

NAIP   Neuronal apoptosis inhibitor protein (NAIP) is the first member of a larger family of proteins called IAP (inhibitor of apoptosis proteins) found in humans. *NAIPs* are predominantly expressed in motor neurons and macrophages and/or immature DCs (101, 102). These proteins all contain a BIR (baculovirus IAP repeat) domain in their N-termini and are known to inhibit cell death (103). In addition to the BIR domain, the NAIP protein also contains a NBD-LRR sequence. The NAIPs group with IPAF (Figure 2), owing primarily to conserved homology in the NACHT domains. Biochemically, NAIP and IPAF function antithetically. Deletion and truncation forms of the gene are genetically associated with autosomal recessive spinal muscular atrophies (SMAs), characterized by the depletion of spinal cord motor neurons and progressive neurodegeneration (103). *NAIP/BIR* genes have also been implicated in host response to bacterial infection. In humans, *Legionella* is capable of intracellular replication in specialized phagosomal compartments in macrophages (104). In contrast, most mouse strains are nonpermissive to bacterial replication (104, 105). In susceptible strains, the *NAIP5/Birc1e* gene is associated with increased *Legionella pneumophila* replication (106).

CARD7/NALP1/DEFCAP/NAC   The CARD7/NALP1 protein is unique in having a N-terminal pyrin domain, followed by NBD-LRR and a C-terminal CARD domain (6, 107–109). The protein is widely expressed but exhibits heightened expression in immune cells. The protein interacts with caspases in overexpression systems, and further interacts with Apaf-1 through a CARD-CARD homotypic interaction (12, 108, 109). Chu et al. (109) have proposed that CARD7/NALP1 interaction with Apaf-1 occurs first, which then recruits caspases to the complex. Overexpressed full-length CARD7/NALP1 enhanced apoptosis and caspase activation induced by exogenously introduced Apaf-1; however, the CARD or NBD domain alone interfered with apoptosis induced by Apaf-1/procaspase-9.

The CARD7/NALP1 protein is a component of two important and large protein complexes: the "apoptosome" (109) and the "inflammasome" complexes (12). The former is a multi-protein complex of >1 MDa that is composed of Apaf-1, caspases, and additional proteins (110). The latter is a cell-free complex composed of caspase-1/5, ASC, and CARD7/NALP1, in addition to other molecules, including CIAS1, which is marked by the processing of procaspases and pro-IL-1β (12, 23). These studies suggest that CARD7/NALP1 plays an important function in both apoptosis and inflammation and forecast a complex array of interplay with molecules found in large complexes.

Disease-Associated Mutations in CATERPILLERs

An understanding of the in vivo role of CLR proteins is aided by the remarkable association of CLR genes with human diseases, creating in vivo experiments of nature. The genes associated with diseases are *MHC2TA* with BLS; *NOD2/CARD15* with CD and BS; *CIAS1* with FCAS (familial cold autoinflammatory syndrome), MWS, and NOMID/CINCA; and *NAIP* with SMA. These diseases have different etiologies and pathologies, underscoring the manifold expression patterns and functions of CLR genes and proteins in human diseases. A summary of the mutations found in these diseases is shown in Figure 3.

BARE LYMPHOCYTE SYNDROME   Various genetic lesions in the *MHC2TA* gene are known to cause type II BLS (complementation group A, MIM no. 209920), an autosomal-recessive immunodeficiency. Known mutations are associated with loss of MHC class II expression. Mutations of CIITA fall into three basic groups: splice site, nonsense, and missense mutations (54). BLS2, BCH1, ATU, and RC$_{paternal}$ mutations result in exon skipping of one of the C-terminal LRRs (24, 111–113) (Figure 3). The BLS2 mutation is shown to affect nuclear localization (114). The molecular mechanisms of the other three exon skipping mutations have not been described. Two nonsense mutations, E381ter and W688ter (BCH2), result in truncated proteins (112, 115). Three missense mutations, F961S, 1027ΔI (RC$_{maternal}$),

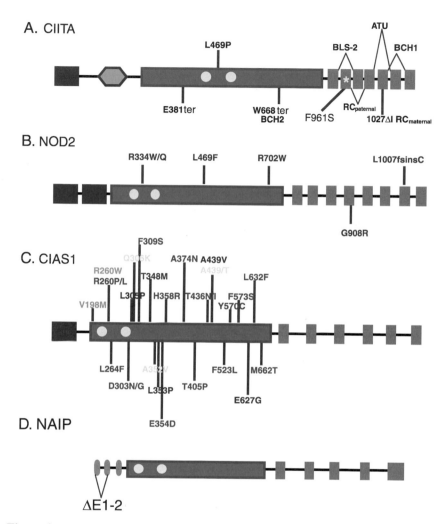

Figure 3 Disease-associated mutations with CLRs. Yellow circles represent Walker A and B motifs. The LRR domain is represented by individual exons. (*A*) *MHC2TA*: mutations in the CIITA gene *MHC2TA* are found in the NACHT or LRR domains. (*B*) *NOD2/CARD15*: CD-associated mutations (*blue*) occur at or near the LRR domain, while BS-associated mutations (*red*) occur in the NACHT domain. (*C*) *CIAS1*: all disease-associated mutations are found within a single exon encoding the NACHT domain (color key: *orange*, FCU and MWS; *light blue*, FCU, MWS, and CINCA; *green*, CINCA; *red*, FCU; *yellow*, MWS; *purple*, MWS and CINCA). (*D*) *NAIP*: deletions associated with SMA are located in the first two BIR domains.

and L469P, have variable phenotypes (113, 116, 117). One BLS patient showed no mutations in the coding and noncoding regions of *MHC2TA* gene, but transcription was significantly lower. Promoter regions that were sequenced were identical to published sequences, suggesting a novel regulatory region or pathway (113).

CROHN'S DISEASE   Mutations in *NOD2/CARD15* have been associated with two phenotypically distinct inflammatory conditions: CD (MIM no. 605956) and BS (MIM no. 186580). CD is characterized by chronic mucosal damage caused by immune cell infiltration, possibly due to an abnormal inflammatory response to bacterial lumenal products. Two groups initially demonstrated via different parameters (87, 88) that mutations in the *NOD2/CARD15* gene conferred a relative risk for simple homozygotes of 38, compound homozygotes of 44, and simple heterozygotes of 3. In Caucasian populations, 8%–17% of patients with CD have two disease-associated alleles (118). Other minor allelic variants do occur, and together 50% of Caucasian CD patients carry at least one mutant allele (119). The *NOD2/CARD15*-associated mutations have been confirmed by others in Caucasian but not in Asian patients (120–124). The lack of simple Mendelian inheritance underscores the genetic and environmental complexity of CD.

The major CD-associated mutations, L1007fsinsC, G908R, and R702W, are typically loss-of-function mutations with regard to peptidoglycan-induced NF-κB signaling. Only R702W falls within the regulatory region located at the carboxy-terminal end of the NBD exon (125), whereas G908R and L1007fsinsC fall in the LRRs. The decreased NF-κB signaling seems paradoxical to the pathophysiology of CD that is characterized by chronic inflammation and increased NF-κB activation. Nonetheless, NOD2/CARD15 might be an antibacterial factor for the intracellular bacterium *Salmonella typhimurium* (126). Introduction of wild-type (but not disease-associated variants) NOD2/CARD15 in cells resulted in decreased viable internalized bacteria (126). This finding, along with a similar finding for CARD4/NOD1 (80), suggests that expression of *NOD2/CARD15* disease-associated mutants might decrease immune responses to certain pathogenic bacteria. Alternatively, *NOD2/CARD15* is expressed in Paneth cells, which secrete antimicrobial factors such as defensins (127). Dysregulation of NOD2/CARD15-dependent pathways might influence the secretion of antimicrobial substances, leading to chronic infection or inflammation (128). This hypothesis is supported by the observation that patients with CD have a paucity of defensin secretion (128). Although NF-κB is known to activate many proinflammatory genes, its role in intraepithelial cells (IECs) remains less clear. Transgenic mice expressing an IEC-specific super-repressor of IκBα display increased sensitivity to dextran sodium sulfate–induced colitis, implying that NF-κB may attenuate incidence of colitis. Therefore, NOD2/CARD15 activation of NF-κB may be protective in the colon (129). Lastly, *NOD2/CARD15* disease-associated mutants expressed by macrophages might lead to inappropriate "conditioning" of the macrophage that in turn influences the effector–regulatory cell balance, tilting the scenario toward chronic inflammation (130). *NOD2/CARD15*$^{-/-}$ mice have a subtle phenotype and initially do not develop colitis, suggesting a role for additional modifier genes (131). However, Watanabe et al. (132) have demonstrated that macrophages from $NOD2/CARD15^{-/-}$ mice in response to TLR2 agonists have increased IL-12 secretion that favors a Th1 response, recapitulating some features of human CD. They conclude that NOD2/CARD15 is a negative regulator of TLR2 responses.

BLAU SYNDROME   BS is characterized by uveitis, arthritis, and dermatitis (133). Disease-associated mutations are located within the central NBD, flanking both sides of the Mg^{+2}-binding site (Walker B) (89). Position R334 is conserved absolutely in vertebrate NOD2/CARD15 proteins, suggesting a role for this residue, but L469 is variable. Nonetheless, teleost NOD2/CARD15 proteins encode a conservative V469 substitution (46). R334W/Q and L469F mutations are associated with increased basal NF-κB activity and might suggest a mechanism for the observed inflammation characteristic of BS and its autosomally dominant mode of inheritance.

CIAS1-LINKED DISORDERS   Mutations of *CIAS1*, a component of the inflammasome (12), are associated with several genetic autoinflammatory conditions: FCU/FCAS (MIM no. 120100), MWS (MIM no. 191900), and NOMID/CINCA (MIM no. 607115) (91, 94). These diseases manifest in recurrent episodes of inflammatory attacks associated with arthritis, fever, and rash (134, 135). Analysis of patients provides clues as to the molecular defect in patients bearing the *CIAS1* variant. Basal levels of cytokines in unstimulated cells, including IL-1β, TNF-α, IL-3, IL-5, and IL-6, were substantially increased in afflicted MWS patients compared with normal controls (136). The importance of the aberrant cytokine expression pattern, in particular IL-1β is underscored by the dramatic response of MWS patients with *CIAS1* mutations to Anakinra, a therapeutic agent consisting of recombinant IL-1R antagonist (137, 138). All 27 of the disease-associated missense mutations lie within the central NACHT exon (139) (Figure 3). The most common mutation, R260W, is associated with all three diseases, implying the role of modifier genes in specific disease phenotypes. This mutation might be analogous to the R334Q mutation in *NOD2/CARD15* that is associated with BS (139). Two recent analyses of variant forms of CIAS1 have provided strong evidence that the disease-associated forms of CIAS1 spontaneously activate proinflammatory responses (23, 140). First, when the disease-associated mutants R260W, D303N, and E637G are introduced into monocytic THP-1 cells, which express the ASC protein, they cause spontaneous IL-1β secretion. In contrast, wild-type CIAS1 does not alter IL-1β production despite the presence of ASC (140). The increased function of the mutants correlates with dramatically increased association of these proteins with ASC (140). Secondly, Agostini et al. (23) demonstrated that CIAS1 is part of the inflammasome complex, and CIAS1 is associated with ASC, caspase-1, and Cardinal. The interaction of these molecules leads to the activation of pro-IL-1β, resulting in the production of mature IL-1β. The same report showed that in monocytes from a MWS patient with the R260W mutation, spontaneous IL-1β

synthesis is significantly enhanced compared with cells bearing a wild-type gene, whereas LPS-stimulated IL-1β synthesis is modestly enhanced. These results are consistent with the conclusion that variant CIAS1 causes spontaneous activation of the inflammatory pathway leading to proinflammatory cytokine synthesis. However, the function of wild-type CIAS1 remains to be fully elucidated.

SPINAL MUSCULAR ATROPHY   *NAIPs* are inhibitors of apoptosis (141, 142). The genomic region containing *NAIP* and *survival motor neuron* (*SMN*) genes is a locus for SMA1 (MIM no. 253300) and is part of a large inverted duplication on human chromosome 5q13.1. Mutations in *NAIP* are associated with a modifying phenotype of SMA in humans (*Birc1*) and susceptibility to *Legionella pneumophila* in certain strains of inbred mice (*Birc1e*) (106, 143). SMA is an autosomally recessive neuronal degenerative disease characterized by atrophy of the voluntary muscles and loss of spinal motor neurons (144). Deletions in the first two exons of *Birc1* are associated with ~67% of type 1 SMA (103) and are concordant with disease severity. The protein not only suppresses apoptosis in neuronal-derived cell lines such as PC12, but when introduced recombinantly into mice, it reduces ischemic damage (145, 146). Because the protein can block apoptosis, it has been proposed that unchecked apoptosis in motor neurons from SMA patients may be responsible for excessive cell death leading to atrophy (147). Several apoptotic mechanisms have been assigned to the protein. One suggests that it blocks caspase activation (141, 147). Another indicates that NAIP mediates anti-apoptosis through a TAK1/JNK1 signaling pathway (142). Finally, NAIP is found to bind hippocalin, a calcium-binding protein restricted to neurons, in a yeast two-hybrid system and protects against calcium-induced caspase activation and cell death (148). The mouse *NAIP* genes are encoded by multiple *NAIP* paralogs (*NAIP1–7*) (149). *NAIP1$^{-/-}$* mice demonstrate increased apoptosis in response to toxin-mediated brain injury (150), suggesting that *NAIP1* is involved in neuroprotection.

Mouse macrophages infected with intracellular bacteria such as *Salmonella* or incubated with latex beads to induce phagocytosis show increased *NAIP* expression (151). Most importantly, the levels of *NAIP* expression segregate with susceptibility to *Legionella pneumophila*. Permissiveness to *Legionella pneumophila* intracellular replication maps to a single locus, *Lgn1* (Chr.13qD1) in mice. A/J, FvB/NJ, C3H/HeJ, BALB/cJ, and 129S1 strains are permissive to *Legionella* replication; C57BL/6J, P/J, and 129X1 strains are nonpermissive (143). The permissive A/J strain expresses a lower quantity of NAIP compared with the resistant C57BL/6 strain (143, 151). Diez et al. (106) have demonstrated that susceptibility in the A/J strain is encoded by the *Birc1e/NAIP5* gene by using BAC (derived from C57BL6 or 129X1 mice) transgenic mice, suggesting possible haploinsufficiency. Genotyping of permissive and nonpermissive strains demonstrates that nonsynonymous mutations in the last two exons in the *Birc1e* gene correlate with permissiveness in all strains (143). However, neither report has found an association between NAIP-induced apoptosis and resistance to *Legionella* infection. The role of NAIP in producing proinflammatory and immune responses in macrophages to counter an infection, or its role as a sensor of bacterial product, remain to be demonstrated but provide intriguing possibilities for its function in the immune system.

Potential of CATERPILLER Proteins in Meeting the Challenges of Immunity

At the beginning of this review, we posed two challenges faced by the immune system: to recognize and respond to a diversity of antigens, and to prevent an overzealous, self-destructive immune response. Although the field is too young to render a final verdict, it is intriguing to consider if CLRs might meet these challenges. Regarding a diversity of immune detection and signals, emerging evidence suggests that some CLR proteins can detect pathogen-derived products ("detect" is used loosely here to reflect direct or indirect recognition of pathogen products with the caveats described earlier). A central issue is whether CLRs that serve this role detect such products with a high degree of specificity, similar to TCR and Ig, or if they recognize invariant molecular patterns similar to TLRs. Regardless, a relevant observation is that many CLR transcripts undergo differential splicing that is translated to a variety of isoforms that might exhibit different detection specificities (Figure 4). This may parallel the diversity generated by V(D)J and the class-switch recombinations, although these recombination events occur at the DNA level, whereas CLRs undergo splicing of exons encoding the LRR, a domain important for the recognition of pathogen-derived products. These splice forms may modulate the function of the full-length form, thus fine-tuning an immune response. In addition, heterodimers among CLR members have been demonstrated, including IPAF interactions with CARD4/NOD1, NOD2/CARD15, and CARD7 (NAC) (17). Hetero-oligomerization may change the specificity of the sensor function, reminiscent of the association of Ig or TCR-heavy and -light chains to form a recognition unit for specific antigen and antigen plus MHC, respectively. Because there are more than 20 members in this family, the combinatorial possibilities should be astronomical. Using Apaf-1 as a model, the Apaf-1 oligomer consists of a heptamer, which can further increase the combinatorial recognition unit. Verification that such hetero-oligomerization does exist under physiologic conditions and different stimuli would be of great importance. In addition, there are a host of non-CLR proteins with CARD, Pyrin, NBD, or LRR domains that potentially can interact with CLR family members to further fine-tune the recognition unit and form large complexes such as apoptosomes, enhanceosomes, or inflammasomes (Figure 4). Although the above discussion focuses on the possibility of CLR proteins as pathogen sensor molecules, all the properties described above may also contribute to a divergence of signaling pathways initiated via CLRs.

Finally, it is of interest that a majority of the human CLR genes are found in the subtelomeric region of the chromosome (3). Although the significance of this location is unclear, some olfactory genes are also predominantly located at this region (152, 153). Considering that both immune detection and odor sensing require the ability to distinguish an enormous array of signals, this shared location

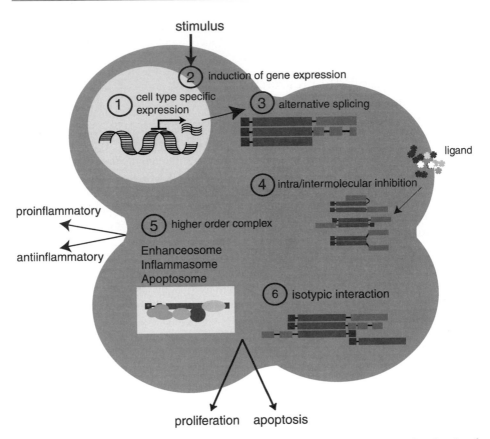

Figure 4 Generating CLR diversity within the immune system. At least five levels of diversity have been described for CLRs. (1) Cell-type-specific expression patterns dictate which CLR and/or adaptor/signaling molecules are expressed coordinately. (2) Stimulation-induced expression further diversifies the response. (3) Alternative splicing has been reported for CLR genes, thus modulating possible interacting molecules. (4) At the protein level, CLRs can be regulated by intra- and intermolecular interactions. (5) Upon the appropriate signal, CLRs can bind different interacting molecules to affect their function. Another level of diversity is hypothesized. (6) Isotypic interactions in which isoforms of CLR proteins can interact with each other, different adaptor molecules, and/or ligands. These interactions can influence or be influenced by any of the other five levels of diversity, creating a large network of CLR communication and possible outcomes for pathogen sensing and/or signal transduction.

may not be coincidental. Recent analyses of the genomic database have found blocks of sequences preferentially found at the subtelomeric or pericentromeric region that share a high degree of identity and are believed to arise by segmental duplication (154, 155). These regions are thought to undergo a high degree of evolutionary turnover. Whether the preponderance of subtelomeric localization provides another means to diversify the CLR gene composition is of obvious importance.

The second challenge that faces the immune system is the capacity to limit an ongoing immune response, and thus limit the destruction of self. In the examples in which mutations in a CLR gene are associated with disease susceptibility, all except for CIITA involve mutations that are associated with autoinflammatory disorders. A hypothesis that is compatible with these observations is that the affected gene product provides a check on a flagrant inflammatory response. Mutation of the gene disrupted this check, thus leading to autoinflammation. Indeed we have found that the CLR protein, Monarch-1, constitutes a negative regulator of NF-κB and AP-1 activation, and further suppresses proinflammatory cytokine production in macrophage cell lines (K. Williams, unpublished observation). Similarly, CLR16.2 constitutes a negative regulator in T cells (B. Conti, unpublished observation). Such negative regulatory function would be pivotal for the prevention of an overzealous inflammatory response, such as those associated with autoimmunity/autoinflammation and with sepsis.

In summary, the CLR family of proteins is a newly discovered family important in controlling inflammation and apoptosis and likely to have wide impact not only in the immune system and organs/tissues rich with inflammatory cells such as the skin, CNS, lung, and gastrointestinal tracts, but also may serve functions in nonimmune cells. Although newly discovered, they appear to have their evolutionary roots in plants and are likely an ancient family of genes. A signature of this family is its association with a number of autoinflammatory, immunologic, and neurologic disorders. As members of this family are likely to interact with each other and with other proteins, the impact on signal transduction and pathogen detection are likely crucial for cells to distinguish distinct signals and fine-tune their responses.

APPENDIX

Abbreviations used: AD, activation domain; ASC, apoptosis-associated speck-like protein containing a CARD; BIR, baculovirus IAP repeat; BLS, bare lymphocyte syndrome; BS, Blau syndrome; CARD, caspase-recruitment domain; CATERPILLER, CARD, transcription enhancer, R-(purine)-binding, pyrin, lots of leucine-rich repeats; CD, Crohn's disease; CIAS, cold-induced autoinflammatory syndrome; CIITA, class II transactivator; CINCA, chronic infantile neurologic cutaneous articular; CLR, CATERPILLER; DAP, diaminopimelic acid; DC, dendritic cell; FCAS, familial cold autoinflammatory syndrome; FCU, familial cold urticaria; HR, hypersensitive response; IAP, inhibitor of apoptosis; IEC, intraepithelial cell; Ig, immunoglobulin; JNK, c-Jun N-terminal kinase; LRR, leucine-rich repeat; MWS, Muckle-Wells syndrome; NACHT, NAIP, CIITA, HET-E and TP1; NAIP, neuronal apoptosis inhibitor protein; NALP, NACHT leucine-rich domain and pyrin-containing protein; NBD, nucleotide-binding domain; NB-ARC, nucleotide-binding, Apaf-1, plant R gene product, CED-4; NOD, nucleotide-binding oligomerization domain; NOMID, neonatal-onset multi-system inflammatory disease; PAAD, pyrin, AIM, ASC, and death domain–like protein; PAMP, pathogen-associated molecular patterns; PAN, PAAD and NACHT; PYD, pyrin domain; PYPAF, pyrin-containing Apaf-1-like protein; SMA, spinal muscular atrophy; TCR, T cell receptor; TIR, Toll and interleukin-1 receptor; TLR, Toll-like receptor.

ACKNOWLEDGMENTS

The authors apologize to those whose citations were omitted owing to space constraints. The authors wish to acknowledge W.J. Brickey, J. Lich, and J. Dangl for critical reading of this manuscript, and J. Harton, K. Williams, and B. Conti for sharing unpublished observations. J. Ting is supported by NIH grants: AI29564, AI54309, AI057175, and DK38108. B. Davis is supported by NIH T32 DK07737 and is a fellow of the Crohn's and Colitis Foundation of America.

**The *Annual Review of Immunology* is online at
http://immunol.annualreviews.org**

LITERATURE CITED

1. Barton GM, Medzhitov R. 2002. Toll-like receptors and their ligands. *Curr. Top. Microbiol. Immunol.* 270:81–92

2. Takeda K, Kaisho T, Akira S. 2003. Toll-like receptors. *Annu. Rev. Immunol.* 21: 335–76

3. Harton JA, Linhoff MW, Zhang J, Ting JP. 2002. Cutting edge: CATERPILLER: a large family of mammalian genes containing CARD, pyrin, nucleotide-binding, and leucine-rich repeat domains. *J. Immunol.* 169:4088–93

4. Inohara N, Nunez G. 2003. NODs: intracellular proteins involved in inflammation and apoptosis. *Nat. Rev. Immunol.* 3:371–82

5. Tschopp J, Martinon F, Burns K. 2003. NALPs: a novel protein family involved in inflammation. *Nat. Rev. Mol. Cell. Biol.* 4:95–104

6. Martinon F, Hofmann K, Tschopp J. 2001. The pyrin domain: a possible member of the death domain-fold family implicated in apoptosis and inflammation. *Curr. Biol.* 11:R118–20

7. Pawlowski K, Pio F, Chu Z, Reed JC, Godzik A. 2001. PAAD—a new protein domain associated with apoptosis, cancer and autoimmune diseases. *Trends Biochem. Sci.* 26:85–87

8. Wang L, Manji GA, Grenier JM, Al-Garawi A, Merriam S, et al. 2002. PYPAF7, a novel PYRIN-containing Apaf1-like protein that regulates activation of NF-κB and caspase-1-dependent cytokine processing. *J. Biol. Chem.* 277:29874–80

9. Liepinsh E, Barbals R, Dahl E, Sharipo A, Staub E, Otting G. 2003. The death-domain fold of the ASC PYRIN domain, presenting a basis for PYRIN/PYRIN recognition. *J. Mol. Biol.* 332:1155–63

10. Inohara N, Koseki T, del Peso L, Hu Y, Yee C, et al. 1999. Nod1, an Apaf-1-like activator of caspase-9 and nuclear factor-κB. *J. Biol. Chem.* 274:14560–67

11. Richards N, Schaner P, Diaz A, Stuckey J, Shelden E, et al. 2001. Interaction between pyrin and the apoptotic speck protein (ASC) modulates ASC–induced apoptosis. *J. Biol. Chem.* 276:39320–29

12. Martinon F, Burns K, Tschopp J. 2002. The inflammasome: a molecular platform triggering activation of inflammatory

caspases and processing of proIL-β. *Mol. Cell* 10:417–26

13. Stehlik C, Krajewska M, Welsh K, Krajewski S, Godzik A, Reed JC. 2003. The PAAD/PYRIN-only protein POP1/ASC2 is a modulator of ASC-mediated nuclear-factor-κB and pro-caspase-1 regulation. *Biochem. J.* 373:101–13

14. Masumoto J, Zhou W, Chen FF, Su F, Kuwada JY, et al. 2003. Caspy, a zebrafish caspase, activated by ASC oligomerization is required for pharyngeal arch development. *J. Biol. Chem.* 278:4268–76

15. Linhoff MW, Harton JA, Cressman DE, Martin BK, Ting JP. 2001. Two distinct domains within CIITA mediate self-association: involvement of the GTP-binding and leucine-rich repeat domains. *Mol. Cell. Biol.* 21:3001–11

16. Aravind L, Dixit VM, Koonin EV. 2001. Apoptotic molecular machinery: vastly increased complexity in vertebrates revealed by genome comparisons. *Science* 291:1279–84

17. Damiano JS, Oliveira V, Welsh K, Reed JC. 2004. Heterotypic interactions among NACHT domains: implications for regulation of innate immune responses. *Biochem. J.* 381:213–19

18. Hake SB, Masternak K, Kammerbauer C, Janzen C, Reith W, et al. 2000. CIITA leucine-rich repeats control nuclear localization, in vivo recruitment to the major histocompatibility complex (MHC) class II enhanceosome, and MHC class II gene transactivation. *Mol. Cell. Biol.* 20:7716–25

19. Harton JA, O'Connor W Jr, Conti BJ, Linhoff MW, Ting JP. 2002. Leucine-rich repeats of the class II transactivator control its rate of nuclear accumulation. *Hum. Immunol.* 63:588–601

20. Camacho-Carvajal MM, Klingler S, Schnappauf F, Hake SB, Steimle V. 2004. Importance of class II transactivator leucine-rich repeats for dominant-negative function and nucleo-cytoplasmic transport. *Int. Immunol.* 16:65–75

21. Zhu XS, Linhoff MW, Li G, Chin KC, Maity SN, Ting JP. 2000. Transcriptional scaffold: CIITA interacts with NF-Y, RFX, and CREB to cause stereospecific regulation of the class II major histocompatibility complex promoter. *Mol. Cell. Biol.* 20:6051–61

22. Masternak K, Muhlethaler-Mottet A, Villard J, Zufferey M, Steimle V, Reith W. 2000. CIITA is a transcriptional coactivator that is recruited to MHC class II promoters by multiple synergistic interactions with an enhanceosome complex. *Genes Dev.* 14:1156–66

23. Agostini L, Martinon F, Burns K, McDermott MF, Hawkins PN, Tschopp J. 2004. NALP3 forms an IL-1β-processing inflammasome with increased activity in Muckle-Wells autoinflammatory disorder. *Immunity* 20:319–25

24. Steimle V, Otten LA, Zufferey M, Mach B. 1993. Complementation cloning of an MHC class II transactivator mutated in hereditary MHC class II deficiency (or bare lymphocyte syndrome). *Cell* 75:135–46

25. Su AI, Cooke MP, Ching KA, Hakak Y, Walker JR, et al. 2002. Large-scale analysis of the human and mouse transcriptomes. *Proc. Natl. Acad. Sci. USA* 99:4465–70

26. Hulbert SH, Webb CA, Smith SM, Sun Q. 2001. Resistance gene complexes: evolution and utilization. *Annu. Rev. Phytopathol.* 39:285–312

27. Nimchuk Z, Eulgem T, Holt BF 3rd, Dangl JL. 2003. Recognition and response in the plant immune system. *Annu. Rev. Genet.* 37:579–609

28. Meyers BC, Dickerman AW, Michelmore RW, Sivaramakrishnan S, Sobral BW, Young ND. 1999. Plant disease resistance genes encode members of an ancient and diverse protein family within the nucleotide-binding superfamily. *Plant J.* 20:317–32

29. Zhou T, Wang Y, Chen JQ, Araki H, Jing Z, et al. 2004. Genome-wide identification

of NBS genes in *japonica* rice reveals significant expansion of divergent non-TIR NBS-LRR genes. *Mol. Genet. Genomics* 271:402–15

30. Staskawicz BJ, Ausubel FM, Baker BJ, Ellis JG, Jones JD. 1995. Molecular genetics of plant disease resistance. *Science* 268:661–67

31. Kjemtrup S, Nimchuk Z, Dangl JL. 2000. Effector proteins of phytopathogenic bacteria: bifunctional signals in virulence and host recognition. *Curr. Opin. Microbiol.* 3:73–78

32. Staskawicz BJ, Mudgett MB, Dangl JL, Galan JE. 2001. Common and contrasting themes of plant and animal diseases. *Science* 292:2285–89

33. Martin GB, Bogdanove AJ, Sessa G. 2003. Understanding the functions of plant disease resistance proteins. *Annu. Rev. Plant. Biol.* 54:23–61

34. Jia Y, McAdams SA, Bryan GT, Hershey HP, Valent B. 2000. Direct interaction of resistance gene and avirulence gene products confers rice blast resistance. *EMBO J.* 19:4004–14

35. Deleted in proof

36. Shao F, Golstein C, Ade J, Stoutemyer M, Dixon JE, et al. 2003. Cleavage of *Arabidopsis* PBS1 by a bacterial type III effector. *Science* 301:1230–33

37. Salmeron JM, Oldroyd GE, Rommens CM, Scofield SR, Kim HS, et al. 1996. Tomato *Prf* is a member of the leucine-rich repeat class of plant disease resistance genes and lies embedded within the *Pto* kinase gene cluster. *Cell* 86:123–33

38. Scofield SR, Tobias CM, Rathjen JP, Chang JH, Lavelle DT, et al. 1996. Molecular basis of gene-for-gene specificity in bacterial speck disease of tomato. *Science* 274:2063–65

39. Tang X, Frederick RD, Zhou J, Halterman DA, Jia Y, Martin GB. 1996. Initiation of plant disease resistance by physical interaction of AvrPto and Pto kinase. *Science* 274:2060–63

40. Mackey D, Holt BF, Wiig A, Dangl JL.

2002. RIN4 interacts with *Pseudomonas syringae* type III effector molecules and is required for RPM1-mediated resistance in *Arabidopsis. Cell* 108:743–54

41. Mackey D, Belkhadir Y, Alonso JM, Ecker JR, Dangl JL. 2003. *Arabidopsis* RIN4 is a target of the type III virulence effector AvrRpt2 and modulates RPS2-mediated resistance. *Cell* 112:379–89

42. Chamaillard M, Hashimoto M, Horie Y, Masumoto J, Qiu S, et al. 2003. An essential role for NOD1 in host recognition of bacterial peptidoglycan containing diaminopimelic acid. *Nat. Immunol.* 4:702–7

43. Girardin SE, Boneca IG, Carneiro LAM, Antignac A, Jehanno M, et al. 2003. Nod1 detects a unique muropeptide from gram-negative bacterial peptidoglycan. *Science* 300:1584–87

44. Girardin SE, Boneca IG, Viala J, Chamaillard M, Labigne A, et al. 2003. Nod2 is a general sensor of peptidoglycan through muramyl dipeptide (MDP) detection. *J. Biol. Chem.* 278:8869–72

45. Inohara N, Ogura Y, Fontalba A, Gutierrez O, Pons F, et al. 2003. Host recognition of bacterial muramyl dipeptide mediated through NOD2. Implications for Crohn's disease. *J. Biol. Chem.* 278:5509–12

46. Ogura Y, Saab L, Chen FF, Benito A, Inohara N, Nunez G. 2003. Genetic variation and activity of mouse Nod2, a susceptibility gene for Crohn's disease. *Genomics* 81:369–77

47. Wienholds E, Schulte-Merker S, Walderich B, Plasterk RH. 2002. Target-selected inactivation of the zebrafish *rag1* gene. *Science* 297:99–102

48. Trede NS, Langenau DM, Traver D, Look AT, Zon LI. 2004. The use of zebrafish to understand immunity. *Immunity* 20:367–79

49. Inohara N, Nunez G. 2000. Genes with homology to mammalian apoptosis regulators identified in zebrafish. *Cell Death Differ.* 7:509–10

50. Vision TJ, Brown DG, Tanksley SD. 2000.

The origins of genomic duplications in *Arabidopsis. Science* 290:2114–17

51. Blanc G, Barakat A, Guyot R, Cooke R, Delseny M. 2000. Extensive duplication and reshuffling in the *Arabidopsis* genome. *Plant Cell* 12:1093–101

52. Michelmore RW, Meyers BC. 1998. Clusters of resistance genes in plants evolve by divergent selection and a birth-and-death process. *Genome Res.* 8:1113–30

53. Accolla RS, Jotterand-Bellomo M, Scarpellino L, Maffei A, Carra G, Guardiola J. 1986. aIr-1, a newly found locus on mouse chromosome 16 encoding a trans-acting activator factor for MHC class II gene expression. *J. Exp. Med.* 164:369–74

54. Reith W, Mach B. 2001. The bare lymphocyte syndrome and the regulation of MHC expression. *Annu. Rev. Immunol.* 19:331–73

55. Ting JP, Trowsdale J. 2002. Genetic control of MHC class II expression. *Cell* 109(Suppl. S):S21–33

56. Boss JM, Jensen PE. 2003. Transcriptional regulation of the MHC class II antigen presentation pathway. *Curr. Opin. Immunol.* 15:105–11

57. Nekrep N, Fontes JD, Greyer M, Peterlin BM. 2003. When the lymphocyte loses its clothes. *Immunity* 18:453–57

58. Raval A, Howcroft TK, Weissman JD, Kirshner S, Zhu XS, et al. 2001. Transcriptional coactivator, CIITA, is an acetyltransferase that bypasses a promoter requirement for TAF(II)250. *Mol. Cell.* 7:105–15

59. Wright KL, Chin KC, Linhoff M, Skinner C, Brown JA, et al. 1998. CIITA stimulation of transcription factor binding to major histocompatibility complex class II and associated promoters in vivo. *Proc. Natl. Acad. Sci. USA* 95:6267–72

60. Martin BK, Chin KC, Olsen JC, Skinner CA, Dey A, et al. 1997. Induction of MHC class I expression by the MHC class II transactivator CIITA. *Immunity* 6:591–600

61. Gobin SJ, Peijnenburg A, Keijsers V, van den Elsen PJ. 1997. Site α is crucial for two routes of IFNγ-induced MHC class I transactivation: the ISRE-mediated route and a novel pathway involving CIITA. *Immunity* 6:601–11

62. Wong AW, Brickey WJ, Taxman DJ, van Deventer HW, Reed W, et al. 2003. CIITA-regulated plexin-A1 affects T-cell-dendritic cell interactions. *Nat. Immunol.* 4:891–98

63. Chang CH, Guerder S, Hong SC, van Ewijk W, Flavell RA. 1996. Mice lacking the MHC class II transactivator (CIITA) show tissue-specific impairment of MHC class II expression. *Immunity* 4:167–78

64. Itoh-Lindstrom Y, Piskurich JF, Felix NJ, Wang Y, Brickey WJ, et al. 1999. Reduced IL-4-, lipopolysaccharide-, and IFN-γ-induced MHC class II expression in mice lacking class II transactivator due to targeted deletion of the GTP-binding domain. *J. Immunol.* 163:2425–31

65. Koonin EV, Aravind L. 2000. The NACHT family—a new group of predicted NTPases implicated in apoptosis and MHC transcription activation. *Trends Biochem. Sci.* 25:223–24

66. Riley JL, Westerheide SD, Price JA, Brown JA, Boss JM. 1995. Activation of class II MHC genes requires both the X box region and the class II transactivator (CIITA). *Immunity* 2:533–43

67. Zhou H, Glimcher LH. 1995. Human MHC class II gene transcription directed by the carboxyl terminus of CIITA, one of the defective genes in type II MHC combined immune deficiency. *Immunity* 2:545–53

68. Nickerson K, Sisk TJ, Inohara N, Yee CSK, Kennell J, et al. 2001. Dendritic cell-specific MHC class II transactivator contains a caspase recruitment domain that confers potent transactivation activity. *J. Biol. Chem.* 276:19089–93

69. Chin KC, Li GG, Ting JP. 1997. Importance of acidic, proline/serine/threonine-rich, and GTP-binding regions in the

major histocompatibility complex class II transactivator: generation of transdominant-negative mutants. *Proc. Natl. Acad. Sci. USA* 94:2501–6

70. Harton JA, Cressman DE, Chin KC, Der CJ, Ting JP. 1999. GTP binding by class II transactivator: role in nuclear import. *Science* 285:1402–5

71. Kretsovali A, Spilianakis C, Dimakopoulos A, Makatounakis T, Papamatheakis J. 2001. Self-association of class II transactivator correlates with its intracellular localization and transactivation. *J. Biol. Chem.* 276:32191–97

72. Sisk TJ, Roys S, Chang CH. 2001. Self-association of CIITA and its transactivation potential. *Mol. Cell. Biol.* 21:4919–28

73. Raval A, Weissman JD, Howcroft TK, Singer DS. 2003. The GTP-binding domain of class II transactivator regulates its nuclear export. *J. Immunol.* 170:922–30

74. Bertin J, Nir WJ, Fischer CM, Tayber OV, Errada PR, et al. 1999. Human CARD4 protein is a novel CED-4/Apaf-1 cell death family member that activates NF-κB. *J. Biol. Chem.* 274:12955–58

75. Zou H, Henzel WJ, Liu X, Lutschg A, Wang X. 1997. Apaf-1, a human protein homologous to *C. elegans* CED-4, participates in cytochrome c-dependent activation of caspase-3. *Cell* 90:405–13

76. Li P, Nijhawan D, Budihardjo I, Srinivasula SM, Ahmad M, et al. 1997. Cytochrome c and dATP-dependent formation of Apaf-1/caspase-9 complex initiates an apoptotic protease cascade. *Cell* 91:479–89

77. Srinivasula SM, Ahmad M, Fernandes-Alnemri T, Alnemri ES. 1998. Autoactivation of procaspase-9 by Apaf-1-mediated oligomerization. *Mol. Cell* 1:949–57

78. Kobayashi K, Inohara N, Hernandez LD, Galan JE, Nunez G, et al. 2002.

RICK/Rip2/CARDIAK mediates signalling for receptors of the innate and adaptive immune systems. *Nature* 416:194–99

79. Chin AI, Dempsey PW, Bruhn K, Miller JF, Xu Y, Cheng GH. 2002. Involvement of receptor-interacting protein 2 in innate and adaptive immune responses. *Nature* 416:190–94

80. Girardin SE, Tournebize R, Mavris M, Page AL, Li XA, et al. 2001. CARD4/Nod1 mediates NF-κB and JNK activation by invasive *Shigella flexneri*. *EMBO Rep.* 2:736–42

81. Inohara N, Ogura Y, Chen FF, Muto A, Nunez G. 2001. Human Nod1 confers responsiveness to bacterial lipopolysaccharides. *J. Biol. Chem.* 276:2551–54

82. Yoo NJ, Park WS, Kim SY, Reed JC, Son SG, et al. 2002. Nod1, a CARD protein, enhances pro-interleukin-1β processing through the interaction with procaspase-1. *Biochem. Biophys. Res. Commun.* 299:652–58

83. Ogura Y, Inohara N, Benito A, Chen FF, Yamaoka S, Nunez G. 2001. Nod2, a Nod1/Apaf-1 family member that is restricted to monocytes and activates NF-κB. *J. Biol. Chem.* 276:4812–18

84. Gutierrez O, Pipaon C, Inohara N, Fontalba A, Ogura Y, et al. 2002. Induction of Nod2 in myelomonocytic and intestinal epithelial cells via nuclear factor-κB activation. *J. Biol. Chem.* 277:41701–5

85. Lala S, Ogura Y, Osbourne C, Hor S-Y, Bromfield A, et al. 2003. Crohn's disease and the NOD2 gene: a role for Paneth cells. *Gastroenterology* 125:47–57

86. Ogura Y, Lala A, Xin W, Smith E, Dowds TZ, et al. 2003. Expression of NOD2 in Paneth cells: a possible link to Crohn's ileitis. *Gut* 52:1591–97

87. Hugot JP, Chamaillard M, Zouali H, Lesage S, Cezard JP, et al. 2001. Association of NOD2 leucine-rich repeat variants

with susceptibility to Crohn's disease. *Nature* 411:599–603

88. Ogura Y, Bonen DK, Inohara N, Nicolae DL, Chen FF, et al. 2001. A frameshift mutation in NOD2 associated with susceptibility to Crohn's disease. *Nature* 411:603–6

89. Miceli-Richard C, Lesage S, Ryobojad M, Prieur AM, Manouvrier-Hanu S, et al. 2001. CARD15 mutations in Blau syndrome. *Nat. Genet.* 29:19–20

90. Chamaillard M, Philpott D, Girardin SE, Zouali H, Lesage S, et al. 2003. Gene-environment interaction modulated by allelic heterogeneity in inflammatory diseases. *Proc. Natl. Acad. Sci. USA* 100:3455–60

91. Hoffman HM, Mueller JL, Broide DH, Wanderer AA, Kolodner RD. 2001. Mutation of a new gene encoding a putative pyrin-like protein causes familial cold autoinflammatory syndrome and Muckle-Wells syndrome. *Nat. Genet.* 29:301–5

92. Manji GA, Wang L, Geddes BJ, Brown M, Merriam S, et al. 2002. PYPAF1, a PYRIN-containing Apaf1-like protein that assembles with ASC and regulates activation of NF-κB. *J. Biol. Chem.* 277:11570–75

93. Aganna E, Martinon F, Hawkins PN, Ross JB, Swan DC, et al. 2002. Association of mutations in the *NALP3/CIAS1/PYPAF1* gene with a broad phenotype including recurrent fever, cold sensitivity, sensorineural deafness, and AA amyloidosis. *Arthritis Rheum.* 46:2445–52

94. Feldmann J, Prieur AM, Quartier P, Berquin P, Certain S, et al. 2002. Chronic infantile neurological cutaneous and articular syndrome is caused by mutations in *CIAS1*, a gene highly expressed in polymorphonuclear cells and chondrocytes. *Am. J. Hum. Genet.* 71:198–203

95. Kikuchi-Yanoshita R, Taketomi Y, Koga K, Sugiki T, Atsumi Y, et al. 2003. Induction of PYPAF1 during in vitro maturation of mouse mast cells. *J. Biochem.* 134:699–709

96. Srinivasula SM, Poyet JL, Razmara M, Datta P, Zhang ZJ, Alnemri ES. 2002. The PYRIN-CARD protein ASC is an activating adaptor for caspase-1. *J. Biol. Chem.* 277:21119–22

97. Dowds TA, Masumoto J, Chen FF, Ogura Y, Inohara N, Nunez G. 2003. Regulation of cryopyrin/Pypaf1 signaling by pyrin, the familial Mediterranean fever gene product. *Biochem. Biophys. Res. Commun.* 302:575–80

98. Stehlik C, Lee SH, Dorfleutner A, Stassinopoulos A, Sagara J, Reed JC. 2003. Apoptosis-associated speck-like protein containing a caspase recruitment domain is a regulator of procaspase-1 activation. *J. Immunol.* 171:6154–63

99. O'Connor WJ, Harton JA, Zhu X, Linhoff M, Ting JP. 2003. Cutting edge: CIAS1/Cryopyrin/PYPAF1/NALP3 is an inducible inflammatory mediator with NF-κB suppressive properties. *J. Immunol.* 171:6329–33

100. Stehlik C, Fiorentino L, Dorfleutner A, Bruey JM, Ariza EM, et al. 2002. The PAAD/PYRIN-family protein ASC is a dual regulator of a conserved step in nuclear factor-κB activation pathways. *J. Exp. Med.* 196:1605–15

101. Liston P, Roy N, Tamai K, Lefebvre C, Baird S, et al. 1996. Suppression of apoptosis in mammalian cells by NAIP and a related family of IAP genes. *Nature* 379:349–53

102. Matsunaga T, Ishida T, Takekawa M, Nishimura S, Adachi M, Imai K. 2002. Analysis of gene expression during maturation of immature dendritic cells derived from peripheral blood monocytes. *Scand. J. Immunol.* 56:593–601

103. Roy N, Mahadevan MS, McLean M, Shutler G, Yaraghi Z, et al. 1995. The gene for neuronal apoptosis inhibitory protein is partially deleted in individuals with spinal muscular atrophy. *Cell* 80:167–78

104. Segal G, Shuman HA. 1998. How is the intracellular fate of the *Legionella*

pneumophila phagosome determined? *Trends Microbiol.* 6:253–55

105. Joshi AD, Sturgill-Koszycki S, Swanson MS. 2001. Evidence that Dot-dependent and -independent factors isolate the *Legionella pneumophila* phagosome from the endocytic network in mouse macrophages. *Cell Microbiol.* 3:99–114

106. Diez E, Lee SH, Gauthier S, Yaraghi Z, Tremblay M, et al. 2003. *Birc1e* is the gene within the *Lgn1* locus associated with resistance to *Legionella pneumophila*. *Nat. Genet.* 33:55–60

107. Bertin J, DiStefano PS. 2000. The PYRIN domain: a novel motif found in apoptosis and inflammation proteins. *Cell Death Differ.* 7:1273–74

108. Hlaing T, Guo RF, Dilley KA, Loussia JM, Morrish TA, et al. 2001. Molecular cloning and characterization of DEFCAP-L and -S, two isoforms of a novel member of the mammalian Ced-4 family of apoptosis proteins. *J. Biol. Chem.* 276:9230–38

109. Chu ZL, Pio F, Xie ZH, Welsh K, Krajewska M, et al. 2001. A novel enhancer of the Apaf1 apoptosome involved in cytochrome c-dependent caspase activation and apoptosis. *J. Biol. Chem.* 276:9239–45

110. Cain K, Bratton SB, Langlais C, Walker G, Brown DG, et al. 2000. Apaf-1 oligomerizes into biologically active approximately 700-kDa and inactive approximately 1.4-MDa apoptosome complexes. *J. Biol. Chem.* 275:6067–70

111. Peijnenburg A, Van den Berg R, Van Eggermond MJ, Sanal O, Vossen JM, et al. 2000. Defective MHC class II expression in an MHC class II deficiency patient is caused by a novel deletion of a splice donor site in the MHC class II trans-activator gene. *Immunogenetics* 51:42–49

112. Bontron S, Steimle V, Ucla C, Eibl MM, Mach B. 1997. Two novel mutations in the MHC class II transactivator CIITA in a second patient from MHC class II deficiency complementation group A. *Hum. Genet.* 99:541–46

113. Dziembowska M, Fondaneche MC, Vedrenne J, Barbieri G, Wiszniewski W, et al. 2002. Three novel mutations of the CIITA gene in MHC class II-deficient patients with a severe immunodeficiency. *Immunogenetics* 53:821–29

114. Cressman DE, Chin KC, Taxman DJ, Ting JP. 1999. A defect in the nuclear translocation of CIITA causes a form of type II bare lymphocyte syndrome. *Immunity* 10:163–71

115. Brown JA, He XF, Westerheide SD, Boss JM. 1996. Characterization of the expressed CIITA allele in the class II MHC transcriptional mutant RJ2.2.5. *Immunogenetics* 43:88–91

116. Quan V, Towey M, Sacks S, Kelly AP. 1999. Absence of MHC class II gene expression in a patient with a single amino acid substitution in the class II transactivator protein CIITA. *Immunogenetics* 49:957–63

117. Wiszniewski W, Fondaneche MC, Le Deist F, Kanariou M, Selz F, et al. 2001. Mutation in the class II trans-activator leading to a mild immunodeficiency. *J. Immunol.* 167:1787–94

118. Bonen DK, Cho JH. 2003. The genetics of inflammatory bowel disease. *Gastroenterology* 124:532–36

119. Lesage S, Zouali H, Cezard JP, Colombel JF, Belaiche J, et al. 2002. CARD15/NOD2 mutational analysis and genotype-phenotype correlation in 612 patients with inflammatory bowel disease. *Am. J. Hum. Genet.* 70:845–57

120. Vermeire S, Wild G, Kocher K, Cousineau J, Dufresne L, et al. 2002. CARD15 genetic variation in a Quebec population: prevalence, genotype-phenotype relationship, and haplotype structure. *Am. J. Hum. Genet.* 71:74–83

121. Guo QS, Xia B, Jiang Y, Qu Y, Li J. 2004. NOD2 3020insC frameshift mutation is not associated with inflammatory bowel

disease in Chinese patients of Han nationality. *World J. Gastroenterol.* 10:1069–71

122. Sugimura M, Kinouchi Y, Takahashi S, Aihara H, Takagi S, et al. 2003. *CARD15/NOD2* mutational analysis in Japanese patients with Crohn's disease. *Clin. Genet.* 63:160–62

123. Yamazaki K, Takazoe M, Tanaka T, Kazumori T, Nakamura Y. 2002. Absence of mutation in the *NOD2/CARD15* gene among 483 Japanese patients with Crohn's disease. *J. Hum. Genet.* 47:469–72

124. Inoue N, Tamura K, Kinouchi Y, Fukuda Y, Takahashi S, et al. 2002. Lack of common *NOD2* variants in Japanese patients with Crohn's disease. *Gastroenterology* 123:86–91

125. Tanabe T, Chamaillard M, Ogura Y, Zhu L, Qiu S, et al. 2004. Regulatory regions and critical residues of NOD2 involved in muramyl dipeptide recognition. *EMBO J.* 23:1587–97

126. Hisamatsu T, Suzuki M, Reinecker HC, Nadeau WJ, McCormick BA, et al. 2003. CARD15/NOD2 functions as an antibacterial factor in human intestinal epithelial cells. *Gastroenterology* 124:993–1000

127. Ayabe T, Satchell DP, Wilson CL, Parks WC, Selsted ME, et al. 2000. Secretion of microbicidal α-defensins by intestinal Paneth cells in response to bacteria. *Nat. Immunol.* 1:113–18

128. Aldhous MC, Nimmo ER, Satsangi J. 2003. NOD2/CARD15 and the Paneth cell: another piece in the genetic jigsaw of inflammatory bowel disease. *Gut* 52:1533–35

129. Russo MP, Boudreau F, Li FL, Panja A, Traber PG, et al. 2001. NF-κB blockade exacerbates experimental colitis in transgenic mice expressing an intestinal epithelial cells specific IκB super-repressor. *Gastroenterology* 120(5):A70. 369 Suppl. 1 (Abstr.)

130. Bouma G, Strober W. 2003. The immunological and genetic basis of inflammatory bowel disease. *Nat. Rev. Immunol.* 3:521–33

131. Pauleau AL, Murray PJ. 2003. Role of Nod2 in the response of macrophages to Toll-like receptor agonists. *Mol. Cell. Biol.* 23:7531–39

132. Watanabe T, Kitani A, Murray PJ, Strober W. 2004. NOD2 is a negative regulator of Toll-like receptor 2-mediated T helper type 1 responses. *Nat. Immunol.* 5:800–8

133. Alonso D, Elgart GW, Schachner LA. 2003. Blau syndrome: a new kindred. *J. Am. Acad. Dermatol.* 49:299–302

134. Kile RL, Rusk HA. 1940. A case of cold urticaria with an unusual family history. *JAMA* 114:1067–68

135. Tindall JP, Beeker SK, Rosse WF. 1969. Familial cold urticaria. A generalized reaction involving leukocytosis. *Arch. Intern. Med.* 124:129–34

136. Aksentijevich I, Nowak M, Mallah M, Chae JJ, Watford WT, et al. 2002. *De novo CIAS1* mutations, cytokine activation, and evidence for genetic heterogeneity in patients with neonatal-onset multisystem inflammatory disease (NOMID): a new member of the expanding family of pyrin-associated autoinflammatory diseases. *Arthritis Rheum.* 46:3340–48

137. Hawkins PN, Lachmann HJ, McDermott MF. 2003. Interleukin-1-receptor antagonist in the Muckle-Wells syndrome. *N. Engl. J. Med.* 348:2583–84

138. Hawkins PN, Lachmann HJ, Aganna E, McDermott MF. 2004. Spectrum of clinical features in Muckle-Wells syndrome and response to anakinra. *Arthritis Rheum.* 50:607–12

139. Neven B, Callebaut I, Prieur AM, Feldmann J, Bodemer C, et al. 2004. Molecular basis of the spectral expression of *CIAS1* mutations associated with phagocytic cell-mediated autoinflammatory disorders CINCA/NOMID, MWS, and FCU. *Blood* 103:2809–15

140. Dowds TA, Masumoto J, Zhu L, Inohara N, Nunez G. 2004. Cryopyrin-induced interleukin 1β secretion in monocytic cells:

enhanced activity of disease-associated mutants and requirement for ASC. *J. Biol. Chem.* 279:21924–28

141. Maier JKX, Lahoua Z, Gendron NH, Fetni R, Johnston A, et al. 2002. The neuronal apoptosis inhibitory protein is a direct inhibitor of caspases 3 and 7. *J. Neurosci.* 22:2035–43

142. Sanna MG, Correia JD, Ducrey O, Lee J, Nomoto K, et al. 2002. IAP suppression of apoptosis involves distinct mechanisms: the TAK1/JNK1 signaling cascade and caspase inhibition. *Mol. Cell. Biol.* 22:1754–66

143. Wright EK, Goodart SA, Growney JD, Hadinoto V, Endrizzi MG, et al. 2003. *Naip5* affects host susceptibility to the intracellular pathogen *Legionella pneumophila. Curr. Biol.* 13:27–36

144. Iannaccone ST, Smith SA, Simard LR. 2004. Spinal muscular atrophy. *Curr. Neurol. Neurosci. Rep.* 4:74–80

145. Gotz R, Karch C, Digby MR, Troppmair J, Rapp UR, et al. 2000. The neuronal apoptosis inhibitory protein suppresses neuronal differentiation and apoptosis in PC12 cells. *Hum. Mol. Genet.* 9:2479–89

146. Xu DG, Crocker SJ, Doucet JP, St-Jean M, Tamai K, et al. 1997. Elevation of neuronal expression of NAIP reduces ischemic damage in the rat hippocampus. *Nat. Med.* 3:997–1004

147. Deveraux QL, Roy N, Stennicke HR, Van Arsdale T, Zhou Q, et al. 1998. IAPs block apoptotic events induced by caspase-8 and cytochrome c by direct inhibition of distinct caspases. *EMBO J.* 17:2215–23

148. Mercer EA, Korhonen L, Skoglosa Y, Olsson PA, Kukkonen JP, et al. 2000. NAIP interacts with hippocalcin and protects neurons against calcium-induced cell death through caspase-3-dependent and -independent pathways. *EMBO J.* 19:3597–607

149. Growney JD, Dietrich WF. 2000. High-resolution genetic and physical map of the *Lgn1* interval in C57BL/6J implicates *Naip2* or *Naip5* in *Legionella pneumophila* pathogenesis. *Genome Res.* 10:1158–71

150. Holcik M, Thompson CS, Yaraghi Z, Lefebvre CA, MacKenzie AE, et al. 2000. The hippocampal neurons of *neuronal apoptosis inhibitory protein 1 (NAIP1)*-deleted mice display increased vulnerability to kainic acid-induced injury. *Proc. Natl. Acad. Sci. USA* 97:2286–90

151. Diez E, Yaraghi Z, MacKenzie A, Gros P. 2000. The neuronal apoptosis inhibitory protein (Naip) is expressed in macrophages and is modulated after phagocytosis and during intracellular infection with *Legionella pneumophila. J. Immunol.* 164:1470–77

152. Linardopoulou E, Mefford HC, Nguyen O, Friedman C, van den Engh G, et al. 2001. Transcriptional activity of multiple copies of a subtelomerically located olfactory receptor gene that is polymorphic in number and location. *Hum. Mol. Genet.* 10:2373–83

153. Mefford HC, Linardopoulou E, Coil D, van den Engh G, Trask BJ. 2001. Comparative sequencing of a multicopy subtelomeric region containing olfactory receptor genes reveals multiple interactions between non-homologous chromosomes. *Hum. Mol. Genet.* 10:2363–72

154. Samonte RV, Eichler EE. 2002. Segmental duplications and the evolution of the primate genome. *Nat. Rev. Genet.* 3:65–72

155. Nahon JL. 2003. Birth of 'human-specific' genes during primate evolution. *Genetica* 118:193–208

156. Wang Y, Hasegawa M, Imamura R, Kinoshita T, Kondo C, et al. 2004. PYNOD, a novel Apaf-1/CED4-like protein is an inhibitor of ASC and caspase-1. *Int. Immunol.* 16:777–86

Annu. Rev. Immunol. 2005. 23:415–45
doi: 10.1146/annurev.immunol.23.021704.115606
Copyright © 2005 by Annual Reviews. All rights reserved
First published online as a Review in Advance on November 29, 2004

B CELL SIGNALING AND TUMORIGENESIS

Hassan Jumaa,[1] Rudolf W. Hendriks,[2] and Michael Reth[1]

[1]Institute for Biology III, Albert-Ludwigs University of Freiburg and Max Planck Institute for Immunobiology, 79108 Freiburg, Germany; email: jumaa@immunbio.mpg.de, reth@immunbio.mpg.de
[2]Department of Immunology, Erasmus MC Rotterdam NL-3000 DR Rotterdam, The Netherlands; email: r.hendriks@erasmusmc.nl

Key Words B cell development, leukemia, SLP-65, BLNK, Btk

■ **Abstract** The proliferation and differentiation of lymphocytes are regulated by receptors localized on the cell surface. Engagement of these receptors induces the activation of intracellular signaling proteins that transmit the receptor signals to distinct targets and control the cellular responses. The first signaling proteins to be discovered in higher organisms were the products of oncogenes. For example, the kinases Src and Abelson (Abl) were originally identified as oncogenes and were later characterized as important proteins for signal transduction in various cell types, including lymphocytes. Now, as many cellular signaling molecules have been discovered and ordered into certain pathways, we can better understand why particular signaling proteins are associated with tumorigenesis. In this review, we discuss recent progress in unraveling the molecular mechanisms of signaling pathways that control the proliferation and differentiation of early B cells. We point out the concepts of auto-inhibition and subcellular localization as crucial aspects in the regulation of B cell signaling.

INTRODUCTION

The development of B lymphocytes from hematopoietic stem cells can be divided into distinct stages on the basis of the sequential expression or loss of cell surface or intracellular proteins and of the rearrangement of the immunoglobulin (Ig) genes (1, 2). The progression from hematopoietic stem cells to mature B cells is regulated by specific signaling mechanisms in which Ig-related receptors play a crucial role (3). In pre-B cells, successful V(D)J rearrangement of the Ig heavy chain (HC) gene results in the expression of membrane-bound μHC protein. This mμHC associates with the pre-existing surrogate light chain (SLC) consisting of λ5 and VpreB and the signaling components Ig-α/Ig-β to form the pre-B cell receptor (pre-BCR). A productive light chain (LC) gene rearrangement leads to the expression of the B cell antigen receptor (BCR), in which the LC replaces the SLC. Thus, the pre-BCR and the BCR serve as critical checkpoints that monitor successful Ig H and Ig L chain recombination, respectively. Therefore, these receptors are the main center of B cell signaling, and they control the progression of B cells through development.

Pre-BCR signaling is essential for the selection, proliferation, and differentiation of pre-B cells. Usually, the pre-BCR is only transiently expressed and therefore barely detectable on the surface of wild-type pre-B cells. Surface pre-BCR expression is associated with rapid pre-B cell expansion. Most likely, the pre-BCR role as a potent stimulator of pre-B cell proliferation is the reason for the stringent regulation of its expression. Interestingly, it is the pre-BCR itself that is responsible for this regulation. For instance, the SLC component $\lambda 5$ induces the internalization of the pre-BCR and leads to the low-level expression of the pre-BCR on the cell surface (4). In addition, a negative feedback loop of pre-BCR signaling leads to the suppression of SLC expression. After a few cycles of cell division, the pre-B cells exhaust their supply of SLC and, therefore, cannot express a pre-BCR (5). To carry on B cell development, the downregulation of SLC expression must be accompanied by the induction of recombination at the loci of the conventional LC, which replaces the SLC and is expressed together with μHC in the context of the BCR. The downregulation of SLC expression and induction of LC recombination can be considered as pre-B cell differentiation markers. Although the importance of pre-BCR signals for proliferation and differentiation is clear, the underlying mechanisms and the molecules involved are still not fully characterized. It is also unclear whether distinct sets of signaling molecules are responsible for the different pre-BCR functions that control pre-B cell proliferation and differentiation.

Activation of the pre-BCR/BCR signaling involves phosphorylation of the cytoplasmic immunoreceptor tyrosine-based activation motifs (ITAMs), which are present in the two Ig superfamily members Ig-α and Ig-β, as a first step in the formation of a lipid-raft-associated calcium-signaling module (6, 7). This complex contains three separate classes of activated protein tyrosine kinases (PTKs), the Src family kinase Lyn, the Syk/ZAP70 kinase, and the Tec-family kinase Btk (Bruton's tyrosine kinase), as well as other proteins, including the adapter molecule SH2-containing leukocyte protein of 65 kDa (SLP-65, also known as BLNK or BASH), phosphoinositide 3-kinase (PI3K), Vav (a guanine nucleotide exchange factor for the Rho/Rac family of GTPases), and phospholipase C-$\gamma 2$ (PLC$\gamma 2$). Targeted disruption of structural components or downstream signaling proteins of the pre-BCR or BCR complex results in characteristic arrests in B cell development (Figure 1). Importantly, the expression and activity of proteins that are critically involved in signal transduction in B cells are strictly regulated. Syk is activated by binding to the phosphorylated ITAM tyrosines of Ig-α or Ig-β and most likely acts as a positive allosteric enzyme that can amplify BCR signals through the initiation of a positive feedback loop (8). The apparent redundancy among the Src family members Lyn, Fyn, and Blk has complicated the clarification of the role of the individual enzymes. Nevertheless, the ability of an activated Blk mutant to increase Ig-β and Syk phosphorylation demonstrated an important capacity of Src family kinases as well as their proximal point of action (9). By analogy with the BCR in mature B cells, it is assumed that activation of PLC$\gamma 2$ by Syk and Btk results in the

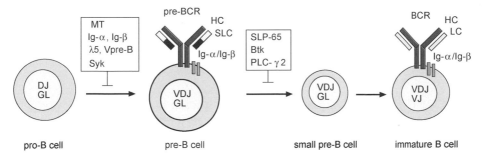

Figure 1   A simplified scheme of B cell development. Productive rearrangement of the HC gene locus in pro-B cells results in pre-BCR expression on pre-B cells. Productive rearrangement of one of the LC gene loci in small pre-B cells leads to BCR expression on immature B cells. Inactivation of the indicated genes results in specific maturation arrests during B cell development. GL, germline configuration of the Ig genes.

production of the second messengers, inositol-1,4,5-trisphosphate (IP3) and diacylglycerol (DAG), which activate calcium signaling, protein kinase C (PKC), and subsequently NF-κB (6, 10–13). However, as this model was recently challenged by the description of a separate pre-BCR signaling route in which the activation of NF-κB signaling is Syk-independent but involves Src family PTKs as well as PKCλ (14), further experiments are required to characterize the pre-BCR signaling pathways in substantial detail.

CONTROL OF B CELL SIGNALING

The phenomena of auto-inhibition and relocalization of signaling proteins to specific subcellular compartments play an important role in the initiation and regulation of signaling, which only recently has become more appreciated (15, 16). The characterization of these mechanisms helps to understand better the deregulation caused by oncogene products. Receptors as well as intracellular signaling proteins should only become active under the right circumstances and at the appropriate place within the cell. To ensure this, the activity and the subcellular localization of signaling proteins are controlled by several mechanisms. One common mechanism involves the intrinsic ability of a signaling molecule to return to a closed, inactive conformation. Such auto-inhibition may be mediated by a regulatory domain, which folds over and blocks the access to the catalytic or effector domain of a signaling protein. Signal transduction requires a shift in the equilibrium between a closed auto-inhibited conformation and an open signaling active conformation. This shift can be mediated either by protein modifications or by binding of a regulatory subunit to its target structures. Therefore, in most cases signals are generated only at certain places inside the cell. The equilibrium between auto-inhibition and activation is also affected by negative regulatory elements like protein tyrosine phosphatases (PTPs) that counteract the activation and allow signal amplification only if critical thresholds are reached.

ABL

The PTK c-Abl and its oncogenic forms v-Abl and BCR-ABL (17) provide good examples of these regulatory principles. The crystal structure of the c-Abl protein shows a conformation in which the SH2 and SH3 domain folds over the catalytic domain of c-Abl, resulting in auto-inhibition of the kinase activity (18, 19). In the case of the c-Abl 1b form, binding of the N-terminal myristoyl modification to the kinase domain further stabilizes the closed and therefore inactive conformation. An N-terminal truncation and fusion with another protein moiety as shown by the oncogenic forms of Abl can prevent the auto-inhibitory conformation and lead to a constitutive activation of the Abl kinase. More importantly, the oncogenic modifications result in a relocalization of the active kinase to a place in the cell where the kinase is presumably protected from the action of negative regulatory PTPs. At these cellular sites, the oncogenic Abl forms can interact with other signaling partners (20). The myristoylated v-Abl is localized in specialized membrane domains such as rafts and the myristoylation anchor of v-Abl is required for the transformation of NIH/3T3 cells (21). The BCR-ABL oncogene product shows an N-terminal deletion interfering with the auto-inhibition of the normal c-Abl protein. In addition, the coiled-coil structure of the BCR part of BCR-ABL mediates tetramerization and presumably a specific relocalization of the deregulated kinase (20).

The Syk Tyrosine Kinase

The importance of auto-inhibition and relocalization has also been recently recognized in signal transductions from the BCR. The engagement of the BCR results in a rapid activation of the Src family kinase Lyn and the cytosolic kinase Syk, both of which are regulated by auto-inhibition (22). In the case of Syk, the two N-terminal tandem SH2 domains inhibit the activity of the kinase domains (23). This auto-inhibition is only released if Syk meets its activation sequence, namely the ITAMs that are located in the cytosolic tails of the Ig-α/Ig-β heterodimer of the BCR (8, 24). The binding to phosphorylated Ig-α or Ig-β places the active Syk in the right position to allow further phosphorylation of neighboring ITAM sequences. This results in further Syk recruitment and activation, which then lead to the amplification of the BCR signal (25). However, the process of Syk recruitment and activation is under tight control of membrane-bound or cytosolic PTPs, which efficiently eliminate the phospho groups at the ITAMs and thus counteract Syk activation (26). Without additional regulation, PTPs prevent the positive amplification loop generated by Syk after binding to phosphorylated ITAMs (8). Therefore, another critical event in B cell activation, apart from the release of Syk from auto-inhibition, is the relocalization of the BCR/Syk complex to a place inside the cells where PTPs are not active. For example, the colocalization of the BCR together with an active oxidase, producing superoxide anions and hydrogen peroxides, should result in the oxidation of a critical cysteine in the catalytic domain of BCR-proximal PTPs and their inactivation (27). Signal transduction from the BCR thus seems to require not only kinase activation but also PTP inhibition via the relocalization of the BCR to subcellular sites with high oxidase activity.

The Lyn Tyrosine Kinase

The Src family kinase Lyn might support BCR activation by phosphorylating the first tyrosine of the ITAM sequence and other BCR proximal signaling elements and presumably by stimulating oxidase activity (8). Apart from its positive effect on BCR signaling, however, Lyn participates in a negative feedback loop that terminates BCR signaling. Upon activation, Lyn phosphorylates inhibitory receptors like CD22 and CD72, which are then bound by phosphatases that dephosphorylate the ITAMs and inhibit signal transduction (28). Indeed, B cells from Lyn-deficient mice do not show drastic developmental defects and are hyperreactive rather than hyporeactive (29, 30). Furthermore, Lyn-deficient mice show a high susceptibility to the development of autoimmune diseases, characterized by circulating autoreactive antibodies and the deposition of IgG immune complexes in the kidney (31). These results demonstrate the importance of Lyn as an inhibitory element of BCR signaling, whereas Lyn's role as a positive signaling element of BCR signaling is only seen if Lyn deficiency is combined with deficiencies of other signaling elements, such as Btk (32).

In the chicken B cell line DT40, Lyn deficiency results in the reduction of both calcium mobilization and tyrosine phosphorylation of substrate proteins. In contrast, Syk deficiency results in a complete loss of calcium mobilization, indicating that Syk plays a dominant role in this context compared with Lyn (22, 33). Similarly, murine B cells deficient for Syk family kinases, namely Syk and ZAP70, show a severe block of early B cell development at the pre-B cell stage and a defective allelic exclusion (34). In addition to its role as a tyrosine kinase, Syk may also perform an adaptor protein function. For example, upon activation, Syk becomes phosphorylated at several tyrosines, which are situated in the linker region between the two SH2 domains or between the SH2 domain and the kinase domain (35, 36). These phosphorylated tyrosines may be required for the binding and recruitment of other signaling proteins that participate in signaling. For instance, phosphorylation of tyrosine 341 of Syk has been implicated as a binding site for SH2 domains of PLCγ2 and Vav (36, 37). The impacts of the adaptor protein function and tyrosine kinase activity of Syk on B cell proliferation and differentiation are currently unclear. Nonetheless, Syk is one of the dominant driving forces for the proliferation and expansion of the early pre-B cells, as murine B cells deficient of Syk kinase activity are blocked at the pro-B cell stage and do not enter the proliferation program of pre-B cells (34).

Pre-B Cell Proliferation

The activation of PI3K and the Ras/Raf/MEK/Erk pathways by Syk may provide the essential mechanisms of Syk-induced proliferation (38). PI3K activation results in the activation of the adaptor protein BAM32 (39) and other effector signaling proteins, including PKB/AKT, which promotes cell proliferation and suppresses apoptosis (40). Indeed, Syk activation was shown to be necessary for PI3K activity in B cells (41). The important role of Syk in the proliferation program of pre-B cells implies that Syk has the potential of an oncogene. However, mutations or translocations affecting the Syk gene have rarely been found in leukemias (42). To prevent transformation by Syk, pre-B cells may have developed several negative regulatory feedback loops to control the proliferation signals provided by Syk. One of these loops clearly involves the adapter protein SLP-65, which leads to the downregulation of the pre-BCR and subsequent limitation of Syk activity (see below). However, Syk activity is also strongly controlled by phosphatases as described above. In addition, the expression level of Syk is strictly controlled by protein degradation. In this context, the proto-oncogene Cbl plays an important role (43, 44). Phosphorylation of Syk at tyrosine 317 provides a binding site for the phosphotyrosine binding (PTB) domain of Cbl (45–47). In addition to the adaptor protein function, Cbl contains a ring domain and functions as an ubiquitin ligase, which is part of a complex mediating the rapid ubiquitination and subsequent degradation of Syk (48). This Cbl-mediated degradation of Syk might be an important negative regulatory loop, which limits the amount and range of active Syk in the B cells. Although Syk itself is only rarely implicated in lymphocyte tumors, two Syk-associated proteins, Cbl and Vav, were first identified as proto-oncogenes, indicating that they are important in the regulation of the Syk-mediated proliferation signals (37, 49).

THE ADAPTOR PROTEIN SLP-65 IS A TUMOR SUPPRESSOR

SLP-65 and Pre-B Cell Differentiation

Since its identification as a signaling component that is phosphorylated upon BCR engagement, SLP-65 has become the central element in pre-BCR/BCR signaling. SLP-65 is one of the most prominent targets of Syk kinase activity, which phosphorylates SLP-65 on several tyrosines following BCR stimulation. Phosphorylated SLP-65 provides docking sites for various signaling proteins, including Grb2, Vav, Nck, PLC-γ2, Btk, and the pre-BCR/BCR subunit Ig-α, thereby coupling the pre-BCR/BCR with downstream signaling elements (50, 51). The central role of SLP-65 in B cell signaling was highlighted by the phenotype of the SLP-65-deficient mice (52–55), which is comparable to the X-linked immunodeficiency (*xid*) phenotype found in mice deficient for Btk (see below). These mice show strongly reduced overall numbers of mature B cells, absence of CD5$^+$ (B1)

B cells, reduced serum levels of IgM and IgG3, impaired responses to thymus-independent antigens, and a reduced capacity of B cells to proliferate in vitro in response to various stimuli (52). The consequences of SLP-65 deficiency are even more severe in humans, leading to agammaglobulinemia similar to XLA (X-linked agammaglobulinemia), which is caused by mutations in Btk (56).

Several lines of evidence suggest that the adaptor protein SLP-65 is a central element in transmitting the differentiation signals of the pre-BCR (Figure 2). For instance, pre-B cells deficient for SLP-65 show a remarkable increase of surface pre-BCR expression and an enhanced proliferation rate. The expression of the pre-BCR is required for the proliferation of SLP-65-deficient pre-B cells because SLP-65-deficient cells lacking components of the pre-BCR display a reduced proliferation rate. Reconstitution of SLP-65 expression results in downregulation of surface pre-BCR expression and enhanced pre-B cell differentiation (57, 58). These data suggest that although SLP-65 is required for the pre-BCR signals that lead to pre-BCR downregulation and pre-B cell differentiation, it is not required for signals inducing pre-B cell proliferation. The essential role of Syk compared with the dispensable role of SLP-65 in pre-B cell proliferation suggests that Syk transmits the pre-BCR signals that induce proliferation via a signaling cascade lacking or independent of SLP-65. In contrast, SLP-65 has a negative effect on pre-B cell proliferation because it causes the downregulation of both pre-BCR and IL-7R expression (57, 59).

It is feasible that activated Syk alone, in the absence of any downstream adapter proteins, is able to induce some PLCγ activation, although this apparently does not result in a full calcium response. However, suboptimal PLCγ activation may produce enough DAG to recruit the GDP/GTP exchange factor Ras-GRP to the membrane, resulting in Ras activation and signal transduction through the Ras/Raf/MEK/Erk pathway (Figure 2). Syk activation in SLP-65-deficient pre-B cells may stimulate the Erk pathway, which is essential for the high proliferation rate of these pre-B cells (57, 60). Although not yet directly shown by genetic or biochemical experiments, it is feasible that the adapter function of Syk is involved in the activation of the Erk pathway.

SLP-65 and Pre-B Cell Leukemia

A main consequence of SLP-65 deficiency is the elevated pre-BCR expression on the cell surface, resulting in a permanent Syk activation and enhanced proliferation of SLP-65-deficient pre-B cells. A further dramatic consequence of SLP-65 deficiency is the development of pre-B cell leukemia. In roughly 6% of these mice at the age of 10 weeks, splenomegaly and occasionally solid tumors were found. The affected mice showed penetration of pre-B cells in all tissues (57). These data suggest that SLP-65 acts as a tumor suppressor that limits the proliferation of pre-B cells. Strong evidence for the tumor suppressor role of SLP-65 is provided by experiments showing that SLP-65-deficient pre-B cells cause leukemia when injected into immune-deficient mice, whereas reconstitution of SLP-65 expression

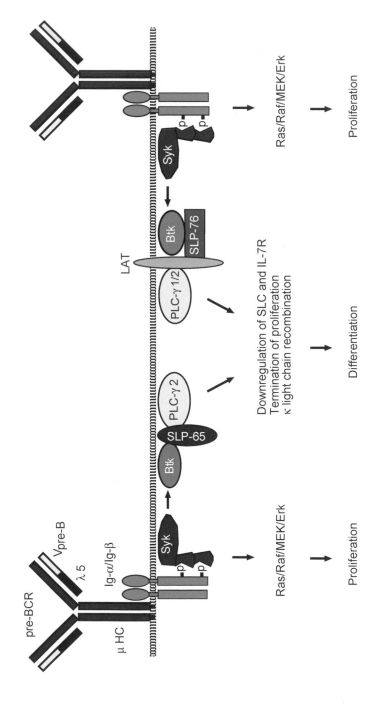

Figure 2   Distinct signaling pathways regulate the proliferation and differentiation of pre-B cells. The adaptor protein SLP-65, in association with Btk, is required for the differentiation signals that downregulate the SLC and induce the recombination of the LC gene locus. An alternative complex containing SLP-76 and LAT participates in the transduction of pre-BCR signals for pre-B cell differentiation. The proliferation of pre-B cells is induced by SLP-65-independent pre-BCR signals, which are supported by signaling from the IL-7 receptor (not depicted).

stimulated the differentiation of these cells and inhibited their potential to cause leukemia (61). Although these data point to a tumor suppressor role of SLP-65, they suggest that SLP-65 deficiency alone is not sufficient to cause leukemia development because the majority of the SLP-65-deficient mice do not develop leukemia. SLP-65 deficiency is rather the first event that requires secondary mutations for the transformation of pre-B cells and leukemia development. Likely targets of these secondary mutations are the signaling proteins involved in pre-B cell differentiation. SLP-65-deficient pre-B cells are only partially blocked in differentiation, which suggests that residual pre-BCR signals are still transmitted, enabling pre-B cell differentiation in the absence of SLP-65. This residual pre-BCR signaling depends on the adaptor proteins LAT (linker for activation of T cells) and SLP-76 (58) (Figure 2). LAT and SLP-76 are well-known adaptor proteins essential for signaling from the T cell receptor (TCR) (62). Mutations affecting the residual pre-BCR signaling and thus the residual differentiation capacity of SLP-65-deficient pre-B cells should increase the frequency of leukemia in SLP-65-deficient mice. Indeed, SLP-65/LAT-double-deficient (and SLP-65/Btk-double-deficient; see below) mice show a severe block of pre-B cell differentiation and an increased incidence of pre-B cell leukemia (58; H. Jumaa, unpublished results). Similarly, SLP-65/CD19-double-deficient mice also show a severe block in B cell differentiation and increased frequency of pre-B cell leukemia compared with SLP-65-deficient mice (63).

Further targets for secondary mutations that transform SLP-65-deficient pre-B cells may belong to the signaling pathway of the IL-7 receptor. SLP-65-deficient pre-B cells require IL-7 for survival and proliferation, although they can proliferate even at low IL-7 concentrations (57). Mutations affecting IL-7 receptor signaling may render SLP-65-deficient pre-B cells independent of IL-7 and result in transformation of these cells. However, it is still unclear which genes are affected by secondary mutations and what mechanisms are responsible for these mutations.

Potential Role of the V(D)J Recombinase in Leukemia Formation

In this context, the finding of expression of the recombination-activating genes RAG-1 and RAG-2, which mediate V(D)J recombination, in strongly proliferating SLP-65-deficient pre-B cells led to the hypothesis that continuous V(D)J recombination activity may contribute to the accumulation of mutations, deletions, and/or chromosomal translocations, and finally result in the oncogenic transformation of pre-B cells (57, 63). Normally, RAG expression is transiently downregulated upon pre-BCR signaling to terminate further Ig H chain rearrangement, thus ensuring that only one functional Ig H chain is synthesized, a phenomenon referred to as allelic exclusion (64). RAG activity is coupled to the cell cycle (65, 66), because the V(D)J recombination process involves DNA cleavage and because the presence of DNA double strand breaks (DSB) during DNA replication or mitosis could interfere with faithful transmission of genetic information to daughter cells.

Moreover, incorrect repair of DNA may give rise to genomic instability, which can result in carcinogenesis through activation of proto-oncogenes or inactivation of tumor suppressor genes (67, 68). The identification, in particular B and T cell lymphomas, of translocation breakpoints in which an Ig or TCR locus was fused with other regions of chromosomal DNA containing oncogene loci first pointed at the involvement of the V(D)J recombinase system in lymphomagenesis. In recent studies, the endonuclease activity of the RAG complex was found to be essential for chromosomal translocations and oncogenic gene amplification (69–72).

Several models have been proposed to explain how the V(D)J recombinase might be involved in such chromosomal rearrangements (reviewed in 73). One model involves erroneous recombination whereby V(D)J recombinase activity results in a DSB in an antigen receptor locus, which is subsequently joined to a DSB outside that locus, generated either by RAG-mediated cleavage at a DNA region that is not a consensus V(D)J recombination signal sequence or by an unrelated RAG-independent means. Another model is that RAG proteins capture exogenous target DNA and carry out transposition-mediated genome rearrangements. Such a transposition reaction could result in chromosomal translocations and may also result in DNA insertion. This transposition reaction was recently shown to occur in vivo when an excised signal-end fragment from the TCRα locus was found to be inserted into the X-linked hypoxanthine–guanine phosphoribosyl transferase locus in human T cells (74).

V(D)J Recombinase Activity in SLP-65-Deficient Pre-B Cells

Several lines of evidence indeed suggest that tumor formation is dependent on the ongoing RAG activity in SLP-65-deficient pre-B cells: (a) RAG expression is detected both in SLP-65-deficient pre-B cells and lymphoma cells (57, 63; R.W. Hendriks, unpublished results); (b) whereas L chain rearrangement is normally only initiated in cells that have terminated SLC expression, SLP-65-deficient pre-B cell lymphomas contain cells that coexpress Ig H chain, SLC, and Ig κ L chain (75); (c) defective SLP-65 expression is associated with secondary, mostly nonproductive, V_H gene rearrangements in most BCR-ABL1 kinase-positive pre-B cell acute lymphoblastic leukemias (pre-B ALL) (76); (d) we did not detect tumor formation in a limited group of Btk/SLP-65-double-deficient mice, which were crossed onto a RAG-1-deficient background, whereby pre-B cellularity was rescued with a pre-rearranged Ig H chain transgene (R.W. Hendriks, unpublished results). Although these results indicate that RAG activity is required for the malignant transformation of SLP-65-deficient pre-B cells, the reason for RAG expression in these cells is still unclear. In particular, it is unclear whether SLP-65-deficient pre-B cells are arrested at a stage where they express the RAG enzymes or whether SLP-65 function is required for the downregulation of RAG expression.

The finding that RAG expression is downregulated in SLP-65-deficient large cycling pre-B cells suggests that RAG downregulation is independent of SLP-65

(57). As RAG downregulation is required for allelic exclusion (64), this finding may explain the intact Ig H allelic exclusion in SLP-65-deficient pre-B cells (63). This might seem contradictory to previous findings that suggested a SLP-65 role in the downregulation of RAG expression (59, 63). However, Schebesta et al. (59) reconstituted Pax-5-deficient pro-B cells with SLP-65, and it may be argued that the regulation of RAG gene expression is different in the absence of this essential transcription factor. Hayashi et al. (63) have compared pre-B cell populations from wild-type mice, SLP-65-deficient mice, and SLP-65/CD19-double-deficient mice. They found increased expression of RAG-2 protein in the absence of SLP-65. These differences do not necessarily point to a role for SLP-65 in RAG downregulation because they might reflect the different cell cycle status or stage of differentiation in these mice. When we introduced SLP-65 expression into SLP-65-deficient pre-B cells and compared them with parental cells, we found the opposite result, as SLP-65 expression induced both RAG expression and germline κ transcription (H. Jumaa, unpublished results). Taken together, the available data suggest that SLP-65-deficient pre-B cells represent a stage in which SLP-65-independent signals have already ensured Ig H allelic exclusion. This stage is characterized by basal levels of RAG expression that seem to be high enough to induce tumor formation. At this stage of development, wild-type pre-B cells downregulate the pre-BCR and become resting cells. However, SLP-65-deficient pre-B cells keep cycling owing to enhanced expression of the pre-BCR and IL-7R (57, 59), both of which induce proliferation. The importance of pre-BCR expression is demonstrated by the fact that all leukemia cells in the SLP-65-deficient mice express the pre-BCR on the cell surface, suggesting a crucial role for the pre-BCR in leukemia development. In agreement with this view, SLP-65/λ5-double-deficient mice incapable of pre-BCR expression show no signs of leukemia development. Pre-B cells from these SLP-65/λ5-double-deficient mice express a surface pre-BCR form lacking an SLC or a conventional LC (77). This LC-deficient pre-BCR seems to be sufficient for inducing allelic exclusion, but insufficient for the stimulation of pre-B cell proliferation (77, 78).

SLP-65 DEFICIENCY IN HUMAN PRE-B CELL ACUTE LYMPHOBLASTIC LEUKEMIA

In mice, SLP-65 deficiency results in a partial block in pre-B cell differentiation, whereas the proliferation capacity is enhanced owing to the increased pre-BCR expression on the cell surface. In contrast to the partial block in murine B cell development, SLP-65 deficiency in humans leads to a complete block of differentiation at the pre-B cell stage (56). A block in differentiation combined with the cell's ability to survive and proliferate is a likely model for the development of leukemia in humans. Because SLP-65 is required for the differentiation of both human and murine pre-B cells, a somatic SLP-65 deficiency in developing human pre-B cells blocks their differentiation but may not affect their survival. Indeed, we found that about half of the analyzed cases of childhood pre-B cell acute lymphoblastic leukemia (pre-B ALL), the most common cancer disease in children, shows a drastic reduction of SLP-65 expression (61). The finding that the SLP-65 gene contains alternative exons (termed exon 3a and 3b) located in intron 3 provides one mechanism to explain the reduction in SLP-65 expression. If exon 3a or 3b are included in the SLP-65 mRNA, a premature stop codon is introduced, which interrupts the open reading frame of SLP-65 and prevents protein expression. Specific splicing factors are most likely required to exclude these alternative exons from the mature SLP-65 mRNA and to allow SLP-65 protein synthesis. Alteration of this splicing program may result in SLP-65 deficiency. Currently, neither the splicing factors required for proper SLP-65 RNA splicing nor the reasons that lead to the deregulation of the splicing machinery are known. Because some viruses can reorganize the splicing machinery, a viral infection may lead to the inclusion of SLP-65 alternative exons, which reduces the ratio of normal transcripts. Consequently, the amount of SLP-65 protein is reduced and pre-B cell differentiation is hindered. In this scenario, not only a complete loss but also a reduction in the amount of SLP-65 protein may be sufficient to impede pre-B cell differentiation. Additional mutations, possibly due to continued RAG expression, would then result in cell transformation and pre-B cell leukemia. The heterogeneity in morphology and cytogenetics of the pre-B ALL lymphoblasts may result from the heterogeneity of secondary mutations that transform the cells. In this view, the postulated differentiation block, which represents the initial step in leukemia development (79), is due to a defect in SLP-65 function. This defect may affect SLP-65 expression or one of its essential interaction partners. Indeed, defective expression of two of these essential partners, Syk and Btk, was reported in the leukemic cells of childhood ALL patients (79, 80). In both cases, aberrant transcripts lacking parts of the coding sequence were found in the leukemic cells.

Two lines of evidence suggest that the inclusion of the alternative exons is the primary cause of SLP-65 deficiency in human pre-B ALL, although additional scenarios are not excluded. First, the oncogene BCR-ABL blocks pre-B cell differentiation by downregulating the expression of proteins involved in pre-BCR signaling such as SLP-65 (76). The downregulation of SLP-65 expression takes place at the level of splicing as high levels of SLP-65 transcripts containing the alternative exon 3b were detected in BCR-ABL-positive cells (76). Incubation of these cells with the BCR-ABL inhibitor STI571 increased the ratio of normal SLP-65 transcripts and induced differentiation from pre-B to the immature B cell stage (76). Similarly, leukemic cells of BCR-ABL-positive pre-B ALL patients express high levels of the exon 3b containing SLP-65 transcripts. Again, STI571 treatment increased the ratio of normal SLP-65 transcripts and induced differentiation (76). The second line of evidence for the notion that alternative splicing (e.g., recognition of exon 3b) is the primary cause for defective SLP-65 expression in pre-B ALL is the finding that a single nucleotide alteration that increases the recognition of exon 3b is more frequently found in the SLP-65 gene of pre-B ALL patients than in the normal population (H. Jumaa, unpublished results). This would be the first human polymorphism, which is correlated with the development of pre-B cell leukemia.

Exon 3b seems to be the most important alternative exon for the splicing machinery in the human SLP-65 gene. In addition to the premature stop codon, the inclusion of exon 3b introduces a downstream in-frame ATG. If included, the downstream ATG in exon 3b might generate a SLP-65 isoform lacking the N-terminus, whereas the normal ATG would, in this case, lead to the production of a protein consisting only of the SLP-65 N-terminus. Such aberrant proteins might interfere with SLP-65 function in a dominant negative fashion because they might sequester SLP-65 interaction partners and inhibit the transmission of differentiation signals from the pre-BCR. Notably, the N-terminus of SLP-65 is highly conserved and contains crucial interaction sites for SLP-65 function because deletion of this region abolishes SLP-65 activity in pre-B cell differentiation (57).

An interesting difference between the murine and human SLP-65-deficient leukemia is the correlation between pre-BCR expression and SLP-65 deficiency. As mentioned above, the increased proliferation capacity of SLP-65-deficient pre-B cells in the mouse is correlated with pre-BCR expression, whereas no such correlation was observed in human pre-B ALL cases (61). A possible explanation for this difference is that pre-BCR expression is required at the initial time of leukemia, whereas an established pre-B ALL tumor no longer needs pre-BCR expression for proliferation. The ongoing RAG activity in SLP-65-deficient pre-B cells may not only result in secondary mutations, but may also lead to secondary V_H rearrangements at the HC gene locus. Such secondary rearrangements occur by replacement of an already rearranged V_H gene segment by another (in most cases upstream) V_H gene segment (81). The phenomenon of V_H gene replacement is well known in murine Abelson murine leukemia virus-transformed pre-B cell lines that frequently gain or lose HC expression owing to secondary V(D)J rearrangements (82). In agreement with this, the frequency of V_H gene replacement by secondary rearrangement in BCR-ABL-positive pre-B ALL is 75%, which is surprisingly high compared with 5% (frequency of V_H gene replacement) in normal human B cells (76).

Although the link between SLP-65 deficiency and leukemia development seems to be established in mice (57, 63), experiments mainly using microarrays for gene expression profiling suggest normal expression of SLP-65 in human pre-B ALL (83). One drawback of this method, however, is that aberrant transcripts and alternatively spliced forms are recognized as normal transcripts, although they are unable to generate a functional protein. Notably, only full-length SLP-65 can fulfill its function in pre-B cell differentiation. To check for full-length SLP-65 expression and confirm the correlation between SLP-65 deficiency and childhood pre-B ALL, we analyzed >100 pre-B ALL samples by western blot. These experiments confirmed the high frequency of deficient SLP-65 protein expression in pre-B ALL cases (H. Jumaa, unpublished results).

BRUTON'S TYROSINE KINASE

X-Linked Agammaglobulinemia and X-Linked Immunodeficiency

Btk (Bruton's tyrosine kinase) is a nonreceptor PTK that was originally identified as the gene defective in the human immunodeficiency disease XLA (84, 85). Btk is a 659 amino acid protein that belongs to the Tec kinase family, which also includes Tec, Itk, Bmx/Etk, and Rlk (86). These tyrosine kinases are structurally similar to Src family kinases in that they consist of an SH3, an SH2, and a catalytic domain. However, they also have a Tec homology (TH) domain, just upstream of the SH3 domain. The TH domain contains a proline-rich sequence implicated in intramolecular interaction with SH3 domains, thereby mediating auto-inhibition by preventing the interaction of these domains with their ligands. Like most Tec kinases (with the exception of Rlk), Btk also has an N-terminal pleckstrin homology (PH) domain that is able to bind phosphatidylinositols, which is essential for the recruitment of Btk to the plasma membrane upon PI3K activation.

Btk is expressed throughout B cell differentiation, but at the transition from mature B cells to plasma cells expression is downregulated (87–89). Although Btk is also present in myeloid and erythroid cells, these cell lineages do not appear to be affected in XLA or *xid*. Btk is not detected in the T cell lineage. In addition to its function in pre-BCR signaling, Btk has been implicated as a mediator of signals from various other receptors, including $Fc\varepsilon R$, IL-5R, IL-6R, IL-10R, collagen receptor, erythropoietin receptor, and Toll-like receptor 4 (90–96).

XLA, which was first described by Bruton in 1952 (97), is characterized by protracted and recurrent bacterial infections (reviewed in 98). Patients have less than 1% of the normal number of peripheral B cells, and the B cells that are present have an immature IgM^{high} phenotype and show an increased κ to λ ratio (99). Serum levels of all Ig classes are very low owing to the lack of plasma cells in the secondary lymphoid organs. When stimulated with anti-CD40 and IL-4, XLA B cells proliferate normally, show CD23 expression, and differentiate into specific Ab-producing cells (100). Heterozygous female XLA carriers do not have clinical or immunological symptoms, but they do manifest a unilateral X chromosome inactivation in the peripheral blood B lymphocyte population because of a selective disadvantage in proliferation, differentiation, and survival of cells that have the defective Btk gene on the active X chromosome (101, 102).

The exact location of the developmental arrest in XLA has been controversial for some time because the numbers of cytoplasmic μHC-expressing pre-B cells in XLA bone marrow are variable (103–105). Nevertheless, by more detailed flow cytometric studies, using antibodies specific for human V_{preB}, Nomura et al. (106) showed that in XLA patients the $c\mu^+SLC^+$ pre-B cell fraction mainly consists of small cells, suggesting that Btk is necessary for the proliferative expansion and the survival of $c\mu^+$ pre-B cells. Because most patients have substantial numbers of pro-B cells in their bone marrow, XLA generally results in an increased ratio of pro-B to pre-B cells. XLA is a heterogeneous disease, even within single families. An international registry for XLA (http://bioinf.uta.fi/BTKbase/) shows that mutations in all domains of the Btk gene cause the disease, although there is a remarkable but unexplained absence of missense mutations in the SH3 domain (107). So far, no correlation has been observed between the position of the mutation and phenotypic variables such as age at time of diagnosis or severity of the clinical or immunological symptoms. Therefore, this heterogeneity might be related to other genetic or environmental factors.

In contrast to XLA, Btk deficiency in the mouse is not associated with a major early B cell developmental block, but rather with impaired maturation and poor survival of peripheral B cells. This *xid* phenotype is present both in the CBA/N strain of mice carrying an Arg28 missense mutation within the Btk PH domain (108–111) and in mice with a targeted disruption of Btk in their germ line (89, 112). Btk-deficient mice have ~50% fewer B cells in the periphery and manifest a specific arrest of peripheral B cell differentiation within the immature B cell pool at the progression of IgM^{high} to $IgM^{low}AA4^+CD23^+$ transitional B cells (113–115). Using in vivo competition assays based on the phenomenon of X chromosome inactivation in $Btk^{+/-}$ or heterozygous *xid* female mice (89, 116, 117), it was shown that the immature $IgM^{high}IgD^{low}$ B cell population in the periphery still contains a substantial proportion of Btk-deficient cells, whereas in the mature $IgM^{low}IgD^{high}$ follicular B cell population these cells are virtually absent. In the peritoneum of Btk-deficient mice, the population of $CD5^+$ B-1 B cells is lacking, whereas marginal zone (MZ) B cells are present in normal numbers in the spleen. As the preferential clonal survival of MZ B cells requires functional Btk, Btk-deficient MZ B cells have a severely reduced life span (118). In $Btk^{+/-}$ female mice, Btk-deficient marginal zone B cells have a strong selective disadvantage in vivo, as $Btk^-/lacZ^+$ cells were undetectable in the $CD23^-CD21^+$ fraction of MZ B cells (R.W. Hendriks, unpublished). *Xid* mice have low levels of serum IgM and IgG3, whereas the levels of other isotypes are normal. They do not respond to thymus-independent type 2 polysaccharide antigens, but respond normally to thymus-dependent antigens (109, 112, 119). Btk is known to have a critical function in BCR-directed cell cycle induction in mature B cells. Anti-IgM-stimulated Btk-deficient B cells do not progress into cell division, exhibiting a high rate of apoptosis owing to a decreased ability to induce the antiapoptosis regulatory protein $Bcl-X_L$ (120–122). Btk-deficient B cells show normal proliferation induced via CD40 (112, 120). As mature B cell differentiation is critically controlled by parallel maturation and survival signals through the BCR and CD40, a profound B cell defect was observed in mice expressing the *xid* mutation and simultaneously lacking T cells or functional CD40 (123–126).

Btk and B Cell Receptor Signaling

Shortly after the identification of Btk, it was demonstrated that Btk is activated by BCR stimulation (127–129). Further biochemical studies in Btk-deficient cells

showed that Btk is an important regulator of BCR-induced calcium mobilization
(10, 130). It is thought that Btk is targeted to the plasma membrane through interactions of its PH domain with phosphatidylinositol-3,4,5-trisphosphate (PtdIns-
3,4,5,-P$_3$), a second messenger that is generated by PI3K (131, 132). Subsequently,
Btk is phosphorylated by Syk or the Src family tyrosine kinase Lyn at position
Y551 in the kinase domain, which promotes the catalytic activity of Btk and
subsequently results in its autophosphorylation at Y223 (133). Although Y223
phosphorylation does not appear to influence the Btk catalytic activity, it prevents
binding to the Wiskott Aldrich syndrome protein (WASP) and increases the affinity
to Syk (134). Concomitantly, Syk activation results in phosphorylation of SLP-65,
thereby providing docking sites for Btk and PLCγ2 SH2 domains. In this pathway,
activated Btk phosphorylates PLCγ2, once it is brought into close proximity of
PLCγ2 by SLP-65 (133, 135–137) (see Figure 3A). Activated PLCγ2 hydrolyzes

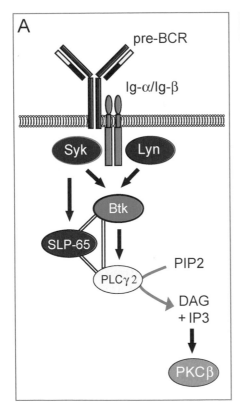
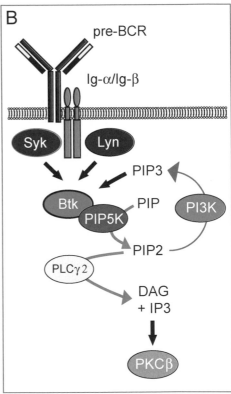

Figure 3   Signaling pathways downstream from the pre-BCR that activate PLCγ2 in the
mouse. (*A*) The classical SLP-65-dependent route, in which SLP-65 connects activated Btk
and PLCγ2. In this pathway, Btk needs its catalytic activity to stimulate PLCγ2. (*B*) The
SLP-65-independent pathway, in which Btk recruits PIP5K. In this pathway, Btk stimulates
PLCγ2 independent of its kinase activity. For details and abbreviations, see text.

its substrate, phosphatidylinositol-4,5-bisphosphate (PtdIns-4,5,-P$_2$), resulting in the production of the secondary messengers DAG and IP3. Consistent with this model, mice with targeted mutations in PI3K, SLP-65, or PLCγ2 all exhibit phenotypes similar to Btk mutant mice (52–55, 138–140).

IP3 mediates the opening of intracellular calcium stores, which subsequently activates PKCβ. Next, activated PKCβ phosphorylates IκB kinase α and thereby induces NF-κB activation, resulting in the upregulation of the antiapoptotic protein Bcl-X$_L$ and cyclin D2 (141–143). At the same time, PKCβ acts as a feedback loop inhibitor of Btk activation by phosphorylating the serine residue at position 180 in the TH domain of Btk. This phosphorylation counteracts Btk activity, as mutation of S180 is associated with hyperphosphorylation, increased membrane localization of Btk, and enhanced BCR-induced Ca^{2+} signaling. Another negative regulatory mechanism of Btk function is provided by SH2-containing inositol phosphatase (SHIP), which is activated upon FcγRIIB coligation to the BCR. By reducing the level of PtdIns-3,4,5,-P$_3$, SHIP regulates the association of Btk with the membrane through PH domain-phosphoinositol lipid interactions (137, 144).

The PH domain gain-of-function mutant E41K (Glu-to-Lys) shows increased membrane localization and phosphorylation of Btk in quiescent cells, independent of PI3K activity, bringing Btk in close proximity of other BCR signaling molecules (132, 145). The E41K mutation, which was isolated using a retroviral random mutagenesis scheme, was shown to induce transformation of NIH 3T3 fibroblasts in soft agar cultures and factor-independent growth of the IL-5-dependent pro-B cell line Y16 (145). The E41K transforming capacity is augmented by mutation of the main auto-phosphorylation site at Y223 in the SH3 domain (146). Expression of E41K-Btk in Ramos B cells enhances the sustained increase in intracellular calcium following BCR cross-linking (130). To analyze whether constitutive activation of Btk results in enhanced proliferation or malignant transformation of cells in the B cell lineage in vivo, transgenic mice were generated that expressed E41K or E41K-Y223F mutant Btk. However, in transgenic mice in which expression of E41K mutant human Btk was driven by the B cell–specific CD19 promoter or the MHC class II Ea locus control region, B cell development was almost completely arrested in the bone marrow or the spleen, respectively (147, 148). Those few residual B cells present were efficiently driven into terminal IgM plasma cell differentiation and did not give rise to B cell lymphoma (147, 148). Nevertheless, expression of E41K Btk enhanced blast formation of splenic B cells in culture, either with or without mitogens. These findings suggest that expression of the E41K-Btk mimics BCR occupancy by autoantigens. We were also unable to detect any in vivo potentiating effects of the Y223F mutation on the phenotype of E41K-Btk mice, as expression of the E41K or E41K-Y223F Btk mutants resulted in parallel phenotypes, whereby the extent of B cell deletion was dose dependent (75). Also, transgenic expression of the Y223F mutant Btk under the control of the CD19 promoter did not result in a phenotype, but could fully correct the features of the Btk-deficient phenotype (149). Because the SH3 domain has specificity for the N-terminal proline-rich region of the Btk TH domain, investigators have hypothesized that intra- or intermolecular interaction between the TH and SH3 domains might have an important regulatory function (150). However, our findings indicate that Y223 autophosphorylation-dependent interactions are not essential for Btk function in B cell development in vivo. This may also explain the remarkable absence of missense mutations in the Btk SH3 domain in a total of 155 missense mutations identified so far in XLA families (107), while on the basis of SH3 domain size about 10 of these should be located within the SH3 domain.

Taken together, in contrast to the ability of Btk mutants to induce transformation of fibroblasts in vitro, there is no evidence for an oncogenic function of Btk in B cells in vivo. In this context, it is remarkable that the Btk family member Bmx/Etk has been implicated in the progression of several tumors. Although Etk did not itself induce transformation, it is a critical mediator of Src-induced cell transformation and STAT-3 activation in liver epithelial cells (151) and controls proliferation and tumorigenic growth of mammary epithelial cancer cells (152).

Btk and Pre-BCR Signaling

Although Btk was found to be phosphorylated after cross-linking of Ig-β on RAG-2-deficient pro-B cells (7), the function of Btk downstream of the pre-B cell receptor in the mouse has been unclear for some time. In general, no striking differences were observed in the absolute numbers, production rate, or kinetics of turnover of pre-B cells, when *xid* or Btk-deficient mice were compared with wild-type control mice (89, 109, 112, 153). Only Cancro et al. (154) reported a diminished pre-B cell production rate in CBA/N *xid* mice, but this was accompanied by an increased proportional survival of pre-B cells, resulting in a normal size of the immature B cell pool. Nevertheless, several lines of evidence point to an important role for Btk at the developmental progression of pre-B cells into immature B cells in the mouse: (*a*) Btk-deficient pre-B cells show an increased proliferative response to IL-7, as detected in long-term Whitlock-Witte bone marrow cultures and in IL-7-driven fetal liver or adult bone marrow cultures (155–157); (*b*) Btk-deficient cells have a selective disadvantage in contributing to the IgM$^+$IgD$^-$ B220$^+$ immature B cell population in the bone marrow of Btk$^{+/-}$ female mice (89); (*c*) during the transition of large cycling to small resting pre-B cells, Btk-deficient cells fail to downregulate efficiently the expression of the sialoglycoprotein CD43, the metallopeptidase BP-1, or SLC, and Btk-deficient cells also show impaired induction of cell surface expression of the CD2 adhesion molecule, the IL-2R and MHC class II (157); (*d*) Btk-deficient cells manifest a specific developmental delay within the small pre-B cell compartment of ∼3 hours when compared with wild-type cells (157); (*e*) Btk-deficient B cells have reduced Ig λ L chain usage, implicating Btk in the activation of gene rearrangements at the λ L chain locus (158); (*f*) pre-B cells that lack both Btk and SLP-65 show an almost complete arrest in development, pointing to a synergistic role for Btk and SLP-65 in the developmental progression of pre-B cells (75, 160); and, lastly, (*g*) Btk cooperates with SLP-65 as a tumor suppressor in pre-B cells (75).

Collectively, these findings on the role of Btk in Btk-deficient mice demonstrate that Btk in human and mouse acts at distinct stages in pre-B cell development. Whereas in human Btk is critical for the induction of pre-B cell expansion, in mouse Btk plays an essential role to limit pre-B cell proliferation. Although more experiments are required to explain the differential role of Btk in the two species, this may well be related to the fact that pre-B cell proliferation in mouse, in contrast to human, is crucially dependent on IL-7. IL-7R signaling activates the Ras/Raf/MEK/MAP kinase pathway independent of Btk (7). To date, no IL-7-like growth factor has been found to regulate early B cell development in human and therefore it is possible that the expansion of pre-BCR positive cells is exclusively dependent on pre-BCR signaling and downstream Btk activation. Another way to explain the differences between XLA and *xid* phenotypes is a differential compensation for the loss of Btk by Tec family members. Although Tec-deficient mice show normal B cell development, an almost complete block at the $CD43^+B220^+$ large pre-B cell stage was reported in Btk/Tec-double-deficient mice (159). Therefore, one can conclude that Tec kinase can partially compensate for the loss of Btk function at the developmental progression of large cycling into small resting pre-B cells. However, the total numbers of pre-B cells in the Btk/Tec-double-mutant mice were similar to those in wild-type or single-mutant mice. Moreover, in vivo BrdU labeling experiments indicate that the proliferative activity of the pre-B cell population is not significantly different among wild-type, Tec-deficient, Btk-deficient, or Tec/Btk-double-deficient mice (W. Ellmeier, personal communication). These findings indicate that, in the mouse, pre-B cell proliferation is intact, even in the absence of both Tec and Btk. In contrast, in XLA pre-B cell proliferation is severely affected, and therefore a differential ability of Tec to compensate for Btk in humans and mice cannot explain the phenotypic differences between XLA and *xid*.

Btk Acts as a Tumor Suppressor in SLP-65-Deficient Pre-B Cells

The model in which the interaction of Btk with phosphorylated SLP-65 is critical to Btk's ability to activate $PLC\gamma2$ was challenged by the finding of a severe phenotype in the SLP-65/Btk-double-mutant mice (160). Whereas mice deficient for SLP-65 or Btk show only a partial arrest at the large cycling pre-B cell stage, a nearly complete block is present in SLP-65/Btk-double-deficient mice. Therefore, the two molecules not only function in a single BCR signal transduction pathway, but they also function independently in parallel pathways. Btk and SLP-65 have a synergistic role in the developmental progression of large cycling pre-B cells, including the downregulation of the expression of the pre-BCR and the induction of CD2, CD25, and MHC class II expression (75). Although Btk-deficient mice do not develop pre-B cell tumors, we observed that Btk cooperates with SLP-65 as a tumor suppressor. The incidence of pre-B cell lymphomas was significantly higher in SLP-65/Btk-double-mutant mice because at 16 weeks of age $\sim$75% of these mice

(12 out of 16) developed a pre-B cell lymphoma, compared with SLP-65-single-deficient mice ($\sim$5%, 3 out of 66). Conversely, transgenic B cell–specific low-level expression of a constitutive active form of human Btk, the E41K-Y223F mutant (see below), prevented tumor formation in SLP-65/Btk-double-mutant mice (75). In the bone marrow, expression of the Btk mutant partially corrected the maturation defects of pre-B cells, including the modulation of SLC expression. These results indicate that constitutively active Btk can compensate for the loss of SLP-65 tumor suppressor function.

The nature of the cooperation of Btk with SLP-65 remains to be identified, although it is conceivable that the increased frequency of pre-B cell lymphoma development in SLP-65/Btk-double-mutant mice may simply reflect the increased pool size of proliferating pre-B cells in double-mutant mice (75, 160). Alternatively, the concomitant absence of Btk may contribute to tumor formation by changing not only the number of cycling pre-B cells but also their properties, such as proliferative capacity, apoptosis susceptibility or V(D)J recombination activity. Btk likely has a role in a SLP-65-independent pathway in pre-B cells. In this context, it is important to note that recent data obtained in the mature B cell line A20 demonstrate that Btk can activate PLCγ2 in such a parallel pathway (161). The PH domain of Btk binds to phosphatidylinositol-4-phosphate-5-kinases (PIP5Ks), the enzymes that synthesize PtdIns-4,5-P2, which is a common substrate shared by both PI3K and PLCγ2 (see Figure 3B). The recruitment of the Btk-PIP5Ks complex to plasma membrane lipid rafts initiates a positive feedback loop that allows Btk to stimulate the production of the substrate for PI3K, leading to continued PtdIns-3,4,5,-P$_3$ synthesis, which is required for sustained Btk localization to the plasma membrane. As PtdIns-4,5-P$_2$ is also a substrate for PLCγ2, the shuttling function of Btk also provides substrate for PLCγ2 in a SLP-65-independent fashion. If the association of Btk with PIP5Ks is also operational in pre-B cells, such a feed-forward PLCγ2 activation loop could explain the synergistic roles of Btk and SLP-65 in these cells.

The shuttling mechanism that allows Btk to stimulate PtdIns-4,5-P$_2$ production does not appear to require Btk kinase activity, as overexpression of kinase-inactive Btk has been shown to stimulate PtdIns-3,4,5,-P$_3$ production by PI3K (137, 161). Moreover, kinase-inactive Btk was able to partially or fully reconstitute BCR-stimulated calcium flux in Btk-deficient DT40 chicken B cells (10, 162) or mouse splenic B cells (163). Moreover, transgenic overexpression of the kinase-inactive human Btk K430R mutant also induced NF-κB activation and Bcl-X$_L$ and cyclin D2 expression upon BCR stimulation in mature B cells (149). Expression of physiological levels of K430R Btk in pre-B cells normalized λ L chain usage and partially reconstituted the impaired pre-B cell maturation and IL-7 responsiveness in Btk-deficient mice. Although these findings imply that in pre-B cells Btk partially functions as an adapter molecule independent of its kinase activity, it remains possible that Btk adapter function depends on the presence of SLP-65, which in this context might serve as a scaffold molecule to bring other kinases, such as Src-like kinases or Syk, in close proximity to Btk and PLCγ2. However, it has recently been reported that the site-specific tyrosine phosphorylation of the PLCγ2 SH2-SH3 linker mediated by Btk cannot be mediated by Syk (164). To establish that SLP-65 is not required for Btk adapter function, we crossed transgenic mice expressing the kinase inactive K430R-Btk mutant onto a SLP-65-deficient background. We observed that kinase-inactive Btk was able to rescue the severe developmental arrest at the pre-B cell stage present in SLP-65/Btk-double-mutant mice (163). Moreover, as the frequencies of pre-B cell tumor development in SLP-65-deficient mice and in K430R-Btk transgenic mice on a SLP-65/Btk-double-deficient background were similar (163), we conclude that Btk exerts its tumor suppressor function in pre-B cells as an adapter protein, independent of its kinase activity. This finding is consistent with two parallel Btk signaling pathways, whereby Btk tumor suppressor activity resides in the SLP-65-independent and kinase-activity-independent PIP5K shuttle function of Btk (see Figure 3A,B).

In addition, Btk/PI3K-double-deficient mice were reported to have more severe defects than either single-mutant mouse in terms of B cell numbers in the spleen and in vitro proliferative capacity of B cells (143). As Btk membrane recruitment or tyrosine phosphorylation appear unaffected by PI3K inhibitors or in PI3K-deficient cells (137, 143, 165), Btk can also be recruited to the plasma membrane through a mechanism independent of interactions between the PH domain and PtdIns-3,4,5,-P$_3$, e.g., by phosphorylated SLP-65 (see Figure 3A).

Although SLP-65 deficiency and pre-BCR expression are required for the development of pre-B cell leukemia, the molecular mechanism of the malignant transformation of SLP-65-deficient pre-B cells and the exact role of RAG in the process of transformation still require further investigations. The fact that mice deficient for other components of the pre-BCR signaling machinery do not develop leukemia suggests a unique role for SLP-65 as the crucial pre-BCR signaling element that mediates differentiation and prevents leukemia. Tumor development is not related to the severity of the pre-B cell block. Mice that are Btk/Tec-double-deficient have an almost complete arrest at the pre-B cell stage, which is more severe than the arrest observed in SLP-65-deficient mice, but they do not appear to develop pre-B cell leukemia (W. Ellmeier, personal communication).

CONCLUDING REMARKS

Proliferation and differentiation are highly coordinated processes during B cell development. This review underlines the fact that independent pre-BCR signal transduction pathways regulate pre-B cell proliferation and differentiation simultaneously. Recent studies reveal that SLP-65 in association with Btk is the central regulator that promotes pre-B cell differentiation. In the SLP-65-deficient pre-B cells, the equilibrium between proliferation and differentiation is shifted toward proliferation, leading to an increased incidence of leukemia development. However, more work is necessary to characterize the downstream effects of SLP-65-mediated signaling and to understand how SLP-65 limits pre-B cell proliferation.

The identification of the signaling proteins and molecular mechanisms that regulate pre-B cell proliferation and differentiation may provide deeper insights into the process of leukemia development and may lead to novel strategies for tumor treatments.

ACKNOWLEDGMENTS

We thank S. Middendorp and P. Nielsen for assistance. This work was partly supported by the Deutsche Forschungsgesellschaft (SFB 620) to H.J. and M.R., and by the Netherlands Organization for Scientific Research to R.W.H. (901-07-209).

The *Annual Review of Immunology* is online at
http://immunol.annualreviews.org

LITERATURE CITED

1. Rolink AG, ten Boekel E, Yamagami T, Ceredig R, Andersson J, Melchers F. 1999. B cell development in the mouse from early progenitors to mature B cells. *Immunol. Lett.* 68:89–93

2. Hardy RR, Li YS, Allman D, Asano M, Gui M, Hayakawa K. 2000. B-cell commitment, development and selection. *Immunol. Rev.* 175:23–32

3. Niiro H, Clark EA. 2002. Regulation of B-cell fate by antigen-receptor signals. *Nat. Rev. Immunol.* 2:945–56

4. Ohnishi K, Melchers F. 2003. The non-immunoglobulin portion of λ5 mediates cell-autonomous pre-B cell receptor signaling. *Nat. Immunol.* 4:849–56

5. Melchers F, ten Boekel E, Seidl T, Kong XC, Yamagami T, et al. 2000. Repertoire selection by pre-B cell receptors and B-cell receptors, and genetic control of B-cell development from immature to mature B cells. *Immunol. Rev.* 175:33–46

6. Guo B, Kato RM, Garcia-Lioret M, Wahl MI, Rawlings DJ. 2000. Engagement of the human pre-B cell receptor generates a lipid raft-dependent calcium signaling complex. *Immunity* 13:243–53

7. Kouro T, Nagata K, Takaki S, Nisitani S, Hirano M, et al. 2001. Bruton's tyrosine kinase is required for signaling the CD79b-mediated pro-B to pre-B cell transition. *Int. Immunol.* 13:485–93

8. Rolli V, Gallwitz M, Wossning T, Flemming A, Schamel WW, et al. 2002. Amplification of B cell antigen receptor signaling by a Syk/ITAM positive feedback loop. *Mol. Cell* 10:1057–69

9. Tretter T, Ross AE, Dordai DI, Desiderio S. 2003. Mimicry of pre-B cell receptor signaling by activation of the tyrosine kinase Blk. *J. Exp. Med.* 198:1863–73

10. Takata M, Kurosaki T. 1996. A role for Bruton's tyrosine kinase in B cell antigen receptor-mediated activation of phospholipase C-γ 2. *J. Exp. Med.* 184:31–40

11. Petro JB, Rahman SM, Ballard DW, Khan WN. 2000. Bruton's tyrosine kinase is required for activation of IκB kinase and nuclear factor κB in response to B cell receptor engagement. *J. Exp. Med.* 191:1745–54

12. Bajpai UD, Zhang K, Teutsch M, Sen R, Wortis HH. 2000. Bruton's tyrosine kinase links the B cell receptor to nuclear factor κB activation. *J. Exp. Med.* 191:1735–44

13. Watanabe D, Hashimito S, Ishiai M, Matsushita M, Baba Y, et al. 2001. Four tyrosine residues in phospholipase C-γ 2,

identified as Btk-dependent phosphorylation sites, are required for B cell antigen receptor-coupled calcium signaling. *J. Biol. Chem.* 276:38595–601

14. Saijo K, Schmedt C, Su IH, Karasuyama H, Lowell CA, et al. 2003. Essential role of Src-family protein tyrosine kinases in NF-κB activation during B cell development. *Nat. Immunol.* 4:274–79

15. Schlessinger J. 2003. Signal transduction. Autoinhibition control. *Science* 300:750–52

16. Dykstra M, Cherukuri A, Sohn HW, Tzeng SJ, Pierce SK. 2003. Location is everything: lipid rafts and immune cell signaling. *Annu. Rev. Immunol.* 21:457–81

17. Wong S, Witte ON. 2004. The BCR-ABL story: bench to bedside and back. *Annu. Rev. Immunol.* 22:247–306

18. Pluk H, Dorey K, Superti-Furga G. 2002. Autoinhibition of c-Abl. *Cell* 108:247–59

19. Nagar B, Hantschel O, Young MA, Scheffzek K, Veach D, et al. 2003. Structural basis for the autoinhibition of c-Abl tyrosine kinase. *Cell* 112:859–71

20. Tauchi T, Miyazawa K, Feng GS, Broxmeyer HE, Toyama K. 1997. A coiled-coil tetramerization domain of BCR-ABL is essential for the interactions of SH2-containing signal transduction molecules. *J. Biol. Chem.* 272:1389–94

21. Varticovski L, Daley GQ, Jackson P, Baltimore D, Cantley LC. 1991. Activation of phosphatidylinositol 3-kinase in cells expressing abl oncogene variants. *Mol. Cell. Biol.* 11:1107–13

22. Kurosaki T. 1999. Genetic analysis of B cell antigen receptor signaling. *Annu. Rev. Immunol.* 17:555–92

23. Wossning T, Reth M. 2004. B cell antigen receptor assembly and Syk activation in the S2 cell reconstitution system. *Immunol. Lett.* 92:67–73

24. Shiue L, Zoller MJ, Brugge JS. 1995. Syk is activated by phosphotyrosine-containing peptides representing the tyrosine-based activation motifs of the high affinity receptor for IgE. *J. Biol. Chem.* 270:10498–502

25. Reth M, Brummer T. 2004. Feedback regulation of lymphocyte signalling. *Nat. Rev. Immunol.* 4:269–77

26. Healy JI, Goodnow CC. 1998. Positive versus negative signaling by lymphocyte antigen receptors. *Annu. Rev. Immunol.* 16:645–70

27. Reth M. 2002. Hydrogen peroxide as second messenger in lymphocyte activation. *Nat. Immunol.* 3:1129–34

28. Cornall RJ, Goodnow CC, Cyster JG. 1999. Regulation of B cell antigen receptor signaling by the Lyn/CD22/SHP1 pathway. *Curr. Top. Microbiol. Immunol.* 244:57–68

29. Chan VW, Meng F, Soriano P, DeFranco AL, Lowell CA. 1997. Characterization of the B lymphocyte populations in Lyn-deficient mice and the role of Lyn in signal initiation and down-regulation. *Immunity* 7:69–81

30. Chan VW, Lowell CA, DeFranco AL. 1998. Defective negative regulation of antigen receptor signaling in Lyn-deficient B lymphocytes. *Curr. Biol.* 8:545–53

31. Blasioli J, Goodnow CC. 2002. Lyn/CD22/SHP-1 and their importance in autoimmunity. *Curr. Dir. Autoimmun.* 5:151–60

32. Whyburn LR, Halcomb KE, Contreras CM, Lowell CA, Witte ON, Satterthwaite AB. 2003. Reduced dosage of Bruton's tyrosine kinase uncouples B cell hyperresponsiveness from autoimmunity in *lyn*$^{-/-}$ mice. *J. Immunol.* 171:1850–58

33. Takata M, Sabe H, Hata A, Inazu T, Homma Y, et al. 1994. Tyrosine kinases Lyn and Syk regulate B cell receptor-coupled Ca2$^+$ mobilization through distinct pathways. *EMBO J.* 13:1341–49

34. Schweighoffer E, Vanes L, Mathiot A, Nakamura T, Tybulewicz VL. 2003. Unexpected requirement for ZAP-70 in pre-B cell development and allelic exclusion. *Immunity* 18:523–33

35. Furlong MT, Mahrenholz AM, Kim KH, Ashendel CL, Harrison ML, Geahlen RL. 1997. Identification of the major sites of autophosphorylation of the murine protein-tyrosine kinase Syk. *Biochim. Biophys. Acta* 1355:177–90

36. Hong JJ, Yankee TM, Harrison ML, Geahlen RL. 2002. Regulation of signaling in B cells through the phosphorylation of Syk on linker region tyrosines. A mechanism for negative signaling by the Lyn tyrosine kinase. *J. Biol. Chem.* 277:31703–14

37. Deckert M, Tartare-Deckert S, Couture C, Mustelin T, Altman A. 1996. Functional and physical interactions of Syk family kinases with the Vav proto-oncogene product. *Immunity* 5:591–604

38. Jiang K, Zhong B, Gilvary DL, Corliss BC, Vivier E, et al. 2002. Syk regulation of phosphoinositide 3-kinase-dependent NK cell function. *J. Immunol.* 168:3155–64

39. Niiro H, Maeda A, Kurosaki T, Clark EA. 2002. The B lymphocyte adaptor molecule of 32 kD (Bam32) regulates B cell antigen receptor signaling and cell survival. *J. Exp. Med.* 195:143–49

40. Marte BM, Downward J. 1997. PKB/Akt: connecting phosphoinositide 3-kinase to cell survival and beyond. *Trends Biochem. Sci.* 22:355–58

41. Beitz LO, Fruman DA, Kurosaki T, Cantley LC, Scharenberg AM. 1999. SYK is upstream of phosphoinositide 3-kinase in B cell receptor signaling. *J. Biol. Chem.* 274:32662–66

42. Kanie T, Abe A, Matsuda T, Kuno Y, Towatari M, et al. 2004. TEL-Syk fusion constitutively activates PI3-K/Akt, MAPK and JAK2-independent STAT5 signal pathways. *Leukemia* 18:548–55

43. Lupher ML Jr, Rao N, Lill NL, Andoniou CE, Miyake S, et al. 1998. Cbl-mediated negative regulation of the Syk tyrosine kinase. A critical role for Cbl phosphotyrosine-binding domain binding to Syk phosphotyrosine 323. *J. Biol. Chem.* 273:35273–81

44. Rao N, Dodge I, Band H. 2002. The Cbl family of ubiquitin ligases: critical negative regulators of tyrosine kinase signaling in the immune system. *J. Leukoc. Biol.* 71:753–63

45. Yankee TM, Keshvara LM, Sawasdikosol S, Harrison ML, Geahlen RL. 1999. Inhibition of signaling through the B cell antigen receptor by the protooncogene product, c-Cbl, requires Syk tyrosine 317 and the c-Cbl phosphotyrosine-binding domain. *J. Immunol.* 163:5827–35

46. Sada K, Zhang J, Siraganian RP. 2000. Point mutation of a tyrosine in the linker region of Syk results in a gain of function. *J. Immunol.* 164:338–44

47. Rao N, Ghosh AK, Ota S, Zhou P, Reddi AL, et al. 2001. The non-receptor tyrosine kinase Syk is a target of Cbl-mediated ubiquitylation upon B-cell receptor stimulation. *EMBO J.* 20:7085–95

48. Sohn HW, Gu H, Pierce SK. 2003. Cbl-b negatively regulates B cell antigen receptor signaling in mature B cells through ubiquitination of the tyrosine kinase Syk. *J. Exp. Med.* 197:1511–24

49. Lupher ML Jr, Andoniou CE, Bonita D, Miyake S, Band H. 1998. The c-Cbl oncoprotein. *Int. J. Biochem. Cell Biol.* 30:439–44

50. Wienands J, Schweikert J, Wollscheid B, Jumaa H, Nielsen PJ, Reth M. 1998. SLP-65: a new signaling component in B lymphocytes which requires expression of the antigen receptor for phosphorylation. *J. Exp. Med.* 188:791–95

51. Fu C, Turck CW, Kurosaki T, Chan AC. 1998. BLNK: a central linker protein in B cell activation. *Immunity* 9:93–103

52. Jumaa H, Wollscheid B, Mitterer M, Wienands J, Reth M, Nielsen PJ. 1999. Abnormal development and function of B lymphocytes in mice deficient for the signaling adaptor protein SLP-65. *Immunity* 11:547–54

53. Pappu R, Cheng AM, Li B, Gong Q, Chiu C, et al. 1999. Requirement for B cell

linker protein (BLNK) in B cell development. *Science* 286:1949–54

54. Hayashi K, Nittono R, Okamoto N, Tsuji S, Hara Y, et al. 2000. The B cell-restricted adaptor BASH is required for normal development and antigen receptor-mediated activation of B cells. *Proc. Natl. Acad. Sci. USA* 97:2755–60

55. Xu S, Tan JE, Wong EP, Manickam A, Ponniah S, Lam KP. 2000. B cell development and activation defects resulting in *xid*-like immunodeficiency in BLNK/SLP-65-deficient mice. *Int. Immunol.* 12:397–404

56. Minegishi Y, Rohrer J, Coustan-Smith E, Lederman HM, Pappu R, et al. 1999. An essential role for BLNK in human B cell development. *Science* 286:1954–57

57. Flemming A, Brummer T, Reth M, Jumaa H. 2003. The adaptor protein SLP-65 acts as a tumor suppressor that limits pre-B cell expansion. *Nat. Immunol.* 4:38–43

58. Su YW, Jumaa H. 2003. LAT links the pre-BCR to calcium signaling. *Immunity* 19:295–305

59. Schebesta M, Pfeffer PL, Busslinger M. 2002. Control of pre-BCR signaling by Pax5-dependent activation of the BLNK gene. *Immunity* 17:473–85

60. Fleming HE, Paige CJ. 2001. Pre-B cell receptor signaling mediates selective response to IL 7 at the pro-B to pre-B cell transition via an ERK/MAP kinase-dependent pathway. *Immunity* 15:521–31

61. Jumaa H, Bossaller L, Portugal K, Storch B, Lotz M, et al. 2003. Deficiency of the adaptor SLP-65 in pre-B cell acute lymphoblastic leukaemia. *Nature* 423:452–56

62. Samelson LE. 2002. Signal transduction mediated by the T cell antigen receptor: The role of adapter proteins. *Annu. Rev. Immunol.* 20:371–94

63. Hayashi K, Yamamoto M, Nojima T, Goitsuka R, Kitamura D. 2003. Distinct signaling requirements for Dmu selection, IgH allelic exclusion, pre-B cell transition, and tumor suppression in B cell progenitors. *Immunity* 18:825–36

64. Grawunder U, Leu TM, Schatz DG, Werner A, Rolink AG, et al. 1995. Down-regulation of RAG1 and RAG2 gene expression in pre-B cells after functional immunoglobulin heavy chain rearrangement. *Immunity* 3:601–8

65. Lin WC, Desiderio S. 1993. Regulation of V(D)J recombination activator protein RAG-2 by phosphorylation. *Science* 260:953–59

66. Li Z, Dordai DI, Lee J, Desiderio S. 1996. A conserved degradation signal regulates RAG-2 accumulation during cell division and links V(D)J recombination to the cell cycle. *Immunity* 5:575–89

67. Cox MM, Goodman MF, Kreuzer KN, Sherratt DJ, Sandler SJ, Marians KJ. 2000. The importance of repairing stalled replication forks. *Nature* 404:37–41

68. Rothstein R, Michel B, Gangloff S. 2000. Replication fork pausing and recombination or "gimme a break." *Genes Dev.* 14:1–10

69. Raghavan SC, Kirsch IR, Lieber MR. 2001. Analysis of the V(D)J recombination efficiency at lymphoid chromosomal translocation breakpoints. *J. Biol. Chem.* 276:29126–33

70. Zhu C, Mills KD, Ferguson DO, Lee C, Manis J, et al. 2002. Unrepaired DNA breaks in p53-deficient cells lead to oncogenic gene amplification subsequent to translocations. *Cell* 109:811–21

71. Difilippantonio MJ, Petersen S, Chen HT, Johnson R, Jasin M, et al. 2002. Evidence for replicative repair of DNA double-strand breaks leading to oncogenic translocation and gene amplification. *J. Exp. Med.* 196:469–80

72. Raghavan SC, Swanson PC, Wu X, Hsieh CL, Lieber MR. 2004. A non-B-DNA structure at the Bcl-2 major breakpoint region is cleaved by the RAG complex. *Nature* 428:88–93

73. Roth DB. 2003. Restraining the V(D)J recombinase. *Nat. Rev. Immunol.* 3:656–66

74. Messier TL, O'Neill JP, Hou SM, Nicklas JA, Finette BA. 2003. In vivo

transposition mediated by V(D)J recombinase in human T lymphocytes. *EMBO J.* 22:1381–88

75. Kersseboom R, Middendorp S, Dingjan GM, Dahlenborg K, Reth M, et al. 2003. Bruton's tyrosine kinase cooperates with the B cell linker protein SLP-65 as a tumor suppressor in pre-B cells. *J. Exp. Med.* 198:91–98

76. Klein F, Feldhahn N, Harder L, Wang H, Wartenberg M, et al. 2004. The BCR-ABL1 kinase bypasses selection for the expression of a pre-B cell receptor in pre-B acute lymphoblastic leukemia cells. *J. Exp. Med.* 199:673–85

77. Su YW, Flemming A, Wossning T, Hobeika E, Reth M, Jumaa H. 2003. Identification of a pre-BCR lacking surrogate light chain. *J. Exp. Med.* 198:1699–706

78. Galler GR, Mundt C, Parker M, Pelanda R, Martensson IL, Winkler TH. 2004. Surface μ heavy chain signals downregulation of the V(D)J-recombinase machinery in the absence of surrogate light chain components. *J. Exp. Med.* 199:1523–32

79. Goodman PA, Wood CM, Vassilev A, Mao C, Uckun FM. 2001. Spleen tyrosine kinase (Syk) deficiency in childhood pro-B cell acute lymphoblastic leukemia. *Oncogene* 20:3969–78

80. Goodman PA, Wood CM, Vassilev AO, Mao C, Uckun FM. 2003. Defective expression of Bruton's tyrosine kinase in acute lymphoblastic leukemia. *Leuk. Lymphoma* 44:1011–18

81. Zhang Z, Zemlin M, Wang YH, Munfus D, Huye LE, et al. 2003. Contribution of Vh gene replacement to the primary B cell repertoire. *Immunity* 19:21–31

82. Reth M, Jackson S, Alt FW. 1986. VHDJH formation and DJH replacement during pre-B differentiation: nonrandom usage of gene segments. *EMBO J.* 5:2131–38

83. Imai C, Ross ME, Reid G, Coustan-Smith E, Schultz KR, et al. 2004. Expression of the adaptor protein BLNK/SLP-65 in

childhood acute lymphoblastic leukemia. *Leukemia* 18:922–25

84. Tsukada S, Saffran DC, Rawlings DJ, Parolini O, Allen RC, et al. 1993. Deficient expression of a B cell cytoplasmic tyrosine kinase in human X-linked agammaglobulinemia. *Cell* 72:279–90

85. Vetrie D, Vorechovsky I, Sideras P, Holland J, Davies A, et al. 1993. The gene involved in X-linked agammaglobulinaemia is a member of the *src* family of protein-tyrosine kinases. *Nature* 361:226–33

86. Smith CI, Islam TC, Mattsson PT, Mohamed AJ, Nore BF, Vihinen M. 2001. The Tec family of cytoplasmic tyrosine kinases: mammalian Btk, Bmx, Itk, Tec, Txk and homologs in other species. *Bioessays* 23:436–46

87. de Weers M, Verschuren MC, Kraakman ME, Mensink RG, Schuurman RK, et al. 1993. The Bruton's tyrosine kinase gene is expressed throughout B cell differentiation, from early precursor B cell stages preceding immunoglobulin gene rearrangement up to mature B cell stages. *Eur. J. Immunol.* 23:3109–14

88. Smith CI, Baskin B, Humire-Greiff P, Zhou JN, Olsson PG, et al. 1994. Expression of Bruton's agammaglobulinemia tyrosine kinase gene, BTK, is selectively down-regulated in T lymphocytes and plasma cells. *J. Immunol.* 152:557–65

89. Hendriks RW, de Bruijn MF, Maas A, Dingjan GM, Karis A, Grosveld F. 1996. Inactivation of Btk by insertion of lacZ reveals defects in B cell development only past the pre-B cell stage. *EMBO J.* 15:4862–72

90. Kawakami Y, Yao L, Miura T, Tsukada S, Witte ON, Kawakami T. 1994. Tyrosine phosphorylation and activation of Bruton tyrosine kinase upon FcεRI cross-linking. *Mol. Cell. Biol.* 14:5108–13

91. Sato S, Katagiri T, Takaki S, Kikuchi Y, Hitoshi Y, et al. 1994. IL-5 receptor-mediated tyrosine phosphorylation of

SH2/SH3-containing proteins and activation of Bruton's tyrosine and Janus 2 kinases. *J. Exp. Med.* 180:2101–11

92. Matsuda T, Takahashi-Tezuka M, Fukada T, Okuyama Y, Fujitani Y, et al. 1995. Association and activation of Btk and Tec tyrosine kinases by gp130, a signal transducer of the interleukin-6 family of cytokines. *Blood* 85:627–33

93. Go NF, Castle BE, Barrett R, Kastelein R, Dang W, et al. 1990. Interleukin 10, a novel B cell stimulatory factor: unresponsiveness of X chromosome-linked immunodeficiency B cells. *J. Exp. Med.* 172:1625–31

94. Quek LS, Bolen J, Watson SP. 1998. A role for Bruton's tyrosine kinase (Btk) in platelet activation by collagen. *Curr. Biol.* 8:1137–40

95. Schmidt U, Van Den Akker E, Parren-Van Amelsvoort M, Litos G, De Bruijn M, et al. 2004. Btk is required for an efficient response to erythropoietin and for SCF-controlled protection against TRAIL in erythroid progenitors. *J. Exp. Med.* 199:785–95

96. Jefferies CA, Doyle S, Brunner C, Dunne A, Brint E, et al. 2003. Bruton's tyrosine kinase is a Toll/interleukin-1 receptor domain-binding protein that participates in nuclear factor κB activation by Toll-like receptor 4. *J. Biol. Chem.* 278:26258–64

97. Bruton OC 1952. Agammaglobulinemia. *Pediatrics* 9:722–28

98. Sideras P, Smith CI. 1995. Molecular and cellular aspects of X-linked agammaglobulinemia. *Adv. Immunol.* 59:135–223

99. Conley ME. 1985. B cells in patients with X-linked agammaglobulinemia. *J. Immunol.* 134:3070–74

100. Nonoyama S, Tsukada S, Yamadori T, Miyawaki T, Jin YZ, et al. 1998. Functional analysis of peripheral blood B cells in patients with X-linked agammaglobulinemia. *J. Immunol.* 161:3925–29

101. Conley ME, Brown P, Pickard AR, Buckley RH, Miller DS, et al. 1986. Expression of the gene defect in X-linked agamma-globulinemia. *N. Engl. J. Med.* 315:564–67

102. Fearon ER, Winkelstein JA, Civin CI, Pardoll DM, Vogelstein B. 1987. Carrier detection in X-linked agammaglobulinemia by analysis of X-chromosome inactivation. *N. Engl. J. Med.* 316:427–31

103. Pearl ER, Vogler LB, Okos AJ, Crist WM, Lawton AR, Cooper MD. 1978. B lymphocyte precursors in human bone marrow: an analysis of normal individuals and patients with antibody-deficiency states. *J. Immunol.* 120:1169–75

104. Landreth KS, Engelhard D, Anasetti C, Kapoor N, Kincade PW, Good RA. 1985. Pre-B cells in agammaglobulinemia: evidence for disease heterogeneity among affected boys. *J. Clin. Immunol.* 5:84–89

105. Campana D, Farrant J, Inamdar N, Webster AD, Janossy G. 1990. Phenotypic features and proliferative activity of B cell progenitors in X-linked agammaglobulinemia. *J. Immunol.* 145:1675–80

106. Nomura K, Kanegane H, Karasuyama H, Tsukada S, Agematsu K, et al. 2000. Genetic defect in human X-linked agamma-globulinemia impedes a maturational evolution of pro-B cells into a later stage of pre-B cells in the B-cell differentiation pathway. *Blood* 96:610–17

107. Vihinen M, Kwan SP, Lester T, Ochs HD, Resnick I, et al. 1999. Mutations of the human BTK gene coding for bruton tyrosine kinase in X-linked agammaglobulinemia. *Hum. Mutat.* 13:280–85

108. Scher I, Ahmed A, Strong DM, Steinberg AD, Paul WE. 1975. X-linked B-lymphocyte immune defect in CBA/HN mice. I. Studies of the function and composition of spleen cells. *J. Exp. Med.* 141:788–803

109. Wicker LS, Scher I. 1986. X-linked immune deficiency (*xid*) of CBA/N mice. *Curr. Top. Microbiol. Immunol.* 124:87–101

110. Rawlings DJ, Saffran DC, Tsukada S, Largaespada DA, Grimaldi JC, et al. 1993. Mutation of unique region of Bruton's

tyrosine kinase in immunodeficient *XID* mice. *Science* 261:358–61

111. Thomas JD, Sideras P, Smith CI, Vorechovsky I, Chapman V, Paul WE. 1993. Colocalization of X-linked agammaglobulinemia and X-linked immunodeficiency genes. *Science* 261:355–58

112. Khan WN, Alt FW, Gerstein RM, Malynn BA, Larsson I, et al. 1995. Defective B cell development and function in Btk-deficient mice. *Immunity* 3:283–99

113. Hardy RR, Hayakawa K, Parks DR, Herzenberg LA. 1983. Demonstration of B-cell maturation in X-linked immunodeficient mice by simultaneous three-colour immunofluorescence. *Nature* 306:270–72

114. Allman D, Lindsley RC, DeMuth W, Rudd K, Shinton SA, Hardy RR. 2001. Resolution of three nonproliferative immature splenic B cell subsets reveals multiple selection points during peripheral B cell maturation. *J. Immunol.* 167:6834–40

115. Su TT, Rawlings DJ. 2002. Transitional B lymphocyte subsets operate as distinct checkpoints in murine splenic B cell development. *J. Immunol.* 168:2101–10

116. Nahm MH, Paslay JW, Davie JM. 1983. Unbalanced X chromosome mosaicism in B cells of mice with X-linked immunodeficiency. *J. Exp. Med.* 158:920–31

117. Forrester LM, Ansell JD, Micklem HS. 1987. Development of B lymphocytes in mice heterozygous for the X-linked immunodeficiency (*xid*) mutation. *xid* inhibits development of all splenic and lymph node B cells at a stage subsequent to their initial formation in bone marrow. *J. Exp. Med.* 165:949–58

118. Martin F, Kearney JF. 2000. Positive selection from newly formed to marginal zone B cells depends on the rate of clonal production, CD19, and btk. *Immunity* 12:39–49

119. Bona C, Mond JJ, Paul WE. 1980. Synergistic genetic defect in B-lymphocyte function. I. Defective responses to B-cell stimulants and their genetic basis. *J. Exp. Med.* 151:224–34

120. Anderson JS, Teutsch M, Dong Z, Wortis HH. 1996. An essential role for Bruton's [corrected] tyrosine kinase in the regulation of B-cell apoptosis. *Proc. Natl. Acad. Sci. USA* 93:10966–71

121. Brorson K, Brunswick M, Ezhevsky S, Wei DG, Berg R, et al. 1997. *xid* affects events leading to B cell cycle entry. *J. Immunol.* 159:135–43

122. Solvason N, Wu WW, Kabra N, Lund-Johansen F, Roncarolo MG, et al. 1998. Transgene expression of bcl-xL permits anti-immunoglobulin (Ig)-induced proliferation in *xid* B cells. *J. Exp. Med.* 187:1081–91

123. Wortis HH, Burkly L, Hughes D, Roschelle S, Waneck G. 1982. Lack of mature B cells in nude mice with X-linked immune deficiency. *J. Exp. Med.* 155:903–13

124. Mond JJ, Scher I, Cossman J, Kessler S, Mongini PK, et al. 1982. Role of the thymus in directing the development of a subset of B lymphocytes. *J. Exp. Med.* 155:924–36

125. Oka Y, Rolink AG, Andersson J, Kamanaka M, Uchida J, et al. 1996. Profound reduction of mature B cell numbers, reactivities and serum Ig levels in mice which simultaneously carry the *XID* and CD40 deficiency genes. *Int. Immunol.* 8:1675–85

126. Khan WN, Nilsson A, Mizoguchi E, Castigli E, Forsell J, et al. 1997. Impaired B cell maturation in mice lacking Bruton's tyrosine kinase (Btk) and CD40. *Int. Immunol.* 9:395–405

127. Aoki Y, Isselbacher KJ, Pillai S. 1994. Bruton tyrosine kinase is tyrosine phosphorylated and activated in pre-B lymphocytes and receptor-ligated B cells. *Proc. Natl. Acad. Sci. USA* 91:10606–9

128. de Weers M, Brouns GS, Hinshelwood S, Kinnon C, Schuurman RK, et al. 1994. B-cell antigen receptor stimulation

activates the human Bruton's tyrosine kinase, which is deficient in X-linked agammaglobulinemia. *J. Biol. Chem.* 269:23857–60

129. Saouaf SJ, Mahajan S, Rowley RB, Kut SA, Fargnoli J, et al. 1994. Temporal differences in the activation of three classes of non-transmembrane protein tyrosine kinases following B-cell antigen receptor surface engagement. *Proc. Natl. Acad. Sci. USA* 91:9524–28

130. Fluckiger AC, Li Z, Kato RM, Wahl MI, Ochs HD, et al. 1998. Btk/Tec kinases regulate sustained increases in intracellular Ca2$^+$ following B-cell receptor activation. *EMBO J.* 17:1973–85

131. Salim K, Bottomley MJ, Querfurth E, Zvelebil MJ, Gout I, et al. 1996. Distinct specificity in the recognition of phosphoinositides by the pleckstrin homology domains of dynamin and Bruton's tyrosine kinase. *EMBO J.* 15:6241–50

132. Varnai P, Rother KI, Balla T. 1999. Phosphatidylinositol 3-kinase-dependent membrane association of the Bruton's tyrosine kinase pleckstrin homology domain visualized in single living cells. *J. Biol. Chem.* 274:10983–89

133. Rawlings DJ, Scharenberg AM, Park H, Wahl MI, Lin S, et al. 1996. Activation of BTK by a phosphorylation mechanism initiated by SRC family kinases. *Science* 271:822–25

134. Morrogh LM, Hinshelwood S, Costello P, Cory GO, Kinnon C. 1999. The SH3 domain of Bruton's tyrosine kinase displays altered ligand binding properties when auto-phosphorylated in vitro. *Eur. J. Immunol.* 29:2269–79

135. Li Z, Wahl MI, Eguinoa A, Stephens LR, Hawkins PT, Witte ON. 1997. Phosphatidylinositol 3-kinase-γ activates Bruton's tyrosine kinase in concert with Src family kinases. *Proc. Natl. Acad. Sci. USA* 94:13820–25

136. Kurosaki T, Kurosaki M. 1997. Trans-phosphorylation of Bruton's tyrosine kinase on tyrosine 551 is critical for B cell antigen receptor function. *J. Biol. Chem.* 272:15595–98

137. Scharenberg AM, El-Hillal O, Fruman DA, Beitz LO, Li Z, et al. 1998. Phosphatidylinositol-3,4,5-trisphosphate (PtdIns-3,4,5-P3)/Tec kinase-dependent calcium signaling pathway: a target for SHIP-mediated inhibitory signals. *EMBO J.* 17:1961–72

138. Suzuki H, Terauchi Y, Fujiwara M, Aizawa S, Yazaki Y, et al. 1999. *Xid*-like immunodeficiency in mice with disruption of the p85α subunit of phosphoinositide 3-kinase. *Science* 283:390–92

139. Wang D, Feng J, Wen R, Marine JC, Sangster MY, et al. 2000. Phospholipase Cγ2 is essential in the functions of B cell and several Fc receptors. *Immunity* 13:25–35

140. Fruman DA, Satterthwaite AB, Witte ON. 2000. *Xid*-like phenotypes: a B cell signalosome takes shape. *Immunity* 13:1–3

141. Saijo K, Mecklenbrauker I, Santana A, Leitger M, Schmedt C, Tarakhovsky A. 2002. Protein kinase Cβ controls nuclear factor κB activation in B cells through selective regulation of the IκB kinase α. *J. Exp. Med.* 195:1647–52

142. Su TT, Guo B, Kawakami Y, Sommer K, Chae K, et al. 2002. PKC-β controls IκB kinase lipid raft recruitment and activation in response to BCR signaling. *Nat. Immunol.* 3:780–86

143. Suzuki H, Matsuda S, Terauchi Y, Fujiwara M, Ohteki T, et al. 2003. PI3K and Btk differentially regulate B cell antigen receptor-mediated signal transduction. *Nat. Immunol.* 4:280–86

144. Bolland S, Pearse RN, Kurosaki T, Ravetch JV. 1998. SHIP modulates immune receptor responses by regulating membrane association of Btk. *Immunity* 8:509–16

145. Li T, Tsukada S, Satterthwaite A, Havlik MH, Park H, Takatsu K, Witte ON. 1995. Activation of Bruton's tyrosine kinase (BTK) by a point mutation in its pleckstrin homology (PH) domain. *Immunity* 2:451–60

146. Park H, Wahl MI, Afar DE, Turck CW, Rawlings DJ, et al. 1996. Regulation of Btk function by a major autophosphorylation site within the SH3 domain. *Immunity* 4:515–25

147. Maas A, Dingjan GM, Grosveld F, Hendriks RW. 1999. Early arrest in B cell development in transgenic mice that express the E41K Bruton's tyrosine kinase mutant under the control of the CD19 promoter region. *J. Immunol.* 162:6526–33

148. Dingjan GM, Maas A, Nawijn MC, Smit L, Voerman JS, et al. 1998. Severe B cell deficiency and disrupted splenic architecture in transgenic mice expressing the E41K mutated form of Bruton's tyrosine kinase. *EMBO J.* 17:5309–20

149. Middendorp S, Dingjan GM, Maas A, Dahlenborg K, Hendriks RW. 2003. Function of Bruton's tyrosine kinase during B cell development is partially independent of its catalytic activity. *J. Immunol.* 171:5988–96

150. Miller AT, Berg LJ. 2002. New insights into the regulation and functions of Tec family tyrosine kinases in the immune system. *Curr. Opin. Immunol.* 14:331–40

151. Tsai YT, Su YH, Fang SS, Huang TN, Qiu Y, et al. 2000. Etk, a Btk family tyrosine kinase, mediates cellular transformation by linking Src to STAT3 activation. *Mol. Cell. Biol.* 20:2043–54

152. Bagheri-Yarmand R, Mandal M, Taludker AH, Wang RA, Vadlamudi RK, et al. 2001. Etk/Bmx tyrosine kinase activates Pak1 and regulates tumorigenicity of breast cancer cells. *J. Biol. Chem.* 276:29403–9

153. Reid GK, Osmond DG. 1985. B lymphocyte production in the bone marrow of mice with X-linked immunodeficiency (*xid*). *J. Immunol.* 135:2299–302

154. Cancro MP, Sah AP, Levy SL, Allman DM, Constantinescu D, et al. 2000. B cell production and turnover in CBA/Ca, CBA/N and CBA/N-bcl-2 transgenic mice: *xid*-mediated failure among pre B cells is unaltered by bcl-2 overexpression.

Curr. Top. Microbiol. Immunol. 252:31–38

155. Hayashi S, Witte PL, Kincade PW. 1989. The *xid* mutation affects hemopoiesis in long term cultures of murine bone marrow. *J. Immunol.* 142:444–51

156. Narendran A, Ramsden D, Cumano A, Tanaka T, Wu GE, Paige CJ. 1993. B cell developmental defects in X-linked immunodeficiency. *Int. Immunol.* 5:139–44

157. Middendorp S, Dingjan GM, Hendriks RW. 2002. Impaired precursor B cell differentiation in Bruton's tyrosine kinase-deficient mice. *J. Immunol.* 168:2695–703

158. Dingjan GM, Middendorp S, Dahlenborg K, Maas A, Grosveld F, Hendriks RW. 2001. Bruton's tyrosine kinase regulates the activation of gene rearrangements at the λ light chain locus in precursor B cells in the mouse. *J. Exp. Med.* 193:1169–78

159. Ellmeier W, Jung S, Sunshine MJ, Hatam F, Xu Y, et al. 2000. Severe B cell deficiency in mice lacking the tec kinase family members Tec and Btk. *J. Exp. Med.* 192:1611–24

160. Jumaa H, Mitterer M, Reth M, Nielsen PJ. 2001. The absence of SLP65 and Btk blocks B cell development at the preB cell receptor-positive stage. *Eur. J. Immunol.* 31:2164–69

161. Saito K, Tolias KF, Saci A, Koon HB, Humphries LA, et al. 2003. BTK regulates PtdIns-4,5-P2 synthesis: importance for calcium signaling and PI3K activity. *Immunity* 19:669–78

162. Tomlinson MG, Woods DB, McMahon M, Wahl MI, Witte ON, et al. 2001. A conditional form of Bruton's tyrosine kinase is sufficient to activate multiple downstream signaling pathways via PLC γ2 in B cells. *BMC Immunol.* 2:4

163. Middendorp S, Zijlstra AJ, Kersseboom R, Dingjan GM, Jumaa H, Hendriks RW. 2005. Tumor suppressor function of Bruton's tyrosine kinase is independent of its catalytic activity. *Blood.* In press

164. Humphries LA, Dangelmaier C, Sommer K, Kipp K, Kato RM, et al. 2004. Tec kinases mediate sustained calcium influx via site-specific tyrosine phosphorylation of the PLCγ SH2-SH3 linker. *J. Biol. Chem.* 279:37651–61

165. Jou ST, Carpino N, Takahashi Y, Piekorz R, Chao JR, et al. 2002. Essential, nonredundant role for the phosphoinositide 3-kinase p110δ in signaling by the B-cell receptor complex. *Mol. Cell. Biol.* 22:8580–91

Annu. Rev. Immunol. 2005. 23:447–85
doi: 10.1146/annurev.immunol.23.021704.115643
Copyright © 2005 by Annual Reviews. All rights reserved
First published online as a Review in Advance on November 29, 2004

THE NOD MOUSE: A Model of Immune Dysregulation

Mark S. Anderson and Jeffrey A. Bluestone

*Diabetes Center, University of California, San Francisco, California 94143;
email: manderson@diabetes.ucsf.edu, jbluest@diabetes.ucsf.edu*

Key Words   autoimmunity, T lymphocytes, animal models, type 1 diabetes,
immunotherapy, tolerance

■ **Abstract**   Autoimmunity is a complex process that likely results from the summation of multiple defective tolerance mechanisms. The NOD mouse strain is an excellent model of autoimmune disease and an important tool for dissecting tolerance mechanisms. The strength of this mouse strain is that it develops spontaneous autoimmune diabetes, which shares many similarities to autoimmune or type 1a diabetes (T1D) in human subjects, including the presence of pancreas-specific autoantibodies, autoreactive CD4$^+$ and CD8$^+$ T cells, and genetic linkage to disease syntenic to that found in humans. During the past ten years, investigators have used a wide variety of tools to study these mice, including immunological reagents and transgenic and knockout strains; these tools have tremendously enhanced the study of the fundamental disease mechanisms. In addition, investigators have recently developed a number of therapeutic interventions in this animal model that have now been translated into human therapies. In this review, we summarize many of the important features of disease development and progression in the NOD strain, emphasizing the role of central and peripheral tolerance mechanisms that affect diabetes in these mice. The information gained from this highly relevant model of human disease will lead to potential therapies that may alter the development of the disease and its progression in patients with T1D.

INTRODUCTION

The nonobese diabetic (NOD) strain of mouse is an increasingly useful and important model of autoimmune type 1 diabetes (T1D). Since its development more than 20 years ago, this strain has provided a wealth of insight into the inherently complex processes involved in autoimmune diseases. Autoimmune diseases are believed to involve the breakdown of multiple tolerance pathways. These pathways are individual complex networks that help control a harmful self-directed immune response, and they can be broadly divided into central and peripheral tolerance mechanisms. It is widely thought that most autoimmune diseases involve the summation of subtle defects in several of these networks. The NOD mouse represents an experiment of nature, where a strain has evolved that harbors defects in

0732-0582/05/0423-0447$14.00

multiple safety nets, thereby allowing autoimmunity to occur spontaneously. This review highlights recent advances in our understanding of these defects in both the central and peripheral tolerance pathways, and it briefly highlights how these findings are affecting the logical development of new therapies for the treatment of autoimmune diabetes.

Strain Origins and Characteristics

Makino and colleagues (1, 2) originally developed the NOD strain in Japan during the selection of a cataract-prone strain derived from the outbred Jcl:ICR line of mice. During the selection of this cataract-prone strain, the NOD strain was established, through repetitive brother-sister mating, as a subline that spontaneously developed diabetes. The incidence of spontaneous diabetes in the NOD mouse is 60% to 80% in females and 20% to 30% in males (2, 3). Interestingly, the incidence of disease is highest when mice are maintained in a relatively germ-free environment but dramatically decreases when mice are maintained in conventional "dirty" housing facilities (3–5). The basis for this effect is unclear, but it has been suggested that it reflects the fine-tuning of the immune system that occurs during exposure to foreign proteins and protects the individual from allergy, autoimmunity, and other diseases of immune dysregulation (6).

Diabetes onset typically occurs at 12 to 14 weeks of age in female mice and slightly later in male mice. Histological studies have shown that few immune cell infiltrates are noted in islets until approximately 3 to 4 weeks of age, when both male and female mice begin to demonstrate mononuclear infiltrates that surround the islet (peri-insulitis). These infiltrates progress and invade the islets (insulitis) over the subsequent few weeks, such that most mice demonstrate severe insulitis by 10 weeks of age. The finding that the reduced incidence in male mice occurs in spite of similar levels of early insulitis suggests that late regulatory events control disease progression. Thus, the autoimmune process in the pancreas of NOD mice includes two checkpoints: checkpoint 1, or insulitis, which is completely penetrant; and checkpoint 2, or overt diabetes, which is not completely penetrant (7). The islet mononuclear infiltrates are complex in their makeup. The majority of cells are $CD4^+$ T cells, and although $CD8^+$ T cells, NK cells, B cells, dendritic cells, and macrophages can also be identified in the lesions (1, 2), NOD disease is primarily dependent on $CD4^+$ and $CD8^+$ T cells (3, 8, 9). Evidence for this includes the ability to transfer disease with purified $CD4^+$ and $CD8^+$ T cells from NOD donors, the ability of individual T cell clones (both class I and class II restricted) derived from NOD islets to passively transfer disease (10, 11), and the fact that T cell modulating therapies inhibit disease incidence (12–16). Whereas diabetes can be transferred from affected animals by passive transfer of splenocytes, it cannot be transferred by autoantibodies from new onset diabetic donors, although B cells are also clearly important for the development of the disease (see below) (17).

NOD mice are also prone to developing other autoimmune syndromes, including autoimmune sialitis (18), autoimmune thyroiditis (19), autoimmune peripheral polyneuropathy (20), a systemic lupus erythematosus–like disease that develops if mice are exposed to killed mycobacterium (21), and prostatitis (in male mice). Although T cells play a primary role in each of these diseases, the relative role of $CD4^+$ and $CD8^+$ T cells, the antigens recognized, and the role of costimulation can be quite variable. For instance, the peripheral neuropathy caused by extensive demyelination of dorsal root ganglia and other peripheral nerves depends on interferon-producing $CD4^+$ T cells, as opposed to diabetes, which is perforin-dependent (22) and results from the recognition of neural antigens (20; J.A. Bluestone & H. Jordan, unpublished observations). Moreover, the selectivity of the disease can be quite impressive as, under certain circumstances, animals protected from diabetes (23) develop pancreatitis, resulting in destruction of the exocrine tissue in close proximity to the protected islets (Q. Tang, T.C. Meagher, M. Li & J.A. Bluestone, unpublished observations). By comparison, there can be an overlap in NOD autoimmunity. Islet-reactive T cells may initially target cells other than the insulin producing β cells, including the nonmyelinated Schwann cells that surround the islets. Winer et al. (24) demonstrated that NOD mice can exhibit spontaneous responses to Schwann cell proteins, including the antigens shared with islets, such as glutamic acid decarboxylase (GAD) 65, as well as neural antigens such as $S100\beta$ and GFAP (glial fibrillary acidic protein). T cell lines to GFAP promote insulitis, whereas antigen-based therapy with $S100\beta$ and GFAP inhibit the development of diabetes in adoptive transfer experiments. Interestingly, these various autoimmune syndromes are not always found in every animal. Recent data from Bach and colleagues (25) and others suggest that the various diseases may be individually regulated, and they may have unique antigen specificities. Finally, the NOD mouse strain is particularly susceptible to certain experimentally induced autoimmune diseases such as experimental autoimmune encephalomyelitis (26). Thus, like some humans with T1D, the NOD mouse combines an overall genetic propensity for multi-organ autoimmunity with specific targets not limited to organs of the endocrine system.

NOD Genetics

Multiple loci control the genetic susceptibility to diabetes in this mouse. NOD mice harbor a unique major histocompatibility complex (MHC) haplotype, termed H-2^{g7}, that is essential and is the highest genetic contributor for disease susceptibility (27, 28). This MHC haplotype does not express an I-E molecule because of a defective Eα locus. Moreover, the unique I-A molecule contains a nonaspartic acid substitution at position 57 of the beta chain (29) that substantially alters the repertoire of MHC binding peptides presented by this allele (30). Strikingly, this substitution is also seen in human T1D MHC susceptibility loci in the DQ beta chain (31). Several studies that examine the MHC requirement in NOD mice for the development of insulitis and diabetes conclude that homozygosity of the H-2^{g7} haplotype may be necessary for diabetes development and that dominant protection may be provided by some MHC manipulations including introducing a functional I-E or non-I-A^{g7} allele but not others (32–37). The mechanism(s) by which MHC both allows for susceptibility and protects remains open to debate, but include skewing of thymic selection processes (38), induction of regulatory cell populations, or skewing of Th1 versus Th2 effector responses (39). Thus, the major contributor to diabetes susceptibility is the MHC class II molecule itself. Its unique structure, its ability to bind an array of low affinity peptides, and its shared structural features in humans susceptible to this and other autoimmune disease suggests that targeting this gene product, both in terms of genetic screening and potential therapy, remains a high priority. Finally, it should be noted that multiple genes are encoded within the MHC loci, many of which have been associated with immune functions. Possibly, the high diabetes susceptibility endowed by the H-2^{g7} MHC may be caused, in part, by polymorphisms in other genes, such as TNF-α, encoded within this chromosomal segment.

In addition to the MHC locus, many other loci contribute to disease development and are termed *Idd* loci. To date, almost 20 potential *Idd* loci have been identified (40), but in most cases, the exact structural or regulatory elements that lie within these loci still await identification. Researchers have discovered some clues about the nature of some of these genetic susceptibilities. In the case of the *Idd*5 locus (which may encode two regulatory elements), a unique polymorphism in the CTLA-4 gene was determined that affects gene splicing (41). Interestingly, CTLA-4 is also a candidate gene in humans susceptible to a variety of autoimmune diseases, although the structural basis for CTLA-4 dysfunction is distinct. Recent evidence suggests that the changes in the CTLA-4 expression pattern may have profound effects on expression of a closely linked molecule, ICOS, which influences the Th balance and cytokine production. Candidate genes have been suggested in other *Idd* loci as well. Vav 3 polymorphisms may account for *Idd*18, CD101 for *Idd*10, and the IL-2 or IL-21 genes for *Idd*3 (L. Wicker, personal communication). However, to date none of these genes have been directly shown to be dysregulated in NOD mice. The existence of multiple susceptibility loci in the NOD strain again highlights the inherent complexity of the autoimmune process and supports the hypothesis that multiple tolerance networks are defective and interact in this strain. In fact, the spontaneous incidence of diabetes in the NOD mouse strain is likely to be a consequence of the absence of protective genes, as well. In a mouse model for lupus, there is already clear evidence of genetic interaction from several resistance and susceptibility loci that affect different tolerance pathways that, when cosegregated, lead to the lupus phenotype (42). It is also likely that even more, as yet unappreciated genes influence this disease. Recent studies by Auchincloss and colleagues (43), as well as Greiner and colleagues (44), show that tolerance induction in NOD in an organ allograft setting is defective. The genetics of this tolerance resistance appears to be distinct from the currently identified *Idd* loci (45).

Pathogenesis of T1D in NOD Mice

NOD mice exhibit a number of immune defects that may contribute to their expression of autoimmunity. Although much of the emphasis in the field (and this review) has been on the role of T cells in the development and progression of the disease, the immune system in NOD mice harbors defects in multiple subsets of leukocytes. These include defective macrophage maturation and function (46), low levels of natural killer (NK) cell activity (47, 48), defects in NKT cells (49, 50), deficiencies in their regulatory $CD4^+CD25^+$ T cell population (51), and the absence of C5a and hemolytic complement (52).

Recent studies have shed some light on NK function, which is impaired in these mice. NK cell–mediated cytotoxicity is reduced in cells from NOD mice compared to other strains when assayed against NK-sensitive targets (53–55). In addition, the *Idd*6 locus maps to a region of the genome containing the multiple NK cell–associated genes (the NK gene complex) on mouse chromosome 6 (27, 56, 57). At least one mechanism contributes to this NK cell defect. Investigators examining the NK activating receptor, NKG2D, which is expressed on the surface of NK cells, $\gamma\delta$ T cells, activated $CD8^+$ T cells, and NKT cells (48, 58), noted that activated NK cells from NOD mice expressed both NKG2D and its ligand(s), RAE-1. This "inappropriate" upregulation of RAE-1 caused the NKG2D receptor to be internalized through ligand interactions with RAE-1, compromising NK activity, which contributes to the NK cell defect observed in NOD mice. In contrast, a recent study suggests that NK cells may contribute to the effector phase of diabetes in the BDC 2.5 T cell receptor (TCR) transgenic model in the C57BL/6 background (59). In this setting, in which NKG2D is expressed normally, investigators observed that the TCR transgenic mice developed more aggressive and destructive insulitis and a higher incidence of diabetes than NOD background transgenic mice. The cells in the more aggressive infiltrates had a higher level of NK-associated genes expressed both at the protein and transcript level. In addition, NK cell levels correlated with disease severity, and NK cell depletion also lessened disease severity in this model.

Studies have shown that B cells are not required at the effector stage of NOD T1D, as T cells from diabetic NOD donors transfer T1D to B cell–depleted NOD mice. However, recent evidence suggests that B cells play an important role in the development of autoreactivity in NOD T1D. NOD mice rendered B cell deficient by antibody treatment are protected from the development of insulitis and diabetes. Using a genetic approach, several groups have shown that NOD mice homozygous for a germline mutation that disables production of membrane-bound IgM, resulting in maturational arrest of B cell development, affords protection against T1D (17, 60). However, the mechanism, or mechanisms, by which B cells affect T1D pathogenesis is unclear. B cells could influence autoimmune disease through autoantibody production or as antigen-presenting cells (APCs) involved in the selection or activation of autoreactive T cells. Although high titers of anti-insulin and anti-GAD autoantibodies are found in prediabetic NOD mice and diabetic humans, transfer of these autoantibodies fails to induce disease in NOD mouse models. However, a recent report suggests that antibodies may influence disease through the passive transfer from mother to offspring (61). Greeley et al. (61) suggest that maternal anti-islet antibodies may help promote the T cell response in the islet, but they also acknowledge that direct testing of antibody specificity for this effect awaits further analysis. By comparison, activated B cells are competent APCs that may capture and present islet antigens to T cells. Thus, B cells could affect susceptibility to and onset of T1D through their APC function. Although one report showed that a B cell–deficient patient (X-linked agammaglobulinemia) developed T1D, this does not rule out either a potential diversity in disease pathogenesis in different patient populations or a potential role for B cells in contributing disease pathogenesis in most patients with T1D (62).

T Cells are the Key

The most proximal and well-studied pathogenic responses are mediated by T cells. Early studies suggested that both CD4$^+$ and CD8$^+$ T cells participate in the development and progression of the disease. CD4$^+$ T cells are essential both early and late in disease development. For instance, several groups have shown that CD4$^+$ T cells can be used to transfer disease and that anti-CD4 mAb therapy prevents diabetes onset in NOD mice (12). Interestingly, Fathman and colleagues (63) have shown that the antigen-specific T cells reside in the CD4^{high} T cells subpopulation in the pancreatic draining lymph nodes. This fits with the genetic linkage to class II. In fact, CD4$^+$ T cells are very much involved in the pathogenesis of disease and can directly mediate islet cell destruction. However, the CD8$^+$ T cells promote the disease as well. Initial studies pointed to a role for CD8$^+$ T cells early in disease development, perhaps by causing sufficient islet cell destruction to prime the more robust CD4$^+$ T cell response (64). CD8$^+$ T cells may also play a role in effector function (11). The NKG2D ligand, RAE-1, is upregulated in the pancreas of prediabetic NOD mice (65). This upregulation occurs in NOD.SCID mice and also correlates with the expression of NKG2D receptors on many CD8$^+$ T cells. Interestingly, anti-NKG2D antibody therapy as late as 12 weeks of age decreased disease development and resulted in a dramatic decrease in insulitis, especially by decreasing a population of autoreactive glucose 6-phosphatase catalytic subunit related protein (IGRP)-reactive CD8$^+$ T cells.

T Cell Antigen Specificity in T1D in NOD Mice

Given the overall importance of T cells in the pathogenesis of the disease, investigators have devoted an extensive amount of work to identifying the antigen specificity of diabetogenic T cells in the NOD mouse. The antigens recognized by CD4$^+$ and CD8$^+$ include insulin, GAD, insulinoma-associated protein 2 (IA-2), and heat shock protein 60 (Hsp60), all of which are produced in pancreatic islets, with only insulin being uniquely expressed in the islets (reviewed in 66). Previous work established that these T cell specificities correlate with autoantibody specificities to these antigens and that there is a pattern to the kinetics of when these reactivities appear in the NOD mouse. However, one difficulty in identifying the antigens important for actually inciting disease is the process of epitope spreading, whereby an initiating response rapidly leads to other antigen responses in the same target tissue. In fact, it is increasingly likely that multiple antigens may be capable of initiating the pathogenic disease process in these immune-dysregulated animals as multiple T cell reactivities to islet antigens have been observed even in normal individuals. Thus, various processes, including antigen mimicry, nonspecific inflammation, and defective tolerogenic processes, may combine to promote responses against a handful of islet expressing autoantigens.

Investigators have identified many islet autoantigens by examining islet-specific $CD4^+$ and $CD8^+$ T cells that have been cloned from inflamed NOD islets. However, the active autoimmune response present in NOD mice has been hampered by the inability to directly examine autoreactive T cell specificities. For example, the presence of a given autoreactive specificity has often been detected by in vitro stimulation assays with a given antigen (i.e., insulin, GAD, etc.), yielding stimulation indices usually less than 5. Two recent developments have fundamentally changed the field. First, a growing number of TCR transgenic mice recognize autoantigens expressed in the NOD pancreas. In addition, soluble MHC complexes bound to a given peptide autoantigen (in dimeric or tetrameric forms) have been developed that can detect a single T cell antigen specificity, providing a critical tool for tracking T cell specificities (67). These complimentary technologies have enabled a better understanding of the kinetics, anatomical location, and functional activities of given autoreactive TCR specificities. As an example, tetramer reagents containing GAD-derived peptides were developed with specificities recognized by T cell clones or T cells from GAD-immunized mice (68, 69). Although these reagents could not reliably detect GAD-reactive cells in nonmanipulated NOD mice, they have been used in patients with new onset diabetes to monitor disease progression (70). Recent studies also report a high frequency of insulin-reactive $CD8^+$ T cell clones in the islets of NOD mice utilizing a tetramer, but again, no detectable cells were found in the peripheral immune system without in vitro expansion (71).

Recently, investigators have reported two additional T cell specificities by tetramer staining in NOD and TCR transgenic mice. Santamaria and colleagues (72) identifed one new class I–restricted autoantigen in the NOD system by determining the antigen specificity of the 8.3 TCR transgenic NOD mice. This $CD8^+$ T cell was originally cloned from an islet infiltrate. By using a library of peptide mimotopes, a reagent was developed that specifically identified T cells and that shares the same antigen specificity as the 8.3 T cell (73). Using this reagent to examine the polyclonal response in intact NOD animals, the investigators observed a remarkably high percentage of peripheral $CD8^+$ T cells bearing this specificity after the initiation of insulitis (74). In fact, detection of this reactivity in the blood of NOD mice was predictive of the subsequent onset of hyperglycemia. The "real" reactivity of this T cell was identified as islet-specific IGRP (75), a β cell specific protein that localizes to the endoplasmic reticulum and that has no known function. Why the autoimmune response in NOD mice targets this antigen at such a high frequency is unknown, but it is of considerable interest and may be a potential avenue for future antigen-based therapies. There are similar data regarding the BDC 2.5 $CD4^+$ autoreactive TCR. Haskins and colleagues (76) originally cloned this pathogenic T cell from an islet infiltrate, and Katz et al. (77) subsequently produced a TCR transgenic mouse. The exact antigen specificity of this islet granule antigen-specific TCR has yet to be determined, but a peptide mimotope was identified that could stimulate this particular TCR (78, 79). Investigators subsequently developed a MHC class II tetramer bound to this mimotope to track T cells that shared the BDC 2.5 specificity (80, 81). T cells with this specificity were identified in the thymus of NOD mice, and they preferentially expand in the pancreatic lymph nodes when compared to other peripheral lymphoid organs. Interestingly, treatment of BDC 2.5 mice with an I-A^{g7}-p31 peptide dimer blocked the development of diabetes (81). Like the 8.3 TCR specificity for CD8$^+$ cells, the overall precursor frequency of cells with this specificity was surprisingly high in NOD mice, making up 0.1% to 0.2% of all CD4$^+$ T cells in the thymus and peripheral lymph nodes. Interestingly, the precursor frequency of these cells was unchanged in B6.H-2^{g7} congenic and NOR mice, suggesting that non-MHC NOD genes must contribute to protection from the onset of insulitis or diabetes, or that the presence of the appropriate MHC and antigen specificity alone is insufficient to promote diabetes. Importantly, T cells against either of these specificities are able to transfer disease. Taken together, it appears that certain autoantigen specificities are not selected against strongly in the thymus and peripheral effects on these T cells help lead to their pathogenicity. Why these cells are detectable in unimmunized mice when compared to other autoantigen specificities remains to be determined. It will also be interesting to learn if there are other islet specificities that can be detected using tetramers or other approaches to further understand how the autoimmune response unfolds in the NOD mouse.

Expansion and Trafficking Contribute to Disease Progression

An important question regarding the autoimmune response in the islet is, where do the initial T cell priming events occur? Naive T cell priming events are generally thought to occur in the secondary lymphoid organs, where antigen is presented by tissue dendritic cells that have migrated from the tissue into the organ (82). After this priming event, newly activated T cells change their surface receptors and homing pattern and gain access to nonlymphoid compartments where their antigen is located. In the NOD system, several studies have demonstrated that the initial priming events occur in the pancreatic lymph node. Data from the NOD TCR transgenics have shown that antigen becomes available for priming between day 15 and day 18 (83, 84). In addition, an increase in activated/memory T cells is observed in NOD mice around this time (85). Finally, selective removal of the pancreatic lymph node before 3 weeks of age completely protects against the development of diabetes in NOD mice, an effect that was not seen with splenectomy (85). The timing of this activation event appears to be related to a wave of β cell death in the islets that occurs at this time. It may be part of normal pancreatic development, but it does not appear to be unique to the NOD strain (86). A recent paper identified the relevant APC as a dendritic cell that is CD11c$^+$CD11b$^+$CD8α^-

in phenotype (87). More work will be needed to determine why this wave of antigen release and presentation provokes an autoimmune response in NOD mice and not in other strains, but it does provide important clues about the timing and location of important initiating events.

Another intrinsic defect in the NOD mouse involving lymphopenia and homeostatic proliferation of naive NOD T cells may also contribute to disease progression (88). T cell numbers are tightly regulated at a steady state in normal hosts, and when naive T cells are transferred into lymphopenic hosts, they undergo an expansion referred to as homeostatic proliferation (reviewed in 89). During this expansion, naive T cells can acquire effector-like characteristics, including cell surface markers and the ability to quickly produce effector cytokines. Previous studies have shown that a rat model of spontaneous autoimmune diabetes, the BB rat, exhibits a profound lymphodeficiency that has been purported to contribute to disease pathogenesis. Recently, King et al. (88) demonstrated that NOD mice have an acquired lymphopenia that evolves as the mice age. This lymphopenia appears to allow homeostatic proliferation to occur when naive T cells are transferred into these hosts; interestingly, the authors show that this process maps to the *Idd*3 locus. The authors suggest that the homeostatic proliferation of self-reactive lymphocytes in this milieu of β cell death helps trigger them to become bona fide effectors. Additional experiments in this study suggested that the defect is due to interactions between IL-21 and the IL-21R; however, other studies have not observed this lymphopenic phenotype (90, 91). We do not know if the problem is lymphopenia itself or a selective deficiency of certain cell subsets, such as regulatory T cells (Tregs). Thus, the role of IL-21 will need confirmation by other approaches such as antibody blocking or gene knockout approaches. The exact identification of what polymorphisms in the *Idd*3 locus cause this process also awaits determination.

An increasing number of studies suggest that cell trafficking may also be intimately involved in disease progression. Regulatory $CD4^+CD25^+$ T cells capable of preventing diabetes express high levels of the chemokine receptors CCR7, CCR6, and CCR4. Furthermore, the development of insulitis and progression to disease correlates with expression of monocyte chemoattractant protein-1 (MCP-1), macrophage inflammatory protein-1α (MIP-1α), MIP-1β, CCR5, RANTES (regulated on activation, normal T cell expressed and secreted), MCP-3, MCP-5, and IFN-inducible protein-10 (IP-10) (92). One striking feature of spontaneous autoimmune diabetes is the prototypic formation of lymphoid follicular structures within the pancreas. Lymphotoxin (LT), a critical cytokine that controls formation of lymphoid follicles in the spleen, is intimately involved in pathogenesis of T1D (92a). An LTα receptor-immunoglobulin fusion protein (LTαR-Ig), administered to NOD mice, prevented insulitis and diabetes. Even late treatment reversed insulitis and prevented diabetes. Expression of the chemokines BLC (B-lymphocyte chemoattractant) in the pancreas promotes lymphoid follicle development (93). Thus, a well-established lymphoid microenvironment in the islets is critical to the development and progression of T1D.

CENTRAL TOLERANCE AND NOD MICE

Given the overwhelming evidence that T cells are intimately involved in the pathogenesis of diabetes in NOD mice, a large body of work has examined whether defects in thymic selection and development are the major cause of autoimmunity. For instance, some studies suggest that NOD mice harbor a unique morphological lesion in the thymus that may somehow alter thymic selection (39, 94–96). Other studies suggest a global defect in thymic negative selection process that may also contribute to diabetes susceptibility (discussed further below) (97). Recent work on the Aire gene highlighted the significance of thymic selection of ectopically expressed antigens and autoimmune endocrine diseases. The Aire gene was originally identified by positional cloning efforts (98, 99) on patients with the clinical syndrome termed APECED (Autoimmune PolyEndocrinopathy, Candidiasis and Ectodermal Dysplasia), which is characterized by the development of spontaneous autoimmunity in multiple endocrine organs (including T1D in many subjects). Studies on Aire-deficient mice have demonstrated that Aire controls the ectopic expression of many self-proteins (including insulin) in medullary epithelial cells of the thymus (100). In the absence of Aire, there is a defect in the negative selection of organ-specific T cells (101), and Aire-deficient thymic stroma is also sufficient for the transfer of the disease into Aire-sufficient B6 nude hosts (100). Thus, the working model is that Aire helps prevent autoimmune disease by helping drive the negative selection of self-reactive thymocytes with specificity for Aire-driven transcripts.

A direct role for Aire in the NOD mouse model has not been reported, but recent studies on the insulin 2 knockout in the NOD mouse lend support to the central tolerance model invoked by Aire (102, 103). In rodents, two independent insulin genes, *ins1* and *ins2*, are located on different chromosomes. Both humans and rodents have detectable insulin transcripts and proteins present in the thymic stroma (100, 104–108), but through mechanisms that are not completely understood, *ins2* is thought to be preferentially expressed over *ins1* in the thymus of mice (107). Therefore, two groups have examined the role of the *ins2* knockout in the NOD background (102, 103). Because the *ins2* mice still have a normal *ins1* gene, they still produce insulin in a glucose-dependent fashion in the pancreas, but with selectively decreased expression of *ins2* in the thymus. *Ins2*-deficient mice exhibit earlier onset of diabetes in the NOD background when compared to wild-type control NOD mice. Parallel studies in humans with T1D mirror this result: individuals with a certain allele in the VNTR (variable number tandem repeat) element of the insulin gene promoter demonstrate decreased thymic expression of the gene and a higher risk for T1D (104, 105). Thus, these data support the notion that thymically expressed insulin does protect against diabetes, but further studies are warranted to determine the exact effect of this expression on the immune system (i.e., induction of regulatory T cells, negative selection of T cells, etc.) and if this pathway of tolerance is truly abnormal in the NOD mouse.

Investigators have also examined the role of GAD65 in the thymus. This autoantigen was originally identified in human subjects with autoimmune diabetes and stiff-man syndrome, a rare condition in which autoantibodies against GAD react with the protein in nerves, causing paralysis (109). Both autoantibody and T cell reactivity to GAD65 occur at a very high frequency in new onset T1D subjects and those at risk for disease. Similar results have been observed in NOD mice where multiple T cell clones and hybridomas have been generated that recognize multiple individual peptides of this autoantigen (110, 111). These reactivities can be observed early during the autoimmune response in these animals, suggesting a seminal role for this antigen in the initiation of disease. Injection of GAD65 into the thymus conferred protection against diabetes onset (112, 113). Another study suggested that GAD65 was of primary importance as an antigenic target in NOD mice using a transgenic system that prevented GAD65 expression in the islet through an antisense transgenic system (114). These data, however, have recently been questioned, given that GAD65 knockout mice develop diabetes normally in the NOD background (115), and a new study shows that induced tolerance to GAD65 does not alter diabetes susceptibility (116). In this study, the investigators overexpressed GAD65 in APCs by using an invariant chain promoter-driven construct. These transgenic mice expressed the transgene in APCs in both the thymus and periphery, and importantly, these mice were tolerant to GAD65. The robust tolerance to GAD65 was mediated through the radio-resistant and thymic compartments of these mice. Strikingly, there was no change in diabetes susceptibility in NOD mice tolerant to GAD65 in this transgenic system. Thus, these data support the notion that endogenous expression of GAD65 in the thymus may not be crucial in diabetes prevention. Several caveats, however, need to be considered. One is that GAD65 is clearly transcribed in the thymus of NOD mice and, as shown in a recently published study using a GAD65 TCR transgenic, likely negatively selects T cells with GAD65 specificity (117). Another caveat in this system is the role of another GAD isoform, GAD67, as it shares several epitopes with the GAD65 isoform and could confound some of these studies. It is possible that GAD67 and not GAD65 is the predominant isoform in mice, and thus induction of tolerance to GAD65 may not be complete for GAD67.

NOD mice may have other generalized defects in thymic selection processes. Recently, several studies have directly examined thymic selection in the NOD mouse and have shown some identifiable lesions. Data from the crystal structure of the NOD I-A^{g7} molecule suggest that the molecule may be intrinsically unstable, resulting in a poor peptide binder; this property may lead to poor negative selection in response to self-peptides in the thymus (30, 118). However, in this model, poor peptide binding to self-antigens also occurs in the periphery, and how this relates to thymic versus peripheral antigen presentation events remains open to debate. Another study demonstrated that mature NOD thymocytes have altered sensitivity to negative selection mediated by either anti-CD3 mAb or superantigen (97) in both in vitro and in vivo assays. This effect was independent of the expression of I-A^{g7} and appeared to involve both Fas-dependent and Fas-independent apoptosis pathways. A third set of studies compared a double TCR transgenic/neo-self-antigen transgenic system in the NOD genetic background versus the B10 genetic background (119). These experiments revealed that the NOD genetic background conferred a decrease in the ability to negatively select neo-self specific TCRs, a decrease that correlated with diabetes susceptibility supporting a generalized thymic defect in NOD mice. This defect mapped to non-MHC genes and was intrinsic to the T cell compartment, but direct identification of these genes awaits further investigation. Finally, NOD thymocytes are more sensitive to γ-irradiation than some other strains of mice, and this effect has been genetically linked to the *Idd6* locus on mouse chromosome 6 (120). Apoptosis defects in thymocytes have also been disputed by others; a recent report shows no difference in the susceptibility of NOD thymocytes to apoptosis when treated with anti-CD3 mAb (121).

In summary, the NOD mouse has several defects in thymic selection processes. However, it remains to be seen if these global defects alter thymic selection in a manner that leads to diabetes. Does resistance to thymocyte apoptosis lead to escape of more islet-specific T cells? The tetramer studies related to the BDC 2.5 specificity and the IGRP specificity discussed above would argue against this because the precursor frequency of these specificities is unchanged in other genetic backgrounds that do not seem to have this apoptosis-resistance phenotype. Is the process of dysfunctional apoptosis and thymocyte cell death involved in central and peripheral tolerance mechanisms and related to diabetes? In terms of self-antigen presentation and selection in the thymus, insulin expression appears to play a role in protecting against diabetes. It remains to be determined, however, if other specificities are also important for thymically imposed tolerance related to diabetes protection. Interestingly, a group has described a defect in Aire expression in the NOD thymus; perhaps this is yet another mechanism by which central tolerance is disrupted in this mouse strain (122). Finally, the role of I-A^{g7} and its unique peptide-binding properties as it relates to thymic selection still remains to be completely unraveled. For example, does this class II molecule allow for poor negative selection in the thymus or does it somehow alter the ultimate T cell repertoire toward low affinity self-reactivity? Ultimately, it will be necessary to sift through a plethora of thymic defects in NOD mice. Many of these may be epiphenomena or differences among inbred mouse strains. In the future, investigators will need to address which of these observations are consistent and meaningful.

PERIPHERAL TOLERANCE AND NOD MICE

Regulation of the immune response to self-antigens is a complex process that depends on maintaining self-tolerance while retaining the capacity to mount a robust immune response. T cells specific for these autoantigens are present in most normal individuals but are kept under control by multiple peripheral tolerance mechanisms. Peripheral tolerance refers to events that occur after lymphocytes have matured in the thymus and bone marrow and trafficked into peripheral tissues and lymphoid organs where they may encounter self-antigens (123). Peripheral mechanisms play an essential role in the maintenance of tolerance and prevention of autoimmune disease, including in the NOD model. First, autoreactive T cells exist in normal healthy subjects (124, 125), suggesting that thymic deletion is not complete in preventing the escape of such populations, and thus other mechanisms must be keeping these cells in check. In addition, knockout mice for genes that are important for peripheral tolerance pathways, such as IL-2, Fas, and CTLA-4 (126, 127), develop spontaneous autoimmune disease. Finally, as is highlighted below, therapeutics that target peripheral immunity can substantially alter the progression of autoimmunity in both NOD mice and patients with T1D. In this section, we highlight studies that have used the NOD mouse as a tool to study peripheral mechanisms, including deletion, anergy, suppression, and ignorance.

Costimulation

Costimulation of naive T cells plays an important role in preventing autoreactive responses. Since the discovery of the requirement for a "second signal" in naive TCR activation by Jenkins & Schwartz (128), interest in costimulation and its role in diabetes onset and progression in the NOD mouse has greatly increased. Early studies in this area focused on the T cell–expressed receptor CD28 and the APC-expressed ligands for these receptors B7-1 (CD80) and B7-2 (CD86). During a normal productive immune response, B7-1 and/or B7-2 are upregulated on APCs and bind to CD28 on naive T cells. This binding results in a number of important events, including stabilization of IL-2 mRNA (129–132), production of an effective immunological synapse (133, 134), and an increase in antiapoptotic factors in stimulated T cells (135, 136). Given the requirement of costimulation for effective naive TCR stimulation, this pathway is an important control in the prevention of untoward autoimmune responses. Excellent examples of this are demonstrated in experimentally induced autoimmune diseases such as experimental autoimmune encephalitis (26) and collagen-induced arthritis (137). However, despite the current dogma of CD28/B7 costimulation, studies in the NOD mouse have highlighted the complexities of these pathways in controlling spontaneous, ongoing autoimmune responses such as NOD diabetes.

In initial studies, we showed (138) disease onset could be blocked in the NOD by treatment with an anti-B7-2 mAb when administered before 10 weeks of age. These results suggested that CD28/B7-2 was the essential costimulatory pathway for inducing autoimmune diabetes in this setting and seemed to rule out a substantial role for B7-1 in this setting. The mechanism of action of this therapy was unclear because there were limited effects on insulitis and no effect if treatment was delayed until later in the disease course (138). Additional studies used a combination of anti-B7-1 plus anti-B7-2 mAbs or the *murine* CTLA4Ig, a fusion protein that functioned as an effective CD28/B7 antagonist. Surprisingly, total blockade of the CD28/B7 pathway with these agents accelerated the development of diabetes and insulitis. Subsequent work showed that CD28-deficient and B7-1/B7-2 double deficient mice had an increased susceptibility to diabetes on the NOD background (139). Several models were proposed to explain this paradoxical finding. First, multiple studies have shown that CD28 costimulation has a profound effect on Th1/Th2 differentiation. In fact, CD28 knockout mice preferentially develop Th1 responses to nominal and autoantigens in normal and NOD mice (139). Thus, the absence of regulatory Th2 cytokines such as IL-4 might have resulted in exacerbated diabetes in the NOD setting. However, studies have suggested that the absence of IL-4 does not alter diabetes in the NOD mouse strain (140). The treatment with CD28/B7 antagonists affected the development of diabetes even when administered quite late, suggesting that ongoing regulatory processes, controlled by the CD28/B7 pathway, were maintaining immune homeostasis, albeit ultimately failing. Recently, an unexpected observation has explained the negative regulatory role of the CD28/B7 pathway in the development of autoimmune diabetes. Detailed analysis of the CD28 knockout NOD mice identified a selective defect in the number and function of $CD4^+CD25^+$ regulatory T cells (51; discussed further below). Thus, the dysregulation of this costimulatory pathway revealed unexpected secondary effects beyond interference with autoreactive T cell responses.

In 1994, we demonstrated (141) that, unlike CD28, CTLA-4 engagement on activated T cells profoundly inhibited T cell proliferation, IL-2 production, and cell cycle progression. CD28 engagement was essential for CTLA-4 upregulation, a finding that supported an intimate connection between the two opposing regulatory pathways. Thus, it seemed likely that CTLA-4 might be intimately involved in disease development. Several studies have supported a direct role for CTLA-4 in NOD disease progression. In the BDC 2.5/NOD TCR transgenic mouse, Luhder et al. (142) tested the effect of anti-CTLA-4 on the incidence of diabetes and showed that if the treatment is given during a narrow window before the initiation of insulitis, a marked acceleration of diabetes occurs. Similarly, anti-CTLA-4 can accelerate insulitis in nontransgenic NOD mice when given at a young age (143). Interestingly, if treatment was delayed after insulitis had been initiated in the transgenic mouse, there was no acceleration of diabetes. These data support the role of CTLA-4 signaling at the very early stages of disease initiation, just before insulitis develops. Most significantly, multiple genetic studies have linked the *CTLA-4* gene locus and autoimmune susceptibility (reviewed in 144). The *CTLA-4* gene lies on chromosome 1 in close proximity to the *CD28* and *ICOS* genes. This region lies in the diabetes susceptibility locus *Idd*5.1, and recent work suggests that a polymorphism in the *CTLA-4* gene contributes to autoimmunity in NOD mice (41). As with many other *Idd* loci, the *Idd*5.1 region was originally identified using a congenic breeding strategy to find loci that control diabetes susceptibility between the B10 and NOD strain of mouse (27). Many polymorphisms (likely hundreds to thousands) that differ between the NOD and B10 strain are located in this large genetic interval (approximately 1.5 centimorgans). Many of these polymorphisms lie in noncoding regions of the locus and may or may not confer any biological significance, leaving the determination of causative polymorphisms a significant challenge. A noncoding change polymorphism was recently examined in the CTLA-4 gene and was shown to have similarity to a splicing silencer polymorphism identified previously in the CD45 gene (145). This polymorphism correlated with the alternative splicing of a ligand independent form of CTLA-4 in the non-NOD background, which suggests that this form of CTLA-4 may affect disease susceptibility (41). Recent work has also shown the ability of the liCTLA-4 to negatively regulate T cell responses and the presence of increased ZAP-70 phosphorylation in CD45RB low cells in NOD versus NOD.Idd5.1 congenic mice (146); the direct role of this effect on in vivo tolerance, however, has not been elucidated. In fact, direct proof that this polymorphism versus other polymorphisms in the *Idd*5.1 region cause this effect also needs to be directly tested. In sum, these genetic data strongly support a role for the CTLA-4 molecule in disease susceptibility in the NOD mouse, but further work on the molecular mechanism(s) and their effects remain to be elucidated.

Recent reports have examined the role of other costimulatory molecules in the NOD system. ICOS is a CD28 family member that is expressed on T cells and binds its ligand ICOSL, which is expressed on both lymphoid and nonlymphoid tissues (147). In the initial description of ICOS, the investigators showed that this costimulatory pathway preferentially promotes IL-10 production (147). Others have suggested that engagement of this costimulatory pathway can selectively regulate Th2 responses (148). So perhaps not surprisingly, Herman et al. (149) showed that treatment with anti-ICOS in the BDC 2.5/NOD TCR transgenic mouse led to the acceleration of diabetes, and this treatment correlated with a decrease in regulatory T cell populations that express ICOS on the cell surface. Another recent report shows a polymorphism in the NOD ICOS gene that may play a role in the disease risk associated with the *Idd*5.1 region (146), although further work needs to be done to confirm this. Another costimulatory molecule pair that has recently been reported in the NOD model is PD-1 and its ligands PD-L1 and PD-L2 (143). Previous work had identified PD-1 as a CD28/CTLA-4 family member present on T cells that could function as a negative regulator of T cell responses (150–152). Supporting a potential role in autoimmune diseases are PD-1-deficient mice that develop spontaneous lupus or cardiomyopathy, depending on the genetic background of the animal (153, 154). Treatment with either anti-PD-1 or anti-PD-L1 to prediabetic NOD mice accelerated the development of diabetes at several ages and accelerated the development of insulitis in young mice (143). Interestingly, PD-L1 was upregulated in inflamed NOD islets, but PD-L2 was not; this may explain the lack of an effect on diabetes or insulitis by PD-L2 blockade.

Recent reports have examined CD40/CD154 and OX40/OX40L interactions in the NOD model. CD154 and its receptor CD40 are expressed on a wide variety of cells and are responsible for an array of activities, including inducing expression of costimulatory molecules on APCs (155). In relation to NOD mice, anti-CD40L mAbs were shown to block insulitis and diabetes when given to young mice before the onset of insulitis (3 weeks of age), but treatment of older mice (9 weeks of age) had no effect on disease (156). This supports a model in which CD40/CD154 interactions are important in the initial priming stages of the disease. Likewise, CD154-deficient mice do not develop insulitis or diabetes (157), and this effect appears to occur through the loss of the ability of CD4$^+$ T cells to effectively prime an autoreactive CD8$^+$ T cell response (158). In addition, data in a NOD TCR transgenic model suggest that the CD154/CD40 pathway (159), as well as the OX40/OX40L pathway (160), may play a direct role in CD4$^+$ T cell activation, because NOD mice deficient for either CD154 or OX40L have a greatly reduced incidence of diabetes and insulitis. However, paradoxically, CD40L knockout mice show signs of enhanced T cell priming in the BDC 2.5/NOD TCR transgenic mouse (161). Finally, investigators have been increasingly interested in the 4-1BB costimulatory pathway primary on activated CD8$^+$ T cells. Using a fine mapping approach by breeding a diabetes resistant mouse strain, C57BL/10, onto a NOD background, Wicker and colleagues have localized the *Idd*9 locus to 4-1BB gene (CD137) (L.S. Wicker, personal communication). Several polymorphic changes between NOD and B10 were identified, including two amino acid changes. This candidate gene fits with the observation that anti-4-1BB treatment of NOD mice resulted in a different therapeutic profile than that predicted from other systems (162). Thus, the role of additional costimulatory pathways remains unclear, perhaps owing to the vagaries of the model systems or to alternative roles for these molecular interactions on pathogenic versus regulatory events.

In summary, there is no doubt that the many positive and negative costimulatory pathways can dramatically influence diabetes development and progression in NOD mice. This occurs in at least three ways: (*a*) initiation of the autoimmune response, (*b*) the target specificity, and (*c*) regulation of the response. However, like most immune responses, the various costimulatory pathways are likely intimately involved in the generation of immunity (in the case of the NOD mouse, autoimmunity), but that, other than serving as targets for immune intervention, most of these pathways do not shed light on the pathogenic basis for this disease. The clear exceptions to this are the CD28/CTLA-4 and 4-1BB pathways, for which a genetically linked susceptibility allele supports a more direct role for these costimulatory pathways in diabetes pathogenesis.

Th1/Th2 Differentiation

T helper responses can be broadly divided on the basis of the array of cytokines produced during their effector response. Th1 T cells produce proinflammatory cytokines like IFN-γ and TNF-α and help promote a cell-mediated immune response and the production of opsonizing IgG antibodies. In contrast, Th2 T cells produce cytokines like IL-4, IL-5, and IL-10 and help promote selected humoral responses (antibodies that do not bind complement and Fc receptors). In addition, both Th1 and Th2 responses reciprocally regulate each other through their respective cytokines. Investigators generally believe that a Th1 effector response is associated with disease progression in NOD mice and that Th2-like responses can help suppress the development of diabetes (39, 163), although this is an oversimplification of the existing data. Many studies have demonstrated that treatment of NOD mice with cytokines that promote or reagents that block Th1 responses help accelerate or block diabetes incidence, respectively. For example, one of the most important inducers of Th1 responses, the cytokine IL-12, has been shown to accelerate disease in NOD mice (164); however, the IL-12 knockout NOD mouse develops diabetes normally (165). Conversely, it appears that deviation to Th2 responses helps protect against diabetes. As an example, injection of IL-4 or other Th2 cytokines or over-expression of Th2 cytokines in the islets can help protect against diabetes in NOD mice (166). But this is, again, an oversimplification, as IL-4 knockout NOD mice have no change in their diabetes incidence (140), and the transfer of Th2 polarized cells into lymphopenic NOD SCID recipients can still induce diabetes (167).

Nonetheless, factors that help promote Th1 over Th2 effector responses or disturb this balance can directly affect diabetes susceptibility. CD28/B7 costimulation interactions appear to regulate the Th1/Th2 balance, as Th2 differentiation from naive T cells is completely dependent on CD28/B7 costimulation, whereas Th1 differentiation is less dependent (168–171). Thus, the finding that the CD28 knockout or B7-1/B7-2 double knockout in the NOD background has aggressive diabetes has been linked to a productive Th1 effector differentiation in the absence of Th2 effector differentiation (139). Likewise, treatment of NOD mice with anti-CD28 mAbs protected against diabetes, and islet-infiltrating T cells produced more IL-4 than in control mice (172). Another cell surface molecule that may affect Th1/Th2 polarization is the recently identified marker Tim-3, which is preferentially expressed on the surface of Th1 effector cells (173). Initial studies with a Tim-3 Ig fusion protein or an anti-Tim-3 mAb in NOD mice show an acceleration of diabetes with both reagents. The mechanism by which this acceleration occurs remains to be thoroughly worked out, but the investigators suggest that the treatment enhanced Th1 activity or a regulatory cell network. Finally, recent studies show that diabetes in the NOD mouse is regulated by transcription factors that control Th1/Th2 development. Disruption of the transcription factor, STAT4, that controls the IFN-γ signalosome significantly reduces T1D by compromising the pathogenic T cell response, as in the STAT4 knockout NOD mouse (174). By comparison, disruption of STAT6, the transcription factor that controls the IL-4 signal, exacerbates diabetes development (175).

NOD mice have also been investigated for intrinsic changes in cytokine production that may alter Th1/Th2 polarization. A number of studies have shown that antigen-presenting cell populations from NOD mice may produce an array of cytokines that promote Th1 responses when compared to other strains of mice (176–179). In addition, dysfunctional cytokine production may be linked to the *Idd*4 genetic region and the *IL-12p40* gene itself (180, 181). Bolstering this genetic data is a study linking a polymorphism in the human *IL-12p40* gene to T1D risk (182). Conflicting reports suggest preferential Th1 differentiation mapping to the CD4$^+$ T cell population and not to APCs in the NOD strain (183). Studies have also shown that the *Idd*9 genetic region may confer diabetes protection through IL-4 production in the islets and the promotion of Th2 polarization (184), perhaps via vav 3 or 4-1BB (see above). Likewise, recent findings show that if the local cytokine environment within the islet is more Th1-like, there is enhanced recruitment of islet-reactive CD4$^+$ T cells (185).

NKT cells are another cell population that has been investigated closely in the Th1/Th2 model and NOD mice. NKT cells are restricted to the non-MHC CD1d molecule and express TCRs that use an invariant $V\alpha14$-$J\alpha1$ chain and a limited number of TCRβ chains ($V\beta8$, $V\beta2$, and $V\beta7$). When stimulated by CD1d-expressing APCs, these cells can produce an array of cytokines early in the immune response that can potentially polarize T cells toward a Th2 phenotype (186, 187). Investigators have thus investigated NOD mice to see if they harbor a defect in the potentially protective cell population. Studies have shown that NOD mice have lower numbers of NKT cells in the thymus and, to a lesser extent, in the periphery than other strains of mice (188–191). In addition, diabetes protection has been observed in NOD mice that have been restored with higher numbers of NKT cells (188, 190, 192, 193). Alternatively, treatment with the α-GalCer reagent that activates NKT cells has also been shown to block diabetes in NOD mice (49, 194, 195). Finally, germline deletion of the CD1d molecule in the NOD background leads to an exacerbation of diabetes (50, 196). The role of NKT cells has been more controversial in human T1D, with some finding a defect (197) and others discounting the possibility (198).

Regulatory T Cells

For at least 30 years, researchers have suggested that, in addition to T cells that mediate effector immune responses to combat infections and mediate graft rejection, classes of regulatory/suppressor T cells exist to control immunity (reviewed in 175). The modern view of CD4$^+$ regulatory T cells began with observations by Sakaguchi and colleagues that the adoptive transfer of T cells depleted of CD4$^+$CD25$^+$ cells induced multi-organ autoimmunity in the recipient animals (199, 200). These and other investigators provided compelling data to support the existence of regulatory T cells in rodents, especially in those animals that had undergone certain immunotherapeutic interventions in the allogeneic transplant or autoimmune setting. Most importantly, Gershon (202), and subsequently Waldman (201), developed the concept of "infectious tolerance," in which cells from tolerant animals could be transferred to naive recipients, suppressing not only the original antigen specificities but other antigens linked through the same APCs. Prominent among the cellular components of this regulatory network are a small population of CD4$^+$ T cells that develop in the thymus and are exported to the periphery earlier in life. The critical importance of this subset has been established in multiple organ-specific autoimmune systems. For example, in rats or mice, thymectomy-induced autoimmunity could be reversed by the adoptive transfer of CD4$^+$CD25$^+$ cells (203, 204). These regulatory T cells, termed Tregs, coexpress a number of cell surface markers including CD25, CTLA-4, and GITR. Recently, the transcription factor FoxP3 has been directly linked to the CD4$^+$CD25$^+$ Treg population. Strikingly, FoxP3-deficient mice and humans have a distinct inability to effectively generate Treg cells (205, 206), and they both succumb to a multi-organ autoimmune disease that includes autoimmune diabetes in the human patients (207). Treatment of FoxP3-deficient mice with syngeneic Treg cells from FoxP3-sufficient donors can protect against the autoimmune disease (206), and transduction of naive CD4$^+$ cells with FoxP3 can induce these cells to take on features of Tregs (208). Together, the data support the notion that CD4$^+$CD25$^+$ Tregs are an important component of peripheral tolerance mechanisms.

The seminal observation that autoimmunity is kept in check by a network of regulatory cells that suppress immune reactivity to self-antigens in the periphery has been exploited during the past ten years in the field of autoimmune diabetes. The early evidence of Tregs in this model system was the observation that the early β cell immune infiltrate in NOD mice remained for weeks to months before the onset of overt diabetes. This observation suggested a battle of an immunoregulatory process in the NOD model. Data supportive of this concept came from transfer experiments, which showed that prediabetic mice harbored a CD4$^+$ T cell population that could suppress the development of diabetes when cotransferred with syngeneic splenocytes from diabetogenic donors (209, 210). Moreover, a short treatment of NOD mice with cyclophosphamide triggered diabetes within two weeks, purportedly caused by destruction of the regulatory network. Subsequent studies showed that depletion of CD62L^{hi} cells from this regulatory population tracked with a loss of suppression and also that CD4$^+$CD62L^{hi} cells were potent inducers of suppression in the transfer model (211). Similar results were also found using CD25 as a marker of the CD4$^+$ T suppressor populations, and the highest regulatory activity tracked with CD4$^+$CD25$^+$CD62L$^+$ cells (51, 212). These regulatory cells originate both from the thymus and through adaptive mechanisms in the periphery. Support for their thymic origin comes from studies showing the ability of thymus-derived CD4$^+$CD25$^+$CD62L$^+$ cells to suppress in transfer experiments and the fact that thymectomy in the NOD leads to an acceleration of disease onset (213, 214). However, it should be noted that thymectomy affected disease onset as late as 3 weeks after birth. This is in contrast to the classic thymectomy experiments by Nishizuka & Sakakura (200), which suggested that autoimmunity in other strains required that the thymectomy be performed at day 3 after birth. Thus, either the time frame for Treg development is distinct in NOD mice or there are distinct subsets of Tregs that may influence the disease. In this regard, recent studies by Bach and colleagues (25) have determined that selective depletion of regulatory populations based on the markers CD4, CD25, CD62L, and CD45RB^{low} in an adoptive transfer system led to differential control of autoimmunity. The conclusion of this study was that CD4$^+$CD62L$^+$ cells controlled diabetes, CD4$^+$CD25$^+$ T cells controlled gastritis and diabetes, and CD4$^+$CD45RB^{low} cells controlled colitis. Why certain markers track with certain diseases still remains to be unraveled, but the data suggest that there may be a unique "imprinting" of disease protection regulatory cells in each target organ (25).

Work in the CD28 and B7-1/B7-2 double knockout mice in the NOD background suggests that effective costimulation through these molecules is necessary for the generation and maintenance of the CD4$^+$CD25$^+$ regulatory population (51). Eliminating CD28 in NOD mice causes Treg depletion by affecting both their thymic development and peripheral homeostasis (215), which leads to an accelerated diabetic phenotype. This exacerbated autoimmunity was rescued when $CD4^+CD25^+CD62L^+$ cells from syngeneic donors were transferred into these mice (51). In fact, NOD mice themselves may have a generalized defect in their ability to generate effective numbers of Tregs; the percentage of Tregs is approximately half that of other autoimmune resistant strains of mice (51), although there are conflicting data on this issue (91). Recent data also suggest that there is a time-dependent change in the ability of $CD4^+CD25^+$ Tregs to suppress in NOD mice and also in the ability of $CD4^+CD25^-$ T effectors to respond to suppression in vitro (216). In terms of effector function, it appears that naturally occurring Tregs in the NOD system can dispense with IL-10 and IL-4 to mediate their suppressive activity. However, the reactivity is dependent on anti-TGFβ although whether the Tregs are making the cytokine directly has not been elucidated in this setting (211, 217). In this regard, a recent study showed that a transient pulse of the cytokine TGFβ when delivered in the islet, was able to induce the expansion of Tregs. This expansion correlated with the ability to suppress diabetes (218) and fits with the observation that TGFβ can induce FoxP3 expression (219). Thus, it appears that certain cytokines may help drive the production or expansion of Tregs and could thus be harnessed as a tool to treat disease. The working model in the NOD system is that Tregs actively suppress the anti-islet response by T effectors, but ultimately this suppression is insufficient to maintain immune homeostasis.

Several questions remain as to how Tregs are generated and how they function. One question concerns the antigen specificity of Tregs and its importance in Treg activity. Although it is quite clear that the induction of Treg activity depends on the engagement of the TCR, the effector function of these cells has been shown to be antigen-nonspecific. The working hypothesis is that Tregs are generated in the thymus in response to self-antigens that are presented to developing thymocytes. As outlined earlier, many self-antigens are present in the thymus, including the autoimmune diabetes antigens like insulin, GAD, and I-A2. Recent data in transgenic systems have shown that self-antigen presentation in the thymus can induce significant numbers of Tregs (220, 221), which suggests that they may preferentially arise from self-antigen selection events in the thymus. Once these cells have been exported to the periphery, they appear to continuously respond to autoantigen exposure. This assertion is based on several observations. First, the peripheral Tregs require continued MHC class II (222) and CD28/B7 engagement to be maintained in the periphery (23, 215). Second, study of adoptively transferred CSFE-labeled Tregs has shown that these cells continually cycle on the basis of exposure to antigen in target tissues (23). Moreover, it is likely that Tregs can develop in the periphery in response to self-antigens. Recent studies have shown that polyclonal T cell activators such as anti-CD3 (223) and low dose of nominal antigen (224) induce the development of FoxP3$^+$ CD4$^+$CD25$^+$ T cells in normal and NOD mice.

The identification of the antigenic specificity of endogenous Treg cells has been hampered by their anergic phenotype, their presumed polyclonal reactivity, and their relatively low precursor frequency. Recently, two studies demonstrated a mechanism by which Treg populations could be expanded ex vivo to generate effective cell numbers to understand more about their function in vivo (23, 225). Tang et al. (23) examined the issue of antigen specificity in Treg function. In this study, it was demonstrated that BDC 2.5/NOD T cells could be expanded ex vivo to produce a Treg population that expressed the unique BDC 2.5 TCR specificity. When these Tregs were cotransferred with diabetogenic cells, they could suppress diabetes at remarkably low cell numbers. Even more impressively, these Tregs could reverse new-onset diabetes in NOD mice. In addition, when compared to polyclonal Tregs that were expanded from NOD mice, BDC 2.5 Tregs were found to be much more potent in their suppressive activity against diabetes. These data are in line with another study that showed that insulin-specific Tregs produced by active immunization could effectively suppress diabetes in a transfer model (226). These data suggest that the antigen specificity of the Tregs plays an important role in the effectiveness of suppression.

Another question about Treg cell suppression concerns the site at which suppression tolerance occurs in vivo. Recent data from Herman et al. (149) suggest that Tregs are active directly in the pancreatic islet. These experiments again used the BDC 2.5/NOD TCR transgenic mouse to analyze this question. Previous work in this system has shown that BDC 2.5 TCR activation occurs primarily in the draining lymph node(s) of the pancreas several weeks after birth (discussed further below) (84). Although this is the active site for initial activation, the recent study by Herman et al. (149) suggests that the majority of Tregs present in the BDC 2.5 TCR transgenic mouse are actively suppressing in the pancreas, rather than the pancreatic lymph node where presumably the initial priming of the autoreactive response is occurring in this system. Like Tang et al. (23), the authors show that protection against diabetes in a BDC 2.5 transfer system could be potently induced by BDC 2.5-derived Tregs.

In summary, there is no doubt that multiple tolerance pathways regulate disease development and progression in the NOD mice. In some instances, the genetics of the NOD mice may be directly linked to these pathways; in most instances, however, the relevant pathways are likely to provide an overlay of basic immune homeostatic mechanisms that, when altered in this highly sensitive system, tip the balance from disease to protection or visa versa (Figure 1). Thus, perhaps the most important consequence of this field of research is the potential to take this new understanding and harness it to develop novel immunotherapeutics to test in patients with T1D.

RATIONALE FOR TREATMENT

Because of its many similarities to the T1D human patient, the NOD mouse has been used extensively as a preclinical tool for the development of new therapeutic strategies. Many therapies that reduce clonal expansion in an antigen-specific

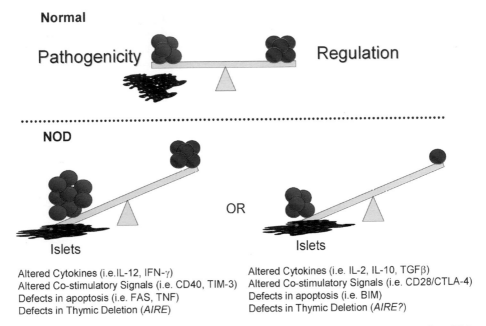

Figure 1   Autoimmunity is a combination of altered pathogenicity and regulation. This figure depicts the importance of the balance between the regulatory cells that control immunity (Tregs, Th2, NKT cells, etc.) and the pathogenic cells that mediate disease. A number of critical biologic parameters are essential for controlling the balance as stated.

manner (GAD, insulin, etc.) have profound effects during the prediabetic stage of disease (227). The selective effects of these therapies on naive antigen-specific cells before the occurrence of epitope spreading significantly expands the antigenic repertoire. By contrast, less than half a dozen therapies have been shown to reverse diabetes once the clinical manifestations of the disease are evident. Moreover, drugs like cyclosporin, which reverse diabetes in mice as well as humans, do not have a durable effect. Although these drugs clear the immune infiltrate in the attacked tissues, once the therapy is discontinued the infiltrates return with increased pathogenic activity and virulence (228). Thus, therapies that induce long-term, durable tolerance depend on the redirection of the immune system to a tolerant state; this state is exemplified by a combination of antigen-specific immune regulation and altered cytokine balance that actively protects the target tissue from destruction. The sheer number of approaches to induce durable tolerance in this animal model is too large to summarize here (for an extensive review see 229), but we would like to highlight a few interesting developments in therapeutic strategies, given the lessons learned in the disease mechanisms discussed above.

Some have questioned the usefulness of the NOD model because so many therapies have been successful as prevention treatments. In fact, more than 175 different agents have been shown to delay or prevent onset of T1D in NOD mice (227). For example, antigen-based therapy of NOD mice with systemically administered insulin was used as a platform for the Diabetes Prevention Trial-1 in patients at high risk for developing T1D. In this study, those high risk patients, treated with insulin, did not show any significant delay in disease onset (230). Similar results have been obtained for other agents like BCG and nicotinamide (231, 232). There are several reasons why the NOD mouse might not be a good model for testing therapies in a prediabetic setting. First, the time course of disease development is quite different; the majority of humans develop the disease at or before puberty, whereas mice develop it much later. This may also explain the skewing of disease incidence between males and females in mice but not in humans. As outlined earlier, the immune system in the young NOD mouse is in a delicate balance that is easily influenced by generalized immunostimulation, which can greatly decrease the incidence of diabetes. Thus, many effective treatments at the prediabetic stage could be preventative because of their direct or secondary effect on immune homeostasis. However, it remains striking how many similarities exist between the disease in rodents and the disease in humans, including the surprising synteny of genetic susceptibility, the fundamental similarity in disease pathogenesis, and the large number of shared autoantigens. Thus, many researchers have suggested that, as a model of human therapy, the NOD mouse is best used after disease onset, either to halt disease progression in the setting of new onset or to reverse the disease in the context of an islet transplant. Using these criteria, many of the reagents that have been shown to be efficacious in prediabetic animals have proven to be ineffective in new onset diabetic mice.

One of the reagents that has shown efficacy in reversing diabetes in NOD mice is anti-CD3 antibody. Anti-CD3 mAbs are potent immunosuppressive agents that have been approved for use in patients undergoing acute kidney allograft rejection. The efficacy of the mAb suggested that it could be effective in a number of other immune disorders such as autoimmunity. In fact, the anti-CD3 mAbs have unique tolerogenic properties (13, 233). Treatment of NOD mice presenting with new-onset diabetes with low doses of anti-CD3 mAbs induced a return to permanent normoglycemia and durable disease remission in 80% of mice. Belghith et al. (217) observed that treatment of mice with the FcR nonbinding anti-CD3 mAb led to a dramatic short-term decrease of pathogenic cells in the inflamed tissue owing to apoptosis of the infiltrating cells. This short-term clonal deletion was followed by a wave of "protective" T cells entering the pancreas, characterized by an increase in IL-10 and TGFβ-producing Tregs, especially in the draining pancreatic lymph nodes of treated animals (217). One unanticipated observation was that the anti-CD3 treatment was equally capable of reversing diabetes in the CD28-deficient NOD mice, which as discussed above, lack Treg cells. These results suggest that the Treg cells can be induced de novo. The precise mechanism of how peripheral engagement of T cells with certain stimuli such as the FcR nonbinding anti-CD3 leads to Treg development and expansion is unknown. However, as suggested by several studies, the same antigen expressed in different sites generates CD4$^+$CD25$^+$ or CD4$^+$CD25$^-$ Treg (220). In addition, presentation of antigenic peptide using a slow releasing pump also leads to Treg development (224). Together, these studies support the concept that either quantitative or qualitative differences in TCR stimulation result in distinct differentiation signals that in some cases promote Treg rather than T effector cell development.

More importantly, in a randomized controlled Phase I/II trial of the FcR non-binding anti-CD3 mAb, hOKT3γ1(Ala-Ala), in newly diagnosed patients with T1D, a single 14-day course decreased the rate of loss of insulin production for over one year and improved glycemic control with concomitant reduction in insulin use. This was achieved without the need for continuous immune suppression and persisted at a time when T cells were quantitatively normal (234). Early studies on the effect of this treatment suggest that it induces a regulatory T cell population that may be responsible for the clinical efficacy of the treatment (235). Thus, anti-CD3 treatment appears to induce its effect by inducing the production of regulatory cell populations that can mediate long-term tolerance. This effect is particularly advantageous because it avoids the long-term immunosuppressive side effects associated with broad spectrum reagents like cyclosporine and T cell depletion treatments.

Given the efficacy of inducing Treg populations with anti-CD3 reagents, it is of interest to develop other techniques that harness these cells. The recent data from Tang et al. (23) have established that islet-specific Tregs can reverse diabetes in NOD mice. This finding provides a platform for future therapy in human subjects, whereby Tregs specific for islet antigens could be selectively expanded ex vivo from new onset T1D patients and used as treatment. This expansion could be facilitated by using multimer reagents that are complexed with known islet-derived antigens. Another recently described protocol using rapamycin/agonist IL-2/antagonist IL-15 seems to selectively deplete T effector populations over Treg populations, and it could be used as a tool in the new onset setting (236). So far, this protocol has been tested in a stringent alloreactive model, but it is a logical choice for therapy. Administration of islet-antigens by oral or other mucosal routes has been shown to induce regulatory cell populations that can mediate diabetes protection (226, 237). Finally, recent data suggest that vitamin D and D3 analogs can be used to induce regulatory cell activity in NOD mice. This is another potential tool for treatment (238), but it has not been directly tested in recent onset diabetes. In sum, the induction and use of Tregs is an exciting new avenue by which antigen-specific tolerance can be induced. Ascertaining what regulates Treg behavior, induction, and activity in T1D will enable investigators to apply this knowledge to the human clinical situation. The NOD mouse will continue to be an indispensable tool for these efforts.

CONCLUSIONS

The NOD mouse has evolved as an important tool that allows researchers to gain insights into tolerance pathways that are active both in the thymus and the periphery. As we have outlined here, autoimmunity in this mouse likely proceeds via the

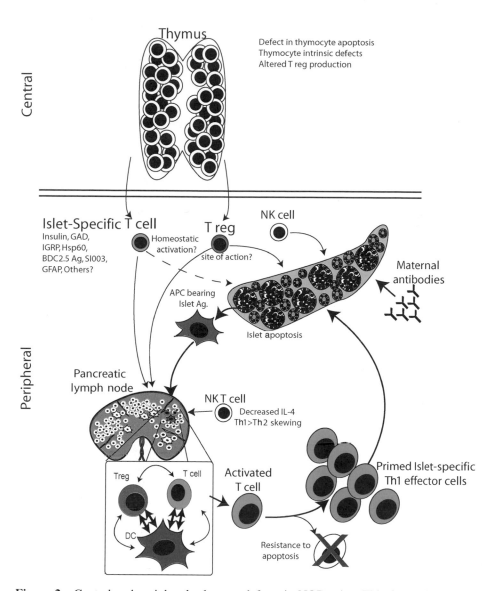

Figure 2   Central and peripheral tolerance defects in NOD mice. This figure depicts the general understanding of potential defects in various tolerogenic processes that might be responsible for the development of diabetes in NOD mice. The figure emphasizes the potential roles of various T cell and other lymphocyte subsets in disease development and progression.

summation of multiple defective tolerance pathways, which are summarized in Figure 2. Thymic development of the NOD T cell repertoire likely harbors defects that allow islet-reactive T cells to escape deletion and prevent the proper generation of regulatory T cells. In the periphery, islet-reactive T cells likely see their antigen in the draining lymph nodes of the pancreas and are inappropriately primed to become effectors. The milieu of cytokines, APCs, innate immune cells, and co-stimulatory molecule interactions that are present during this step likely leads to the initial priming and expansion of an anti-islet response that manifests itself as insulitis. Subsequently, this anti-islet response proceeds over an extended period in a complex immunoregulatory battle involving (but not limited to) Treg cells, NK cells, and Th1 effector skewing that ends in an improper effector response to the islets and the development of diabetes. As demonstrated here, autoimmunity is an incredibly complex process, and the NOD mouse has proved to be an important tool for dissecting both the central and peripheral tolerance mechanisms that contribute to spontaneous autoimmune disease.

ACKNOWLEDGMENTS

The authors thank Todd Eagar for his expertise in preparing the figures and Dr. Abul Abbas, Kevan Herold, and Jeffrey Matthews for reading and critiquing the manuscript and for ongoing discussion and collaborative efforts. M.S.A. was supported by NIH grant 5K08DK059958, the Pew Scholars Program in the Biomedical Sciences, and the Sandler Family Supporting Foundation. J.A.B. was supported by NIH grants U19 AI56388, P30 DK63720, and R01 AI50834. Finally, we thank the Juvenile Diabetes Research Foundation for their ongoing financial support (JDRF Center Grant # 4–2004–372) and continued commitment to research in type 1 diabetes.

The *Annual Review of Immunology* is online at
http://immunol.annualreviews.org

LITERATURE CITED

1. Makino S, Kunimoto K, Muraoka Y, Mizushima Y, Katagiri K, et al. 1980. Breeding of a non-obese, diabetic strain of mice. *Jikken Dobutsu* 29:1–13
2. Kikutani H, Makino S. 1992. The murine autoimmune diabetes model: NOD and related strains. *Adv. Immunol.* 51:285–322
3. Bach JF. 1994. Insulin-dependent diabetes mellitus as an autoimmune disease. *Endocr. Rev.* 15:516–42
4. Singh B, Rabinovitch A. 1993. Influence of microbial agents on the development

and prevention of autoimmune diabetes. *Autoimmunity* 15:209–13
5. Bowman MA, Leiter EH, Atkinson MA. 1994. Prevention of diabetes in the NOD mouse: implications for therapeutic intervention in human disease. *Immunol. Today* 15:115–20
6. Bach JF. 2002. The effect of infections on susceptibility to autoimmune and allergic diseases. *N. Engl. J. Med.* 347:911–20
7. Andre I, Gonzalez A, Wang B, Katz J, Benoist C, et al. 1996. Checkpoints in

the progression of autoimmune disease: lessons from diabetes models. *Proc. Natl. Acad. Sci. USA* 93:2260–63

8. Wicker LS, Miller BJ, Mullen Y. 1986. Transfer of autoimmune diabetes mellitus with splenocytes from nonobese diabetic (NOD) mice. *Diabetes* 35:855–60

9. Bendelac A, Carnaud C, Boitard C, Bach JF. 1987. Syngeneic transfer of autoimmune diabetes from diabetic NOD mice to healthy neonates. Requirement for both L3T4+ and Lyt-2+ T cells. *J. Exp. Med.* 166:823–32

10. Haskins K, Wegmann D. 1996. Diabetogenic T-cell clones. *Diabetes* 45:1299–305

11. Wong FS, Visintin I, Wen L, Flavell RA, Janeway CA Jr. 1996. CD8 T cell clones from young nonobese diabetic (NOD) islets can transfer rapid onset of diabetes in NOD mice in the absence of CD4 cells. *J. Exp. Med.* 183:67–76

12. Shizuru JA, Taylor-Edwards C, Banks BA, Gregory AK, Fathman CG. 1988. Immunotherapy of the nonobese diabetic mouse: treatment with an antibody to T-helper lymphocytes. *Science* 240:659–62

13. Chatenoud L, Thervet E, Primo J, Bach JF. 1994. Anti-CD3 antibody induces long-term remission of overt autoimmunity in nonobese diabetic mice. *Proc. Natl. Acad. Sci. USA* 91:123–27

14. Kurasawa K, Sakamoto A, Maeda T, Sumida T, Ito I, et al. 1993. Short-term administration of anti-L3T4 MoAb prevents diabetes in NOD mice. *Clin. Exp. Immunol.* 91:376–80

15. Wang B, Gonzalez A, Benoist C, Mathis D. 1996. The role of CD8+ T cells in the initiation of insulin-dependent diabetes mellitus. *Eur. J. Immunol.* 26:1762–69

16. Mori Y, Suko M, Okudaira H, Matsuba I, Tsuruoka A, et al. 1986. Preventive effects of cyclosporin on diabetes in NOD mice. *Diabetologia* 29:244–47

17. Serreze DV, Fleming SA, Chapman HD, Richard SD, Leiter EH, et al. 1998. B lymphocytes are critical antigen-presenting cells for the initiation of T cell-mediated autoimmune diabetes in nonobese diabetic mice. *J. Immunol.* 161:3912–18

18. Hu Y, Nakagawa Y, Purushotham KR, Humphreys-Beher MG. 1992. Functional changes in salivary glands of autoimmune disease-prone NOD mice. *Am. J. Physiol. Endocrinol. Metab.* 263:E607–14

19. Many MC, Maniratunga S, Denef JF. 1996. The non-obese diabetic (NOD) mouse: an animal model for autoimmune thyroiditis. *Exp. Clin. Endocrinol. Diabetes* 104:17–20

20. Salomon B, Rhee L, Bour-Jordan H, Hsin H, Montag A, et al. 2001. Development of spontaneous autoimmune peripheral polyneuropathy in B7-2- deficient NOD mice. *J. Exp. Med.* 194:677–84

21. Silveira PA, Baxter AG. 2001. The NOD mouse as a model of SLE. *Autoimmunity* 34:53–64

22. Kagi D, Odermatt B, Seiler P, Zinkernagel RM, Mak TW, et al. 1997. Reduced incidence and delayed onset of diabetes in perforin-deficient nonobese diabetic mice. *J. Exp. Med.* 186:989–97

23. Tang QZ, Henriksen KJ, Bi MY, Finger EB, Szot G, et al. 2004. In vitro-expanded antigen-specific regulatory T cells suppress autoimmune diabetes. *J. Exp. Med.* 199:1455–65

24. Winer S, Tsui H, Lau A, Song AH, Li XM, et al. 2003. Autoimmune islet destruction in spontaneous type 1 diabetes is not β-cell exclusive. *Nat. Med.* 9:198–205

25. Alyanakian MA, You S, Damotte D, Gouarin C, Esling A, et al. 2003. Diversity of regulatory CD4+ T cells controlling distinct organ-specific autoimmune diseases. *Proc. Natl. Acad. Sci. USA* 100: 15806–11

26. Girvin AM, Dal Canto MC, Rhee L, Salomon B, Sharpe A, et al. 2000. A critical role for B7/CD28 costimulation in experimental autoimmune encephalomyelitis: a comparative study using costimulatory molecule-deficient mice and monoclonal

antibody blockade. *J. Immunol.* 164:136–43

27. Wicker LS, Todd JA, Peterson LB. 1995. Genetic control of autoimmune diabetes in the NOD mouse. *Annu. Rev. Immunol.* 13:179–200

28. Tisch R, McDevitt H. 1996. Insulin-dependent diabetes mellitus. *Cell* 85:291–97

29. Acha-Orbea H, McDevitt HO. 1987. The first external domain of the nonobese diabetic mouse class II I-A beta chain is unique. *Proc. Natl. Acad. Sci. USA* 84:2435–39

30. Kanagawa O, Martin SM, Vaupel BA, Carrasco-Marin E, Unanue ER. 1998. Autoreactivity of T cells from nonobese diabetic mice: an I-Ag7-dependent reaction. *Proc. Natl. Acad. Sci. USA* 95:1721–24

31. Todd JA, Bell JI, McDevitt HO. 1987. HLA-DQ beta gene contributes to susceptibility and resistance to insulin-dependent diabetes mellitus. *Nature* 329:599–604

32. Nishimoto H, Kikutani H, Yamamura K, Kishimoto T. 1987. Prevention of autoimmune insulitis by expression of I-E molecules in NOD mice. *Nature* 328:432–34

33. Uehira M, Uno M, Kurner T, Kikutani H, Mori K, et al. 1989. Development of autoimmune insulitis is prevented in E alpha d but not in A beta k NOD transgenic mice. *Int. Immunol.* 1:209–13

34. Lund T, O'Reilly L, Hutchings P, Kanagawa O, Simpson E, et al. 1990. Prevention of insulin-dependent diabetes mellitus in non-obese diabetic mice by transgenes encoding modified I-A beta-chain or normal I-E alpha-chain. *Nature* 345:727–29

35. Bohme J, Schuhbaur B, Kanagawa O, Benoist C, Mathis D. 1990. MHC-linked protection from diabetes dissociated from clonal deletion of T cells. *Science* 249:293–95

36. Podolin PL, Pressey A, DeLarato NH, Fischer PA, Peterson LB, et al. 1993. I-E+

nonobese diabetic mice develop insulitis and diabetes. *J. Exp. Med.* 178:793–803

37. Wicker LS, Appel MC, Dotta F, Pressey A, Miller BJ, et al. 1992. Autoimmune syndromes in major histocompatibility complex (MHC) congenic strains of nonobese diabetic (NOD) mice. The NOD MHC is dominant for insulitis and cyclophosphamide-induced diabetes. *J. Exp. Med.* 176:67–77

38. Schmidt D, Verdaguer J, Averill N, Santamaria P. 1997. A mechanism for the major histocompatibility complex-linked resistance to autoimmunity. *J. Exp. Med.* 186:1059–75

39. Delovitch TL, Singh B. 1997. The nonobese diabetic mouse as a model of autoimmune diabetes: immune dysregulation gets the NOD. *Immunity* 7:727–38

40. Todd JA, Wicker LS. 2001. Genetic protection from the inflammatory disease type 1 diabetes in humans and animal models. *Immunity* 15:387–95

41. Ueda H, Howson JM, Esposito L, Heward J, Snook H, et al. 2003. Association of the T-cell regulatory gene CTLA4 with susceptibility to autoimmune disease. *Nature* 423:506–11

42. Bolland S, Yim YS, Tus K, Wakeland EK, Ravetch JV. 2002. Genetic modifiers of systemic lupus erythematosus in FcγRIIB$^{-/-}$ mice. *J. Exp. Med.* 195:1167–74

43. Makhlouf L, Yamada A, Ito T, Abdi R, Ansari MJ, et al. 2003. Allorecognition and effector pathways of islet allograft rejection in normal versus nonobese diabetic mice. *J. Am. Soc. Nephrol.* 14:2168–75

44. Pearson T, Markees TG, Serreze DV, Pierce MA, Wicker LS, et al. 2003. Genetic separation of the transplantation tolerance and autoimmune phenotypes in NOD mice. *Rev. Endocr. Metab. Disord.* 4:255–61

45. Pearson T, Weiser P, Markees TG, Serreze DV, Wicker LS, et al. 2004. Islet allograft

survival induced by costimulation blockade in NOD mice is controlled by allelic variants of *Idd3*. *Diabetes* 53(8):1972–78

46. Serreze DV, Gaedeke JW, Leiter EH. 1993. Hematopoietic stem-cell defects underlying abnormal macrophage development and maturation in NOD/Lt mice: defective regulation of cytokine receptors and protein kinase C. *Proc. Natl. Acad. Sci. USA* 90:9625–29

47. Kataoka S, Satoh J, Fujiya H, Toyota T, Suzuki R, et al. 1983. Immunologic aspects of the nonobese diabetic (NOD) mouse. Abnormalities of cellular immunity. *Diabetes* 32:247–53

48. Ogasawara K, Hamerman JA, Hsin H, Chikuma S, Bour-Jordan H, et al. 2003. Impairment of NK cell function by NKG2D modulation in NOD mice. *Immunity* 18:41–51

49. Naumov YN, Bahjat KS, Gausling R, Abraham R, Exley MA, et al. 2001. Activation of CD1d-restricted T cells protects NOD mice from developing diabetes by regulating dendritic cell subsets. *Proc. Natl. Acad. Sci. USA* 98:13838–43

50. Wang B, Geng YB, Wang CR. 2001. CD1-restricted NK T cells protect nonobese diabetic mice from developing diabetes. *J. Exp. Med.* 194:313–20

51. Salomon B, Lenschow DJ, Rhee L, Ashourian N, Singh B, et al. 2000. B7/CD28 costimulation is essential for the homeostasis of the CD4+CD25+ immunoregulatory T cells that control autoimmune diabetes. *Immunity* 12:431–40

52. Baxter AG, Cooke A. 1993. Complement lytic activity has no role in the pathogenesis of autoimmune diabetes in NOD mice. *Diabetes* 42:1574–78

53. Carnaud C, Gombert J, Donnars O, Garchon H, Herbelin A. 2001. Protection against diabetes and improved NK/NKT cell performance in NOD.NK1.1 mice congenic at the NK complex. *J. Immunol.* 166:2404–11

54. Kataoka S, Satoh J, Fujiya H, Toyota T, Suzuki R, et al. 1983. Immunologic aspects of the nonobese diabetic (NOD) mouse. Abnormalities of cellular immunity. *Diabetes* 32:247–53

55. Poulton LD, Smyth MJ, Hawke CG, Silveira P, Shepherd D, et al. 2001. Cytometric and functional analyses of NK and NKT cell deficiencies in NOD mice. *Int. Immunol.* 13:887–96

56. Rogner UC, Boitard C, Morin J, Melanitou E, Avner P. 2001. Three loci on mouse chromosome 6 influence onset and final incidence of type I diabetes in NOD.C3H congenic strains. *Genomics* 74:163–71

57. Yokoyama WM, Seaman WE. 1993. The Ly-49 and NKR-P1 gene families encoding lectin-like receptors on natural killer cells: the NK gene complex. *Annu. Rev. Immunol.* 11:613–35

58. Bauer S, Groh V, Wu J, Steinle A, Phillips JH, et al. 1999. Activation of NK cells and T cells by NKG2D, a receptor for stress-inducible MICA. *Science* 285:727–29

59. Poirot L, Benoist C, Mathis D. 2004. Natural killer cells distinguish innocuous and destructive forms of pancreatic islet autoimmunity. *Proc. Natl. Acad. Sci. USA* 101:8102–7

60. Yang M, Charlton B, Gautam AM. 1997. Development of insulitis and diabetes in B cell-deficient NOD mice. *J. Autoimmun.* 10:257–60

61. Greeley SA, Katsumata M, Yu L, Eisenbarth GS, Moore DJ, et al. 2002. Elimination of maternally transmitted autoantibodies prevents diabetes in nonobese diabetic mice. *Nat. Med.* 8:399–402

62. Martin S, Wolf-Eichbaum D, Duinkerken G, Scherbaum WA, Kolb H, et al. 2001. Development of type 1 diabetes despite severe hereditary B-lymphocyte deficiency. *N. Engl. J. Med.* 345:1036–40

63. Lejon K, Fathman CG. 1999. Isolation of self antigen-reactive cells from inflamed islets of nonobese diabetic mice using CD4 high expression as a marker. *J. Immunol.* 163:5708–14

64. Wang B, Gonzalez A, Benoist C, Mathis D. 1996. The role of CD8+ T cells in the

initiation of insulin-dependent diabetes mellitus. *Eur. J. Immunol.* 26:1762–69

65. Ogasawara K, Hamerman JA, Ehrlich LR, Bour-Jordan H, Santamaria P, et al. 2004. NKG2D blockade prevents autoimmune diabetes in NOD mice. *Immunity* 20:757–67

66. Lieberman SM, DiLorenzo TP. 2003. A comprehensive guide to antibody and T-cell responses in type 1 diabetes. *Tissue Antigens* 62:359–77

67. Altman JD, Moss PA, Goulder PJ, Barouch DH, McHeyzer-Williams MG, et al. 1996. Phenotypic analysis of antigen-specific T lymphocytes. *Science* 274:94–96

68. Liu CP, Jiang K, Wu CH, Lee WH, Lin WJ. 2000. Detection of glutamic acid decarboxylase-activated T cells with I-Ag7 tetramers. *Proc. Natl. Acad. Sci. USA* 97:14596–601

69. Jang MH, Seth NP, Wucherpfennig KW. 2003. Ex vivo analysis of thymic CD4 T cells in nonobese diabetic mice with tetramers generated from I-A(g7)/class II-associated invariant chain peptide precursors. *J. Immunol.* 171:4175–86

70. Reijonen H, Novak EJ, Kochik S, Heninger A, Liu AW, et al. 2002. Detection of GAD65-specific T-cells by major histocompatibility complex class II tetramers in type 1 diabetic patients and at-risk subjects. *Diabetes* 51:1375–82

71. Wong FS, Karttunen J, Dumont C, Wen L, Visintin I, et al. 1999. Identification of an MHC class I-restricted autoantigen in type 1 diabetes by screening an organ-specific cDNA library. *Nat. Med.* 5:1026–31

72. Verdaguer J, Schmidt D, Amrani A, Anderson B, Averill N, et al. 1997. Spontaneous autoimmune diabetes in monoclonal T cell nonobese diabetic mice. *J. Exp. Med.* 186:1663–76

73. Anderson B, Park BJ, Verdaguer J, Amrani A, Santamaria P. 1999. Prevalent CD8[+] T cell response against one peptide/MHC complex in autoimmune dia-

betes. *Proc. Natl. Acad. Sci. USA* 96:9311–16

74. Trudeau JD, Kelly-Smith C, Verchere CB, Elliott JF, Dutz JP, et al. 2003. Prediction of spontaneous autoimmune diabetes in NOD mice by quantification of autoreactive T cells in peripheral blood. *J. Clin. Invest.* 111:217–23

75. Lieberman SM, Evans AM, Han B, Takaki T, Vinnitskaya Y, et al. 2003. Identification of the β cell antigen targeted by a prevalent population of pathogenic CD8[+] T cells in autoimmune diabetes. *Proc. Natl. Acad. Sci. USA* 100:8384–88

76. Haskins K, Portas M, Bradley B, Wegmann D, Lafferty K. 1988. T-lymphocyte clone specific for pancreatic islet antigen. *Diabetes* 37:1444–48

77. Katz JD, Wang B, Haskins K, Benoist C, Mathis D. 1993. Following a diabetogenic T cell from genesis through pathogenesis. *Cell* 74:1089–100

78. Judkowski V, Pinilla C, Schroder K, Tucker L, Sarvetnick N, et al. 2001. Identification of MHC class II-restricted peptide ligands, including a glutamic acid decarboxylase 65 sequence, that stimulate diabetogenic T cells from transgenic BDC2.5 nonobese diabetic mice. *J. Immunol.* 166:908–17

79. Yoshida K, Martin T, Yamamoto K, Dobbs C, Munz C, et al. 2002. Evidence for shared recognition of a peptide ligand by a diverse panel of non-obese diabetic mice-derived, islet-specific, diabetogenic T cell clones. *Int. Immunol.* 14:1439–47

80. Stratmann T, Martin-Orozco N, Mallet-Designe V, Poirot L, McGavern D, et al. 2003. Susceptible MHC alleles, not background genes, select an autoimmune T cell reactivity. *J. Clin. Invest.* 112:902–14

81. Masteller EL, Warner MR, Ferlin W, Judkowski V, Wilson D, et al. 2003. Peptide-MHC class II dimers as therapeutics to modulate antigen-specific T cell responses in autoimmune diabetes. *J. Immunol.* 171:5587–95

82. Jenkins MK, Khoruts A, Ingulli E,

Mueller DL, McSorley SJ, et al. 2001. In vivo activation of antigen-specific CD4 T cells. *Annu. Rev. Immunol.* 19:23–45

83. Zhang Y, O'Brien B, Trudeau J, Tan R, Santamaria P, Dutz JP. 2002. In situ β cell death promotes priming of diabetogenic CD8 T lymphocytes. *J. Immunol.* 168:1466–72

84. Hoglund P, Mintern J, Waltzinger C, Heath W, Benoist C, et al. 1999. Initiation of autoimmune diabetes by developmentally regulated presentation of islet cell antigens in the pancreatic lymph nodes. *J. Exp. Med.* 189:331–39

85. Gagnerault MC, Luan JJ, Lotton C, Lepault F. 2002. Pancreatic lymph nodes are required for priming of β cell reactive T cells in NOD mice. *J. Exp. Med.* 196:369–77

86. Trudeau JD, Dutz JP, Arany E, Hill DJ, Fieldus WE, et al. 2000. Neonatal β-cell apoptosis: a trigger for autoimmune diabetes? *Diabetes* 49:1–7

87. Turley S, Poirot L, Hattori M, Benoist C, Mathis D. 2003. Physiological β cell death triggers priming of self-reactive T cells by dendritic cells in a type-1 diabetes model. *J. Exp. Med.* 198:1527–37

88. King C, Ilic A, Koelsch K, Sarvetnick N. 2004. Homeostatic expansion of T cells during immune insufficiency generates autoimmunity. *Cell* 117:265–77

89. Jameson SC. 2002. Maintaining the norm: T-cell homeostasis. *Nat. Rev. Immunol.* 2: 547–56

90. Satoh J, Shintani S, Nobunaga T, Sugawara S, Makino S, et al. 1988. NOD mice with high incidence of type 1 diabetes are not T lymphocytopenic. *Tohoku J. Exp. Med.* 155:151–58

91. Berzins SP, Venanzi ES, Benoist C, Mathis D. 2003. T-cell compartments of prediabetic NOD mice. *Diabetes* 52:327–34

92. Atkinson MA, Wilson SB. 2002. Fatal attraction: chemokines and type 1 diabetes. *J. Clin. Invest.* 110:1611–13

92a. Wu Q, Salomon B, Chen M, Wang Y, Hoffman L, et al. 2001. Reversal of spontaneous autoimmune insulitis in NOD mice by soluble lymphotoxin receptor. *J. Exp. Med.* 193:1327–32

93. Wu Q, Salomon B, Chen M, Wang Y, Hoffman LM, et al. 2001. Reversal of spontaneous autoimmune insulitis in nonobese diabetic mice by soluble lymphotoxin receptor. *J. Exp. Med.* 193:1327–32

94. Savino W, Carnaud C, Luan JJ, Bach JF, Dardenne M. 1993. Characterization of the extracellular matrix-containing giant perivascular spaces in the NOD mouse thymus. *Diabetes* 42:134–40

95. Atlan-Gepner C, Naspetti M, Valero R, Barad M, Lepault F, et al. 1999. Disorganization of thymic medulla precedes evolution towards diabetes in female NOD mice. *Autoimmunity* 31:249–60

96. Colomb E, Savino W, Wicker L, Peterson L, Dardenne M, et al. 1996. Genetic control of giant perivascular space formation in the thymus of NOD mice. *Diabetes* 45:1535–40

97. Kishimoto H, Sprent J. 2001. A defect in central tolerance in NOD mice. *Nat. Immunol.* 2:1025–31

98. Consortium TF-GA. 1997. An autoimmune disease, APECED, caused by mutations in a novel gene featuring two PHD-type zinc-finger domains. The Finnish-German APECED Consortium. Autoimmune Polyendocrinopathy-Candidiasis-Ectodermal Dystrophy. *Nat. Genet.* 17:399–403

99. Nagamine K, Peterson P, Scott HS, Kudoh J, Minoshima S, et al. 1997. Positional cloning of the APECED gene. *Nat. Genet.* 17:393–98

100. Anderson MS, Venanzi ES, Klein L, Chen Z, Berzins SP, et al. 2002. Projection of an immunological self shadow within the thymus by the aire protein. *Science* 298:1395–401

101. Liston A, Lesage S, Wilson J, Peltonen L, Goodnow CC. 2003. Aire regulates

negative selection of organ-specific T cells. *Nat. Immunol.* 4:350–54

102. Moriyama H, Abiru N, Paronen J, Sikora K, Liu E, et al. 2003. Evidence for a primary islet autoantigen (preproinsulin 1) for insulitis and diabetes in the nonobese diabetic mouse. *Proc. Natl. Acad. Sci. USA* 100:10376–81

103. Thebault-Baumont K, Dubois-Laforgue D, Krief P, Briand JP, Halbout P, et al. 2003. Acceleration of type 1 diabetes mellitus in proinsulin 2-deficient NOD mice. *J. Clin. Invest.* 111:851–57

104. Pugliese A, Zeller M, Fernandez A Jr, Zalcberg LJ, Bartlett RJ, et al. 1997. The insulin gene is transcribed in the human thymus and transcription levels correlated with allelic variation at the INS VNTR-IDDM2 susceptibility locus for type 1 diabetes. *Nat. Genet.* 15:293–97

105. Vafiadis P, Bennett ST, Todd JA, Nadeau J, Grabs R, et al. 1997. Insulin expression in human thymus is modulated by INS VNTR alleles at the IDDM2 locus. *Nat. Genet.* 15:289–92

106. Hanahan D. 1998. Peripheral-antigen-expressing cells in thymic medulla: factors in self-tolerance and autoimmunity. *Curr. Opin. Immunol.* 10:656–62

107. Chentoufi AA, Polychronakos C. 2002. Insulin expression levels in the thymus modulate insulin-specific autoreactive T-cell tolerance: the mechanism by which the IDDM2 locus may predispose to diabetes. *Diabetes* 51:1383–90

108. Derbinski J, Schulte A, Kyewski B, Klein L. 2001. Promiscuous gene expression in medullary thymic epithelial cells mirrors the peripheral self. *Nat. Immunol.* 2:1032–39

109. Baekkeskov S, Aanstoot HJ, Christgau S, Reetz A, Solimena M, et al. 1990. Identification of the 64K autoantigen in insulin-dependent diabetes as the GABA-synthesizing enzyme glutamic acid decarboxylase. *Nature* 347:151–56

110. Quinn A, Sercarz EE. 1996. T cells with multiple fine specificities are used by non-obese diabetic (NOD) mice in the response to GAD(524–543). *J. Autoimmun.* 9:365–70

111. Chao CC, McDevitt HO. 1997. Identification of immunogenic epitopes of GAD 65 presented by Ag7 in non-obese diabetic mice. *Immunogenetics* 46:29–34

112. Tisch R, Yang XD, Singer SM, Liblau RS, Fugger L, et al. 1993. Immune response to glutamic acid decarboxylase correlates with insulitis in non-obese diabetic mice. *Nature* 366:72–75

113. Kaufman DL, Clare-Salzler M, Tian J, Forsthuber T, Ting GS, et al. 1993. Spontaneous loss of T-cell tolerance to glutamic acid decarboxylase in murine insulin-dependent diabetes. *Nature* 366:69–72

114. Yoon JW, Yoon CS, Lim HW, Huang QQ, Kang Y, et al. 1999. Control of autoimmune diabetes in NOD mice by GAD expression or suppression in β cells. *Science* 284:1183–87

115. Kash SF, Condie BG, Baekkeskov S. 1999. Glutamate decarboxylase and GABA in pancreatic islets: lessons from knock-out mice. *Horm. Metab. Res.* 31:340–44

116. Jaeckel E, Klein L, Martin-Orozco N, von Boehmer H. 2003. Normal incidence of diabetes in NOD mice tolerant to glutamic acid decarboxylase. *J. Exp. Med.* 197:1635–44

117. Tarbell KV, Lee M, Ranheim E, Chao CC, Sanna M, et al. 2002. CD4+ T cells from glutamic acid decarboxylase (GAD)65-specific T cell receptor transgenic mice are not diabetogenic and can delay diabetes transfer. *J. Exp. Med.* 196:481–92

118. Ridgway WM, Fasso M, Fathman CG. 1999. A new look at MHC and autoimmune disease. *Science* 284:749–51

119. Lesage S, Hartley SB, Akkaraju S, Wilson J, Townsend M, et al. 2002. Failure to censor forbidden clones of CD4 T cells in autoimmune diabetes. *J. Exp. Med.* 196:1175–88

120. Bergman ML, Duarte N, Campino S,

Lundholm M, Motta V, et al. 2003. Diabetes protection and restoration of thymocyte apoptosis in NOD Idd6 congenic strains. *Diabetes* 52:1677–82

121. Villunger A, Marsden VS, Strasser A. 2003. Efficient T cell receptor-mediated apoptosis in nonobese diabetic mouse thymocytes. *Nat. Immunol.* 4:717

122. Zuklys S, Balciunaite G, Agarwal A, Fasler-Kan E, Palmer E, Hollander GA. 2000. Normal thymic architecture and negative selection are associated with aire expression, the gene defective in the autoimmune-polyendocrinopathy-candidiasis-ectodermal dystrophy (APECED). *J. Immunol.* 165:1976–83

123. Walker LS, Abbas AK. 2002. The enemy within: keeping self-reactive T cells at bay in the periphery. *Nat. Rev. Immunol.* 2:11–19

124. Lohmann T, Leslie RD, Londei M. 1996. T cell clones to epitopes of glutamic acid decarboxylase 65 raised from normal subjects and patients with insulin-dependent diabetes. *J. Autoimmun.* 9:385–89

125. Semana G, Gausling R, Jackson RA, Hafler DA. 1999. T cell autoreactivity to proinsulin epitopes in diabetic patients and healthy subjects. *J. Autoimmun.* 12:259–67

126. Tivol EA, Borriello F, Schweitzer AN, Lynch WP, Bluestone JA, et al. 1995. Loss of CTLA-4 leads to massive lymphoproliferation and fatal multiorgan tissue destruction, revealing a critical negative regulatory role of CTLA-4. *Immunity* 3:541–47

127. Waterhouse P, Penninger JM, Timms E, Wakeham A, Shahinian A, et al. 1995. Lymphoproliferative disorders with early lethality in mice deficient in CTLA-4. *Science* 270:985–88

128. Jenkins MK, Schwartz RH. 1987. Antigen presentation by chemically modified splenocytes induces antigen-specific T cell unresponsiveness in vitro and in vivo. *J. Exp. Med.* 165:302–19

129. Jenkins MK, Taylor PS, Norton SD, Urdahl KB. 1991. CD28 delivers a costimulatory signal involved in antigen-specific IL-2 production by human T cells. *J. Immunol.* 147:2461–66

130. Lindstein T, June CH, Ledbetter JA, Stella G, Thompson CB. 1989. Regulation of lymphokine messenger RNA stability by a surface-mediated T cell activation pathway. *Science* 244:339–43

131. Fraser JD, Irving BA, Crabtree GR, Weiss A. 1991. Regulation of interleukin-2 gene enhancer activity by the T cell accessory molecule CD28. *Science* 251:313–16

132. Norton SD, Zuckerman L, Urdahl KB, Shefner R, Miller J, et al. 1992. The CD28 ligand, B7, enhances IL-2 production by providing a costimulatory signal to T cells. *J. Immunol.* 149:1556–61

133. Wulfing C, Davis MM. 1998. A receptor/cytoskeletal movement triggered by costimulation during T cell activation. *Science* 282:2266–69

134. Viola A, Schroeder S, Sakakibara Y, Lanzavecchia A. 1999. T lymphocyte costimulation mediated by reorganization of membrane microdomains. *Science* 283:680–82

135. Boise LH, Minn AJ, Noel PJ, June CH, Accavitti MA, et al. 1995. CD28 costimulation can promote T cell survival by enhancing the expression of Bcl-XL. *Immunity* 3:87–98

136. Sperling AI, Auger JA, Ehst BD, Rulifson IC, Thompson CB, et al. 1996. CD28/B7 interactions deliver a unique signal to naive T cells that regulates cell survival but not early proliferation. *J. Immunol.* 157:3909–17

137. Webb LM, Walmsley MJ, Feldmann M. 1996. Prevention and amelioration of collagen-induced arthritis by blockade of the CD28 co-stimulatory pathway: requirement for both B7-1 and B7-2. *Eur. J. Immunol.* 26:2320–28

138. Lenschow DJ, Ho SC, Sattar H, Rhee L, Gray G, et al. 1995. Differential effects of anti-B7-1 and anti-B7-2 monoclonal antibody treatment on the development of

diabetes in the nonobese diabetic mouse. *J. Exp. Med.* 181:1145–55

139. Lenschow DJ, Herold KC, Rhee L, Patel B, Koons A, et al. 1996. CD28/B7 regulation of Th1 and Th2 subsets in the development of autoimmune diabetes. *Immunity* 5:285–93

140. Wang B, Gonzalez A, Hoglund P, Katz JD, Benoist C, et al. 1998. Interleukin-4 deficiency does not exacerbate disease in NOD mice. *Diabetes* 47:1207–11

141. Walunas TL, Lenschow DJ, Bakker CY, Linsley PS, Freeman GJ, et al. 1994. CTLA-4 can function as a negative regulator of T cell activation. *Immunity* 1:405–13

142. Luhder F, Hoglund P, Allison JP, Benoist C, Mathis D. 1998. Cytotoxic T lymphocyte-associated antigen 4 (CTLA-4) regulates the unfolding of autoimmune diabetes. *J. Exp. Med.* 187:427–32

143. Ansari MJ, Salama AD, Chitnis T, Smith RN, Yagita H, et al. 2003. The programmed death-1 (PD-1) pathway regulates autoimmune diabetes in nonobese diabetic (NOD) mice. *J. Exp. Med.* 198:63–69

144. Kristiansen OP, Larsen ZM, Pociot F. 2000. CTLA-4 in autoimmune diseases–a general susceptibility gene to autoimmunity? *Genes Immun.* 1:170–84

145. Lynch KW, Weiss A. 2001. A CD45 polymorphism associated with multiple sclerosis disrupts an exonic splicing silencer. *J. Biol. Chem.* 276:24341–47

146. Vijayakrishnan L, Slavik JM, Illes Z, Greenwald RJ, Rainbow D, et al. 2004. An autoimmune disease-associated CTLA-4 splice variant lacking the B7 binding domain signals negatively in T cells. *Immunity* 20:563–75

147. Hutloff A, Dittrich AM, Beier KC, Eljaschewitsch B, Kraft R, et al. 1999. ICOS is an inducible T-cell co-stimulator structurally and functionally related to CD28. *Nature* 397:263–66

148. Tesciuba AG, Subudhi S, Rother RP, Faas SJ, Frantz AM, et al. 2001. Inducible cos-timulator regulates Th2-mediated inflammation, but not Th2 differentiation, in a model of allergic airway disease. *J. Immunol.* 167:1996–2003

149. Herman AE, Freeman GJ, Mathis D, Benoist C. 2004. CD4$^+$CD25$^+$ T regulatory cells dependent on ICOS promote regulation of effector cells in the prediabetic lesion. *J. Exp. Med.* 199:1479–89

150. Ishida Y, Agata Y, Shibahara K, Honjo T. 1992. Induced expression of PD-1, a novel member of the immunoglobulin gene superfamily, upon programmed cell death. *EMBO J.* 11:3887–95

151. Agata Y, Kawasaki A, Nishimura H, Ishida Y, Tsubata T, et al. 1996. Expression of the PD-1 antigen on the surface of stimulated mouse T and B lymphocytes. *Int. Immunol.* 8:765–72

152. Freeman GJ, Long AJ, Iwai Y, Bourque K, Chernova T, et al. 2000. Engagement of the PD-1 immunoinhibitory receptor by a novel B7 family member leads to negative regulation of lymphocyte activation. *J. Exp. Med.* 192:1027–34

153. Nishimura H, Nose M, Hiai H, Minato N, Honjo T. 1999. Development of lupus-like autoimmune diseases by disruption of the PD-1 gene encoding an ITIM motif-carrying immunoreceptor. *Immunity* 11:141–51

154. Nishimura H, Okazaki T, Tanaka Y, Nakatani K, Hara M, et al. 2001. Autoimmune dilated cardiomyopathy in PD-1 receptor-deficient mice. *Science* 291:319–22

155. Grewal IS, Flavell RA. 1998. CD40 and CD154 in cell-mediated immunity. *Annu. Rev. Immunol.* 16:111–35

156. Balasa B, Krahl T, Patstone G, Lee J, Tisch R, et al. 1997. CD40 ligand-CD40 interactions are necessary for the initiation of insulitis and diabetes in nonobese diabetic mice. *J. Immunol.* 159:4620–27

157. Green EA, Wong FS, Eshima K, Mora C, Flavell RA. 2000. Neonatal tumor necrosis factor α promotes diabetes in nonobese diabetic mice by CD154-independent

antigen presentation to CD8$^+$ T cells. *J. Exp. Med.* 191:225–38

158. Eshima K, Mora C, Wong FS, Green EA, Grewal IS, et al. 2003. A crucial role of CD4 T cells as a functional source of CD154 in the initiation of insulin-dependent diabetes mellitus in the non-obese diabetic mouse. *Int. Immunol.* 15:351–57

159. Amrani A, Serra P, Yamanouchi J, Han B, Thiessen S, et al. 2002. CD154-dependent priming of diabetogenic CD4$^+$ T cells dissociated from activation of antigen-presenting cells. *Immunity* 16:719–32

160. Weinberg AD, Vella AT, Croft M. 1998. OX-40: life beyond the effector T cell stage. *Semin. Immunol.* 10:471–80

161. Martin-Orozco N, Chen Z, Poirot L, Hyatt E, Chen A, et al. 2003. Paradoxical dampening of anti-islet self-reactivity but promotion of diabetes by OX40 ligand. *J. Immunol.* 171:6954–60

162. Sytwu HK, Lin WD, Roffler SR, Hung JT, Sung HS, et al. 2003. Anti-4-1BB-based immunotherapy for autoimmune diabetes: lessons from a transgenic non-obese diabetic (NOD) model. *J. Autoimmun.* 21:247–54

163. Rabinovitch A. 1994. Immunoregulatory and cytokine imbalances in the pathogenesis of IDDM. Therapeutic intervention by immunostimulation? *Diabetes* 43:613–21

164. Trembleau S, Penna G, Bosi E, Mortara A, Gately MK, et al. 1995. Interleukin 12 administration induces T helper type 1 cells and accelerates autoimmune diabetes in NOD mice. *J. Exp. Med.* 181:817–21

165. Trembleau S, Penna G, Gregori S, Chapman HD, Serreze DV, et al. 1999. Pancreas-infiltrating Th1 cells and diabetes develop in IL-12-deficient nonobese diabetic mice. *J. Immunol.* 163:2960–68

166. Falcone M, Sarvetnick N. 1999. Cytokines that regulate autoimmune responses. *Curr. Opin. Immunol.* 11:670–76

167. Pakala SV, Kurrer MO, Katz JD. 1997. T helper 2 (Th2) T cells induce acute pancreatitis and diabetes in immune-compromised nonobese diabetic (NOD) mice. *J. Exp. Med.* 186:299–306

168. Schweitzer AN, Sharpe AH. 1998. Studies using antigen-presenting cells lacking expression of both B7-1 (CD80) and B7-2 (CD86) show distinct requirements for B7 molecules during priming versus restimulation of Th2 but not Th1 cytokine production. *J. Immunol.* 161:2762–71

169. Rulifson IC, Sperling AI, Fields PE, Fitch FW, Bluestone JA. 1997. CD28 costimulation promotes the production of Th2 cytokines. *J. Immunol.* 158:658–65

170. Salomon B, Bluestone JA. 1998. LFA-1 interaction with ICAM-1 and ICAM-2 regulates Th2 cytokine production. *J. Immunol.* 161:5138–42

171. Rogers PR, Croft M. 2000. CD28, OX-40, LFA-1, and CD4 modulation of Th1/Th2 differentiation is directly dependent on the dose of antigen. *J. Immunol.* 164:2955–63

172. Arreaza GA, Cameron MJ, Jaramillo Λ, Gill BM, Hardy D, et al. 1997. Neonatal activation of CD28 signaling overcomes T cell anergy and prevents autoimmune diabetes by an IL-4-dependent mechanism. *J. Clin. Invest.* 100:2243–53

173. Sanchez-Fueyo A, Tian J, Picarella D, Domenig C, Zheng XX, et al. 2003. Tim-3 inhibits T helper type 1-mediated auto- and alloimmune responses and promotes immunological tolerance. *Nat. Immunol.* 4:1093–101

174. Yang Z, Chen M, Ellett JD, Fialkow LB, Carter JD, et al. 2004. Autoimmune diabetes is blocked in Stat4-deficient mice. *J. Autoimmun.* 22:191–200

175. Chatenoud L, Salomon B, Bluestone JA. 2001. Suppressor T cells—they're back and critical for regulation of autoimmunity! *Immunol. Rev.* 182:149–63

176. Marleau AM, Singh B. 2002. Myeloid dendritic cells in non-obese diabetic mice have elevated costimulatory and T helper-1-inducing abilities. *J. Autoimmun.* 19:23–35

177. Liu J, Beller DI. 2003. Distinct pathways

for NF-κB regulation are associated with aberrant macrophage IL-12 production in lupus- and diabetes-prone mouse strains. *J. Immunol.* 170:4489–96

178. Poligone B, Weaver DJ Jr, Sen P, Baldwin AS Jr, Tisch R. 2002. Elevated NF-κB activation in nonobese diabetic mouse dendritic cells results in enhanced APC function. *J. Immunol.* 168:188–96

179. Weaver DJ Jr, Poligone B, Bui T, Abdel-Motal UM, Baldwin AS Jr, et al. 2001. Dendritic cells from nonobese diabetic mice exhibit a defect in NF-κB regulation due to a hyperactive IκB kinase. *J. Immunol.* 167:1461–68

180. Simpson PB, Mistry MS, Maki RA, Yang W, Schwarz DA, et al. 2003. Cutting edge: diabetes-associated quantitative trait locus, Idd4, is responsible for the IL-12p40 overexpression defect in nonobese diabetic (NOD) mice. *J. Immunol.* 171:3333–37

181. Ymer SI, Huang D, Penna G, Gregori S, Branson K, et al. 2002. Polymorphisms in the Il12b gene affect structure and expression of IL-12 in NOD and other autoimmune-prone mouse strains. *Genes Immun.* 3:151–57

182. Morahan G, Huang D, Ymer SI, Cancilla MR, Stephen K, et al. 2001. Linkage disequilibrium of a type 1 diabetes susceptibility locus with a regulatory IL12B allele. *Nat. Genet.* 27:218–21

183. Koarada S, Wu Y, Olshansky G, Ridgway WM. 2002. Increased nonobese diabetic Th1:Th2 (IFN-γ:IL-4) ratio is CD4$^+$ T cell intrinsic and independent of APC genetic background. *J. Immunol.* 169:6580–87

184. Lyons PA, Hancock WW, Denny P, Lord CJ, Hill NJ, et al. 2000. The NOD Idd9 genetic interval influences the pathogenicity of insulitis and contains molecular variants of Cd30, Tnfr2, and Cd137. *Immunity* 13:107–15

185. Hill NJ, Van Gunst K, Sarvetnick N. 2003. Th1 and Th2 pancreatic inflammation differentially affects homing of islet-reactive CD4 cells in nonobese diabetic mice. *J. Immunol.* 170:1649–58

186. Bendelac A, Rivera MN, Park SH, Roark JH. 1997. Mouse CD1-specific NK1 T cells: development, specificity, and function. *Annu. Rev. Immunol.* 15:535–62

187. MacDonald HR. 2002. Development and selection of NKT cells. *Curr. Opin. Immunol.* 14:250–54

188. Hammond KJ, Pellicci DG, Poulton LD, Naidenko OV, Scalzo AA, et al. 2001. CD1d-restricted NKT cells: an interstrain comparison. *J. Immunol.* 167:1164–73

189. Gombert JM, Herbelin A, Tancrede-Bohin E, Dy M, Chatenoud L, et al. 1996. Early defect of immunoregulatory T cells in autoimmune diabetes. *C. R. Acad. Sci. III* 319:125–29

190. Baxter AG, Kinder SJ, Hammond KJ, Scollay R, Godfrey DI. 1997. Association between $\alpha\beta$TCR$^+$CD4-CD8- T-cell deficiency and IDDM in NOD/Lt mice. *Diabetes* 46:572–82

191. Godfrey DI, Kinder SJ, Silvera P, Baxter AG. 1997. Flow cytometric study of T cell development in NOD mice reveals a deficiency in $\alpha\beta$TCR$^+$CDR-CD8- thymocytes. *J. Autoimmun.* 10:279–85

192. Lehuen A, Lantz O, Beaudoin L, Laloux V, Carnaud C, et al. 1998. Overexpression of natural killer T cells protects Vα14-Jα281 transgenic nonobese diabetic mice against diabetes. *J. Exp. Med.* 188:1831–39

193. Hammond KJ, Poulton LD, Palmisano LJ, Silveira PA, Godfrey DI, et al. 1998. α/β-T cell receptor (TCR)$^+$CD4$^-$CD8$^-$ (NKT) thymocytes prevent insulin-dependent diabetes mellitus in nonobese diabetic (NOD)/Lt mice by the influence of interleukin (IL)-4 and/or IL-10. *J. Exp. Med.* 187:1047–56

194. Sharif S, Arreaza GA, Zucker P, Mi QS, Sondhi J, et al. 2001. Activation of natural killer T cells by alpha-galactosylceramide treatment prevents the onset and recurrence of autoimmune Type 1 diabetes. *Nat. Med.* 7:1057–62

195. Hong S, Wilson MT, Serizawa I, Wu L, Singh N, et al. 2001. The natural killer T-cell ligand alpha-galactosylceramide prevents autoimmune diabetes in non-obese diabetic mice. *Nat. Med.* 7:1052–56

196. Shi FD, Flodstrom M, Balasa B, Kim SH, Van Gunst K, et al. 2001. Germ line deletion of the CD1 locus exacerbates diabetes in the NOD mouse. *Proc. Natl. Acad. Sci. USA* 98:6777–82

197. Wilson SB, Kent SC, Patton KT, Orban T, Jackson RA, et al. 1998. Extreme Th1 bias of invariant $V\alpha24J\alpha Q$ T cells in type 1 diabetes. *Nature* 391:177–81

198. Lee PT, Putnam A, Benlagha K, Teyton L, Gottlieb PA, et al. 2002. Testing the NKT cell hypothesis of human IDDM pathogenesis. *J. Clin. Invest.* 110:793–800

199. Sakaguchi S, Takahashi T, Nishizuka Y. 1982. Study on cellular events in post-thymectomy autoimmune oophoritis in mice. II. Requirement of Lyt-1 cells in normal female mice for the prevention of oophoritis. *J. Exp. Med.* 156:1577–86

200. Nishizuka Y, Sakakura T. 1969. Thymus and reproduction: sex-linked dysgenesia of the gonad after neonatal thymectomy in mice. *Science* 166:753–55

201. Cobbold S, Waldmann H. 1998. Infectious tolerance. *Curr. Opin. Immunol.* 10: 518–24

202. Gershon RK, Kondo K. 1971. Infectious immunological tolerance. *Immunology* 21:903–14

203. Asano M, Toda M, Sakaguchi N, Sakaguchi S. 1996. Autoimmune disease as a consequence of developmental abnormality of a T cell subpopulation. *J. Exp. Med.* 184:387–96

204. Stephens LA, Mason D. 2000. CD25 is a marker for $CD4^+$ thymocytes that prevent autoimmune diabetes in rats, but peripheral T cells with this function are found in both $CD25^+$ and $CD25^-$ subpopulations. *J. Immunol.* 165:3105–10

205. Khattri R, Cox T, Yasayko SA, Ramsdell F. 2003. An essential role for Scurfin in $CD4^+CD25^+$ T regulatory cells. *Nat. Immunol.* 4:337–42

206. Fontenot JD, Gavin MA, Rudensky AY. 2003. Foxp3 programs the development and function of $CD4^+CD25^+$ regulatory T cells. *Nat. Immunol.* 4:330–36

207. Bennett CL, Christie J, Ramsdell F, Brunkow ME, Ferguson PJ, et al. 2001. The immune dysregulation, polyendocrinopathy, enteropathy, X-linked syndrome (IPEX) is caused by mutations of FOXP3. *Nat. Genet.* 27:20–21

208. Hori S, Nomura T, Sakaguchi S. 2003. Control of regulatory T cell development by the transcription factor Foxp3. *Science* 299:1057–61

209. Hutchings PR, Cooke A. 1990. The transfer of autoimmune diabetes in NOD mice can be inhibited or accelerated by distinct cell populations present in normal splenocytes taken from young males. *J. Autoimmun.* 3:175–85

210. Boitard C, Yasunami R, Dardenne M, Bach JF. 1989. T cell-mediated inhibition of the transfer of autoimmune diabetes in NOD mice. *J. Exp. Med.* 169:1669–80

211. Lepault F, Gagnerault MC. 2000. Characterization of peripheral regulatory $CD4^+$ T cells that prevent diabetes onset in nonobese diabetic mice. *J. Immunol.* 164: 240–47

212. Szanya V, Ermann J, Taylor C, Holness C, Fathman CG. 2002. The subpopulation of $CD4^+CD25^+$ splenocytes that delays adoptive transfer of diabetes expresses L-selectin and high levels of CCR7. *J. Immunol.* 169:2461–65

213. Dardenne M, Lepault F, Bendelac A, Bach JF. 1989. Acceleration of the onset of diabetes in NOD mice by thymectomy at weaning. *Eur. J. Immunol.* 19:889–95

214. Herbelin A, Gombert JM, Lepault F, Bach JF, Chatenoud L. 1998. Mature mainstream TCR $\alpha\beta^+CD4^+$ thymocytes expressing L-selectin mediate "active tolerance" in the nonobese diabetic mouse. *J. Immunol.* 161:2620–28

215. Tang QZ, Henriksen KJ, Boden EK,

Tooley AJ, Ye JQ, et al. 2003. Cutting edge: CD28 controls peripheral homeostasis of CD4+CD25+ regulatory T cells. *J. Immunol.* 171:3348–52

216. Gregori S, Giarratana N, Smiroldo S, Adorini L. 2003. Dynamics of pathogenic and suppressor T cells in autoimmune diabetes development. *J. Immunol.* 171:4040–47

217. Belghith M, Bluestone JA, Barriot S, Megret J, Bach JF, et al. 2003. TGF-β-dependent mechanisms mediate restoration of self-tolerance induced by antibodies to CD3 in overt autoimmune diabetes. *Nat. Med.* 9:1202–8

218. Peng Y, Laouar Y, Li MO, Green EA, Flavell RA. 2004. TGF-β regulates in vivo expansion of Foxp3-expressing CD4+CD25+ regulatory T cells responsible for protection against diabetes. *Proc. Natl. Acad. Sci. USA* 101:4572–77

219. Fantini MC, Becker C, Monteleone G, Pallone F, Galle PR, et al. 2004. Cutting edge: TGF-β induces a regulatory phenotype in CD4+CD25− T cells through Foxp3 induction and down-regulation of Smad7. *J. Immunol.* 172:5149–53

220. Apostolou I, Sarukhan A, Klein L, von Boehmer H. 2002. Origin of regulatory T cells with known specificity for antigen. *Nat. Immunol.* 3:756–63

221. Jordan MS, Boesteanu A, Reed AJ, Petrone AL, Holenbeck AE, et al. 2001. Thymic selection of CD4+CD25+ regulatory T cells induced by an agonist self-peptide. *Nat. Immunol.* 2:301–6

222. Gavin MA, Clarke SR, Negrou E, Gallegos A, Rudensky A. 2002. Homeostasis and anergy of CD4+CD25+ suppressor T cells in vivo. *Nat. Immunol.* 3:33–41

223. Walker MR, Kasprowicz DJ, Gersuk VH, Benard A, Van Landeghen M, et al. 2003. Induction of FoxP3 and acquisition of T regulatory activity by stimulated human CD4+CD25− T cells. *J. Clin. Invest.* 112:1437–43

224. Apostolou I, Von Boehmer H. 2004. In vivo instruction of suppressor commitment in naive T cells. *J. Exp. Med.* 199:1401–8

225. Tarbell KV, Yamazaki S, Olson K, Toy P, Steinman RM. 2004. CD25+ CD4+ T cells, expanded with dendritic cells presenting a single autoantigenic peptide, suppress autoimmune diabetes. *J. Exp. Med.* 199:1467–77

226. Mukherjee R, Chaturvedi P, Qin HY, Singh B. 2003. CD4+CD25+ regulatory T cells generated in response to insulin B:9–23 peptide prevent adoptive transfer of diabetes by diabetogenic T cells. *J. Autoimmun.* 21:221–37

227. Atkinson MA, Leiter EH. 1999. The NOD mouse model of type 1 diabetes: as good as it gets? *Nat. Med.* 5:601–4

228. Bougneres PF, Landais P, Boisson C, Carel JC, Frament N, et al. 1990. Limited duration of remission of insulin dependency in children with recent overt type I diabetes treated with low-dose cyclosporin. *Diabetes* 39:1264–72

229. Bach JF. 2002. Immunotherapy of type 1 diabetes: lessons for other autoimmune diseases. *Arthritis. Res.* 4(Suppl. 3):S3–15

230. Diabetes Prevention Trial-Type 1 Diabetes Study Group. 2002. Effects of insulin in relatives of patients with type 1 diabetes mellitus. *N. Engl. J. Med.* 346:1685–91

231. Allen HF, Klingensmith GJ, Jensen P, Simoes E, Hayward A, et al. 1999. Effect of Bacillus Calmette-Guerin vaccination on new-onset type 1 diabetes. A randomized clinical study. *Diabetes Care* 22:1703–7

232. Gale EA, Bingley PJ, Emmett CL, Collier T. 2004. European Nicotinamide Diabetes Intervention Trial (ENDIT): a randomised controlled trial of intervention before the onset of type 1 diabetes. *Lancet* 363:925–31

233. Chatenoud L, Primo J, Bach JF. 1997. CD3 antibody-induced dominant self tolerance in overtly diabetic NOD mice. *J. Immunol.* 158:2947–54

234. Herold KC, Hagopian W, Auger JA, Poumian-Ruiz E, Taylor L, et al. 2002. Anti-CD3 monoclonal antibody in new-onset type 1 diabetes mellitus. *N. Engl. J. Med.* 346:1692–98

235. Herold KC, Burton JB, Francois F, Poumian-Ruiz E, Glandt M, et al. 2003. Activation of human T cells by FcR non-binding anti-CD3 mAb, hOKT3γ1(Ala-Ala). *J. Clin. Invest.* 111:409–18

236. Zheng XX, Sanchez-Fueyo A, Sho M, Domenig C, Sayegh MH, et al. 2003. Favorably tipping the balance between cy-topathic and regulatory T cells to cre-ate transplantation tolerance. *Immunity* 19:503–14

237. Hanninen A, Harrison LC. 2000. $\gamma\delta$ T cells as mediators of mucosal toler-ance: the autoimmune diabetes model. *Immunol. Rev.* 173:109–19

238. Gregori S, Giarratana N, Smiroldo S, Uskokovic M, Adorini L. 2002. A 1alpha,25-dihydroxyvitamin D(3) analog enhances regulatory T-cells and arrests au-toimmune diabetes in NOD mice. *Diabetes* 51:1367–74

Annu. Rev. Immunol. 2005. 23:487–513
doi: 10.1146/annurev.immunol.23.021704.115732
Copyright © 2005 by Annual Reviews. All rights reserved
First published online as a Review in Advance on November 29, 2004

ANTIGEN-SPECIFIC MEMORY B CELL DEVELOPMENT

Louise J. McHeyzer-Williams and
Michael G. McHeyzer-Williams
*The Scripps Research Institute, Department of Immunology, La Jolla,
CA 92037; email: louisemw@scripps.edu; mcheyzer@scripps.edu*

Key Words   adaptive immunity, germinal centers, plasma cells, memory B cells, multiple myeloma

■ **Abstract**   Helper T (Th) cell–regulated B cell immunity progresses in an ordered cascade of cellular development that culminates in the production of antigen-specific memory B cells. The recognition of peptide MHC class II complexes on activated antigen-presenting cells is critical for effective Th cell selection, clonal expansion, and effector Th cell function development (Phase I). Cognate effector Th cell–B cell interactions then promote the development of either short-lived plasma cells (PCs) or germinal centers (GCs) (Phase II). These GCs expand, diversify, and select high-affinity variants of antigen-specific B cells for entry into the long-lived memory B cell compartment (Phase III). Upon antigen rechallenge, memory B cells rapidly expand and differentiate into PCs under the cognate control of memory Th cells (Phase IV). We review the cellular and molecular regulators of this dynamic process with emphasis on the multiple memory B cell fates that develop in vivo.

INTRODUCTION

As outlined in 1949 by Burnet & Fenner (1), heightened reactivity to antigen recall is the central defining characteristic of adaptive immunity. It was not until 1957 that Talmage (2) and Burnet (3) postulated that it was the cells of the immune system that produced the antibodies and that they were the fundamental unit of selection for the immune response (4). Identification of cells that contained antibody (5) and the specificity of the antibody produced by individual cells (6, 7) provided experimental support for clonal selection as the driving force in adaptive immunity.

By the mid-1960s, Miller's studies of neonatal thymectomy (8) identified an essential role of the thymus for efficient adaptive immunity, and Claman's (9) transfers of bone marrow and thymus cell mixtures suggested that these cells worked together. However, it took a series of transfer studies by Mitchell & Miller (10) to establish that it was the bone marrow that produced antibody-forming cell (AFC) precursors and that the thymus-derived cells could be primed to enhance the B cell response. Subsequent studies of the hapten-carrier effect began to probe the mechanisms of T cell–B cell collaboration (11–13) with the idea of an antigen bridge formulated by Rajewsky et al. (14). In this manner, B cell clonal selection and differentiation into plasma cells (PCs) could be controlled in an antigen-specific manner by Th cells.

These classical cellular studies provide the foundations for our understanding of cognate regulation in adaptive immunity. The role of dendritic cells (DCs) as specialized subsets of antigen-presenting cells (APCs) is now very clear, but the differential impact of the various DC subsets on adaptive immunity remains controversial. The level of functional subspecialization in the helper T cell and B cell compartments is also far greater than initially anticipated. As direct experimental access improves, we further resolve our understanding of the cellular and molecular events that shape antigen-specific immunity. Furthermore, cognate regulation begins with T cell receptor (TCR)-peptide MHC class II (pMHCII), but is modified by many molecular interactions that organize at cellular interfaces, now called the immunological synapse. We organize this review across the four major phases in Th cell–regulated development and function of antigen-specific memory B cells.

PHASE I: DEVELOPMENT OF pMHCII-SPECIFIC EFFECTOR TH CELLS

Antigen Experience in the Innate Immune System

The DC compartment is uniquely efficient at protein antigen uptake, processing and presentation (15). Conserved motifs on pathogens trigger innate activation through pattern recognition receptors (PRR), such as the IL-1R/Toll-like receptor family of receptors (16, 17). In protein vaccination strategies, immune adjuvants are needed to activate APCs through these PRR (18). Activated DCs also upregulate costimulatory molecules such as CD40, CD80, and CD86 and chemokine receptors such as CCR7, to relocate from sites of inflammation to the T cell areas of draining lymph nodes (15, 18–20). The rapid shut-down of cellular egress from lymph nodes (21) has also been attributed to local DC activity (22). Thus, antigen-experienced DCs are the critical initiators of Th cell–regulated adaptive immune responses (Figure 1: Phase I).

The type of inflammatory stimulus used for protein vaccination substantially impacts the quality of the subsequent adaptive immune response (18). Although all DCs derive from bone marrow precursors, they pre-exist antigen challenge as an array of different cellular subtypes (15, 18–20). There are three main CD11c$^+$ DC populations (CD8α^- DC, CD8α^+ DC, and plasmacytoid DC), generally referred to as blood-derived DCs that are found in differing proportions across all secondary lymphoid tissue. In lymph nodes draining the skin, there are two further CD11c$^+$ DC subtypes, the Langerhans cells and dermal DC (dDC) (15, 18–20). There are also reports of CD11c$^-$ monocyte-derived DCs (23) that can effectively present antigen to naive Th cells. Although the mechanisms remain poorly resolved,

A

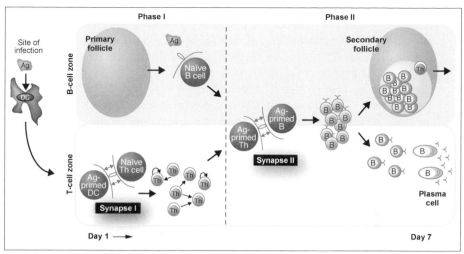

B

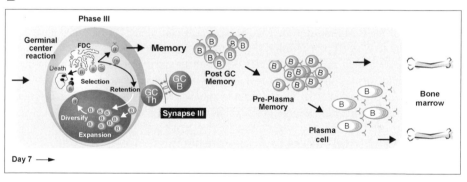

Figure 1   Th cell–regulated B cell memory development. (*A*) A schematic of the cellular interactions that proceed in secondary lymphoid organs toward development of antigen-specific effector Th cells (Phase I) and effector B cells (Phase II). (*B*) A schematic of cellular activity in the GC cycle (Phase III) that leads to the development of antigen-specific memory B cell subsets. The three main cellular products of the GC are depicted.

differential activation of DC subtypes provides one powerful means for controlling cell fate decisions in the development of adaptive immunity.

Direct Experimental Access to pMHCII^{+} DCs

The extent and dynamics of pMHCII expression and its cellular distribution and molecular context in vivo serve to define the innate to adaptive regulatory interface in vivo. Gaining experimental access to pMHCII^{+} DCs in vivo has been technically challenging. A number of monoclonal antibodies have been generated against specific pMHC complexes from self and foreign protein antigens (24–26). These reagents produce clear and reliable signals in vitro and label well in situ for detecting self-pMHC complexes (27, 28). Studies of antigen presentation and adjuvant function in vivo (25, 29) were informative but suffered substantial background owing to self-peptide cross reactivity. Jenkins and colleagues (30) used peptide fused to fluorescent protein to demonstrate the capacity of pMHCII$^+$ dDCs to activate naive Th cells in vivo. These powerful strategies can be broadly used for direct quantitative cellular and molecular assessment of antigen presentation in vivo.

Immune Synapse I: Cognate Priming of pMHCII-Specific Th Cells

The recognition of pMHCII by the TCR of specific Th cells is central to the development of adaptive immunity (31–33). Successful cognate interactions occur through organized rearrangement of cell surface molecules at the cellular interface, now commonly referred to as the immunological synapse (34, 35). Specific TCR-pMHCII interactions cluster toward the center of the immune synapse surrounded by complementary adhesion molecule interactions and excluding negative regulators of TCR signaling (34, 35). At least 2 h conjugate formation is necessary to promote Th cell proliferation (36) with antigen-specific signaling evident up to 10 h (37). Direct imaging provides outstanding clarity to the dynamic nature of conjugate formation (38, 39), resolving the timescale and quality of APC–T cell interactions in vivo (40). Thus, immune synapse formation acts as the first major checkpoint in the development of Th cell–regulated B cell immunity.

Direct Experimental Access to Antigen-Specific Effector Th Cells

Activated DC–naive Th cell conjugate formation results in extensive antigen-specific Th clonal expansion and the differentiation of effector Th cells. As with pMHCII$^+$ DCs, direct experimental access to antigen-specific effector Th cells was a substantial technical barrier. The Th1/Th2 paradigm for Th cell function emerged from studies of Th cell lines propagated long-term in vitro (41–43). These lines and hybrids of antigen-specific Th cells served as useful models for the functional potential of Th cells and have been extraordinarily valuable for dissecting the molecular mechanisms driving functional commitment (44). Adoptive transfer of TCR transgenic Th cells has been another valuable method for accessing many facets of dynamic Th cell behavior in vivo (45–47). Our approach has been to retain the TCR diversity present in wild-type mice and isolate the antigen-specific compartment once expanded with antigen in vivo (48–52).

The first generation of the isolation strategy relied upon known V region gene expression and the modulation of cell surface molecules upon antigen-specific activation in vivo (48). This strategy revealed the presence and dynamics of clonal selection based on TCR expression (53) and the impact of thymic selection on the emergence of clonal dominance (54). Functional studies directly ex vivo revealed a surprisingly high level of heterogeneity for cytokine production (55) and demonstrated a substantial change in Th cell physiology that accompanies antigen experience (56). These approaches laid the foundations for the pMHCII tetramer technology that was developed by John Altman and Michael McHeyzer-Williams while postdoctoral fellows with Mark Davis (49–52). This new class of reagents provided direct access to antigen-specific Th cells in a manner that was also a quantitative functional assay. The impact of this approach is most noticeable in the analysis of CD8 T cell responses and has been adapted in many forms to directly access TCR binding kinetics in the Th cell compartment (57) allowing TCR structure function connections (58) with single cell resolution (59).

Using a combination of these approaches, we have recently identified a preexisting functional division in the naive Th cell compartment (60). In these studies, half of the naive Th cell compartment of B10.BR mice was shown to express Ly6C, a GPI-anchored glycoprotein. This Ly6C^{hi} naive Th cell compartment expresses distinct pMHCII-specific TCR repertoires imprinted during thymic selection. Interestingly, the Ly6C^{hi} Th cell subset was subspecialized for PC production in vivo across two separate adoptive transfer models for thymus-dependent immunity. Thus, we reveal a level of cellular diversity in the naive Th cell compartment that directly impacts B cell fate in vivo.

Activation of Naive Antigen-Specific B Cells

Lanzavecchia (61) experimentally reconciled the idea of an antigen bridge between B cells and Th cells into two sets of signals, one involving native antigen and B cell receptor (BCR) recognition and the other processing antigen and MHC class II. More recently, Neuberger and colleagues (62) argued that native antigen may be tethered by FcR or complement receptors to cells in vivo. When antigen is presented by APC to B cells, there is central focusing of BCR and intracellular signaling intermediates on the B cells (62). Adhesion molecules form peripheral rings, and negative regulators, such as CD45 and CD22, are excluded from the cellular interfaces. These APC–B cell immune synapses decrease B cell activation thresholds and promote the uptake and processing of the cell-associated antigen (62). There have also been reports of soluble IL-4 in vitro (63) and myeloid cell–associated IL-4 production in vivo (64) that condition the naive B cell compartment to receive signals through MHC class II molecules. Although these signals have global effects on naive B cells as a consequence of certain immune adjuvants, they do not appear to impact the production of antigen-specific IgG1 (64). Nevertheless, adjuvant-activated cells of the innate immune system appear to have the capacity to impact early B cell fate in ways that still remain poorly understood.

PHASE II: DEVELOPMENT OF EFFECTOR B CELL RESPONSES

Immune Synapse II: Cognate Priming of Antigen-Experienced B Cells

The immune synapse between effector Th cells and antigen-experienced B cells is quantitatively and qualitatively distinct from Immune Synapse I. Besides the TCR-pMHCII requirement, there are a large and ever increasing number of cell surface molecules known to play a role in this second major checkpoint in the development of B cell memory (65). CD40 is constitutively expressed by B cells and CD40L is upregulated on activated Th cells and known to play an essential role in class switch recombination (CSR) and GC formation (66–68). Lack of OX40 (CD134) and/or OX40L (CD134L) interferes with CSR but leaves GC formation intact (65). CD27-CD70 appears to promote PC formation, whereas CD30-CD153 interactions have an inhibitory effect on CSR and limit antibody production in vivo (65). Although it is not clearly resolved when and where these specific interactions occur, many of these interactions are likely to modify B cell fate at Immune Synapse II.

Lymphotoxin (LT)-α (69), LTβ (70), tumor necrosis factor receptor (TNFR)-I (71), and LTβR (72, 73) have important roles in the developmental organization of lymphoid tissue at homeostasis that indirectly impacts B cell development. B cell activating factor (BAFF) and a proliferation-inducing ligand (APRIL) and their receptors, BAFFR, TACI, and BCMA, have substantial effects on B cell development (74) but are also implicated in the regulation of B cell immune responses (75, 76). CD95 and CD95L have well-characterized effects on the B cell response, with deficiencies causing lympho-proliferative disorders and autoimmune susceptibility, but they may act later during the GC reaction with impact on antigen-driven selection (77–79). Whether these TNFR/TNFL family members are expressed on separate subsets of effector Th and activated B cells, at quantitatively distinct levels, at precise times after immunization, or in precise locations within the secondary lymphoid tissues still remains to be clearly determined.

More recently, inducible costimulator ligand (ICOSL), constitutively expressed on B cells, and ICOS, on activated Th cells, have been suggested as acting upstream of CD40-CD40L interactions (80–82). Other members of this B7-CD28 family clearly indicate a temporal preference of action in vivo (83). Although CD28 signals to naive Th cells through CD80 and CD86 on activated DCs have substantial impact on activation and clonal expansion (83), their influence at Immune Synapse II is less well established. CTLA4 is another well-characterized example of a late acting effect that regulates the necessary decline in immune activation and clonal expansion (84, 85). These spatio-temporal levels of molecular control may have substantial impact on the outcome of the adaptive response effecting the quality and quantity of the primary and memory B cell response.

Class-Switch Recombination (CSR)

The magnitude and isotype spectrum of antibodies expressed and secreted by antigen-specific B cells provides the most sensitive and quantitative measure of cognate T cell help in vivo. Cell-associated signals, such as CD40L to CD40 (66–68), are necessary to initiate antibody isotype switch in vivo, with some other signals, such as BAFF-BAFFR (75), able to compensate. However, the impact of Th cell–derived cytokines has been more closely scrutinized and generally considered the more influential regulators of CSR in vivo.

IL-4 drives the switch to IgG1 (86–88) and in a stepwise manner through IgG1 to IgE (89). Animals lacking IL-4 (90) or STAT-6 to transduce IL-4 signals (91, 92) switch to IgG1 with a lowered efficiency while ablating IgE production. Animals lacking the IL-21R also have lowered IgG1, but exhibit increased levels of IgE (93). Double deficiency of IL-4 and IL-21R has a broader effect on all IgG subclasses as well as IgE, suggesting a more fundamental role for IL-21 in B cell responses (93). IFN-γ is implicated in the switch to the IgG2a subclass (86) and away from IgG1 as a counter-balance to the influence of IL-4. B cell–specific ablation of TGFβRII has implicated TGFβ in the induction of IgA (94). IL-2 and IL-5 also augment IgA production, but do so by preferentially supporting IgA$^+$ B cells rather than promoting CSR (95, 96). A similar indirect action may be attributed to IL-6, whose absence in vivo (97, 98) results in the selective loss of IgG2a and IgG2b in thymus-dependent immune responses.

Hence, the induction of isotype switch recombination, the propagation and survival of isotype-switched B cells, and their development into short-lived PCs may be imprinted at first contact between antigen-specific effector Th cells and antigen-experienced B cells. The switch to downstream isotypes apparent in the GC reaction and into the memory B cell compartment may also have its origins at this early developmental stage. The isotype-switched prememory B cells may also be subject to separate and perhaps distinct levels of cellular and molecular control at this later stage in development. The long-term survival of isotype-switched memory B cells and the control of their response to antigen recall may not be related to the initial induction signals for CSR, and they remain important variables in the efficacy of long-term humoral protection.

Non-GC Development of Short-Lived Plasma Cells

In general, all rapidly emerging antigen-specific PCs in the primary response that develop without entering into GCs are thought to be short-lived (99). These PCs express and secrete germline-encoded antigen-specific antibodies (100) and have half-lives of 3–5 days in vivo (99). They first appear in the T cell zones and migrate to the red pulp of the spleen (101). This migration pattern in vivo appears to be controlled by increased responsiveness to the CXCR4 ligand CXCL12 and the decreased expression of CXCR5 and CCR7 (102). Most in vitro models of PC formation likely produce the equivalent of short-lived non-GC PCs. Although a

PC is considered terminally differentiated, some activated B cells can be shown to secrete antibody and still be able to divide. These cells are referred to as plasmablasts and can be considered a transient stage of PC development in vivo and in vitro.

Differential antibody isotype expression is a level of functional diversity that indicates different modes of cognate Th cell regulation. These differences in isotype emerge across all subtypes of antigen-specific PC, and the developmental impact outside antibody isotype itself remains poorly understood. What controls the expansion of particular precursors, the migration patterns of their progeny, or the potentially different requirements for survival and death across different isotype-specific PC subpopulations is still unclear.

Calame and colleagues (103) recently produced a mouse with a B cell selective ablation of *Prdm1* (encodes Blimp-1) that displayed a substantial deficit of serum antibody before intentional immunization, with little to no specific antibody production in thymus-independent and thymus-dependent immune responses (103). To ascertain whether this was a defect in antibody secretion or a defect in the development of PCs, we directly monitored the 4-hydroxy-3-nitrophenyl acetyl (NP)-specific B cell response in these animals (103). In the spleens at day 7 of the primary response, short-lived non-GC B cells were largely absent. Blimp-1 is known to promote cell cycle arrest directly through *c-myc* repression, or indirectly through upregulation of cdk inhibitors *p18* and *p21* (104, 105). Blimp-1 may also directly repress *Pax-5* to release its control over the X-box binding protein, XBP-1 (106, 107). This transcription factor, XBP-1, is also necessary for PC development in vivo (108) through its control of the unfolded protein response (109) and many secretory pathway components (107). However, it remains unclear which of these pathways more directly causes the PC developmental defect in these mice.

PHASE III: DEVELOPMENT OF MEMORY B CELLS

The Germinal Center (GC) Reaction

Secondary follicle formation is the alternate B cell fate at Immune Synapse II (Figure 1: Phase II). This massive and rapid clonal expansion displaces resting follicular B cells, creating the dynamic cellular underpinnings of the GC reaction (110, 111). There is evidence for pre-GC clonal selection based on germline encoded BCR to initiate secondary follicle formation (112, 113). Polarization of secondary follicles into a T cell proximal zone of expanding centroblasts (the dark zone) and a T cell distal zone of noncycling centrocytes (the light zone) signifies the beginning of the GC reaction (Figure 1: Phase III). The GC reaction is a cycle of cellular activity and molecular change that regulates antigen-specific clonal evolution during the development of B cell memory (114–116). Clonal expansion followed by BCR diversification and affinity-based selection results in either retention and re-entry into a second GC cycle of events, or exit from the GC and entry into the long-lived memory B cell compartment.

Somatic Hypermutation

Antigen-specific B cells that initially enter the GC cycle expand rapidly and down-regulate their germline-encoded BCR (110, 111). Clonal expansion is coupled to BCR diversification through somatic hypermutation (SHM) (117, 118). Although microdissection provided access to GC B cells, these population-based repertoire analyses generated a PCR recombination artifact in vitro (119). Hence, single cell resolution is necessary for these types of BCR repertoire studies. SHM has also been demonstrated outside GC (69, 120); however, in these examples it is difficult to exclude the presence of ectopic GC outside secondary lymphoid tissue (121). Thus, under normal physiological conditions and acute reaction to antigen exposure, the GC is the most likely location to support SHM.

SHM is seen through the introduction of single base-pair substitutions, with rare insertions and deletions into the variable regions of antibody gene segments. The recent discovery of the activation-induced cytidine deaminase (AID) (122, 123) represents a major breakthrough in our understanding of this diversification mechanism. However, investigators still debate whether AID acts on an RNA intermediate or directly on a DNA substrate (124, 125). Nevertheless, double-stranded DNA breaks with some sequence preference appear to be intermediates in this process (126), together with error-prone DNA polymerases, to introduce mismatched nucleotides into these lesions (127, 128). There must also be some means to subvert mismatch repair mechanisms in these GC B cells, but the genetic ablation of most known systems has no substantial influence on SHM patterns (129). The details of this multistep mechanism are of great importance to our appreciation of BCR repertoire development in vivo.

Antigen-Driven Affinity Maturation

Approximately one mutation is introduced into the BCR with each cell division. The variant BCR are then expressed on the surface of noncycling centrocytes that are selected on the basis of the affinity of the BCR binding to antigen (130). Follicular dendritic cells (131, 132) have been implicated in this antigen-driven selection mechanism owing to their presence at high density in the light zone of GC with $Fc\gamma R$ and complement receptors that trap and display native antigen as immune complexes (IC) (133, 134). One model proposes competitive binding for antigen between germline-encoded antibody in the IC and variant antibody expressed by the newly emergent centrocyte. To test this model, Shlomchik and colleagues (135) developed an animal that can only express membrane but no secreted antibody. These animals still produce GCs with evidence for affinity maturation, indicating that there is no requirement for IC during affinity maturation. Hence, it seems clear that the processes controlling affinity maturation in the GC reaction do not require secreted antibody. As the selection mechanism must clearly use native antigen as a template, the means for presenting this antigen, its local depot, and the cells involved in regulating this process remain important open question in the field.

Immune Synapse III: Regulated Exit from the Germinal Center Reaction

The majority of centrocytes expressing variant BCR die in situ. Overexpression of antiapoptotic molecules, such as Bcl-2 or Bcl-xL, results in the accumulation of low affinity B cells in vivo, arguing for apoptosis as the clearance mechanism (79, 136). Centrocytes that express higher affinity BCR receive a productive antigen signal with costimulation that rescues them from apoptosis (137). This positive selection mechanism may be regulated in a cognate manner by GC Th cells (138, 139). GC Th cells express antigen-specific TCR (53, 140, 141) and distinct cell surface phenotype (142) and may undergo their own level of antigen-driven selection in the GC microenvironment (141). Interestingly, based on expressed TCR, not all antigen-specific Th cells enter the GC reaction. Furthermore, a GC phase in development is not necessary for the generation of Th cell memory (143), an important developmental process about which very little is known.

After positive selection in the GC cycle, the higher affinity variant centrocytes can return to the dark zone. Here, a second round of clonal expansion introduces a new set of point mutations in the progeny that will again be tested for higher affinity (144). Hence, reiterative GC cycles of expansion, diversification, and selection rapidly amplify high-affinity variants of the original antigen-specific B cell compartment.

At some stage, variant centrocytes are exported from the GC reaction to enter the memory B cell compartment (115, 145). Very little is understood of the differential signals required at this stage of development. Interestingly, in the absence of AID (123) the GC reaction contains significantly greater numbers of B cells. It is possible that delayed or distorted antigen-specific selection processes may have caused the cellular congestion in this case. GC congestion is also seen in the absence of Blimp-1 (103). The absence of this transcriptional repressor may have delayed GC exit in this model. Although the highest detectable levels of Blimp-1 are found in PCs, there are reports of small fractions of GC B cells also containing Blimp-1 protein (146). Although there are still many alternate explanations, these trends indicate the existence of B cell intrinsic signals in the regulation of prememory B cells' exit from the GC cycle.

PHASE IV: THE MEMORY B CELL RESPONSE TO ANTIGEN RECALL

Antigen-Specific Memory B Cell Subsets

Exit from the GC reaction signifies entry into the long-lived memory B cell compartment. Early studies indicate that memory B cells are persistent, long-lived, antigen-specific B cells (147), with new models that indicate this survival is not dependent on signals through the BCR on antigen-experienced B cells (148). Experimental access to the antigen-specific B cell compartment in non-BCR transgenic animals has the longest history of the three antigen-experienced cellular subsets considered in this review. As soluble antigen is the ligand for the BCR, all approaches use variations of labeled antigen to identify antigen-specific B cells. Although panning techniques used gel-associated antigen (149, 150), flow cytometry provided the most reliable access to antigen-specific B cells (151, 152). These earliest studies by Herzenberg and colleagues (151, 152) coupled cell sorting technology and direct labeling to enrich antigen-specific B cells for adoptive transfer. These early studies helped to demonstrate that B cells with receptors for antigen were the precursors for AFCs.

This approach has been adopted by many groups (147, 153–155), with the subsequent evaluation of specificity and purity demonstrated by the frequency for AFCs or the enrichment for production of antigen-specific antibodies in vitro. McHeyzer-Williams et al. (156) adopted this approach to isolate NP-specific memory B cells directly ex vivo. We focused on the NP-specific memory response and evaluated target cell purities based on single cell cloning of memory B cells in vitro (156). Further, we devised the first single cell RT-PCR analysis in lymphocytes and used this technique to estimate the extent of SHM in the individual progeny of memory B cell clones (156). Subsequently, we applied single cell RT-PCR directly ex vivo to analyze BCR repertoires with single cell resolution (112, 157). As discussed above, we have extended this approach to Th cells using V region–based strategies (48) or pMHCII-tetramers (51) with similar applications for the study of TCR repertoire development in vivo (53).

There are multiple subtypes of antigen-specific memory B cells. As discussed previously, antibody isotype itself defines a major developmental and functional subdivision in the memory B cell compartment. The spectrum of isotype produced depends on the quality of cognate Th cell regulation, which itself depends on the antigen, its dose, route of entry, and adjuvant context. How different isotype-specific prememory B cells are controlled at the final stages of GC exit and how they are differentially maintained in the memory B cell compartment are not clearly understood.

At a more fundamental level of function, there is general consensus for at least one other major subdivision in the memory B cell compartment. One subtype of affinity-matured memory B cells persists as nonsecreting cells that are the precursors of the rapid cellular response to antigen recall. Long-lived PCs that are terminally differentiated, affinity-matured, and home to the bone marrow are the second category of post-GC B cells that can be considered a subtype of memory B cells and that contribute to humoral or serological memory.

Post-GC and Pre-Plasma Memory B Cell Subsets

Memory response precursors have been typically defined as IgM⁻IgD⁻6B2⁺ (6B2 recognizes the B cell form of CD45) antigen-binding B cells (154, 156, 158, 159) that do not secrete antibody until expansion and differentiation into PC after rechallenge with antigen. These 6B2⁺ memory B cells express mutated receptors and can be found in late primary and secondary responses to antigen (112, 156, 157). More recently, we have identified a separate, phenotypically distinct 6B2⁻ memory B cell compartment using NP-conjugated keyhole limpet hemocyanin (NP-KLH) and the Ribi adjuvant system (160). Both 6B2⁺ and 6B2⁻ memory subsets rapidly re-emerge upon antigen recall as IgM⁻IgD⁻ NP-binding cells, easily distinguished from memory response PCs through lack of CD138 (Syndecan 1) expression (112, 157) (see Figure 2 for a summary of phenotype and genotype). Both subsets persist at substantial numbers for at least eight weeks postrecall and do not secrete antibody in ELISPOT assays directly ex vivo. Both compartments express the lambda light chain, with demonstrable levels of IgG isotype and the Igβ BCR coreceptor (CD79b) present in at least half of the 6B2⁻ NP-binding memory B cells (160). Single cell RT-PCR analysis demonstrated the presence of somatically mutated Vλ mRNA in both subsets with evidence for antigen-driven selection.

The responsiveness of each memory subset upon adoptive transfer and antigen recall, the parent-to-progeny relationship, and the capacity to produce PCs and antibody in the serum allowed us to propose a model of linear development to connect these memory response precursors and terminally differentiated PCs (160). We proposed that 6B2⁺ post-GC memory B cells were developmentally upstream of 6B2⁻ pre-plasma memory B cells that were a nonsecreting stable cell fate and developmentally upstream of memory response PCs. Our phenotypic and molecular analysis of the primary response to NP-KLH (161) identified similar subtypes of NP-specific B cells that emerged during the first weeks after initial priming and persisted up to eight weeks without rechallenge. These data were consistent with our linear development model in which the 6B2⁺ post-GC memory B cells were the main cellular product of the GC reaction that gave rise to 6B2⁻ pre-plasma memory B cells and long-lived PCs once outside the GC reaction (see Figure 1B for the schematic).

Memory B Cells with Atypical Cell Surface Phenotype

There is evidence for this atypical 6B2⁻ memory B cell compartment in studies using the NP-specific BCR transgenic quasimonoclonal (QM) mouse model (162). Wabl and colleagues (163) identified 6B2⁻CD19⁻CD138⁻ B cells in the peripheral blood of these animals, expressing downstream antibody isotypes that contained rearranged and mutated IgH and IgL mRNA. Noelle and colleagues (164) identified a similar 6B2$^{low/-}$ antigen-experienced B cell compartment upon adoptive transfer of these QM B cells and antigen exposure in vivo. The low CD138 levels, nonsecreting status, and bone marrow homing propensity of this QM B cell subset (164) closely resembled the 6B2⁻ pre-plasma memory compartment described in the non-BCR transgenic model (103, 160, 161). These 6B2$^{low/-}$ QM B cells were considered plasma cell precursors because they could give rise to antigen-specific PCs upon adoptive transfer, without secondary exposure to antigen (164). However, proliferation was required before differentiation into PCs, hence the distinction from PCs themselves (164). Nevertheless, the B cells that persist

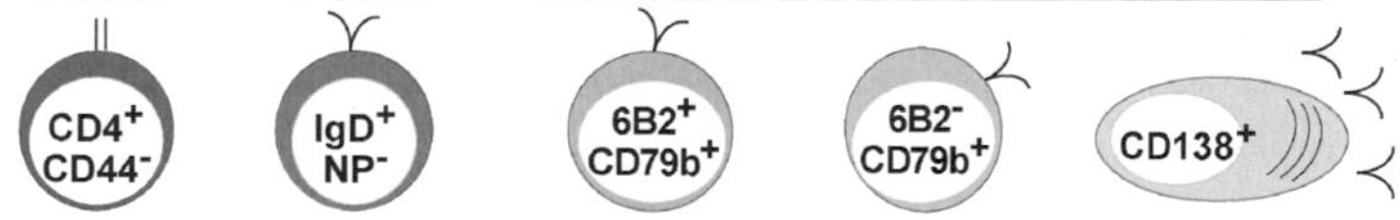

Cell Surface	Naive T cells CD4+ CD44-	Naive B cells IgD+ NP-	Day 5 Memory Response NP-specific 6B2+ CD79b+	6B2- CD79b+	CD138+
NP	-	-	++	++	++
IgD [11.26]	-	+++	+	+	-
λ-1 [JC5.1]	-	+	++	++	++
CD79b [HM79]	-	++	++	+++	+
B220 [6B2]	-	++	++	-	+
CD138 [281.2]	-	-	-	-	++++
CD19 [1D3]	-	+++	+++	-	++
CD22 [Cy34.1]	-	+++	++	-	-
CD24 [M1/69]	-	++	++++	++	+++
CD40 [3/23]	-	++	+	-	-
CD9 [KMC3]	-	+	+	++	+
CD43 [S7]	+++	+	-	+++	+++
CD11b [M1/70]	-	+	-	++	-
Gene					
Igl-V1 [λ-1]	-	++	++++	++++	++++
Cd79b [Igβ]	-	+++	++++	++	++
Sdc1 [Cd138]	-	-	-	-	++
Cd19	-	++	++	+	+
Cd22	-	++++	+++	++	-
Cd24a	-	+++	+++	+	+++
Tnfrsf5 [Cd40]	-	++	+	+	-
Cd9	-	-	-	++	+
prdm1 [Blimp-1]	-	-	-	-	++
xbp1	-	+	+	++	++++

Figure 2   Phenotype and genotype of NP-specific memory B cell subsets. Cells were analyzed directly by flow cytometry and isolated directly ex vivo for Affymetrix gene expression analysis. For cell surface analysis a protein signal of (–) equals an MFI of 0–20, (+) is 21–100, (++) is 101–500, (+++) is 501–1000, (++++) >1000. For Affymetrix microarray analysis an mRNA signal of (–) equals a fluorescence of 0–200, (+) is 201–1000, (++) is 1001–5000, (+++) is 5001–10000, (++++) >10000.

long-term in this model are clearly post-GC, isotype-switched, and antigen-experienced B cells, and thus may be considered cellular components of the memory B cell compartment.

Diamond and colleagues (165) developed a peptide tetramer-based method for detecting peptide-specific B cells in vivo. They demonstrate a substantial number of 6B2$^-$ and CD19$^-$ peptide-binding cells in immunized BALB/c mice (165). Specificity is demonstrated for peptide-binding cells after sorting and culture by ELISPOT; however, CD138 is not used to exclude peptide-binding PCs, and phenotype (either 6B2 or CD19 separation) is not used before assay of function. However, this group demonstrates the presence of CD79b mRNA in both 6B2$^+$ and 6B2$^-$ putative B cell subsets. Cambier and colleagues (166) also noted 6B2$^{low/-}$ cells accumulate to ~50% of Id$^-$ B cells in aged 3–83$\mu\delta$ BCR transgenic mice. Although CD45 is expressed by the Id$^-$ B cells, the high molecular weight isoform detected by 6B2 was absent (166). Using this same antibody (>95% of naive human B cells labeled with 6B2), Bleesing & Fleisher (167) demonstrated that most CD27$^+$ memory B cells in human peripheral blood (168, 169) had lost 6B2 binding (167). The 6B2 distribution was similar for IgM and downstream non-IgM CD27$^+$ memory B cells (167). Thus, there is evidence for the pre-plasma memory B cells as a persistent antigen-experienced B cell in both mouse and human.

Pre-Plasma Memory B Cells and the Multiple Myeloma Progenitor

One may reasonably speculate that if pre-plasma memory B cells comprise a substantial fraction of B cell memory then they should be represented among the many different varieties of mature B cell leukemias and lymphomas. The myelomagenic progenitor in multiple myeloma (MM) may be one such candidate (164, 170). MM is an incurable malignancy characterized by accumulations of clonal PCs in the bone marrow (171, 172). Although disease pathology is largely due to the dysregulated turnover and overgrowth of long-lived PCs, populations of antigen-experienced, somatically mutated non-PC B cell progenitors appear to underlie disease etiology (170, 173). Accumulating evidence implicates a circulating post-GC B cell subtype that expresses low molecular weight isoforms of CD45, bimodal expression of CD19, low to negative CD20, CD21, and CD22, and no expression of CD138 (170, 173, 174). These putative progenitor cells also express elevated levels of the adhesion molecule CD11b, not typically found on conventional B cells in human or mouse (170) or on naive, post-GC memory B cells or PCs in mouse, but found at high levels on pre-plasma memory B cells (160, 161) (see Figure 2). Thus, the MM progenitor may represent a malignant transformation of cells from the pre-plasma memory B cell compartment.

Monocytes Masquerading as Memory B Cells

Bell & Gray (175) recently raised the possibility that the pre-plasma memory B cells were actually monocytes that had captured specific antibody, masquerading as antigen-binding 6B2⁻ memory B cells. These studies used a three-color flow cytometric strategy without assessing CD79b expression on their putative 6B2⁻ B cell compartment. Using immunized serum transfer in a variety of experimental situations, FcγR ablated animals (RIII and common γ chain), and PE-specific memory responses, we found little evidence of monocytes that interfered with our specific analysis (103; L. McHeyzer-Williams & M. McHeyzer-Williams, unpublished data). Conversely, we found 6B2⁻ pre-plasma memory B cells that also expressed CD79b in both FcγR-knockout mice and the PE-memory response (L. McHeyzer-Williams & M. McHeyzer-Williams, unpublished). One may be misled by background staining of non-B cells when relying on antigen binding alone to identify memory B cells. Also, obtaining purified populations of B cells in the absence of typical B cell–associated markers is difficult, as we found in our original studies. There were many CD79b⁻ cells within the 6B2⁻ fraction of NP-binding events that we also inadvertently selected for our original studies. However, our functional assays outside of flow cytometry (BCR repertoire studies and adoptive transfer) detected the presence of B cell activity within these putative memory B cell populations, even without the CD79b selection that we now use for all our isolation procedures involving the 6B2⁻ pre-plasma memory compartment.

Extended Phenotype and Genotype of Memory B Cell Subsets

Figure 2 summarizes the cell surface phenotype of the two memory response precursors, compared quantitatively with naive B cells and memory response PCs. The first section of phenotype (Figure 2, upper 6 rows) emphasizes the main selection criterion to use when purifying the NP-specific memory B cell subsets. We have now expanded the molecular analyses of both NP-specific memory B cell subsets to quantify more clearly the levels of the most critical and only reliable B cell lineage marker, rearranged immunoglobulin genes. Affymetrix microarray assessment direct ex vivo (Figure 2, lower half) and Q-PCR confirmation of lambda light chain expression (data not shown) from equivalent numbers of 6B2⁺ post-GC memory cells and 6B2⁻ pre-plasma memory B cells indicate equivalent amounts of mRNA in these putative memory populations. Although surface-expressed CD79b protein is even higher in the 6B2⁻ memory subset (Figure 2, upper panel), CD79b mRNA levels are present in all subsets but lower in the pre-plasma memory cells (Figure 2, lower panel). These microarray data for CD79b were also confirmed using Q-PCR (data not shown). A series of other typical and atypical cell surface molecules found to change across the proposed cellular development program, have mRNA levels that are broadly concordant with the protein expression (Figure 2).

The original single cell RT-PCR repertoire analysis of the pre-plasma memory compartment (160, 161) was criticized (175) as having a low success rate for obtaining sequence (60%, 30%, 15% across PC, post-GC, and pre-plasma memory for Vλ mRNA, respectively). Using CD79b as an extra selection criterion (compared with the initial study) and a redesigned single cell RT-PCR, we can now amplify rearranged lambda light chain mRNA from 45%–50% of single memory B cells from either population (data not shown). The PCs from the same D5 memory timepoint still achieve 60% efficiency in these experiments and represent the higher end of efficiency for the current system.

Thus, regardless of the unique cell surface phenotype expressed, we believe that the current flow strategy focuses on NP-specific memory B cell populations. The schematic presented in Figure 2 should allow purification of these separate cellular compartments through application of the extended phenotype and evaluation through genotypic population and single cell analysis.

Long-Lived Plasma Cells as a Memory B Cell Compartment

Long-lived antibody-secreting B cells can also be considered part of the memory B cell compartment. The long-lived PCs secrete isotype-switched antibody and display evidence of SHM with affinity-increasing mutation patterns, but they do not self-replenish through turnover (114, 176, 177). This post-GC antigen-specific B cell compartment appears during the second week after initial antigen exposure (112) and preferentially homes to the bone marrow for growth factor support of stromal cells (178). On the basis of gene ablation studies, investigators have concluded that these cells use a variety of redistribution mechanisms, such as upregulation of CXCR4 and $\alpha4\beta1$ integrin binding to its ligand VCAM-1 (102), to get to the bone marrow, where they can persist for the life of the animal (99, 179–183). In the bone marrow, long-lived PCs need signals through the TNFR family member, BCMA for survival (184). Investigators have also proposed that a pre-plasma cell precursor (164) or memory cells themselves (185) produce PCs in a non-antigen-dependent manner as a means of maintaining serum antibody levels for extended periods.

The extended longevity of the long-lived PC can be demonstrated using BrdU incorporation and adoptive transfer (180–183). The extinguished gene programs associated with PC development (106, 107, 186) support a terminally differentiated end stage cell that needs to arrest cell cycle progression (187) and that will not be reactivated upon antigen recall. Nevertheless, on the basis of the evidence from a GC phase in development, of the extended longevity of these PCs, and of the continued production of high-affinity antibody, we consider these cells to belong to the memory B cell compartment.

Immune Synapse IV: Cognate Regulation of Memory B Cell Responses

Persistent high-affinity serum antibody provides the first layer of protection against antigen rechallenge. Although binding to antigen is a clearance mechanism, it may also serve to increase the efficiency of antigen presentation to memory B cells through rapid IC formation and binding to FcR or complement receptors on cells of the innate system. In this manner, antibody may amplify the sensitivity of the memory B cell response to antigen recall. Memory B cells to thymus-dependent antigens require cognate Th cell regulation (110, 111). Although the details on memory Th cells remain poorly resolved, the quality of immune synapse formation between memory Th cells and memory B cells is distinct from any of the preceding exchanges. The level of cellular heterogeneity on both sides of this interaction can substantially impact the developmental choices available to the memory responders.

Blimp-1 Impacts Memory B Cell Development

As previously discussed, in the absence of Blimp-1, primary response GCs are oversized (103). Surprisingly, by day 14 after priming, there is also an obvious deficit in the development of 6B2⁻ pre-plasma memory B cells. Although the phenotype in the spleen was somewhat variable, the propensity of the pre-plasma memory B cell to home to the bone marrow (160, 161) displayed a clear and dramatic quantitative developmental phenotype (103). Furthermore, long-lived PCs that dominate at day 14 of the primary response were also missing in the absence of Blimp-1. Thus, the oversized GCs may reflect the accumulation of cells whose differentiation was blocked, consistent with the proposed linear development model.

Upon reimmunization, there was an exaggerated and equivalent expansion of NP-binding B cells in the presence or absence of Blimp-1 (103). Hence, by this criterion, memory B cells had developed in the absence of Blimp-1 during the primary response GC reaction. However, the developmental progression was again dramatically blocked at the 6B2⁺ post-GC memory B cell stage. Many of the NP-specific 6B2⁺ B cells also expressed the GC marker GL7 (tenfold greater than wild type), but there were negligible numbers of 6B2⁻ pre-plasma memory B cells or memory response PCs (103). The bone marrow was also devoid of pre-plasma memory cells after antigen recall. Thus, the primary response GC produced B cells with the capability of rapid expansion upon antigen recall, but no ability to produce pre-plasma memory B cells or memory response PCs.

CONCLUDING REMARKS

Humoral immunity considers specific serum antibody as the effector element of long-term B cell responses. In this review, we emphasize memory B cells and their subspecialized activities as the key regulators of the response to antigen recall. Th cell–regulated memory B cell development is an emergent cellular behavior regulated through an ordered series of cellular and molecular changes in vivo. We now have experimental access to the cells involved at each stage of this process to probe the molecular regulators of these critical cell fate decisions in vivo. Cellular heterogeneity at all stages is extensive. Direct quantitative cellular and molecular analysis offers new standards for evaluating vaccine efficacy, while transformed equivalents of memory B cell subtypes provide new targets for therapeutic intervention in disease.

The *Annual Review of Immunology* is online at
http://immunol.annualreviews.org

LITERATURE CITED

1. Burnet FM, Fenner F. 1949. *The Production of Antibodies*. Melbourne: Macmillan
2. Talmage DW. 1957. Allergy and immunology. *Annu. Rev. Med.* 8:239–56
3. Burnet FM. 1957. A modification of Jerne's theory of antibody production using the concept of clonal selection. *Aust. J. Sci.* 20:67–69
4. Burnet FM. 1958. *Clonal Selection Theory of Acquired Immunity*. Cambridge, UK: Cambridge Univ. Press
5. Fagraeus A. 1948. The plasma cell reaction and its relation to the formation of antibodies in vitro. *J. Immunol.* 58:1–3
6. Nossal GJ. 1959. Antibody production by single cells. III. The histology of antibody production. *Br. J. Exp. Pathol.* 40:301–11
7. Raff MC, Feldmann M, De Petris S. 1973. Monospecificity of bone marrow-derived lymphocytes. *J. Exp. Med.* 137:1024–30
8. Miller JF. 1961. Immunological function of the thymus. *Lancet* 2:748–49
9. Claman HN, Chaperon EA, Triplett RF. 1966. Thymus-marrow cell combinations. Synergism in antibody production. *Proc. Soc. Exp. Biol. Med.* 122:1167–71
10. Miller JF, Mitchell GF. 1967. The thymus and the precursors of antigen reactive cells. *Nature* 216:659–63
11. Paul WE, Siskind GW, Benacerraf B. 1966. Studies on the effect of the carrier molecule on antihapten antibody synthesis. II. Carrier specificity of anti-2,4-dinitrophenyl-poly-l-lysine antibodies. *J. Exp. Med.* 123:689–705
12. Katz DH, Paul WE, Goidl EA, Benacerraf B. 1970. Carrier function in anti-hapten immune responses. I. Enhancement of primary and secondary anti-hapten antibody responses by carrier preimmunization. *J. Exp. Med.* 132:261–82
13. Mitchison NA. 1971. The carrier effect in the secondary response to hapten-protein conjugates. I. Measurement of the effect with transferred cells and objections to the local environment hypothesis. *Eur. J. Immunol.* 1:10–17
14. Rajewsky K, Schirrmacher V, Nase S, Jerne NK. 1969. The requirement of more than one antigenic determinant for immunogenicity. *J. Exp. Med.* 129:1131–43
15. Banchereau J, Steinman RM. 1998. Dendritic cells and the control of immunity. *Nature* 392:245–52
16. Aderem A, Ulevitch RJ. 2000. Toll-like receptors in the induction of the innate immune response. *Nature* 406:782–87
17. Janeway CA Jr, Medzhitov R. 2002. Innate immune recognition. *Annu. Rev. Immunol.* 20:197–216
18. Pulendran B. 2004. Modulating vaccine responses with dendritic cells and Toll-like receptors. *Immunol. Rev.* 199:227–50
19. Shortman K, Liu YJ. 2002. Mouse and human dendritic cell subtypes. *Nat. Rev. Immunol.* 2:151–61
20. Itano AA, Jenkins MK. 2003. Antigen presentation to naive CD4 T cells in the lymph node. *Nat. Immunol.* 4:733–39
21. Mandala S, Hajdu R, Bergstrom J, Quackenbush E, Xie J, et al. 2002. Alteration of lymphocyte trafficking by sphingosine-1-phosphate receptor agonists. *Science* 296:346–49
22. Martin-Fontecha A, Sebastiani S, Hopken UE, Uguccioni M, Lipp M, et al. 2003. Regulation of dendritic cell migration to the draining lymph node: impact on T lymphocyte traffic and priming. *J. Exp. Med.* 198:615–21
23. Randolph GJ, Inaba K, Robbiani DF, Steinman RM, Muller WA. 1999. Differentiation of phagocytic monocytes into

lymph node dendritic cells in vivo. *Immunity* 11:753–61

24. Dadaglio G, Nelson CA, Deck MB, Petzold SJ, Unanue ER. 1997. Characterization and quantitation of peptide-MHC complexes produced from hen egg lysozyme using a monoclonal antibody. *Immunity* 6:727–38

25. Zhong G, Reis e Sousa C, Germain RN. 1997. Production, specificity, and functionality of monoclonal antibodies to specific peptide-major histocompatibility complex class II complexes formed by processing of exogenous protein. *Proc. Natl. Acad. Sci. USA* 94:13856–61

26. Reay PA, Matsui K, Haase K, Wulfing C, Chien YH, Davis MM. 2000. Determination of the relationship between T cell responsiveness and the number of MHC-peptide complexes using specific monoclonal antibodies. *J. Immunol.* 164:5626–34

27. Inaba K, Pack M, Inaba M, Sakuta H, Isdell F, Steinman RM. 1997. High levels of a major histocompatibility complex II-self peptide complex on dendritic cells from the T cell areas of lymph nodes. *J. Exp. Med.* 186:665–72

28. Inaba K, Turley S, Yamaide F, Iyoda T, Mahnke K, et al. 1998. Efficient presentation of phagocytosed cellular fragments on the major histocompatibility complex class II products of dendritic cells. *J. Exp. Med.* 188:2163–73

29. Zhong G, Reis e Sousa C, Germain RN. 1997. Antigen-unspecific B cells and lymphoid dendritic cells both show extensive surface expression of processed antigen-major histocompatibility complex class II complexes after soluble protein exposure in vivo or in vitro. *J. Exp. Med.* 186:673–82

30. Itano AA, McSorley SJ, Reinhardt RL, Ehst BD, Ingulli E, et al. 2003. Distinct dendritic cell populations sequentially present antigen to CD4 T cells and stimulate different aspects of cell-mediated immunity. *Immunity* 19:47–57

31. Norcross MA. 1984. A synaptic basis for T-lymphocyte activation. *Ann. Immunol.* 135D:113–34

32. Bromley SK, Burack WR, Johnson KG, Somersalo K, Sims TN, et al. 2001. The immunological synapse. *Annu. Rev. Immunol.* 19:375–96

33. Iezzi G, Karjalainen K, Lanzavecchia A. 1998. The duration of antigenic stimulation determines the fate of naive and effector T cells. *Immunity* 8:89–95

34. Monks CR, Freiberg BA, Kupfer H, Sciaky N, Kupfer A. 1998. Three-dimensional segregation of supramolecular activation clusters in T cells. *Nature* 395:82–86

35. Grakoui A, Bromley SK, Sumen C, Davis MM, Shaw AS, et al. 1999. The immunological synapse: a molecular machine controlling T cell activation. *Science* 285:221–27

36. Lee KH, Holdorf AD, Dustin ML, Chan AC, Allen PM, Shaw AS. 2002. T cell receptor signaling precedes immunological synapse formation. *Science* 295:1539–42

37. Huppa JB, Gleimer M, Sumen C, Davis MM. 2003. Continuous T cell receptor signaling required for synapse maintenance and full effector potential. *Nat. Immunol.* 4:749–55

38. Stoll S, Delon J, Brotz TM, Germain RN. 2002. Dynamic imaging of T cell-dendritic cell interactions in lymph nodes. *Science* 296:1873–76

39. Miller MJ, Wei SH, Parker I, Cahalan MD. 2002. Two-photon imaging of lymphocyte motility and antigen response in intact lymph node. *Science* 296:1869–73

40. Mempel TR, Henrickson SE, Von Andrian UH. 2004. T-cell priming by dendritic cells in lymph nodes occurs in three distinct phases. *Nature* 427:154–59

41. Mosmann TR, Cherwinski H, Bond MW, Giedlin MA, Coffman RL. 1986. Two types of murine helper T cell clone. I. Definition according to profiles of lymphokine activities and secreted proteins. *J. Immunol.* 136:2348–57

42. Mosmann TR, Coffman RL. 1989. TH1 and TH2 cells: different patterns of lymphokine secretion lead to different functional properties. *Annu. Rev. Immunol.* 7: 145–73

43. Seder RA, Paul WE. 1994. Acquisition of lymphokine-producing phenotype by CD4+ T cells. *Annu. Rev. Immunol.* 12:635–73

44. Szabo SJ, Sullivan BM, Peng SL, Glimcher LH. 2003. Molecular mechanisms regulating Th1 immune responses. *Annu. Rev. Immunol.* 21:713–58

45. Kearney ER, Pape KA, Loh DY, Jenkins MK. 1994. Visualization of peptide-specific T cell immunity and peripheral tolerance induction in vivo. *Immunity* 1: 327–39

46. Reinhardt RL, Jenkins MK. 2003. Whole-body analysis of T cell responses. *Curr. Opin. Immunol.* 15:366–71

47. Jenkins MK, Khoruts A, Ingulli E, Mueller DL, McSorley SJ, et al. 2001. In vivo activation of antigen-specific CD4 T cells. *Annu. Rev. Immunol.* 19:23–45

48. McHeyzer-Williams MG, Davis MM. 1995. Antigen-specific development of primary and memory T cells in vivo. *Science* 268:106–11

49. McHeyzer-Williams MG, Altman JD, Davis MM. 1996. Enumeration and characterization of memory cells in the TH compartment. *Immunol. Rev.* 150:5–21

50. McHeyzer-Williams MG, Altman JD, Davis MM. 1996. Tracking antigen-specific helper T cell responses. *Curr. Opin. Immunol.* 8:278–84

51. Altman JD, Moss PA, Goulder PJ, Barouch DH, McHeyzer-Williams MG, et al. 1996. Phenotypic analysis of antigen-specific T lymphocytes. *Science* 274:94–96

52. Davis MM, Lyons DS, Altman JD, McHeyzer-Williams M, Hampl J, et al. 1997. T cell receptor biochemistry, repertoire selection and general features of TCR and Ig structure. *Ciba Found. Symp.* 204:94–100

53. McHeyzer-Williams LJ, Panus JF, Mikszta JA, McHeyzer-Williams MG. 1999. Evolution of antigen-specific T cell receptors in vivo: preimmune and antigen-driven selection of preferred complementarity-determining region 3 (CDR3) motifs. *J. Exp. Med.* 189:1823–37

54. Lu FW, Yasutomo K, Goodman GB, McHeyzer-Williams LJ, McHeyzer-Williams MG, et al. 2000. Thymocyte resistance to glucocorticoids leads to antigen-specific unresponsiveness due to "holes" in the T cell repertoire. *Immunity* 12:183–92

55. Panus JF, McHeyzer-Williams LJ, McHeyzer-Williams MG. 2000. Antigen-specific T helper cell function: differential cytokine expression in primary and memory responses. *J. Exp. Med.* 192:1301–16

56. Bikah G, Pogue-Caley RR, McHeyzer-Williams LJ, McHeyzer-Williams MG. 2000. Regulating T helper cell immunity through antigen responsiveness and calcium entry. *Nat. Immunol.* 1:402–12

57. Crawford F, Kozono H, White J, Marrack P, Kappler J. 1998. Detection of antigen-specific T cells with multivalent soluble class II MHC covalent peptide complexes. *Immunity* 8:675–82

58. Savage PA, Boniface JJ, Davis MM. 1999. A kinetic basis for T cell receptor repertoire selection during an immune response. *Immunity* 10:485–92

59. Savage PA, Davis MM. 2001. A kinetic window constricts the T cell receptor repertoire in the thymus. *Immunity* 14:243–52

60. McHeyzer-Williams LJ, McHeyzer-Williams MG. 2004. Developmentally distinct Th cells control plasma cell production in vivo. *Immunity* 20:231–42

61. Lanzavecchia A. 1985. Antigen-specific interaction between T and B cells. *Nature* 314:537–39

62. Batista FD, Iber D, Neuberger MS. 2001. B cells acquire antigen from target cells

after synapse formation. *Nature* 411:489–94

63. Rudge EU, Cutler AJ, Pritchard NR, Smith KG. 2002. Interleukin 4 reduces expression of inhibitory receptors on B cells and abolishes CD22 and Fcγ RII-mediated B cell suppression. *J. Exp. Med.* 195:1079–85

64. Jordan MB, Mills DM, Kappler J, Marrack P, Cambier JC. 2004. Promotion of B cell immune responses via an alum-induced myeloid cell population. *Science* 304:1808–10

65. Bishop GA, Hostager BS. 2001. B lymphocyte activation by contact-mediated interactions with T lymphocytes. *Curr. Opin. Immunol.* 13:278–85

66. Armitage RJ, Fanslow WC, Strockbine L, Sato TA, Clifford KN, et al. 1992. Molecular and biological characterization of a murine ligand for CD40. *Nature* 357:80–82

67. Banchereau J, Bazan F, Blanchard D, Briere F, Galizzi JP, et al. 1994. The CD40 antigen and its ligand. *Annu. Rev. Immunol.* 12:881–922

68. Quezada SA, Jarvinen LZ, Lind EF, Noelle RJ. 2004. CD40/CD154 interactions at the interface of tolerance and immunity. *Annu. Rev. Immunol.* 22:307–28

69. Matsumoto M, Lo SF, Carruthers CJ, Min J, Mariathasan S, et al. 1996. Affinity maturation without germinal centres in lymphotoxin-α-deficient mice. *Nature* 382:462–66

70. Koni PA, Sacca R, Lawton P, Browning JL, Ruddle NH, Flavell RA. 1997. Distinct roles in lymphoid organogenesis for lymphotoxins α and β revealed in lymphotoxin β-deficient mice. *Immunity* 6:491–500

71. Fu YX, Huang G, Matsumoto M, Molina H, Chaplin DD. 1997. Independent signals regulate development of primary and secondary follicle structure in spleen and mesenteric lymph node. *Proc. Natl. Acad. Sci. USA* 94:5739–43

72. Futterer A, Mink K, Luz A, Kosco-Vilbois MH, Pfeffer K. 1998. The lymphotoxin β receptor controls organogenesis and affinity maturation in peripheral lymphoid tissues. *Immunity* 9:59–70

73. Rennert PD, James D, Mackay F, Browning JL, Hochman PS. 1998. Lymph node genesis is induced by signaling through the lymphotoxin β receptor. *Immunity* 9:71–79

74. Mackay F, Schneider P, Rennert P, Browning J. 2003. BAFF and APRIL: a tutorial on B cell survival. *Annu. Rev. Immunol.* 21:231–64

75. Litinskiy MB, Nardelli B, Hilbert DM, He B, Schaffer A, et al. 2002. DCs induce CD40-independent immunoglobulin class switching through BLyS and APRIL. *Nat. Immunol.* 3:822–29

76. von Bulow GU, van Deursen JM, Bram RJ. 2001. Regulation of the T-independent humoral response by TACI. *Immunity* 14:573–82

77. Shlomchik MJ, Marshak-Rothstein A, Wolfowicz CB, Rothstein TL, Weigert MG. 1987. The role of clonal selection and somatic mutation in autoimmunity. *Nature* 328:805–11

78. Smith KG, Nossal GJ, Tarlinton DM. 1995. FAS is highly expressed in the germinal center but is not required for regulation of the B-cell response to antigen. *Proc. Natl. Acad. Sci. USA* 92:11628–32

79. Takahashi Y, Cerasoli DM, Dal Porto JM, Shimoda M, Freund R, et al. 1999. Relaxed negative selection in germinal centers and impaired affinity maturation in bcl-xL transgenic mice. *J. Exp. Med.* 190:399–410

80. McAdam AJ, Greenwald RJ, Levin MA, Chernova T, Malenkovich N, et al. 2001. ICOS is critical for CD40-mediated antibody class switching. *Nature* 409:102–5

81. Dong C, Juedes AE, Temann UA, Shresta S, Allison JP, et al. 2001. ICOS costimulatory receptor is essential for T-cell activation and function. *Nature* 409:97–101

82. Tafuri A, Shahinian A, Bladt F, Yoshinaga

SK, Jordana M, et al. 2001. ICOS is essential for effective T-helper-cell responses. *Nature* 409:105–9

83. Sharpe AH, Freeman GJ. 2002. The B7-CD28 superfamily. *Nat. Rev. Immunol.* 2: 116–26

84. Walunas TL, Lenschow DJ, Bakker CY, Linsley PS, Freeman GJ, et al. 1994. CTLA-4 can function as a negative regulator of T cell activation. *Immunity* 1:405–13

85. Waterhouse P, Penninger JM, Timms E, Wakeham A, Shahinian A, et al. 1995. Lymphoproliferative disorders with early lethality in mice deficient in CTLA-4. *Science* 270:985–88

86. Snapper CM, Paul WE. 1987. Interferon-γ and B cell stimulatory factor-1 reciprocally regulate Ig isotype production. *Science* 236:944–47

87. Snapper CM, Finkelman FD, Paul WE. 1988. Regulation of IgG1 and IgE production by interleukin 4. *Immunol. Rev.* 102:51–75

88. McHeyzer-Williams MG. 1989. Combinations of interleukins 2, 4 and 5 regulate the secretion of murine immunoglobulin isotypes. *Eur. J. Immunol.* 19:2025–30

89. Yoshida K, Matsuoka M, Usuda S, Mori A, Ishizaka K, Sakano H. 1990. Immunoglobulin switch circular DNA in the mouse infected with *Nippostrongylus brasiliensis*: evidence for successive class switching from μ to ε via γ 1. *Proc. Natl. Acad. Sci. USA* 87:7829–33

90. Kuhn R, Rajewsky K, Muller W. 1991. Generation and analysis of interleukin-4 deficient mice. *Science* 254:707–10

91. Takeda K, Tanaka T, Shi W, Matsumoto M, Minami M, et al. 1996. Essential role of Stat6 in IL-4 signalling. *Nature* 380:627–30

92. Shimoda K, van Deursen J, Sangster MY, Sarawar SR, Carson RT, et al. 1996. Lack of IL-4-induced Th2 response and IgE class switching in mice with disrupted Stat6 gene. *Nature* 380:630–33

93. Ozaki K, Spolski R, Feng CG, Qi CF,

Cheng J, et al. 2002. A critical role for IL-21 in regulating immunoglobulin production. *Science* 298:1630–34

94. Cazac BB, Roes J. 2000. TGF-β receptor controls B cell responsiveness and induction of IgA in vivo. *Immunity* 13:443–51

95. Coffman RL, Lebman DA, Shrader B. 1989. Transforming growth factor β specifically enhances IgA production by lipopolysaccharide-stimulated murine B lymphocytes. *J. Exp. Med.* 170:1039–44

96. Sonoda E, Matsumoto R, Hitoshi Y, Ishii T, Sugimoto M, et al. 1989. Transforming growth factor β induces IgA production and acts additively with interleukin 5 for IgA production. *J. Exp. Med.* 170:1415–20

97. Kopf M, Baumann H, Freer G, Freudenberg M, Lamers M, et al. 1994. Impaired immune and acute-phase responses in interleukin-6-deficient mice. *Nature* 368:339–42

98. Kopf M, Herren S, Wiles MV, Pepys MB, Kosco-Vilbois MH. 1998. Interleukin 6 influences germinal center development and antibody production via a contribution of C3 complement component. *J. Exp. Med.* 188:1895–906

99. Ho F, Lortan JE, MacLennan ICM, Khan M. 1986. Distinct short-lived and long-lived antibody-producing cell populations. *Eur. J. Immunol.* 16:1297–301

100. Jacob J, Kelsoe G. 1992. In situ studies of the primary immune response to (4-hydroxy-3-nitrophenyl)acetyl. II. A common clonal origin for periarteriolar lymphoid sheath-associated foci and germinal centers. *J. Exp. Med.* 176:679–87

101. Jacob J, Kassir R, Kelsoe G. 1991. In situ studies of the primary immune response to (4-hydroxy-3-nitrophenyl)acetyl. I. The architecture and dynamics of responding cell populations. *J. Exp. Med.* 173:1165–75

102. Hargreaves DC, Hyman PL, Lu TT, Ngo VN, Bidgol A, et al. 2001. A coordinated change in chemokine responsiveness

guides plasma cell movements. *J. Exp. Med.* 194:45–56

103. Shapiro-Shelef M, Lin KI, McHeyzer-Williams LJ, Liao J, McHeyzer-Williams MG, Calame K. 2003. Blimp-1 is required for the formation of immunoglobulin secreting plasma cells and pre-plasma memory B cells. *Immunity* 19:607–20

104. Calame KL, Lin KI, Tunyaplin C. 2003. Regulatory mechanisms that determine the development and function of plasma cells. *Annu. Rev. Immunol.* 21:205–30

105. Shapiro-Shelef M, Calame K. 2004. Plasma cell differentiation and multiple myeloma. *Curr. Opin. Immunol.* 16:226–34

106. Shaffer AL, Lin KI, Kuo TC, Yu X, Hurt EM, et al. 2002. Blimp-1 orchestrates plasma cell differentiation by extinguishing the mature B cell gene expression program. *Immunity* 17:51–62

107. Shaffer AL, Shapiro-Shelef M, Iwakoshi NN, Lee A-H, Qian S-B, et al. 2004. XBP1, downstream of Blimp-1, expands the secretory apparatus and other organelles, and increases protein synthesis in plasma cell differentiation. *Immunity* 21:81–93

108. Reimold AM, Iwakoshi NN, Manis J, Vallabhajosyula P, Szomolanyi-Tsuda E, et al. 2001. Plasma cell differentiation requires the transcription factor XBP-1. *Nature* 412:300–7

109. Iwakoshi NN, Lee AII, Vallabhajosyula P, Otipoby KL, Rajewsky K, Glimcher LH. 2003. Plasma cell differentiation and the unfolded protein response intersect at the transcription factor XBP-1. *Nat. Immunol.* 4:321–19

110. MacLennan ICM. 1994. Germinal centers. *Annu. Rev. Immunol.* 12:117–39

111. MacLennan ICM, Gray D. 1986. Antigen-driven selection of virgin and memory B cells. *Immunol. Rev.* 91:61–85

112. McHeyzer-Williams MG, McLean MJ, Lalor PA, Nossal GJV. 1993. Antigen-driven B cell differentiation in vivo. *J. Exp. Med.* 178:295–307

113. Shih TA, Meffre E, Roederer M, Nussen-zweig MC. 2002. Role of BCR affinity in T cell dependent antibody responses in vivo. *Nat. Immunol.* 3:570–75

114. McHeyzer-Williams MG, Ahmed R. 1999. B cell memory and the long-lived plasma cell. *Curr. Opin. Immunol.* 11:172–79

115. McHeyzer-Williams LJ, Driver DJ, McHeyzer-Williams MG. 2001. Germinal center reaction. *Curr. Opin. Hematol.* 8:52–59

116. Wolniak KL, Shinall SM, Waldschmidt TJ. 2004. The germinal center response. *Crit. Rev. Immunol.* 24:39–65

117. Jacob J, Kelsoe G, Rajewsky K, Weiss U. 1991. Intraclonal generation of antibody mutants in germinal centres. *Nature* 354:389–92

118. Berek C, Berger A, Apel M. 1991. Maturation of the immune response in germinal centers. *Cell* 67:1121–29

119. Ford JE, McHeyzer-Williams MG, Lieber MR. 1994. Analysis of individual immunoglobulin lambda light chain genes amplified from single cclls is inconsistent with variable region gene conversion in germinal-center B cell somatic mutation. *Eur. J. Immunol.* 24:1816–22

120. William J, Euler C, Christensen S, Shlomchik MJ. 2002. Evolution of autoantibody responses via somatic hypermutation outside of germinal centers. *Science* 297:2066–70

121. de Boer BA, Voigt I, Kim HJ, Camacho SA, Lipp M, et al. 2000. Affinity maturation in ectopic germinal centers. *Curr. Top. Microbiol. Immunol.* 251:191–95

122. Revy P, Muto T, Levy Y, Geissmann F, Plebani A, et al. 2000. Activation-induced cytidine deaminase (AID) deficiency causes the autosomal recessive form of the Hyper-IgM syndrome (HIGM2). *Cell* 102:565–75

123. Muramatsu M, Kinoshita K, Fagarasan S, Yamada S, Shinkai Y, Honjo T. 2000. Class switch recombination and hypermutation require activation-induced cytidine

deaminase (AID), a potential RNA editing enzyme. *Cell* 102:553–63

124. Honjo T, Kinoshita K, Muramatsu M. 2002. Molecular mechanism of class switch recombination: linkage with somatic hypermutation. *Annu. Rev. Immunol.* 20:165–96

125. Petersen-Mahrt SK, Harris RS, Neuberger MS. 2002. AID mutates *E. coli* suggesting a DNA deamination mechanism for antibody diversification. *Nature* 418:99–103

126. Bross L, Fukita Y, McBlane F, Demolliere C, Rajewsky K, Jacobs H. 2000. DNA double-strand breaks in immunoglobulin genes undergoing somatic hypermutation. *Immunity* 13:589–97

127. Zan H, Komori A, Li Z, Cerutti A, Schaffer A, et al. 2001. The translesion DNA polymerase ζ plays a major role in Ig and bcl-6 somatic hypermutation. *Immunity* 14:643–53

128. Gearhart PJ, Wood RD. 2001. Emerging links between hypermutation of antibody genes and DNA polymerases. *Nat. Rev. Immunol.* 1:187–92

129. Jacobs H, Fukita Y, van der Horst GTJ, de Boer J, Weeda G, et al. 1998. Hypermutation of immunoglobulin genes in memory B cells of DNA repair-deficient mice. *J. Exp. Med.* 187:1735–43

130. Rajewsky K. 1996. Clonal selection and learning in the antibody system. *Nature* 381:751–58

131. Tew JG, Kosco MH, Burton GF, Szakal AK. 1990. Follicular dendritic cells as accessory cells. *Immunol. Rev.* 117:185–211

132. Kosco-Vilbois MH. 2003. Are follicular dendritic cells really good for nothing? *Nat. Rev. Immunol.* 3:764–69

133. Barrington RA, Pozdnyakova O, Zafari MR, Benjamin CD, Carroll MC. 2002. B lymphocyte memory: role of stromal cell complement and FcγRIIB receptors. *J. Exp. Med.* 196:1189–99

134. Szakal AK, Kosco MH, Tew JG. 1988. A novel in vivo follicular dendritic cell-dependent iccosome-mediated mechanism for delivery of antigen to antigen-processing cells. *J. Immunol.* 140:341–53

135. Hannum LG, Haberman AM, Anderson SM, Shlomchik MJ. 2000. Germinal center initiation, variable gene region hypermutation, and mutant B cell selection without detectable immune complexes on follicular dendritic cells. *J. Exp. Med.* 192:931–42

136. Smith KG, Light A, O'Reilly LA, Ang SM, Strasser A, Tarlinton D. 2000. bcl-2 transgene expression inhibits apoptosis in the germinal center and reveals differences in the selection of memory B cells and bone marrow antibody-forming cells. *J. Exp. Med.* 191:475–84

137. Liu YJ, Joshua DE, Williams GT, Smith CA, Gordon J, MacLennan IC. 1989. Mechanism of antigen-driven selection in germinal centres. *Nature* 342:929–31

138. Campbell DJ, Kim CH, Butcher EC. 2001. Separable effector T cell populations specialized for B cell help or tissue inflammation. *Nat. Immunol.* 2:876–81

139. Kim CH, Rott LS, Clark-Lewis I, Campbell DJ, Wu L, Butcher EC. 2001. Subspecialization of CXCR5+ T cells: B helper activity is focused in a germinal center-localized subset of CXCR5+ T cells. *J. Exp. Med.* 193:1373–81

140. Gulbranson-Judge A, MacLennan I. 1996. Sequential antigen-specific growth of T cells in the T zones and follicles in response to pigeon cytochrome c. *Eur. J. Immunol.* 26:1830–37

141. Zheng B, Han S, Zhu Q, Goldsby R, Kelsoe G. 1996. Alternative pathways for the selection of antigen-specific peripheral T cells. *Nature* 384:263–66

142. Zheng B, Han S, Kelsoe G. 1996. T helper cells in murine germinal centers are antigen-specific emigrants that downregulate Thy-1. *J. Exp. Med.* 184:1083–91

143. Mikszta JA, McHeyzer-Williams LJ, McHeyzer-Williams MG. 1999. Antigen-driven selection of TCR in vivo: related TCR α-chains pair with diverse TCR β-chains. *J. Immunol.* 163:5978–88

144. Kepler TB, Perelson AS. 1993. Somatic hypermutation in B cells: an optimal control treatment. *J. Theor. Biol.* 164:37–64

145. McHeyzer-Williams MG. 2003. B cells as effectors. *Curr. Opin. Immunol.* 15:354–61

146. Angelin-Duclos C, Cattoretti G, Lin KI, Calame K. 2000. Commitment of B lymphocytes to a plasma cell fate is associated with Blimp-1 expression in vivo. *J. Immunol.* 165:5462–71

147. Gray D, Skarvall H. 1988. B-cell memory is short-lived in the absence of antigen. *Nature* 336:70–73

148. Maruyama M, Lam KP, Rajewsky K. 2000. Memory B-cell persistence is independent of persisting immunizing antigen. *Nature* 407:636–42

149. Nossal GJ, Pike BL, Battye FL. 1978. Sequential use of hapten-gelatin fractionation and fluorescence-activated cell sorting in the enrichment of hapten-specific B lymphocytes. *Eur. J. Immunol.* 8:151–57

150. Noelle RJ, Snow EC, Uhr JW, Vitetta ES. 1983. Activation of antigen-specific B cells: role of T cells, cytokines, and antigen in induction of growth and differentiation. *Proc. Natl. Acad. Sci. USA* 80:6628–31

151. Bonner WA, Hulett HR, Sweet RG, Herzenberg LA. 1972. Fluorescence activated cell sorting. *Rev. Sci. Instrum.* 43:404–9

152. Julius MH, Masuda T, Herzenberg LA. 1972. Demonstration that antigen-binding cells are precursors of antibody-producing cells after purification with a fluorescence-activated cell sorter. *Proc. Natl. Acad. Sci. USA* 69:1934–38

153. Greenstein JL, Leary J, Horan P, Kappler JW, Marrack P. 1980. Flow sorting of antigen-binding B cell subsets. *J. Immunol.* 124:1472–81

154. Hayakawa K, Ishii R, Yamasaki K, Kishimoto T, Hardy RR. 1987. Isolation of high-affinity memory B cells: phycoerythrin as a probe for antigen-binding cells. *Proc. Natl. Acad. Sci. USA* 84:1379–83

155. Kodituwakku AP, Jessup C, Zola H, Roberton DM. 2003. Isolation of antigen-specific B cells. *Immunol. Cell Biol.* 81:163–70

156. McHeyzer-Williams MG, Nossal GJV, Lalor PA. 1991. Molecular characterization of single memory B cells. *Nature* 350:502–5

157. Lalor PA, Nossal GJV, Sanderson RD, McHeyzer-Williams MG. 1992. Functional and molecular characterization of single, (4-hydroxy-3-nitrophenyl)acetyl (NP)-specific, IgG1+ B cells from antibody-secreting and memory B cell pathways in the C57BL/6 immune response to NP. *Eur. J. Immunol.* 22:3001–11

158. Black SJ, van der Loo W, Loken MR, Herzenberg LA. 1978. Expression of IgD by murine lymphocytes. Loss of surface IgD indicates maturation of memory B cells. *J. Exp. Med.* 147:984–96

159. Herzenberg LA, Black SJ, Tokuhisa T. 1980. Memory B cells at successive stages of differentiation. Affinity maturation and the role of IgD receptors. *J. Exp. Med.* 151:1071–87

160. McHeyzer-Williams LJ, Cool M, McHeyzer-Williams MG. 2000. Antigen-specific B cell memory: expression and replenishment of a novel B220− memory B cell compartment. *J. Exp. Med.* 191:1149–66

161. Driver DJ, McHeyzer-Williams LJ, Cool M, Stetson DB, McHeyzer-Williams MG. 2001. Development and maintenance of a B220− memory B cell compartment. *J. Immunol.* 167:1393–405

162. Cascalho M, Ma A, Lee S, Masat L, Wabl M. 1996. A quasi-monoclonal mouse. *Science* 272:1649–52

163. Cascalho M, Wong J, Brown J, Jack HM, Steinberg C, Wabl M. 2000. A B220−, CD19− population of B cells in the peripheral blood of quasimonoclonal mice. *Int. Immunol.* 12:29–35

164. O'Connor BP, Cascalho M, Noelle RJ. 2002. Short-lived and long-lived bone

marrow plasma cells are derived from a novel precursor population. *J. Exp. Med.* 195:737–45

165. Newman J, Rice JS, Wang C, Harris SL, Diamond B. 2003. Identification of an antigen-specific B cell population. *J. Immunol. Methods* 272:177–87

166. Johnson SA, Rozzo SJ, Cambier JC. 2002. Aging-dependent exclusion of antigen-inexperienced cells from the peripheral B cell repertoire. *J. Immunol.* 168:5014–23

167. Bleesing JJ, Fleisher TA. 2003. Human B cells express a CD45 isoform that is similar to murine B220 and is downregulated with acquisition of the memory B-cell marker CD27. *Cytometr. B* 51:1–8

168. Tangye SG, Liu YJ, Aversa G, Phillips JH, de Vries JE. 1998. Identification of functional human splenic memory B cells by expression of CD148 and CD27. *J. Exp. Med.* 188:1691–703

169. Klein U, Rajewsky K, Kuppers R. 1998. Human immunoglobulin (Ig)M$^+$IgD$^+$ peripheral blood B cells expressing the CD27 cell surface antigen carry somatically mutated variable region genes: CD27 as a general marker for somatically mutated (memory) B cells. *J. Exp. Med.* 188:1679–89

170. Pilarski LM, Seeberger K, Coupland RW, Eshpeter A, Keats JJ, et al. 2002. Leukemic B cells clonally identical to myeloma plasma cells are myelomagenic in NOD/SCID mice. *Exp. Hematol.* 30:221–28

171. Billadeau D, Quam L, Thomas W, Kay N, Greipp P, et al. 1992. Detection and quantitation of malignant cells in the peripheral blood of multiple myeloma patients. *Blood* 80:1818–24

172. Hallek M, Bergsagel PL, Anderson KC. 1998. Multiple myeloma: increasing evidence for a multistep transformation process. *Blood* 91:3–21

173. Szczepek AJ, Seeberger K, Wizniak J, Mant MJ, Belch AR, Pilarski LM. 1998. A high frequency of circulating B cells share clonotypic Ig heavy-chain VDJ rearrangements with autologous bone marrow plasma cells in multiple myeloma, as measured by single-cell and in situ reverse transcriptase-polymerase chain reaction. *Blood* 92:2844–55

174. Bergsagel PL, Smith AM, Szczepek A, Mant MJ, Belch AR, Pilarski LM. 1995. In multiple myeloma, clonotypic B lymphocytes are detectable among CD19$^+$ peripheral blood cells expressing CD38, CD56, and monotypic Ig light chain. *Blood* 85:436–47

175. Bell J, Gray D. 2003. Antigen-capturing cells can masquerade as memory B cells. *J. Exp. Med.* 197:1233–44

176. Smith KG, Light A, Nossal GJV, Tarlinton DM. 1997. The extent of affinity maturation differs between the memory and antibody-forming cell compartments in the primary immune response. *EMBO J.* 16:2996–3006

177. Takahashi Y, Dutta PR, Cerasoli DM, Kelsoe G. 1998. In situ studies of the primary immune response to (4-hydroxy-3-nitrophenyl)acetyl. V. Affinity maturation develops in two stages of clonal selection. *J. Exp. Med.* 187:885–95

178. Minges Wols HA, Underhill GH, Kansas GS, Witte PL. 2002. The role of bone marrow-derived stromal cells in the maintenance of plasma cell longevity. *J. Immunol.* 169:4213–21

179. Benner R, Hijmans W, Haaijman JJ. 1981. The bone marrow: the major source of serum immunoglobulins, but still a neglected site of antibody formation. *Clin. Exp. Immunol.* 46:1–8

180. Manz RA, Thiel A, Radbruch A. 1997. Lifetime of plasma cells in the bone marrow. *Nature* 388:133–34

181. Manz RA, Lohning M, Cassese G, Thiel A, Radbruch A. 1998. Survival of long-lived plasma cells is independent of antigen. *Int. Immunol.* 11:1703–11

182. Slifka MK, Matloubian M, Ahmed R. 1995. Bone marrow is a major site of long-term antibody production after acute viral infection. *J. Virol.* 69:1895–902

183. Slifka MK, Antia R, Whitmire JK, Ahmed R. 1998. Humoral immunity due to long-lived plasma cells. *Immunity* 8:363–72

184. O'Connor BP, Raman VS, Erickson LD, Cook WJ, Weaver LK, et al. 2004. BCMA is essential for the survival of long-lived bone marrow plasma cells. *J. Exp. Med.* 199:91–98

185. Bernasconi NL, Traggiai E, Lanzavecchia A. 2002. Maintenance of serological memory by polyclonal activation of human memory B cells. *Science* 298:2199–202

186. Underhill GH, George D, Bremer EG, Kansas GS. 2003. Gene expression profiling reveals a highly specialized genetic program of plasma cells. *Blood* 101:4013–21

187. Tourigny MR, Ursini-Siegel J, Lee H, Toellner KM, Cunningham AF, et al. 2002. CDK inhibitor p18(INK4c) is required for the generation of functional plasma cells. *Immunity* 17:179–89

Annu. Rev. Immunol. 2005. 23:515–48
doi: 10.1146/annurev.immunol.23.021704.115611
Copyright © 2005 by Annual Reviews. All rights reserved
First published online as a Review in Advance on January 19, 2005

THE B7 FAMILY REVISITED

Rebecca J. Greenwald,[1] Gordon J. Freeman,[2] and Arlene H. Sharpe[1]

[1]Department of Pathology, Harvard Medical School and Brigham and Women's Hospital, Boston, Massachusetts 02115; email: rgreenwald@rics.bwh.harvard.edu, asharpe@rics.bwh.harvard.edu
[2]Department of Medical Oncology, Dana-Farber Cancer Institute, Department of Medicine, Harvard Medical School, Boston, Massachusetts 02115; email: gordon_freeman@dfci.harvard.edu

Key Words   costimulation, B7, CD28, tolerance

■ **Abstract**   The discovery of new functions for the original B7 family members, together with the identification of additional B7 and CD28 family members, have revealed new ways in which the B7:CD28 family regulates T cell activation and tolerance. B7-1/B7-2:CD28 interactions not only promote initial T cell activation but also regulate self-tolerance by supporting $CD4^+CD25^+$ T regulatory cell homeostasis. CTLA-4 can exert its inhibitory effects in both B7-1/B7-2 dependent and independent fashions. B7-1 and B7-2 can signal bidirectionally by engaging CD28 and CTLA-4 on T cells and by delivering signals into B7-expressing cells. The five new B7 family members, ICOS ligand, PD-L1 (B7-H1), PD-L2 (B7-DC), B7-H3, and B7-H4 (B7x/B7-S1) are expressed on professional antigen-presenting cells as well as on cells within nonlymphoid organs, providing new means for regulating T cell activation and tolerance in peripheral tissues. The new CD28 families members, ICOS, PD-1, and BTLA, are inducibly expressed on T cells, and they have important roles in regulating previously activated T cells. PD-1 and BTLA also are expressed on B cells and may have broader immunoregulatory functions. The ICOS:ICOSL pathway appears to be particularly important for stimulating effector T cell responses and T cell–dependent B cell responses, but it also has an important role in regulating T cell tolerance. In addition, the PD-1:PD-L1/PD-L2 pathway plays a critical role in regulating T cell activation and tolerance. In this review, we revisit the roles of the B7:CD28 family members in regulating immune responses, and we discuss their therapeutic potential.

INTRODUCTION

Pathways in the B7:CD28 family have key roles in regulating T cell activation and tolerance and are promising therapeutic targets. These pathways not only provide critical positive second signals that promote and sustain T cell responses, but they also contribute critical negative second signals that downregulate T cell responses (1–7). These negative signals function to limit, terminate, and/or attenuate T cell responses, and they appear to be especially important for regulating

T cell tolerance and autoimmunity. The B7-1/B7-2:CD28/CTLA-4 (cytotoxic T lymphocyte-associated antigen 4) pathway is the best characterized T cell costimulatory pathway, but it is complex because of the dual specificity of B7-1 (CD80) and B7-2 (CD86) for the stimulatory receptor CD28 and the inhibitory receptor CTLA-4 (CD152). CD28 delivers signals important for T cell activation and survival, whereas CTLA-4 inhibits T cell responses and regulates peripheral T cell tolerance (for recent reviews, please see References 1–3, 6, 8). Researchers have delineated two new pathways in the B7:CD28 family: one involving ICOS (inducible costimulator) (9) and ICOS ligand [B7h (10), GL50 (11), B7RP-1 (12), LICOS (13), B7-H2 (14)]; the other involving the PD-1 (15) receptor and its ligands, PD-L1 (16) [B7-H1 (17)] and PD-L2 (18) [B7-DC (19)]. Two additional B7 homologs, B7-H3 (20) and B7-H4 (21) [B7x (22), B7S1 (23)], and another CD28 homolog, BTLA (B and T lymphocyte attenuator) (24), also have been identified, indicating that there are still additional pathways within the B7:CD28 superfamily to be characterized (see Tables 1 and 2).

This review focuses on recent advances in our understanding of the functions of pathways in the B7:CD28 family. First, we discuss recently identified novel immune and nonimmune functions of B7-1 and B7-2. Next, we will summarize our current understanding of the ICOS:ICOS ligand and PD-1:PD-1 ligand pathways in regulating T cell activation and tolerance and consider their therapeutic potential. Finally, we discuss recent studies on B7-H3, B7-H4, and BTLA.

NEW FUNCTIONS FOR THE ORIGINAL B7s

The B7-1/B7-2:CD28/CTLA-4 pathway consists of two B7 family members, B7-1 and B7-2, that bind to the same two receptors, CD28 and CTLA-4 (1, 6, 25). These receptors have distinct kinetics of expression and affinities for B7-1 and

TABLE 1   Comparison of CD28 family of receptors

	CD28	CTLA-4	ICOS	PD-1	BTLA
% identity	100%	30%	27%	23%	23%
Chromosome					
Human	2q33	2q33	2q33	2q37	3q13.2
Mouse	1C1, 30.1 cM	1C2, 30.1 cM	1C2, 32 cM	1D, 55 cM	16A1
Structure					
Ligand binding motif	MYPPPY	MYPPPY	FDPPPF	?	?
Cytoplasmic domain	PI3K motif, PP2A	PI3K motif, PP2A, ?SHP2	PI3K	ITIM motif, SHP2 ITSM motif, SHP1	Two ITIM motifs
Expression					
Cell type	T	T	T, NK	T, B, M	T, B

TABLE 2 Comparison of B7 family of costimulatory molecules

	B7-1 (CD80)	B7-2 (CD86)	ICOSL (B7h, B7-H2; B7RP-1)	PD-L1 (B7-H1)	PD-L2 (B7-DC)	B7-H3	B7-H4 (B7x; B7S1)
% identity of extracellular domain	100%	27%	27%	25%	23%	29%	21%
Chromosome							
Human	3q13	3q21	21q22	9p24	9p24	15q24	1p13.1
Mouse	16B, 32.8	16B, 26.9	10C1	19B	19B	9A	3F2.2
Expression[a]							
Lymphoid[b]	B, M, DC, T	B, M, DC, T	B, M, DC, T	B, M, DC, T	DC, M	B, T, M, DC, NK	T, B, M, DC
Non-lymphoid	Rare; including podocyte	Rare	Fibroblast Endothelial Epithelial	Endothelial, Tissues (including placenta); Tumors (including many T cell lymphomas, carcinomas, melanomas, glioblastoma)	Some B cell lymphomas	Bone Marrow	Lung and ovarian tumors
Receptor	CD28 CTLA-4	CD28 CTLA-4	ICOS	PD-1	PD-1	?	?

[a]Protein, but not mRNA expression is summarized; see text for regulation of expression.

[b]B = B cell; M = macrophage; DC = dendritic cell; T = T cell; NK = natural killer cell.

B7-2 (26). CD28 is constitutively expressed on the surface of T cells, whereas CTLA-4 expression is rapidly upregulated following T cell activation. CTLA-4 is the higher affinity receptor for both B7-1 and B7-2. The kinetics of expression of B7-1 and B7-2 also differ. B7-2 is constitutively expressed at low levels and rapidly upregulated, whereas B7-1 is inducibly expressed later than B7-2. Recent work has revealed novel immune (27–30) and nonimmune (31, 32) functions for B7-1 and B7-2. Additional recent studies also indicate that CTLA-4 can exert inhibitory functions independent of B7-1 and B7-2 (33). Thus, investigators continue to discover important biological functions for this key immunoregulatory pathway.

New Immune Functions for B7-1 and B7-2

Although the role of B7:CD28 interactions in promoting initial T cell activation is well established, a role for B7:CD28 interactions in promoting T cell tolerance has been appreciated more recently. Investigation of the severe and accelerated diabetes that develops in $CD28^{-/-}$ and $B7\text{-}1/B7\text{-}2^{-/-}$ NOD (nonobese diabetic) mice (34) revealed that B7:CD28 interactions control T regulatory cells (Treg). $CD28^{-/-}$ and $B7\text{-}1/B7\text{-}2^{-/-}$ NOD mice have markedly reduced numbers of $CD4^{+}CD25^{+}$ Treg compared with wild-type NOD mice. The regulatory function of $CD28^{-/-}$ $CD4^{+}CD25^{+}$ Treg is not impaired in vitro and in vivo. Recent work indicates that CD28:B7 interactions are needed for development and maintenance of $CD4^{+}CD25^{+}$ Treg (29). When wild-type T cells are transferred into $B7\text{-}1/B7\text{-}2^{-/-}$ recipients and primed with antigen-pulsed wild-type dendritic cells (DC), these T cells have markedly increased responses compared with T cells primed in wild-type recipients (35). These enhanced responses are not due to CTLA-4, because increased effector cytokine responses are not affected by CTLA-4 blockade. However, the transfer of $CD4^{+}CD25^{+}$ Treg inhibits these enhanced T cell responses, suggesting that the reduced numbers of $CD4^{+}CD25^{+}$ Treg in the $B7\text{-}1/B7\text{-}2^{-/-}$ recipients leads to the increased T cell responses. Thus, B7:CD28 interactions have a critical role in the homeostasis of $CD4^{+}CD25^{+}$ regulatory T cells, which play an essential role in regulating self-tolerance and T cell activation.

A role for B7-1 and B7-2 on T cells also may contribute to downregulation of immune responses. Although B7-1 and B7-2 on antigen-presenting cells (APCs) have well-recognized roles as T cell costimulatory molecules, the functional significance of B7-1 and B7-2 expression on T cells is not well understood. B7-2 is constitutively expressed on some resting T cells, whereas B7-1 is not present on resting T cells (27). Both B7-1 and B7-2 can be upregulated on T cells. T cells that constitutively overexpress B7-2 on T cells have dramatically reduced alloresponses and graft-versus-host disease (GVHD) mortality. Conversely, $B7\text{-}1/B7\text{-}2^{-/-}$ T cells led to significantly accelerated alloresponses compared with wild-type T cells, as measured by graft-versus-host disease mortality. Further studies indicate that B7 expression on T cells downregulates alloresponses via a T:T interaction with CTLA-4. These findings suggest that upregulation of B7 on T cells may be important for in vivo T cell homeostasis. B7-1 and B7-2 on T cells also may be important for transmission of an inhibitory signal by $CD4^+CD25^+$ Treg cells (28). $B7\text{-}1/B7\text{-}2^{-/-}$ $CD4^+CD25^-$ T cells were resistant to suppression by concentrations of $CD4^+CD25^+$ Treg that suppressed wild-type $CD4^+CD25^-$ T effector cells. Intriguingly, suppression was restored by expression of full length but not B7-1 or B7-2 truncation mutants that lack the transmembrane and cytoplasmic domains but are costimulation-competent. These studies suggest that there may be bidirectional functions for B7 on T cells. B7 may not only engage CTLA-4 on T cells but also deliver signals into the T cell.

Another means by which B7-1 and B7-2 may influence immune responses is through reverse signaling into B7-expressing APC (30, 36, 37). Recent studies indicate that B7 can transmit suppressive signals into DC, following engagement of CTLA-4. Both a soluble form of CTLA-4 (CTLA-4Ig) and a membrane-anchored form of CTLA-4 on Treg can activate the immunosuppressive pathway of tryptophan catabolism in DC. Initial studies show that engagement of B7-1/B7-2 on murine DC by CTLA-4Ig activates a signaling pathway that stimulates DC to produce IFN-γ, which acts in an autocrine or paracrine fashion to induce indoleamine 2,3-dioxygenase (IDO), an enzyme that degrades tryptophan to byproducts that inhibit T cell proliferation (30). Murine models point to an important role for IDO in maintaining maternal-fetal tolerance and suppressing T cell responses to MHC-mismatched allografts, tumors, and self-antigens (37). Pharmacologic inhibition of IDO abrogated the protective effects of CTLA-Ig in a mouse islet cell transplant model, indicating an important role for IDO in mediating the effects of CTLA-4Ig in vivo. Further studies indicate that CTLA-4 on mouse $CD4^+CD25^+$ Treg can mediate the same IDO-inducing effect in vitro (36). Ligation of B7-1/B7-2 on human monocyte-derived DC by CTLA-4/CD28 on human $CD4^+$ T cells appears to be necessary for triggering IDO (37). These studies suggest that bidirectional B7:CTLA-4 interactions may participate in downregulation of T cell responses and induction of T cell tolerance. Therefore, CTLA-4 not only regulates T cell receptor (TCR) and CD28 signals in T cells but also delivers signals via B7s into DC to induce IDO.

Emerging data indicate that B7-2 on B cells can signal bidirectionally. B7-2 stimulates CD28 on T cells and transduces positive signals into B cells that increase IgG1 and IgE production (38, 39). This may be particularly important for memory B cells in which B7-2 is upregulated. In vitro studies show that cross-linking of B7-2 on CD40 ligand and IL-4-activated B cells increases the level and rate of IgG1 transcription. B7-2 stimulated nuclear localization of the NF-κB p50 subunit, phosphorylation of RelA (p65) and IkB-α, and increased Oct-2 expression and binding to the 3'IgH enhancer. These effects do not occur in $B7\text{-}2^{-/-}$ B cells. These findings, together with the studies of DC and T cells discussed above, suggest that reverse signaling of B7-1 or B7-2 into B7-1/B7-2 expressing cells is a novel aspect of B7-1/B7-2 function and may cause a variety of biological effects.

B7-1/B7-2 Independent Function of CTLA-4

A number of autoimmune diseases, including insulin-dependent diabetes mellitus (IDDM), Grave's disease, Hashimoto's thyroiditis, Addison's disease, rheumatoid arthritis, and multiple sclerosis, have shown genetic linkage to the CTLA-4 locus. Researchers have identified splice variants of CTLA-4 as candidates for risk of Grave's disease, autoimmune hypothyroidism, and type 1 diabetes (40). In the NOD mouse model of type 1 diabetes, increased risk for disease was correlated with a novel alternatively spliced form of CTLA-4 called ligand independent CTLA-4 (liCTLA-4). The liCTLA-4 variant lacks the IgV-like exon 2 that includes the MYPPPY motif required for binding to B7-1 and B7-2. Whereas full length CTLA-4 (flCTLA-4) is upregulated in T cells following activation, liCTLA-4 is expressed in resting T cells and rapidly downregulated early during T cell activation (33). On the mRNA and protein levels, liCTLA-4 is expressed at the highest levels on $CD4^+CD45Rb^{lo}$ T cells, suggesting that expression is derived from the memory and/or Treg population. Despite missing the extracellular ligand binding domain, liCTLA-4 inhibits both T cell proliferation and cytokine production, leading to dephosphorylation of TCR ζ chain (33). This suggests that the cytoplasmic tail of CTLA-4, independent of extracellular B7 binding domain, is capable of delivering a negative signal. Expression of liCTLA-4, but not flCTLA-4, is increased in $CD4^+CD45Rb^{lo}$ memory/regulatory cells from diabetes-resistant NOD Idd5.1 congenic mice by four-fold compared with diabetes-susceptible NOD mice. $CD4^+CD45Rb^{lo}$ NOD Idd5.1 cells exhibit decreased phosphorylation of the TcR ζ chain and zap70 activity compared with $CD4^+CD45Rb^{lo}$ NOD cells. Taken together, these findings suggest that liCTLA-4 may function to prevent activation of memory/effector T cells to weak stimuli and thereby regulate susceptibility to T cell–mediated autoimmune diseases. In contrast, the expression of flCTLA-4 in the immunological synapse is proportional to the strength of the TCR stimulus and may serve as a mechanism for inhibiting high-affinity T cells (41).

Non-Immune Functions for B7-1 and B7-2

New research shows that B7-1 in the kidney serves as an inducible regulator of the glomerular filtration apparatus (32). B7-1 expression can be upregulated in genetic and induced experimental models of nephrotic syndrome on kidney podocytes, which create the final barrier to urinary protein loss. The B7-1 expressed in podocytes is a novel splice variant of B7-1 that has the same coding sequence but an alternative 3' untranslated exon 7 with multiple ATTTA motifs that should lead to rapid mRNA turnover. Podocyte expression of B7-1 correlated with the severity of murine and human lupus nephritis. B7-1 expression in podocytes is induced by lipopolysaccharide (LPS) through TLR-4 and leads to reorganization of the actin cytoskeleton in vitro. $B7-1^{-/-}$ mice are protected from LPS-induced nephrotic syndrome, suggesting a link between podocyte B7-1 expression and proteinuria. LPS also induces B7-1 expression and proteinuria in SCID mice, indicating that B7-1 induction may be a direct action of LPS on podocytes and not secondary to activation of T or B cells. These findings suggest B7-1 can be upregulated in nonimmune cells by danger signals and may contribute to proteinuria by reorganizing the actin cytoskeleton and disrupting function of the glomerular filter.

Recent studies also have identified B7-1 and B7-2 as cellular attachment receptors for adenovirus serotype 3 (31). Adenoviruses, nonenveloped DNA viruses that have a capsid with icosahedral symmetry, bind to cellular attachment receptors via the distal knob domain of the 12 fiber proteins that extend from the vertices of the capsid. The knob domain of the adenovirus type 3 fiber protein binds to the extracellular portion of B7-1 and B7-2. The identification of B7-1 and B7-2 as receptors for adenovirus type 3 explains the distinct tropism of adenovirus serotype 3 and adenoviral vectors derived from adenovirus serotype 3. Most of the 51 adenovirus serotypes, including the adenovirus serotype 2 and 5 (the most common adenovirus serotypes used for gene therapy approaches), use the coxsackie and adenovirus receptor (CAR) as their major cellular attachment receptor. CAR has weak homology to B7, and it is a cell adhesion molecule and tumor suppressor molecule that is downregulated in tumors. The discovery of B7-1 and B7-2 as receptors for adenovirus type 3 suggests that adenovirus type 3 vectors may be useful in cancer gene therapy approaches to target tumors. Whether adenovirus infection influences the function of B7-1 and B7-2 remains to be determined.

Functions of the B7-1/B7-2:CD28/CTLA-4 Pathway Revisited

Recent studies have revealed additional means by which B7-1/B7-2: CD28/CTLA-4 interactions regulate T cell activation and tolerance, and they lead to a revised view of the pathway's functions. Basal or constitutive expression of B7 appears to be key for maintaining regulatory T cell homeostasis and preventing immune responses against self-antigens. The high expression of liCTLA-4 in resting T cells also may prevent T cell activation. Following exposure to inflammatory stimuli, B7-1/B7-2 expression on APC is upregulated, and B7:CD28 signals promote T cell activation in concert with signals through the TCR. LiCTLA is rapidly downregulated in T cells early during T cell activation. Later, following induction of flCTLA-4, B7:CTLA-4 interactions downregulate T cell responses. B7 on T cells, as well as on APC's, may serve to terminate T cell responses. It is not yet clear how signals through CD28 and CTLA-4 are coordinated. Fl CTLA-4 may inhibit CD28-mediated T cell activation by outcompeting CTLA-4 for B7-1/B7-2 binding at the cell surface, by directly antagonizing TCR or CD28 signals within the cell, by engaging B7 on T cells, and/or by signaling through B7-1/B7-2 into the APC to induce IDO.

THE ICOSL:ICOS PATHWAY

Structure and Expression of ICOS and ICOS Ligand

The CD28 homolog ICOS is upregulated on T cells after activation (12, 42). Like CD28 and CTLA-4, ICOS is a glycosylated disulfide-linked homodimer (43). Structurally, several distinct regions between ICOS and CD28 may enable key functional differences for these receptors (9, 11, 12, 44). The ICOS cytoplasmic tail contains a YMFM motif that binds the p85 subunit of PI3K, similar to the YMNM motif of CD28 (42). ICOS stimulates greater PI3K activity than CD28 costimulation (45, 46). However, in contrast to CD28, the ICOS YMFM motif does not allow for binding to Grb2, which is critical for IL-2 production (46, 47). ICOS also lacks a PXXP site that is critical for SH3-kinase binding, and it does not activate c-jun N-terminal kinase (45). ICOS signals lead to effector cytokine production and can be inhibited by CTLA-4 engagement (48).

ICOS is upregulated on CD4$^+$ T and CD8$^+$ T following activation and is present on effector and memory T cells (12, 42). ICOS expression is stimulated on T cells by both TCR and CD28 signals (42, 44, 49, 50). Importantly, ICOS expression is not solely dependent on CD28 signals, because blockade of ICOS in CD28$^{-/-}$ mice further inhibited Th1/Th2 differentiation (51). Both Th1 and Th2 cells express ICOS during T cell differentiation; however, ICOS levels persist at higher levels on Th2 cells than they do on Th1 cells (42, 50). In humans, IL-12 and IL-23, cytokines that stimulate Th1 responses, also enhance ICOS expression on activated Th cells (52). ICOS is also upregulated on activated NK cells, and it promotes NK cell function (53).

ICOSL mRNA is expressed constitutively in lymphoid and nonlymphoid tissues including kidney, liver, peritoneum, lung, and testes (10–14, 54, 55). Fibroblasts express ICOSL mRNA after culture with TNF-α and IFN-γ (10). ICOSL has been detected on the surface of B cells, macrophages, dendritic cells, a subset of CD3$^+$ T cells, and other cell types including endothelial cells and some epithelial cells (10–12, 56–58). In contrast to B7-1 and B7-2, the expression of ICOSL is not dependent on NF-κB and is not enhanced by cross-linking of CD40 or Ig (56). Signaling through the B cell receptor and IL-4 receptor downregulate expression of ICOSL on B cells (59). Further studies are required to understand the function of ICOSL expression in nonlymphoid tissues.

Functional Studies of ICOS

REGULATION OF T HELPER CELL DIFFERENTIATION BY ICOS   ICOS   and   CD28 have unique and overlapping functions that synergize to regulate CD4$^+$ T cell differentiation. Like CD28, ICOS augments T cell differentiation and cytokine production and provides critical signals for immunoglobulin production (1, 60). CD28, but not ICOS, regulates the early production of IL-2 by naive T cells. ICOS is expressed on a proportion of T cells obtained from unmanipulated mice. It is not clear whether these cells are memory, regulatory, or naive T cells. ICOS engagement was shown initially to selectively produce high levels of IL-10 and IL-4, but in vivo studies in several different model systems have demonstrated that ICOS can stimulate production of both Th1 and Th2 cytokines during initial priming and during effector T cell responses (9, 50). ICOS-expressing cells were analyzed from secondary lymphoid tissues of untreated mice by flow cytometry and categorized into low, medium, or high expressors of ICOS (61). Intriguingly, ICOS^{high} T cells were linked to IL-10 production, ICOS^{medium} T cells secreted IL-4, IL-5, and IL-13, and ICOS^{low} T cells were associated with IL-2, IL-3, IL-6, and IFN-γ production. These findings describe the phenotype of resting T cells and do not consider the possibility that activated or memory T cells expressing ICOS under Th1- and Th2-priming conditions may have a different cytokine profile. In fact, high expression of ICOS has been correlated with production of IFN-γ during *Toxoplasma gondii* infection and inflammatory bowel disease (62, 63) and with the Th2 cytokines IL-4, IL-5, IL-13, and IL-10 in *Schistosoma mansoni* infection and asthma (64, 65). ICOS has been shown to regulate Th2 differentiation at the transcriptional level (43, 66). ICOS$^{-/-}$ T cells have reduced c-maf expression and IL-4 production (66, 67). ICOS can regulate cytokine production in activated Th1 and Th2 cells and Treg cells in vivo, as discussed below.

REGULATION OF HUMORAL IMMUNE RESPONSES   Costimulatory signals through ICOS provide critical T cell help to B cells (9, 20, 42, 68, 69). Studies using pathway antagonists, transgenic mice, and knockout mice have revealed the important role of ICOS in B cell differentiation, immunoglobulin class switching, germinal center formation, and memory B cell development. Histologically, ICOS is expressed on T cells in the germinal centers and T cell zones of spleen, lymph nodes, and Peyer's patches (44, 49). ICOSL can be detected in the B cell areas of lymphoid tissue and in the follicles in the spleen and Peyer's patches (55). Transgenic mice expressing ICOSL-Ig fusion protein exhibit lymphoid hyperplasia in the B and T cell areas of the spleen, lymphoid nodes, and Peyer's patches, and they have increased levels of circulating IgG (12). The high expression of ICOS on germinal center T cells provides critical signals to B cells that lead to the formation of germinal centers and antibody maturation. Studies in ICOS$^{-/-}$ and ICOSL$^{-/-}$ mice have shown that ICOS is required for T cell–dependent B cell responses (20, 68–70). Mice lacking ICOS exhibit reduced germinal centers in response to primary immunization, profound defects in germinal center formation upon secondary challenge, and defects in IgG class switching. Researchers revealed a critical role for ICOS in human T:B collaboration when they identified an adult onset common variable immunodeficiency disease with the homozygous loss of ICOS on T cells in four patients (71). Although normal ex vivo T cell responses were observed, naive and memory B cell development were markedly impaired, suggesting the importance of ICOS in providing T cell help to B cells in humans. The analysis of humoral responses in CD28/ICOS$^{-/-}$ mice to environmental antigens, T-dependent protein antigens, and vesicular stomatitis virus demonstrated profound defects in immunoglobulin responses, much greater than those observed in CD28$^{-/-}$ mice, suggesting synergistic and distinct roles for CD28 and ICOS (72).

Therapeutic Manipulation of the ICOSL:ICOS Pathway in Disease Models

AUTOIMMUNITY   ICOS regulates autoimmune diseases in several model systems. ICOS regulates the outcome of disease in the murine model of multiple sclerosis, experimental allergic encephalomyelitis (EAE) but appears to have distinct roles at different times during the pathogenesis of EAE (20, 73, 74). Blockade of ICOS during induction of EAE exacerbated disease, whereas ICOS blockade during the effector phase of EAE ameliorated disease (74, 75). When $ICOS^{-/-}$ mice were primed with myelin oligodendrocyte glycoprotein (MOG), increases in IFN-γ and defects in IL-13 production were observed and correlated with more severe disease (20). ICOS also provides signals to T cells that are required for their encephalitogenicity. Activation of myelin basic protein-reactive TCR transgenic T cells in vitro in the presence of ICOS-Ig prevented these T cells from transferring EAE to recipients (73). ICOS blockade was associated with decreased T cell IFN-γ and IL-10 production. Intriguingly, the TCR transgenic cells were able to enter the brain; however, these cells showed increased apoptosis. These studies highlight the importance of understanding how ICOS regulates T cell responses during different phases of an immune response.

Disruption of the ICOSL:ICOS pathway improved the clinical course of collagen-induced arthritis. In a murine model of collagen-induced arthritis, administration of anti-ICOSL mAb during the initiation and effector phase ameliorated disease, as demonstrated by reduced joint swelling and lower clinical arthritis scores (76). When draining lymph node cells from mice given anti-ICOSL mAb were restimulated in vitro with collagen antigen, IFN-γ and IL-10 levels were decreased. Reduced levels of collagen-specific IgG1, IgG2a, and IgG2b also were seen. Similar findings were reported in $ICOS^{-/-}$ mice, where resistance to disease was associated with decreases in the proinflammatory cytokine IL-17 (77). The expression of ICOS has been detected on peripheral blood mononuclear cells and synovial fluid mononuclear cells of patients with rheumatoid arthritis (78). Analysis of stimulated synovial fluid $CD4^+$ T cells for cytokines showed elevated levels of IFN-γ, IL-10, and IL-4. Thus, the ICOSL:ICOS pathway appears to regulate both Th1 and Th2 responses and critically regulates the pathogenesis of collagen-induced arthritis.

Recent evidence shows that more ICOS is expressed on activated autoimmune-prone NOD T cells than on C57Bl/6 T cells (79). ICOS also may control Treg function in autoimmune disease, particularly IL-10-producing Treg cells. In a murine model of type 1 diabetes, Treg played a critical role in regulating the progression of diabetes from a prediabetic lesion (80). In the pancreatic lymph nodes, ICOS and IL-10 transcripts were highly expressed on Treg cells. Significantly, blockade of ICOS alters the balance between T effector and Treg, resulting in progression from a prediabetic insulitis to diabetes. These findings suggest that Treg cells regulate autoimmune development in an ICOS-dependent manner directly in the prediabetic lesion.

ASTHMA AND ALLERGY   Investigators have observed unique roles for CD28 and ICOS in asthma and allergy models in which CD28 may be critical for antigen priming and Th differentiation, whereas ICOS regulates Th2 effector function. ICOS has a key role in regulating Th2 responses that mediate asthma and allergy

(81). In mice lacking ICOS, marked defects in humoral responses (antigen-specific IgG1 and IgE) and Th2 cytokines (IL-4, IL-13) were observed in a murine asthma model (82). ICOS appears to regulate ongoing Th2 responses. ICOS blockade reduced lung inflammation and airway hyper-reactivity following adoptive transfer of highly polarized Th2 cells into naive mice (42). By delaying ICOS blockade until 21 days after airway priming, researchers significantly reduced lung inflammation after airway challenge (83). Thus, blockade of ICOS inhibited Th2 effector function but not Th2 differentiation. In contrast, similar blockade of the B7:CD28/CTLA-4 pathway after priming had no impact on Th2 effector responses. In a model of allergic airway disease in which mice are sensitized with *S. mansoni* eggs and later challenged with parasite antigen in the airways, blockade of ICOS signaling with ICOS-Ig reduced airway inflammation (84). The decreased airway inflammation was accompanied by a reduction in inflammatory cells infiltrating the lungs and decreased IL-5 production. Blockade of ICOS had no effect on Th2 differentiation in this system; however, blockade of ICOS inhibited Th2 cytokine production during restimulation of bronchial lymph node cultures containing Th2 effector cells. Thus, CD28 appears to have a predominant role in priming T cells during the Th2 immune response, whereas ICOS regulates effector T cell responses.

ICOS may also be important in the generation of Treg. Tregs can suppress the development of asthma-associated airway hyperreactivity. Culture of mature bronchial lymph node dendritic cells from animals primed with a respiratory allergen stimulated the generation of Treg cells (64). The development of these IL-10-producing Treg cells was dependent on ICOSL:ICOS interactions. Airway hyperreactivity could be inhibited by adoptive transfer of these Treg cells into sensitized mice. These findings suggest a novel mechanism by which ICOS and IL-10 reduce airway inflammation associated with asthma and implicate ICOS in regulating respiratory tolerance.

INFECTIOUS DISEASE   Recent studies have demonstrated an important role for ICOS in regulating the development of both Th1 and Th2 responses during infection. The protective Th1 response to the intracellular bacterium *Listeria monocytogenes* is impaired following blockade of ICOS (85). The development of *Listeria*-specific CD4$^+$ and CD8$^+$ T cells is inhibited by ICOS-Ig treatment, resulting in decreased IFN-γ production, increased bacterial titers, and progression of disease. ICOS signaling also dramatically regulates the immune response to cutaneous leishmaniasis and *Nippostrongylus brasiliensis*, which both elicit dominant Th2 responses (51, 86, 87). ICOS$^{-/-}$ mice exhibit resistance to *L. mexicana* with decreases in both Th1 and Th2 cytokines resulting in less severe disease compared with wild-type mice (86). During infection with *L. major*, inhibition of ICOS signals by administration of anti-ICOSL mAb or infection of ICOS$^{-/-}$ mice markedly decreased footpad swelling in normally susceptible BALB/c mice, inhibited IL-4, IL-5, and IL-10 secretion from local lymph nodes, and reduced serum IgE and IgG1 levels (87). Treatment of *N. brasiliensis*-infected ICOS$^{-/-}$ mice or wild-type mice with anti-ICOSL mAb inhibited serum IgE production and eosinophilia, and adult worm counts were reduced compared with wild-type controls (87). Thus, ICOS is a critical regulator of the Th1/Th2 balance in vivo.

The relative role of ICOS in regulating IFN-γ versus IL-10 production is not clear, but it may influence the outcome of infection. In wild-type C57Bl/6 mice infected with *S. mansoni*, the immune response to schistosome egg antigens is predominantly a Th1 response during the first seven weeks of infection and a Th2 response during the chronic phase of the disease after seven weeks in which small granulomas form (88). When anti-ICOS mAb were administered four weeks after *S. mansoni* infection, mice developed exacerbated hepatic immunopathology, which was associated with markedly enhanced IFN-γ production by schistosoma egg granuloma cells and CD4$^+$ T cells from the mesenteric lymph nodes, and decreased IL-10 production by the granuloma cells. Further studies are required to understand the underlying mechanism by which ICOS can positively and negatively regulate cytokine responses.

The CD28 and ICOS pathways have unique, synergistic roles in promoting antimicrobial immunity. Elimination of CD28 can impair, but not block, immune responses to lymphocytic choriomeningitis (LCMV), vesicular stomatitis virus (VSV), *T. gondii*, *Heligsomoides polygyrus*, and *N. brasiliensis* (51, 62, 89). ICOS blockade or elimination reduced immunoglobulin production and Th cytokines during primary responses to VSV, LCMV, and influenza (90). Similarly, blockade of ICOS can inhibit CD4 T cell responses to HIV-1 in human peripheral blood mononuclear cells (91). In contrast to the effects of ICOS on CD4 T cell differentiation, ICOS blockade had no impact on viral CTL responses during the immune responses to VSV, LCMV, and influenza; however, humoral responses were more greatly inhibited in CD28/ICOS$^{-/-}$ mice than in CD28$^{-/-}$ mice following VSV infection (51, 72, 90). In CD28$^{-/-}$ mice infected with *T. gondii*, blockade of ICOS resulted in decreased IFN-γ production, increased parasite burdens, and mortality (62). When ICOS-Ig is administered to CD28$^{-/-}$ mice at the time of inoculation with *N. brasiliensis*, both Th1 (IFN-γ) and Th2 (IL-4, IL-5) cytokines were reduced further than in CD28$^{-/-}$ mice, suggesting that the ICOS pathway regulates both Th1 and Th2 cytokine production in vivo (51). Further understanding the interplay between the CD28 and ICOS pathways during infection will be critical for designing therapeutic approaches to ameliorate chronic infections.

TRANSPLANTATION   ICOS has an important role in mediating transplant rejection and is a new potential therapeutic target. Much attention has focused on blocking the B7:CD28 and/or CD40:CD40L pathways to prevent transplant rejection (92). Although these studies have shown promising results in preventing initial graft rejection, in most cases the graft is eventually destroyed by chronic rejection. Thus, researchers are actively investigating other costimulatory pathways for their potential role in regulating ongoing immune responses that contribute to both acute and chronic transplant rejection.

Transplants are often rejected when graft tissue is destroyed by Th1-dependent inflammatory responses. Treatment of recipients of mismatched cardiac allografts with anti-ICOS mAb or an ICOS-Ig fusion protein, or transfer of grafts into ICOS$^{-/-}$ recipient mice, prolonged graft survival, although to a lesser degree than CTLA-4Ig or anti-CD40L mAb therapy (93). Chronic rejection developed with each of these treatments. However, treatment of cardiac allograft recipients with ICOS-Ig plus CTLA-4Ig resulted in long-term survival of the allograft and donor-specific tolerance (94). Likewise, administration of anti-ICOS and anti-CD40L mAb inhibited the development of chronic rejection that developed with either antibody alone. Administration of anti-ICOS mAb with the immunosuppressive agent cyclosporine A also resulted in permanent cardiac graft survival (93), but did not improve islet allograft survival (95). These findings suggest that coblockade of ICOS:ICOSL and the CD40:CD40L or CD28: B7 pathways can have synergistic effects in preventing transplant rejection.

The timing of ICOS blockade significantly influences therapeutic effects. In a cardiac allograft model, delayed ICOS blockade prolonged allograft survival into mismatched recipients compared with early ICOS blockade in which rejection was accelerated (96). Delayed ICOS blockade resulted in a reduction in the number of allospecific IL-10 secreting cells and an increase in both IFN-γ and IL-4 secreting cells. Delayed blockade of ICOS prevented both alloreactive CD4$^+$ and CD8$^+$ T cell expansion, whereas early blockade inhibited only CD4$^+$ T cell expansion. Therefore, the timing for manipulation of the ICOS pathway may be an important consideration for therapy.

Summary of Functions of the ICOSL:ICOS Pathway

Taken together, these studies indicate that the ICOS:ICOSL pathway provides key positive second signals that promote T cell activation, differentiation and effector responses, and T cell-dependent B cell responses. Both CD28 and ICOS signaling upregulate Th1 as well as Th2 cytokines; however, ICOS does not upregulate IL-2 production. Thus, ICOS stimulates T cell effector function but not T cell expansion. CD28 and ICOS contribute unique, synergistic signals that promote humoral immunity. The role of ICOS in stimulating IL-10 production may contribute to its role in regulating Treg, T cell tolerance, and autoimmunity. The function of ICOS during in vivo immune responses appears to depend on timing/stage of immune response as well as microenvironment, because ICOSL can be expressed on endothelial and epithelial cells as well as professional antigen-presenting cells.

THE PD-1L: PD-1 PATHWAY

Structure and Expression of PD-1 and Its Ligands PD-L1 and PD-L2

PD-1 (Programmed death-1) (15, 97, 98) is an Ig superfamily member related to CD28 and CTLA-4, but it lacks the membrane proximal cysteine that allows these molecules to homodimerize. PD-1 is monomeric (16, 18, 99). The PD-1 cytoplasmic domain has two tyrosines, one that constitutes an immunoreceptor tyrosine-based inhibition motif (ITIM), and the other an immunoreceptor tyrosine-based switch motif (ITSM) (100). PD-1 is expressed during thymic development primarily on CD4$^-$CD8$^-$ (double negative) cells and double negative $\gamma\delta$ thymocytes (101) and induced on peripheral CD4$^+$ and CD8$^+$ T cells, B cells, and monocytes upon activation (102). NK-T cells express low levels of PD-1 (101). The broader expression of PD-1 contrasts with restricted expression of other CD28 family members to T cells. Preliminary studies with dimeric Ig fusion proteins suggest that PD-L2 has a two- to six-fold higher affinity for PD-1 than does PD-L1 (99). Although both tyrosines are phosphorylated following engagement, mutagenesis studies indicate that the tyrosine within the ITSM motif is required for the inhibitory activity of PD-1, as opposed to the tyrosine in the ITIM that is more typically associated with inhibitory signaling (103).

The PD-1 ligands exhibit distinct patterns of expression; PD-L1 is expressed more broadly than is PD-L2 (16–19). PD-L1 is expressed on resting and upregulated on activated B, T, myeloid, and dendritic cells (104). PD-L1 is expressed on CD4$^+$ CD25$^+$ T cells, but whether it has a role in function of this regulatory population in not yet clear. In contrast to B7-1 and B7-2, PD-L1 is expressed in nonhematopoietic cells including microvascular endothelial cells and in nonlymphoid organs including heart, lung, pancreas, muscle, and placenta (58, 104–107). The expression of PD-L1 within nonlymphoid tissues suggests that PD-L1 may regulate self-reactive T or B cells in peripheral tissues and/or may regulate inflammatory responses in the target organs. However, the roles of PD-L1 on T cells, APCs, and host tissues are not yet clear. There are many potential bidirectional interactions between PD-L1 and PD-1 owing to the broad expression of PD-L1 and the expression of PD-1 on T cells, B cells, and macrophages. In contrast, PD-L2 is induced by cytokines only on macrophages and DCs. The relatively greater role of IFN-γ in stimulating PD-L1 expression and IL-4 in stimulating PD-L2 expression suggests that PD-L1 and PD-L2 may have distinct functions in regulating Th1 and Th2 responses (104, 108).

Functional Studies of PD-1:PD-L Pathway

Investigators initially identified the PD-1 receptor by subtractive hybridization studies using a T cell hybridoma undergoing programmed cell death, hence its name (102). Subsequent studies have not shown a direct role for PD-1 in cell death; however, an indirect role via downregulation of growth factor production is possible. Like CTLA-4, very low levels of PD-1 are sufficient for potent inhibition of the earliest stages of T cell activation (109). Co-localization of PD-1 with TCR/CD28 is necessary for PD-1-mediated inhibition. In contrast to CTLA-4, PD-1 inhibits expression of the cell survival gene bcl-x$_L$ (110). Both CTLA-4 and PD-1 limit glucose metabolism and Akt activation, but by different mechanisms. CTLA-4 inhibited Akt activation via protein phosphatase 2a, whereas PD-1 blocked CD28-mediated activation of PI3K. In primary human T cells, crosslinking of PD-1 leads to phosphorylation of both cytoplasmic tyrosines; however, only mutation of the

ITSM leads to loss of inhibitory activity. In T cells, the phosphorylated ITSM recruits both SHP-2 and SHP-1, whereas in B cells, only SHP-2 was recruited (109).

Studies are just beginning to elucidate PD-L1 and PD-L2 function. Initial in vitro functional studies suggested that PD-L1 and PD-L2 have overlapping functions during T cell responses. Some in vitro studies have demonstrated that PD-L1 and PD-L2 can inhibit T cell proliferation and cytokine production; others showed that the PD-1 ligands enhance T cell activation. Anti-CD3 mAb plus either PD-L1 or PD-L2-Ig proteins linked to beads inhibited T cell proliferation and cytokine production by both resting and previously activated $CD4^+$ and $CD8^+$ T cells and even by naive T cells from cord blood (110). Inhibition was not seen when $PD-1^{-/-}$ T cells were incubated with anti-CD3 plus PD-L1-Ig, indicating that the inhibitory signal was transduced by PD-1. Studies using Chinese hamster ovary (CHO) cells transfected with MHC class II, and PD-L1 or PD-L2 in the presence or absence of B7-2 also support an inhibitory role for PD-L1 and PD-L2 (16, 18). When previously activated TCR transgenic $CD4^+$ T cells were cultured with peptide and CHO cells expressing PD-L1 or PD-L2, T proliferation and cytokine production were markedly reduced. T cell proliferation and cytokine production also were strongly reduced when the TCR transgenic T cells were cultured with CHO transfectants expressing B7-2 and PD-L1 or PD-L2 at low antigen concentrations. At high antigen concentrations, these transfectants reduced cytokine production but did not inhibit T cell proliferation. The PD-1 ligands exert these effects by causing cell cycle arrest in G_0/G_1 but not cell death. Engagement of PD-1 also can inhibit B cell cycle progression. These studies demonstrate overlapping functions of PD-L1 and PD-L2 and support a role for the PD-L:PD-1 pathway in downregulating T cell responses.

Other studies, however, indicate that PD-L1 and PD-L2 also can stimulate T cell proliferation. When resting T cells were stimulated with low levels of anti-CD3 and immobilized B7-H1-Ig (PD-L1-Ig), T cell proliferation was modestly enhanced, IL-10 production was markedly increased, and IFN-γ and granulocyte monocyte colony stimulating factor (GM-CSF) were modestly elevated, but there was little effect on IL-2 or IL-4 production (17, 111). $CD28^{-/-}$ T cells were stimulated similarly to wild-type cells. When resting $CD4^+$ T cells were incubated with immobilized anti-CD3 plus B7-DC-Ig (PD-L2-Ig), proliferation and IFN-γ production were strongly increased, but there was little effect on IL-2, IL-4, or IL-10 production. Little effect was observed on $CD8^+$ T cell responses (19).

The reasons for the contradictory results of functional studies with PD-1 ligands are not clear. Differential functions for PD-L1 and PD-L2 may not only relate to differences in expression but also may reflect distinct interactions of PD-L1 and/or PD-L2 with a second, as yet to be defined, receptor. A putative second receptor for PD-1 ligands might deliver a stimulatory signal similar to that of CD28. Recent data suggest the existence of another receptor that binds PD-L1 and PD-L2; mutants of PD-L1 and PD-L2, which lose their ability to bind PD-1, retain costimulatory activity for T cells (112). Alternatively, the ITSM motif in the cytoplasmic domain of PD-1 may provide a means for PD-1 to interact with different phosphatases, perhaps depending upon the activation history of the T cell. These differential interactions through PD-1 could deliver either positive or negative signals. Finally, PD-L1 and/or PD-L2 may signal bidirectionally.

Therapeutic Manipulation of the PD-L:PD-1 Pathway in Disease Models

AUTOIMMUNITY   The phenotype of PD-1$^{-/-}$ mice first suggested a role for PD-1 in regulating T cell tolerance and autoimmunity (113, 114). A proportion of PD-1$^{-/-}$ mice on the C57Bl/6 background develop a late-onset, progressive arthritis and lupus-like glomerulonephritis. Introduction of the lpr (fas gene) mutation into PD-1$^{-/-}$ mice accelerates disease. In contrast, PD-1$^{-/-}$ BALB/c mice develop a dilated cardiomyopathy in which autoantibodies to troponin-1 arise (115). The expression of PD-L1 and PD-L2 at high levels in the heart suggests a role for PD-1 ligands in preventing potentially self-reactive lymphocytes from causing tissue injury. PD-1$^{-/-}$ mice further show that PD-1 negatively regulates CD8^{+} T cells in vivo.

The roles of PD-1 and its ligands in regulating autoimmune disease have been investigated in animal models of diabetes, colitis, and multiple sclerosis. Administration of anti-PD-1 or anti-PD-L1 mAb to one- to ten-week-old prediabetic NOD female mice and to male NOD mice (usually resistant to diabetes) led to the rapid onset of diabetes, and it was associated with increased IFN-γ producing GAD-reactive splenocytes but not anti-insulin antibodies (116). The broad temporal range of the effects of anti-PD-1 and anti-PD-L1 contrasts with the diabetes-provoking effects of anti-CTLA-4 mAb only in neonatal female NOD mice (117). These distinct effects suggest that CTLA-4 regulates the initial phase of disease, whereas PD-1: PD-L1 interactions regulate both the initiation and progression of autoimmune diabetes in NOD mice. Anti-PD-L2, in contrast to anti-PD-L1, did not alter diabetes in NOD mice. The diabetes-promoting effects of PD-L1, but not PD-L2, correlate with the expression of PD-L1 on inflammatory cells infiltrating islets and on islet cells in diabetic NOD mice (104, 116). The expression of PD-L1 on islet cells suggests that PD-L1 may critically control the responses of self-reactive T cells in the target organ.

The role of PD-L1 on the islet appears to be complex; recent studies have shown that 7–14% of C57BL/6 transgenic mice that constitutively express PD-L1 in pancreatic islet β cells (RIP.B7-H1 mice) spontaneously develop T cell-mediated autoimmune diabetes at three to six weeks of age (118). In the RIP.mOva T cell adoptive transfer model of diabetes, PD-L1 expression on islets enhanced CD8^{+} T cell expansion and induction of autoimmune diabetes. PD-L1 expressing islets did not appear to be more susceptible to apoptosis or cytotoxicity and did not produce IL-10 upon in vitro culture. Anti-PD-1 mAb did not block the accelerated T cell responses, suggesting that islet-specific expression of PD-L1 can promote T cell responses in a PD-1 independent fashion. Further studies are needed to dissect how PD-L1 expression on islet cells, as well as T cells, APC, and endothelial cells, regulates responses of self-reactive T cells. Timing and location of PD-L1 expression may be important. These seemingly contradictory data also might reflect the consequences of bidirectional signaling of PD-L1. Alternatively, PD-L1 may interact with a second, as yet to be identified, positive receptor when it is basally or constitutively expressed. However, following induction of a T cell response and PD-1 upregulation, PD-L1:PD-1 interactions predominate and downregulate T cells.

PD-L1 and its ligands have a negative regulatory role in EAE (119, 120). PD-1, PD-L1, and PD-L2 are expressed on infiltrating inflammatory cells in the brains of mice with EAE (104, 119). PD-L1 is also expressed on vascular endothelial cells, astrocytes, and microglia. Anti-PD-1 administration during the induction of EAE accelerated the onset and increased the severity of EAE, and it led to increased frequency of IFN-γ producing MOG-reactive T cells and higher serum levels of anti-MOG antibodies. Anti-PD-L2, but not anti-PD-L1, accelerated and exacerbated MOG-induced EAE in C57BL/6 wild-type mice. However, recent studies suggest that anti-PD-L1 and anti-PD-L2 mAb may have different functions, depending on the strain of mice studied. Both anti-PD-L1 and anti-PD-L2 worsened PLP-induced EAE in NOD mice (2).

A role for PD-L1 in controlling the responses of self-reactive T cells is further indicated by the severe clinical EAE that develops following immunization of PD-L1$^{-/-}$ mice with MOG$_{35-55}$ or following the adoptive transfer of MOG$_{35-55}$-specific T cells into PD-L1$^{-/-}$ recipients (120). PD-L1 deficiency converted the 129Sv strain from a resistant strain to an EAE susceptible strain. Transfer of wild-type or PD-L1$^{-/-}$ encephalitogenic T cells into PD-L1$^{-/-}$ recipients demonstrated a critical role for PD-L1 in limiting pathogenic effector T cell responses and revealed that PD-L1 on both the T cell and in the recipient control encephalitogenic T cell responses. PD-L1$^{-/-}$ C57BL/6 mice also developed more severe MOG-induced EAE than wild-type controls. The increased MOG-specific CD4$^+$ T cell responses in PD-L1$^{-/-}$ mice may reflect multiple negative regulatory functions for PD-L1 by limiting expansion and/or Th1 differentiation of naive CD4$^+$ T cells, negatively regulating reactivation of MOG-specific effector CD4$^+$ T cells in the target organ, or limiting expansion of antigen-specific T cells through engagement of PD-1 on Tregs. Upregulation of PD-L1 during Th1-driven inflammation might serve as a negative feedback mechanism for limiting pathogenic T cell responses in the brain. The distinct effects seen in anti-PD-L1 mAb treated mice and PD-L1$^{-/-}$ mice may reflect differences in timing of PD-L1 blockade or elimination. In the studies using anti-PD-L1, the anti-PD-L1 mAb was administered beginning on the day of immunization and continued on alternate days for ten days. Because in PD-L1$^{-/-}$ mice, PD-L1 is absent throughout the induction and effector phases of the immune response, the antibody administration may not have been sufficient to block PD-L1:PD-1 interactions throughout the response.

PD-1 and PD-L1 also regulate the pathogenesis of colitis (121). In a mouse model of inflammatory bowel disease induced by adoptive transfer of CD4$^+$ CD45RB^{hi} T cells to SCID mice, administration of anti-PD-L1, but not anti-PD-L2, after the transfer of CD4$^+$CD45RB^{hi} T cells ameliorated colitis and reduced

CD4$^+$ recovery from the spleen and lamina propria. CD4$^+$ lamina propria T cells isolated from anti-PD-L1-treated mice seven weeks after T cell transfer produced less IFN-γ, IL-2, and TNF-α, but not IL-4 or IL-10 compared with controls when stimulated with anti-CD3 and anti-CD28 in vitro. Treatment with anti-PD-L2 reduced IL-4 and IL-10 production. These findings suggest that PD-L1, but not PD-L2, promotes mucosal inflammation. Further studies are needed to analyze whether PD-L1 on the T cell or other cells regulates the expansion, differentiation, and/or migration of the CD4$^+$CD45RB^{hi} T cells into the colon and whether PD-1: PD-L1 interactions mediate these effects. Experimentally induced autoimmune hepatitis also is accelerated in mice lacking PD-L1 (122).

Studies in humans with autoimmune disease also suggest a regulatory role for PD-1. Significantly increased expression of PD-1 on T cells and of PD-L1 on T, B, and macrophage/dendritic cells is seen in inflamed colon from inflammatory bowel disease patients (57). Researchers have observed increased expression of PD-1 on CD4$^+$ T cells in synovial fluid from patients with rheumatoid arthritis. These PD-1 expressing CD4$^+$ T cells also expressed CTLA-4 and produced IL-10 (123). An intronic single nucleotide polymorphism (SNP) in PD-1 has been associated with development of SLE in Europeans (124), and the same SNP has also been associated with increased risk of diabetes (125). In the associated SNP, the binding site for the runt-related transcription factor (RUNX-1, also called AML-1) is altered. Investigators have found autoantibodies against PD-L1 in sera of 29% of patients with rheumatoid arthritis compared with 4% in healthy controls, correlating with active disease (126). Immobilized autoantibodies to PD-L1 stimulated CD4$^+$ T cell proliferation, IL-10 production, and programmed cell death.

ASTHMA   Following allergen challenge, PD-L1 is markedly elevated on DC, macrophages, and B cells in the lungs; PD-L2 expression is significantly increased on lung and draining lymph node DC and macrophages; and PD-1 is upregulated on T cells in the lung and draining lymph node (127). Administration of anti-PD-L2 at the time of allergen challenge, but not at the time of sensitization, increased airway hyper-reactivity, the number of eosinophils, and IL-5 and IL-13 in the bronchoalveolar lavage fluid (127). This suggests that PD-L2 regulates the effector phase of the response. When restimulated with OVA in vitro, CD4$^+$ and CD8$^+$ draining lymph node cells from PD-L2-treated mice showed reduced expression of IFN-γ by intracellular staining. Neutralization of IFN-γ by anti-IFN-γ pretreatment did not affect airway hyperreactivity in controls, but it diminished the effects of anti-PD-L2 treatment, suggesting that PD-L2 regulates asthma by an IFN-γ–dependent mechanism. Neither anti-PD-L1 nor anti-PD-1 affected asthmatic responses (127). Further work is needed to determine whether anti-PD-L2 treatment blocked PD-L2 interactions with receptor or cross-linked PD-L2 on DC or macrophages.

INFECTIOUS DISEASE   PD-1: PD-L1 interactions may be important for controlling antiviral CD8$^+$ T cell responses. Following infection with adenovirus, PD-1$^{-/-}$

mice exhibited increased proliferation of effector T cells in the liver and enhanced clearance of the virus (128). The enhanced $CD8^+$ T cell expansion in $PD-L1^{-/-}$ mice implicate PD-L1 engagement of PD-1 in regulating antiviral immunity (120). Chronic viral infections are often associated with suppressed T cell responses. PD-1:PD-L1 interactions may contribute to the functional inactivation of virus-specific $CD8^+$ T cells during chronic viral infection. Blockade of the PD-L1:PD-1 pathway may provide a means to boost antiviral immunity. A role for PD-L1 in pathogen immune evasion strategies is suggested by recent work showing that *S. mansoni* worms induce T cell anergy by upregulating PD-L1 expression on macrophages (129). Blocking PD-L1, but not PD-L2, on schistosome worm-modulated macrophages prevents them from inducing $CD4^+$ and $CD8^+$ T cell anergy.

TRANSPLANTATION   The role of PD-1, PD-L1, and PD-L2 has been investigated in models of cardiac and islet transplantation. PD-1, PD-L1, and PD-L2 expression are induced within cardiac allografts undergoing rejection (130). Neither PD-L1Ig nor PD-L2Ig alone prolonged cardiac allograft survival. However, PD-L1Ig, but not PD-L2Ig, plus cyclosporine A significantly enhanced allograft survival over that of cyclosporine A or PD-L1Ig alone and led to decreased intragraft expression of IFN-γ as well as CCR5 and CXCR3 mRNA. Similarly, PD-L1Ig had synergistic effects when given with rapamycin and led to permanent survival of fully MHC-disparate cardiac allografts. PD-L1Ig also promoted long-term graft survival in $CD28^{-/-}$ recipients (130) and markedly reduced cardiac transplant arteriosclerosis when given in conjunction with anti-CD154 mAb (130). PD-L1Ig and anti-CD154 similarly synergized and induced long-term survival of islet allografts, whereas either alone failed to prolong islet allograft survival (131). These findings suggest that PD-1 targeting, when used together with agents in current clinical use or in clinical trails, may strikingly improve the survival of solid organ transplantation. The exact mechanism by which PD-L1Ig exerts protective effects in these models is not clear; PD-L1Ig could be triggering a negative signal through PD-1 or blocking a positive signal for T cell activation and function. The accelerated rejection of PD-L1–expressing pancreatic islet allografts suggests that PD-L1 expression in pancreatic islets may promote, rather than inhibit, T cell responses (118).

In a murine acute graft-versus-host disease (GVHD) model, GVHD lethality is accelerated when PD-1 engagement is prevented (132). GVHD was markedly accelerated by a blocking anti-PD-1 mAb or PD-L1Ig fusion protein. The magnitude of GVHD acceleration was similar when $PD-1^{-/-}$ $CD4^+$ or $CD8^+$ T cells were infused into sublethally irradiated recipients. Neither perforin nor fas ligand were required for GVHD acceleration, but donor IFN-γ production was necessary. Co-blockade of CTLA-4 and PD-1 synergized and further accelerated GVHD, indicating that the effects of PD-1 and CTLA-4 act independently to downregulate GVHD lethality. Together, these findings demonstrate that PD-1 ligation down-regulates GVHD by modulating IFN-γ production, and they suggest that PD-1 ligation may provide a novel approach for preventing GVHD lethality.

PD-1:PD-L1 interactions also may influence alloresponses by inducing regulatory cells (133). Anti-PD-1 and anti-PD-L1 abrogate the prolonged cardiac survival that is induced by intratracheal delivery of allogeneic splenocytes. Anti-PD-1 mAb and anti-PD-L1 mAb, but not anti-PD-L2 mAb, prevented induction of regulatory cells by intratracheal alloantigen delivery. The regulatory population induced by intratracheal antigen administration is not well-characterized in this model, and the regulatory cells may not only be $CD4^+CD25^+$ cells but also DC.

TUMOR IMMUNITY   PD-L1 and PD-L2 are expressed on a variety of tumors. PD-L1 is expressed on many murine tumor cell lines, and IFN-γ enhanced PD-L1 expression on murine tumor cell lines (134). PD-L1 is highly expressed on many human carcinomas (135, 136), including those of the breast, cervix, lung, ovary, and colon, as well as on melanomas (136) and glioblastomas (137). PD-L1 is not expressed on B cell hematologic malignancies but is strongly expressed in some primary T cell lymphomas (136). PD-L1 also is expressed on most thymic epithelial tumors, including benign and invasive thymomas as well as thymic carcinoma. PD-L2 has been identified as the gene that best discriminates primary mediastinal B cell lymphoma (PMBL) from other diffuse large B cell lymphomas, and it may be a useful molecular diagnostic marker (138). PD-L2 also is highly expressed in Hodgkin lymphoma cell lines (138). The genomic locus containing PD-L1, PD-L2, and several adjacent genes is amplified in PMBL and Hodgkin lymphoma.

The upregulation of PD-L1 on tumors has led to the hypothesis that PD-L1 on tumors may be a means by which tumors evade T cell recognition. Indeed, animal models have shown that PD-L1 expression on tumor cells inhibits T cell tumor immunity. Tumor cells that express PD-L1 grow in wild-type mice but are suppressed in PD-1$^{-/-}$ mice (139). Primed 2C RAG-2$^{-/-}$ PD-1$^{-/-}$ T cells exhibit increased cytokine production, proliferation, and cytolytic activity against tumors compared with wild-type 2C cells in vitro, and they promote tumor rejection in vivo under circumstances in which wild-type 2C cells did not reject (134). Anti-PD-L1 increased 2C T effector, but not priming responses. Expression of PD-L1 on tumor cells promotes tumor growth and increased apoptosis of tumor-reactive T cells (135). Tumor-associated DC express higher levels of PD-L1, and T cells cultured with myeloid dendritic cells in the presence of anti-PD-L1 had a greater ability to prevent autologous human ovarian carcinoma growth in NOD-SCID mice (140). Similarly, anti-PD-L1 administration enhanced survival of mice given PD-L1-expressing tumor cells (141). These findings suggest that PD-L1: PD-1-mediated inhibitory signals give tumors a selective advantage for growth by inhibiting CD8$^+$ T cell responses, and that PD-L1 blockade may be a valuable approach for cancer immunotherapy. Because a goal of many tumor immunotherapy protocols is to induce a Th1 phenotype and because IFN-γ stimulates PD-L1 expression on tumor cells as well as APC and endothelial cells, PD-L1 upregulation may diminish the success of tumor immunotherapy.

In contrast, PD-L2 expression on J558 plasmacytoma cells promotes CD8-mediated antitumor immunity. PD-L2 expression led to rapid tumor rejection and development of immunity to subsequent tumor challenge. PD-L2 enhanced tumor-reactive T cell priming and effector function. Intriguingly, the function of wild-type and PD-1$^{-/-}$ T cell were similarly enhanced by PD-L2 transfected tumor cells, suggesting that PD-L2 cells promote CTL killing by a receptor other than PD-1 (142). Treatment of mouse DC with a novel human IgM antibody that can bind and crosslink both mouse and human PD-L2 on DC stimulates DC functions, including antigen acquistion and IL-12 production in vitro, and promotes antitumor immunity in vivo (143). This novel antibody was efficacious when given at the time of B16 melanoma tumor cell administration or after tumors were established in the lungs. This tumor resistance is mediated by CD8^{+} T cells and depends on perforin and granzyme B. These studies suggest that PD-L2 may function, in part, by signaling into PD-L2 expressing cells.

Summary of Functions of the PD-L: PD-1 Pathway

The PD-1:PD-L1/PD-L2 pathway has critical roles in regulating T cell activation and tolerance. CTLA-4 and PD-1 have important nonredundant inhibitory functions. CTLA-4 appears to have a more central role in the lymphoid organs, whereas PD-1 has an important role in regulating inflammatory responses in peripheral tissues. The broad expression of PD-L1 in lymphoid and nonlymphoid organs and the more restricted, but overlapping, expression of PD-L2 in DC and macrophages may explain, in part, how these B7 family members can have overlapping and distinct biological functions. PD-1 and PD-L1 also negatively regulate CD8^{+} T cell responses. PD-L1 clearly has an important role in peripheral T cell tolerance and has been exploited by tumors and microbes to evade T cell–mediated antitumor and antimicrobial responses. The contribution of PD-L1 on lymphoid, endothelial, and other cells in controlling the T cell responses to foreign and self-antigens remains to be determined. Further studies also are needed to understand how PD-L1 and PD-L2 can mediate both positive and negative signals.

B7-H3 (B7RP-2)

Structure and Expression

Human and mouse B7-H3 (B7RP-2) have ~88% amino acid identity (20, 144). Differential splicing of human B7-H3 leads to a 4Ig domain (VCVC) transcript [also called B7-H3b (144) and 4Ig-B7-H3 (145)] and a 2Ig domain (containing V1 and C2) transcript (144, 146). In contrast, the mouse B7-H3 gene gives rise to only one single VC domain form of B7-H3. Both human and mouse B7-H3 mRNA are expressed broadly in lymphoid and non-lymphoid organs (20, 144, 146). The 4Ig transcript is the dominant form in human tissues (144–146). B7-H3 mRNA is not detectable in human peripheral blood mononuclear cells (20, 145). B7-H3 mRNA is induced on human T cells cocultured with DC (147) and constitutively expressed in freshly isolated and cultured nasal epithelial cells (148). Human B7-H3 protein is not expressed constitutively on monocytes, B cells, T cells or NK cells, but it can be induced on these cell types (20, 145). B7-H3 is induced on monocytes by GM-CSF, or LPS, and on T cells, B cells, and NK cells by phorbol myristate acetate (PMA) plus ionomycin (145). B7-H3 is expressed on immature and mature human myeloid DC. Murine B7-H3 mRNA expression is stimulated in mouse DC by IFN-γ, but suppressed by IL-4 (70). LPS stimulates B7-H3 protein expression on murine DC, B cells, and macrophages (70); cell surface expression was seen early after stimulation and maintained over time. Anti-IgM and anti-CD40 also promote B7-H3 expression on mouse B cells, whereas anti-CD40 can induce B7-H3 expression on mouse macrophages (70).

The receptor for B7-H3 has not yet been identified but is distinct from known CD28 family members. B7-H3Ig binds to activated but not resting CD4$^+$ and CD8$^+$ T cells (20, 144).

Functional Studies

Recent studies support roles for B7-H3 as a stimulator and inhibitor of T cell responses. Initial studies showed that in conjunction with anti-CD3, human B7-H3Ig fusion protein (B7-H3VC-Ig) costimulated human CD4$^+$ and CD8$^+$ T cell proliferation, although less than B7-1Ig, and stimulated IFN-γ production and CD8 lytic activity (20). In a model of EL-4 lymphoma, injection of B7-H3 expression plasmid into the tumor resulted in complete regression of 50% of tumors, a response that depended upon CD8 T cells and NK cells (149). However, several recent studies have indicated that B7-H3 has an inhibitory function. Activation of purified human CD4 T cells by anti-CD3 and anti-CD28 was inhibited by addition of CHO. HLA-DR2 transfectants expressing either human B7-H3VC or B7-H3VCVC (146). Reduced proliferation and IFN-γ, TNF-α, IL-10, and GM-CSF production were observed. These results indicate that the B7-H3 VC and B7-H3 VCVC forms have similar functions and can downregulate T cell responses. Immobilized mouse B7-H3Ig inhibited mouse CD4$^+$ and CD8$^+$ cell proliferation and IL-2 and IFN-γ production mediated by anti-CD3 in vitro (70). Anti-CD28 could overcome the B7-H3-mediated inhibition, suggesting that B7-H3 may exert greater effects when CD28-mediated costimulation is limited.

Studies in B7-H3$^{-/-}$ mice also support an inhibitory function for B7-H3 (70). B7-H3$^{-/-}$ APC showed a two-fold increase in alloreactive T cell proliferation in a MLR response. Under Th1 but not Th2 polarizing conditions, B7-H3$^{-/-}$ mice developed more severe airway inflammation than wild-type control mice, and showed a three- to six-fold increase in T cell responses. B7-H3$^{-/-}$ mice developed EAE two days earlier than wild-type mice, but disease severity and incidence were comparable to wild-type. Aged ($\sim$17-month-old) B7-H3$^{-/-}$ mice developed serum antibodies to ssDNA, but there was no evidence of immune complex deposition in glomeruli or lymphocytic infiltrates in organs. CTL responses to LCMV and influenza virus were comparable in wild-type and B7-H3$^{-/-}$ mice. Taken together, studies in B7-H3$^{-/-}$ mice suggest that B7-H3 negatively regulates T cell responses that occur under Th1 polarizing conditions. Because IFN-γ promotes B7-H3 expression on DC, investigators have suggested that B7-H3 may provide a negative feedback mechanism during the amplification phase of Th1 responses. The absence of an effect of B7-H3 in Th2 conditions may be explained by IL-4 suppression of B7-H3 expression. The modest increase in susceptibility to autoimmune disease and lack of effect on CTL responses suggest that B7-H3 may have overlapping functions with other B7 family members expressed in APC and nonlymphoid organs, particularly PD-L1, PD-L2, or B7-H4.

Further studies are needed to reconcile the results of studies showing inhibitory and stimulatory functions for B7-H3. Such results could be explained by the existence of two receptors for B7-H3 with opposing functions, similar to CD28 and CTLA-4. Alternatively, these differential results may reflect the outcome of B7-H3–mediated inhibitory signals in different cell types.

B7-H4(B7x/B7S1)

Structure and Expression

The newest member of the B7 family, B7-H4(B7x/B7S1) (21–23), is a negative regulator of T cell responses. The structure of B7-H4 as a gpi-linked molecule distinguishes it from other B7 family members. The 87% amino acid identity between mouse and human B7-H4 suggests an important evolutionarily conserved function. Human and mouse B7-H4 mRNAs are expressed broadly in both lymphoid (spleen and thymus) and nonlymphoid organs (including lung, liver, testis, ovary, placenta, skeletal muscle, pancreas, and small intestine). Limited studies of B7-H4 protein expression indicate that B7-H4 is not expressed on freshly isolated human T cells, B cells, DC, and monocytes, but it can be induced on these cell types after in vitro stimulation. In mice, B7-H4 protein is expressed constitutively on B220$^+$ B cells, and it can be induced on peritoneal macrophages and some bone marrow–derived CD11c$^+$ DC. B7-H4 is not detected in normal human tissues by immunohistochemistry. It is not clear whether this difference in mRNA and protein expression reflects low levels of protein expression that are below the limit of detection by immunohistochemistry or regulation of B7-H4 expression at the translational level. Immunohistochemical staining shows that B7-H4 is highly expressed in lung and ovarian tumors, and real-time polymerase chain reaction (PCR) analyses indicate that mouse B7-H4 also is highly expressed in a number of tumor cell lines, including prostate, lung, and colon carcinomas.

B7-H4Ig binds to a receptor on activated but not naive T cells. The receptor is distinct from CTLA-4, ICOS and PD-1, and the receptor for B7-H3. Although initial studies indirectly implicated B7-H4 as the ligand for BTLA, based upon the binding of B7-H4Ig to wild-type, but not BTLA$^{-/-}$ cells, more recent studies indicate that BTLA is not likely to be the receptor for B7-H4 and that HVEM is the unique BTLA ligand (152). The receptor for B7-H4 remains to be identified.

Functional Studies

Functional studies using B7-H4 transfectants and immobilized B7-H4Ig demonstrate that B7-H4 delivers a signal that inhibits TCR-mediated CD4$^+$ and CD8$^+$ T proliferation, cell-cycle progression in the G0/G1phase, and IL-2 production (21–23). B7-1 costimulation cannot overcome B7-H4-Ig-induced inhibition. Administration of B7-H4Ig to mice reduced T cell proliferation and CTL activity and extended survival of mice in a GVHD model. Anti-B7-H4 blocking mAb increased T cell proliferation and IL-2 production in vitro. In vivo administration of the anti-B7-H4 blocking mAb at the time of immunization with keyhole limpet hemacyanin (KLH) in complete Freund's adjuvant (CFA) led to a modest increase in anti-KLH antibody IgM production and a two- to three-fold increase in T cell proliferation and IL-2 production upon in vitro restimulation with KLH, suggesting greater T cell priming in vivo in the presence of anti-B7-H4. Anti-B7-H4 blocking mAb markedly accelerated the onset and severity of EAE and increased CD4$^+$ and CD8$^+$ T cells and CD11b$^+$ macrophages in the brain of anti-B7-H4-treated mice. The broad and inducible expression of B7-H4, together with these functional studies, suggest that B7-H4 may serve to downregulate immune responses in peripheral tissues and play a role in regulating T cell tolerance. Expression of B7-H4 on tumors suggests that B7-H4 may play a role in evasion of tumor immunity (150).

BTLA

Structure and Expression

The CD28 family member BTLA (24) is similar functionally to PD-1 and CTLA-4. BTLA lacks the cysteine needed for dimerization and is monomeric. Identified initially as a molecule selectively expressed on Th1 cells, BTLA is expressed only on lymphocytes. Similar to CTLA-4, ICOS, and PD-1, BTLA is induced on T cells during activation. BTLA remains expressed on Th1 but not Th2 cells, suggesting that BTLA may specifically downregulate Th1-mediated inflammatory responses. This expression pattern contrasts with ICOS, which remains elevated on Th2 cells, but is downregulated on Th1 cells. BTLA also is expressed on B cells (151), similar to PD-1. However, BTLA is expressed on resting and activated B cells, whereas PD-1 is upregulated on activated B cells. BTLA has two ITIM motifs. Similar to PD-1, cross-linking BTLA with antigen receptors stimulates its tyrosine phosphorylation and leads to recruitment of SHP-1 and SHP-2, providing a mechanism for BTLA-mediated inhibition.

Functional Studies

BTLA exerts inhibitory effects on B and T lymphocytes (24). BTLA$^{-/-}$ B cells show modestly increased responses to anti-IgM, and BTLA$^{-/-}$ T cells show an increased response to anti-CD3 in vitro. Polarized BTLA$^{-/-}$ Th1 cells have about a two-fold increase in proliferation to antigen. Whether BTLA specifically regulates Th1 effector function is not yet clear. BTLA$^{-/-}$ mice show a three-fold increase in hapten-specific antibody responses and enhanced susceptibility to EAE (24). The relative roles of BTLA in negatively regulating T cell and B cell responses and peripheral B and T cell tolerance remain to be determined. The phenotype of the $BTLA^{-/-}$ mice resembles the phenotype of $PD-1^{-/-}$ mice; both strains exhibit increased susceptibility to autoimmunity, and both have more subtle phenotypes than $CTLA-4^{-/-}$ mice. It is not yet clear whether $BTLA^{-/-}$ mice spontaneously develop signs of autoimmune disease as they age or on particular genetic backgrounds, similar to $PD-1^{-/-}$ mice. Researchers have suggested that PD-1 and BTLA may have redundant inhibitory functions directed toward maintaining peripheral tolerance and attenuating inflammatory responses. Further work is needed to analyze the functions of BTLA in vivo and to determine whether it has distinct or overlapping roles with PD-1 and CTLA-4. Additional understanding of BTLA should provide insight into the therapeutic potential of BTLA manipulation; blockade of BTLA may be useful for enhancing antimicrobial and antitumor immunity.

CONCLUDING REMARKS

The balance between stimulatory and inhibitory signals is required for effective immune responses to pathogens and for maintaining self-tolerance. Signals through the B7:CD28 family are major regulators of this critical balance because the growing number of pathways in the B7:CD28 family provide second signals that can regulate the activation, inhibition, and fine tuning of T cell responses. It is not yet clear whether these pathways provide redundant positive and negative signals or whether there is some hierarchy in the orchestration of their signals. CD28 and ICOS synergize to promote the activation of T cell responses, with CD28 having a predominant role during initial T cell activation and ICOS regulating antigen-experienced T cells. B7:CD28 family members provide an abundance of inhibitory signals that can attenuate T cell responses and promote T cell tolerance. CTLA-4 is the predominant inhibitory pathway, but it has synergistic nonredundant inhibitory functions with PD-1. The more subtle inhibitory functions of BTLA, B7-H3, and B7-H4 suggest that these new CD28 and B7 family members may have functions that overlap with each another and/or with PD-1 ligands, PD-1, and CTLA-4. The expression of the newer B7 family members within nonlymphoid as well as lymphoid organs suggests that newer B7 family members may regulate immune responses uniquely in periphery tissues. Further study of the functions of B7:C28 family members individually and their interplay should provide insights into mechanisms of T cell activation and tolerance; this study has great therapeutic potential for controlling T cell responses.

ACKNOWLEDGMENTS

This work was supported by grants from NIH (to R.J.G., G.J.F., and A.H.S.) and National MS Society (to A.H.S.). We thank M. Keir for thoughtful discussions and helpful suggestions for this review. Because of space restrictions, we were able to cite only a fraction of the relevant literature and apologize to any colleagues whose contributions may not be appropriately acknowledged in this review.

The *Annual Review of Immunology* is online at
http://immunol.annualreviews.org

LITERATURE CITED

1. Sharpe AH, Freeman GJ. 2002. The B7-CD28 superfamily. *Nat. Rev. Immunol.* 2:116–26

2. Khoury SJ, Sayegh MH. 2004. The roles of the new negative T cell costimulatory pathways in regulating autoimmunity. *Immunity* 20:529–38

3. Chen LP. 2004. Co-inhibitory molecules of the B7-CD28 family in the control of T-cell immunity. *Nat. Rev. Immunol.* 4:336–47

4. Abbas AK. 2003. The control of T cell activation vs. tolerance. *Autoimmun. Rev.* 2:115–18

5. Carreno BM, Collins M. 2002. The B7 family of ligands and its receptors: new pathways for costimulation and inhibition of immune responses. *Annu. Rev. Immunol.* 20:29–53

6. Chikuma S, Bluestone JA. 2003. CTLA-4 and tolerance: the biochemical point of view. *Immunol. Res.* 28:241–53

7. Coyle AJ, Gutierrez-Ramos JC. 2003. More negative feedback? *Nat. Immunol.* 4:647–48

8. Greenwald RJ, Latchman YE, Sharpe AH. 2002. Negative co-receptors on lymphocytes. *Curr. Opin. Immunol.* 14:391–96

9. Hutloff A, Dittrich AM, Beier KC, Eljaschewitsch B, Kraft R, et al. 1999. ICOS is an inducible T-cell co-stimulator structurally and functionally related to CD28. *Nature* 397:263–66

10. Swallow MM, Wallin JJ, Sha WC. 1999. B7h, a novel costimulatory homolog of B7.1 and B7.2, is induced by TNF α. *Immunity* 11:423–32

11. Ling V, Wu PW, Finnerty HF, Bean KM, Spaulding V, et al. 2000. Cutting edge: identification of GL50, a novel B7-like protein that functionally binds to ICOS receptor. *J. Immunol.* 164:1653–57

12. Yoshinaga SK, Whoriskey JS, Khare SD, Sarmiento U, Guo J, et al. 1999. T-cell costimulation through B7RP-1 and ICOS. *Nature* 402:827–32

13. Brodie D, Collins AV, Iaboni A, Fennelly JA, Sparks LM, et al. 2000. LICOS, a primordial costimulatory ligand? *Curr. Biol.* 10:333–36

14. Wang SD, Zhu GF, Chapoval AI, Dong H, Tamada K, et al. 2000. Costimulation of T cells by B7-H2, a B7-like molecule that binds ICOS. *Blood* 96:2808–13

15. Ishida Y, Agata Y, Shibahara K, Honjo T. 1992. Induced expression of PD-1, a novel member of the immunoglobulin gene superfamily, upon programmed cell death. *EMBO J.* 11:3887–95

16. Freeman GJ, Long AJ, Iwai Y, Bourque K, Chernova T, et al. 2000. Engagement of the PD-1 immunoinhibitory receptor by a novel B7 family member leads to negative regulation of lymphocyte activation. *J. Exp. Med.* 192:1027–34

17. Dong HD, Zhu GF, Tamada K, Chen LP. 1999. B7-H1, a third member of the B7 family, co-stimulates T-cell proliferation and interleukin-10 secretion. *Nat. Med.* 5:1365–69

18. Latchman Y, Wood CR, Chernova T, Chaudhary D, Borde M, et al. 2001. PD-L2 is a second ligand for PD-1 and inhibits T cell activation. *Nat. Immunol.* 2:261–68

19. Tseng SY, Otsuji M, Gorski K, Huang X, Slansky JE, et al. 2001. B7-DC, a new dendritic cell molecule with potent

costimulatory properties for T cells. *J. Exp. Med.* 193:839–46

20. Chapoval AI, Ni J, Lau JS, Wilcox RA, Flies DB, et al. 2001. B7-H3: a costimulatory molecule for T cell activation and IFN-γ production. *Nat. Immunol.* 2:269–74

21. Sica GL, Choi IH, Zhu GF, Tamada K, Wang SD, et al. 2003. B7-H4, a molecule of the B7 family, negatively regulates T cell immunity. *Immunity* 18:849–61

22. Zang XX, Loke P, Kim J, Murphy K, Waitz R, Allison JP. 2003. B7x: a widely expressed B7 family member that inhibits T cell activation. *Proc. Natl. Acad. Sci. USA* 100:10388–92

23. Prasad DVR, Richards S, Mai XM, Dong C. 2003. B7S1, a novel B7 family member that negatively regulates T cell activation. *Immunity* 18:863–73

24. Watanabe N, Gavrieli M, Sedy JR, Yang JF, Fallarino F, et al. 2003. BTLA is a lymphocyte inhibitory receptor with similarities to CTLA-4 and PD-1. *Nat. Immunol.* 4:670–79

25. Coyle AJ, Gutierrez-Ramos JC. 2001. The expanding B7 superfamily: increasing complexity in costimulatory signals regulating T cell function. *Nat. Immunol.* 2:203–9

26. van der Merwe PA, Davis SJ. 2003. Molecular interactions mediating T cell antigen recognition. *Annu. Rev. Immunol.* 21:659–84

27. Taylor PA, Lees CJ, Fournier S, Allison JP, Sharpe AH, Blazar BR. 2004. B7 expression on T cells down-regulates immune responses through CTLA-4 ligation via T-T interactions. *J. Immunol.* 172:34–39

28. Paust S, Lu LR, McCarty N, Cantor H. 2004. Engagement of B7 on effector T cells by regulatory T cells prevents autoimmune disease. *Proc. Natl. Acad. Sci. USA* 101:10398–403

29. Tang QZ, Henriksen KJ, Boden EK, Tooley AJ, Ye JQ, et al. 2003. Cutting edge: CD28 controls peripheral homeostasis of CD4$^+$CD25$^+$ regulatory T cells. *J. Immunol.* 171:3348–52

30. Grohmann U, Orabona C, Fallarino F, Vacca C, Calcinaro F, et al. 2002. CTLA-4-Ig regulates tryptophan catabolism in vivo. *Nat. Immunol.* 3:1097–101

31. Short JJ, Pereboev AV, Kawakami Y, Vasu C, Holterman MJ, Curiel DT. 2004. Adenovirus serotype 3 utilizes CD80 (B7.1) and CD86 (B7.2) as cellular attachment receptors. *Virology* 322:349–59

32. Reiser J, von Gersdorff G, Loos M, Oh J, Asanuma K, et al. 2004. Induction of B7-1 in podocytes is associated with nephrotic syndrome. *J. Clin. Invest.* 113:1390–97

33. Vijayakrishnan L, Slavik JM, Illes Z, Greenwald RJ, Rainbow D, et al. 2004. An autoimmune disease-associated CTLA-4 splice variant lacking the B7 binding domain signals negatively in T cells. *Immunity* 20:563–75

34. Salomon B, Lenschow DJ, Rhee L, Ashourian N, Singh B, et al. 2000. B7/CD28 costimulation is essential for the homeostasis of the CD4$^+$CD25$^+$ immunoregulatory T cells that control autoimmune diabetes. *Immunity* 12:431–40

35. Lohr J, Knoechel B, Jiang S, Sharpe AH, Abbas AK. 2003. The inhibitory function of B7 costimulators in T cell responses to foreign and self-antigens. *Nat. Immunol.* 4:664–69

36. Fallarino F, Grohmann U, Hwang KW, Orabona C, Vacca C, et al. 2003. Modulation of tryptophan catabolism by regulatory T cells. *Nat. Immunol.* 4:1206–12

37. Munn DH, Sharma MD, Mellor AL. 2004. Ligation of B7-1/B7-2 by human CD4$^+$ T cells triggers indoleamine 2,3-dioxygenase activity in dendritic cells. *J. Immunol.* 172:4100–10

38. Podojil JR, Kin NW, Sanders VM. 2004. CD86 and β2-adrenergic receptor signaling pathways, respectively, increase Oct-2 and OCA-B Expression and binding to the 3'-IgH enhancer in B cells. *J. Biol. Chem.* 279:23394–404

39. Podojil JR, Sanders VM. 2003. Selective

regulation of mature IgG1 transcription by CD86 and β 2-adrenergic receptor stimulation. *J. Immunol.* 170:5143–51

40. Ueda H, Howson JM, Esposito L, Heward J, Snook H, et al. 2003. Association of the T-cell regulatory gene CTLA4 with susceptibility to autoimmune disease. *Nature* 423:506–11

41. Egen JG, Kuhns MS, Allison JP. 2002. CTLA-4: new insights into its biological function and use in tumor immunotherapy. *Nat. Immunol.* 3:611–18

42. Coyle AJ, Lehar S, Lloyd C, Tian J, Delaney T, et al. 2000. The CD28-related molecule ICOS is required for effective T cell-dependent immune responses. *Immunity* 13:95–105

43. Rudd CE, Schneider H. 2003. Unifying concepts in CD28, ICOS and CTLA4 coreceptor signalling. *Nat. Rev. Immunol.* 3:544–56

44. Beier KC, Hutloff A, Dittrich AM, Heuck C, Rauch A, et al. 2000. Induction, binding specificity and function of human ICOS. *Eur. J. Immunol.* 30:3707–17

45. Parry RV, Rumbley CA, Vandenberghe LH, June CH, Riley JL. 2003. CD28 and inducible costimulatory protein Src homology 2 binding domains show distinct regulation of phosphatidylinositol 3-kinase, Bcl-xL, and IL-2 expression in primary human CD4 T lymphocytes. *J. Immunol.* 171:166–74

46. Okamoto N, Tezuka K, Kato M, Abe R, Tsuji T. 2003. PI3-kinase and MAP-kinase signaling cascades in AILIM/ICOS- and CD28-costimulated T-cells have distinct functions between cell proliferation and IL-10 production. *Biochem. Biophys. Res. Commun.* 310:691–702

47. Harada Y, Tanabe E, Watanabe R, Weiss BD, Matsumoto A, et al. 2001. Novel role of phosphatidylinositol 3-kinase in CD28-mediated costimulation. *J. Biol. Chem.* 276:9003–8

48. Riley JL, Blair PJ, Musser JT, Abe R, Tezuka K, et al. 2001. ICOS costimula-

tion requires IL-2 and can be prevented by CTLA-4 engagement. *J. Immunol.* 166:4943–48

49. Mages HW, Hutloff A, Heuck C, Buchner K, Himmelbauer H, et al. 2000. Molecular cloning and characterization of murine ICOS and identification of B7h as ICOS ligand. *Eur. J. Immunol.* 30:1040–47

50. McAdam AJ, Chang TT, Lumelsky AE, Greenfield EA, Boussiotis VA, et al. 2000. Mouse inducible costimulatory molecule (ICOS) expression is enhanced by CD28 costimulation and regulates differentiation of CD4$^+$ T cells. *J. Immunol.* 165:5035–40

51. Kopf M, Coyle AJ, Schmitz N, Barner M, Oxenius A, et al. 2000. Inducible costimulator protein (ICOS) controls T helper cell subset polarization after virus and parasite infection. *J. Exp. Med.* 192:53–61

52. Wassink L, Vieira PL, Smits HH, Kingsbury GA, Coyle AJ, et al. 2004. ICOS expression by activated human Th cells is enhanced by IL-12 and IL-23: increased ICOS expression enhances the effector function of both Th1 and Th2 cells. *J. Immunol.* 173:1779–86

53. Ogasawara K, Yoshinaga SK, Lanier LL. 2002. Inducible costimulator costimulates cytotoxic activity and IFN-γ production in activated murine NK cells. *J. Immunol.* 169:3676–85

54. Richter G, Hayden-Ledbetter M, Irgang M, Ledbetter JA, Westermann J, et al. 2001. Tumor necrosis factor-α regulates the expression of inducible costimulator receptor ligand on CD34$^+$ progenitor cells during differentiation into antigen presenting cells. *J. Biol. Chem.* 276:45686–93

55. Yoshinaga SK, Zhang M, Pistillo J, Horan T, Khare SD, et al. 2000. Characterization of a new human B7-related protein: B7RP-1 is the ligand to the co-stimulatory protein ICOS. *Int. Immunol.* 12:1439–47

56. Aicher A, Hayden-Ledbetter M, Brady WA, Pezzutto A, Richter G, et al. 2000. Characterization of human inducible

costimulator ligand expression and function. *J. Immunol.* 164:4689–96

57. Nakazawa A, Dotan I, Brimnes J, Allez M, Shao L, et al. 2004. The expression and function of costimulatory molecules B7H and B7-H1 on colonic epithelial cells. *Gastroenterology* 126:1347–57

58. Wiendl H, Mitsdoerffer M, Schneider D, Melms A, Lochmuller H, et al. 2003. Muscle fibres and cultured muscle cells express the B7.1/2-related inducible costimulatory molecule, ICOSL: implications for the pathogenesis of inflammatory myopathies. *Brain* 126:1026–35

59. Liang L, Porter EM, Sha WC. 2002. Constitutive expression of the B7h ligand for inducible costimulator on naive B cells is extinguished after activation by distinct B cell receptor and interleukin 4 receptor-mediated pathways and can be rescued by CD40 signaling. *J. Exp. Med.* 196:97–108

60. Sperling AI, Bluestone JA. 2001. ICOS costimulation: It's not just for TH2 cells anymore. *Nat. Immunol.* 2:573–74

61. Lohning M, Hutloff A, Kallinich T, Mages HW, Bonhagen K, et al. 2003. Expression of ICOS in vivo defines CD4+ effector T cells with high inflammatory potential and a strong bias for secretion of interleukin 10. *J. Exp. Med.* 197:181–93

62. Villegas EN, Lieberman LA, Mason N, Blass SL, Zediak VP, et al. 2002. A role for inducible costimulator protein in the CD28-independent mechanism of resistance to *Toxoplasma gondii*. *J. Immunol.* 169:937–43

63. Kanai T, Totsuka T, Tezuka K, Watanabe M. 2002. ICOS costimulation in inflammatory bowel disease. *J. Gastroenterol.* 37(Suppl. 14):78–81

64. Akbari O, Freeman GJ, Meyer EH, Greenfield EA, Chang TT, et al. 2002. Antigen-specific regulatory T cells develop via the ICOS-ICOS-ligand pathway and inhibit allergen-induced airway hyperreactivity. *Nat. Med.* 8:1024–32

65. Bonhagen K, Liesenfeld O, Stadecker MJ, Hutloff A, Erb K, et al. 2003. ICOS+ Th cells produce distinct cytokines in different mucosal immune responses. *Eur. J. Immunol.* 33:392–401

66. Nurieva RI, Duong J, Kishikawa H, Dianzani U, Rojo JM, et al. 2003. Transcriptional regulation of th2 differentiation by inducible costimulator. *Immunity* 18:801–11

67. Nurieva RI, Mai XM, Forbush K, Bevan MJ, Dong C. 2003. B7h is required for T cell activation, differentiation, and effector function. *Proc. Natl. Acad. Sci. USA* 100:14163–68

68. McAdam AJ, Greenwald RJ, Levin MA, Chernova T, Malenkovich N, et al. 2001. ICOS is critical for CD40-mediated antibody class switching. *Nature* 409:102–5

69. Tafuri A, Shahinian A, Bladt F, Yoshinaga SK, Jordana M, et al. 2001. ICOS is essential for effective T-helper-cell responses. *Nature* 409:105–9

70. Suh WK, Gajewska BU, Okada H, Gronski MA, Bertram EM, et al. 2003. The B7 family member B7-H3 preferentially down-regulates T helper type 1-mediated immune responses. *Nat. Immunol.* 4:899–906

71. Grimbacher B, Hutloff A, Schlesier M, Glocker E, Warnatz K, et al. 2003. Homozygous loss of ICOS is associated with adult-onset common variable immunodeficiency. *Nat. Immunol.* 4:261–68

72. Suh WK, Tafuri A, Berg-Brown NN, Shahinian A, Plyte S, et al. 2004. The inducible costimulator plays the major costimulatory role in humoral immune responses in the absence of CD28. *J. Immunol.* 172:5917–23

73. Sporici RA, Beswick RL, von Allmen C, Rumbley CA, Hayden-Ledbetter M, et al. 2001. ICOS ligand costimulation is required for T-cell encephalitogenicity. *Clin. Immunol.* 100:277–88

74. Rottman JB, Smith T, Tonra JR, Ganley K, Bloom T, et al. 2001. The costimulatory molecule ICOS plays an important role in the immunopathogenesis of EAE. *Nat. Immunol.* 2:605–11

75. Dong C, Nurieva RI. 2003. Regulation of immune and autoimmune responses by ICOS. *J. Autoimmun.* 21:255–60

76. Iwai H, Kozono Y, Hirose S, Akiba H, Yagita H, et al. 2002. Amelioration of collagen-induced arthritis by blockade of inducible costimulator-B7 homologous protein costimulation. *J. Immunol.* 169:4332–39

77. Nurieva RI, Treuting P, Duong J, Flavell RA, Dong C. 2003. Inducible costimulator is essential for collagen-induced arthritis. *J. Clin. Invest.* 111:701–6

78. Okamoto T, Saito S, Yamanaka H, Tomatsu T, Kamatani N, et al. 2003. Expression and function of the co-stimulator H4/ICOS on activated T cells of patients with rheumatoid arthritis. *J. Rheumatol.* 30:1157–63

79. Greve B, Vijayakrishnan L, Kubal A, Sobel RA, Peterson LB, et al. 2004. The diabetes susceptibility locus Idd5.1 on mouse chromosome 1 regulates ICOS expression and modulates murine experimental autoimmune encephalomyelitis. *J. Immunol.* 173:157–63

80. Herman AE, Freeman GJ, Mathis D, Benoist C. 2004. CD4$^+$CD25$^+$ T regulatory cells dependent on ICOS promote regulation of effector cells in the prediabetic lesion. *J. Exp. Med.* 199:1479–89

81. Coyle AJ, Gutierrez-Ramos JC. 2004. The role of ICOS and other costimulatory molecules in allergy and asthma. *Springer Semin. Immunopathol.* 25:349–59

82. Dong C, Juedes AE, Temann UA, Shresta S, Allison JP, et al. 2001. ICOS costimulatory receptor is essential for T-cell activation and function. *Nature* 409:97–101

83. Gonzalo JA, Tian J, Delaney T, Corcoran J, Rottman JB, et al. 2001. ICOS is critical for T helper cell-mediated lung mucosal inflammatory responses. *Nat. Immunol.* 2:597–604

84. Tesciuba AG, Subudhi S, Rother RP, Faas SJ, Frantz AM, et al. 2001. Inducible cos-timulator regulates Th2-mediated inflammation, but not Th2 differentiation, in a model of allergic airway disease. *J. Immunol.* 167:1996–2003

85. Mittrucker HW, Kursar M, Kohler A, Yanagihara D, Yoshinaga SK, Kaufmann SH. 2002. Inducible costimulator protein controls the protective T cell response against *Listeria* monocytogenes. *J. Immunol.* 169:5813–17

86. Greenwald RJ, McAdam AJ, Van der Woude D, Satoskar AR, Sharpe AH. 2002. Cutting edge: inducible costimulator protein regulates both Th1 and Th2 responses to cutaneous leishmaniasis. *J. Immunol.* 168:991–95

87. Miyahira Y, Akiba H, Ogawa SH, Ishi T, Watanabe S, et al. 2003. Involvement of ICOS-B7RP-1 costimulatory pathway in the regulation of immune responses to *Leishmania major* and *Nippostrongylus brasiliensis* infections. *Immunol. Lett.* 89:193–99

88. Rutitzky LI, Ozkaynak E, Rottman JB, Stadecker MJ. 2003. Disruption of the ICOS-B7RP-1 costimulatory pathway leads to enhanced hepatic immunopathology and increased γ interferon production by CD4 T cells in murine schistosomiasis. *Infect. Immun.* 71:4040–44

89. Gause WC, Chen SJ, Greenwald RJ, Halvorson MJ, Lu P, et al. 1997. CD28 dependence of T cell differentiation to IL-4 production varies with the particular type 2 immune response. *J. Immunol.* 158:4082–87

90. Bertram EM, Tafuri A, Shahinian A, Chan VS, Hunziker L, et al. 2002. Role of ICOS versus CD28 in antiviral immunity. *Eur. J. Immunol.* 32:3376–85

91. Zhou X, Kubo M, Nishitsuji H, Kurihara K, Ikeda T, et al. 2004. Inducible-costimulator-mediated suppression of human immunodeficiency virus type 1 replication in CD4$^+$ T lymphocytes. *Virology* 325:252–63

92. Rothstein DM, Sayegh MH. 2003. T-cell costimulatory pathways in allograft

rejection and tolerance. *Immunol. Rev.* 196:85–108

93. Ozkaynak E, Gao W, Shemmeri N, Wang C, Gutierrez-Ramos JC, et al. 2001. Importance of ICOS-B7RP-1 costimulation in acute and chronic allograft rejection. *Nat. Immunol.* 2:591–96

94. Kosuge H, Suzuki J, Gotoh R, Koga N, Ito H, et al. 2003. Induction of immunologic tolerance to cardiac allograft by simultaneous blockade of inducible co-stimulator and cytotoxic T-lymphocyte antigen 4 pathway. *Transplantation* 75:1374–79

95. Nanji SA, Hancock WW, Anderson CC, Adams AB, Luo B, et al. 2004. Multiple combination therapies involving blockade of ICOS/B7RP-1 costimulation facilitate long-term islet allograft survival. *Am. J. Transplant.* 4:526–36

96. Salama AD, Yuan X, Nayer A, Chandraker A, Inobe M, et al. 2003. Interaction between ICOS-B7RP1 and B7-CD28 costimulatory pathways in alloimmune responses in vivo. *Am. J. Transplant.* 3:390–95

97. Vibhakar R, Juan G, Traganos F, Darzynkiewicz Z, Finger LR. 1997. Activation-induced expression of human programmed death-1 gene in T-lymphocytes. *Exp. Cell. Res.* 232:25–28

98. Shinohara T, Taniwaki M, Ishida Y, Kawaichi M, Honjo T. 1994. Structure and chromosomal localization of the human PD-1 gene (PDCD1). *Genomics* 23:704–6

99. Zhang XW, Schwartz JCD, Guo XL, Bhatia S, Cao EH, et al. 2004. Structural and functional analysis of the costimulatory receptor programmed death-1. *Immunity* 20:337–47

100. Shlapatska LM, Mikhalap SV, Berdova AG, Zelensky OM, Yun TJ, et al. 2001. CD150 association with either the SH2-containing inositol phosphatase or the SH2-containing protein tyrosine phosphatase is regulated by the adaptor protein SH2D1A. *J. Immunol.* 166:5480–87

101. Nishimura H, Honjo T, Minato N. 2000.

Facilitation of β selection and modification of positive selection in the thymus of PD-1-deficient mice. *J. Exp. Med.* 191:891–98

102. Agata Y, Kawasaki A, Nishimura H, Ishida Y, Tsubata T, et al. 1996. Expression of the PD-1 antigen on the surface of stimulated mouse T and B lymphocytes. *Int. Immunol.* 8:765–72

103. Okazaki T, Maeda A, Nishimura H, Kurosaki T, Honjo T. 2001. PD-1 immunoreceptor inhibits B cell receptor-mediated signaling by recruiting src homology 2-domain-containing tyrosine phosphatase 2 to phosphotyrosine. *Proc. Natl. Acad. Sci. USA* 98:13866–71

104. Liang SC, Latchman YE, Buhlmann JE, Tomczak MF, Horwitz BH, et al. 2003. Regulation of PD-1, PD-L1, and PD-L2 expression during normal and autoimmune responses. *Eur. J. Immunol.* 33:2706–16

105. Rodig N, Ryan T, Allen JA, Pang H, Grabie N, et al. 2003. Endothelial expression of PD-L1 and PD-L2 down-regulates CD8$^+$ T cell activation and cytolysis. *Eur. J. Immunol.* 33:3117–26

106. Petroff MG, Chen LP, Phillips TA, Azzola D, Sedlmayr P, Hunt JS. 2003. B7 family molecules are favorably positioned at the human maternal-fetal interface. *Biol. Reprod.* 68:1496–504

107. Ishida M, Iwai Y, Tanaka Y, Okazaki T, Freeman GJ, et al. 2002. Differential expression of PD-L1 and PD-L2, ligands for an inhibitory receptor PD-1, in the cells of lymphohematopoietic tissues. *Immunol. Lett.* 84:57–62

108. Loke P, Allison JP. 2003. PD-L1 and PD-L2 are differentially regulated by Th1 and Th2 cells. *Proc. Natl. Acad. Sci. USA* 100:5336–41

109. Chemnitz JM, Parry RV, Nichols KE, June CH, Riley JL. 2004. SHP-1 and SHP-2 associate with immunoreceptor tyrosine-based switch motif of programmed death 1 upon primary human T cell stimulation, but only receptor

ligation prevents T cell activation. *J. Immunol.* 173:945–54

110. Carter LL, Fouser LA, Jussif J, Fitz L, Deng B, et al. 2002. PD-1:PD-L inhibitory pathway affects both CD4$^+$ and CD8$^+$ T cells and is overcome by IL-2. *Eur. J. Immunol.* 32:634–43

111. Tamura H, Dong H, Zhu G, Sica GL, Flies DB, et al. 2001. B7-H1 costimulation preferentially enhances CD28-independent T-helper cell function. *Blood* 97:1809–16

112. Wang SD, Bajorath J, Flies DB, Dong HD, Honjo T, Chen LP. 2003. Molecular modeling and functional mapping of B7-H1 and B7-DC uncouple costimulatory function from PD-1 interaction. *J. Exp. Med.* 197:1083–91

113. Nishimura H, Nose M, Hiai H, Minato N, Honjo T. 1999. Development of lupus-like autoimmune diseases by disruption of the PD-1 gene encoding an ITIM motif-carrying immunoreceptor. *Immunity* 11:141–51

114. Nishimura H, Okazaki T, Tanaka Y, Nakatani K, Hara M, et al. 2001. Autoimmune dilated cardiomyopathy in PD-1 receptor-deficient mice. *Science* 291:319–22

115. Okazaki T, Tanaka Y, Nishio R, Mitsuiye T, Mizoguchi A, et al. 2003. Autoantibodies against cardiac troponin I are responsible for dilated cardiomyopathy in PD-1-deficient mice. *Nat. Med.* 9:1477–83

116. Ansari MJ, Salama AD, Chitnis T, Smith RN, Yagita H, et al. 2003. The programmed death-1 (PD-1) pathway regulates autoimmune diabetes in nonobese diabetic (NOD) mice. *J. Exp. Med.* 198:63–69

117. Luhder F, Hoglund P, Allison JP, Benoist C, Mathis D. 1998. Cytotoxic T lymphocyte-associated antigen 4 (CTLA-4) regulates the unfolding of autoimmune diabetes. *J. Exp. Med.* 187:427–32

118. Subudhi SK, Zhou P, Yerian LM, Chin RK, Lo JC, et al. 2004. Local expression of B7-H1 promotes organ-specific

autoimmunity and transplant rejection. *J. Clin. Invest.* 113:694–700

119. Salama AD, Chitnis T, Imitola J, Ansari MJ, Akiba H, et al. 2003. Critical role of the programmed death-1 (PD-1) pathway in regulation of experimental autoimmune encephalomyelitis. *J. Exp. Med.* 198:71–78

120. Latchman YE, Liang SC, Wu Y, Chernova T, Sobel RA, et al. 2004. PD-L1-deficient mice show that PD-L1 on T cells, antigen-presenting cells, and host tissues negatively regulates T cells. *Proc. Natl. Acad. Sci. USA* 101:10691–96

121. Kanai T, Totsuka T, Uraushihara K, Makita S, Nakamura T, et al. 2003. Blockade of B7-H1 suppresses the development of chronic intestinal inflammation. *J. Immunol.* 171:4156–63

122. Dong HD, Zhu GF, Tamada K, Flies DB, van Deursen JMA, Chen LP. 2004. B7-H1 determines accumulation and deletion of intrahepatic CD8$^+$ T lymphocytes. *Immunity* 20:327–36

123. Hatachi S, Iwai Y, Kawano S, Morinobu S, Kobayashi M, et al. 2003. CD4$^+$ PD-1$^+$ T cells accumulate as unique anergic cells in rheumatoid arthritis synovial fluid. *J. Rheumatol.* 30:1410–19

124. Prokunina L, Castillejo-Lopez C, Oberg F, Gunnarsson I, Berg L, et al. 2002. A regulatory polymorphism in PDCD1 is associated with susceptibility to systemic lupus erythematosus in humans. *Nat. Genet.* 32:666–69

125. Nielsen C, Hansen D, Husby S, Jacobsen BB, Lillevang ST. 2003. Association of a putative regulatory polymorphism in the PD-1 gene with susceptibility to type 1 diabetes. *Tissue Antigens* 62:492–97

126. Dong H, Strome SE, Matteson EL, Moder KG, Flies DB, et al. 2003. Costimulating aberrant T cell responses by B7-H1 autoantibodies in rheumatoid arthritis. *J. Clin. Invest.* 111:363–70

127. Matsumoto K, Inoue H, Nakano T, Tsuda M, Yoshiura Y, et al. 2004. B7-DC regulates asthmatic response by an

IFN-γ-dependent mechanism. *J. Immunol.* 172:2530–41

128. Iwai Y, Terawaki S, Ikegawa M, Okazaki T, Honjo T. 2003. PD-1 inhibits antiviral immunity at the effector phase in the liver. *J. Exp. Med.* 198:39–50

129. Smith P, Walsh CM, Mangan NE, Fallon RE, Sayers JR, et al. 2004. *Schistosoma mansoni* worms induce anergy of T cells via selective up-regulation of programmed death ligand 1 on macrophages. *J. Immunol.* 173:1240–48

130. Ozkaynak E, Wang L, Goodearl A, McDonald K, Qin S, et al. 2002. Programmed death-1 targeting can promote allograft survival. *J. Immunol.* 169:6546–53

131. Gao W, Demirci G, Strom TB, Li XC. 2003. Stimulating PD-1-negative signals concurrent with blocking CD154 costimulation induces long-term islet allograft survival. *Transplantation* 76:994–99

132. Blazar BR, Carreno BM, Panoskaltsis-Mortari A, Carter L, Iwai Y, et al. 2003. Blockade of programmed death-1 engagement accelerates graft-versus-host disease lethality by an IFN-γ-dependent mechanism. *J. Immunol.* 171:1272–77

133. Aramaki O, Shirasugi N, Takayama T, Shimazu M, Kitajima M, et al. 2004. Programmed death-1-programmed death-L1 interaction is essential for induction of regulatory cells by intratracheal delivery of alloantigen. *Transplantation* 77:6–12

134. Blank C, Brown I, Peterson AC, Spiotto M, Iwai Y, et al. 2004. PD-L1/B7H-1 inhibits the effector phase of tumor rejection by T cell receptor (TCR) transgenic CD8$^+$ T cells. *Cancer Res.* 64:1140–45

135. Dong H, Strome SE, Salomao DR, Tamura H, Hirano F, et al. 2002. Tumor-associated B7-H1 promotes T-cell apoptosis: a potential mechanism of immune evasion. *Nat. Med.* 8:793–800

136. Brown JA, Dorfman DM, Ma FR, Sullivan EL, Munoz O, et al. 2003. Blockade of programmed death-1 ligands on dendritic cells enhances T cell activation and cytokine production. *J. Immunol.* 170:1257–66

137. Wintterle S, Schreiner B, Mitsdoerffer M, Schneider D, Chen LP, et al. 2003. Expression of the B7-related molecule B7-H1 by glioma cells: a potential mechanism of immune paralysis. *Cancer Res.* 63:7462–67

138. Rosenwald A, Wright G, Leroy K, Yu X, Gaulard P, et al. 2003. Molecular diagnosis of primary mediastinal B cell lymphoma identifies a clinically favorable subgroup of diffuse large B cell lymphoma related to Hodgkin lymphoma. *J. Exp. Med.* 198:851–62

139. Iwai Y, Ishida M, Tanaka Y, Okazaki T, Honjo T, Minato N. 2002. Involvement of PD-L1 on tumor cells in the escape from host immune system and tumor immunotherapy by PD-L1 blockade. *Proc. Natl. Acad. Sci. USA* 99:12293–97

140. Curiel TJ, Wei S, Dong HD, Alvarez X, Cheng P, et al. 2003. Blockade of B7-H1 improves myeloid dendritic cell-mediated antitumor immunity. *Nat. Med.* 9:562–67

141. Strome SE, Dong H, Tamura H, Voss SG, Flies DB, et al. 2003. B7-H1 blockade augments adoptive T-cell immunotherapy for squamous cell carcinoma. *Cancer Res.* 63:6501–5

142. Liu XL, Gao JX, Wen J, Yin LJ, Li O, et al. 2003. B7DC/PDL2 promotes tumor immunity by a PD-1-independent mechanism. *J. Exp. Med.* 197:1721–30

143. Radhakrishnan S, Nguyen LT, Ciric B, Flies D, Van Keulen VP, et al. 2004. Immunotherapeutic potential of B7-DC (PD-L2) cross-linking antibody in conferring antitumor immunity. *Cancer Res.* 64:4965–72

144. Sun MY, Richards S, Prasad DVR, Mai XM, Rudensky A, Dong C. 2002. Characterization of mouse and human B7-H3 genes. *J. Immunol.* 168:6294–97

145. Steinberger P, Majdic O, Derdak SV, Pfistershammer K, Kirchberger S, et al. 2004. Molecular characterization of human 4Ig-B7-H3, a member of the B7

family with four Ig-like domains. *J. Immunol.* 172:2352–59

146. Ling V, Wu PW, Spaulding V, Kieleczawa J, Luxenberg D, et al. 2003. Duplication of primate and rodent B7-H3 immunoglobulin V- and C-like domains: divergent history of functional redundancy and exon loss. *Genomics* 82:365–77

147. Ferlazzo G, Semino C, Meta M, Procopio F, Morandi B, Melioli G. 2002. T lymphocytes express B7 family molecules following interaction with dendritic cells and acquire bystander costimulatory properties. *Eur. J. Immunol.* 32:3092–101

148. Saatian B, Yu XY, Lane AP, Doyle T, Casolaro V, Spannhake EW. 2004. Expression of genes for B7-H3 and other T cell ligands by nasal epithelial cells during differentiation and activation. *Am. J. Physiol. Lung Cell. Mol. Physiol.* 287: L217–25

149. Sun X, Vale M, Leung E, Kanwar JR, Gupta R, Krissansen GW. 2003. Mouse B7-H3 induces antitumor immunity. *Gene Ther.* 10:1728–34

150. Choi IH, Zhu G, Sica GL, Strome SE, Cheville JC, et al. 2003. Genomic organization and expression analysis of B7-H4, an immune inhibitory molecule of the B7 family. *J. Immunol.* 171:4650–54

151. Gavrieli M, Watanabe N, Loftin SK, Murphy TL, Murphy KM. 2003. Characterization of phosphotyrosine binding motifs in the cytoplasmic domain of B and T lymphocyte attenuator required for association with protein tyrosine phosphatases SHP-1 and SHP-2. *Biochem. Biophys. Res. Commun.* 312:1236–43

152. Sedy JR, Gavrieli M, Potter KG, Hurchla MA, Lindsley RC, et al. 2004. B and T lymphocyte attenuator regulates T cell activation through interaction with herpesvirus entry mediator. *Nat. Immunol.* 6:90–98

Annu. Rev. Immunol. 2005. 23:549–600
doi: 10.1146/annurev.immunol.22.012703.104743
Copyright © 2005 by Annual Reviews. All rights reserved
First published online as a Review in Advance on December 8, 2004

TEC FAMILY KINASES IN T LYMPHOCYTE DEVELOPMENT AND FUNCTION[*]

Leslie J. Berg,[1] Lisa D. Finkelstein,[2] Julie A. Lucas,[1] and Pamela L. Schwartzberg[2]

[1]*Department of Pathology, University of Massachusetts Medical School, Worcester, Massachusetts 01655; email: Leslie.Berg@umassmed.edu*
[2]*National Human Genome Research Institute, National Institutes of Health, Bethesda, Maryland 20892; email: pams@nhgri.nih.gov*

Key Words Itk/Emt/Tsk, Rlk/Txk, Tec, phospholipase C-γ, actin

■ **Abstract** The Tec family tyrosine kinases are now recognized as important mediators of antigen receptor signaling in lymphocytes. Three members of this family, Itk, Rlk, and Tec, are expressed in T cells and activated in response to T cell receptor (TCR) engagement. Although initial studies demonstrated a role for these proteins in TCR-mediated activation of phospholipase C-γ, recent data indicate that Tec family kinases also regulate actin cytoskeletal reorganization and cellular adhesion following TCR stimulation. In addition, Tec family kinases are activated downstream of G protein–coupled chemokine receptors, where they play parallel roles in the regulation of Rho GTPases, cell polarization, adhesion, and migration. In all these systems, however, Tec family kinases are not essential signaling components, but instead function to modulate or amplify signaling pathways. Although they quantitatively reduce proximal signaling, mutations that eliminate Tec family kinases in T cells nonetheless qualitatively alter T cell development and differentiation.

INTRODUCTION

The Tec family nonreceptor tyrosine kinases have recently emerged as key regulators of signaling pathways in T lymphocytes. The importance of this family was first established in 1993 when mutations affecting Btk were found to be associated with the human genetic disorder X-linked agammaglobulinemia (XLA) and the murine mutant X-linked immunodeficiency (*xid*), immunodeficiencies associated with decreased serum immunoglobulins and impaired B cell development (1–4).[1] XLA provided the first example of mutations affecting a tyrosine kinase linked to a primary human immunodeficiency, highlighting the importance of tyrosine kinases

---

[*]The U.S. Government has the right to retain a nonexclusive, royalty-free license in and to any copyright covering this paper.
[1]See Appendix for a full list of abbreviations used.

for antigen receptor signaling pathways and their roles in lymphocyte development and function.

The Tec family of kinases now consists of five family members, which are expressed primarily in hematopoietic cells: Tec, Btk, Itk (also known as Tsk and Emt), Rlk (also known as Txk), and Bmx (also known as Etk). Additional related Tec family kinases have been found in *Drosophila melanogaster*, zebrafish (*Danio rerio*), skate (*Raja eglanteria*), and sea urchin (*Anthocidaris crassispina*) (5). Although the Tec family kinases resemble Src family kinases, having tyrosine kinase catalytic and Src homology protein interaction domains, they are notable in that most family members possess a pleckstrin homology (PH) domain that binds to the products of phosphoinositide 3-kinase (PI3K). The Tec family kinases are the only tyrosine kinases that possess PH domains and that can be regulated by PI3K. In T lymphocytes, three major Tec kinases are expressed: Itk, Rlk, and Tec, all of which are tyrosine phosphorylated upon T cell receptor (TCR) stimulation (6–9).

Although mutations of the Tec family kinases have not yet been associated with T cell defects in humans, in mice mutations affecting Itk or Itk and Rlk lead to decreased responses to TCR stimulation, including proliferation, IL-2 production, and production of effector cytokines (10–14). Mutations affecting these kinases are thus associated with a variety of biochemical defects downstream of TCR signaling (10, 11, 13, 15), as well as with impaired thymic development (12, 16, 17) and altered mature T cell effector functions (14, 17, 18). In this review, we cover the structure and mechanism of activation of Tec family kinases, the roles of Tec kinases in T lymphocyte signaling pathways, and the functional importance of these molecules for lymphocyte development and immune responses.

EXPRESSION OF THE TEC KINASES IN LYMPHOCYTES

T lymphocytes express at least three Tec family kinases: Itk, Rlk, and Tec. Additionally, one report (19) mentions that Bmx/Etk expression can be detected in the Jurkat lymphoma cell line. Each of the three major T cell Tec family kinases exhibits distinct patterns and levels of expression that may reflect their functional importance in different T cell subsets and stages of development.

Itk (inducible T cell kinase; also known as Emt, expressed in mast cells and T lymphocytes, and Tsk, T cell–specific kinase) is the predominant Tec kinase in T cells and was first cloned by degenerate PCR of T cell–specific tyrosine kinases (20–24). At least two forms of Itk have been cloned from mouse, which vary by inclusion or deletion of a sequence encoding six amino acids (20, 21, 24). The longer version, which appears to be a splice variant, is not detected in human cells. Itk expression is found in thymocytes and mature T cells, mast cells, natural killer cells, and NKT cells, with the highest levels of expression in the mature adult thymus (20, 21, 23, 24). Expression of Itk is induced upon T cell activation and treatment with IL-2 (20, 22, 23). Two recent reports demonstrate higher levels of Itk mRNA and protein in Th2 cells relative to Th1 cells, perhaps reflecting Itk's importance in the development of Th2 responses (25, 26). Mature T cells and thymocytes from mice deficient in Itk show impaired activation of phospholipase C-γ (PLC-γ), defective actin reorganization, and multiple functional defects in response to TCR stimulation (10–15, 17, 27, 28).

Rlk (resting lymphocyte kinase; also known as Txk) was also cloned in degenerate PCR screens for novel tyrosine kinases expressed in T lymphocytes (29–32). Like Itk, Rlk expression is found in thymocytes, mature resting T cells, and mast cells (31, 32). Real-time RT-PCR demonstrates that Rlk mRNA is expressed at 3- to 10-fold lower levels than Itk in resting mature T cells (25, 26). Expression of Rlk drops dramatically upon T cell receptor stimulation (31, 32). Rlk expression increases again in primary differentiated Th1 cells and Th1 cell clones, but it remains very low in differentiated Th2 cells and cell clones (25, 26, 31, 33), suggesting that Rlk is functionally more important for Th1 cell function. Consistent with these observations, IL-12 was shown to increase and IL-4 to decrease expression of Rlk in peripheral blood CD4$^+$ cells (33). Although two forms of Rlk have been detected, there are no clear differences in the ratio of these isoforms in different T cell populations (6). Mutation of *Rlk* leads to minimal T cell defects, yet it can exacerbate defects observed in Itk-deficient T cells (10, 11).

Tec (tyrosine kinase expressed in hepatocellular carcinoma), the founding member of this family, was originally cloned from a mouse liver cDNA library. Tec has a more broad pattern of expression both in hematopoietic and other cell types (34). Tec is expressed at relatively low levels in resting T cells. Real-time RT-PCR studies suggest its mRNA is 100-fold lower than that of Itk. However, Tec expression is induced after stimulation of T cells for 2–3 days (35), suggesting that it may be more important for effector cell function or upon restimulation of preactivated cells. Like Itk, Tec is expressed at slightly higher levels (twofold) in Th2 cells than in Th1 cells (35). No functional defects have been reported to date in Tec-deficient T cells. However, in mouse B cells, mutation of Tec worsens defects associated with Btk deficiency (36), suggesting functional redundancy with other family members. Multiple splice forms of Tec have been reported (37), but their functional differences in T cells remain unknown.

Of note, Btk, the most famous Tec family kinase, is broadly expressed in most hematopoietic cells, but it is not expressed in T cells. For excellent reviews of the Tec kinases in other cell types, we refer the readers to References 38–40.

DOMAIN STRUCTURES OF TEC KINASE FAMILY MEMBERS

The five mammalian Tec kinases share an overall similar domain organization that closely resembles the organization of the Src family tyrosine kinases (5) (Figure 1). Starting at the carboxy-terminus is the kinase domain, followed by a single Src homology (SH)-2 and then a single SH3 domain. At this point, the Tec kinase structures diverge from the Src family kinases. Specifically, at the amino-terminal

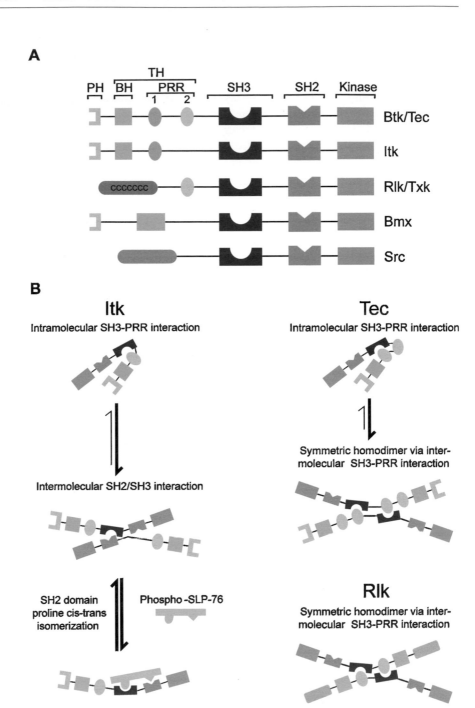

side of the SH3 domain, all Tec kinases except Bmx have a proline-rich region (PRR). Btk and Tec share a second tandem PRR, adjacent to a Zn^{2+}-binding region known as the Btk homology (BH) motif. The BH motif is also found in Itk, adjacent to its single PRR. For Itk, Btk, and Tec, the combined Btk motif and the single or double PRRs are often referred to as the Tec homology (TH) domain. Finally, at the very amino-terminus of the protein, Itk, Btk, Tec, and Bmx share a PH domain, whereas Rlk contains a cysteine-string motif.

The individual functions of each of these protein domains are well established. The kinase domains have catalytic activity for transferring phosphate onto tyrosine residues of substrate proteins. These domains share the conserved structural features of all catalytically active kinases, and in the cases of Btk and Itk, X-ray crystallographic data confirm the close similarity between the Btk and Itk kinase domains and those of the Src family kinases (41, 42).

The SH2, SH3, PRR, and BH domains all mediate protein-protein interactions that regulate the binding partners of the Tec kinases and thus determine their proximity to signaling complexes and potential substrates. Numerous independent biochemical approaches have been used to identify binding partners for these Tec family kinase domains, including pull-down assays with GST-fusion proteins, yeast two-hybrid assays, and the testing of candidate molecules initially identified as binding partners of proteins with related domains (Table 1). Overall, these strategies have yielded a substantial list of proteins that can interact with individual domains of Tec kinase family members, or in some cases with full-length Tec kinase proteins. Although not all these potential binding partners have been confirmed in

---

←

Figure 1 Domain structures and domain interactions of Tec family tyrosine kinases. (*A*) Tec family tyrosine kinases share an overall similar organizational structure to kinases of the Src family (*bottom*). (*B*) Among the Tec family kinases found in T cells, Itk has the most well-characterized domain structures and interactions. An intramolecular interaction between the Itk SH3 domain and PRR can occur. At higher protein concentrations, an intermolecular dimer formed by reciprocal interactions between the Itk SH2 and SH3 domains is favored over the intramolecular interaction seen in the monomer. In addition, the SH2 domain of Itk contains a proline residue that undergoes *cis-trans* isomerization, causing a global conformational change in the SH2 domain structure. In the *cis* form, the SH2 domain interacts preferentially with the Itk SH3 domain; in the *trans* form, the SH2 domain binds preferentially to phosphotyrosine-containing ligands, such as phospho-SLP-76, which also binds cooperatively to the Itk SH3 domain. Similarly to Itk, Tec can undergo an intramolecular association involving the Tec SH3 and PRR domains. However, the preferred structure for Tec is an intermolecular dimer formed by reciprocal interactions between SH3 and PRR regions on two different Tec molecules. For Rlk, intramolecular interaction between the SH3 and PRR regions does not occur; instead, Rlk only forms a symmetric homodimer via intermolecular SH3-PRR interactions. The arrows represent likely interconversions between protein conformations, with the dark arrow indicating the more favored conformation.

TABLE 1   Interactions of Tec kinase domains with other proteins

PH	TH	SH3	SH2	Kinase (substrate)
PIP3	LAT (Itk)	Vav (Itk)	SLP-76 (Itk)	PLC-γ (Itk, Rlk, Btk)
PKCβ1	Vav (Tec)	Sam68 (Itk)	Vav (Itk)	CD28 (Itk)
G$\beta\gamma$	GRB-2 (Itk, Rlk)	WASP (Btk, Itk)	Dok1 (Tec)	Vav (Tec)
PIP5K	Dok1 (Tec)	c-Cbl (Itk, Btk)	Cyclophilin (Itk)	SLP-76 (Rlk)
	c-kit (Tec)	CD28 (Itk, Tec)		Dok1,2 (Tec)
	Src kinases (Itk Rlk, Btk, Tec)	SLP-76 (Itk)		LAT (Itk)
		Fyn (Itk)		BRDG1 (Tec)
		PLC-γ (Itk)		LARG (Tec)

physiologically relevant assays, a significant number have. In the sections below, this review highlights the interactions that have garnered additional support from functional, as well as biochemical, assays.

The amino-terminal domains of all five mammalian Tec family kinases contain the major determinants of the subcellular localization of the proteins. For Itk, Btk, Tec, and Bmx, this region includes a PH domain that preferentially binds to phosphatidylinositol (3,4,5) trisphosphate ($PI_{(3,4,5)}P_3$) (43–46). As a result, the PH domain–containing Tec kinases are predominantly cytosolic in resting lymphocytes, where levels of $PI_{(3,4,5)}P_3$ are low. However, following activation, $PI_{(3,4,5)}P_3$ levels in the plasma membrane increase dramatically, leading to the recruitment of these kinases to the membrane. In contrast, Rlk lacks a PH domain; in addition, two isoforms of the Rlk protein are expressed in cells (6). The longer Rlk isoform contains a cysteine-string motif that becomes palmitoylated and recruits Rlk to the lipid raft compartment of the plasma membrane. The shorter form of Rlk lacks both a PH domain as well as the cysteine-string motif; this isoform of Rlk is constitutively localized in the nucleus when expressed in isolation.

RECEPTOR-MEDIATED ACTIVATION OF
TEC KINASES IN T CELLS

Itk is Activated by Signaling through Multiple
T Cell Surface Receptors

Tec kinases have been implicated in signaling downstream of a variety of receptors in multiple cell types. In T cells, the pathway most heavily studied is the activation of Tec kinases via signaling through the TCR. Initial studies, performed in Jurkat cells, demonstrated that Itk is tyrosine phosphorylated following TCR crosslinking (7, 9). Although the relevance of this phosphorylation could not be discerned from these studies, the conclusion that Itk is involved in TCR signaling was generally accepted on the basis of the known role of Btk in BCR signaling (47). More definitive evidence that Itk functions as a transducer of TCR signals came from biochemical and cellular studies performed on T cells from Itk-deficient mice (12, 13). As shown first by D. Littman and colleagues (12), T cells lacking Itk are impaired in proliferative responses to TCR crosslinking but respond normally to pharmacological stimulation with a phorbol ester plus a calcium ionophore. These findings were then complemented by a later study demonstrating that TCR-mediated phosphorylation and activation of PLC-γ1 are defective in T cells lacking Itk, firmly establishing Itk as an intermediate in the pathway from the TCR to PLC-γ1 (13).

In addition to a role in TCR signaling, Itk may be important in signaling downstream of the T cell costimulatory receptor CD28, according to several reports (48–53). These data primarily demonstrate biochemical interactions between Itk and CD28. The initial study on this topic showed that, following CD28 stimulation of Jurkat T cells, Itk binds to CD28 and becomes tyrosine phosphorylated (48). Further in vitro studies using recombinant proteins concluded that Itk binding to CD28 requires the presence of the Src family tyrosine kinase p56lck (Lck) (49), a finding that was then confirmed using Lck-deficient Jurkat T cells (50). Structure-function analysis of the tyrosine residues in the CD28 cytoplasmic tail also provided support for the close association between Lck and Itk activities following CD28 stimulation (51).

In an effort to map the binding interaction between Itk and CD28, R. Rottapel and colleagues (52) showed that the SH3 domain of Itk binds to proline-rich sequences in the CD28 cytoplasmic tail. Interestingly, this study also indicated that peptides corresponding to this region of CD28 would activate Itk kinase activity in vitro, providing a potential mechanism by which CD28 stimulation might activate a downstream tyrosine kinase (52). Finally, Itk was shown to phosphorylate all four tyrosine residues of the CD28 cytoplasmic tail in in vitro kinase assays (53), providing evidence for another potential role of Itk in CD28 signaling. However, despite this wealth of biochemical data, evidence substantiating a functional role for Itk in CD28 signaling is still lacking (see below).

Itk is also implicated in signaling downstream of the T cell surface receptor CD2. Like the studies of CD28 signaling, studies of Itk signaling demonstrate that Itk is tyrosine phosphorylated following CD2 crosslinking on Jurkat cells or peripheral blood T cells (54). Furthermore, Itk activation following CD2 stimulation requires the activity of Lck (54) and depends on the PRR of the CD2 cytoplasmic tail (55). Finally, studies in transfected Jurkat cells indicate that a kinase-inactive mutant of Itk can inhibit CD2-mediated activation of the nuclear factor of activated T cells (NFAT) transcription factor, as assessed by a reporter assay (56). Nonetheless, functional data substantiating a role for Itk in CD2 signaling in primary T cells is still lacking.

Two recent studies also report a role for Itk in signaling downstream of the chemokine receptor CXCR4 (57, 58). Itk and Rlk tyrosine phosphorylation, as well as Itk translocation to the plasma membrane, are induced following chemokine stimulation of T cells (57, 58). Similar to the activation of Itk downstream of the TCR, chemokine-induced Itk phosphorylation and membrane localization are inhibited by Src family kinase and PI3K inhibitors, respectively (57, 58). Moreover, these studies demonstrate defective cell migration, as well as impaired actin polymerization, in Itk-deficient T cells responding to SDF-1α (CXCL12). Interestingly, these defects are further diminished in the absence of both Itk and Rlk (58), suggesting that both Tec kinase family members contribute to chemokine responses in T cells.

Rlk is Activated by TCR and Chemokine Receptor Signaling

Unlike Itk, Rlk's precise role in T cell signaling has been more difficult to discern. $Rlk^{-/-}$ T cells show only mild impairments in TCR signaling, but the absence of both Itk and Rlk leads to a dramatic deficiency in TCR signaling compared with that observed in T cells lacking Itk alone (10, 11). These genetic data, suggesting that Rlk can contribute to the TCR signal transduction pathway, are complemented by biochemical data, indicating that Rlk is tyrosine phosphorylated in response to TCR stimulation and that this phosphorylation depends on a Src family kinase such as Lck (6, 59). Rlk has also been shown to phosphorylate SLP-76, a T cell adapter protein required for TCR signal transduction (60). Additional genetic data also indicate that ectopic expression of Rlk can replace Itk or Btk and restore functional antigen receptor signaling in either T cells or B cells, respectively (61, 62). However, as described above, $Rlk^{-/-}Itk^{-/-}$ T cells show greatly impaired responses to the chemokines SDF-1α and MIP3-β compared with $Itk^{-/-}$ T cells, suggesting an additional role for Rlk in chemokine receptor signaling (58).

In T Cells, Tec is Activated by TCR and CD28 Signaling

To date, experiments to determine the role of Tec in T cells have not provided a clear answer regarding whether Tec is required for TCR and CD28 signaling. Biochemical studies and assays based on transfection of Tec into Jurkat cells indicate that Tec is activated in response to TCR stimulation, and that Tec overexpression can potentiate TCR-mediated PLC-γ1 phosphorylation and NFAT activation (8, 35, 63). Like Itk, Tec is phosphorylated in response to CD28 crosslinking and associates with CD28 via an interaction between the Tec SH3 domain and a PRR in the CD28 cytoplasmic tail (8, 64). One functional study using an antisense approach showed that primary T cells that express reduced amounts of Tec produced less IL-2 than control antisense-treated T cells (63). Despite these data, T cells from Tec-deficient mice have no detectable defects in TCR or CD28 signaling (36). Thus, a more definitive conclusion concerning the role of Tec in T cells may require the generation and analysis of mice lacking both Tec and Itk, or Tec and Rlk.

Although the role of Tec in T cells has remained elusive, numerous studies have documented an important role of Tec in signaling downstream of cytokine receptors in other cell types. These data indicate that Tec is involved in signaling downstream of the IL-3 receptor, the IL-5 receptor, the prolactin receptor, the erythropoietin receptor, the G-CSF receptor, c-kit, and the IL-6 family of receptors (using the shared receptor subunit gp130) (reviewed in 38–40, 65). Several studies have also indicated that Tec is phosphorylated and activated by the Jak kinases that are associated with these cytokine receptors (66, 67). One potential function of Tec downstream of cytokine receptors is the activation of the guanine nucleotide exchange factor (GEF), Vav1, suggesting a role for Tec in cytoskeletal reorganization in response to cytokines (68, 69). Interestingly, additional Tec kinase family members, such as Btk and Bmx, are also implicated in cytokine receptor signaling pathways (38, 39). Thus, the investigation of Tec kinases as potential mediators of cytokine receptor signaling in T cells may be a fruitful area for future research.

REGULATION OF TEC KINASE ACTIVITY BY SUBCELLULAR LOCALIZATION

Several critical components are required for the activation of Tec kinases downstream of cell surface receptors (Figure 2). These components include recruitment of the kinase to the plasma membrane at the site of the activated receptor, colocalization of the kinase with receptor associated adapter proteins and substrates, and, finally, tyrosine phosphorylation of the kinase by an upstream activator, most frequently a Src family kinase. As far as is known, membrane recruitment is the first step of activation.

Membrane Localization via Pleckstrin Homology (PH) Domains is Regulated by PI3K Activity

For two of the Tec kinases present in T cells, Itk and Tec, membrane recruitment is mediated by their amino-terminal PH domains. The importance of the PH domain was highlighted by the discovery that the naturally occurring *xid* defect in mice results from a point mutation in the Btk PH domain (3, 4), a conclusion subsequently reinforced by the finding of similar PH domain mutations as genetic defects resulting in XLA in humans (70).

The PH domain generally consists of a β-barrel formed by two β-sheets, followed by a carboxy-terminal α-helix (43, 71). As first shown for the PH domain of Btk (43–45, 72), the PH domains of both Itk and Tec also bind to phosphoinositides, with a preference for inositides phosphorylated at the D3 position of the inositol ring (19, 43, 46). These findings initially suggested that Tec kinases may be regulated by the activity of PI3K, a suggestion that has been verified in a number of studies (19, 46, 63, 73–75). The importance of PI3K activity for Itk and Tec activation in response to TCR stimulation is also highlighted by the requirement for the Rho family GTP exchange factor Vav1 in this process (76). This requirement is attributed to the role of Vav1 in TCR-induced PI3K activation, which is potentially mediated by the small GTPase Rac1, a known target of the Vav1 exchange factor activity (76).

A

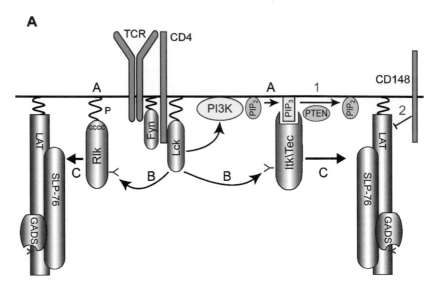

Figure 2 Mechanisms of activation and inactivation of Tec family kinases downstream of surface receptors, such as the TCR. The activation of Tec family tyrosine kinases downstream of T cell surface receptors requires at least three distinct steps: (*A*) Localization of the kinase to the plasma membrane at the site of the activated receptor. For Itk and Tec, this localization requires the PH domain and depends on receptor-mediated activation of PI3K and generation of $PI_{(3,4,5)}P_3$. For Rlk, membrane localization is mediated by palmitoylation of the cysteine-string motif and is independent of PI3K activity; (*B*) transphosphorylation of the kinase by a Src family kinase, such as Lck; (*C*) association of the kinase with adapter proteins, such as SLP-76, GADS, and LAT, that form a complex in response to receptor stimulation. The precise order of these steps in the activation process has not been established. Potential mechanisms by which Tec family tyrosine kinases are inactivated include (*numbers in red*) (1) PTEN, a lipid phosphatase that hydrolyzes $PI_{(3,4,5)}P_3$ into $PI_{(4,5)}P_2$, and SHIP (not shown), which hydrolyzes $PI_{(3,4,5)}P_3$ into $PI_{(3,4)}P_2$; and (2) CD148, a protein tyrosine phosphatase that has been implicated in dephosphorylation of T cell signaling proteins such as SLP-76 and LAT, which would eliminate the docking sites for Tec family kinases.

Together, these data lead to a model wherein receptor stimulation leads to activation of PI3K, resulting in the accumulation of $PI_{(3,4,5)}P_3$ in the plasma membrane. The PH domain–containing Tec kinases are then recruited to the membrane at the site of the activated receptor. This localization is essential for the subsequent phosphorylation and activation of the Tec family kinase (3, 4, 46, 63, 77, 78). Furthermore, replacement of the Itk PH domain with an alternative membrane localization signal, such as a myristoylation and acylation target sequence, produces an Itk protein that can localize to the plasma membrane but cannot be tyrosine phosphorylated following TCR stimulation (78). These data indicate a critical role for the PH domain in Itk activation beyond simple membrane recruitment. Furthermore, recent data on the membrane localization of Tec indicates an important role for the SH2 and SH3 domains in addition to the Tec PH domain (63, 79, 80).

Additional differences in the functional properties of the distinct Tec family kinase PH domains have also been observed. For instance, an activating mutation was identified in the Btk PH domain involving substitution of glutamic acid with lysine at residue 41 (81). This activating mutation (E41K) leads to increased $PI_{(3,4,5)}P_3$-binding of the mutant PH domain (63) and thus generates a Btk protein that exhibits increased localization to the membrane compared with wild-type Btk (81). In contrast, however, the comparable amino acid substitution in the Tec PH domain (E42K) leads to reduced binding to $PI_{(3,4,5)}P_3$ in vitro and reduced functional activity in T cells (63), indicating a significant structural difference between the Btk and Tec PH domains.

The dependence of Tec kinase activation on $PI_{(3,4,5)}P_3$ levels in the plasma membrane also implicates additional regulators of inositol phosphates in the modulation of Tec kinase activity (Figure 2). For instance, in B cells, Btk activity is downregulated by the enzyme SHIP, an SH2-containing inositol phosphatase that catalyzes the hydrolysis of $PI_{(3,4,5)}P_3$ to $PI_{(3,4)}P_2$ (73). SHIP may also contribute to the regulation of Tec in T cells (81a). A second mechanism that downregulates Tec kinase activity is the hydrolysis of $PI_{(3,4,5)}P_3$ into $PI_{(4,5)}P_2$ by the dual specificity phosphatase, PTEN. This pathway's importance in T cells was demonstrated by the discovery that the Jurkat tumor line, commonly used for signal transduction studies, has a naturally occurring deficiency in PTEN (82, 83); interestingly, this lack of PTEN leads to constitutively high levels of $PI_{(3,4,5)}P_3$ in Jurkat cells and, consequently, to a constitutive localization of Itk to the plasma membrane in these cells (77, 82).

A very recent study has also provided intriguing evidence that in B cells, Btk participates in a positive feedback loop to promote the production of $PI_{(4,5)}P_2$, the substrate for both PI3K and PLC-γ (84). In this pathway, Btk binds to PIP5 kinase and shuttles this enzyme to the plasma membrane where it converts $PI_{(4)}P$ into $PI_{(4,5)}P_2$. By this mechanism, the activated B cell is ensured of an ongoing supply of $PI_{(4,5)}P_2$ to drive the further production of $PI_{(3,4,5)}P_3$, as well as the second messengers, diacylglycerol (DAG) and inositol (1,4,5) trisphosphate (IP_3). To date, no similar mechanism has been described for a Tec kinase in T cells.

One final mechanism regulating Tec family kinase membrane localization mediated by the PH domain is the phosphorylation of this domain by protein kinase C (PKC). Early studies first indicated that the PH domains of Btk and Itk directly bind to PKCβ, and that the association between Btk or Itk and PKCβ could be detected by coimmunoprecipitation from mast cells (85, 86). The Btk and Itk PH domains were then shown to be substrates for PKC phosphorylation in vitro (85, 86). A functional connection between Tec kinases and PKC was first suggested by data showing that PKC depletion in mast cells led to increased phosphorylation of Btk but to decreased phosphorylation of Itk following FcεRI crosslinking (85, 86). The findings on Btk were further reinforced by genetic data indicating that targeted mutation of the PKCβ gene in mice results in a B cell immunodeficiency remarkably similar to that seen in the absence of Btk activity (87). Paradoxically, biochemical studies demonstrate that PKC phosphorylation of Btk leads to enhanced Btk membrane localization and tyrosine phosphorylation and to augmented antigen receptor signaling in both B cells and mast cells (88). Together, these data suggest that precise modulation of Tec kinase membrane localization is critical for optimal levels of antigen receptor signaling. Whether Itk and Tec are similarly regulated by PKC phosphorylation in T cells remains to be determined.

Membrane Localization of Rlk is Mediated by a Palmitoylated Cysteine-String Motif

Two distinct isoforms of the Rlk protein have been identified that arise by translation initiation from two different sites on the same cDNA molecule (6). Interestingly, both isoforms of Rlk lack the amino-terminal PH domain found in Itk and Tec. Instead, the larger isoform of Rlk contains an amino-terminal cysteine-string motif that directs palmitoylation of the protein (6), leading to constitutive localization of Rlk to the membrane and, specifically, to lipid rafts (59). The shorter isoform of Rlk lacks the cysteine-string motif and fatty acid modification. This shorter isoform colocalizes with the longer isoform when the two proteins are coexpressed, but it constitutively translocates to the nucleus when expressed alone (6). The precise function of the nuclear form of Rlk is not known, but one report indicates that Rlk may function as a transcription factor for the IFN-γ gene (89). Interestingly, Itk has also been reported to localize to the nucleus, a process that is enhanced by its interaction with the nuclear import chaperone, karyopherin α (Rch1α) (90).

REGULATION OF TEC FAMILY KINASE ACTIVITY BY COLOCALIZATION WITH RECEPTOR-ASSOCIATED ADAPTER PROTEINS AND SUBSTRATES

A second major mechanism for regulating Tec family kinase activity downstream of activated receptors in T cells is via the localization of the kinase with receptor-associated adapter proteins and substrates. On this topic, the majority of data focus on Itk and its interaction with proteins in the TCR signaling pathway. Several studies have demonstrated that Itk binds directly to SLP-76 via the Itk-SH2 domain, binding to phosphorylated tyrosine residues in SLP-76 (77, 91). In addition, the Itk-SH3 domain and the PRR of SLP-76 also interact, providing cooperative binding of two domains of Itk to SLP-76, thus potentially increasing the stability of this interaction (77). Interestingly, the Itk-SH2 domain appears to be remarkably selective, as it binds only SLP-76 in activated T cells; similarly, the Btk-SH2 domain also selectively binds to the SLP-65 adapter protein in activated B cells (91, 92). Because a functional SH2 domain is critical for TCR-mediated phosphorylation and activation of Itk, the localization of Itk to the SLP-76 adapter protein is an essential aspect of the signal transduction pathway (93).

Itk also interacts with the adapter protein LAT (linker for activation of T cells) (77, 93, 94). Currently, it is not clear whether this interaction is direct or indirect. If indirect, the binding of Itk to LAT may be mediated via the adapter protein GRB-2, which binds to the Itk PRR and also to tyrosine-phosphorylated LAT (77, 95, 95a). Alternatively, Itk binding to SLP-76 may be required for its interaction with LAT. Regardless of the detailed mechanism, the association of Itk with LAT is clearly a critical component of the signal transduction pathway leading from the TCR to Itk. This conclusion is supported by studies performed in Jurkat T cells lacking LAT, in which TCR stimulation fails to activate Itk (93, 94).

Tyrosine phosphorylation of Itk in response to TCR stimulation also depends on the tyrosine kinase Zap-70 (94). Because Zap-70 does not directly phosphorylate Itk (94), this requirement is most likely indirect, via the need to recruit Itk to the Zap-70-dependent SLP-76/LAT adapter complex (77, 93, 94). The requirement for Itk to colocalize with the LAT/SLP-76 adapter complex also provides a potential mechanism to terminate Itk signaling. For instance, overexpression of the tyrosine phosphatase CD148 leads to reduced phosphorylation of LAT and PLC-γ1 in activated Jurkat T cells; this pathway is also expected to downregulate Itk activity, further attenuating the signals downstream of the TCR (96) (Figure 2).

In addition to interactions with the LAT/SLP-76 adapter complex, Tec kinases bind to other T cell signaling proteins that may regulate their activity in response to receptor stimulation. For instance, Itk binds directly to PLC-γ1 (97), its most well-documented substrate following TCR stimulation (10, 13, 98). A T cell adapter protein, RIBP, has been identified on the basis of a screen for Rlk-binding proteins (99). RIBP, which also binds to Itk, plays a role in T cell activation, based on the findings that RIBP-deficient T cells show reduced proliferation and IL-2 secretion following TCR plus CD28 stimulation (99). Another interesting set of Tec kinase–interacting proteins is the heterotrimeric G proteins. G$\beta\gamma$ subunits of heterotrimeric G proteins bind to PH domains, as first described for the β-adrenergic receptor kinase (100) and for Btk (101). Subsequently, the G$\beta\gamma$ subunits were shown to bind to Itk and to stimulate Itk kinase activity in vitro (102). These findings were then extended to Gα subunits of the Gq class, which were shown to bind to Btk and to stimulate Btk activity both in vitro and in intact chicken DT-40 B cells (103). Given the suggestive data that TCR signaling leads to heterotrimeric G protein activation (104), and further that this pathway regulates TCR proximal events such as TCRζ, CD3ε, as well as Zap-70 phosphorylation (105), the interactions of Tec kinases with these proteins may be important components of the TCR signaling pathway.

REGULATION OF TEC FAMILY KINASE ACTIVITY
BY PHOSPHORYLATION

The third mechanism regulating Tec family kinase activity downstream of receptor stimulation in T cells is through the tyrosine phosphorylation of the enzyme. As was first demonstrated for Btk (106–109), Tec kinases are phosphorylated on a conserved activation loop tyrosine in the kinase domain, and this phosphorylation enhances enzymatic activity of the kinase. This mechanism, which is common to multiple families of protein kinases, results in a conformational change in the kinase domain that provides substrates access to the catalytic site (110). However, unlike the closely related Src family tyrosine kinases, Tec kinases do not autophosphorylate this activation loop tyrosine. Instead, phosphorylation of Y551 in Btk (107, 109), Y511 in Itk (9), and Y420 in Rlk (6, 59) are mediated by Src family tyrosine kinases in a transphosphorylation reaction. Tec has also been shown to be directly phosphorylated and activated by the Src family tyrosine kinase Lyn, although the identity of the activating tyrosine in Tec has not been rigorously identified (111).

Transphosphorylation of Tec family kinases on the activation loop tyrosine in the kinase domain leads to increased Tec kinase activity in vitro and is critical for Tec kinase–mediated signal transduction in intact T cells. For Itk and Rlk, substitution of Y511 or Y420, respectively, with phenylalanine produces a protein that has impaired in vitro kinase activity (9, 59). In contrast, phosphorylation of the wild-type Itk protein at Y511 by Lck, or of the wild-type Rlk protein at Y420 by Fyn, increases Itk and Rlk in vitro kinase activity (9, 59). Furthermore, Jurkat T cells lacking Lck show no TCR-induced tyrosine phosphorylation of Itk, indicating a critical role for Lck in Itk activation in intact cells (7, 9). For Rlk, Y420 is critical for tyrosine phosphorylation of Rlk following TCR stimulation (59).

The functional significance of phosphorylation on the activation loop tyrosine has been demonstrated for Btk as well as Itk. For Btk, a study using the chicken DT-40 B cell tumor line showed that Y551 in Btk is essential for Btk-mediated calcium mobilization downstream of the B cell antigen receptor (112). Interestingly, this study also demonstrated that functional Btk activity depends on the presence of both the Lyn and Syk tyrosine kinases (112), suggesting a common mechanism for activating Btk and Itk in response to antigen receptor stimulation in B and T cells, respectively. In the case of T cells, data addressing the functional significance of tyrosine phosphorylation sites is restricted to Itk, where Y511 was shown to be essential for Itk-dependent signaling downstream of the TCR (98).

Following transphosphorylation by a Src family kinase, Tec kinases then autophosphorylate on a conserved tyrosine in the SH3 domain, as has been most notably demonstrated for Btk and Itk (98, 108, 109, 113, 114). Although well-documented at the biochemical level, the functional significance of this autophosphorylation activity has been more difficult to discern. For Btk, mutation of the autophosphorylation site Y223 to phenylalanine has little effect on the ability of

Btk to restore normal calcium mobilization, IP3 production, or PLC-γ2 phosphorylation responses to Btk-deficient DT-40 chicken B cells (112), although it potentiated Btk activity in fibroblasts (108). In contrast, in primary T cells, mutation of the Itk autophosphorylation site Y180 leads to partially impaired Itk activity in response to TCR stimulation (98). Interestingly, these tyrosines are positioned within the substrate-binding surface of the SH3 domains of Btk and Itk (115, 116). This intriguing location suggests that autophosphorylation at this site may be more critical for modulating protein-protein interactions with the Tec kinases, rather than as a mechanism to regulate enzymatic activity. Support for this notion is provided by one study documenting altered ligand-binding properties of the phosphorylated versus nonphosphorylated Btk SH3 domain (117). For instance, c-cbl binding to the Btk SH3 domain is unaffected by phosphorylation at Y223, whereas binding of the Wiskott-Aldrich syndrome protein (WASP) is completely restricted to the nonphosphorylated Btk SH3 domain. In contrast, only the phosphorylated Btk SH3 domain binds to the tyrosine kinase Syk in lysates from activated B cells (117).

REGULATION OF TEC FAMILY KINASE ACTIVITY BY INTRA- AND INTERMOLECULAR INTERACTIONS AMONG TEC KINASE PROTEIN DOMAINS

One additional mechanism regulating Tec family kinase activity is reversible alterations in the tertiary structure of the enzyme. Conformational changes play a critical role in regulating the activities of Src family tyrosine kinases as well as Syk family tyrosine kinases in lymphocytes (118, 119). The most well-characterized of these conformational changes are those described for the Src family tyrosine kinases, where multiple intramolecular interactions serve to stabilize the binding of the C-terminal negative regulatory phosphotyrosine to the SH2 domain of the enzyme (118). In this way, the Src family kinases are maintained in a folded, inactive state prior to receptor stimulation. For Tec family kinases, the regulation of kinase activity by intramolecular domain associations is likely to be distinct from that of Src family kinases, as Tec kinases lack the conserved carboxy-terminal negative regulatory tyrosine phosphorylation site common to Src family kinases. Nonetheless, several pieces of evidence suggest that Tec kinases may also be regulated by conformational changes following receptor stimulation (Figure 1B).

The original finding that suggested an important role for conformational changes regulating Tec kinase activity was the observation that the Itk SH3 and PRR domains fold into an intramolecular structure (115). This intramolecular interaction between the Itk SH3 and PRR regions was also shown to prevent the binding of each domain to its respective ligands (115). Subsequent structural studies demonstrated that Btk and Tec also form intramolecular SH3-PRR complexes, whereas Rlk does not. However, for Btk, Tec, and Rlk, the preferred structure is a homodimer formed via reciprocal SH3-PRR intermolecular interactions, a structure that is not formed by the Itk SH3-PRR protein fragment (120–125). Further complicating this issue, a fragment of Itk containing both the SH2 and SH3 domains, rather than the SH3 and PRR domains, does dimerize in solution in a manner that would preclude the intramolecular association of the Itk PRR to the SH3 domain aromatic binding pocket (126). Thus, for Itk these data suggest the possibility that the dimerization of two Itk molecules by reciprocal SH2-SH3 domain interactions may be an intermediate step in activating the kinase, by displacing the intramolecular SH3 domain–PRR interaction (126).

Alternatively, for Itk as well as for the other Tec kinases, dimerization via reciprocal SH3-SH2 or SH3-PRR associations may represent the inactive state of the enzyme. This latter possibility is supported by data indicating that, for both Btk and Tec, deletion of the SH3 domain results in a dramatic increase in kinase activity (81, 127). Additionally, the PRR regions of Btk, Itk, and Rlk bind to SH3 domains of Src family kinases such as Fyn (59, 77, 128, 129). This interaction is also predicted to disrupt intra- and intermolecular interactions, potentially providing an activation signal. However, unlike Btk and Tec, deletion of the Itk SH3 domain has only a modest effect on Itk kinase activity (130), and mutation of the conserved tryptophan (Itk-W208) that is essential for SH3 domain interactions with PRR ligands has little or no impact on Itk kinase activity (93, 98). An overall view of the domain interactions that regulate Tec kinase activity requires structural data on the full-length proteins to complement the structures already reported on individual Tec kinase domains (41, 42, 71, 115, 116, 120, 122, 123, 125, 126, 131–134).

Another interesting difference between Itk and the other Tec kinase family members is the recent description of a proline-dependent conformational switch within the Itk SH2 domain (132, 135). Surprisingly, the proline involved in this switch is not conserved in any of the other Tec kinase family members (132). However, for the Itk SH2 domain, this conformational switch mediates interconversion of the SH2 domain between one isomer that binds phosphotyrosine-containing ligands and the other isomer that undergoes intermolecular association with the Itk SH3 domain (126, 132, 135, 136). Consequently, this conformational switch has the potential to be a critical element in the regulation of Itk function by modulating the ability of Itk to bind ligands such as SLP-76 and thus to participate in the TCR signaling pathway. Of further interest, Itk was also recently shown to bind to the peptidyl-prolyl isomerase cyclophilin A, an enzyme that catalyzes *cis-trans* proline isomerization, such as that described within the Itk SH2 domain (135). Itk kinase activity is also inhibited by this interaction with cyclophilin A, an effect that could be reversed by treatment with cyclosporine A (135). Consistent with this, T cells from cyclophilin A–deficient mice are hyperresponsive to TCR stimulation and show increased phosphorylation of PLC-γ1 (25). These data suggest another level at which Itk activity might be regulated in T cells.

An X-ray crystal structure of the isolated Itk kinase domain has recently been reported (42). Structures of both the nonphosphorylated and phosphorylated (Y511) kinase domain bound to the broadly active kinase inhibitor staurosporine were determined, in addition to a structure of the unliganded nonphosphorylated kinase domain (42). These data revealed several surprising aspects of the Itk kinase domain structure. First, investigators did not observe any major conformational differences among these three structures of the Itk kinase domain, which indicates that, for Itk, phosphorylation of a residue on the activation loop does not induce a conformational change. However, because Y511 of Itk is absolutely essential for Itk functional activity in primary T cells (98), and phosphorylation of this residue enhances Itk kinase activity (9), there is likely an alternative role for this phosphorylation site in Itk activation.

A second surprising aspect of the Itk kinase domain structures is that all three of these structures resemble the active forms of other protein kinase domains, yet the isolated Itk kinase domain is catalytically inactive (42, 137). Similarly, the isolated kinase domain of Btk is also catalytically inactive (138), an obvious difference from that observed with Src family tyrosine kinases. Additionally, the X-ray crystal structure of the isolated nonphosphorylated Btk kinase domain is strikingly similar to those reported for the Itk kinase domain (41). Together these data suggest a role for additional Tec family kinase protein domains in the formation of a catalytically active enzyme. This notion is consistent with biochemical studies demonstrating that deletion of the Itk PH domain and part of the TH domain reduces Itk kinase activity by 10-fold, whereas mutation of two conserved prolines in the Itk PRR reduces Itk kinase activity by 100-fold (137). Resolution of the three-dimensional structure of the full-length Itk protein would likely explain these surprising findings.

FUNCTIONS OF TEC FAMILY KINASES IN T CELL SIGNALING PATHWAYS

Mutations affecting the Tec family kinases Itk and Rlk lead to impaired responses to TCR stimulation, including proliferation, IL-2 production, and production of effector cytokines (10, 12–15, 25, 26). For proliferation and IL-2 production, defects are minimal in Rlk-deficient cells, moderately severe in $Itk^{-/-}$ cells, and most severe in $Rlk^{-/-}Itk^{-/-}$ cells (10). The rescue of these phenotypes by stimulation with phorbol esters and calcium ionophores suggests that these cells have relatively proximal defects in TCR signaling (10, 12, 13). Accordingly, mutation of these kinases is associated with a variety of biochemical defects downstream of the TCR (Tables 2, 3).

TCR Signaling

Upon TCR stimulation, there is a rapid sequential activation of the Lck and Zap-70 tyrosine kinases, which in turn phosphorylate a number of molecules, including the adapter proteins LAT and SLP-76. These two key adapters serve as a platform for the recruitment of molecules into a signaling complex, including PLC-γ, GRB-2, GADS, ADAP, Vav, Nck, and the Tec kinase Itk (Figure 3) (reviewed in 95,

TABLE 2 Characteristics of the Tec family kinases expressed in T cells[a]

Gene	Localization	TCR	CD28	Chemokines	Substrates	Important for		Rescuing B cell apoptosis
						PLC-γ phosph	NFAT activation	
Itk	Cyto $\rightarrow$ mb via PH; nuclear	Activates[b]	Binds, activates	Activates	PLC-γ, CD28, LAT	Yes	Overexpressed—no; KD blocks; required in vivo	Yes
Rlk	Membrane via palmitoylation; nuclear	Activates	ND	Activates	PLC-γ, SLP-76, CTLA-4?	Yes	ND	No
Tec	Cyto $\rightarrow$ mb via PH and SH3	Activates	Binds, activates	Activates	PLC-γ, Dok1, 2, LARG	Yes	Overexpressed—yes antisense or KD blocks	Yes

[a]ND, not done; KD, kinase dead.
[b]Indicates that TCR, CD28, and chemokines activate these kinases.

TABLE 3 Similar phenotypes of mice deficient in T cell signaling proteins[a]

	Development		Proximal Events			Biochemical Defects			Distal Events	In vivo phenotype					
	Defects in pre-TCR signaling	Defects in repertoire selection	Defects in PLC-g activation	Defects in actin polymerization	Defects in calcium flux	Defects in ERK activation	Defects in NFAT activation	Alterations in cytokine production	Defects in integrin adhesion	CD4+ cells have activated phenotype	CD4+ cells produce Th2-type cytokines	Defects in AICD	Increase in serum IgE/IgG1 levels	Eosinophilia	References
Itk-/-	Mild	Yes	Yes	Yes	Yes	Yes	Yes	IL-2, IL-4, and IFNg ↑	Yes[b]	Yes	reduced	Yes	IgG1: small IgE: 5X	Mild	10–17
Rlk-/-Itk-/-	Mild	Yes	Yes	Yes	Yes	Yes	Yes	Multiple cytokines defective	Yes[b]	Yes	Yes	Yes	IgG1: 5X IgE: 20X	ND	10, 11, 17
SLP-76-/-	Blocked	NA	Yes[c]	Yes[c]	Yes[c]	Yes[c]	Yes[c]	NA	ND	NA	NA	NA	NA	NA	95a
Vav1-/-	Yes	Yes	Yes	Yes	Yes	Yes	Yes	IL-2 →	Yes	ND	Reduced mRNA	ND	ND	ND	168, 204
LATY136F	Blocked	NA	Yes	ND	Yes	No	ND	Most cells produce Th2 cytokines	ND	Yes	80% cells produced IL-4	Yes	IgG1: 200X IgE: 10,000X	Yes	205, 206
PKCq-/-	ND	ND	Yes	Yes	Yes	No	Yes/No	IL-2, IL-4 ↑	ND	ND	No	ND	ND	ND	207–209
WASP-/-	Mild	ND	ND	Yes	Mild	No	Yes	IL-2 →	No	Mild[d]	Yes[e]	ND	ND	ND	210, 211
NFATc1-/-	Yes	ND	NA	NA	NA	NA	ND	IL-4 and IL-6 ↑	ND	No	No	No	No	No	143
NFATc2-/-	No	No	NA	NA	NA	NA	Defective NFATc1 activation	IL-4 ↑	ND	Yes	Yes	Yes	both increased	Yes	143
NFATc3-/-	ND	Yes	NA	NA	NA	NA	ND	No	ND	Yes	No	No, increased AICD	No	ND	143
NFATc1/c2 DKO	ND	ND	NA	NA	NA	NA	No	Multiple cytokines defective	ND	Yes	Yes	Yes	IgG1: 10X IgE: 500X	ND	143
NFATc2/c3 DKO	ND	ND	NA	NA	NA	NA	ND	IL-4 ←	ND	Yes	Yes	Yes	IgG1: 400X IgE: 5,000X	Yes	143

[a] Yellow, shows a defect; grey, not tested (not done, ND); blue, not applicable (NA) (i.e., there are no mature T cells); red, no defect.
[b] L.D. Finkelstein & P. L. Schwartzberg, unpublished results.
[c] In Jurkat J14 SLP-76-deficient cell line.
[d] J. Aoki & P.L. Schwartzberg, unpublished results.
[e] But cytokine not secreted.

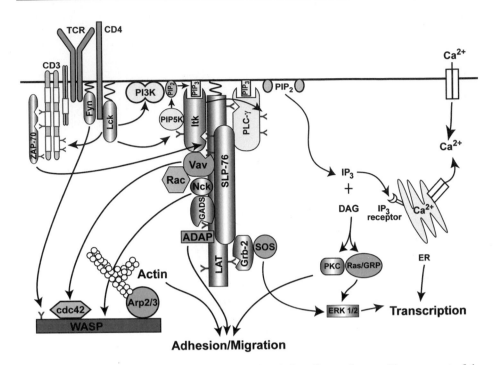

Figure 3   Tec kinases contribute to TCR-mediated signaling pathways. Engagement of the TCR leads to rapid activation of Lck and Zap-70, which phosphorylate numerous downstream targets, including the adapter molecules LAT and SLP-76. Together, these adapters form a platform for the accumulation of molecules into a signaling complex that includes PLC-γ, GRB-2, GADS, Nck, Vav1, ADAP, WASP, Tec family kinases, and other associated molecules. Itk and probably other Tec kinases physically interact with SLP-76 and possibly LAT, bringing it into this complex where it can phosphorylate PLC-γ. Recent data also suggest a role for Itk in regulating Vav1 localization, which further suggests that Itk supports the integrity of the TCR-induced signaling complex. This complex is important for transducing signals that regulate Ca^{2+} mobilization (via PLC-γ and IP_3), PKC and MAPK activation (via DAG and GRB-2-SOS pathways), transcriptional activation, and actin reorganization and cell adhesion (via Vav and its effectors, Rac, Cdc42, and Rho).

95a). For simplicity, we refer to this as one signaling complex, although there are likely multiple independent or linked complexes containing subsets of these and additional proteins. This T cell signaling complex is required for downstream activation of Ca^{2+} mobilization and MAP kinases via activation of PLC-γ and GRB-2-SOS pathways. Mutations affecting the proximal kinases Lck and Zap-70 or the adapters LAT and SLP-76 effectively prevent activation of Ca^{2+} and extracellular-signal-regulated kinase (ERK) pathways downstream of the TCR in cell lines and block T cell development in mice (reviewed in 139). In addition, components of this complex contribute to the regulation of the actin cytoskeleton (95).

In vitro and in vivo studies have demonstrated a number of potential interactions between the Tec family kinases and other components of this signaling complex, including an inducible interaction between the SH2 and SH3 domains of Itk and SLP-76 (77, 91) and interactions with LAT via SH2- and PRR-mediated mechanisms (77, 93, 94). Evidence also suggests potential interactions between Tec family kinases and Vav [via both the Tec TH (69) and Itk SH2 and SH3 domains (77)], GRB-2 [via the Itk and Rlk PRR domains (59, 77)], and PLC-γ [via the Itk SH2 and SH3 domains (97)].

Consistent with a role for Tec kinases in the LAT-SLP-76 signaling complex, initial phosphorylation events, including tyrosine phosphorylation of the TCRζ chain and Zap-70, are normal in $Itk^{-/-}$ and $Rlk^{-/-}Itk^{-/-}$ cells (10, 13). Gross patterns of phosphorylation of many components of this signaling complex, including Vav, SLP-76, Cbl, and WASP, are also normal in these mutant cells (11, 140; L.D. Finkelstein, unpublished). However, the Tec family kinases play a role in the phosphorylation and regulation of PLC-γ1 (10, 13). Accordingly, stimulation of $Itk^{-/-}$ or $Rlk^{-/-}Itk^{-/-}$ T cells with a phorbol ester plus Ca^{2+} ionophore rescues many of their functional defects (10, 13).

REGULATION OF PLC-γ AND Ca^{2+} MOBILIZATION   PLC-γ is a key cellular enzyme that cleaves $PI_{(4,5)}P_2$ to generate two key second messengers, IP_3 and DAG (141). IP_3 binds to receptors on intracellular organelles, leading to the release of intracellular Ca^{2+} stores, which then, via a poorly understood process, triggers the store-operated or Ca^{2+}-release-activated Ca^{2+} channels (CRAC) on the plasma membrane, leading to a prolonged phase of Ca^{2+} influx from extracellular stores (142). This prolonged influx is required for activation of downstream effectors, including the NFAT transcription factors (143). Accordingly, kinase-inactive mutants of either Itk or Tec, or antisense to Tec, block TCR-induced NFAT reporter activation (8, 56, 63, 77) (see Table 2).

Initial studies of B cells deficient in Btk or T cells deficient in Itk or Rlk and Itk suggest that these kinases play a major role in the regulation of PLC-γ and IP_3 production. Btk-deficient clones of the DT-40 cell line show absent tyrosine phosphorylation of PLC-γ2 (the major isoform in B cells) (144). Although cells from XLA patients do not necessarily show reduced levels of total tyrosine phosphorylation of PLC-γ2, they do show defective phosphorylation of Y753 and Y759, two critical regulatory tyrosines (145, 146). Both thymocytes and mature T cells from $Itk^{-/-}$ and $Rlk^{-/-}Itk^{-/-}$ cells show reduced phosphorylation of PLC-γ1, particularly on the regulatory tyrosine Y783 (10, 11, 13, 98; P.L. Schwartzberg, unpublished). Moreover, studies in heterologous cells argue that Rlk, Itk, and Btk can all directly phosphorylate PLC-γ1 (98, 145, 147).

Accordingly, T cells that are deficient in Itk or Itk and Rlk show reduced TCR-induced IP_3 production and Ca^{2+} mobilization. In both thymocytes and mature T cells, Ca^{2+} mobilization appears to be most affected in the late stage of prolonged

Ca^{2+} influx from extracellular stores (10, 11, 13). Stimulation in the presence of EGTA leads to similar intracellular Ca^{2+} levels in wild-type and mutant cells, parallel to findings in Btk-deficient B cells (145). Internal stores of Ca^{2+} appear to be intact, at least in Itk-deficient T cells (13), as demonstrated by studies using EGTA plus thapsigargan, an inhibitor of Ca^{2+} reuptake by the ER Ca^{2+}-sensitive ATPase (148). Moreover, depletion of intracellular stores of Ca^{2+} with thapsigargan alone, which can stimulate CRAC channels and lead to an influx from extracellular sources, also gave similar responses in $Itk^{-/-}$, $Rlk^{-/-}Itk^{-/-}$, and wild-type T cells (13; E.M. Schaeffer & P.S. Schwartzberg, unpublished), suggesting that there is not a defect in the mechanism of coupling of intracellular Ca^{2+} stores to extracellular influx. The defect in Ca^{2+} influx has therefore been attributed to the decreased IP_3 production (13), which may not be sufficient to maintain depletion of intracellular stores required for prolonged triggering of CRAC channels in these cells (149).

Although studies of $Itk^{-/-}$ T cells argue that Itk is the major kinase involved in PLC-γ regulation, mutation of both Rlk and Itk can worsen the Ca^{2+} defect in Itk-deficient cells, even though Rlk-deficient cells show little if any effects on Ca^{2+} in response to TCR stimulation (10). Similarly, overexpression of Rlk can partially rescue the Ca^{2+} defect in Itk-deficient cells, suggesting that there is some degree of functional redundancy between these kinases (61).

How Tec contributes to these pathways in T cells remains less clear. However, a recent paper argued that in preactivated cells, Tec participates in regulation of PLC-γ1 and Ca^{2+} mobilization downstream of PKCθ (150). Whether such a pathway operates in naive cells is not clear.

DAG-MEDIATED PATHWAYS   The second major product of PLC-γ is DAG, which can activate members of the PKC family (151). In B cells, numerous cross-regulatory connections between Btk and PKC family members have been demonstrated (see above). Although PKC activation has not been directly examined in T cells from $Itk^{-/-}$ and $Rlk^{-/-}Itk^{-/-}$ mice, PMA plus anti-CD3 stimulation can rescue proliferation of T cells from $Itk^{-/-}$ and $Rlk^{-/-}Itk^{-/-}$ mice, evidence of a major role for DAG-mediated defects in their phenotypes (10). As discussed above, a recent paper argues that Tec is involved in the impaired activation PLC-γ1 observed in $PKC\theta^{-/-}$ T cells (150). This same paper describes a downstream defect in the activation of PKCα in $PKC\theta^{-/-}$ cells, which the authors attribute to the defective PLC-γ activation.

In T cells, another important effector of DAG is Ras-GRP, a novel activator of the Ras/Raf/MAPK pathway in T cells (95). Consistent with a predicted decrease in DAG production, T cells deficient in Itk or Rlk and Itk show reduced activation of ERK in response to either anti-CD3 or antigen stimulation (10, 11, 15). JNK activation was also abnormal in $Itk^{-/-}$ mature T lymphocytes after stimulation with antigen (15). In contrast, activation of the p38 MAPK, which may rely more on GRB-2-mediated pathways, appeared relatively normal in thymocytes of $Rlk^{-/-}Itk^{-/-}$ mice (11), although this has not been examined in mature cells or under conditions of antigen stimulation.

Mutational analyses argue that kinase activity, the major Src family phosphorylation site in the kinase domain, and SH3 domains are all required for Itk function, including ERK activation and IL-2 production downstream of TCR signaling (98). Overexpression of kinase-inactive Itk constructs can block activation of a NFAT reporter construct and phosphorylation of PLC-γ1 (58, 77). Moreover, the autophosphorylation site contributes to the efficiency of proper Itk function (98). Together these data support the critical function of tyrosine phosphorylation for Itk function. For Btk, function of the SH2 domain, which interacts with BLNK/SLP-65, is also required for rescue of Btk-deficient cells (144). This is also likely to be the case for Itk, which requires a functional SH2 domain for its activation (93), suggesting that both phosphorylation and protein interactions are critical for Itk function.

OTHER CONTRIBUTIONS TO PLC-γ ACTIVATION   Phosphorylation may not be the only mechanism by which Tec family kinases regulate PLC-γ. In B cells, overexpression of a kinase-inactive Btk can increase Ca^{2+} mobilization in cell lines (152, 153). The recent finding that the PH domain of Btk can assist in the shuttling of phosphatidylinositol 4-phosphate 5-kinase (PIP5K) to the plasma membrane suggests that the Tec kinases may potentiate signaling by providing more $PI_{(4,5)}P_2$, the substrate for PLC-γ (84). In this study, the PH domain of Tec was also found to bind PIP5K in vitro, suggesting that multiple Tec kinases may be able to influence this pathway of phosphoinositide regulation.

Tec kinases may also contribute to phosphorylation of other components in LAT-SLP-76 signaling complexes. Overexpression studies suggest that Rlk can phosphorylate SLP-76 and potentiate SLP-76-mediated activation of ERK and expression of an NFAT/AP1 reporter construct (60). In vitro expression studies suggest that Itk can phosphorylate LAT on Y171 and Y191, two distal tyrosines that may be involved in recruitment of Vav and GRB-2 (154). Expression of a kinase-inactive Itk decreased phosphorylation of LAT and the amount of Vav in LAT coimmunoprecipitates. These observations, combined with the multiple potential interactions of Tec kinases with other components of TCR signaling, suggest that the Tec kinases contribute to the integrity of signaling complexes, an idea that is revisited below in the discussion of actin cytoskeleton regulation.

Tec FAMILY KINASES AS MODULATORS OF TCR SIGNALING   Mutations   affecting both Rlk and Itk do not eliminate PLC-γ phosphorylation and Ca^{2+} mobilization but rather reduce the efficiency of these processes. These data may result from functional redundancy between Tec family kinases and the presence of Tec in the $Rlk^{-/-}Itk^{-/-}$ cells. Alternatively, there may be multiple kinases that contribute to these activation pathways, including Lck, Fyn, and Zap-70. These observations have generated the notion that Tec kinases do not act as triggers of TCR signaling like the more proximal kinases Lck and Zap-70, nor as gatekeepers like the adapter molecules LAT and SLP-76. Rather, Tec family kinases modulate or amplify the efficiency of downstream TCR signaling (155, 156). Indeed, one study using single-cell imaging of cells that express kinase-inactive mutants of Lck or Itk found that expression of these mutants produced very different responses. Cells that express kinase-inactive Lck either did not flux Ca^{2+} or fully fluxed Ca^{2+}, depending on the amount of kinase-inactive Lck expressed (157). In contrast, cells that express kinase-inactive Itk had reduced Ca^{2+} flux per cell. Thus, Tec kinases may be seen as modulators of T cell responses, a view that is consistent with their effects on T cell development and mature T helper cell differentiation (see below).

There is some degree of functional redundancy among the Tec family kinases in the activation of PLC-γ, but evidence nonetheless suggests that Itk, Rlk, and Tec each have distinct properties and mechanisms of activation (Table 2). Rlk, Itk, Tec, and Bmx can all rescue PLC-γ phosphorylation and Ca^{2+} mobilization to varying degrees in Btk-deficient DT-40 cells, yet Rlk fails to rescue BCR-induced apoptosis, highlighting the differences between this kinase and the other Tec family members (62). Moreover, overexpression of Tec but not Itk can activate an NFAT reporter construct in Jurkat cells, and can do so independently of the LAT and SLP-76 adapters, which supports the view that Tec may interact in these pathways via different intermediates (8, 35). Such a view is consistent with the distinct patterns of localization and substrates for these kinases, including SLP-76 for Rlk and Dok1 and Dok2 for Tec (6, 8, 35, 60). A recent paper also raises the possibility that differential sensitivities to the inhibitors PTEN and SHIP may contribute to functional differences between Itk and Tec (81a).

Tec Kinases and Actin Cytoskeletal Reorganization

Another major function of TCR signaling is the reorganization of the actin cytoskeleton, which contributes to the accumulation of signaling molecules to the site of TCR stimulation and the generation of the immune synapse (158). Several recent reports have demonstrated that the Tec family kinase Itk is required for actin polymerization and polarization downstream of TCR engagement.

An initial study showed that expression of mutant forms of Itk, including a kinase-inactive mutant and the isolated PH domain, blocked anti-CD3-stimulated actin polymerization in Jurkat T cells (19). Similar results were reported for a mutant affecting the Itk SH2 domain (27). Importantly, actin polymerization and polarization to either anti-TCR-coated beads or peptide-pulsed antigen presenting cells (APCs) were markedly impaired in T cells from both $Itk^{-/-}$ and $Rlk^{-/-}Itk^{-/-}$ mice (27, 28). In these systems, both $Itk^{-/-}$ and $Rlk^{-/-}Itk^{-/-}$ T cells are equally defective, evidence that these phenotypes are attributable to the lack of Itk (28). Interestingly, these phenotypes appear more severe than the Ca^{2+} mobilization defects in $Itk^{-/-}$ cells, with virtually no increase in actin polarization observed upon exposure to antigen. Whether this is due to differences in the sensitivities of the actin polarization and Ca^{2+} assays remains to be evaluated.

The requirement of Itk for TCR-mediated actin polarization suggests that Itk deficiency may affect other actin-dependent processes, including the recruitment of proteins required for formation of the immune synapse. Indeed, polarization of Vav1 to the site of contact with peptide-pulsed APCs was abnormal in $Itk^{-/-}$ T cells (28). In addition, studies using $Itk^{-/-}$ T cells conjugated to anti-TCR-coated beads reveal defective localization of multiple synapse-associated proteins, including PKCθ, the β2 integrin LFA-1, and the cytoskeletal protein talin (L.D. Finkelstein & P.L. Schwartzberg, unpublished).

Another process that requires an intact actin cytoskeleton is the TCR-mediated increase in integrin adhesion. Upon engagement of the TCR, integrin-mediated adhesion is upregulated via a poorly understood process known as "inside-out" signaling, which involves PI3K, PKCs, the adapter molecule ADAP, the GTPase Rap1, Vav1, and actin cytoskeletal reorganization (159). Recent data also implicate the Tec family kinase Itk in this process. Jurkat T cells expressing either a kinase-inactive mutant or the PH domain of Itk were blocked in anti-CD3-stimulated β1 adhesion to the extracellular matrix protein fibronectin (19). Expression of a membrane-targeted mutant of Itk could stimulate adhesion in cells stimulated with anti-CD4, which activates Lck but does not stimulate adhesion on its own. Conversely, expression of kinase-inactive Itk blocked adhesion that was stimulated by expression of an activated p110 PI3K construct in conjunction with anti-CD4 stimulation, evidence that Itk is a major effector of PI3K-mediated increases in adhesion. Itk is also critical for TCR-induced integrin adhesion in primary mouse T cells. Itk-deficient T cells show defective conjugate formation to antigen-pulsed APCs (28) and anti-CD3-stimulated upregulation of β2 integrin adhesion (L.D. Finkelstein & P.L. Schwartzberg, unpublished). Similarly, Btk is required for integrin-mediated adhesion downstream of the B cell receptor by a process involving cytoskeletal reorganization (160). A role for Tec kinases in signaling to the actin cytoskeleton downstream from integrins is also suggested from studies of Etk/Bmx in other cell types (161, 162).

BIOCHEMICAL REQUIREMENTS FOR ACTIN CYTOSKELETON REGULATION: EFFECTS ON THE WISKOTT-ALDRICH SYNDROME PROTEIN (WASP)   Evidence suggests that Tec kinases can interact with several proteins involved in assembly of the actin cytoskeleton. WASP is a key actin regulatory protein. WASP activates the Arp2/3 complex that helps nucleate new actin filaments (163). In vitro data demonstrate that the SH3 domains of both Itk and Btk can interact with the PRR of WASP (117, 164, 165). Additionally, Btk was found to phosphorylate WASP in a Cdc42-dependent fashion, suggesting that WASP was a downstream effector of Tec family kinases (166, 167).

Evidence suggests that WASP may be activated by two mechanisms: (a) binding of WASP to activated Cdc42-GTP, which induces an open conformation of the protein that can then bind to Arp2/3 (163); and/or (b) phosphorylation of tyrosine 291 (140). A recent study demonstrated that $Itk^{-/-}$ T cells stimulated with APCs plus peptide show reduced binding to an antibody that recognizes the open conformation of WASP. Stimulated $Itk^{-/-}$ T cells also show defective activation of Cdc42 at the site of contact with the APC, as detected with a GFP fusion of the WASP GTPase-binding domain (28). However, another study has demonstrated normal phosphorylation of tyrosine 291 of WASP in $Itk^{-/-}$ T cells, suggesting that WASP activation is intact in these cells (140). Although the contributions of Cdc42 and tyrosine phosphorylation for activation of WASP in T cells merit further study, the data above suggest that Itk is unlikely to act directly on WASP but rather contributes to the regulation of Cdc42.

EFFECTS ON Vav   In T cells, a critical factor for Cdc42 activation is the guanine nucleotide exchange factor Vav1, which is rapidly activated by tyrosine phosphorylation upon TCR stimulation (168). Vav1-deficient T cells have defective TCR-mediated activation of Rac and Cdc42 and, like $Itk^{-/-}$ cells, show defects in both TCR-driven actin polarization and integrin adhesion (76, 169, 170). In contrast, in at least one study, WASP was dispensable for regulation of integrin-mediated adhesion and clustering of integrins (169). Vav1 interacts with several signaling proteins involved in the T cell signaling complex, including SLP-76, LAT, and the Tec kinases (77, 95, 95a, 154). Data in other cell types suggest that Tec binds to Vav via its TH domain and can phosphorylate Vav, resulting in enhanced GEF activity for Rac (68, 69).

Although $Itk^{-/-}$ and $Rlk^{-/-}Itk^{-/-}$ T cells show normal gross patterns of tyrosine phosphorylation of Vav (11), studies of $Itk^{-/-}$ and $Rlk^{-/-}Itk^{-/-}$ T cells demonstrated a failure of Vav to localize to the site of contact with the APC (28). These data suggest that Itk may help control the recruitment or stabilization of Vav1 into the TCR signaling complex. Expression of a membrane-targeted prenylated mutant of Vav1 can partially rescue the actin polarization defect in Jurkat T cells treated with siRNA to Itk (212), supporting the idea that the defect in Vav1 localization directly contributes to the actin defects in Itk-deficient cells. Whether this altered localization affects activity or phosphorylation of specific tyrosine residues of Vav1 in Itk-deficient cells remains to be determined.

Itk may assist in the regulation of Vav1 localization by several potential mechanisms. One study argues that Itk can phosphorylate LAT on tyrosines 171 and 191, thus promoting a Vav1-LAT interaction, which is impaired in cells expressing a kinase-inactive mutant of Itk (154). However, the requirement for Itk kinase catalytic activity in TCR-mediated actin polymerization is not clear (19, 27). One study reported that a kinase-inactivating point mutant of Itk blocks actin polymerization (19), while two other studies argue that kinase-inactivating point mutants do not block actin polarization and polymerization (27, 157). Indeed, such data was originally used to argue that Itk was not involved in regulation of the actin cytoskeleton (157). Although it remains unclear why these studies vary from each other, differences may reflect levels of Itk mutants expressed or the cell lines and actual mutant constructs used.

The recent demonstration that an SH2 mutant of Itk can efficiently block actin polarization suggests that protein interactions may be important for Itk's functions in regulating the actin cytoskeleton (27). Itk can interact with SLP-76 and potentially with LAT via its SH2 domain (95, 95a, 154). Vav also interacts with these molecules, raising the possibility that Itk functions as an adapter, helping to stabilize interactions of Vav within this signaling complex. Vav and Itk directly bind each other, as do Vav and Tec (212). Whether Itk deficiency alters the interactions of Vav1 with another protein in this signaling complex awaits further experimental investigation.

OTHER POTENTIAL EFFECTORS OF ACTIN AND ADHESION DEFECTS   Whether mislocalization of Vav is the only cause of the actin and adhesion defects in Itk-deficient cells remains unclear. As discussed above, Tec kinases can also influence activation of PKCs, members of which affect actin cytoskeleton dynamics and T cell adhesion (86). Tec kinases also contribute to the regulation of PIP5K (84). Intriguingly, many actin regulatory proteins, including WASP, gelsolin, α-actinin, and profilin, are regulated by binding of $PI_{(4,5)}P_2$, the product of PIP5K (171). Recruitment of PIP5K via its interactions with a Tec kinase could help recruit and locally activate actin-binding proteins at the site of TCR stimulation, thereby contributing to the establishment and stabilization of cell polarization (172).

Finally, the role of Ca^{2+} in these processes cannot be underestimated. Intracellular Ca^{2+} levels contribute to the regulation of actin reorganization and integrin adhesion, in part through the activation of the Ca^{2+}-sensitive protease calpain. Calpain can cleave actin-binding proteins, which permits reorganization of the actin cytoskeleton and clustering of integrins and thereby increases adhesive contacts (173). How Itk deficiency affects these processes has not yet been evaluated.

CONSEQUENCES FOR T CELL PHENOTYPES   The regulation of the actin cytoskeleton and adhesion by Itk suggests that the phenotypes of Itk-deficient cells may not solely arise from biochemical defects in PLC-γ activation. Although the biochemical defects in Itk-deficient T cells are less severe, they resemble those observed in Vav1-deficient T cells, including decreased activation of PLC-γ, ERK, and downstream transcription factors (168) (see Table 3). Moreover, many of the phenotypes of Itk-deficient T cells, including impaired thymic selection, altered CD4:CD8 ratios, and decreased proliferation and cytokine production (10–12, 15, 16), may be accounted for by decreased duration of signaling that results from decreased actin polarization and integrin-mediated adhesion (Figure 4). Nonetheless, Itk activation is also impaired in Vav-deficient cells (76), highlighting the many levels of feedback among molecules in TCR signaling, where linear relationships are not always easily drawn. Whether Tec kinases contribute to the regulation of Vav family members in B cells and how this may influence the phenotype of Btk-deficient B cells remains an intriguing question. Overexpression of activated Btk, Itk, or Tec can increase membrane ruffle/lamellopodia and actin stress fiber formation (82, 174, 175). Evidence from *Drosophila* also demonstrates a role for Tec29 in formation of an actin-based structure, the ring canal (176). Finally, Btk can associate with F-actin itself via basic residues in the Btk PH domain (177).

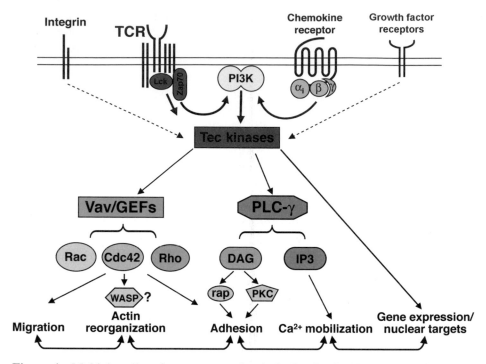

Figure 4   Multiple cell surface receptors signal via Tec family kinases. Tec kinases are activated downstream of antigen receptors (TCR and surface immunoglobulin) and G protein–coupled chemokine receptors through the actions of PI3K and Src family kinases. In other cell types, Tec family kinases are also activated by integrins and growth factor receptors. Tec kinases regulate multiple cellular functions, including activation of PLC-γ and actin cytoskeleton reorganization, which in turn help to regulate Ca^{2+} mobilization, activation of PKCs, MAPK, and downstream transcription factors, as well as cell adhesion and migration.

CD28 Signaling

As with TCR engagement, stimulation through the CD28 receptor induces tyrosine phosphorylation and activation of Itk (see above and Table 2) (48–51). A recent study suggests that Itk activation downstream of CD28 is involved in the amplification of TCR-mediated signals, leading to Ca^{2+} mobilization (178). Stimulation of Jurkat cells expressing a tail-less mutant of CD28 led to impaired PLC-γ phosphorylation and Ca^{2+} mobilization, which correlated with decreased phosphorylation of Itk and could be partially overcome by overexpression of Itk. Nonetheless, data from another study showed increased responsiveness of Itk-deficient T cells to anti-CD28 stimulation, supporting the idea that Itk plays a negative regulatory role in CD28 signaling (179). Although this study did not examine the biochemical mechanism of this response, this work suggests that Itk may have distinct roles downstream of CD3 and CD28. However, interpretations of this study may be complicated by the high numbers of previously activated or memory (i.e., CD44^{hi}) CD4$^+$ T cells present in $Itk^{-/-}$ compared with wild-type mice. CD44^{hi} CD4$^+$ T cells are hyperresponsive to stimulation relative to naive CD4$^+$ T cells, and may thus have biased the outcome of the proliferation assays performed in this study (C.M. Li & L.J. Berg, unpublished observation). Thus, the precise role of Itk in CD28 signaling awaits further study.

Although an initial study cited normal responses to CD28 costimulation in Tec-deficient T cells (36), other reports have shown that Tec, like Itk, is capable of binding CD28 and is activated upon CD28 engagement (8, 64) (see Table 2). One of the proteins phosphorylated in response to CD28 stimulation is p62 Dok (Dok1), a RasGAP-associated adapter (8). Tec and Dok1 interact in heterologous cells, and kinase-inactive Tec can block tyrosine phosphorylation of Dok1 downstream of growth factor receptors and the BCR (180, 181). Recent data suggest that Dok1 may participate in negative feedback regulation of Tec (80). Co-expression in heterologous cells demonstrates that Tec but not Itk can tyrosine phosphorylate Dok1 (8). Overexpression of Tec, but not Itk, also enhances transcription of an IL-2 reporter construct in response to anti-CD28 plus PMA stimulation (8). Moreover, only kinase-inactive Tec, not kinase-inactive Itk, could block expression of the IL-2 reporter construct and IL-2 production in response to anti-CD28 plus PMA stimulation. Thus, Tec kinases are implicated in signaling pathways emanating from both the TCR and costimulatory receptors, although their actions may differ downstream in these signaling pathways.

Finally, there are conflicting reports on the ability of Rlk to phosphorylate CTLA-4 in in vitro and coexpression systems (60, 182). As discussed above, Itk is also activated in response to CD2 and may participate in NFAT activation downstream of this adhesive receptor (54, 56). However, the in vivo functional correlates of these observations are unclear.

Effects on Transcription

As described above, T cells containing mutations of Itk or Itk and Rlk exhibit defective activation of TCR signaling intermediates. Accordingly, these mutant T cells also display defective nuclear localization and activation of multiple transcription factors. Consistent with their defects in prolonged Ca^{2+} mobilization, both $Itk^{-/-}$ and $Rlk^{-/-}Itk^{-/-}$ T cells show decreased activation of the Ca^{2+}-sensitive NFAT transcription factors (14, 17). In particular, activation of both NFATc1, which is important for Th2 cytokine production, and NFATc2, which regulates transcription of the Egr family of transcription factors are severely impaired in both $Itk^{-/-}$ and $Rlk^{-/-}Itk^{-/-}$ T cells. Indeed, phenotypes of $Itk^{-/-}$ and $Rlk^{-/-}Itk^{-/-}$ mice resemble those of mice harboring mutations in some NFAT family members (183) (Table 3). Consistent with the decreased ERK and JNK phosphorylation observed in $Itk^{-/-}$ and $Rlk^{-/-}Itk^{-/-}$ T cells (15, 17), decreased activation of AP-1 has also been observed (17).

Although activation of NF-κB is defective in Btk-deficient B cells (38), the role of Tec kinases in activation of NF-κB in T lymphocytes is less clear. Two groups have reported relatively normal activation of this transcription factor in $Itk^{-/-}$ and $Rlk^{-/-}Itk^{-/-}$ T cells, which has been attributed to their less severe effects on early Ca^{2+} mobilization (10, 14). However, this question may need to be readdressed under different conditions of stimulation given defective localization of PKCθ observed in $Itk^{-/-}$ cells (L.D. Finkelstein & P.L. Schwartzberg, unpublished) and the importance of PKCθ for NF-κB activation in T cells (95, 95a).

A recent paper has demonstrated that Tec kinases also contribute to the BCR-mediated activation of serum response factor (SRF) in B cells via a Lyn-Syk-Btk-PLC-γ-mediated pathway that requires Rho family GTPases (184). The role of Tec kinases in regulation of SRF in T cells has not yet been examined.

Finally, studies of T helper cell differentiation have implicated both Itk and Rlk in the regulation of GATA-3 and T-bet (see below), although these effects are likely to be secondary to their effects on activation of the above transcriptional pathways (17, 26).

DIRECT EFFECTS ON TRANSCRIPTION   In addition to these indirect effects on transcription factor activation, Tec kinases may also directly influence transcription in the nucleus. Upon TCR stimulation, a major portion of Rlk traffics to the nucleus (6). Kashiwakura and colleagues (33, 185) have found that overexpression of Rlk can transactivate an IFN-γ reporter construct, an effect that requires nuclear localization and phosphorylation of Rlk. A subsequent study from this group has demonstrated direct binding of Rlk to a region of the IFN-γ promoter (89). Whether Rlk phosphorylates another protein binding to the IFN-γ promoter or has a direct effect on transcription is not clear.

Although nuclear localization is most dramatic for Rlk, other studies have suggested that both Btk and Itk can also translocate to the nucleus (90, 186). For Itk, an interaction with the nuclear import chaperone karyopherin/Rch1α has been demonstrated (90). This interaction requires proline 242 of Rch1α. Expression of a P242A mutant of Rch1α decreased both nuclear localization of Itk and CD3-mediated IL-2 production. Btk has been shown to phosphorylate two transcription factors, the basal transcription factor TF-IIi and Bright, which contributes to Ig gene transcription (186, 187).

Chemokine Signaling

Recent studies have demonstrated that stimulation of cells with the chemokine SDF-1α or the chemoattractant fMet-Leu-Phe (fMLP) can induce translocation and activation of Tec kinases, including Btk, Tec, and Itk (57, 58, 174, 188, 189). Accordingly, Itk is required for T cell migration and increased adhesion in response to SDF-1α (57, 58). Defects in migration are worsened by lack of both Itk and Rlk, similar to findings in TCR signaling (58). In vivo data demonstrate defective recruitment of Itk-deficient cells into airways in an allergic asthma model or in response to SDF-1α (18, 57). Other data show defective localization of $Rlk^{-/-}$ $Itk^{-/-}$ cells in lymphoid organs upon transfer to intact wild-type animals (58). Moreover, although $Rlk^{-/-} Itk^{-/-}$ mice have normal numbers of thymocytes, they show decreased T cell numbers in peripheral lymph nodes (58), supporting a defect in T cell migration in vivo. Similarly, a Btk inhibitor decreases neutrophil migration in response to fMLP (188).

Cellular and biochemical studies have demonstrated that overexpression of a kinase-inactive mutant of Itk in Jurkat cells blocked SDF-1α-induced cell polarization and activation of Rac and Cdc42 (58). Thus, Tec kinases play a role in regulating Rho family GTPases, cell polarization, and adhesion downstream of chemokine receptors as well as the TCR. These data are consistent with previous studies demonstrating a role for Tec kinases in regulating Rho family GTPases during chemotaxis, collagen signaling, and integrin signaling in non-T cell systems, such as neutrophils and platelets (65). Although it is not clear how Tec kinases influence activation of Rho family GTPases in chemokine signaling, it is of interest whether this involves the regulation of Vav or another GEF. Tec is implicated in the activation of the leukemia-associated RhoGEF (LARG) (190), suggesting that Tec kinases contribute to the regulation of multiple Rho family GTPases.

TEC KINASES IN T CELL DEVELOPMENT

A critical role for Tec family kinases in lymphocyte development first became evident with the discovery of Btk. Although investigators have not found naturally occurring mutations in Itk, Rlk, or Tec, mice deficient in one or more of these Tec kinase family members have been generated, confirming a role for these proteins in T cell development (10–13).

Roles in Positive Selection

The generation of mice deficient in Itk, (12, 13), Rlk (10), or Tec (36) demonstrate that Itk is the dominant Tec kinase in T cell development and function. Initial analyses of Itk-deficient mice revealed a normal distribution of all T cell subsets, except for a smaller percentage and total number of CD4$^+$ T cells in both the thymus and periphery (12). Thus, there were not any profound blocks in T cell development in the absence of Itk. However, when Itk-deficient mice were crossed to either AND (H2^b) or H-Y TCR transgenic lines, very few CD4 or CD8 single positive (SP) thymocytes, respectively, developed, indicating a role for Itk in positive selection events in the thymus (12). Mice deficient in both Itk and Rlk were subsequently crossed to the same TCR transgenic lines. In this case, an even more profound defect in CD4 or CD8 SP maturation was observed, providing evidence that a deficiency in Rlk exacerbates the defects in positive selection seen in the absence of Itk (11). A later study examining the role of Itk in the thymic selection of a wider array of TCR specificities confirmed that positive selection into the CD4 lineage is always less efficient in the absence of Itk than in its presence, although the magnitude of the defect varied with the avidity of each TCR analyzed (16).

Roles in Negative Selection

Several independent lines of evidence indicate that Tec family kinases are also important for TCR signaling, leading to negative selection in the thymus. The first studies of this issue examined H-Y TCR transgenic male mice, in which the MHC class I–restricted male-specific antigen is ubiquitously expressed. Examination of Itk-deficient H-Y TCR transgenic male mice initially suggested that the absence of Itk had virtually no effect on negative selection (12). However, a subsequent study of $Itk^{-/-}$ and $Rlk^{-/-}Itk^{-/-}$ H-Y TCR transgenic male mice indicated that, in the absence of Itk or both Itk and Rlk, there is a decreased efficiency of negative selection (11). This latter study demonstrated that the absolute numbers of $CD8^+$ $H\text{-}Y^+$ peripheral T cells increased in $Rlk^{-/-}Itk^{-/-}$ mice compared with controls, indicating a true failure of negative selection. Overall, these data suggest that in the absence of both Itk and Rlk, reduced TCR signaling results in a switch from negative selection to positive selection of $H\text{-}Y^+$ thymocytes (11).

The results of studies on negative selection were less clear-cut for several MHC class II–specific systems. For example, several $V\beta3^+$ TCR transgenic lines (AND, 2B4, 5C.C7) were crossed to $Itk^{-/-}$ mice, and negative selection mediated by an endogenous mouse mammary tumor virus superantigen was examined (183). In addition, negative selection of 5C.C7 TCR transgenic thymocytes was examined in $Itk^{-/-}$ mice that were also expressing a low level of the cognate antigen for this TCR, moth cytochrome c (183, 191). In none of these cases did the number of TCR transgenic peripheral $CD4^+$ T cells ever increase in mice lacking Itk compared with wild-type controls. These findings indicated that, for the MHC class II–specific self-reactive TCRs examined, a deficiency in Itk may delay, but does not block, negative selection. Clear defects in negative selection may only result from the simultaneous absence of Itk and Rlk.

The defects in both positive and negative selection observed in the absence of Itk and/or Rlk are consistent with the known functions of Tec family kinases in T cell signaling and the role of these signaling pathways in thymic selection. As had first been described for peripheral T cells, $Itk^{-/-}$ and $Rlk^{-/-}Itk^{-/-}$ thymocytes have impaired calcium mobilization and reduced activation of the ERK MAP-kinases in response to TCR stimulation (11). Optimal calcium signaling is required for both positive and negative selection, whereas the activation of ERK1/2 is essential only for positive selection (139). Interestingly, the activation of another MAP-kinase, p38, is important for negative selection, but not positive selection (192). In contrast to the ERK MAP-kinases, p38 activation in response to TCR stimulation in thymocytes does not require the Tec family kinases Itk or Rlk (11). Overall, these data predict that positive selection is more impaired than negative selection in Tec family kinase–deficient mice, a prediction that seems supported by the available data on this topic.

Effects on Lineage Development and Commitment

Concurrent with repertoire selection, signaling through the TCR is also thought to influence the commitment of thymocytes to either the CD8 or CD4 lineage, depending on the MHC class I versus class II specificity of their TCR. Signaling proteins both upstream and downstream of Itk, such as Lck and ERK1/2, respectively, are important in the CD4/CD8 lineage decision (193). These data, along with the observation that $Itk^{-/-}$ and $Rlk^{-/-}Itk^{-/-}$ mice have altered CD4:CD8 ratios in the thymus and periphery (10, 12, 13, 155), raise the question of whether Tec family kinases are involved in this developmental process. However, in five separate model systems studied, researchers did not detect any alterations in CD4/CD8 lineage commitment (16).

Aspects of T cell differentiation other than CD4/CD8 lineage commitment are altered in $Itk^{-/-}$ and $Rlk^{-/-}Itk^{-/-}$ mice. For instance, $Itk^{-/-}$ mice have roughly one half the normal numbers of CD4$^+$ T cells (12). In light of recent evidence that CD4$^+$ T cell differentiation depends not only on the strength of the TCR signal but also on the consistency and duration of that signal (194), the disruption of this process in the absence of Itk seems reasonable. However, $Rlk^{-/-}Itk^{-/-}$ mice have no reductions in the percentage or numbers of CD4$^+$ T cells compared with wild-type mice (10). This latter observation may reflect that defects in negative selection balance out defects in CD4$^+$ T cell selection and differentiation in $Rlk^{-/-}Itk^{-/-}$ mice, which results in an overall similar frequency of selectable TCRs in these mice compared with wild-type controls. This notion also predicts that the CD4$^+$ T cells present in $Rlk^{-/-}Itk^{-/-}$ mice are comprised of a different repertoire of TCR specificities than is seen in wild-type mice. In contrast, $Itk^{-/-}$ mice have near-normal numbers of CD8$^+$ peripheral T cells and a higher percentage and total number of CD8 SP cells in the thymus. Even more strikingly, $Rlk^{-/-}Itk^{-/-}$ mice have increased numbers of CD8$^+$ thymocytes and peripheral T cells. Furthermore, the phenotypes of the CD8$^+$ thymocytes and T cells in both $Itk^{-/-}$ and $Rlk^{-/-}Itk^{-/-}$ mice are unique in that they have a memory or previously activated T cell phenotype (16). These latter findings indicate that Itk and/or Rlk play an as-yet-undefined role in CD8$^+$ T cell differentiation and homeostasis.

A role for Itk and/or Rlk in CD4$^+$ T cell homeostasis is also likely as $Itk^{-/-}$ and $Rlk^{-/-}Itk^{-/-}$ mice have two- to threefold increases in the percentage of memory/activated-phenotype peripheral CD4$^+$ T cells (15, 183). One recent study reports that the development and survival of a nonconventional T cell subset, NKT cells, is also impaired in the absence of Itk (195). Interestingly, this defect manifested as an accumulation of immature NKT cells in $Itk^{-/-}$ mice. This study also concluded that Itk may be important in the peripheral homeostasis of

NKT cells, on the basis of the findings that NKT cells are progressively lost as $Itk^{-/-}$ mice age.

Effects on Pre-TCR Signaling

Although an important role for Tec family kinases in the later, TCR-dependent stages of T cell development in the thymus has been clearly demonstrated, no obvious defects in pre-TCR signaling have been observed in the absence of Itk and/or Rlk (10, 12, 16, 155). At the $CD3^-CD4^-CD8^-$ (triple negative; TN) stage of thymocyte development, proper signals downstream of the pre-TCR are required for cells to progress to the double positive (DP) stage. Numerous signaling proteins, such as Lck, LAT, and SLP-76, all of which are part of the same TCR signaling pathway as the Tec family kinases, are crucial for proper T cell development at this stage (196). Interference with, or elimination of, any of these proteins generally leads to a severe block in T cell development at the TN-DP transition (Table 3). In both $Itk^{-/-}$ and $Rlk^{-/-}Itk^{-/-}$ mice, approximately normal numbers of DP thymocytes are observed; furthermore, closer inspection of the TN stages of thymocyte development in these mice reveals a normal distribution of four described TN subsets (TN1–TN4). An impairment in pre-TCR-dependent thymocyte maturation signals is only detected in mixed bone marrow chimeras, in which $Itk^{-/-}$ or $Rlk^{-/-}Itk^{-/-}$ bone marrow is competing with wild-type bone marrow to repopulate the thymus of an irradiated host. However, even in these latter experiments, the defect observed in the $Itk^{-/-}$ or $Rlk^{-/-}Itk^{-/-}$ thymocytes is not absolute but rather results in a selective reduction of the Tec family kinase–deficient cells at the TN-DP transition (J.A. Lucas & L.J. Berg, unpublished observation).

One potential explanation for why pre-TCR signaling is not significantly impaired in the absence of Itk and/or Rlk is that Tec family kinase–dependent signaling may not be completely abolished in these cells, owing to the presence of Tec. An alternative explanation is that an independent pathway for PLC-γ1 activation, such as potential phosphorylation by the Syk tyrosine kinase, may be upregulated in TN thymocytes compared with later stages of T cell development.

ROLE OF TEC FAMILY KINASES IN T CELL EFFECTOR FUNCTIONS

Proliferation and IL-2 Production

The importance of the Tec kinases in T cells is underscored by the effects of these kinases on mature T cell function. In particular, mutations affecting Itk reduce T cell proliferation in response to anti-CD3 antibodies, concanavalin A, allogeneic MHC, or peptide antigen (for TCR transgenic cells) (10, 12, 13, 15). Decreased IL-2 production from $Itk^{-/-}$ T cells has been documented in response to anti-CD3 antibodies or upon antigen stimulation (10, 13, 15, 98). Accordingly, IL-2 can substantially rescue proliferative defects in Itk-deficient T cells (10, 12). Defects in proliferation and IL-2 production are worse in T cells lacking both Itk and Rlk, supporting a degree of genetic redundancy between these two kinases (10). In contrast to observations with $Itk^{-/-}$ cells, however, high-dose IL-2 failed to rescue fully the proliferative defects of $Rlk^{-/-}Itk^{-/-}$ splenocytes. This observation likely results from the more severe defects in CD25 induction in $Rlk^{-/-}Itk^{-/-}$ T cells, even in the presence of exogenous IL-2 (10).

Nonetheless, costimulation with anti-CD28 can improve many of these responses, particularly in $Itk^{-/-}$ cells. Indeed, stimulation of total splenocytes with anti-CD3 minimizes the proliferative defects associated with Itk deficiency (compare References 10 and 12). Similarly, stimulation of Itk-deficient T cells with antigen in the context of APCs reveals less severe reductions in proliferation than is seen with anti-CD3 stimulation of purified CD4 cells, again supporting the role of costimulation in rescuing defects associated with Itk deficiency (15).

Tec Family Kinases and T Helper Cell Differentiation

As discussed above, mutations affecting the Tec kinases do not prevent T cell development or T cell responses, but instead appear to modify or decrease the efficiency of activation, leading to altered development and function. Whether this is solely due to genetic redundancy between the kinases is not known. However, in mature $CD4^+$ T helper cell effector functions, distinct phenotypes associated with the individual kinases have emerged (Table 3).

Rlk AND Th1 DIFFERENTIATION   A role for Tec kinases in T helper cell differentiation and function was first suggested by the expression pattern of Rlk, which is preferentially found in both mouse and human Th1 but not Th2 cell clones (31, 33). This finding has been recently confirmed by real-time PCR and protein analyses in primary mouse T helper cells differentiated in culture (25, 26). Further experiments have shown that overexpression of Rlk can activate an IFN-γ reporter construct and increase expression of IFN-γ but not IL-4 in Jurkat cells (33). Conversely, antisense oligonucleotides to the Rlk message reduced IFN-γ production in peripheral blood T cells and T cell clones. Induction of IFN-γ required nuclear translocation and phosphorylation of Rlk. Moreover, a second paper from this group demonstrated that Rlk could directly bind to a sequence upstream of the IFN-γ gene start site, as well as to a related sequence in the promoters of CCR5 and TNF-α (89). Intriguingly, gene delivery of a Rlk expression plasmid with a hemagglutinin virus of Japan (HVJ) envelope vector in mice was found to increase expression of IFN-γ, but not of IL-4 or IL-2, from splenocytes and to decrease IgE production (197). However, comparisons with other Tec family kinases were not reported in these studies. One should note that $Rlk^{-/-}$ mouse T cells do not exhibit obvious defects in IFN-γ production or responses to a Th1-inducing pathogen, *Toxoplasma gondii* (10, 17). Mutation of the adapter molecule RIBP/TSAd/LAD, which interacts with both Rlk and Itk, decreases production of IL-2 and IFN-γ, but not of IL-4 (99).

Itk AND Th2 DIFFERENTIATION   In vitro stimulation of cells from Tec family kinase–deficient mice initially suggested that $Itk^{-/-}$ and $Rlk^{-/-}Itk^{-/-}$ T cells exhibit global defects in cytokine production (10, 17; J. Debnath & P.L. Schwartzberg, unpublished). Moreover, TGF-β treatment of T cells, which represses expression of both Th1 and Th2 cytokines, is associated with decreased Ca^{2+} mobilization and phosphorylation of Itk (198). However, several studies now argue that Itk plays a specific role in regulating Th2 cytokine production. Stimulation of naive CD4 cells from Itk-deficient mice demonstrates reduced production of the Th2 cytokine IL-4 (14, 26). Conversely, T cells from mice deficient in cyclophilin A, a negative regulator of Itk activity, exhibit increased production of Th2 cytokines, although increased Itk activity in these T cells has not been directly demonstrated (25). Under certain conditions, including stimulation with low-dose antigen or altered peptide ligands, Itk-deficient cells show increased production of IFN-γ (26). A recent study suggests that this increase in IFN-γ may result from abnormal regulation of T-bet expression, which is elevated after stimulation of Itk-deficient CD4 cells (26).

Multiple examples of defective Th2 responses in vivo have been reported in Itk-deficient mice. These include challenge with Th2-inducing parasites such as *Nippostrongylus brasiensis*, *Leishmania major*, and *Shistosome mansoni* (14, 17). For both *L. major* and *S. mansoni*, Itk deficiency was associated with a change to a Th1 response, consistent with the in vitro T-bet findings. This defect in Th2 responses is not limited to responses to parasitic infections; $Itk^{-/-}$ animals also show impaired responses, including decreased T cell infiltration, mucus production, and local Th2 cytokine production in an inhaled Ova-induced model of allergic asthma (18). A recently described inhibitor of Itk decreased lung inflammation in a mouse model of ovalbumin-induced allergy/asthma (198a). Increased Itk expression has also been observed in humans with atopic dermatitis (199).

Surprisingly, mutation of both Rlk and Itk reverses the Itk Th2 defect in response to *S. mansoni* eggs (17). A clue to understanding this observation came from the finding that $Rlk^{-/-}Itk^{-/-}$ cells appear to have a defect in GATA-3 regulation and fail to downregulate GATA-3 upon TCR stimulation (17). Stimulation of cells with PMA and ionomycin can rescue GATA-3 repression, suggesting that the impaired GATA-3 regulation is secondary to their TCR signaling defects.

Nonetheless, the roles of the Tec family kinases in T helper cell responses may be more complex. A recent paper demonstrates that Itk can phosphorylate T-bet and that mutation of this T-bet phosphorylation site prevents the ability of T-bet to bind to GATA-3 and repress its DNA binding activity (199a). Phosphorylation of T-bet was reduced in Itk-deficient T cells. Although it is difficult to resolve these data with the Th2 defect in Itk-deficient mice, both $Itk^{-/-}$ and $Rlk^{-/-}Itk^{-/-}$ mice have many mature cells that express memory phenotype markers (16; P.L. Schwartzberg, unpublished) and these cells can produce elevated levels of Th2 cytokines. The regulation of cytokine production by these cells and its influence on in vivo responses remains to be evaluated. $Itk^{-/-}$ and $Rlk^{-/-}Itk^{-/-}$ mice show increased IgE levels both at baseline and after challenge (17, 18), and $Itk^{-/-}$ mice show evidence of eosinophilia, suggesting complex effects that may influence multiple cell types. Whether defects in cytokine production from naive cells are the only cause of the altered responses to Th2-inducing agents in $Itk^{-/-}$ mice is also unclear. Two recent reports demonstrate defective recruitment of Itk-deficient T cells into the lung either in response to inhaled Ova or SDF-1α, suggesting that migration defects could contribute to the Th2 defects in these mice (18, 57). Nonetheless, on the basis of in vitro migration results, one might predict even more impaired migration of $Rlk^{-/-} Itk^{-/-}$ T cells (58). Yet these cells do mount some Th2 responses.

The effects of other cell types on these phenotypes also remain to be addressed. In particular, Itk-deficient mice have altered development and decreased numbers of NKT cells, a known early source of IL-4 production (195). Altered responses of NK cells and mast cells could also contribute to these defects in vivo (183). Thus, at this time, it remains unclear whether the Th2 defect in Itk-deficient cells result from a specific function of Itk required for Th2 differentiation, the distinct patterns of expression of Rlk and Itk in T helper cells, or other factors.

Finally, there is increased expression of Tec in Th2 cells compared with Th1 cells (35). Interestingly, overexpression of Tec can enhance, and kinase-inactive Tec can inhibit, PMA or PMA plus CD28-induced activation of both IL-2 and IL-4 reporter constructs (64), again supporting distinct functions for this family member.

Effects on CD8 Cell Function and Responses to Viral Infection

Although most studies have concentrated on the role of the Tec family kinases in CD4 effector cells, CD8-mediated cytotoxic T lymphocyte (CTL) responses are also impaired by mutations affecting the Tec kinases. Again, Itk appears to be the major player, with reduced cytotoxicity to allogeneic splenocytes that is worsened by mutation of both Rlk and Itk (P.L. Schwartzberg & J. Debnath, unpublished). An initial report suggested that after infection with viral agents, including lymphocytic choriomeningitis virus (LCMV), vaccinia, and vesicular stomatitis virus (VSV), Itk-deficient animals show a two- to sixfold decrease in antiviral cytolytic activity (200). Defects were most pronounced in response to VSV, which is less virulent and more dependent on IL-2 and CD28 stimulation for optimal response. In vitro proliferation assays reveal that defects could be partially rescued with addition of IL-2. Despite the defects in CTL activity, clearance of LCMV appeared normal, whereas clearance of vacinnia was more variable. A more recent study of LCMV infection, however, suggests that viral clearance is delayed (L. Atherly & L.J. Berg, unpublished). Moreover, this study showed no difference in the cytolytic activity of $Itk^{-/-}$ and $Rlk^{-/-} Itk^{-/-}$ cells relative to wild-type cells on a per cell basis, but rather showed decreased expansion of viral-specific cells and IFN-γ production in response to infection. Surprisingly, in the initial study, anti-VSV-specific antibody titres and VSV clearance appeared normal in $Itk^{-/-}$ mice, suggesting normal T cell help for immunoglobulin production (200).

Effects on Cell Survival

In B and mast cells, multiple lines of evidence suggest that Btk participates in cell survival pathways. Btk-deficient cells show reduced susceptibility to BCR-, IL-3-withdrawal-, and radiation-induced apoptosis but increased susceptibility to anti-Fas-mediated apoptosis (201). These findings may seem paradoxical, but they likely result from the effects of Btk on multiple signaling pathways. Thus, defects in BCR signaling in Btk-deficient cells likely prevent effective BCR-induced apoptosis. In contrast, a direct influence on Fas-mediated pathways is suggested by a study showing that Btk can bind Fas and prevent interaction of Fas with FADD (Fas-associated death domain protein) (202). Given recent evidence for defective TCR signaling and Ca^{2+} mobilization in patients harboring a mutation of caspase 8 (203), it is intriguing to speculate that Tec family kinases may be involved in common pathways downstream from antigen and TNF family receptors.

In T cells, deficiency of Itk or both Itk and Rlk decreases TCR-stimulated or antigen-induced cell death of mature cells (10, 15). Similar findings were reported for SEB-induced deletion of peripheral T cells in $Itk^{-/-}$ animals (15). For $Itk^{-/-}$ and $Rlk^{-/-} Itk^{-/-}$ thymocytes, investigators have also reported defective anti-CD3- plus anti-CD28-mediated killing of DP cells, an in vitro model of thymocyte deletion (11). $Rlk^{-/-} Itk^{-/-}$ T cells and thymocytes exhibited the most severe defects in these processes. The defect in activation-induced cell death in mature cells has been extensively examined in Itk-deficient cells and correlates with abnormal induction of FasL, which is likely to be secondary to decreased induction of NFATc2 and altered regulation of Egr2 and Egr3 (15). Investigators have not observed defects in response to anti-Fas engagement in either mature cells from Itk-deficient mice or DP thymocytes from $Itk^{-/-}$ or $Rlk^{-/-} Itk^{-/-}$ mice, suggesting that, in T cells, these Tec family kinases do not directly affect Fas signaling (11, 15). How these defects in activation-induced cell death and survival contribute to the phenotypes associated with mutations of these kinases, particularly in T helper cell differentiation and abnormal responses to infectious agents, has not been examined. Furthermore, whether defects in antigen-induced cell death contribute to the generation of the large population of "memory" phenotype cells in $Itk^{-/-}$ and $Rlk^{-/-} Itk^{-/-}$ mice is not known.

CONCLUDING REMARKS

Over the past several years, Tec family kinases have emerged as important regulators of TCR signaling that contribute to the activation of PLC-γ1. Recent studies suggest that these kinases also play important roles in pathways controlling actin cytoskeleton reorganization and adhesion (Figure 4, Table 3). In these pathways, Itk appears to be the major player, perhaps reflecting its high levels of expression in T cells. However, unlike the proximal kinases and adapters, Tec kinases are not absolutely required for T cell development or signaling, giving rise to the idea that

Tec kinases are modulators or amplifiers of these signals. This type of modulatory effect on signaling could result in part from the requirement for Tec kinases for prolonged Ca^{2+} influx, actin reorganization, and adhesion, all of which can influence the duration of TCR contacts and signaling.

Mutations affecting Tec kinases, therefore, do not prevent T cell development nor block TCR signaling but rather reduce TCR signaling in a manner that can alter thymocyte development and mature T cell differentiation and function. Indeed, perhaps some of the most interesting aspects of Tec family kinase biology in T cells are their effects on T helper cells. Although these kinases are at least partially functionally redundant for Ca^{2+} signaling pathways, an emerging theme is that each of these kinases also has distinct roles in T cell biology, particularly in T helper cell differentiation, where Itk has emerged as an important regulator of Th2 differentiation and Rlk as a potential regulator of Th1 differentiation. Although the effects of these kinases are complex, these studies suggest that Tec family kinases are potential targets for therapeutic interventions.

Finally, although in T cells the roles of Tec kinases have been best studied in TCR and costimulatory pathways, new data suggest that these kinases also participate in similar signaling pathways regulating Rho GTPases, cell polarization, and migration downstream from G protein–coupled chemokine receptors (Figure 4). The functions of Tec family kinases in other signaling pathways, including those from growth factor and cytokine receptors, and how these may affect T cell functional responses, await further study.

APPENDIX

Abbreviations used: ADAP, adhesion and degranulation adaptor protein; APC, antigen presenting cell; BH, Btk homology; BLNK, B cell linker protein; CRAC, Ca^{2+}-release-activated Ca^{2+} channel; CTL, cytotoxic T lymphocyte; DAG, diacylglycerol; DP, double positive; Emt, expressed in mast cells and T lymphocytes; ERK, extracellular-signal-regulated kinase; FADD, Fas-associated death domain protein; fMLP, fMet-Leu-Phe; GADS, Grb2-related adaptor downstream of Shc; GEF, guanine nucleotide exchange factor; GRB, growth factor receptor-bound protein; GTP, guanosine triphosphate; HVJ, hemagglutinin virus of Japan; IP_3, inositol (1,4,5) trisphosphate; Itk, inducible T cell kinase; JNK, c-jun aminoterminal kinase; LARG, leukemia-associated RhoGEF; LAT, linker for activation of T cells; LCMV, lymphocytic choriomeningitis virus; MAPK, mitogen-activated protein kinase; NFAT, nuclear factor of activated T cells; NKT cell, natural killer T cell; PCR, polymerase chain reaction; PH, pleckstrin homology; $PI_{(3,4,5)}P_3$, phosphatidylinositol (3,4,5) trisphosphate; $PI_{(3,4)}P_2$, phosphatidylinositol (3,4) bisphosphate; $PI_{(4,5)}P_2$, phosphatidylinositol (4,5) bisphosphate; $PI_{(4)}P$, phosphatidylinositol 4-monophosphate; PI3K, phosphoinositide 3-kinase; PIP5K, phosphatidylinositol 4-phosphate 5-kinase; PKC, protein kinase C; PLC-γ, phospholipase C-γ; PMA, phorbol myristate acetate; PRR, proline-rich region; PTEN, phosphatase and tensin homolog; RIBP, Rlk- and Itk-binding protein; Rlk, resting lymphocyte kinase; SEB, Staphylococcus aureus enterotoxin B; SH, Src homology; SHIP, SH2-containing inositol phosphatase; SLP-76, SH2-containing leukocyte protein of 76 kD; SP, single positive; TCR, T cell receptor; Tec, tyrosine kinase expressed in hepatocellular carcinoma; TH, Tec homology; TN, triple negative; Tsk, T cell specific kinase; VSV, vesicular stomatitis virus; WASP, Wiskott-Aldrich syndrome protein; *xid*, murine mutant X-linked immunodeficiency; XLA, X-linked agammaglobulinemia.

ACKNOWLEDGMENTS

The authors apologize to those whose work we were unable to cite owing to space considerations. We thank Mike Cichanowksi for graphics assistance, Amy Andreotti for critical reading of the manuscript, and members of our laboratories for helpful comments. L.J.B. acknowledges support from the NIH and the Center for Disease Control (AI37584 and CI000101). P.L.S. acknowledges support from the Chicago Community Trust/Searle Scholars Program.

The *Annual Review of Immunology* is online at
http://immunol.annualreviews.org

LITERATURE CITED

1. Tsukada S, Saffran DC, Rawlings DJ, Parolini O, Allen RC, et al. 1993. Deficient expression of a B cell cytoplasmic tyrosine kinase in human X-linked agammaglobulinemia. *Cell* 72:279–90

2. Vetrie D, Vorechovsky I, Sideras P, Holland J, Davies A, et al. 1993. The gene involved in X-linked agammaglobulinaemia is a member of the *src* family of protein tyrosine kinases. *Nature* 361:226–32

3. Thomas JD, Sideras P, Smith CIE, Vorechovsky I, Chapman V, et al. 1993. Colocalization of X-linked agammaglobulinemia and X-linked immunodeficiency genes. *Science* 261:355–58

4. Rawlings DJ, Saffran DC, Tsukada S, Largaespada DA, Grimaldi JC, et al. 1993. Mutation of unique region of Bruton's tyrosine kinase in immunodeficient XID mice. *Science* 261:358–61

5. Smith CI, Islam TC, Mattsson PT, Mohamed AJ, Nore BF, et al. 2001. The Tec family of cytoplasmic tyrosine kinases: mammalian Btk, Bmx, Itk, Tec, Txk and

homologs in other species. *Bioessays* 23:436–46

6. Debnath J, Chamorro M, Czar MJ, Schaeffer EM, Lenardo MJ, et al. 1999. *rlk/TXK* encodes two forms of a novel cysteine string tyrosine kinase activated by Src family kinases. *Mol. Cell. Biol.* 19:1498–507

7. Gibson S, August A, Kawakami Y, Kawakami T, Dupont B, et al. 1996. The EMT/ITK/TSK (EMT) tyrosine kinase is activated during TCR signaling: LCK is required for optimal activation of EMT. *J. Immunol.* 156:2716–22

8. Yang WC, Ghiotto M, Barbarat B, Olive D. 1999. The role of Tec protein-tyrosine kinase in T cell signaling. *J. Biol. Chem.* 274:607–17

9. Heyeck SD, Wilcox HM, Bunnell SC, Berg LJ. 1997. Lck phosphorylates the activation loop tyrosine of the Itk kinase domain and activates Itk kinase activity. *J. Biol. Chem.* 272:25401–8

10. Schaeffer EM, Debnath J, Yap G, McVicar D, Liao XC, et al. 1999.

Requirement for Tec kinases Rlk and Itk in T cell receptor signaling and immunity. *Science* 284:638–41

11. Schaeffer EM, Broussard C, Debnath J, Anderson S, McVicar DW, et al. 2000. Tec family kinases modulate thresholds for thymocyte development and selection. *J. Exp. Med.* 192:987–1000

12. Liao XC, Littman DR. 1995. Altered T cell receptor signaling and disrupted T cell development in mice lacking Itk. *Immunity* 3:757–69

13. Liu KQ, Bunnell SC, Gurniak CB, Berg LJ. 1998. T cell receptor-initiated calcium release is uncoupled from capacitative calcium entry in Itk-deficient T cells. *J. Exp. Med.* 187:1721–27

14. Fowell DJ, Shinkai K, Liao XC, Beebe AM, Coffman RL, et al. 1999. Impaired NFATc translocation and failure of Th2 development in Itk-deficient CD4+ T cells. *Immunity* 11:399–409

15. Miller A, Berg L. 2002. Defective Fas ligand expression and activation-induced cell death in the absence of IL-2-inducible T cell kinase. *J. Immunol.* 168:2163–72

16. Lucas JA, Atherly LO, Berg LJ. 2002. The absence of Itk inhibits positive selection without changing lineage commitment. *J. Immunol.* 168:6142–51

17. Schaeffer E, Yap G, Lewis CM, Czar MJ, McVicar DW, et al. 2001. Mutation of Tec family kinases alters T helper cell differentiation. *Nat. Immunol.* 2:1183–88

18. Mueller C, August A. 2003. Attenuation of immunological symptoms of allergic asthma in mice lacking the tyrosine kinase Itk. *J. Immunol.* 170:5056–63

19. Woods ML, Kivens WJ, Adelsman MA, Qiu Y, August A, et al. 2001. A novel function for the Tec family tyrosine kinase Itk in activation of $\beta 1$ integrins by the T-cell receptor. *EMBO J.* 20:1232–44

20. Siliciano JD, Morrow TA, Desiderio SV. 1992. *itk*, a T-cell-specific tyrosine kinase gene inducible by interleukin 2.

Proc. Natl. Acad. Sci. USA 89:11194–98

21. Heyeck SD, Berg LJ. 1993. Developmental regulation of a murine T-cell-specific tyrosine kinase gene, Tsk. *Proc. Natl. Acad. Sci. USA* 90:669–73

22. Gibson S, Leung B, Squire JA, Hill M, Arima N, et al. 1993. Identification, cloning, and characterization of a novel human T-cell-specific tyrosine kinase located at the hematopoietin complex on chromosome 5q. *Blood* 82:1561–72

23. Tanaka N, Asao H, Ohtani K, Nakamura M, Sugamura K. 1993. A novel human tyrosine kinase gene inducible in T cells by interleukin 2. *FEBS Lett.* 324:1–5

24. Yamada N, Kawakami Y, Kimura H, Fukamachi H, Baier G, et al. 1993. Structure and expression of novel protein-tyrosine kinases, Emb and Emt, in hematopoietic cells. *Biochem. Biophys. Res. Commun.* 192:231–40

25. Colgan J, Asmal M, Neagu M, Yu B, Schneidkraut J, et al. 2004. Cyclophilin A regulates TCR signal strength in CD4+ T cells via a proline-directed conformational switch in Itk. *Immunity* 21:189–201

26. Miller AT, Wilcox HM, Lai Z, Berg LJ. 2004. Signaling through Itk promotes T helper 2 differentiation via negative regulation of T-bet. *Immunity* 21:67–80

27. Grasis JA, Browne CD, Tsoukas CD. 2003. Inducible T cell tyrosine kinase regulates actin-dependent cytoskeletal events induced by the T cell antigen receptor. *J. Immunol.* 170:3971–76

28. Labno CM, Lewis CM, You D, Leung DW, Takesono A, et al. 2003. Itk functions to control actin polymerization at the immune synapse through localized activation of Cdc42 and WASP. *Curr. Biol.* 13:1619–24

29. Haire RN, Litman GW. 1995. The murine form of TXK, a novel TEC kinase expressed in thymus maps to chromosome 5. *Mamm. Genome* 6:476–80

30. Haire RN, Ohta Y, Lewis JE, Fu SM,

Kroisel P, et al. 1994. TXK, a novel human tyrosine kinase expressed in T cells shares sequence identity with Tec family kinases and maps to 4p12. *Hum. Mol. Genet.* 3:897–901

31. Hu Q, Davidson D, Schwartzberg PL, Macchiarini F, Lenardo MJ, et al. 1995. Identification of Rlk, a novel protein tyrosine kinase with predominant expression in the T cell lineage. *J. Biol. Chem.* 270:1928–34

32. Sommers CL, Huang K, Shores EW, Grinberg A, Charlick DA, et al. 1995. Murine *txk*: a protein tyrosine kinase gene regulated by T cell activation. *Oncogene* 11:245–51

33. Kashiwakura J, Suzuki N, Nagafuchi H, Takeno M, Takeba Y, et al. 1999. Txk, a nonreceptor tyrosine kinase of the Tec family, is expressed in T helper type 1 cells and regulates interferon γ production in human T lymphocytes. *J. Exp. Med.* 190:1147–54

34. Mano H, Ishikawa F, Nishida J, Hirai H, Takaku F. 1990. A novel protein-tyrosine kinase, tec, is preferentially expressed in liver. *Oncogene* 5:1781–86

35. Tomlinson MG, Kane LP, Su J, Kadlecek TA, Mollenauer MN, et al. 2004. Expression and function of Tec, Itk, and Btk in lymphocytes: evidence for a unique role for Tec. *Mol. Cell. Biol.* 24:2455–66

36. Ellmeier W, Jung S, Sunshine MJ, Hatam F, Xu Y, ct al. 2000. Severe B cell deficiency in mice lacking the Tec kinase family members Tec and Btk. *J. Exp. Med.* 192:1611–24

37. Merkel AL, Atmosukarto II, Stevens K, Rathjen PD, Booker GW. 1999. Splice variants of the mouse Tec gene are differentially expressed in vivo. *Cytogenet. Cell Genet.* 84:132–39

38. Qiu Y, Kung HJ. 2000. Signaling network of the Btk family kinases. *Oncogene* 19:5651–61

39. Mano H. 1999. Tec family of protein-tyrosine kinases: an overview of their structure and function. *Cytokine Growth Factor Rev.* 10:267–80

40. Kawakami Y, Kitaura J, Hata D, Yao L, Kawakami T. 1999. Functions of Bruton's tyrosine kinase in mast and B cells. *J. Leukoc. Biol.* 65:286–90.

41. Mao C, Zhou M, Uckun FM. 2001. Crystal structure of Bruton's tyrosine kinase domain suggests a novel pathway for activation and provides insights into the molecular basis of X-linked agammaglobulinemia. *J. Biol. Chem.* 276:41435–43

42. Brown K, Long JM, Vial SC, Dedi N, Dunster NJ, et al. 2004. Crystal structures of interleukin-2 tyrosine kinase and their implications for the design of selective inhibitors. *J. Biol. Chem.* 279:18727–32

43. Kojima T, Fukuda M, Watanabe Y, Hamazato F, Mikoshiba K. 1997. Characterization of the pleckstrin homology domain of Btk as an inositol polyphosphate and phosphoinositide binding domain. *Biochem. Biophys. Res. Commun.* 236:333–39

44. Rameh LE, Arvidsson A, Carraway KL III, Couvillon AD, Rathbun G, et al. 1997. A comparative analysis of the phosphoinositide binding specificity of pleckstrin homology domains. *J. Biol. Chem.* 272:22059–66

45. Salim K, Bottomley MJ, Querfurth E, Zvelebil MJ, Gout I, et al. 1996. Distinct specificity in the recognition of phosphoinositides by the pleckstrin homology domains of dynamin and Bruton's tyrosine kinase. *EMBO J.* 15:6241–50

46. August A, Sadra A, Dupont B, Hanafusa H. 1997. Src-induced activation of inducible T cell kinase (ITK) requires phosphatidylinositol 3-kinase activity and the Pleckstrin homology domain of inducible T cell kinase. *Proc. Natl. Acad. Sci. USA* 94:11227–32

47. Satterthwaite AB, Li Z, Witte ON. 1998. Btk function in B cell development and response. *Semin. Immunol.* 10:309–16

48. August A, Gibson S, Kawakami Y, Kawakami T, Mills GB, et al. 1994. CD28 is associated with and induces the immediate tyrosine phosphorylation and activation of the Tec family kinase ITK/EMT in the human Jurkat leukemic T-cell line. *Proc. Natl. Acad. Sci. USA* 91:9347–51

49. Raab M, Cai YC, Bunnell SC, Heyeck SD, Berg LJ, et al. 1995. p56Lck and p59Fyn regulate CD28 binding to phosphatidylinositol 3-kinase, growth factor receptor-bound protein GRB-2, and T cell-specific protein-tyrosine kinase ITK: implications for T-cell costimulation. *Proc. Natl. Acad. Sci. USA* 92: 8891–95

50. Gibson S, August A, Branch D, Dupont B, Mills GM. 1996. Functional LCK is required for optimal CD28-mediated activation of the TEC family tyrosine kinase EMT/ITK. *J. Biol. Chem.* 271: 7079–83

51. Gibson S, Truitt K, Lu Y, Lapushin R, Khan H, et al. 1998. Efficient CD28 signalling leads to increases in the kinase activities of the TEC family tyrosine kinase EMT/ITK/TSK and the SRC family tyrosine kinase LCK. *Biochem. J.* 330:1123–28

52. Marengere LE, Okkenhaug K, Clavreul A, Couez D, Gibson S, et al. 1997. The SH3 domain of Itk/Emt binds to proline-rich sequences in the cytoplasmic domain of the T cell costimulatory receptor CD28. *J. Immunol.* 159:3220–29

53. King PD, Sadra A, Teng JM, Xiao-Rong L, Han A, et al. 1997. Analysis of CD28 cytoplasmic tail tyrosine residues as regulators and substrates for the protein tyrosine kinases, EMT and LCK. *J. Immunol.* 158:580–90

54. King PD, Sadra A, Han A, Liu XR, Sunder-Plassmann R, et al. 1996. CD2 signaling in T cells involves tyrosine phosphorylation and activation of the Tec family kinase, EMT/ITK/TSK. *Int. Immunol.* 8:1707–14

55. King PD, Sadra A, Teng JM, Bell GM, Dupont B. 1998. CD2-mediated activation of the Tec-family tyrosine kinase ITK is controlled by proline-rich stretch-4 of the CD2 cytoplasmic tail. *Int. Immunol.* 10:1009–16

56. Tanaka N, Abe H, Yagita H, Okumura K, Nakamura M, et al. 1997. Itk, a T cell-specific tyrosine kinase, is required for CD2-mediated interleukin-2 promoter activation in the human T cell line Jurkat. *Eur. J. Immunol.* 27:834–41

57. Fischer AM, Mercer JC, Iyer A, Ragin MJ, August A. 2004. Regulation of CXC chemokine receptor 4-mediated migration by the Tec family tyrosine kinase ITK. *J. Biol. Chem.* 479:29816–20

58. Takesono A, Horai R, Mandai M, Dombroski D, Schwartzberg PL. 2004. Requirement for Tec kinases in chemokine-induced migration and activation of Cdc42 and Rac. *Curr. Biol.* 14:917–22

59. Chamorro M, Czar MJ, Debnath J, Cheng G, Lenardo MJ, et al. 2001. Requirements for activation and RAFT localization of the T-lymphocyte kinase Rlk/Txk. *BMC Immunol.* 2:3

60. Schneider H, Guerette B, Guntermann C, Rudd CE. 2000. Resting lymphocyte kinase (Rlk/Txk) targets lymphoid adaptor SLP-76 in the cooperative activation of interleukin-2 transcription in T-cells. *J. Biol. Chem.* 275:3835–40

61. Sommers CL, Rabin RL, Grinberg A, Tsay HC, Farber J, et al. 1999. A role for the Tec family tyrosine kinase Txk in T cell activation and thymocyte selection. *J. Exp. Med.* 190:1427–38

62. Tomlinson MG, Kurosaki T, Berson AE, Fujii GH, Johnston JA, et al. 1999. Reconstitution of Btk signaling by the atypical Tec family tyrosine kinases Bmx and Txk. *J. Biol. Chem.* 274:13577–85

63. Yang WC, Ching KA, Tsoukas CD, Berg LJ. 2001. Tec kinase signaling in T cells is regulated by phosphatidylinositol 3-kinase and the Tec pleckstrin homology domain. *J. Immunol.* 166:387–95

64. Yang WC, Olive D. 1999. Tec kinase is involved in transcriptional regulation of IL-2 and IL-4 in the CD28 pathway. *Eur. J. Immunol.* 29:1842–49

65. Takesono A, Finkelstein LD, Schwartzberg PL. 2002. Beyond calcium: new signaling pathways for Tec family kinases. *J. Cell Sci.* 115:3039–48

66. Takahashi-Tezuka M, Hibi M, Fujitani Y, Fukada T, Yamaguchi T, et al. 1997. Tec tyrosine kinase links the cytokine receptors to PI-3 kinase probably through JAK. *Oncogene* 14:2273–82

67. Yamashita Y, Watanabe S, Miyazato A, Ohya K, Ikeda U, et al. 1998. Tec and Jak2 kinases cooperate to mediate cytokine-driven activation of c-fos transcription. *Blood* 91:1496–507

68. Kline JB, Moore DJ, Clevenger CV. 2001. Activation and association of the Tec tyrosine kinase with the human prolactin receptor: mapping of a Tec/Vav1-receptor binding site. *Mol. Endocrinol.* 15:832–41

69. Machide M, Mano H, Todokoro K. 1995. Interleukin 3 and erythropoietin induce association of Vav with Tec kinase through Tec homology domain. *Oncogene* 11:619–25

70. Vihinen M, Brandau O, Branden LJ, Kwan SP, Lappalainen I, et al. 1998. BTKbase, mutation database for X-linked agammaglobulinemia (XLA). *Nucleic Acids Res.* 26:242–47

71. Hyvonen M, Saraste M. 1997. Structure of the PH domain and Btk motif from Bruton's tyrosine kinase: molecular explanations for X-linked agammaglobulinaemia. *EMBO J.* 16:3396–404

72. Fukuda M, Kojima T, Kabayama H, Mikoshiba K. 1996. Mutation of the pleckstrin homology domain of Bruton's tyrosine kinase in immunodeficiency impaired inositol 1,3,4,5-tetrakisphosphate binding capacity. *J. Biol. Chem.* 271:30303–6

73. Bolland S, Pearse RN, Kurosaki T, Ravetch JV. 1998. SHIP modulates immune receptor responses by regulating membrane association of Btk. *Immunity* 8:509–16

74. Li Z, Wahl MI, Eguinoa A, Stephens LR, Hawkins PT, et al. 1997. Phosphatidylinositol 3-kinase-γ activates Bruton's tyrosine kinase in concert with Src family kinases. *Proc. Natl. Acad. Sci. USA* 94:13820–25

75. Lu Y, Cuevas B, Gibson S, Khan H, LaPushin R, et al. 1998. Phosphatidylinositol 3-kinase is required for CD28 but not CD3 regulation of the TEC family tyrosine kinase EMT/ITK/TSK: functional and physical interaction of EMT with phosphatidylinositol 3-kinase. *J. Immunol.* 161:5404–12

76. Reynolds LF, Smyth LA, Norton T, Freshney N, Downward J, et al. 2002. Vav1 transduces T cell receptor signals to the activation of phospholipase C-γ1 via phosphoinositide 3-kinase-dependent and -independent pathways. *J. Exp. Med.* 195:1103–14

77. Bunnell SC, Diehn M, Yaffe MB, Findell PR, Cantley LC, et al. 2000. Biochemical interactions integrating Itk with the T cell receptor-initiated signaling cascade. *J. Biol. Chem.* 275:2219–30

78. Ching KA, Kawakami Y, Kawakami T, Tsoukas CD. 1999. Emt/Itk associates with activated TCR complexes: role of the pleckstrin homology domain. *J. Immunol.* 163:6006–13

79. Garcon F, Bismuth G, Isnardon D, Olive D, Nunes JA. 2004. Tec kinase migrates to the T cell-APC interface independently of its pleckstrin homology domain. *J. Immunol.* 173:770–75

80. Garcon F, Ghiotto M, Gerard A, Yang WC, Olive D, et al. 2004. The SH3 domain of Tec kinase is essential for its targeting to activated CD28 costimulatory molecule. *Eur. J. Immunol.* 34:1972–80

81. Li T, Tsukada S, Satterthwaite A, Havlik MH, Park H, et al. 1995. Activation of Bruton's tyrosine kinase (BTK) by a point mutation in its pleckstrin

homology (PH) domain. *Immunity* 2: 451–60

81a. Tomlinson MG, Heath VL, Turck CW, Watson SP, Weiss A. 2004. SHIP family inositol phosphatases interact with and negatively regulate the Tec tyrosine kinase. *J. Biol. Chem.* 279:55089–96

82. Shan X, Czar MJ, Bunnell SC, Liu P, Liu Y, et al. 2000. Deficiency of PTEN in Jurkat T cells causes constitutive localization of Itk to the plasma membrane and hyperresponsiveness to CD3 stimulation. *Mol. Cell. Biol.* 20:6945–57

83. Xu Z, Stokoe D, Kane LP, Weiss A. 2002. The inducible expression of the tumor suppressor gene PTEN promotes apoptosis and decreases cell size by inhibiting the PI3K/Akt pathway in Jurkat T cells. *Cell Growth Differ.* 13:285–96

84. Saito K, Tolias KF, Saci A, Koon HB, Humphries LA, et al. 2003. BTK regulates PtdIns-4,5-P2 synthesis: importance for calcium signaling and PI3K activity. *Immunity* 19:669–78

85. Kawakami Y, Yao L, Tashiro M, Gibson S, Mills GB, et al. 1995. Activation and interaction with protein kinase C of a cytoplasmic tyrosine kinase, Itk/Tsk/Emt, on FcεRI cross-linking on mast cells. *J. Immunol.* 155:3556–62

86. Yao L, Kawakami Y, Kawakami T. 1994. The pleckstrin homology domain of Bruton tyrosine kinase interacts with protein kinase C. *Proc. Natl. Acad. Sci. USA* 91:9175–79

87. Leitges M, Schmedt C, Guinamard R, Davoust J, Schaal S, et al. 1996. Immunodeficiency in protein kinase Cβ-deficient mice. *Science* 273:788–91

88. Kang SW, Wahl MI, Chu J, Kitaura J, Kawakami Y, et al. 2001. PKCβ modulates antigen receptor signaling via regulation of Btk membrane localization. *EMBO J.* 20:5692–702

89. Takeba Y, Nagafuchi H, Takeno M, Kashiwakura J, Suzuki N. 2002. Txk, a member of nonreceptor tyrosine kinase of Tec family, acts as a Th1 cell-specific transcription factor and regulates IFN-γ gene transcription. *J. Immunol.* 168:2365–70

90. Perez-Villar JJ, O'Day K, Hewgill DH, Nadler SG, Kanner SB. 2001. Nuclear localization of the tyrosine kinase Itk and interaction of its SH3 domain with karyopherin α (Rch1α). *Int. Immunol.* 13:1265–74

91. Su YW, Zhang Y, Schweikert J, Koretzky GA, Reth M, et al. 1999. Interaction of SLP adaptors with the SH2 domain of Tec family kinases. *Eur. J. Immunol.* 29:3702–11

92. Hashimoto S, Iwamatsu A, Ishiai M, Okawa K, Yamadori T, et al. 1999. Identification of the SH2 domain binding protein of Bruton's tyrosine kinase as BLNK—functional significance of Btk-SH2 domain in B-cell antigen receptor-coupled calcium signaling. *Blood* 94:2357–64

93. Ching KA, Grasis JA, Tailor P, Kawakami Y, Kawakami T, et al. 2000. TCR/CD3-Induced activation and binding of Emt/Itk to linker of activated T cell complexes: requirement for the Src homology 2 domain. *J. Immunol.* 165:256–62

94. Shan X, Wange RL. 1999. Itk/Emt/Tsk activation in response to CD3 cross-linking in Jurkat T cells requires ZAP-70 and Lat and is independent of membrane recruitment. *J. Biol. Chem.* 274:29323–30

95. Weiss A, Samelson LE. 2003. T-lymphocyte activation. In *Fundamental Immunology*, ed. WE Paul, pp. 321–63. New York: Lippincott-Raven

95a. Samelson LE. 2003. Signal transduction mediated by the T cell antigen receptor: the role of adapter molecules. *Annu. Rev. Immunol.* 20:371–94

96. Baker JE, Majeti R, Tangye SG, Weiss A. 2001. Protein tyrosine phosphatase CD148-mediated inhibition of T-cell receptor signal transduction is associated with reduced LAT and phospholipase

Cγ1 phosphorylation. *Mol. Cell. Biol.* 21:2393–403

97. Perez-Villar JJ, Kanner SB. 1999. Regulated association between the tyrosine kinase Emt/Itk/Tsk and phospholipase-Cγ1 in human T lymphocytes. *J. Immunol.* 163:6435–41

98. Wilcox HM, Berg LJ. 2003. Itk phosphorylation sites are required for functional activity in primary T cells. *J. Biol. Chem.* 278:37112–21

99. Rajagopal K, Sommers CL, Decker DC, Mitchell EO, Korthauer U, et al. 1999. RIBP, a novel Rlk/Txk- and Itk-binding adaptor protein that regulates T cell activation. *J. Exp. Med.* 190:1657–68

100. Touhara K, Inglese J, Pitcher JA, Shaw G, Lefkowitz RJ. 1994. Binding of G protein βγ-subunits to pleckstrin homology domains. *J. Biol. Chem.* 269:10217–20

101. Tsukada S, Simon MI, Witte ON, Katz A. 1994. Binding of βγ subunits of heterotrimeric G proteins to the PH domain of Bruton tyrosine kinase. *Proc. Natl. Acad. Sci. USA* 91:11256–60

102. Langhans-Rajasekaran SA, Wan Y, Huang XY. 1995. Activation of Tsk and Btk tyrosine kinases by G protein βγ subunits. *Proc. Natl. Acad. Sci. USA* 92: 8601–5

103. Bence K, Ma W, Kozasa T, Huang XY. 1997. Direct stimulation of Bruton's tyrosine kinase by G(q)-protein α-subunit. *Nature* 389:296–99

104. Harnett M, Rigley K. 1992. The role of G-proteins versus protein tyrosine kinases in the regulation of lymphocyte activation. *Immunol. Today* 13:482–86

105. Stanners J, Kabouridis PS, McGuire KL, Tsoukas CD. 1995. Interaction between G proteins and tyrosine kinases upon T cell receptor·CD3-mediated signaling. *J. Biol. Chem.* 270:30635–42

106. Afar DEH, Park H, Howell BW, Rawlings DJ, Cooper J, et al. 1996. Regulation of Btk by Src family tyrosine kinases. *Mol. Cell Biol.* 16:3465–71

107. Mahajan S, Fargnoli J, Burkhardt AL,

Kut SA, Saouaf SJ, et al. 1995. Src family protein tyrosine kinases induce autoactivation of Bruton's tyrosine kinase. *Mol. Cell. Biol.* 15:5304–11

108. Park H, Wahl MI, Afar DE, Turck CW, Rawlings DJ, et al. 1996. Regulation of Btk function by a major autophosphorylation site within the SH3 domain. *Immunity* 4:515–25

109. Rawlings DJ, Scharenberg AM, Park H, Wahl MI, Lin S, et al. 1996. Activation of BTK by a phosphorylation mechanism initiated by SRC family kinases. *Science* 271:822–25

110. Johnson LN, Noble MEM, Owen DJ. 1996. Active and inactive protein kinases: structural basis for regulation. *Cell* 85:149–58

111. Mano H, Yamashita Y, Miyazato A, Miura Y, Ozawa K. 1996. Tec protein-tyrosine kinase is an effector molecule of Lyn protein-tyrosine kinase. *FASEB J.* 10:637–42

112. Kurosaki T, Kurosaki M. 1997. Trans-phosphorylation of Bruton's tyrosine kinase on tyrosine 551 is critical for B cell antigen receptor function. *J. Biol. Chem.* 272:15595–98

113. Nore BF, Mattsson PT, Antonsson P, Backesjo CM, Westlund A, et al. 2003. Identification of phosphorylation sites within the SH3 domains of Tec family tyrosine kinases. *Biochim. Biophys. Acta* 1645:123–32

114. Wahl MI, Fluckiger AC, Kato RM, Park H, Witte ON, et al. 1997. Phosphorylation of two regulatory tyrosine residues in the activation of Bruton's tyrosine kinase via alternative receptors. *Proc. Natl. Acad. Sci. USA* 94:11526–33

115. Andreotti AH, Bunnell SC, Feng S, Berg LJ, Schreiber SL. 1997. Intramolecular association of two domains in a Tec family tyrosine kinase influences binding of signaling proteins. *Nature* 385:93–97

116. Hansson H, Mattsson PT, Allard P, Haapaniemi P, Vihinen M, et al. 1998. Solution structure of the SH3 domain from

Bruton's tyrosine kinase. *Biochemistry* 37:2912–24

117. Morrogh LM, Hinshelwood S, Costello P, Cory GO, Kinnon C. 1999. The SH3 domain of Bruton's tyrosine kinase displays altered ligand binding properties when auto-phosphorylated in vitro. *Eur. J. Immunol.* 29:2269–79

118. Sicheri F, Kuriyan J. 1997. Structures of Src-family tyrosine kinases. *Curr. Opin. Struct. Biol.* 7:777–85

119. Folmer RH, Geschwindner S, Xue Y. 2002. Crystal structure and NMR studies of the apo SH2 domains of ZAP-70: two bikes rather than a tandem. *Biochemistry* 41:14176–84

120. Hansson H, Okoh MP, Smith CI, Vihinen M, Hard T. 2001. Intermolecular interactions between the SH3 domain and the proline-rich TH region of Bruton's tyrosine kinase. *FEBS Lett.* 489:67–70

121. Hansson H, Smith CI, Hard T. 2001. Both proline-rich sequences in the TH region of Bruton's tyrosine kinase stabilize intermolecular interactions with the SH3 domain. *FEBS Lett.* 508:11–15

122. Laederach A, Cradic KW, Brazin KN, Zamoon J, Fulton DB, et al. 2002. Competing modes of self-association in the regulatory domains of Bruton's tyrosine kinase: intramolecular contact versus asymmetric homodimerization. *Protein Sci.* 11:36–45

123. Laederach A, Cradic KW, Fulton DB, Andreotti AH. 2003. Determinants of intra-versus intermolecular self-association within the regulatory domains of Rlk and Itk. *J. Mol. Biol.* 329:1011–20

124. Okoh MP, Vihinen M. 2002. Interaction between Btk TH and SH3 domain. *Biopolymers* 63:325–34

125. Pursglove SE, Mulhern TD, Mackay JP, Hinds MG, Booker GW. 2002. The solution structure and intramolecular associations of the Tec kinase SRC homology 3 domain. *J. Biol. Chem.* 277:755–62

126. Brazin KN, Fulton DB, Andreotti AH.

2000. A specific intermolecular association between the regulatory domains of a Tec family kinase. *J. Mol. Biol.* 302:607–23

127. Yamashita Y, Miyazato A, Ohya K, Ikeda U, Shimada K, et al. 1996. Deletion of Src homology 3 domain results in constitutive activation of Tec protein-tyrosine kinase. *Jpn. J. Cancer Res.* 87:1106–10

128. Cheng G, Ye ZS, Baltimore D. 1994. Binding of Bruton's tyrosine kinase to Fyn, Lyn, or Hck through a Src homology 3 domain-mediated interaction. *Proc. Natl. Acad. Sci. USA* 91:8152–55

129. Yang W, Malek SN, Desiderio S. 1995. An SH3-binding site conserved in Bruton's tyrosine kinase and related tyrosine kinases mediates specific protein interactions in vitro and in vivo. *J. Biol. Chem.* 270:20832–40

130. Hao S, August A. 2002. The proline rich region of the Tec homology domain of ITK regulates its activity. *FEBS Lett.* 525:53–58

131. Baraldi E, Carugo KD, Hyvonen M, Surdo PI, Riley AM, et al. 1999. Structure of the PH domain from Bruton's tyrosine kinase in complex with inositol 1,3,4,5-tetrakisphosphate. *Structure Fold Des.* 7:449–60

132. Mallis RJ, Brazin KN, Fulton DB, Andreotti AH. 2002. Structural characterization of a proline-driven conformational switch within the Itk SH2 domain. *Nat. Struct. Biol.* 9:900–5

133. Okoh MP, Vihinen M. 1999. Pleckstrin homology domains of Tec family protein kinases. *Biochem. Biophys. Res. Commun.* 265:151–57

134. Tzeng SR, Lou YC, Pai MT, Jain ML, Cheng JW. 2000. Solution structure of the human BTK SH3 domain complexed with a proline-rich peptide from p120cbl. *J. Biomol. NMR* 16:303–12

135. Brazin KN, Mallis RJ, Fulton DB, Andreotti AH. 2002. Regulation of the tyrosine kinase Itk by the peptidyl-prolyl

isomerase cyclophilin A. *Proc. Natl. Acad. Sci. USA* 99:1899–904

136. Breheny PJ, Laederach A, Fulton DB, Andreotti AH. 2003. Ligand specificity modulated by prolyl imide bond cis/trans isomerization in the Itk SH2 domain: a quantitative NMR study. *J. Am. Chem. Soc.* 125:15706–7

137. Hawkins J, Marcy A. 2001. Characterization of Itk tyrosine kinase: contribution of noncatalytic domains to enzymatic activity. *Protein Expr. Purif.* 22:211–19

138. Lowry WE, Huang J, Lei M, Rawlings D, Huang XY. 2001. Role of the PHTH module in protein substrate recognition by Bruton's agammaglobulinemia tyrosine kinase. *J. Biol. Chem.* 276:45276–81

139. Starr TK, Jameson SC, Hogquist KA. 2003. Positive and negative selection of T cells. *Annu. Rev. Immunol.* 21:139–76

140. Badour K, Zhang J, Shi F, Leng Y, Collins M, et al. 2004. Fyn and PTP-PEST-mediated regulation of Wiskott-Aldrich syndrome protein (WASp) tyrosine phophorylation is required for coupling T cell antigen receptor engagement to WASp effector function and T cell activation. *J. Exp. Med.* 199:99–111

141. Rhee SG. 2001. Regulation of phosphoinositide-specific phospholipase C. *Annu. Rev. Biochem.* 70:281–312

142. Lewis RS, Cahalan MD. 1995. Potassium and calcium channels in lymphocytes. *Annu. Rev. Immunol.* 13:623–53

143. Crabtree GR, Olson EN. 2002. NFAT signaling: choreographing the social lives of cells. *Cell* 109:S67–79

144. Takata M, Kurosaki T. 1996. A role for Bruton's tyrosine kinase in B cell antigen receptor-mediated activation of phospholipase C-γ2. *J. Exp. Med.* 184:31–40

145. Fluckiger AC, Li Z, Kato RM, Wahl MI, Ochs HD, et al. 1998. Btk/Tec kinases regulate sustained increases in intracellular Ca^{2+} following B-cell receptor activation. *EMBO J.* 17:1973–85

146. Humphries LA, Dangelmaier C, Sommer K, Kipp K, Kato RM, et al. 2004. Tec kinases mediate sustained calcium influx via site-specific tyrosine phosphorylation of the PLCγ SH2-SH3 linker. *J. Biol. Chem.* 279:37651–61

147. Veri MC, DeBell KE, Seminario MC, DiBaldassarre A, Reischl I, et al. 2001. Membrane raft-dependent regulation of phospholipase Cγ-1 activation in T lymphocytes. *Mol. Cell. Biol.* 21:6939–50

148. Thastrup O, Cullen PJ, Drobak BK, Hanley MR, Dawson AP. 1990. Thapsigargin, a tumor promoter, discharges intracellular Ca^{2+} stores by specific inhibition of the endoplasmic reticulum Ca^{2+}-ATPase. *Proc. Natl. Acad. Sci. USA* 87:2466–70

149. Parekh AB, Fleig A, Penner R. 1997. The store-operated calcium current I (CRAC): nonlinear activation by InsP3 and dissociation from calcium release. *Cell* 89:973–80

150. Altman A, Kaminski S, Busuttil V, Droin N, Hu J, et al. 2004. Positive feedback regulation of PLCγ1/Ca^{2+} signaling by PKCθ in restimulated T cells via a Tec kinase-dependent pathway. *Eur. J. Immunol.* 34:2001–11

151. Newton AC. 2004. Diacylglycerol's affair with protein kinase C turns 25. *Trends Pharmacol. Sci.* 25:175–77

152. Scharenberg AM, El-Hillal O, Fruman DA, Beitz LO, Li Z, et al. 1998. Phosphatidylinositol-3,4,5-trisphosphate (PtdIns-3,4,5-P3)/Tec kinase-dependent calcium signaling pathway: a target for SHIP-mediated inhibitory signals. *EMBO J.* 17:1961–72

153. Tomlinson MG, Woods DB, McMahon M, Wahl MI, Witte ON, et al. 2001. A conditional form of Bruton's tyrosine kinase is sufficient to activate multiple downstream signaling pathways via PLCγ 2 in B cells. *BMC Immunol.* 2:4

154. Perez-Villar J, Whitney G, Sitnick M, Dunn R, Venkatesan S, et al. 2002. Phosphorylation of the linker for activation

of T-cells by Itk promotes recruitment of Vav. *Biochemistry* 41:10732–40

155. Schaeffer EM, Schwartzberg PL. 2000. Tec family kinases in lymphocyte signaling and function. *Curr. Opin. Immunol.* 12:282–88

156. August A, Fischer A, Hao S, Mueller C, Ragin M. 2002. The Tec family of tyrosine kinases in T cells, amplifiers of T cell receptor signals. *Int. J. Biochem. Cell Biol.* 34:1184–89

157. Donnadieu E, Lang V, Bismuth G, Ellmeier W, Acuto O, et al. 2001. Differential roles of Lck and Itk in T cell response to antigen recognition revealed by calcium imaging and electron microscopy. *J. Immunol.* 166:5540–49

158. Kupfer A, Kupfer H. 2003. Imaging immune cell interactions and functions: SMACs and the immunological synapse. *Semin. Immunol.* 15:295–300

159. Pribila JT, Quale AC, Mueller KL, Shimizu Y. 2004. Integrins and T cell-mediated immunity. *Annu. Rev. Immunol.* 22:157–80

160. Spaargaren M, Beuling EA, Rurup ML, Meijer HP, Klok MD, et al. 2003. The B cell antigen receptor controls integrin activity through Btk and PLCγ2. *J. Exp. Med.* 198:1539–50

161. Chen R, Kim O, Li M, Xiong X, Guan JL, et al. 2001. Regulation of the PH-domain-containing tyrosine kinase Etk by focal adhesion kinase through the FERM domain. *Nat. Cell Biol.* 3:439–44

162. Abassi Y, Rehn M, Ekman N, Alitalo K, Vuori K. 2003. p130Cas couples the tyrosine kinase Bmx/Etk with regulation of the actin cytoskeleton and cell migration. *J. Biol. Chem.* 278:35636–43

163. Snapper SB, Rosen FS. 1999. The Wiskott-Aldrich syndrome protein (WASP): roles in signaling and cytoskeletal organization. *Annu. Rev. Immunol.* 17:905–29

164. Bunnell SC, Henry PA, Kolluri R, Kirchhausen T, Rickles RJ, et al. 1996. Identification of Itk/Tsk Src homology 3 do-

main ligands. *J. Biol. Chem.* 271:25646–56

165. Cory GO, MacCarthy-Morrogh L, Banin S, Gout I, Brickell PM, et al. 1996. Evidence that the Wiskott-Aldrich syndrome protein may be involved in lymphoid cell signaling pathways. *J. Immunol.* 157:3791–95

166. Baba Y, Nonoyama S, Matsushita M, Yamadori T, Hashimoto S, et al. 1999. Involvement of Wiskott-Aldrich syndrome protein in B-cell cytoplasmic tyrosine kinase pathway. *Blood* 93:2003–12

167. Guinamard R, Aspenstrom P, Fougereau M, Chavrier P, Guillemot JC. 1998. Tyrosine phosphorylation of the Wiskott-Aldrich syndrome protein by Lyn and Btk is regulated by CDC42. *FEBS Lett.* 434:431–36

168. Tybulewicz V, Ardouin L, Prisco A, Reynolds L. 2003. Vav1: a key signal transducer downstream of the TCR. *Immunol. Rev.* 192:42–52

169. Krawczyk C, Oliveira-Dos-Santos AJ, Sasaki T, Griffiths EK, Ohashi PS, et al. 2002. Vav1 controls integrin clustering and MHC/peptide-specific cell adhesion to antigen-presenting cells. *Immunity* 16:331–43

170. Fischer KD, Kong YY, Nishina H, Tedford K, Marengere LE, et al. 1998. Vav is a regulator of cytoskeletal reorganization mediated by the T-cell receptor. *Curr. Biol.* 8:554–62

171. Takenawa T, Itoh T. 2001. Phosphoinosites, key molecules for regulation of actin cytoskeletal organization and membrane traffic from the plasma membrane. *Biochim. Biophys. Acta* 1533:190–206

172. Schwartzberg P. 2003. Amplifying Btk's signal. *Immunity* 19:634–36

173. Stewart MP, McDowall A, Hogg N. 1998. LFA-1-mediated adhesion in regulated by cytoskeletal restraint and by a Ca^{2+}-dependent protease, calpain. *J. Cell Bio.* 140:699–707

174. Nore BF, Vargas L, Mohamed AJ, Branden LJ, Backesjo CM, et al. 2000.

Redistribution of Bruton's tyrosine kinase by activation of phosphatidylinositol 3-kinase and Rho-family GTPases. *Eur. J. Immunol.* 30:145–54

175. Mao J, Xie W, Yuan H, Simon MI, Mano H, et al. 1998. Tec/Bmx non-receptor tyrosine kinases are involved in regulation of Rho and serum response factor by $G\alpha 12/13$. *EMBO J.* 17:5638–46

176. Roulier EM, Panzer S, Beckendorf SK. 1998. The Tec29 tyrosine kinase is required during *Drosophila* embryogenesis and interacts with Src64 in ring canal development. *Mol. Cell* 1:819–29

177. Yao L, Janmey P, Frigeri LG, Han W, Fujita J, et al. 1999. Pleckstrin homology domains interact with filamentous actin. *J. Biol. Chem.* 274:19752–61

178. Michel F, Attal-Bonnefoy G, Mangino G, Mise-Omata S, Acuto O. 2001. CD28 as a molecular amplifier extending TCR ligation and signaling capabilities. *Immunity* 15:935–45

179. Liao XC, Fournier S, Killeen N, Weiss A, Allison JP, et al. 1997. Itk negatively regulates induction of T cell proliferation by CD28 costimulation. *J. Exp. Med.* 186:221–28

180. van Dijk TB, van Den Akker E, Amelsvoort MP, Mano H, Lowenberg B, et al. 2000. Stem cell factor induces phosphatidylinositol 3′-kinase-dependent Lyn/Tec/Dok-1 complex formation in hematopoietic cells. *Blood* 96:3406–13

181. Yoshida K, Yamashita Y, Miyazato A, Ohya K, Kitanaka A, et al. 2000. Mediation by the protein-tyrosine kinase Tec of signaling between the B cell antigen receptor and Dok-1. *J. Biol. Chem.* 275:24945–52

182. Ellis JH, Sutmuller RP, Sims MJ, Cooksley S. 1998. Functional analysis of the T-cell-restricted protein tyrosine kinase Txk. *Biochem. J.* 335:277–84

183. Lucas JA, Miller AT, Atherly LO, Berg LJ. 2003. The role of Tec family kinases in T cell development and function. *Immunol. Rev.* 191:119–38

184. Hao S, Kurosaki T, August A. 2003. Differential regulation of NFAT and SRF by the B cell receptor via a $PLC\gamma$-Ca^{2+}-dependent pathway. *EMBO J.* 22:4166–77

185. Kashiwakura J, Suzuki N, Takeno M, Itoh S, Oku T, et al. 2002. Evidence of autophosphorylation in Txk: Y91 is an autophosphorylation site. *Biol. Pharm. Bull.* 25:718–21

186. Webb CF, Yamashita Y, Ayers N, Evetts S, Paulin Y, et al. 2000. The transcription factor *Bright* associates with Bruton's tyrosine kinase, the defective protein in immunodeficiency disease. *J. Immunol.* 165:6956–65

187. Yang W, Desiderio S. 1997. BAP-135, a target for Bruton's tyrosine kinase in response to B cell receptor engagement. *Proc. Natl. Acad. Sci. USA* 94:604–9

188. Gilbert C, Levasseur S, Desaulniers P, Dusseault AA, Thibault N, et al. 2003. Chemotactic factor-induced recruitment and activation of Tec family kinases in human neutrophils. II. Effects of LFM-A13, a specific Btk inhibitor. *J. Immunol.* 170:5235–43

189. Lachance G, Levasseur S, Naccache PH. 2002. Chemotactic factor-induced recruitment and activation of Tec family kinases in human neutrophils. Implication of phosphatidynositol 3-kinases. *J. Biol. Chem.* 277:21537–41

190. Suzuki N, Nakamura S, Mano H, Kozasa T. 2003. $G\alpha 12$ activates Rho GTPase through tyrosine-phosphorylated leukemia-associated RhoGEF. *Proc. Natl. Acad. Sci. USA* 100:733–38

191. Ho WY, Cooke MP, Goodnow CC, Davis MM. 1994. Resting and anergic B cells are defective in CD28-dependent costimulation of naive $CD4^+$ T cells. *J. Exp. Med.* 179:1539–49

192. Sugawara T, Moriguchi T, Nishida E, Takahama Y. 1998. Differential roles of ERK and p38 MAP kinase pathways in

positive and negative selection of T lymphocytes. *Immunity* 9:565–74

193. Germain RN. 2002. T-cell development and the CD4-CD8 lineage decision. *Nat. Rev. Immunol.* 2:309–22

194. Singer A. 2002. New perspectives on a developmental dilemma: the kinetic signaling model and the importance of signal duration for the CD4/CD8 lineage decision. *Curr. Opin. Immunol.* 14:207–15

195. Gadue P, Stein PL. 2002. NK T cell precursors exhibit differential cytokine regulation and require Itk for efficient maturation. *J. Immunol.* 169:2397–406

196. Borowski C, Martin C, Gounari F, Haughn L, Aifantis I, et al. 2002. On the brink of becoming a T cell. *Curr. Opin. Immunol.* 14:200–6

197. Takeno M, Yoshikawa H, Kurokawa M, Takeba Y, Kashiwakura JI, et al. 2004. Th1-dominant shift of T cell cytokine production, and subsequent reduction of serum immunoglobulin E response by administration in vivo of plasmid expressing Txk/Rlk, a member of Tec family tyrosine kinases, in a mouse model. *Clin. Exp. Allergy* 34:965–70

198a. Lin TA, McIntyre KW, Das J, Liu C, O'Day KD, et al. 2004. Selective Itk inhibitors block T-cell activation and murine lung inflammation. *Biochemistry* 43:11056–62

198. Chen CH, Seguin-Devaux C, Burke NA, Oriss TB, Watkins SC, et al. 2003. Transforming growth factor β blocks Tec kinase phosphorylation, Ca^{2+} influx, NFATc translocation causing inhibition of T cell differentiation. *J. Exp. Med.* 197:1689–99

199. Matsumoto Y, Oshida T, Obayashi I, Imai Y, Matsui K, et al. 2002. Identification of highly expressed genes in peripheral blood T cells from patients with atopic dermatitis. *Int. Arch. Allergy Immunol.* 129:327–40

199a. Hwang ES, Szabo S, Schwartzberg PL, Glimcher LH. 2005. Silencing of the Th2

program in the T helper progenitor cell by ITK regulated interaction of T-bet with GATA-3. *Science.* In press

200. Bachmann MF, Littman DR, Liao XC. 1997. Antiviral immune responses in Itk-deficient mice. *J. Virol.* 71:7253–57

201. Uckun FM. 1998. Bruton's tyrosine kinase (BTK) as a dual-function regulator of apoptosis. *Biochem. Pharmacol.* 56:683–91

202. Vassilev A, Ozer Z, Navara C, Mahajan S, Uckun FM. 1999. Bruton's tyrosine kinase as an inhibitor of the Fas/CD95 death-inducing signaling complex. *J. Biol. Chem.* 274:1646–56

203. Chun HJ, Zheng L, Ahmad M, Wang J, Speirs CK, et al. 2002. Pleiotropic defects in lymphocyte activation caused by caspase-8 mutations lead to human immunodeficiency. *Nature* 419:395–99

204. Gulbranson-Judge A, Tybulewicz VL, Walters AE, Toellner K-M, MacLennan ICM, et al. 1999. Defective immunoglobulin class switching in Vav-deficient mice is attributable to compromised T cell help. *Eur. J. Immunol.* 29:477–87

205. Sommers CL, Park CS, Lee J, Feng C, Fuller CL, et al. 2002. A LAT mutation that inhibits T cell development yet induces lymphoproliferation. *Science* 296:2040–43

206. Aguado E, Richelme S, Nunez-Cruz S, Miazek A, Mura AM, et al. 2002. Induction of T helper type 2 immunity by a point mutation in the LAT adaptor. *Science* 296:2036–40

207. Marsland BJ, Soos TJ, Spath G, Littman DR, Kopf M. 2004. Protein kinase C θ is critical for the development of in vivo T helper (Th)2 cell but not Th1 cell responses. *J. Exp. Med.* 19:181–89

208. Pfeifhofer C, Kofler K, Gruber T, Tabrizi NG, Lutz C, et al. 2003. Protein kinase C θ affects Ca^{2+} mobilization and NFAT cell activation in primary mouse T cells. *J. Exp. Med.* 197:1525–35

209. Sun Z, Arendt CW, Ellmeier W, Schaeffer EM, Sunshine MJ, et al. 2000. PKC-θ is required for TCR-induced NF-κB activation in mature but not immature T lymphocytes. *Nature* 404:402–7

210. Badour K, Zhang J, Siminovitch KA. 2003. The Wiskott-Aldrich syndrome protein: forging the link between actin and cell activation. *Immunol. Rev.* 192: 98–112

211. Morales-Tirado V, Johannson S, Hanson E, Howell A, Zhang J, et al. 2004. Cutting edge: selective requirement for the Wiskott-Aldrich syndrome protein in cytokine, but not chemokine, secretion by CD4$^+$ T cells. *J. Immunol.* 173:726–30

212. Dombroski D, Houghtling RA, Labno CM, Precht P, Takesono A, et al. 2005. Kinase-independent functions for Itk in TCR-induced regulation of Vav and the actin cytoskeleton. *J. Immunol.* In press

Annu. Rev. Immunol. 2005. 23:601–49
doi: 10.1146/annurev.immunol.23.021704.115737
Copyright © 2005 by Annual Reviews. All rights reserved
First published online as a Review in Advance on December 10, 2004

MOLECULAR GENETICS OF T CELL DEVELOPMENT

Ellen V. Rothenberg and Tom Taghon

*Division of Biology, California Institute of Technology, Pasadena, California 91125;
email: evroth@its.caltech.edu, ttaghon@caltech.edu*

Key Words thymus, transcription factor, Notch, lineage commitment, β-selection

■ **Abstract** T cell development is guided by a complex set of transcription factors that act recursively, in different combinations, at each of the developmental choice points from T-lineage specification to peripheral T cell specialization. This review describes the modes of action of the major T-lineage-defining transcription factors and the signal pathways that activate them during intrathymic differentiation from pluripotent precursors. Roles of Notch and its effector RBPSuh (CSL), GATA-3, E2A/HEB and Id proteins, c-Myb, TCF-1, and members of the Runx, Ets, and Ikaros families are critical. Less known transcription factors that are newly recognized as being required for T cell development at particular checkpoints are also described. The transcriptional regulation of T cell development is contrasted with that of B cell development, in terms of their different degrees of overlap with the stem-cell program and the different roles of key transcription factors in gene regulatory networks leading to lineage commitment.

OVERVIEW OF T CELL DEVELOPMENT AND ITS REQUIREMENTS

T cells are the only hematopoietic cells that are not generated in the bone marrow. Instead, virtually all circulating T lymphocytes are generated in the thymus, and many different types exist. T cells are further distinguished among hematopoietic cells by their potentially infinite proliferative life spans and by their capacity for differentiative specialization even after their mature features are in place. Some of this specialization is triggered by environmental signals from antigen recognition and/or other ligand/receptor interactions. Thus T cell development, as a process, incorporates multiple stages at which different choices are available to the cells, extending over many cell cycles and a long period of time. In spite of this complexity, the T cell program as a whole is unified by the identities of the key regulators throughout the process: Many of the same regulatory factors and growth factor receptors are used again and again at different stages. This review focuses on the roles of these factors in establishing T cell identity as they guide uncommitted hematopoietic precursors into, and through, thymic differentiation.

0732-0582/05/0423-0601$14.00

A Map of the Terrain: Stages of T Cell Development

At least five stages have been defined in which specific regulators are needed for T cell development to proceed. First, there is the specification process, through which multipotent precursors first enter the T cell pathway, usually as they first immigrate to the thymus. Second is the complex process in which proliferative expansion and T cell receptor (TCR) gene rearrangement are combined with commitment to the T lineage within the thymus. These first stages are examined closely at the end of this review. Third is β-selection, which is a cascade of differentiation and proliferation events triggered specifically by "pre-TCR" signaling in precursors of TCR$\alpha\beta$ T cells, after successful rearrangement of the TCRβ gene. Fourth is TCR-dependent positive selection, a major physiological transition, which is coupled with developmental divergence between CD4 and CD8 lineages of T cells. Fifth is the continuing differentiation of T cells in the periphery, which occurs upon stimulation with antigen, antigen-presenting cells, and cytokines. This has been most closely studied for the divergence of Th1 and Th2 CD4 cell types. These stages are diagrammed in Figure 1.

The β-selection and positive selection checkpoints make production of mature T cells depend on successful rearrangement of the T cell receptor genes, either TCRγ and TCRδ or TCRα and TCRβ. Rearrangement is made possible by the expression of the linked RAG-1 and RAG-2 recombinase genes and by the accessibility of the TCR-coding loci in chromatin at the appropriate stages. Transcriptional induction of RAG genes and transcription factor-mediated opening of the TCR loci thus constitute aspects of T cell specification. TCRγ, δ, and β rearrangement all occur during the early DN (double negative) stages (Figure 1), whereas TCRα rearrangement is only permitted in cells that have reached the DP (CD4$^+$ CD8$^+$ TCR^{low}) stage. The cell can sense the success of these rearrangements in encoding a translatable protein because there is also transcriptional activation of the genes encoding the signaling components of the TCR complex, from the earliest stages, and these proteins enable products of newly recombined TCR genes to assemble into functional signaling complexes. Successful TCRβ rearrangement entitles the cell to pass through the β-selection checkpoint and become eligible for differentiation

Figure 1   Outline of T cell development: landmark stages, checkpoints, and developmental choices. Right side: cell-surface markers used in combination to distinguish specific developmental stages. DN: double negative for CD4 and CD8, and as used in this figure, implied to be negative for cell-surface T cell receptor complex expression as well. TCR$\gamma\delta$ and NKT cells are also commonly CD4$^-$ CD8$^-$ but are mature TCR$^+$ subsets that are presented separately. DN1, DN2, DN3, and DN4 stages of DN cell differentiation are distinguished by CD44, c-Kit, and CD25 expression as indicated. DP: CD4$^+$ CD8$^+$ TCR$\alpha\beta$-low. CD4 SP: CD4$^+$ CD8$^-$ TCR$\alpha\beta$-high. CD8 SP: CD4$^-$ CD8$^+$ TCR$\alpha\beta$-high. Branch points from the TCR$\alpha\beta$ mainstream for NKT and T-reg lineages of TCR$\alpha\beta$ cells are incompletely defined.

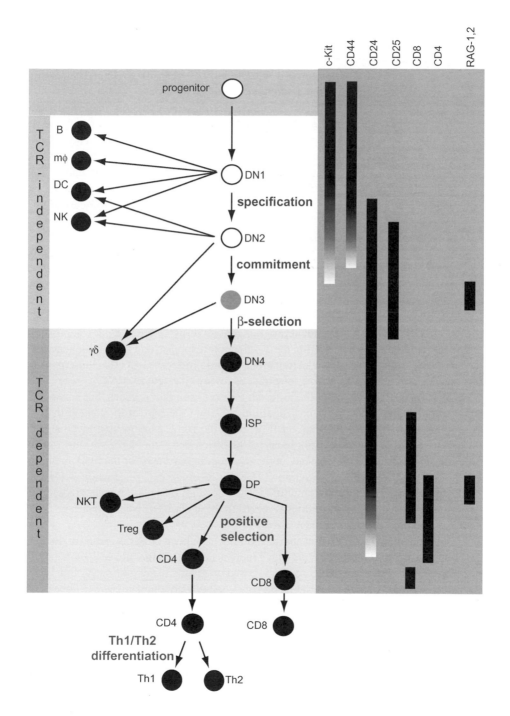

in the TCR$\alpha\beta$ lineage, including the activation of TCRα gene rearrangement. As an alternative to β-selection, successful rearrangement of TCRγ and TCRδ together enables the cell to differentiate as a TCR$\gamma\delta$ cell instead. Cells failing at both will die. Only after successful generation of a TCR$\alpha\beta$ receptor with appropriate specificity are TCR$\alpha\beta$ lineage cells able to pass through a second checkpoint, i.e., positive selection, and then complete their maturation.

TCR-dependent signaling in thymocyte development not only determines survival versus death, but also acts more subtly in other kinds of lineage choice, as discussed in recent reviews (1–5). The quality of signaling at these checkpoints can have a strong influence on the choice of developmental paths that follow. A particularly clear case is at positive selection, when the strength and duration of signaling induced by TCR/ligand interaction in the thymus not only determines which cells will be positively selected, but also guides them to differentiate into either CD4 T cells or CD8 T cells (3–5). For the purposes of this review, most notable about these TCR-dependent events is how very similar signals, from variants of the same receptor, trigger radically different regulatory consequences. In positive selection, for example, this trigger is a transient interaction, and yet CD4 cell and CD8 cell positive selection processes elicit divergent developmental cascades that result in numerous long-term differences in mature cell function and effector potential, which will be maintained through many cell divisions in the periphery. The TCR-dependent program that governs TCR$\gamma\delta$ cell development is also remarkably different from the β-selection response, and the consequences of pre-TCR triggering at β-selection are also quite different from the consequences of TCR triggering at positive selection, as reviewed elsewhere (6).

The explanations lie in the different transcription factor genes that are specifically induced under different conditions (5), and the regulatory context that influences which of these genes will be available for activation by a given signal. Thus in this review, we do not focus on the differences among the various triggering signals as such, but instead, review the regulatory basis for the fundamentally different developmental programs (TCR$\gamma\delta$ development, β-selection, CD4 cell maturation, and CD8 cell maturation) that they call into play. A remarkable fraction of the regulatory molecules involved in these choices also play roles in T cell development from the earliest stages.

The genetic manipulation approaches that have been most powerful for dissecting regulatory relationships are much more accessible in the mouse than in human systems, and so most of this review is based on results in the murine system. However, where evidence is available, human T cell development appears to depend on the same regulators, and some clues suggest that the roles of key factors in T cell development may be broadly conserved among jawed vertebrates.

Critical Regulators: Introductory Overview

Gene knockout experiments have shown that T cell development depends from its earliest stages on at least a half dozen transcription factors, one "instructive" signaling system, and at least three other signaling systems used for growth and survival at particular points. Nearly all of these regulators play ongoing roles in T cell development, although their specific effects shift from one stage to another. They are introduced briefly here, and in the following sections, the roles of each of the transcriptional regulators are discussed in detail.

T cell gene expression and even the first recognizable stages of T cell development depend on the transcription factors GATA-3, c-Myb, members of the Runx family, members of the E2A/HEB family, and members of the Ikaros family. In fetal life, appearance of specified pre-T cells also depends on the Ets-family transcription factor PU.1. Most of these factors are needed for other hematopoietic fates besides the T cell fate. Hunchback-class zinc finger factors of the Ikaros family are needed for all lymphocyte lineages, and the E2A/HEB class of bHLH transcription factors is absolutely essential for B cell development as well as for T cell development. Other factors, such as c-Myb, PU.1, and Runx1, are required to generate the multipotent hematopoietic progenitors of T cells, in addition to playing specific roles in early T cell functions proper. The one transcription factor that appears to be T cell specific is GATA-3. However, this too is a close relative of the stem-cell factor GATA-2. The ability of these molecules to turn on T cell genes as opposed to non-T cell genes is therefore likely to represent target-gene specificity emerging from combinatorial transcription factor action.

T cell development also depends on two other transcription factors that represent dedicated effectors of cell-surface receptor signaling, TCF-1 (Tcf7) and RBPSuh (a.k.a. RBP-Jκ, or CBF/Suppressor of Hairless/Lag-1 = CSL). These factors are distinctive because they are repressors by default but are changed into activators by signaling cascades in response to environmental signals. TCF-1 is the effector of the Wnt/frz/β-catenin signaling cascade, and RBPSuh is the effector of the Notch signaling cascade. The exact roles that these factors play in T cell development appear to be different, as described below, but they share the critical feature that their presence in the precursors of T cells imposes a dichotomous switch-like behavior on every function they control. The same genes that they activate in the presence of a signal, they repress in the absence of a signal. The Notch signaling cascade is the unique "instructive" signaling system used for T cell specification, whereas the Wnt/TCF signaling system has an important role in proliferation coupled with differentiation.

Other genes that are essential for T cell development encode cytokine receptors as well as pre-TCR/TCR components that are needed for survival and proliferation. Early in T cell development the IL-7 receptor complex (IL7Rα/γc = CD127/CD132) is most important, while survival and proliferation are dominated later by signals from different versions of the TCR complex (pre-TCR, TCR$\gamma\delta$, or TCR$\alpha\beta$ associated with CD4 or CD8 coreceptors). These signal-dependent receptors all differ from the Notch system in that they primarily trigger the de novo appearance or nuclear localization of transcription factors, rather than conversion of a repressor to an activator. They thus lend themselves more to promoting graded responses, such as proliferation and activation, rather than the kinds of all-or-none dichotomous effects of Notch/RBPSuh. The transcription factors mobilized include STAT5, NF-κB, NF-AT, and AP-1 in different combinations, with greater or lesser contributions from the PI-3 kinase, Akt/PKB, and Ras/MAP kinase signaling pathways (see 1–5). The survival and proliferative (trophic) effects of these receptor systems are well explained by the activation of these mediators.

Triggering of cytokine receptors, like the triggering of TCR complexes, can also have developmental effects that are specific to different stages. Whereas the receptors are lineage-specific in their expression, the factors they activate are not. Without minimizing the importance of these pathways, the developmental consequences of their triggering must be heavily influenced by changes in the "regulatory contexts" within which they are activated. In this review, therefore, we focus primarily on the transcription factors themselves and the transcription-linked signaling systems that set these different regulatory contexts.

REPERTORY PLAYERS: T CELL IDENTITY FACTORS IN RECURRENT ROLES

A particular set of T cell transcription factors and signaling molecules is used repeatedly throughout T cell development to establish T cell identity and then to make choices between successive T-lineage subspecializations. These recurrent players include Notch molecules and their direct transcriptional effector RBPSuh (CSL); GATA-3; the bHLH factors E2A and HEB and their antagonists Id2 and Id3; Runx1 and Runx3; and possibly also members of the Ikaros family. These factors can be viewed as central to T cell identity, somewhat analogous to the B cell factors EBF and Pax5 (7), which are compared in more detail below. However, in the case of T cell development, the individual functions that these factors perform are discontinuous, stage-specific, and even subject to alternation between activating and inhibitory effects from one stage to the next. These "identity factors" are described here in detail.

Notch and its Mediators

The transmembrane signaling receptor Notch1 is a representative of an ancient, evolutionarily conserved family of developmental regulators that was first noted for its importance for neurogenesis in embryos of *Drosophila melanogaster*. In the mouse, Notch1 is essential for embryonic viability also, and it is expressed at a particularly high level in the thymus. In the late 1990s, Notch gain of function was shown to have powerful influences on TCR-dependent selection events in the thymus. Then with the advent of conditional knockout technology, it became possible to remove Notch1 function, and this revealed that T cell development is intensely and specifically dependent on Notch1 in the pluripotent precursor stage (reviewed in 8–10). Without Notch1, precursors cannot develop into T cells at all, and B cells develop in the thymus instead. At the same time, retroviral

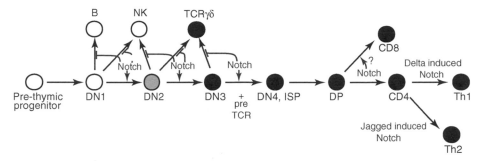

Figure 2   Roles of Notch and its transcriptional effectors in T cell specification and developmental choices. Stages at which T cell development is affected by gain or loss of function of Notch1, other Notch proteins, or the Notch transcriptional mediator RBPSuh (CSL) are indicated. See text for details and review citations.

transduction of constitutively active Notch (Notch1IC) into pluripotent precursors showed that Notch gain of function could also enhance T cell development while blocking B cell development (Figure 2). As noted above, one major pathway of Notch signaling involves cleavage of the Notch cytoplasmic domain to generate a transcriptional activation domain, which migrates to the nucleus and converts a default repressor, RBPSuh, into an activator. Knockout experiments indicate that this is the pathway through which Notch promotes T cell development and suppresses B cell development (11, 12). Notch1/RBPSuh are the first, and so far the only, regulators in which gain and loss of function have been shown to have simple reciprocal effects on initial T cell specification.

Notch family molecules also play more complex roles later, both in TCR-dependent selection events and in peripheral T cell differentiation. Conditional knockout studies with deletion in intrathymic DN cells have shown that Notch1 is needed for TCRβ gene rearrangement; also, in vitro assay systems show that Notch/Delta interactions are needed to sustain T cells through the proliferation and differentiation events of β-selection, complementing signals from the pre-TCR (13–16) (Figure 2). Deletion of RBPSuh between T-lineage specification and β-selection favors development of TCR$\gamma\delta$ lineage T cells at the expense of TCR$\alpha\beta$ T cells (12) (Figure 2). Normally, Notch1 and the genes that it immediately activates are expressed at the highest levels in DN (double negative) thymocytes prior to β-selection, and substantially downregulated thereafter (14, 17). Constitutive expression of activated Notch perturbs the gene expression setpoints in DP (double positive) cells that emerge from β-selection (14, 18) and can lead to leukemias that resemble cells frozen in mid-β-selection (19–21). Thus, not only Notch activation but also its correctly regulated deactivation are important to generate the pool of TCR$\alpha\beta^+$ thymocytes from which positive selection and maturation will occur.

Alterations of Notch activation in thymocytes at later stages can sharply perturb positive selection and the CD4/CD8 lineage choice as well (Figure 2). However, the exact effects seen vary substantially in different experimental tests (reviewed in 8–10, 22–24). In overexpression studies the result depends on the exact form of the constitutively activated Notch molecule, since the intracellular domain of Notch contains a number of separate domains mediating interactions with different coeffectors (see reviews, above). Most gain-of-function studies have shown an enhancement of CD8 cell development, though this is not uniform, and whether this is due to trophic effects, alteration of signaling, or developmental programming is subject to debate. Loss-of-function studies have been complicated by the ability of multiple Notch family members to contribute to thymocyte responses at these late stages and by uncertainties about the specificities of pharmacological inhibitors of Notch signaling and the exact modes of action of endogenous signaling modulators. Also complicating the interpretation of all the transgenic and knockout experiments is an intrinsic aspect of thymocyte population dynamics, namely the small number of cell division cycles between the end of β-selection and the start of positive selection. This means that Notch manipulation might affect positive selection indirectly through perturbations of the β-selection process, and its impact may appear different in kinetic than in steady-state analyses.

Some clarification may emerge eventually from identification of the ligands for Notch during positive selection. Notch receptors interact with two different kinds of ligands, Delta-like and Jagged family molecules, and although they both activate RBPSuh, they promote distinct developmental responses through additional pathways that are still under investigation (25–27). Very recently, it has emerged that the differential signaling capacities of Notch family members interacting with Delta-like versus Jagged family ligands are probably quite significant in peripheral T cell differentiation (Figure 2). Differential uses of these classes of Notch ligands, and perhaps Notch family members, in contacts between mature peripheral T cells and antigen-presenting cells, act as instructive signals to bias the subsequent differentiation of the T cells into specialized effectors of the Th1, Th2, or T-reg classes (27–30). Although RBPSuh seems to have a direct involvement in the Notch/Jagged pathway that favors the Th2 fate, other Notch/Delta-like signaling pathways appear to contribute to the Th1 fate (27). Thus Notch signaling underlies a succession of divergent choices in T cell differentiation that continue long after its initial role in T- versus B-lineage specification.

GATA-3

GATA-3 is the one transcription factor that appears to be expressed in a completely T cell–specific way among all hematopoietic cell types. While it is also needed for many nonhematopoietic cell types, and GATA-3 mutants do not survive midgestation, the only hematopoietic effects seen are a reduction in hematopoietic progenitor cells, complete loss of T cell development, and a late defect in the final maturation of NK cells (31–33). GATA-3 expression rises as T-lineage differentiation begins (T. Taghon, E.-S. David, J.C. Zúñiga-Pflücker & E.V. Rothenberg, submitted; 34) and peaks in the thymus during the proliferation at β-selection

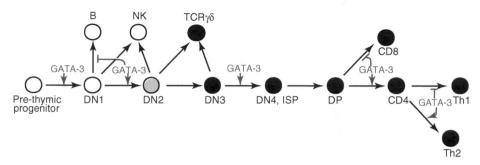

Figure 3   Roles of GATA-3 in support of T cell development. Stages at which loss of GATA-3 function affects T lineage differentiative progression and developmental choices are shown with the implied direction of the normal GATA-3 effect as indicated. Within the T lineage, overexpression of GATA-3 or a GATA-3 hypomorphic mutant has similar effects to those indicated; however, in prethymic precursors, GATA-3 overexpression causes a paradoxical deviation away from all lymphoid fates (not shown in figure).

and again, later, in cells undergoing positive selection to the CD4 SP thymocyte fate (32, 35, 36). Expression drops again in resting peripheral T cells, but can be reinduced specifically upon antigen activation. GATA-3 plays critical functional roles in all of these stages, as summarized in Figure 3.

GATA-3 is implicated in regulating the genes that are needed in multiple stages of T cell development, from intrathymic targets such as RAG-2, TCR gene enhancers, and CD8, to the peripheral T cell effector IL-4 (37–41). Germline knockout experiments show that it is critical for the generation of any identifiable T cell precursors, either in vivo (in chimeras) or in vitro. Conditional knockout experiments, which delete GATA-3 only after the cells immigrate to the thymus, show that it is also needed for normal β-selection and proliferation in the DN to DP transition (36). Then it has a prominent role at positive selection, promoting the development of CD4 SP cells and blocking the development of CD8 SP cells (35, 36, 42). In peripheral T cells, it modulates cell survival and migration behavior (43) and plays a dominant role in the differentiation of CD4 T cells to a Th2 fate (reviewed in 44, 45).

In spite of its vital regulatory involvement in T cell developmental progression, GATA-3 is not a simple equivalent of dominant lineage regulators like erythroid GATA-1 or B cell EBF or Pax5. Forced expression of GATA-3 in nonthymic hematopoietic precursors does not enhance or accelerate T cell specification. Instead, it completely aborts T cell specification, and this shocking result is a consistent finding both in vivo and in vitro (T. Taghon, M. De Smedt, T. Kerre, J. Plum, E.V. Rothenberg & G. LeClercq, submitted for publication; T. Taghon & E.V. Rothenberg, in preparation; 46, 47) (Figure 3). These severely discordant results for gain and loss of function of GATA-3 are a hallmark of the T cell specification process (discussed below). If retroviral transduction is used to elevate GATA-3 expression later, in thymocytes, it continues to show inappropriately inhibitory effects, although GATA-3 effects on developmental choice at these later stages at least display the same sign as indicated in loss-of-function studies (35, 42, 47, 48). In mature peripheral T cells, on the other hand, gain and loss of function of GATA-3 give concordant results for the role of this factor in the Th1/Th2-lineage choice (44, 45, 49–51). This implies that T cell development not only relies repeatedly on GATA-3 but also continually adjusts the regulatory context of the cells to become more and more tolerant of GATA-3 at a wide range of doses.

A possible explanation for the difficult behavior of GATA-3 is that, like other GATA factors, it can have a wide range of biochemically distinct activities (40, 52, 53). It can carry out chromatin remodeling (IL-4), overt transcriptional activation (IL-5), and repression (IFNγ). Although the mechanisms through which GATA-3 represses are poorly characterized (54, 55), one mechanism is suggested by the presence of functional GATA-3 sites intermixed with SATB1 sites in a nuclear matrix attachment region of the CD8 locus, i.e., a locus that is turned off when GATA-3 expression promotes CD4 cell development (41). Different domains of the GATA-3 molecule are implicated in these different activities (52, 56, 57), supporting the idea that distinct functions are based on interactions with different sets of collaborating factors. This makes it plausible that developmental changes in the expression of other specific, potentially collaborating factors during T cell maturation could gradually disfavor access to non-T cell genes and protect critical T cell genes from inappropriate actions of GATA-3.

One intriguing potential cofactor for GATA-3 could be FOG-1, better known for its cooperative role with GATA-1 during erythrocyte and megakaryocyte differentiation. FOG-1 is expressed within the thymus and required for normal T cell development, since FOG-1-deficient thymocytes are unable to progress through β-selection (58), when GATA-3 activity levels appear to be high. However, it is still unclear how FOG-1 behaves in this setting as a GATA-3 cofactor. FOG-1 can inhibit GATA-3 activity in a Th2-promoting assay (58, 59), and thus its potential role might involve reducing GATA-3 activity at specific stages of T cell development. Titration of FOG-1 could potentially explain the toxicity of high level GATA-3 expression at an early stage. In any case, it is striking how subtly GATA-3 must be deployed during the time of its most critical T cell role, at the start of T cell development.

E2A/HEB

T cells share with B cells a reliance on type I bHLH transcription factors (E proteins) for their development from an early stage (60–62). Thymocytes express not only E2A, the family member that is most important in B cell development, but also the closely related factors HEB (Tcf12) and E2-2 (Tcf4) (63). A number of T cell target genes are known to be positively regulated by this class of factors, including CD4 and the surrogate light chain gene pTα (64–66), and E protein binding sites are prominent in regulatory elements of RAG-1/RAG-2 recombinase genes that are active in DN stages and in TCR gene enhancers. E2A also provides a unique survival function in conjunction with IL-7-dependent growth (67). Moreover, E2A/HEB dimers appear to act as positive regulators for another critical T cell transcription factor, GATA-3 (68).

Thus it is not surprising that forced expression of any of the Id factors (Idb, inhibitors of DNA binding), which heterodimerize with E2A-class bHLH factors to block their DNA binding, completely aborts early T cell specification (69, 70). In fact, forced expression of Id proteins can direct precursors into the NK lineage instead, a developmental pathway that in normal conditions is completely dependent on the Id2 gene (63). The E proteins are therefore among the essential directors of T-lineage development, and the balance between E protein and Id activity in multipotent precursors is critical to arbitrate the lineage choice between T/B and NK/DC/myeloid fates, as discussed below.

The functions of E proteins are discontinuous, however, even within the thymus (Figure 4). E2A in particular is most essential prior to the DP stage (71). Dominant negative mutants of HEB that interfere with all E proteins also block T cell development, no later than the DN to DP transition (72). However, as T cell precursors pass through alternating periods of proliferative expansion (DN2), stasis (DN3), and reactivation (DN4/ISP), E protein activation alternates with periods of inhibition, as pre-TCR- or TCR-triggered activation results in waves of Id3 induction that are functionally important for the success of selection (73–75). While Id proteins can support proliferation and other activation responses (76), E proteins actively promote G_1 arrest at developmental checkpoints (77). Thus, although the loss of E protein function blocks T cell development completely, overexpression of E proteins in experimental systems does not perceptibly drive precursors into the T cell pathway.

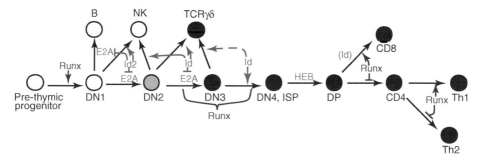

Figure 4   Roles of Runx factors and the E protein/Id ratios in T cell development. The figure combines data for stages of action by Runx1 and Runx3, and the roles of Id2 and Id3 as antagonists of the E2A and HEB (E protein) bHLH factors. Note the alternating phases of E protein and Id dominance that are required for T cell development and the roles of Runx factors acting parallel to GATA-3 at β-selection and in opposition to GATA-3 at positive selection (see Figure 3).

NONLINEAGE-SPECIFIC REGULATORS WITH ESSENTIAL ROLES IN T CELL SPECIFICATION

The context in which the T-lineage identity factors operate is greatly affected by the action of additional factors of different structural groups. These other factors are just as critical for the generation of T cells as those discussed above, but they are not yet shown to be implicated in the T-lineage choice as compared with other cell fates. However, these factors continue to play important roles at specific choice points within the T lineage.

Runx Factors

The three mammalian Runx factors are all expressed in the thymus and used throughout T cell development, although they are not T cell specific in expression or function (reviewed in 78, 79). GATA-3 and Runx3 are probably associated with thymocyte differentiation throughout the jawed vertebrates, as shown by the high-level coexpression of these factors specifically in the thymus of the cartilaginous fish *Raja eglanteria* (80). The most abundant Runx factor in the thymus (Runx1) is expressed as a legacy from hematopoietic stem cells, where it plays an indispensable role (81, 82). This early role dominates the phenotype of Runx1 germline knockout animals, since there is no development of any kind of lymphocytes when generation of definitive hematopoietic precursors is blocked. However, evidence from conditional Runx knockouts, domain-specific Runx knockouts, Runx transgenics, and regulatory mutations in specific T-lineage target genes together unambiguously indicates that Runx factors play specific, central roles in positive and negative gene regulation within the T cell differentiation program (79, 83–88). Runx factors promote DN cell expansion and β-selection, expression of CD8 in the DN to DP transition, and the selection and maturation of CD8 SP cells (Figure 4). The mechanisms involved may be complex, since thymocytes express a variety of splice and promoter-use isoforms of Runx genes that are predicted to encode functionally heterogeneous proteins (84, 89, 90).

Runx factors are poor transactivators alone, but capable of activating when they collaborate with partners binding to the same *cis*-regulatory module, such as Ets family factors or c-Myb. In the TCRα and TCRβ *cis*-regulatory elements, Runx/Ets collaboration provides essential positive regulatory function, while Runx/Myb collaboration activates the TCRγ and TCRδ *cis*-regulatory elements (91–96). Runx factors also provide substantial repressor activity at other target sites, recruiting Groucho/TLE/Grg family proteins or Sin3A by interaction with different C-terminal domains, and this is also important in T cell development. Runx1 activity in the expansion and differentiation of DN thymocytes depends, at least in part, on the Groucho-interaction domain (83).

Two specific targets of Runx repression have been analyzed in elegant detail. The CD4 gene turns out to be silenced by Runx1 in late DN thymocytes, before β-selection, and by Runx3 in CD8 SP thymocytes, after positive selection

(84–86). Furthermore, Runx-dependent repression appears to be important for correct regulation of the RAG-1/2 locus (97). The mode of action in the case of RAG-1/2 is interesting because it imposes a default condition of repression, starting at β-selection, which is conditionally alleviated by factors binding a distal "antisilencing element." This element is specific for permitting expression in DP thymocytes, and it is active only until positive selection occurs. If there must be a DP-specific mechanism for antagonizing Runx repression, this implies that Runx factors are present and active throughout the DP stage, as well as in DN and SP thymocytes.

Evidence now accumulating indicates that Runx factors (most likely Runx3) probably have a positive role in CD8 SP cell maturation (Figure 4), beyond their ability to repress CD4 (85, 88, 98, 99, 99a). Exactly how this works is not yet known. When overexpressed from the DN stage, any of the three Runx family members appears to accelerate β-selection to the CD8$^+$ ISP stage, but then to block the CD4 expression that normally results in a DP phenotype (84, 87). It is not clear whether the strong Lck-dependent signals needed to induce positive selection to the CD4 lineage can be delivered to the cells in the face of this global CD4 repression. Thus Runx factors might drive positive selection toward the CD8 SP pathway not only through their positive effects on CD8 and their negative effects on CD4, but also through the indirect consequences of these alterations on strength of Lck signaling. Even independently of CD4 expression, TCR specificity, or duration of signaling, however, Runx3 appears to promote CD8 SP lineage development, suggesting a central role in developmental programming of cytolytic T cells (99a; T. Sato, S.-i. Ohno, T. Hayashi, C. Sato, K. Hayashi, K. Kohu, M. Satake & S. Habu, submitted for publication; Sonoko Habu, personal communication).

The reciprocal effects of Runx and GATA-3 in CD4/CD8 differentiation raise the question of whether these factors antagonize each other during positive selection. So far, one report (100) suggests that forced expression of Runx blocks GATA-3 upregulation in peripheral T cells and thus biases the Th1/Th2 choice against the Th2 fate. However, both GATA-3 and Runx1 are needed for efficient β-selection. The mechanisms through which GATA-3 and Runx factors could interact in the thymus remain to be explored.

Ikaros Family Transcription Factors

Ikaros and its family members were the first transcription factors found to be essential for lymphocyte development, as distinct from development of other hematopoietic cell types (reviewed in 101). At least three members of the family are expressed in the thymus, in part continuing expression from earlier hematopoietic precursors. Ikaros itself is essential for B cell and fetal T cell development, and inhibition of the whole family by dominant-negative transgene expression eliminates T and NK cell development as well. While many hematopoietic genes possess Ikaros binding sites, there has been controversy about the mode of action of this regulator and whether it is predominantly activating or repressive (102, 103; reviewed in 104).

Much remains unresolved about the exact ways in which it interacts with the inputs from other lymphoid transcriptional regulators. However, the Ikaros family factors are demonstrably important at a number of successive stages: hematopoietic stem-cell maintenance, development of common lymphoid progenitors, β-selection and activation of CD8 expression, and the setting of thresholds for mitogenic activation of immature and mature T cells (103, 105–108). Recent data suggest that Ikaros could also have a role in determining when strong TCR signaling should lead to negative selection, rather than to CD4 SP positive selection (109).

One Ikaros family member, Helios, is expressed selectively in stem cells and in cells of the T cell lineage, with increasing expression during T cell specification and decreasing expression during B cell development. T-lineage-specific Helios expression is conserved, like GATA-3 and Runx3 expression, from mammals to cartilaginous fish (80). This suggests that Helios could play an important and specific role in T cell development, but the functional data needed to address this question are lacking.

At positive selection, the effects of Ikaros and the effects of Runx factors appear to be exerted in the same direction, generally facilitating CD8 expression and/or CD8 cell differentiation (85, 86, 88, 103). The ability of Ikaros factors to associate with chromatin-remodeling complexes (104) could be implicated in these actions, since the chromatin-remodeling component Brg appears to participate in some of the same regulatory events (110). Thus, future genetic and biochemical evidence may reveal that the driver of the positive actions of Ikaros factors in T cell development could be a complex involving Ikaros, together with Runx and Brg proteins.

Critical Growth-Promoting Factors: TCF/LEF-1

TCF/LEF factors, the nuclear effectors of the Wnt pathway, are essential both at β-selection and at an earlier stage of IL-7-dependent expansion in the DN1 to DN2 transition (111–114). TCF-1 (Tcf7) is one of the most highly expressed transcription factors in developing thymocytes (E.-S. David & E.V. Rothenberg, unpublished data), with partially redundant expression of a closely related factor, LEF-1, in the fetal thymus. Antisense oligonucleotides against TCF-1 inhibit T cell generation from prethymic progenitors in fetal thymic organ culture (34). Normally, TCF-1 is converted from a repressor to a transcriptional activator by interaction with β-catenin (or the related protein plakoglobin), and it is the activating roles of TCF-1 that appear to be most important for T cell development, based on genetic manipulations of the TCF-1/β-catenin interaction interface (114). However, these effects appear primarily to reflect an essential role in proliferation, which is normally very extensive in T cell development, rather than in lineage decisions per se (115). Members of the TCF family including TCF-1 itself are shared between developing T cells and adult hematopoietic stem cells, where they play important roles in proliferation prior to differentiation (116). In mice, TCF-1 becomes increasingly important as a function of age for the waves of T cell precursors that differentiate after birth, in order for these cells to reach the DN2 stage (112).

c-Myb

The proto-oncogene c-Myb is also essential for T cell development, as well as essential for B cell development and for definitive hematopoietic stem-cell generation (117–119). Molecular evidence indicates complex, context-dependent roles for c-Myb in c-Kit, CD4, TCRγ, and TCRδ gene expression (120–122). It is most obviously involved in proliferative phases such as β-selection (123). Recently, through conditional inactivation at different stages of T cell development, the critical role for c-Myb has been confirmed at β-selection (124), in part associated with reduced rearrangement at the TCR-β locus. Furthermore, c-Myb is important for survival of DP thymocytes and specifically for the development of CD4 SP thymocytes (124).

Hit-and-Run Specification Factors: PU.1

The last group of essential T cell regulators is different in that it both supports and constrains T-lineage development. This group is represented by PU.1, a divergent Ets subfamily member, which is expressed only in the earliest stages of T cell development, along with other stem-cell legacy genes such as GATA-2 and SCL/Tal-1 (125–127; T. Taghon, R. Pant & E.V. Rothenberg, unpublished data). A close relative of PU.1, Spi-B, is also expressed in DN thymocytes and then shut off at β-selection (125, 128). PU.1 is not expressed in mature T cells, and instead plays continuing roles in macrophage, granulocyte, and B cell development (129, 130). It is possible that the role of PU.1 for T cell precursors is mainly to provide a general proliferative function prior to specification; there is evidence that PU.1 acts this way in the erythroid lineage, where it also has a hit-and-run role (131). In early B cell precursors, PU.1 is important for IL-7Rα expression (132), and, conceivably, some of these cells are uncommitted precursors of T cells as well. PU.1 function is most important for the earliest precursors of the fetal cohorts of T cells (133). If its role is basically proliferative in these cells, it is curious that these are pre-T cell populations in which TCF/LEF function seems to be less critical (112). Conceivably, there could be a fetal-specific proliferative mechanism dependent on PU.1 that is replaced in postnatal lymphopoiesis by one dependent on Wnt/TCF-1.

While PU.1 gene disruption destroys fetal T cell development (126, 133), forced maintenance of PU.1 expression in precursors also blocks T cell development at early stages (134). Thus, PU.1 support of fetal T cell development is dose dependent, and also, obligatorily, a hit-and-run role. Besides supporting the proliferation of multilineage lymphoid precursors, PU.1 and Spi-B may in fact maintain the non-T-cell developmental options of these precursors, prior to T-lineage commitment (134, 135). The linkage between acquisition of T cell characteristics and closure of alternative options is discussed in detail below.

OTHER TRANSCRIPTION FACTORS WITH SPECIALIZED ROLES IN T CELL DEVELOPMENT

The factors already listed do not fully account for all the lineage-specific aspects of T cell development. There are additional regulators that have potent impacts on a few selective aspects of T cell development in the thymus, or which are less well characterized in this context than those we have already introduced. Two widely used classes of transcription factors, Ets family factors and HOX cluster factors, are used in developing T cells, although the coexpression of multiple family members with overlapping functions makes it harder to use genetics to distinguish all the roles of individual genes. Another group consists of the T-box factors T-bet and eomesodermin and their collaborator Hlx. These are factors that are well known in peripheral T cell differentiation in response to antigen, but which may also play a role in the intrathymic differentiation of particular T and NK cell lineages. There are also a number of dedicated transcriptional repressors and nuclear localization-directing factors whose roles will eventually need to be explained.

Ets Family Transcription Factors: Continuing Roles, Multiple Players

Transcription factors of the Ets family are strongly implicated in early T cell gene regulation. Binding sites for these factors are found in the regulatory regions of multiple lymphocyte differentiation genes, often linked to Runx sites and/or overlapping with Ikaros sites (92, 94, 95, 136). In the T cell lineage, Ets family function is guaranteed by redundancy. Ets-1, Ets-2, Fli, Tel, Elf, and GABPα are among the members of this family that are expressed throughout most of T cell development, with Erg and members of the divergent PU.1/Spi subfamily expressed for more limited periods (125). The overlapping expression patterns of these factors and their redundant DNA-binding specificities make it easy to underestimate their regulatory importance for T cell development if one only considers results of single-gene mutants (137). The effects of Ets-1 knockouts are sharper in NK cells, which do not express such high levels of other Ets family members (138). However, recent data indicate that GABPα may play a specific role in IL-7Rα gene expression in T-lineage cells (139).

HOX Genes

Homeodomain-containing HOX genes are crucial mediators of patterning of the anterior/posterior axis during embryonic development, and increasing evidence points to their role as mediators of hematopoiesis. Primarily, genes of the HOX-A cluster seem to be expressed in hematopoietic cells (140). There is some evidence for a developmental expression pattern colinear with the order of genes in the cluster, as during embryogenesis, in some hematopoietic lineages and also during T cell development (141). Little functional evidence is available from HOX knockout studies yet due to their lethality, and T-lineage conditional inactivation studies are lacking. HOX-A9, however, has been shown to be crucial for T cell development, as well as for certain other hematopoietic lineages. Mice deficient for this gene display a severe reduction in DN2 and DN3 thymocytes, possibly due to a lack of IL-7R expression (142).

T-box Factors T-bet (Tbx21) and Eomesodermin, and their Collaborators

Functional maturation of multiple T cell subsets depends upon the Tbx-family factors, T-bet (Tbx21, Tbt-1) and Eomesodermin, which promote the ability to express IFN-γ, and may also activate granzyme B and perforin (55, 143–147). T-bet is expressed alone in activated CD4 conventional Th1 and NKT cells, whereas Eomesodermin contributes a partially redundant function in CD8 conventional T cells and in NK cells. In mature conventional TCR$\alpha\beta$ CD4 cells, T-bet represents a critical node in a bistable regulatory network, where it promotes the establishment of Th1-type function in opposition to GATA-3 (reviewed in 44, 45). Not only is T-bet essential for postthymic differentiation of Th1 cells, but it also is specifically required for intrathymic generation of the whole NKT lineage of T cells (147).

To activate differentiation to a Th1 effector fate, T-bet induces expression of another factor, the divergent homeodomain transcription factor Hlx, which then collaborates with it to turn on IFNγ (148–150). Recent data suggest that T-bet can also activate one of the promoters of Runx1 (147), which could provide an indirect mechanism for it to inhibit GATA-3 expression in some contexts, as described above (100). In T cell subsets other than conventional TCR$\alpha\beta$ cells, however, T-bet and GATA-3 appear to be mutually compatible in their contributions to function, as for example in TCR$\gamma\delta$ cells, NK cells, and NKT cells (55, 147). (For excellent discussion of the other factors used for NK and NKT cell development, see 147, 151).

Although T-bet and eomesodermin are not T-lineage specific and are not yet known to play any early role in T cell precursor specification, there is early, regulated expression of T-bet in DN thymocytes (F.-S. David & E.V. Rothenberg, unpublished data). Direct perturbation experiments will be needed to determine whether precocious induction of these genes could play a role in the T/NK or the TCR$\alpha\beta$/TCR$\gamma\delta$ lineage choices.

TOX: A New HMG Box Factor

Both β-selection and positive selection are induced by TCR-mediated signaling, and a new transcription factor has been identified as a target of this signaling that plays a role in both processes. TOX is a novel member of the family of HMG box containing transcription factors that also comprises other important mediators of T cell development, such as TCF-1 and LEF-1 (152). TOX is specifically upregulated following pre-TCR signaling and positive selection, but, strikingly, does not seem to be involved in TCR-mediated activation of mature, peripheral T cells. Transgenic mice that express TOX under the control of the Lck promoter show an increase in both ISP (post β-selection) and SP (post positive selection) CD8$^+$ thymocytes. TOX induction during positive selection is calcineurin dependent and results in Runx3 upregulation, which in turn downregulates CD4 (153). This cascade can be counteracted by strong or sustained TCR signaling, a process that involves upregulation of GATA-3. Thus, the strength of TCR-mediated signaling at positive selection seems to change GATA-3 versus TOX ratios to result in CD4 versus CD8 lineage development (153), though this model awaits confirmation by knockout studies.

Essential Repressors: Gfi-1, N-CoR1, and δEF1

Mutations in several genes coding for dedicated transcriptional repressors suggest that repression may be an essential aspect of T cell specification, at least at particular stages. The repressors analyzed to date are not T-lineage-specific in their expression and their roles in T cell development have mostly emerged as incidental features of a more global phenotype. But there is compelling evidence that losses of function of the repressors Gfi-1, N-CoR1, or δEF1 (ZEB, AREB6, Zfh, TCF-8) can each severely distort T cell development at specific stages. All three are normally expressed throughout most of intrathymic development, but the target genes that they must repress are not defined yet. While one can speculate that genes such as PU.1 should be important targets of stage-specific repression, very little is clear yet about the way these factors actually work to promote T cell development. The stages affected by loss of function of these three repressors are apparently different, although they have not been fully characterized to date.

Either a partial or a complete loss of function of the zinc finger-homeodomain repressor δEF1 causes a severe loss of thymic cellularity, with a particularly strong decrease in the earliest c-kit$^+$ intrathymic populations and the DP cells (154). Some recovery occurs in later stages. The severity of this phenotype appears paradoxical, because δEF1 (ZEB) is capable of competing with E proteins to interfere with activation at E-box sites, and loss of δEF1 should favor activity of E proteins in T cell gene expression. There is even evidence that this repressor could downregulate GATA-3 expression itself (68). However, recall that both GATA-3 and E proteins can only promote T cell development when they themselves are under tight regulation (see above). A tonic level of repression of critical genes by δEF1 may also be important to maintain expression within tolerable limits (as for GATA-3) or to enforce specificity by requiring concerted action by positively regulating factors (155). δEF1 mutants also show derepressed integrin α4 expression, which could affect migration among appropriate zones of the thymus (154).

The nuclear receptor corepressor N-CoR1 has a strikingly important role in enabling thymocytes to develop through β-selection. In an N-CoR1 knockout, thymocytes are blocked almost completely at the DN to DP transition (156). Unfortunately, no further characterization is available. The DN to DP transition is a time of very rapid proliferation and rapid shifts in the requirements for E box proteins, their Id antagonists, TCF, and c-Myb, as described above. Availability of this general-purpose repressive cofactor may be essential to mediate these regulatory shifts. Alternatively, the lack of N-CoR may have resulted in a failure to generate a pre-TCR in the first place, e.g., by interfering with TCR gene rearrangement.

The mutants of Gfi-1 have a subtler phenotype that affects particular stages of development both before and after β-selection. Gfi-1 is a repressor with 6 zinc fingers and a SNAG repression domain, and it is needed for normal development of neutrophils but not of granulocyte-macrophage precursors or of erythroid cells. In Gfi-1$^{-/-}$ mutants, B cell development and T cell development are both partially inhibited, with clear bottlenecks in the progression of DN thymocytes to normal DN2 and DN3 states, depressed CD4 SP-cell production, and enhanced CD8-cell production (157, 158). These perturbations are consistent with the developmental pattern of Gfi-1 expression in the thymus, which is turned on in the DN2 stage and persists through the DP stage (159). Gfi-1 may be important to repress the bHLH antagonist Id proteins at the correct stages, since Id2 and Id1 are aberrantly highly expressed in the Gfi-1$^{-/-}$ thymus (158). However, this could also be an indirect effect of abnormal precursor utilization in the thymus, since the DN1 subset in these mutants appears abnormal (158), lacking the c-kit$^+$ IL-7R^{low} cells that are the most potent T cell precursors in a normal thymus (108).

Some ambiguity attends the role of Gfi-1, in part because it has a close relative that is also expressed in the thymus, Gfi-1B. This repressor is similar in overall structure to Gfi-1, but diverges in sequence, and its effects are either redundant or antagonistic to those of Gfi-1 depending on the developmental context. Gfi-1B is expressed more narrowly in hematopoiesis, preferentially in erythroid lineage cells, where it is required (159–161). In thymocytes, Gfi-1B is reportedly expressed only in a sharp spike in the DN3 stage, where it may play a role in β-selection (159). It is not clear which factor, Gfi-1 or Gfi-1B, is more important during β-selection in vivo. However, there is evidence from a peripheral T cell system that Gfi-1 has another, distinctive function that could make it valuable in the T-lineage specification process. In mature peripheral T cells undergoing stimulation under Th2 conditions, Gfi-1 is induced in parallel with GATA-3. Then Gfi-1 permits efficient cell proliferation to proceed, counteracting the cytostatic effects of GATA-3 while preserving differentiative functions of GATA-3 (162). As noted above, prethymic T cell precursors can only tolerate low levels of GATA-3 (47), even though they cannot develop further without it. Thus the Gfi-1 expression could be important to provide a protective function for DN2/DN3 thymocytes, enabling them to couple strong proliferation with their differentiation in response to GATA-3.

Chromatin Modifier SATB1

T cell development appears to require not only a multitude of repressors but also at least one factor that associates specific DNA sequences with the nuclear matrix, the Special AT-rich Binding protein SATB1. SATB1 is a two-Cut domain-Homeodomain protein that is expressed preferentially in thymocytes, and T cell development is severely deranged, though not completely blocked, in SATB1 mutants (163). The activation properties of SATB1$^{-/-}$ peripheral T cells are also defective, resembling those of DP thymocytes or cells just undergoing positive selection, suggesting that the loss of SATB1 allows them to emigrate to the periphery without actually having matured. Although it does not act like a conventional sequence-specific transcription factor, SATB1 appears to be needed to choreograph a range of distinct gene regulation transitions during development. This factor is primarily known as a negative regulator, as it is essential for the correct timing of repression of the CD25 (IL-2Rα) and CD127 (IL-7Rα) genes in DP thymocytes. However, it is also needed for correct positive as well as negative regulation of the CD2, CD5, GABPα, CD8α, and c-Myc genes (41, 163, 164).

It now appears that the role of SATB1 is to propagate a particular chromatin configuration over a broad domain that can extend tens of kilobases from the SATB1 binding site itself (164, 165). The nuclear matrix interaction capability of SATB1 may play a physical part in this role, as recent evidence shows that a number of lymphocyte gene expression choices involve compartmentalizing nonexpressed alleles to the nuclear periphery (reviewed in 166). This makes SATB1 a very important effector of regulatory information-processing "decisions." It is very provocative that developing thymocytes should require a dedicated, cell type–specific factor of this type. However, the very permissive sequence specificity of SATB1 and the situation-dependent way in which it engages different subsets of its target genes make it in some ways more akin to a general chromatin remodeling factor than to a sequence-specific transcription factor. These characteristics strongly imply that interactions with other, highly specific factor complexes are required to deploy SATB1 to the correct sites and perhaps to select its correct functions.

PATTERNS OF COMBINATORIAL TRANSCRIPTION FACTOR ACTION IN T VERSUS B CELL DEVELOPMENT

We have already considered the activities of individual factors, "longitudinally" through T cell development. However, none of them work solo at any T cell developmental stage or choice point. The same factors used in specification are also used later in T cell differentiation, in combinations that shift from stage to stage, giving each choice point and checkpoint of T cell development a distinct regulatory signature. Each of these transitions can only be dissected mechanistically with reference to the combination of factors that acts at that point. To put the complexity of the T cell developmental process in perspective, it is helpful to compare it with the regulatory cascade that is now thought to specify the B lymphocyte lineage.

A Comparative Model: The B Cell Gene Regulatory Network

The molecular genetics of B cell development have been elucidated dramatically since the late 1990s, as summarized in Figure 5 (reviewed in 7, 167–169). B cell

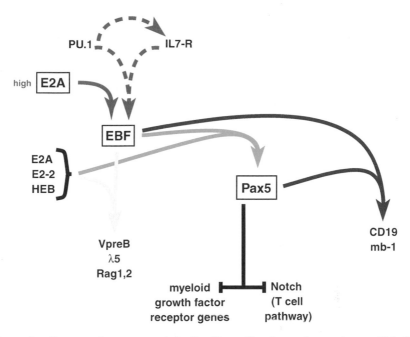

Figure 5   Gene regulatory network for B cell specification and commitment. This figure is based on the body of work cited in the text, in which B cell development depends on the combined action of three factors, E2A, EBF, and Pax-5. The figure highlights the network topology that is supported thus far by genetic epistasis experiments, as well as the distinctive roles of E2A, EBF, and Pax-5 in the positive and negative gene expression required for B-lineage commitment. Some evidence exists to link PU.1 action with the initiation of EBF expression, possibly involving the expression of IL-7Rα for optimized growth under permissive signaling conditions.

development from pluripotent hematopoietic precursors is guided by the three transcription factors E2A, EBF (Early B cell factor, a.k.a. Olf-1), and Pax5. These factors act in a relatively simple gene regulatory cascade in the initial stages of B cell specification. The precursor in which the specification process will unfold is normally rendered competent by its expression of PU.1 and Ikaros, without which B cell development does not begin (108, 132, 170). Increasing levels of E2A in such a precursor turn on EBF expression (171), possibly in collaboration with PU.1. In turn, EBF then collaborates with E2A, and/or with other bHLH factors of the same class if necessary (HEB, E2-2), to turn on expression of additional downstream genes and of Pax5 (169, 172, 173). Pax5 is not needed for the initiation of B cell gene expression, but it activates definitive B cell genes and locks down the committed B cell state by foreclosing other developmental options. It can directly block T cell specification, in part through downregulation of Notch (174), and it can interfere with correct regulation of myeloid target genes by PU.1 to disfavor additional options.

The polarity of this network is shown by the effects of knockouts and by the epistatic rescue of PU.1 or E2A mutants when EBF expression is turned on artificially (169, 173). Just as loss of expression of any of the B cell regulators interferes with B cell development, gain of expression of EBF or Pax5 enhances B cell development (172, 174, 175). Notably, these increases in B cell development in response to either EBF or Pax5 are primarily at the expense of T cell development. In general, the B cell–specific trio of E2A, EBF, and Pax5 are expressed and control gene expression throughout precursor differentiation to maturity. E2A and Pax5 then continue to be required in mature peripheral B cells, until Pax5 is shut off during the antigen-dependent terminal differentiation of B cells into plasma cells. The continued function of the B cell transcriptional cascade reflects the fact that these factors regulate not only the expression of genes used in particular stages of B cell development—surrogate light chains, RAG genes, and Activation Induced Deaminase (AID) at different stages—but also the transcriptional accessibility of the immunoglobulin genes in chromatin (176–179). These activities make the B cell–specification factors important for somatic hypermutation and heavy chain class-switching in mature, activated B cells as well as for initial VDJ rearrangement in their early precursors.

T Lineage Versus B Lineage: An Overview

The paradigm developed for B cell development includes several features in common with T cell development. These are (a) the absolute requirements for bHLH factors (E2A, and/or HEB, E2-2) and for Ikaros family factors (Ikaros, Aiolos, Helios), and (b) the derivation of both B and T cells (at least in fetal life) from PU.1-expressing progenitors. Genes active in B cell precursors also share with those active in T cell precursors the importance of combinations of Runx and Ets transcription factor binding sites (95). Together, these observations implicate bHLH, Ikaros, PU.1, and Runx expression in shared aspects of T and B cell development. However, the two pathways differ markedly in the other specific factors that become activated in these precursors: EBF and Pax5 as opposed to GATA-3, TCF-1, and Notch/RBPSuh. More provocatively, they may differ also in the regulatory relationships among these factors and the developmental mechanisms used for T and B cell specification.

In comparison with B cell development, several process components appear to be lacking during T-lineage specification. There is no factor expressed selectively in T cell precursors that has an unequivocal positive role, an equivalent of EBF or Pax5 in B cell development. None of the T cell transcription factors has yet been able, when overexpressed, to drive the development of multipotent progenitors instructively into the T cell pathway, except the activation of Notch/RBPSuh activity, which is not T-lineage specific (180). There is also no clear identification yet of the factor(s) playing a lineage-specific commitment role through direct or indirect repression, a role that is played in B cell development by Pax5.

The T-lineage program itself includes multiple discontinuities and branch points, as shown in Figure 1, and the developmental choices that remain open each require divergent actions of different transcription factor coalitions. Thus the transcription factors used in specification are repeatedly brought back into play, but with shifting patterns of cooperation and antagonism as maturation proceeds.

A Succession of Different Regulatory Coalitions at Different Stages of T Cell Development

Figure 6 broadly summarizes major phases of action of key T cell transcription factors. The factors that work positively to establish T-lineage identity as distinct from other hematopoietic cell types, from the earliest stages, include Notch/RBPSuh, GATA-3, TCF/LEF factors, and E proteins such as E2A and HEB. As we discuss below in detail, levels of Notch, E protein, and GATA-3 activity as opposed to Id and PU.1 activity seem to be crucial to decide whether precursors will choose T as opposed to B, NK, or dendritic cell (DC) lineage fates. These factors collaborate with a broader group that establish the precursor subset(s) from which T-lineage specification can occur: c-Myb, Runx factors, Ikaros, and PU.1 and/or other Ets factors.

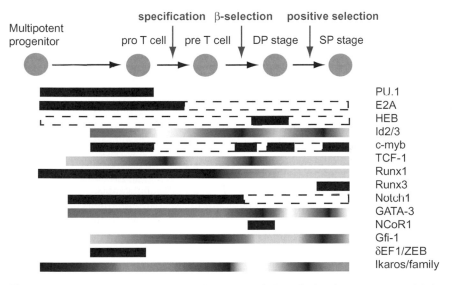

Figure 6 Complex regulatory requirements of T cell development at multiple T-lineage checkpoints. The figure summarizes genetic analyses showing functional dependence of T cell development on shifting combinations of multiple specific transcription factors, loss of any of which blocks at the indicated stages. Events occurring in the periphery are not included. For details, see text. Black, extreme dependence (knockout has severe effect). Gray, moderate or uncertain dependence. White, no dependence, possible antagonist effect. Broken lines indicate stages when factors are likely expressed but genetic evidence for functional dependence is lacking.

The pausing of T cell precursors at the DN3 stage, and the enforcement of the β-selection checkpoint, involve both Ikaros family and E proteins. The cells express a particularly high level of active Notch and its target genes. In agreement with the high E protein activity, this is the period when the most active TCR gene rearrangement is unleashed by the highest RAG gene expression, and when the highest levels of pTα are expressed, favoring TCR$\alpha\beta$ precursor differentiation. Meanwhile, PU.1 and other non-T regulators are shut off at this point.

For TCR$\alpha\beta$ precursors, β-selection depends on a particularly broad coalition of transcriptional regulators. One set of factors is activated simply by the pre-TCR signal itself: This set includes immediate early Zn finger transcription factors of the Egr family, NF-AT, and NF-κB (181–183). However, this is not simply an activation event; it is a mini-differentiation cascade that recalls virtually all the T cell identity-determining factors to participate in some kind of genetically required role.

To initiate β-selection, Notch signaling seems to be essential (15), though the Notch-activated target gene Hes-1 declines in expression throughout the DN to DP transition, suggesting that this signaling is transient. Meanwhile, E protein roles shift rapidly from the E protein–mediated DN3 arrest, through an Id3-dependent proliferative phase, then back to a phase when a particular E protein (HEB) becomes essential, as the cells approach the DP postmitotic state (74, 184). β-selection causes GATA-3 levels to rise, and GATA-3 activity becomes rate-limiting at least for the early phases of the DN to DP transition (32, 35, 36). At the same time, c-Myb becomes a critical proliferative driver (118, 123), Runx1 continues to be important for full population expansion (86), and TCF-1 or its relative LEF-1 becomes indispensable, especially in the later phases of the β-selection response (111, 113, 114). However, this is not a regulatory free-for-all. β-selection terminates the expression of the last PU.1/Spi family member, Spi-B, and the expression of other specific Ets and bHLH transcription factor variants that added to the regulatory complexity of the precursor stages (125; M.K. Anderson & E.V. Rothenberg, unpublished results). Conceivably, the repressors such as Gfi-1 and N-CoR that are required at this stage play a role in execution of these silencing events.

After β-selection, DP cells have a short default lifetime that can only be extended by successful positive selection to the CD4 or CD8 lineage. TCF-1 and c-Myb appear to act as viability factors (114, 124). At this point, regulatory requirements for further differentiation appear much simplified. TCR-activated signaling factors such as NF-AT family members, AP-1 and NF-κB, are undoubtedly involved in the transient positive selection signal. There is evidence that strong, sustained signaling in positive selection directly activates the GATA-3 gene (35), whereas transient signaling selectively activates Runx3 expression (99). GATA-3 activity supports the differentiation of cells that are selected to the CD4-cell fate (35, 36). Conversely, when Runx3 is activated together with Ikaros it directs or sustains cells that proceed to the CD8-cell fate (84–86, 98, 99a, 103), with a possible contribution from Notch mediators as well (185).

In peripheral CD4 cells, GATA-3 and Runx again appear to be in opposition, but now they are associated with different collaborators than in the CD4/CD8 lineage choice. Recent evidence suggests that for Th2 differentiation, GATA-3 once again works in parallel with some form of Notch signaling, as in the earliest stages of thymocyte specification (27), but in apparent contrast to the CD4/CD8 choice in positive selection. Meanwhile, in Th1 differentiation, Runx factors are presumably activated by T-bet (147) and act in collaboration with T-bet and Hlx.

Another important developmental branch point that is only starting to be explained is in the DN2 and DN3 stages, when TCR$\gamma\delta$ cells diverge from the TCR$\alpha\beta$ lineage. These two major subdivisions of T cells are biologically distinct throughout most vertebrates (186–188) and differ in a significant number of respects, only the first of which is the ability of TCR$\gamma\delta$ cells to mature successfully without undergoing the regulatory upheaval of β-selection or the proliferative burst that accompanies it (189–193). TCR$\gamma\delta$ cells differ from TCR$\alpha\beta$ cells in their developmental responses to levels of E protein activity and to increases or decreases in Notch signaling levels (12, 13, 72, 194–198). Both Notch signaling and E protein activity are essential throughout the DN period for all T cell precursors, but the lower levels that seem to be acceptable for TCR$\gamma\delta$ cell development could form a continuum with the levels that are permissive only for NK-cell development. The window of opportunity for the NK- and DC-lineage options stays open long enough to raise a question as to whether it overlaps with the branch point between TCR$\alpha\beta$ and TCR$\gamma\delta$ pathways of T cell development (196, 199). Thus it is possible that the choice between TCR$\alpha\beta$ and TCR$\gamma\delta$ T cell fates is mechanistically intertwined with the choice between T, NK, and DC fates.

Several other T-lineage choice points remain poorly explained. NKT cells depend on a constellation of regulators more typical of NK cells than of T cells (147, 200–203), and it is intriguing but obscure how this alternative program is accessed from precursors that presumably diverge only after β-selection (204). T_{reg} cells, active guardians of tolerance, also appear to emerge in the thymus and begin to express the transcription factor Foxp3, but the intrathymic stimuli that direct this program likewise remain to be defined (205).

T CELL LINEAGE SPECIFICATION AND COMMITMENT

Initial T cell specification and its relationship to commitment define an important frontier. This is the process that first demands the great regulatory complexity of T cell development that we have just reviewed, invoking the aid of a large fraction of the regulators that will be used in all subsequent steps of T cell development combined. Also, the regulatory properties of the earliest T cell precursors often appear close to those of leukemic cells, suggesting that enforcement of the correct regulatory relationships in this process may be critical to prevent malignant transformation. The last section of this review is therefore focused on what is known about the molecular mechanisms that initially establish T-lineage identity.

To date, it has not yet been possible to demonstrate a straightforward regulatory cascade, with clear polarity and epistasis relationships, for the transcription factors involved in T cell development. There are several reasons for this, not merely technical but reflecting significant aspects of the T cell specification mechanism. First, the T cell development program can have multiple, diverse points of entry, in regulatory terms. Second, there is a massive overlap between the regulatory requirements of T cell specification and the hematopoietic stem-cell program. Third, there is the strikingly prolonged and flexible specification and commitment process itself. Finally, as a result, early T-lineage differentiation is intensely dependent on environmental conditions to maintain not only viability but also T-lineage identity.

A Pathway with Multiple Entry Points

The first important step for T cell development to occur is the migration of a multipotent progenitor toward the thymus. Thymic immigration places the precursors in an environment rich with the Delta-like Notch ligands that are critical for T cell development (25, 26), and indeed this entry triggers a burst of Notch activation (206). Another feature that may be specific to the thymic microenvironment is high oxygen tension, which may be essential for T cell development (34, 207). Finally, the thymus is a rich source of ligands for the two growth factor receptors expressed on early T cell precursors, c-kit and IL-7, as well as Wnt factors that activate TCF-1/LEF-1 transcription factors. These distinctive microenvironmental features are important to initiate and sustain the specification process.

Recent evidence shows that the most likely cell to migrate from the bone marrow to the thymus under normal conditions has a Lin^- $Sca-1^+c-Kit^+$ (LSK) phenotype (208) (Figure 7). Cells with this phenotype, also found in the bone marrow, include self-renewing HSCs and multipotential progenitors. The thymus can thus initiate T cell development in cells that have diverse developmental alternatives. Moreover, this is not the only class of cells that is poised to respond to the thymic microenvironment.

There is now evidence for at least four different kinds of murine prethymic cells that can give rise to T cells when introduced into an appropriate environment, as shown in Figure 7 (209–213). Virtually all uncommitted T cell precursors are capable of differentiating into NK cells as well (16, 214), but they are distinguished in terms of their retention of B and/or myeloid potential. One is the Common Lymphoid Progenitor (CLP), a $Sca-1^{lo}$ $c-kit^{lo}$ $IL-7R\alpha^+$ Lin^- bone marrow cell type. CLPs are also efficient B cell precursors but lack myeloid potential (215). A variant CLP (CLP-2) is also found in the bone marrow, with a $c-kit^{lo}$ $B220^+$ phenotype and the capacity to generate both B and T cells (216). A different kind of precursor is an Early T cell Progenitor (ETP), first characterized among the highly immature cells in the thymus and thus part of the DN1 compartment. The ETP is a less efficient B cell precursor than the CLP, in agreement with its intrathymic appearance, but it is a better myeloid precursor (108). The ETP is $Sca-1^+$ $c-kit^+$ $IL-7R\alpha^-$ Lin^- and differs from the CLP in that its generation and developmental capacities do not depend on Ikaros (108). Cells resembling ETP can be found in the bone marrow, where they represent a T lineage–biased, efficient source of

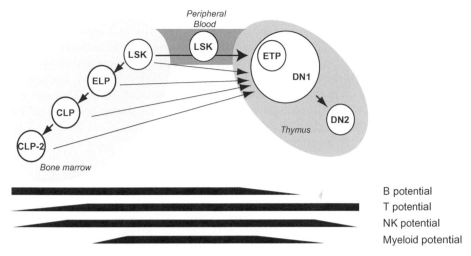

Figure 7   Distinct precursor cell types with the shared competence to generate T cells in the thymus. The figure summarizes the studies reviewed in the text, where a variety of different adult cell types with different combinations of other developmental potentials are all capable of responding to the thymic microenvironment and differentiating into T cells. LSK: the Lin^- $Sca-1^+$ $c-Kit^+$ bone marrow cell fraction, highly pluripotent and recently shown to be the most prevalent source of thymus immigrating cells in normal animals. ETP: first defined as a partially restricted intrathymic subset of Early T cell Progenitors within the DN1 population, which appears to represent an early derivative of the immigrants after arrival in the thymus. ELP: the Early Lymphoid Precursor, a population with excellent T- and B-lineage potential that retains some myeloid potential but with much reduced nonlymphoid activity as compared with LSK cells. CLP and CLP-2: two distinct types of Common Lymphoid Progenitors, with strong B-lineage potential as well as T potential but little or no myeloid potential.

thymus-populating cells (217). Yet another cell type that may represent the precursor of both the ETP and the CLP, called the Early Lymphoid Precursor (ELP), has been described in the adult bone marrow and identified by its expression of a RAG1-GFP knock-in gene. The ELP can generate T, B, NK, and myeloid cells with different efficiencies (218) (Figure 7).

A somewhat different hierarchy of shared developmental potentials is found in prethymic cells in the fetus (not shown). In the fetal liver, the $Sca-1^+$ $c-kit^+$ Lin^- cells that give rise to T cell precursors generally exhibit substantial myeloid potential, and myeloid and T potentials are maintained together even when B cell potential is lost. The fetal precursors also differ in other respects from the prethymic cells in the adult (219–222).

While a simpler, more linear scheme for stepwise commitment might be more appealing, the variable order in which B versus myeloid potentials are lost among precursors appears to be a genuine feature of the cells competent to undertake the T cell developmental pathway. Even within the adult thymus, phenotypically diverse T-lineage precursors can be found that give rise to T cells with different kinetics and with different combinations of alternative B, NK, and myeloid developmental capabilities (223). The predictable, robust differences in developmental potential among these precursors imply that they express different transcription factor combinations that situate them in distinct regulatory states. Thus, the gene regulatory network that operates in T-lineage specification must be capable of funneling this whole range of different input regulatory states into a common T cell developmental progression.

Similarities Between Stem-Cell and T Cell Regulatory Programs

One way to force diverse precursors into a common program would be to express dominant transcriptional regulators that actively repress alternative, pluripotent states. However, this is not the way that T-lineage specification seems to proceed. Instead, there is a striking overlap between the factors required for the T-lineage specification process and factors known to be used, even required, in multipotent hematopoietic stem cells. Ikaros, PU.1, Runx1, and c-Myb are required not only for T cell specification; they are also important for stem-cell specification, maintenance, or self-renewal (106, 119, 224, 225). Notch pathway and Wnt/TCF signaling may also be used to promote stem-cell self-renewal (116, 226). Even GATA-3 is structurally very similar to the essential stem-cell factor GATA-2. These overlapping regulatory requirements obviously pose technical problems for gene knockout strategies to investigate the modes of action of these factors in early stages of T cell specification. More interestingly, though, they bring into sharp focus a global regulatory similarity between the stem-cell state and the state of a T cell precursor even after specification and commitment (Figure 8).

The number of regulatory changes needed to bridge the gap from stem cell/multipotent progenitor to DN2 thymocyte could be small. Among the obvious candidates, lymphoid precursors might diverge from multipotent progenitors by altering the relative activities of different bHLH heterodimers and their interaction partners (e.g., via downregulation of Id1, SCL/Tal-1, and Lmo1/2); but the essential positive bHLH factors, E2A and HEB, are expressed in stem cells as well. One clear difference is that GATA-3 is induced, whereas GATA-2 is downregulated. Furthermore, GATA-3 might be an important mediator in the migration of LSK cells to the thymus, since GATA-3 deficiency results in the absence of even the earliest, DN1-stage thymocytes (32). Thus, if not important for migration, it at least is required for the survival of the earliest thymocytes. However, if GATA-3 can serve any of the same functions as GATA-2, then the continuities between early stage T cells and stem cells are even more impressive (Figure 8). It should not be surprising, therefore, that the T cell pathway is also accessible from a number of different, separable pathways from the multipotent LSK cell (Figure 7).

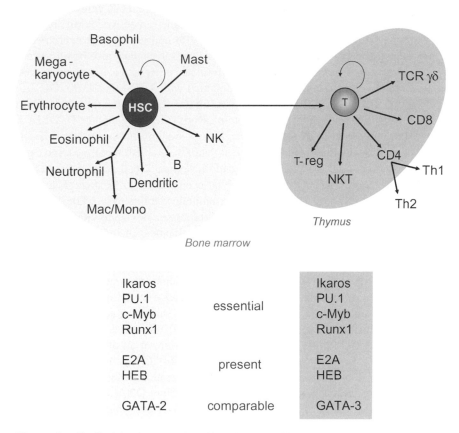

Figure 8 Similarities between T cell and stem-cell regulatory states. In comparison with hematopoietic stem cells (*center cell, left*), committed T cell precursors also remain "pluripotent" (*center cell, right*) insofar as they still face a succession of developmental choices that determine divergent functions, gene expression programs, and physiological setpoints within the T lineage. Transcription factors that are genetically shown to be important for development or maintenance of definitive HSC (*bottom left*) define a very similar set to those that are important for T-lineage specification (*bottom right*).

Timing of Specification and Lineage Choice Events

Specification involves the activation of a first tier of T-lineage genes, and this must be one of the key roles of the combinations of factors involved in this process. The genes that need to be turned on in order to qualify a precursor cell for success in early T-lineage development include those encoding RAG-1 and RAG-2 recombinase components, the CD3γ and ε chains of the TCR and pre-TCR complexes, lineage-specific signaling molecules such as LAT and Lck, and for future TCR$\alpha\beta$

cells, the surrogate α chain pTα. Also required for TCR gene rearrangement is the transcription factor-mediated opening of the respective loci in chromatin, and for survival through the initial stages IL-7Rα and γc expression are needed. The T-lineage-required transcription factors themselves must also be turned on, at the correct times and levels, to regulate these and other, as yet unknown, target genes. Certain *cis*-regulatory elements associated with TCR (38, 91, 93, 94, 227), pTα (65, 66, 228), Lck (229, 230), and RAG (39, 97, 231) genes appear to include targets for RBPSuh, c-Myb, bHLH E proteins, Runx1, GATA-3, and/or TCF/LEF factors. However, remarkably few of the regulatory systems that control early T cell genes have been characterized in sufficient detail to establish factor-specific causality.

Another regulatory feature needed for optimal T cell development is extensive proliferation. For the proliferation that occurs in the DN2 stage, E proteins must collaborate with IL-7Rα signaling to maintain viability (67), while TCF-1, c-Myb, and the Notch-activated transcriptional repressor Hes-1 are vital to sustain clonal expansion (112, 118, 232). "Normal" development of individual precursors can involve $\sim 10^5$-fold expansion, with $\sim 10^3$-fold expansion prior to β-selection (233). Thus, another requirement of the specification process may be a surprising one: to delay terminal differentiation, while proliferation continues.

Indeed, a remarkable feature about T-lineage commitment is how late it can occur, even relative to specification. Figure 1 shows the approximate windows of opportunity for development into B, myeloid, NK, and dendritic cells as alternatives to T cell development. The full foreclosure of all of these alternatives does not appear to occur until the DN3 (c-kit$^-$ CD44$^-$ CD25$^+$) stage (reviewed in 211; 16, 234). This can take 7–10 rounds of proliferation in the fetal thymus (233) and nearly two weeks in the adult thymus (235). Thus, DN3-stage commitment is late in terms of the onset of T-lineage gene expression, which is clearly under way by the DN2 stage; it is late relative to the beginning to TCR gene rearrangement; and in the adult thymus, it is late in terms of the absolute number of days and cell cycles elapsed since the entry of the cells into the thymus (reviewed by 212, 235, 236).

Whereas other potentials are eliminated earlier, both postnatal and fetal thymocytes remain capable of differentiating into dendritic cells and/or NK cells instead of T cells throughout the DN1 and DN2 stages (63, 234, 237–240) (Figure 1). In the fetal thymus, these subsets are capable of macrophage differentiation as well (241). B cell potential is lost much earlier within the thymus and is undetectable among most of the subsets within the DN1 population (212, 223), presumably as a result of direct inhibition via Notch/Delta signaling in the thymic microenvironment (206). Both the NK and the dendritic cell fates, though less favored by Notch/Delta signaling than the T cell fate, are substantially more tolerant of this than the B cell fate (25, 197, 242). These alternatives can be elicited simply by incubation of the DN1 or DN2 thymocytes under appropriate growth conditions, i.e., by moving them into an irradiated host or into in vitro conditions that differ from those presented by the thymic microenvironment. As the DN1 and DN2 stages include the highest frequencies of proliferating cells in the thymus except for those immediately responding to β-selection, this implies that the uncommitted state is actively maintained.

At the individual cell level, even turning on T cell genes does not guarantee commitment. RAG-negative NK cells can develop from RAG1-expressing precursors (218). Myeloid-like dendritic cells can develop from cells that have previously turned on pTα, the component of the pre-TCR, or active RAG recombinase, as shown by the presence of limited lymphoid-type gene rearrangements in their DNA (243). The likelihood of *trans*-specification during the DN1 and DN2 stages can also be boosted dramatically by delivering artificial stimulation to the immature thymocytes. Signals delivered through an ectopically expressed IL-2 receptor or GM-CSF receptor complex can convert most DN2 cells quickly to myeloid cells, even if they have already undergone significant TCR gene rearrangement (244, 245). Once the cells are committed, in the DN3 stage, this response is no longer seen. The exceptional plasticity of DN1 and DN2 cells shows that the early stages of the T-lineage program are compatible with expression of regulatory factors that can execute alternative developmental programs.

Coexpression of Potentially Antagonistic Transcription Factors During Specification

Many of the factors required for T cell specification have spectra of activity that can include inhibitory as well as stimulatory effects on T cell development. The extended window of opportunity for developmental alternatives could be the result of potentially antagonistic activities among these delicately balanced factors (211) (Figure 9).

From the prethymic stages through the DN2 stage, cells have to depend on GATA-3, Notch1/RBPSuh, E box proteins, c-Myb, and Ikaros in order to carry out T-lineage specification, while Ets factors, TCF-1 or LEF-1, Runx factors, and probably PU.1 are used in essential supporting roles. Initially, Id2 is expressed as well, particularly in fetal T cell precursors (63). In other contexts, GATA and PU.1 factors are mutually antagonistic for erythroid versus myeloid development (246–248); Notch and E box proteins are antagonists with respect to B cell development (249, 250); and Runx and GATA-3 appear to have antagonistic effects in CD4/CD8 lineage divergence and possibly Th1/Th2 divergence as well, as described above. The prolonged coexpression of potential antagonists makes a sharp contrast with the kind of positive feedback networks seen to drive terminal differentiation in Th1 or Th2 cells, or in certain embryonic systems (251). However, these factors are all used together, and are all genetically required, during these critical but unstable stages of T cell development.

Overexpression of many of these factors can tilt the balance to a non-T developmental fate or else block proliferation (Figure 9). As already discussed, the E protein/Id balance is critical for T cells to develop instead of NK cells, with Id2 normally promoting the NK fate. However, E proteins block proliferation. Id2 is essential for NK-cell development, and loss-of-function experiments show

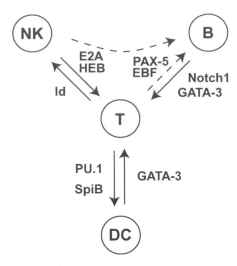

Figure 9 T-lineage specification by regulatory balance among drivers of competing developmental options. As discussed in the text, T-lineage specification in the thymus requires coexpression of factors that promote (PU.1) and inhibit (GATA-3?) the dendritic cell or myeloid program, and factors that promote (Id2) and inhibit (E2A/HEB) the NK cell program, while Notch signaling with a possible contribution from GATA-3 blocks a B cell program that would otherwise be accessible. Of the regulators shown on this diagram, only EBF and Pax-5 are normally not expressed in early thymocytes, possibly due to a direct inhibitory influence from Notch/Delta interaction (T. Taghon, E.-S. David, J.C. Zúñiga-Pflücker & E.V. Rothenberg, submitted). See text for details.

that it is responsible for the NK developmental potential of the most immature thymocyte subsets (63, 151). Id2 is also associated with development of monocyte/macrophages and certain classes of dendritic cells, fates that could be promoted by PU.1 (252–254). Either PU.1 or its relative Spi-B can support dendritic cell development. Forced expression of PU.1 blocks T cell development in thymic organ cultures, with cells arresting in the DN stages and most of the surviving cells showing a myeloid-like phenotype (134; A.H. Weiss & E.V. Rothenberg, unpublished data). The close relative of PU.1, Spi-B, is highly expressed in dendritic cells, and its overexpression redirects T cell precursors to full dendritic-cell differentiation (135; J.M. Lefebvre, M.C. Haks, M.O. Carleton, M. Rhodes, G. Sinnathamby, L.A. Garrett-Sinha, M.C. Simon, L.C. Eisenlohr, D.L. Wiest, submitted for publication; D.L. Wiest, personal communication). Notch signaling in some hematopoietic progenitors actually upregulates PU.1 and thus promotes myeloid development (180), a response that must be restrained in the Notch-dependent T cell precursors.

Even GATA-3 can be problematic for early T cell development. Whereas GATA-3 may be useful as an antagonist of the dendritic cell and B cell pathways, when expressed at high levels, it can also be "read" in uncommitted prethymic cells as a driver of a non-T-lineage fate. In murine bone marrow stem cells, it promotes megakaryocyte development inappropriately, while blocking all lymphoid development (46), suggesting that it cross-reacts with GATA-1 or GATA-2 target genes. Not all of these alternative cell types can be kept viable in the thymic microenvironment, but it is likely that the developmental choices observed there emerge from fluctuations in the balance of the regulators that are used for T-lineage specification as well.

In summary, the combination of transcription factors employed for the establishment of T-lineage identity can be seen as establishing a kind of regulatory tug-of-war during the stages of initial proliferation. The balance among these factors itself appears to be critical to maintain the combination of early T cell gene expression and optimal proliferation. In addition, these cells relinquish their pluripotentiality only by degrees, and even then, give up non-T alternatives only to remain capable of a multiplicity of developmental choices within the T lineage, at later stages of differentiation (Figure 1).

Role of the Microenvironment as a Guide to Commitment

During early T cell development, these potentially diversionary transcription factors are normally limited to low levels of expression that are not sufficient to redirect too many thymocytes from the T cell pathway. However, they create a potential regulatory "hazard" for T-lineage fidelity that can be exacerbated by stimulation. PU.1 and Spi-B, for example, are strongly enhanced in their transcriptional activity by phosphorylation or by association with the activation-dependent transcription factor c-Jun (255–259). Id2 can be induced to high levels by certain kinds of mitogenic stimulation (reviewed in 260). This could be the mechanism through which stimulation of fetal thymocytes via FcR crosslinking drives them to differentiate into NK cells (261).

How do rapidly proliferating DN2 thymocytes avoid these liabilities? Notably, the IL-7R complex that normally drives most thymocyte expansion prior to commitment is a receptor that is particularly weak at MAP kinase activation (262, 263). In contrast, the IL-2 receptor β chain CD122, which activates MAP kinases much better, is confined to precursors that are strongly biased to an NK fate (151, 264). As a result, IL-2/IL-15R or certain other kinds of growth factor stimulation may substantially enhance the likelihood of diversion. Stimulation through ectopically expressed IL-2Rβ (CD122) or GM-CSF receptors can drive the PU.1[+] subsets of thymocytes to monocytic or granulocytic differentiation, without any direct manipulation of PU.1 expression (244, 245). Such extracellular signals only determine cell fate in convergence with the intracellular regulatory environment, however, because the PU.1-negative subsets of thymocytes do not respond. Thus, maintaining repression of IL-2Rβ and GM-CSF receptors may be critical throughout the PU.1-positive stages to keep T-lineage commitment available. At the same time, maintenance of strong Notch/Delta signaling appears to be important to avoid diversion to the NK cell lineage throughout the DN1 and DN2 stages, possibly due to the expression of Id2 by these cells (16).

Commitment is the stage at which this hazard is finally removed. Ultimately, the committed cells are ones in which genes such as PU.1 are turned off. Presumably by this stage at the latest, some of the interaction partners that facilitate inappropriate effects of GATA-3 are also permanently repressed. Commitment is also the stage when a new criterion for survival and proliferation is imposed: The cells lose their ability to survive without signaling through the TCR$\gamma\delta$ or pre-TCR complex. It thus coincides with the forcible end of the TCR-independent phase of T cell development. While the basis for this change is not clear yet, it is tempting to connect it with the extinction of certain stem-cell or pluripotent progenitor functions. Conversely, the shift in survival requirements can also act as a built-in quality control for lineage fidelity, for any regulatory perturbation from this point on that happens to interfere with the TCR complex components or their signal transduction mediators will now cause cell death.

NEW OPPORTUNITIES: ACCESS TO THE
SPECIFICATION PROCESS IN THE ABSENCE
OF A THYMUS

T-lineage specification emerges from a complex interaction of multiple regulators of which none plays a simple, dominant role. The gene regulatory network that controls this process can be clarified only when it is possible to test the effects of individual perturbations in a focused, stage-specific way. In the past, this has been a practical challenge due to "black box" aspects of the closed thymic microenvironment in which so much of T cell specification must take place. Now, however, a new approach opens up access to cellular and molecular mechanisms operating in these early stages.

The increased understanding of cues supplied by the thymic microenvironment has made possible an exciting advance in T cell developmental biology. The OP9-DL1 stromal cell system developed by Zúñiga-Pflücker and coworkers is a monolayer culture transfected to express Delta-like 1, providing an environment that supports T cell precursors in the presence of IL-7 and Flt3L. This system promotes T cell development all the way to positive selection from the most primitive precursors, even from embryonic stem cell lines (16, 26, 265). In this system, the time course of gene activation from the earliest stages can be tracked and linked with the time course of developmental potential change (265; T. Taghon, E.-S. David, J.C. Zúñiga-Pflücker & E.V. Rothenberg, submitted). The reversibility of these events can be probed as a function of time (T. Taghon, E.-S. David, J.C. Zúñiga-Pflücker & E.V. Rothenberg, submitted), and the cells can be accessed for perturbation of the process at any stage.

The quantitative recovery and easy accessibility of precursors in cultures like these makes it possible for the first time to dissect the molecular control of T-lineage specification in real time. With the studies based on this new system, future reviews of the molecular genetics of T cell development will at last be able to illuminate the network of specific interactions among regulators and their causal impacts on developmental change.

ACKNOWLEDGMENTS

Any review like this embodies insights drawn from many people besides the authors themselves. The bibliography understates this debt. We are grateful to many colleagues for sharing their results and interpretations prior to publication, and we apologize to the many whose work we were not able to cite, or could cite only in secondary references. Work in the Rothenberg lab on transcriptional regulation of T cell development and its evolution was supported by grants from the NIH (R01 CA90233, R01 CA98925) and from NASA (NAG2-1588), with previous support from NSF (MCB-9983129) and the Stowers Institute for Medical Research.

The *Annual Review of Immunology* is online at
http://immunol.annualreviews.org

LITERATURE CITED

1. Borowski C, Martin C, Gounari F, Haughn L, Aifantis I, et al. 2002. On the brink of becoming a T cell. *Curr. Opin. Immunol.* 14:200–6

2. Cantrell DA. 2002. Transgenic analysis of thymocyte signal transduction. *Nat. Rev. Immunol.* 2:20–27

3. Singer A. 2002. New perspectives on a developmental dilemma: the kinetic signaling model and the importance of signal duration for the CD4/CD8 lineage decision. *Curr. Opin. Immunol.* 14:207–15

4. Alberola-Ila J, Hernández-Hoyos G. 2003. The Ras/MAPK cascade and the control of positive selection. *Immunol. Rev.* 191:79–96

5. Bosselut R. 2004. CD4/CD8-lineage differentiation in the thymus: from nuclear effectors to membrane signals. *Nat. Rev. Immunol.* 4:529–40

6. Rothenberg EV, Yui MA, Telfer JC. 2003. T-cell developmental biology. In *Fundamental Immunology*, ed. WE Paul, pp. 259–301. Philadelphia: Lippincott, Williams & Wilkins

7. Busslinger M. 2004. Transcriptional control of early B cell development. *Annu. Rev. Immunol.* 22:55–79

8. Pear WS, Radtke F. 2003. Notch signaling in lymphopoiesis. *Semin. Immunol.* 15:69–79

9. Robey EA, Bluestone JA. 2004. Notch signaling in lymphocyte development and function. *Curr. Opin. Immunol.* 16:360–66

10. Radtke F, Wilson A, Mancini SJ, MacDonald HR. 2004. Notch regulation of lymphocyte development and function. *Nat. Immunol.* 5:247–53

11. Han H, Tanigaki K, Yamamoto N, Kuroda K, Yoshimoto M, et al. 2002. Inducible gene knockout of transcription factor recombination signal binding protein-J reveals its essential role in T versus B lineage decision. *Int. Immunol.* 14:637–45

12. Tanigaki K, Tsuji M, Yamamoto N, Han H, Tsukada J, et al. 2004. Regulation of $\alpha\beta/\gamma\delta$ T cell lineage commitment and peripheral T cell responses by Notch/RBP-J signaling. *Immunity* 20:611–22

13. Wolfer A, Wilson A, Nemir M, MacDonald HR, Radtke F. 2002. Inactivation of Notch1 impairs VDJβ rearrangement and allows pre-TCR-independent survival of early $\alpha\beta$ lineage thymocytes. *Immunity* 5:869–79

14. Huang EY, Gallegos AM, Richards SM, Lehar SM, Bevan MJ. 2003. Surface expression of Notch1 on thymocytes: correlation with the double-negative to double-positive transition. *J. Immunol.* 171:2296–304

15. Ciofani M, Schmitt TM, Ciofani A, Michie AM, Cuburu N, et al. 2004. Obligatory role for cooperative signaling by pre-TCR and Notch during thymocyte differentiation. *J. Immunol.* 172:5230–39

16. Schmitt TM, Ciofani M, Petrie HT, Zúñiga-Pflücker JC. 2004. Maintenance of T cell specification and differentiation requires recurrent Notch receptor-ligand interactions. *J. Exp. Med.* 200:469–79

17. Choi JW, Pampeno C, Vukmanovic S, Meruelo D. 2002. Characterization of the transcriptional expression of Notch-1 signaling pathway members, Deltex and HES-1, in developing mouse thymocytes. *Dev. Comp. Immunol.* 26:575–88

18. Deftos ML, Huang E, Ojala EW, Forbush KA, Bevan MJ. 2000. Notch1 signaling promotes the maturation of CD4 and CD8 SP thymocytes. *Immunity* 13:73–84

19. Bellavia D, Campese AF, Alesse E, Vacca A, Felli MP, et al. 2000. Constitutive activation of NF-κB and T-cell leukemia/lymphoma in Notch3 transgenic mice. *EMBO J.* 19:3337–48

20. Aster JC, Xu L, Karnell FG, Patriub V, Pui JC, Pear WS. 2000. Essential roles for ankyrin repeat and transactivation domains in induction of T-cell leukemia by Notch1. *Mol. Cell. Biol.* 20:7505–15

21. Allman D, Karnell FG, Punt JA, Bakkour S, Xu L, et al. 2001. Separation of Notch1 promoted lineage commitment and expansion/transformation in developing T cells. *J. Exp. Med.* 194:99–106

22. Deftos ML, Bevan MJ. 2000. Notch signaling in T cell development. *Curr. Opin. Immunol.* 12:166–72

23. Basson MA, Zamoyska R. 2000. The CD4/CD8 lineage decision: integration of signalling pathways. *Immunol. Today* 21:509–14

24. Hernández-Hoyos G, Alberola-Ila J. 2003. A Notch so simple influence on T cell development. *Semin. Cell Dev. Biol.* 14:121–25

25. Jaleco AC, Neves H, Hooijberg E, Gameiro P, Clode N, et al. 2001. Differential effects of Notch ligands Delta-1 and Jagged-1 in human lymphoid differentiation. *J. Exp. Med.* 194:991–1002

26. Schmitt TM, Zúñiga-Pflücker JC. 2002. Induction of T cell development from hematopoietic progenitor cells by Delta-like-1 in vitro. *Immunity* 17:749–56

27. Amsen D, Blander JM, Lee GR, Tanigaki K, Honjo T, Flavell RA. 2004. Instruction of distinct CD4 T helper cell fates by different Notch ligands on antigen-presenting cells. *Cell* 117:515–26

28. Yvon ES, Vigouroux S, Rousseau RF, Biagi E, Amrolia P, et al. 2003. Over expression of the Notch ligand, Jagged-1 induces alloantigen-specific human regulatory T cells. *Blood* 102:3815–21

29. Maekawa Y, Tsukumo S, Chiba S, Hirai H, Hayashi Y, et al. 2003. Delta1-Notch3 interactions bias the functional differentiation of activated CD4$^+$ T cells. *Immunity* 19:549–59

30. Palaga T, Miele L, Golde TE, Osborne BA. 2003. TCR-mediated Notch signaling regulates proliferation and IFN-γ production in peripheral T cells. *J. Immunol.* 171:3019–24

31. Ting C-N, Olson MC, Barton KP, Leiden JM. 1996. Transcription factor GATA-3 is required for development of the T-cell lineage. *Nature* 384:474–78

32. Hendriks RW, Nawijn MC, Engel JD, van Doorninck H, Grosveld F, Karis A. 1999. Expression of the transcription factor GATA-3 is required for the development of the earliest T cell progenitors and correlates with stages of cellular proliferation in the thymus. *Eur. J. Immunol.* 29:1912–18

33. Samson SI, Richard O, Tavian M, Ranson T, Vosshenrich CA, et al. 2003. GATA-3 promotes maturation, IFN-γ production,

and liver-specific homing of NK cells. *Immunity* 19:701–11

34. Hattori N, Kawamoto H, Fujimoto S, Kuno K, Katsura Y. 1996. Involvement of transcription factors TCF-1 and GATA-3 in the initiation of the earliest step of T cell development in the thymus. *J. Exp. Med.* 184:1137–47

35. Hernández-Hoyos G, Anderson MK, Wang C, Rothenberg EV, Alberola-Ila J. 2003. GATA-3 expression is controlled by TCR signals and regulates CD4/CD8 differentiation. *Immunity* 19:83–94

36. Pai SY, Truitt ML, Ting CN, Leiden JM, Glimcher LH, Ho IC. 2003. Critical roles for transcription factor GATA-3 in thymocyte development. *Immunity* 19:863–75

37. Zhang D-H, Yang L, Ray A. 1998. Cutting edge: differential responsiveness of the IL-5 and IL-4 genes to transcription factor GATA-3. *J. Immunol.* 161:3817–21

38. Tripathi RK, Mathieu N, Spicuglia S, Payet D, Verthuy C, et al. 2000. Definition of a T-cell receptor β gene core enhancer of V(D)J recombination by transgenic mapping. *Mol. Cell. Biol.* 20: 42–53

39. Kishi H, Wei X-C, Jin Z-X, Fujishiro Y, Nagata T, et al. 2000. Lineage specific regulation of the murine RAG-2 promoter: GATA-3 in T cells and Pax-5 in B cells. *Blood* 95:3845–52

40. Lee GR, Fields PE, Flavell RA. 2001. Regulation of IL-4 gene expression by distal regulatory elements and GATA-3 at the chromatin level. *Immunity* 14:447–59

41. Kieffer LJ, Greally JM, Landres I, Nag S, Nakajima Y, et al. 2002. Identification of a candidate regulatory region in the human *CD8* gene complex by colocalization of DNase I hypersensitive sites and matrix attachment regions which bind SATB1 and GATA-3. *J. Immunol.* 168:3915–22

42. Nawijn MC, Ferreira R, Dingjan GM, Kahre O, Drabek D, et al. 2001. Enforced expression of GATA-3 during T cell development inhibits maturation of CD8

single-positive cells and induces thymic lymphoma in transgenic mice. *J. Immunol.* 167:715–23

43. Yamagata T, Mitani K, Oda H, Suzuki T, Honda H, et al. 2000. Acetylation of GATA-3 affects T-cell survival and homing to secondary lymphoid organs. *EMBO J.* 19:4676–87

44. Murphy KM, Reiner SL. 2002. The lineage decisions of helper T cells. *Nat. Rev. Immunol.* 2:933–44

45. Ho IC, Glimcher LH. 2002. Transcription: tantalizing times for T cells. *Cell* 109(Suppl.):S109–20

46. Chen D, Zhang G. 2001. Enforced expression of the GATA-3 transcription factor affects cell fate decisions in hematopoiesis. *Exp. Hematol.* 29:971–80

47. Anderson MK, Hernandez-Hoyos G, Dionne CJ, Arias A, Chen D, Rothenberg EV. 2002. Definition of regulatory network elements for T-cell development by perturbation analysis with PU.1 and GATA-3. *Dev. Biol.* 246:103–21

48. Taghon T, De Smedt M, Stolz F, Cnockaert M, Plum J, Leclercq G. 2001. Enforced expression of GATA-3 severely reduces human thymic cellularity. *J. Immunol.* 167:4468–75

49. Nawijn MC, Dingjan GM, Ferreira R, Lambrecht BN, Karis A, et al. 2001. Enforced expression of GATA-3 in transgenic mice inhibits Th1 differentiation and induces the formation of a T1/ST2-expressing Th2-committed T cell compartment in vivo. *J. Immunol.* 167:724–32

50. Pai SY, Truitt ML, Ho IC. 2004. GATA-3 deficiency abrogates the development and maintenance of T helper type 2 cells. *Proc. Natl. Acad. Sci. USA* 101:1993–98

51. Skapenko A, Leipe J, Niesner U, Devriendt K, Beetz R, et al. 2004. GATA-3 in human T cell helper type 2 development. *J. Exp. Med.* 199:423–28

52. Ranganath S, Murphy KM. 2001. Structure and specificity of GATA proteins in Th2 development. *Mol. Cell Biol.* 21: 2716–25

53. Klein-Hessling S, Jha MK, Santner-Nanan B, Berberich-Siebelt F, et al. 2003. Protein kinase A regulates GATA-3-dependent activation of IL-5 gene expression in Th2 cells. *J. Immunol.* 170:2956–61

54. Usui T, Nishikomori R, Kitani A, Strober W. 2003. GATA-3 suppresses Th1 development by downregulation of Stat4 and not through effects on IL-12Rβ2 chain or T-bet. *Immunity* 18:415–28

55. Yin Z, Chen C, Szabo SJ, Glimcher LH, Ray A, Craft J. 2002. T-Bet expression and failure of GATA-3 cross-regulation lead to default production of IFN-γ by $\gamma\delta$ T cells. *J. Immunol.* 168:1566–71

56. Lee HJ, Takemoto N, Kurata H, Kamogawa Y, Miyatake S, et al. 2000. GATA-3 induces T helper cell type 2 (Th2) cytokine expression and chromatin remodeling in committed Th1 cells. *J. Exp. Med.* 192:105–15

57. Takemoto N, Arai K, Miyatake S. 2002. Cutting edge: the differential involvement of the N-finger of GATA-3 in chromatin remodeling and transactivation during Th2 development. *J. Immunol.* 169:4103–7

58. Zhou M, Ouyang W, Gong Q, Katz SG, White JM, et al. 2001. Friend of GATA-1 represses GATA-3-dependent activity in CD4$^+$ T cells. *J. Exp. Med.* 194:1461–71

59. Kurata H, Lee H-J, McClanahan T, Coffman RL, O'Garra A, Arai N. 2002. Friend of GATA is expressed in naive Th cells and functions as a repressor of GATA-3-mediated Th2 cell development. *J. Immunol.* 168:4538–45

60. Staal FJT, Weerkamp F, Langerak AW, Hendriks RW, Clevers HC. 2001. Transcriptional control of T lymphocyte differentiation. *Stem Cells* 19:165–79

61. Greenbaum S, Zhuang Y. 2002. Regulation of early lymphocyte development by E2A family proteins. *Semin. Immunol.* 14:405–14

62. Engel I, Murre C. 2001. The function of E- and Id proteins in lymphocyte development. *Nat. Rev. Immunol.* 1:193–99

63. Ikawa T, Fujimoto S, Kawamoto H, Katsura Y, Yokota Y. 2001. Commitment to natural killer cells requires the helix-loop-helix inhibitor Id2. *Proc. Natl. Acad. Sci. USA* 98:5164–69

64. Sawada A, Littman DR. 1993. A heterodimer of HEB and an E12-related protein interacts with the CD4 enhancer and regulates its activity in T-cell lines. *Mol. Cell. Biol.* 13:5620–28

65. Petersson K, Ivars F, Sigvardsson M. 2002. The pTα promoter and enhancer are direct targets for transactivation by E box-binding proteins. *Eur. J. Immunol.* 32:911–20

66. Tremblay M, Herblot S, Lecuyer E, Hoang T. 2003. Regulation of pTα gene expression by a dosage of E2A, HEB and SCL. *J. Biol. Chem.* 278:12680–87

67. Kee BL, Bain G, Murre C. 2002. IL-7Rα and E47: independent pathways required for development of multipotent lymphoid progenitors. *EMBO J.* 21:103–13

68. Grégoire J-M, Roméo P-H. 1999. T-cell expression of the human *GATA-3* gene is regulated by a non-lineage specific silencer. *J. Biol. Chem.* 274:6567–78

69. Heemskerk MHM, Blom B, Nolan G, Stegmann APA, Bakker AQ, et al. 1997. Inhibition of T cell and promotion of natural killer cell development by the dominant negative helix loop helix factor Id3. *J. Exp. Med.* 186:1597–602

70. Kim D, Peng X-C, Sun X-H. 1999. Massive apoptosis of thymocytes in T-cell-deficient Id1 transgenic mice. *Mol. Cell. Biol.* 19:8240–53

71. Pan L, Hanrahan J, Li J, Hale LP, Zhuang Y. 2002. An analysis of T cell intrinsic roles of E2A by conditional gene disruption in the thymus. *J. Immunol.* 168:3923–32

72. Barndt RJ, Dai M, Zhuang Y. 2000. Functions of E2A-HEB heterodimers in T-cell development revealed by a dominant

negative mutation of HEB. *Mol. Cell. Biol.* 20:6677–85

73. Rivera RR, Johns CP, Quan J, Johnson RS, Murre C. 2000. Thymocyte selection is regulated by the helix-loop-helix inhibitor protein, Id3. *Immunity* 12:17–26

74. Engel I, Johns C, Bain G, Rivera RR, Murre C. 2001. Early thymocyte development is regulated by modulation of E2A protein activity. *J. Exp. Med.* 194:733–46

75. Bain G, Cravatt CB, Loomans C, Alberola-Ila J, Hedrick SM, Murre C. 2001. Regulation of the helix-loop-helix proteins, E2A and Id3, by the Ras-ERK MAPK cascade. *Nat. Immunol.* 2:165–71

76. Morrow MA, Mayer EW, Perez CA, Adlam M, Siu G. 1999. Overexpression of the helix-loop-helix protein Id2 blocks T cell development at multiple stages. *Mol. Immunol.* 36:491–503

77. Engel I, Murre C. 2004. E2A proteins enforce a proliferation checkpoint in developing thymocytes. *EMBO J.* 23:202–11

78. Levanon D, Groner Y. 2004. Structure and regulated expression of mammalian RUNX genes. *Oncogene* 23:4211–19

79. Ichikawa M, Asai T, Saito T, Yamamoto G, Seo S, et al. 2004. AML-1 is required for megakaryocytic maturation and lymphocytic differentiation, but not for maintenance of hematopoietic stem cells in adult hematopoiesis. *Nat. Med.* 10:299–304

80. Anderson MK, Pant R, Miracle AL, Sun X, Luer CA, et al. 2004. Evolutionary origins of lymphocytes: ensembles of T cell and B cell transcriptional regulators in a cartilaginous fish. *J. Immunol.* 172:5851–60

81. Tracey WD, Speck NA. 2000. Potential roles for RUNX1 and its orthologs in determining hematopoietic cell fate. *Semin. Cell Dev. Biol.* 11:337–42

82. Ling KW, Dzierzak E. 2002. Ontogeny and genetics of the hemato/lymphopoietic system. *Curr. Opin. Immunol.* 14:186–91

83. Nishimura M, Fukushima-Nakase Y, Fujita Y, Nakao M, Toda S, et al. 2004. VWRPY motif-dependent and -independent roles of AML1/Runx1 transcription factor in murine hematopoietic development. *Blood* 103:562–70

84. Telfer JC, Hedblom EE, Anderson MK, Laurent MN, Rothenberg EV. 2004. Localization of the domains in Runx transcription factors required for the repression of CD4 in thymocytes. *J. Immunol.* 172:4359–70

85. Woolf E, Xiao C, Fainaru O, Lotem J, Rosen D, et al. 2003. Runx3 and Runx1 are required for CD8 T cell development during thymopoiesis. *Proc. Natl. Acad. Sci. USA* 100:7731–36

86. Taniuchi I, Osato M, Egawa T, Sunshine MJ, Bae S-C, et al. 2002. Differential requirements for Runx proteins in *CD4* repression and epigenetic silencing during T lymphocyte development. *Cell* 111:621–33

87. Vaillant F, Blyth K, Andrew L, Neil JC, Cameron ER. 2002. Enforced expression of *Runx2* perturbs T cell development at a stage coincident with β-selection. *J. Immunol.* 169:2866–74

88. Hayashi K, Abe N, Watanabe T, Obinata M, Ito M, et al. 2001. Overexpression of AML1 transcription factor drives thymocytes into the CD8 single-positive lineage. *J. Immunol.* 167:4957–65

89. Satake M, Nomura S, Yamaguchi-Iwai Y, Takahama Y, Hashimoto Y, et al. 1995. Expression of the Runt domain-encoding *PEBP2α* genes in T cells during thymic development. *Mol. Cell. Biol.* 15:1662–70

90. Telfer JC, Rothenberg EV. 2001. Expression and function of a stem-cell promoter for the murine CBFα2 gene: distinct roles and regulation in natural killer and T cell development. *Dev. Biol.* 229:363–82

91. Hsiang YH, Spencer D, Wang S, Speck NA, Raulet DH. 1993. The role of viral enhancer "core" motif-related sequences in regulating T cell receptor-γ and -δ gene expression. *J. Immunol.* 150:3905–16

92. Wotton D, Ghysdael J, Wang S, Speck

NA, Owen MJ. 1994. Cooperative binding of Ets-1 and core binding factor to DNA. *Mol. Cell. Biol.* 14:840–50

93. Hernandez-Munain C, Krangel MS. 1994. Regulation of the T-cell receptor δ enhancer by functional cooperation between c-Myb and core-binding factors. *Mol. Cell. Biol.* 14:473–83

94. Giese K, Kingsley C, Kirshner JR, Grosschedl R. 1995. Assembly and function of a TCRα enhancer complex is dependent on LEF-1-induced DNA bending and multiple protein-protein interactions. *Genes Dev.* 9:995–1008

95. Erman B, Cortes M, Nikolajczyk BS, Speck NA, Sen R. 1998. ETS-core binding factor: a common composite motif in antigen receptor gene enhancers. *Mol. Cell. Biol.* 18:1322–30

96. Kim W-Y, Sieweke M, Ogawa E, Wee H-J, Englmeier U, et al. 1999. Mutual activation of Ets-1 and AML1 DNA binding by direct interaction of their autoinhibitory domains. *EMBO J.* 18:1609–20

97. Yannoutsos N, Barreto V, Misulovin Z, Gazumyan A, Yu W, et al. 2004. A *cis* element in the recombination activating gene locus regulates gene expression by counteracting a distant silencer. *Nat. Immunol.* 5:443–50

98. Ehlers M, Laule-Kilian K, Petter M, Aldrian CJ, Grueter B, et al. 2003. Morpholino antisense oligonucleotide-mediated gene knockdown during thymocyte development reveals role for Runx3 transcription factor in CD4 silencing during development of CD4⁻/CD8⁺ thymocytes. *J. Immunol.* 171:3594–604

99. Liu X, Bosselut R. 2004. Duration of TCR signaling controls CD4-CD8 lineage differentiation in vivo. *Nat. Immunol.* 5:280–88

99a. Kohu K, Sato T, Ohno S-i, Hayashi K, Uchino R, et al. 2005. Over-expression of the Runx3 transcription factor increases the proportion of mature thymocytes of the CD8 single positive lineage. *J. Immunol.* In press

100. Komine O, Hayashi K, Natsume W, Watanabe T, Seki Y, et al. 2003. The Runx1 transcription factor inhibits the differentiation of naive CD4⁺ T cells into the Th2 lineage by repressing *GATA3* expression. *J. Exp. Med.* 198:51–61

101. Cortes M, Wong E, Koipally J, Georgopoulos K. 1999. Control of lymphocyte development by the Ikaros gene family. *Curr. Opin. Immunol.* 11:167–71

102. Brown KE, Guest SS, Smale ST, Hahm K, Merkenschlager M, Fisher AG. 1997. Association of transcriptionally silent genes with Ikaros complexes at centromeric heterochromatin. *Cell* 91:845–54

103. Harker N, Naito T, Cortes M, Hostert A, Hirschberg S, et al. 2002. The CD8α gene locus is regulated by the Ikaros family of proteins. *Mol. Cell* 10:1403–15

104. Georgopoulos K. 2002. Haematopoietic cell-fate decisions, chromatin regulation and Ikaros. *Nat. Rev. Immunol.* 2:162–74

105. Winandy S, Wu L, Wang J-H, Georgopoulos K. 1999. Pre-T cell receptor (TCR) and TCR-controlled checkpoints in T cell differentiation are set by Ikaros. *J. Exp. Med.* 190:1039–48

106. Nichogiannopoulou A, Trevisan M, Neben S, Friedrich C, Georgopoulos K. 1999. Defects in hemopoietic stem cell activity in *Ikaros* mutant mice. *J. Exp. Med.* 190:1201–14

107. Papathanasiou P, Perkins AC, Cobb BS, Ferrini R, Sridharan R, et al. 2003. Widespread failure of hematolymphoid differentiation caused by a recessive niche-filling allele of the Ikaros transcription factor. *Immunity* 19:131–44

108. Allman D, Sambandam A, Kim S, Miller JP, Pagan A, et al. 2003. Thymopoiesis independent of common lymphoid progenitors. *Nat. Immunol.* 4:168–74

109. Urban JA, Winandy S. 2004. Ikaros null mice display defects in T cell selection and CD4 versus CD8 lineage decision. *J. Immunol.* 173:4470–78

110. Chi TH, Wan M, Zhao K, Taniuchi I, Chen L, et al. 2002. Reciprocal regulation of

CD4/CD8 expression by SWI/SNF-like BAF complexes. *Nature* 418:195–99

111. Okamura RM, Sigvardsson M, Galceran J, Verbeek S, Clevers H, Grosschedl R. 1998. Redundant regulation of T cell differentiation and TCRα gene expression by the transcription factors LEF-1 and TCF-1. *Immunity* 8:11–20

112. Schilham MW, Wilson A, Moerer P, Benaissa-Trouw BJ, Cumano A, Clevers HC. 1998. Critical involvement of Tcf-1 in expansion of thymocytes. *J. Immunol.* 161:3984–91

113. Gounari F, Aifantis I, Khazaie K, Hoeflinger S, Harada N, et al. 2001. Somatic activation of β-catenin bypasses pre-TCR signaling and TCR selection in thymocyte development. *Nat. Immunol.* 2:863–69

114. Ioannidis V, Beermann F, Clevers H, Held W. 2001. The β-catenin–TCF-1 pathway ensures CD4$^+$CD8$^+$ thymocyte survival. *Nat. Immunol.* 2:691–97

115. Staal FJT, Weerkamp F, Baert MR, van den Burg CM, van Noort M, et al. 2004. Wnt target genes identified by DNA microarrays in immature CD34$^+$ thymocytes regulate proliferation and cell adhesion. *J. Immunol.* 172:1099–108

116. Reya T, Duncan AW, Ailles L, Domen J, Scherer DC, et al. 2003. A role for Wnt signalling in self-renewal of haematopoietic stem cells. *Nature* 423:409–14

117. Allen RD, III, Bender TP, Siu G. 1999. c-Myb is essential for early T cell development. *Genes Dev.* 13:1073–78

118. Emambokus N, Vegiopoulos A, Harman B, Jenkinson E, Anderson G, Frampton J. 2003. Progression through key stages of haemopoiesis is dependent on distinct threshold levels of c-Myb. *EMBO J.* 22:4478–88

119. Mukouyama Y, Chiba N, Mucenski ML, Satake M, Miyajima A, et al. 1999. Hematopoietic cells in cultures of the murine embryonic aorta-gonad-mesonephros region are induced by c-Myb. *Curr. Biol.* 9:833–36

120. Hsiang YH, Goldman JP, Raulet DH. 1995. The role of c-Myb or a related factor in regulating the T cell receptor γ gene enhancer. *J. Immunol.* 154:5195–204

121. Allen RD, III, Kim HK, Sarafova SD, Siu G. 2001. Negative regulation of CD4 gene expression by a HES-1-c-Myb complex. *Mol. Cell. Biol.* 21:3071–82

122. Hernández-Munain C, Krangel MS. 2002. Distinct roles for c-Myb and core binding factor/polyoma enhancer-binding protein 2 in the assembly and function of a multiprotein complex on the TCR δ enhancer in vivo. *J. Immunol.* 169:4362–69

123. Pearson R, Weston K. 2000. c-Myb regulates the proliferation of immature thymocytes following β-selection. *EMBO J.* 19:6112–20

124. Bender TP, Kremer CS, Kraus M, Buch T, Rajewsky K. 2004. Critical functions for c-Myb at three checkpoints during thymocyte development. *Nat. Immunol.* 5:721–29

125. Anderson MK, Hernandez-Hoyos G, Diamond RA, Rothenberg EV. 1999. Precise developmental regulation of Ets family transcription factors during specification and commitment to the T cell lineage. *Development* 126:3131–48

126. Spain LM, Guerriero A, Kunjibettu S, Scott EW. 1999. T cell development in PU.1-deficient mice. *J. Immunol.* 163:2681–87

127. Herblot S, Steff AM, Hugo P, Aplan PD, Hoang T. 2000. SCL and LMO1 alter thymocyte differentiation: inhibition of E2A-HEB function and pre-Tα chain expression. *Nat. Immunol.* 1:138–44

128. Su GH, Ip HS, Cobb BS, Lu M-M, Chen H-M, Simon MC. 1996. The Ets protein Spi-B is expressed exclusively in B cells and T cells during development. *J. Exp. Med.* 184:203–14

129. Lloberas J, Soler C, Celada A. 1999. The key role of PU.1/SPI-1 in B cells, myeloid cells and macrophages. *Immunol. Today* 20:184–89

130. Dahl R, Simon MC. 2003. The importance of PU.1 concentration in hematopoietic lineage commitment and maturation. *Blood Cells Mol. Dis.* 31:229–33

131. Back J, Dierich A, Bronn C, Kastner P, Chan S. 2004. PU.1 determines the self-renewal capacity of erythroid progenitor cells. *Blood* 103:3615–23

132. DeKoter RP, Lee H-J, Singh H. 2002. PU.1 regulates expression of the Interleukin-7 receptor in lymphoid progenitors. *Immunity* 16:297–309

133. McKercher SR, Torbett BE, Anderson KL, Henkel GW, Vestal DJ, et al. 1996. Targeted disruption of the *PU.1* gene results in multiple hematopoietic abnormalities. *EMBO J.* 15:5647–58

134. Anderson MK, Weiss A, Hernandez-Hoyos G, Dionne CJ, Rothenberg EV. 2002. Constitutive expression of PU.1 in fetal hematopoietic progenitors blocks T-cell development at the pro-T stage. *Immunity* 16:285–96

135. Schotte R, Rissoan MC, Bendriss-Vermare N, Bridon JM, Duhen T, et al. 2003. The transcription factor Spi-B is expressed in plasmacytoid DC precursors and inhibits T-, B-, and NK-cell development. *Blood* 101:1015–23

136. Trinh LA, Ferrini R, Cobb BS, Weinmann AS, Hahm K, et al. 2001. Down-regulation of TDT transcription in $CD4^+CD8^+$ thymocytes by Ikaros proteins in direct competition with an Ets activator. *Genes Dev.* 15:1817–32

137. Bories J-C, Willerford DM, Grévin D, Davidson L, Camus A, et al. 1995. Increased T-cell apoptosis and terminal B-cell differentiation induced by inactivation of the Ets-1 proto-oncogene. *Nature* 377:635–38

138. Barton K, Muthusamy N, Fischer C, Ting C-N, Walunas TL, et al. 1998. The Ets-1 transcription factor is required for the development of natural killer cells in mice. *Immunity* 9:555–63

139. Xue H-H, Bollenbacher J, Rovella V, Tripuraneni R, Du Y-B, et al. 2004. GA binding protein regulates interleukin 7 receptor α-chain gene expression in T cells. *Nat. Immunol.* 5:1036–44

140. Sauvageau G, Lansdorp PM, Eaves CJ, Hogge DE, Dragowska WH, et al. 1994. Differential expression of homeobox genes in functionally distinct $CD34^+$ subpopulations of human bone marrow cells. *Proc. Natl. Acad. Sci. USA* 91:12223–27

141. Taghon T, Thys K, De Smedt M, Weerkamp F, Staal FJ, et al. 2003. Homeobox gene expression profile in human hematopoietic multipotent stem cells and T-cell progenitors: implications for human T-cell development. *Leukemia* 17:1157–63

142. Izon DJ, Rozenfeld S, Fong ST, Komuves L, Largman C, Lawrence HJ. 1998. Loss of function of the homeobox gene *Hoxa-9* perturbs early T-cell development and induces apoptosis in primitive thymocytes. *Blood* 92:383–93

143. Szabo SJ, Kim ST, Costa GL, Zhang X, Fathman CG, Glimcher LH. 2000. A novel transcription factor, T-bet, directs Th1 lineage commitment. *Cell* 100:655–69

144. Shier P, Hofstra CL, Ma XJ, Wu Y, Ngo K, Fung-Leung WP. 2000. Tbt-1, a new T-box transcription factor induced in activated Th1 and $CD8^+$ T cells. *Immunogenetics* 51:771–78

145. Mullen AC, High FA, Hutchins AS, Lee HW, Villarino AV, et al. 2001. Role of T-bet in commitment of T_H1 cells before IL-12-dependent selection. *Science* 292:1907–10

146. Pearce EL, Mullen AC, Martins GA, Krawczyk CM, Hutchins AS, et al. 2003. Control of effector $CD8^+$ T cell function by the transcription factor *Eomesodermin*. *Science* 302:1041–43

147. Townsend MJ, Weinmann AS, Matsuda JL, Salomon R, Farnham PJ, et al. 2004. T-bet regulates the terminal maturation and homeostasis of NK and $V\alpha14_i$ NKT Cells. *Immunity* 20:477–94

148. Allen JD, Harris AW, Bath ML, Strasser

A, Scollay R, Adams JM. 1995. Perturbed development of T and B cells in mice expressing an Hlx homeobox transgene. *J. Immunol.* 154:1531–42

149. Mullen AC, Hutchins AS, High FA, Lee HW, Sykes KJ, et al. 2002. Hlx is induced by and genetically interacts with T-bet to promote heritable T_H1 gene induction. *Nat. Immunol.* 3:652–58

150. Zheng WP, Zhao Q, Zhao X, Li B, Hubank M, et al. 2004. Up-regulation of Hlx in immature Th cells induces IFN-γ expression. *J. Immunol.* 172:114–22

151. Lian RH, Kumar V. 2002. Murine natural killer cell progenitors and their requirements for development. *Semin. Immunol.* 14:453–60

152. Wilkinson B, Chen JY, Han P, Rufner KM, Goularte OD, Kaye J. 2002. TOX: an HMG box protein implicated in the regulation of thymocyte selection. *Nat. Immunol.* 3:272–80

153. Aliahmad P, O'Flaherty E, Han P, Goularte OD, Wilkinson B, et al. 2004. TOX provides a link between calcineurin activation and CD8 lineage commitment. *J. Exp. Med.* 199:1089–99

154. Higashi Y, Moribe H, Takagi T, Sekido R, Kawakami K, et al. 1997. Impairment of T cell development in $\delta EF1$ mutant mice. *J. Exp. Med.* 185:1467–79

155. Postigo AA, Sheppard AM, Mucenski ML, Dean DC. 1997. c-Myb and Ets proteins synergize to overcome transcriptional repression by ZEB. *EMBO J.* 16: 3924–34

156. Jepsen K, Hermanson O, Onami TM, Gleiberman AS, Lunyak V, et al. 2000. Combinatorial roles of the nuclear receptor corepressor in transcription and development. *Cell* 102:753–63

157. Hock H, Hamblen MJ, Rooke HM, Traver D, Bronson RT, et al. 2003. Intrinsic requirement for zinc finger transcription factor Gfi-1 in neutrophil differentiation. *Immunity* 18:109–20

158. Yücel R, Karsunky H, Klein-Hitpass L, Möröy T. 2003. The transcriptional repressor Gfi1 affects development of early, uncommitted c-Kit$^+$ T cell progenitors and CD4/CD8 lineage decision in the thymus. *J. Exp. Med.* 197:831–44

159. Doan LL, Kitay MK, Yu Q, Singer A, Herblot S, et al. 2003. Growth factor independence-1B expression leads to defects in T cell activation, IL-7 receptor α expression, and T cell lineage commitment. *J. Immunol.* 170:2356–66

160. Osawa M, Yamaguchi T, Nakamura Y, Kaneko S, Onodera M, et al. 2002. Erythroid expansion mediated by the Gfi-1B zinc finger protein: role in normal hematopoiesis. *Blood* 100:2769–77

161. Saleque S, Cameron S, Orkin SH. 2002. The zinc-finger proto-oncogene *Gfi-1b* is essential for development of the erythroid and megakaryocytic lineages. *Genes Dev.* 16:301–6

162. Zhu J, Guo L, Min B, Watson CJ, Hu-Li J, et al. 2002. Growth factor independent-1 induced by IL-4 regulates Th2 cell proliferation. *Immunity* 16:733–44

163. Alvarez JD, Yasui DH, Niida H, Joh T, Loh DY, Kohwi-Shigematsu T. 2000. The MAR-binding protein SATB1 orchestrates temporal and spatial expression of multiple genes during T-cell development. *Genes Dev.* 14:521–35

164. Cai S, Han H-J, Kohwi-Shigematsu T. 2003. Tissue-specific nuclear architecture and gene expression regulated by SATB1. *Nat. Genet.* 34:42–51

165. Yasui D, Miyano M, Cai S, Varga-Weisz P, Kohwi-Shigematsu T. 2002. SATB1 targets chromatin remodelling to regulate genes over long distances. *Nature* 419:641–45

166. Fisher AG, Merkenschlager M. 2002. Gene silencing, cell fate and nuclear organisation. *Curr. Opin. Genet. Dev.* 12: 193–97

167. Hardy RR. 2003. B-cell commitment: deciding on the players. *Curr. Opin. Immunol.* 15:158–65

168. Maier H, Hagman J. 2002. Roles of EBF and Pax-5 in B lineage commitment and

development. *Semin. Immunol.* 14:415–22

169. Medina KL, Pongubala JMR, Reddy KL, Lancki DW, DeKoter R, et al. 2004. Assembling a gene regulatory network for specification of the B cell fate. *Dev. Cell* 7:607–17

170. Rosenbauer F, Wagner K, Kutok JL, Iwasaki H, Akashi K, et al. 2003. Myeloid and B-lymphoid development require high PU.1 expression by a distal element in vivo. *Blood* 102:342A

171. Ikawa T, Kawamoto H, Wright LY, Murre C. 2004. Long-term cultured E2A-deficient hematopoietic progenitor cells are pluripotent. *Immunity* 20:349–60

172. Cotta CV, Zhang Z, Kim HG, Klug CA. 2003. Pax5 determines B- versus T-cell fate and does not block early myeloid-lineage development. *Blood* 101:4342–46

173. Seet CS, Brumbaugh RL, Kee BL. 2004. Early B Cell Factor promotes B lymphopoiesis with reduced Interleukin 7 responsiveness in the absence of E2A. *J. Exp. Med.* 199:1689–700

174. Souabni A, Cobaleda C, Schebesta M, Busslinger M. 2002. Pax5 promotes B lymphopoiesis and blocks T cell development by repressing *Notch1*. *Immunity* 17:781–93

175. Zhang Z, Cotta CV, Stephan RP, deGuzman CG, Klug CA. 2003. Enforced expression of EBF in hematopoietic stem cells restricts lymphopoiesis to the B cell lineage. *EMBO J.* 22:4759–69

176. Goebel P, Janney N, Valenzuela JR, Romanow WJ, Murre C, Feeney AJ. 2001. Localized gene-specific induction of accessibility to V(D)J recombination induced by E2A and early B cell factor in nonlymphoid cells. *J. Exp. Med.* 194:645–56

177. Smith EM, Gisler R, Sigvardsson M. 2002. Cloning and characterization of a promoter flanking the early B cell factor (EBF) gene indicates roles for E-proteins and autoregulation in the control of EBF expression. *J. Immunol.* 169:261–70

178. Gisler R, Sigvardsson M. 2002. The human V-preB promoter is a target for coordinated activation by early B cell factor and E47. *J. Immunol.* 168:5130–38

179. Sayegh CE, Quong MW, Agata Y, Murre C. 2003. E-proteins directly regulate expression of activation-induced deaminase in mature B cells. *Nat. Immunol.* 4:586–93

180. Schroeder T, Kohlhof H, Rieber N, Just U. 2003. Notch signaling induces multilineage myeloid differentiation and upregulates PU.1 expression. *J. Immunol.* 170:5538–48

181. Aifantis I, Gounari F, Scorrano L, Borowski C, von Boehmer H. 2001. Constitutive pre-TCR signaling promotes differentiation through Ca^{2+} mobilization and activation of NF-κB and NFAT. *Nat. Immunol.* 2:403–9

182. Carleton M, Haks MC, Smeele SA, Jones A, Belkowski SM, et al. 2002. Early growth response transcription factors are required for development of $CD4^-CD8^-$ thymocytes to the $CD4^+CD8^+$ stage. *J. Immunol.* 168:1649–58

183. Xi H, Kersh GJ. 2004. Early growth response gene 3 regulates thymocyte proliferation during the transition from $CD4^-CD8^-$ to $CD4^+CD8^+$. *J. Immunol.* 172:964–71

184. Barndt R, Dai MF, Zhang Y. 1999. A novel role for HEB downstream or parallel to the pre-TCR signaling pathway during $\alpha\beta$ thymopoiesis. *J. Immunol.* 163:3331–43

185. Yasutomo K, Doyle C, Miele L, Germain RN. 2000. The duration of antigen receptor signalling determines $CD4^+$ versus $CD8^+$ T-cell lineage fate. *Nature* 404:506–10

186. Dunon D, Courtois D, Vainio O, Six A, Chen CH, et al. 1997. Ontogeny of the immune system: γ/δ and α/β T cells migrate from thymus to the periphery in alternating waves. *J. Exp. Med.* 186:977–88

187. Rast JP, Litman GW. 1998. Towards understanding the evolutionary origins and

early diversification of rearranging antigen receptors. *Immunol. Rev.* 166:79–86

188. Fehling HJ, Gilfillan S, Ceredig R. 1999. $\alpha\beta/\gamma\delta$ lineage commitment in the thymus of normal and genetically manipulated mice. *Adv. Immunol.* 71:1–76

189. Bruno L, Fehling HJ, von Boehmer H. 1996. The $\alpha\beta$ T cell receptor can replace the $\gamma\delta$ receptor in the development of $\gamma\delta$ lineage cells. *Immunity* 5:343–52

190. Dave VP, Cao Z, Browne C, Alarcon B, Fernandez-Miguel G, et al. 1997. CD3δ deficiency arrests development of the $\alpha\beta$ but not the $\gamma\delta$ T cell lineage. *EMBO J.* 16:1360–70

191. Terrence K, Pavlovich CP, Matechak EO, Fowlkes BJ. 2000. Premature expression of T cell receptor (TCR)$\alpha\beta$ suppresses TCR$\gamma\delta$ gene rearrangement but permits development of $\gamma\delta$ lineage T cells. *J. Exp. Med.* 192:537–48

192. Lee PP, Fitzpatrick DR, Beard C, Jessup HK, Lehar S, et al. 2001. A critical role for Dnmt1 and DNA methylation in T cell development, function, and survival. *Immunity* 15:763–74

193. Pennington DJ, Silva-Santos B, Shires J, Theodoridis E, Pollitt C, et al. 2003. The inter-relatedness and interdependence of mouse T cell receptor $\gamma\delta^+$ and $\alpha\beta^+$ cells. *Nat. Immunol.* 4:991–98

194. Washburn T, Schweighoffer E, Gridley T, Chang D, Fowlkes BJ, et al. 1997. Notch activity influences the $\alpha\beta$ versus $\gamma\delta$ T cell lineage decision. *Cell* 88:833–43

195. Bain G, Romanow WJ, Albers K, Havran WL, Murre C. 1999. Positive and negative regulation of V(D)J recombination by the E2A proteins. *J. Exp. Med.* 189:289–300

196. Blom B, Heemskerk MHM, Verschuren MCM, van Dongen JJM, Stegmann APA, et al. 1999. Disruption of $\alpha\beta$ but not of $\gamma\delta$ T cell development by overexpression of the helix-loop-helix protein Id3 in committed T cell progenitors. *EMBO J.* 18:2793–802

197. De Smedt M, Reynvoet K, Kerre T, Taghon T, Verhasselt B, et al. 2002. Active form of Notch imposes T cell fate in human progenitor cells. *J. Immunol.* 169:3021–29

198. Garcia-Peydro M, de Yebenes VG, Toribio ML. 2003. Sustained Notch1 signaling instructs the earliest human intrathymic precursors to adopt a $\gamma\delta$ T cell fate in fetal thymus organ culture. *Blood* 102:2444–51

199. Lee C-K, Kim K, Geiman TM, Murphy WJ, Muegge K, Durum SK. 1999. Cloning thymic precursor cells: demonstration that individual pro-T1 cells have dual T-NK potential and individual pro-T2 cells have dual $\alpha\beta - \gamma\delta$ T cell potential. *Cell Immunol.* 191:139–44

200. Lacorazza HD, Miyazaki Y, Di Cristofano A, Deblasio A, Hedvat C, et al. 2002. The ETS protein MEF plays a critical role in perforin gene expression and the development of Natural Killer and NK-T cells. *Immunity* 17:437–49

201. Ohteki T, Ho S, Suzuki H, Mak TW, Ohashi PS. 1997. Role for IL-15/IL-15 receptor β-chain in Natural Killer 1.1$^+$ T cell receptor-$\alpha\beta^+$ cell development. *J. Immunol.* 159:5931–35

202. Ohteki T, Yoshida H, Matsuyama T, Duncan GS, Mak TW, Ohashi PS. 1998. The transcription factor interferon regulatory factor 1 (IRF-1) is important during the maturation of Natural Killer 1.1$^+$ T cell receptor α/β^+ (NK1$^+$ T) cells, natural killer cells, and intestinal intraepithelial T cells. *J. Exp. Med.* 187:967–72

203. Walunas TL, Wang B, Wang CR, Leiden JM. 2000. Cutting edge: The Ets1 transcription factor is required for the development of NK T cells in mice. *J. Immunol.* 164:2857–60

204. MacDonald HR. 2002. Development and selection of NKT cells. *Curr. Opin. Immunol.* 14:250–54

205. Ramsdell F. 2003. Foxp3 and natural regulatory T cells: key to a cell lineage? *Immunity* 19:165–68

206. Harman BC, Jenkinson EJ, Anderson G.

2003. Entry into the thymic microenvironment triggers Notch activation in the earliest migrant T cell progenitors. *J. Immunol.* 170:1299–303

207. Ivanov V, Merkenschlager M, Ceredig R. 1993. Antioxidant treatment of thymic organ cultures decreases NF-κB and TCF1(α) transcription factor activities and inhibits $\alpha\beta$ T cell development. *J. Immunol.* 151:4694–704

208. Schwarz BA, Bhandoola A. 2004. Circulating hematopoietic progenitors with T lineage potential. *Nat. Immunol.* 9:953–60

209. Kincade PW, Igarashi H, Medina KL, Kouro T, Yokota T, et al. 2002. Lymphoid lineage cells in adult murine bone marrow diverge from those of other blood cells at an early, hormone-sensitive stage. *Semin. Immunol.* 14:385–94

210. Prohaska SS, Scherer DC, Weissman IL, Kondo M. 2002. Developmental plasticity of lymphoid progenitors. *Semin. Immunol.* 14:377–84

211. Rothenberg EV, Dionne CJ. 2002. Lineage plasticity and commitment in T-cell development. *Immunol. Rev.* 187:96–115

212. Bhandoola A, Sambandam A, Allman D, Meraz A, Schwarz B. 2003. Early T lineage progenitors: New insights, but old questions remain. *J. Immunol.* 171:5653–58

213. Wang H, Spangrude GJ. 2003. Aspects of early lymphoid commitment. *Curr. Opin. Hematol.* 10:203–7

214. Douagi I, Colucci F, Di Santo JP, Cumano A. 2002. Identification of the earliest prethymic bipotent T/NK progenitor in murine fetal liver. *Blood* 99:463–71

215. Kondo M, Weissman IL, Akashi K. 1997. Identification of clonogenic common lymphoid progenitors in mouse bone marrow. *Cell* 91:661–72

216. Martin CH, Aifantis I, Scimone ML, von Andrian UH, Reizis B, et al. 2003. Efficient thymic immigration of B220$^+$

lymphoid-restricted bone marrow cells with T precursor potential. *Nat. Immunol.* 4:866–73

217. Perry SS, Wang H, Pierce LJ, Yang AM, Tsai S, Spangrude GJ. 2004. L-Selectin defines a bone marrow analogue to the thymic early T-lineage progenitor. *Blood* 103:2990–96

218. Igarashi H, Gregory SC, Yokota T, Sakaguchi N, Kincade PW. 2002. Transcription from the RAG1 locus marks the earliest lymphocyte progenitors in bone marrow. *Immunity* 17:117–30

219. Katsura Y. 2002. Redefinition of lymphoid progenitors. *Nat. Rev. Immunol.* 2:127–32

220. Mebius RE, Miyamoto T, Christensen J, Domen J, Cupedo T, et al. 2001. The fetal liver counterpart of adult common lymphoid progenitors gives rise to all lymphoid lineages, CD45$^+$CD4$^+$CD3$^-$ cells, as well as macrophages. *J. Immunol.* 166:6593–601

221. Lu M, Kawamoto H, Katsube Y, Ikawa T, Katsura Y. 2002. The common myelolymphoid progenitor: a key intermediate stage in hemopoiesis generating T and B cells. *J. Immunol.* 169:3519–25

222. Yokota T, Kouro T, Hirose J, Igarashi H, Garrett KP, et al. 2003. Unique properties of fetal lymphoid progenitors identified according to RAG1 gene expression. *Immunity* 19:365–75

223. Porritt HE, Rumfelt LL, Tabrizifard S, Schmitt TM, Zúñiga-Pflücker JC, Petrie HT. 2004. Heterogeneity among DN1 prothymocytes reveals multiple progenitors with different capacities to generate T cell and non-T cell lineages. *Immunity* 20:735–45

224. Fisher RC, Lovelock JD, Scott EW. 1999. A critical role for PU.1 in homing and long-term engraftment by hematopoietic stem cells in the bone marrow. *Blood* 94:1283–90

225. North TE, de Bruijn MF, Stacy T, Talebian L, Lind E, et al. 2002. Runx1 expression marks long-term repopulating

hematopoietic stem cells in the midgesta-tion mouse embryo. *Immunity* 16:661–72

226. Varnum-Finney B, Xu L, Brashem-Stein C, Nourigat C, Flowers D, et al. 2000. Pluripotent, cytokine-dependent, hematopoietic stem cells are immortal-ized by constitutive Notch1 signaling. *Nat. Med.* 6:1278–81

227. Sikes ML, Gomez RJ, Song J, Oltz E. 1998. A developmental stage-specific promoter directs germline transcription of DβJβ gene segments in precursor T lym-phocytes. *J. Immunol.* 161:1399–405

228. Reizis B, Leder P. 2002. Direct induction of T lymphocyte-specific gene expression by the mammalian Notch signaling path-way. *Genes Dev.* 16:295–300

229. Allen JM, Forbush KA, Perlmutter RM. 1992. Functional dissection of the *lck* proximal promoter. *Mol. Cell. Biol.* 12: 2758–68

230. McCracken S, Leung S, Bosselut R, Ghys-dael J, Miyamoto NG. 1994. Myb and Ets related transcription factors are required for activity of the human *lck* type I pro-moter. *Oncogene* 9:3609–15

231. Wang Q-F, Lauring J, Schlissel MS. 2000. c-Myb binds to a sequence in the proximal region of the RAG-2 promoter and is es-sential for promoter activity in T-lineage cells. *Mol. Cell. Biol.* 20:9203–11

232. Tomita K, Hattori M, Nakamura E, Nakanishi S, Minato N, Kageyama R. 1999. The bHLH gene *Hes1* is essential for expansion of early T cell precursors. *Genes Dev.* 13:1203–10

233. Kawamoto H, Ohmura K, Fujimoto S, Lu M, Ikawa T, Katsura Y. 2003. Extensive proliferation of T cell lineage-restricted progenitors in the thymus: an essential process for clonal expression of diverse T cell receptor beta chains. *Eur. J. Im-munol.* 33:606–15

234. Shen HQ, Lu M, Ikawa T, Masuda K, Ohmura K, et al. 2003. T/NK bipotent progenitors in the thymus retain the po-tential to generate dendritic cells. *J. Im-munol.* 171:3401–6

235. Petrie HT. 2003. Cell migration and the control of post-natal T-cell lymphopoiesis in the thymus. *Nat. Rev. Immunol.* 3:859–66

236. Rothenberg EV. 2000. Stepwise specifi-cation of lymphocyte developmental lin-eages. *Curr. Opin. Genet. Dev.* 10:370–79

237. Wu L, Li C-L, Shortman K. 1996. Thymic dendritic cell precursors: relationship to the T lymphocyte lineage and phenotype of the dendritic cell progeny. *J. Exp. Med.* 184:903–11

238. Spits H, Blom B, Jaleco AC, Weijer K, Verschuren MC, et al. 1998. Early stages in the development of human T, natural killer and thymic dendritic cells. *Immunol. Rev.* 165:75–86

239. Ikawa T, Kawamoto H, Fujimoto S, Katsura Y. 1999. Commitment of com-mon T/natural killer (NK) progenitors to unipotent T and NK progenitors in the murine fetal thymus revealed by a single progenitor assay. *J. Exp. Med.* 190:1617–25

240. Michie AM, Carlyle JR, Schmitt TM, Lju-tic B, Cho SK, et al. 2000. Clonal charac-terization of a bipotent T cell and NK cell progenitor in the mouse fetal thymus. *J. Immunol.* 164:1730–33

241. Lee C-K, Kim JK, Kim Y, Lee MK, Kim K, et al. 2001. Generation of macrophages from early T progenitors in vitro. *J. Im-munol.* 166:5964–69

242. Ohishi K, Varnum-Finney B, Serda RE, Anasetti C, Bernstein ID. 2001. The Notch ligand, Delta-1, inhibits the differentia-tion of monocytes into macrophages but permits their differentiation into dendritic cells. *Blood* 98:1402–7

243. Corcoran L, Ferrero I, Vremec D, Lu-cas K, Waithman J, et al. 2003. The lym-phoid past of mouse plasmacytoid cells and thymic dendritic cells. *J. Immunol.* 170:4926–32

244. King AG, Kondo M, Scherer DC, Weiss-man IL. 2002. Lineage infidelity in myeloid cells with TCR gene rearrange-ment: a latent developmental potential of

proT cells revealed by ectopic cytokine receptor signaling. *Proc. Natl. Acad. Sci. USA* 99:4508–13

245. Iwasaki-Arai J, Iwasaki H, Miyamoto T, Watanabe S, Akashi K. 2003. Enforced Granulocyte/Macrophage Colony-Stimulating Factor signals do not support lymphopoiesis, but instruct lymphoid to myelomonocytic lineage conversion. *J. Exp. Med.* 197:1311–22

246. Rekhtman N, Radparvar F, Evans T, Skoultchi A. 1999. Direct interaction of hematopoietic transcription factors PU.1 and GATA-1: functional antagonism in erythroid cells. *Genes Dev.* 13:1398–411

247. Zhang P, Behre G, Pan J, Iwama A, Wara-Aswapati N, et al. 1999. Negative cross-talk between hematopoietic regulators: GATA proteins repress PU.1. *Proc. Natl. Acad. Sci. USA* 96:8705–10

248. Nerlov C, Querfurth E, Kulessa H, Graf T. 2000. GATA-1 interacts with the myeloid PU.1 transcription factor and represses PU.1-dependent transcription. *Blood* 95:2543–51

249. Izon DJ, Aster JC, He Y, Weng A, Karnell FG, et al. 2002. Deltex1 redirects lymphoid progenitors to the B cell lineage by antagonizing Notch1. *Immunity* 16:231–43

250. Nie L, Xu M, Vladimirova A, Sun X-H. 2003. Notch-induced E2A ubiquitination and degradation are controlled by MAP kinase activities. *EMBO J.* 22:5780–92

251. Davidson EH, McClay DR, Hood L. 2003. Regulatory gene networks and the properties of the developmental process. *Proc. Natl. Acad. Sci. USA* 100:1475–80

252. Hacker C, Kirsch RD, Ju X-S, Hieronymus T, Gust TC, et al. 2003. Transcriptional profiling identifies Id2 function in dendritic cell development. *Nat. Immunol.* 4:380–86

253. Ishiguro A, Spirin KS, Shiohara M, Tobler A, Gombart AF, et al. 1996. Id2 expression increases with differentiation of human myeloid cells. *Blood* 87:5225–31

254. Cooper CL, Brady G, Bilia F, Iscove

NN, Quesenberry PJ. 1997. Expression of the Id family helix-loop-helix regulators during growth and development in the hematopoietic system. *Blood* 89:3155–65

255. Mao C, Ray-Gallet D, Tavitian A, Moreau-Gachelin F. 1996. Differential phosphorylations of Spi-B and Spi-1 transcription factors. *Oncogene* 12:863–73

256. Rieske P, Pongubala JM. 2001. AKT induces transcriptional activity of PU.1 through phosphorylation-mediated modifications within its transactivation domain. *J. Biol. Chem.* 276:8460–68

257. Wang J-M, Lai M-Z, Yang-Yen H-F. 2003. Interleukin-3 stimulation of *mcl-1* gene transcription involves activation of the PU.1 transcription factor through a p38 mitogen-activated protein kinase-dependent pathway. *Mol. Cell. Biol.* 23:1896–909

258. Mazzi P, Donini M, Margotto D, Wientjes F, Dusi S. 2004. IFN-γ induces gp91^{phox} expression in human monocytes via protein kinase C-dependent phosphorylation of PU.1. *J. Immunol.* 172:4941–47

259. Behre G, Whitmarsh AJ, Coghlan MP, Hoang T, Carpenter CL, et al. 1999. c-Jun is a c-Jun NH$_2$-terminal kinase-independent coactivator of the PU.1 transcription factor. *J. Biol. Chem.* 274:4939–46

260. Yokota Y, Mori S. 2002. Role of Id family proteins in growth control. *J. Cell. Physiol.* 190:21–28

261. Durum SK, Lee C, Geiman TM, Murphy WJ, Muegge K. 1998. CD16 cross-linking blocks rearrangement of the TCRβ locus and development of $\alpha\beta$ T cells and induces development of NK cells from thymic progenitors. *J. Immunol.* 161:3325–29

262. Gadina M, Sudarshan C, Visconti R, Zhou YJ, Gu H, et al. 2000. The docking molecule gab2 is induced by lymphocyte activation and is involved in signaling by interleukin-2 and interleukin-15 but not other common γ chain-using cytokines. *J. Biol. Chem.* 275:26959–66

263. Kovanen PE, Rosenwald A, Fu J, Hurt EM, Lam LT, et al. 2003. Analysis of γc-family cytokine target genes. Identification of dual-specificity phosphatase 5 (DUSP5) as a regulator of mitogen-activated protein kinase activity in interleukin-2 signaling. *J. Biol. Chem.* 278:5205–13

264. Rosmaraki EE, Douagi I, Roth C, Colucci F, Cumano A, Di Santo JP. 2001. Identification of committed NK cell progenitors in adult murine bone marrow. *Eur. J. Immunol.* 31:1900–9

265. Schmitt TM, De Pooter RF, Gronski MA, Cho SK, Ohashi PS, Zúñiga-Pflücker JC. 2004. Induction of T cell development and establishment of T cell competence from embryonic stem cells differentiated in vitro. *Nat. Immunol.* 5:410–17

Annu. Rev. Immunol. 2005. 23:651–82
doi: 10.1146/annurev.immunol.23.021704.115702
First published online as a Review in Advance on December 10, 2004

Understanding Presentation of Viral Antigens to CD8$^+$ T Cells In Vivo: The Key to Rational Vaccine Design*

Jonathan W. Yewdell and S.M. Mansour Haeryfar

Laboratory of Viral Diseases, National Institute of Allergy and Infectious Diseases, National Institutes of Health, Bethesda, Maryland 20892-0440; email: jyewdell@niaid.nih.gov

Key Words antigen presentation, CTL, virus, MHC

■ **Abstract** CD8$^+$ T cells play a critical role in antiviral immunity by exerting direct antiviral activity against infected cells. Because of their ability to recognize all types of viral proteins, they offer the promise of providing broad immunity to viruses that evade humoral immunity by varying their surface proteins. Consequently, there is considerable interest in developing vaccines that elicit effective antiviral T_{CD8+} responses. Generating optimal vaccines ultimately requires rational design based on detailed knowledge of how T_{CD8+} are activated in vivo under natural circumstances. Here we review recent progress obtained largely by in vivo studies in mice to understand the mechanistic basis for activation of naive T_{CD8+} in virus infections. These studies point the way to detailed understanding and provide some key information for vaccine development, although much remains to be learned to enable truly rational vaccine design.

INTRODUCTION: CELLULAR IMMUNITY TO VIRUSES

As Éli Metchnikoff predicted, cellular elements play a critical role in the immunity of multicellular organisms to pathogens (1). The macrosized cells "phaging" rose thorns first spied by Metchnikoff in starfish larvae have been joined by many other cell types. The complexity, dexterity, and subtleties of the vertebrate cellular immune system would undoubtedly astound and delight Metchnikoff, particularly the major protagonists of this review, T cells, which are thoroughly incapable of dealing with thorns. Still, Paul Ehrlich, Metchnikoff's nemesis and champion of the humoral arm of immunity, would also take great pleasure in the exquisite antigen specificity of T cells and particularly in the fact that it is based on the same principle as the binding of his beloved "Antikörper" to their antigens.

---

*The U.S. Government has the right to retain a nonexclusive, royalty-free license in and to any copyright covering this paper.

0732-0582/05/0423-0651$14.00

T cells owe their specificity to the T cell receptor (TCR). The TCR interacts with MHC class I or II molecules bearing short peptides snug in their eponymous, now-famous groove. In this review, we use "determinant" to refer to antigenic peptides in place of "epitope," which has gained wide usage. [Jerne coined "epitope" to specifically designate the surface region of a protein (hence *epi-*) that interacts with a complementary antibody *paratope* (2)]. Thanks to thymic selection events, the TCR works in conjunction with one of two coreceptors, CD4 or CD8, whose mutually exclusive expression in mature T cells limits T cell interactions to MHC class II or class I molecules, respectively. Additional molecules function to transduce the signals generated by the interaction of TCR and coreceptors with appropriate MHC-peptide complexes to activate the previously inert T cell. The sensitivity of T cells to their cognate antigens is nothing short of astounding: Compelling evidence suggests that T cells can be activated by antigen-presenting cells (APCs) displaying a single agonistic MHC-peptide complex (hereafter referred to simply as "complexes") present in a sea of tens of thousands of complexes with nonantigenic peptides (3, 4). Although this level of sensitivity may be atypical, it is likely that T cells routinely recognize APCs bearing 10–100 complexes.

The high sensitivity of T cells is essential to their function. To maintain a TCR repertoire of sufficient complexity to counter the universe of potential antigens, clones of any given specificity must be present at low copy numbers. Although they can divide faster than any other vertebrate cell (a complete cell cycle in 6 to 8 h), T cells still must respond rapidly to reach the numbers required to mount an effective response to pathogens. Indeed, many pathogens multiply so briskly (some viruses can generate more than 1000 progeny in less than 6 h after contacting a suitable host cell), the innate immune system must perform a critical holding action for 3 to 5 days until T cells (and B cells) attain fighting strength. Of equal or perhaps even greater importance, sensitive triggering enables earlier and more effective detection of pathogen-infected cells by T cells, which is of paramount importance for viruses with rapid replication cycles.

The job of exerting direct antipathogen activity falls largely to $CD8^+$ T cells (T_{CD8+}). This task is enabled by the constitutive expression of class I molecules in nearly all tissue types (class II molecules are constitutively expressed only by a subset of cells of immune lineage). T_{CD8+} principally function to control and eradicate intracellular pathogens, particularly the thousands of virus types capable of infecting a given vertebrate species. T_{CD8+} limit virus replication by either killing virus-infected cells or by releasing cytokines that induce an antiviral state in cells. There is great hope that vaccines that induce T_{CD8+} will be useful in preventing or ameliorating infections with viruses that are resistant to traditional antiviral vaccines geared toward induction of antibodies with virus-neutralizing activity. These include viruses that are intrinsically resistant to antibody neutralization (e.g., human immunodeficiency virus), viruses whose antigen variability makes them elusive targets [e.g., influenza A virus (IAV)], and chronic viruses that exhaust otherwise normal T_{CD8+} responses (e.g., hepatitis B virus).

It has proven more difficult than many anticipated to develop vaccines that elicit T_{CD8+} responses effective against such viruses. Although in the end, these difficulties may reflect intrinsic features of virus-host relationships that cannot be surmounted, there is considerable room for improvement in our ability to manipulate T_{CD8+} responses. Further, such knowledge would have a positive impact on developing vaccines effective in treating established tumors and treatments for T_{CD8+}-based autoimmune conditions.

Nature is frequently the best teacher. A more detailed understanding of how viral antigens are naturally presented to T_{CD8+} is essential to the rational design of T_{CD8+} vaccines. Although in vitro experiments provide insight into natural processes, they cannot substitute for in vivo investigation. Consequently, we heavily weight this review to experiments performed in vivo. Nearly all of the studies we discuss have been performed using mouse model systems. Some immunologists who are focused on the workings of the human immune system question the relevance of mouse model systems. Although mice and human immune systems demonstrate a number of important differences, these constitute a tiny fraction of their common features. One of the most important results to emerge from complete sequencing of human and mouse genomes is their astonishing similarity. Indeed, from a pragmatic standpoint, a more significant hurdle in generalizing findings from mouse model systems occurs between mouse and human viruses. Most viruses that infect humans either do not infect mice or do so in fundamentally different ways than they infect humans. Even closely related mouse and human viruses exhibit significant differences in their routes of transmission, target tissues, and interference with host immunity. Although this limits the direct applicability of any given mouse-virus system to understanding human immunity, clearly mouse models will continue to be the principal source of insight into the workings of the human immune system.

CRITICAL QUESTIONS: THE FOUR Ws

Understanding of antiviral T_{CD8+} responses requires answering the following questions.

1. What cell types do the presenting?
2. Where does presentation occur?
3. When does presentation occur?
4. What form of antigen is used to generate complexes recognized by T_{CD8+}?

The answers to these questions will vary considerably, depending on the exact circumstances of the system under investigation.

One variable is the differentiation status of T_{CD8+} to be activated. Two states can be distinguished. Naive T_{CD8+} are those that have yet to be activated by antigen since their emergence from the thymus. Their initial activation is termed priming. Memory T_{CD8+} are those T_{CD8+} generated by priming that persist after the original priming event has terminated. Their reactivation upon secondary exposure to antigen is termed boosting. In this review we focus on T_{CD8+} priming, which is more important for preventive vaccines, which, by definition, must activate naive T_{CD8+}. In any event, researchers have done far more work on activation of naive T_{CD8+} than on reactivation of memory T_{CD8+}, about which very little is known.

Another critical variable is viral tropism, that is, the ability of the virus to infect various cell types, particularly professional APCs (pAPCs; see below), because this will obviously have a great impact on antigen presentation. Other important factors include:

1. route and dose of infection;
2. viral replication kinetics, particularly whether the virus establishes chronic/latent infections;
3. exact nature of the determinant studied (e.g., the folding efficiency, expression kinetics, abundance of protein in which the determinant resides, and even the properties of the peptide itself with regard to its generation by cellular proteases and stability); and
4. the effects of VIPRs (viral proteins interfering with antigen presentation) (5).

Even within a given virus-host system, there will be multiple answers to each of these questions. The trick, generalizable to all of biology, is to determine the relative overall importance of the various mechanisms in play. This requires detailed analysis of multiple systems. Even then, it is essential to recognize that any new system may not conform to the consensus mechanisms generally employed. Although scientists are trained to simplify, the glory of biology truly resides in its rich complexity.

Some Antigen Processing Essentials

Before leaping into the jaws of the four Ws, we provide some basic information on antigen processing. Class I molecules can be loaded with peptide ligands in three locations: the endoplasmic reticulum (ER), the endosomal/lysosomal compartment, or the cell surface. Cell surface loading is limited to preprocessed peptides, and its physiological relevance is probably extremely limited. Endosomal/lysosomal processing is relevant for exogenous protein antigens that can be processed into class I binding peptides by the proteases present in this compartment. This pathway is probably restricted largely to pAPCs, that is, to cells of bone marrow (BM) origin whose routine job descriptions include activating T_{CD8+} (and T_{CD4+}). pAPCs consist of dendritic cells (DCs), macrophages (Mϕs), and B cells. The heightened ability of B cells in antigen presentation depends on their highly efficient internalization of antigens that associate with surface Ig. In most circumstances, it is unlikely that sufficient numbers of naive B cells specific for a given virus are present to play a role in primary immune responses, although B cells could play a role in secondary responses. Moreover, B cells probably don their pAPC hats most frequently for activating T_{CD4+}. Similarly, Fc-receptor-mediated internalization and processing of antigens by pAPCs is probably relevant only for secondary responses to viruses or responses in chronic virus infections, because levels of virus-specific antibodies are too low when the priming of naive T_{CD8+} occurs.

Most class I molecules acquire their peptide ligands in the ER, and most of these peptides are generated from cytosolic substrates. Proteins can reach the cytosol either by being synthesized by ribosomes or by penetrating the plasma membrane or internal membranes after being internalized. Endogenous peptides appear to derive primarily from defective forms of nascent proteins (termed DRiPs, for defective ribosomal products) that are rapidly degraded by proteasomes. Exogenous proteins that reach the cytosol are also initially degraded into fragments, principally by proteasomes. Additional cytosolic proteases can further cut and trim proteasome-generated peptides. Peptides normally enter the ER courtesy of TAP (transporter associated with antigen processing), but they can also gain entry via the translocon, particularly if the peptide is part of a minigene product with an appended ER-targeting sequence. TAP-independent transport of non-ER-targeted peptides occurs via an undefined route, but at a much lower efficiency. The ER has limited endoproteolytic activity and virtually no capacity for COOH-terminal trimming. It does, however, have aminopeptidases that are regulated in parallel with antigen processing components.

To understand in vivo processing of viral antigens by pAPCs, the first and most important distinction is whether antigens are processed via the endosomal or via the classical cytosolic pathway. These can be distinguished by using chemical or genetic inhibitors that are specific (more or less) for the two processes. The most precise information comes from the use of proteasome inhibitors, particularly if two chemically distinct, highly specific inhibitors (e.g., lactacystin and epoxomicin) yield concordant results. Proteasome inhibitors have proven to be of great use in vitro. Although they could potentially be used for in vivo antigen presentation studies (a proteasome inhibitor is now used clinically to treat certain cancers), this has not been reported and would be complicated by their effects on non-pAPCs, including T cells.

Distinguishing presentation pathways in vivo has therefore largely fallen to genetic manipulation in the form of $TAP^{0/0}$ mice, mice with a targeted disruption of the TAP1 gene, one of the two essential subunits of TAP. The absence of functional TAP profoundly decreases the efficiency of the cytosolic processing pathway (though not completely), but it also affects the endosomal pathway and cell surface loading by *reducing* the number of peptide-receptive class I molecules available for binding extracellular or endosomally generated peptides (6, 7). Consequently, the effects of TAP knockout must be interpreted cautiously, particularly when using semiquantitative readouts based on T cell activation where partial effects on presentation can appear to be complete if limiting numbers of complexes are generated by APCs.

WHICH CELLS PRESENT ANTIGEN? WHERE AND WHEN DOES THIS OCCUR?

A glimpse at any immunology textbook will inform the reader that naive T_{CD8+} are exclusively activated by DCs. This statement is largely based on evidence using isolated DCs to activate T_{CD8+} in vitro, where DCs are extremely potent stimulators of T_{CD8+} activation relative to other cells, particularly amateur APCs (aAPCs). Even if we accept the validity of in vitro activation assays, which aAPCs are used as straw cells? Typically they will be established cell lines that bear only a vague relationship to the tissues of their origin, and they may have unusual properties that interfere with APC activity. The statement is also based on an assumed requirement for help/costimulation provided by T_{CD4+}/pAPCs, also inferred from in vitro systems or highly contrived in vivo situations. Yet T_{CD8+} responses to many viruses demonstrate a robust component that is independent of T_{CD4+}-mediated help or costimulation (8). Further, there is solid evidence for priming of T_{CD8+} responses by aAPCs in the form of syngeneic tumor cells expressing viral proteins, whose ability to activate T_{CD8+} in vivo is TAP-dependent (9). Such priming correlates with the ability of tumor cells to enter lymph nodes (10), suggesting a direct interaction between tumor cells and T_{CD8+} (although in neither of the studies was the possible exchange of preformed peptide-class I complexes to pAPCs completely ruled out).

Rather than blithely assume that antiviral T_{CD8+} priming is accomplished by DCs, researchers must rigorously test this hypothesis. Fortunately, several groups have taken up the bit. A number of approaches have been used to study priming of antiviral T_{CD8+}.

1. Manipulate the properties of pAPCs and determine the effect on priming.
2. Isolate cells from virus-infected animals and determine which are able to activate naive T_{CD8+} in vitro, or better yet, in recipient mice if it is possible to determine that activation is based on interaction with the transferred cells themselves.
3. Directly visualize the interaction of T_{CD8+} with APCs leading to T_{CD8+} activation.

Despite dogmatic textbook entries to the contrary, the extent to which DCs shoulder the burden of activating naive T_{CD8+} remains very much up in the air.

Manipulating APCs in vivo

Early studies by Staerz and colleagues (11) demonstrated that T_{CD8+} priming to IAV in mice is eradicated by carrageenan-mediated depletion of phagocytic cells and can be restored by administration of peritoneal exudate cells or a macrophage-like cell line. This pioneering study established the role of pAPCs in priming of antiviral T_{CD8+}. Similarly, mice treated with clodronate liposomes to eradicate phagocytic cells fail to mount T_{CD8+} responses to vesicular stomatitis virus (VSV), although it was not established that responses could be restored by replenishing APCs (12).

Sigal et al. (13) used BM radiation chimeric mice to identify APCs required for priming of virus-specific T_{CD8+}. Most BM-derived cells are highly sensitive to γ-irradiation [but some are resistant, e.g., skin Langerhans cells (LCs) (14)], whereas the thymic epithelial cells that mediate positive selection of T cells are radiation resistant (and of nonmarrow origin). By transplanting irradiated mice with marrow from donor mice, investigators can manipulate the APC population. A crucial issue with this approach is the degree to which the T_{CD8+} repertoire is functionally reconstituted relative to control mice, particularly in its ability to respond to pAPCs expressing the low numbers of complexes typical of physiological presentation of viral proteins. Thus, it is not sufficient to demonstrate a response in reconstituted mice using immunogens that generate superphysiological numbers of complexes (e.g., peptide saturated splenocytes or viruses expressing ER-targeted minigene). Sigal et al. (13) squarely addressed this issue by demonstrating equivalent responses in experimental and control mice to cells pulsed with limiting amounts of synthetic peptides.

Sigal et al. irradiated B6 mice and reconstituted them with BM derived from $TAP1^{0/0}$ mice. Following infection with a recombinant vaccinia virus (rVV) encoding chicken ovalbumin (OVA), such $TAP^{0/0} \rightarrow$ B6 mice fail to mount T_{CD8+} responses to VV antigens or the well-defined OVA K^b-restricted determinant corresponding to residues 257–264 ($OVA_{257-264}$). By contrast, chimeric mice responded to a rVV encoding ER-targeted $OVA_{257-264}$. B6$\rightarrow$B6 control chimeras mounted responses to all of the OVA-expressing rVVs tested. VV is able to infect most cell types, including Mϕs and DCs, and it is well established that TAP is required for presentation of VV-encoded antigens (including OVA) processed by the classical cytosolic pathway (15). This experiment therefore demonstrates that:

1. bone marrow–derived cells are required for presentation of typical VV antigens; and

2. such presentation requires TAP, implying that their presentation occurs via the classical cytosolic pathway.

Lenz et al. (16) confirmed the requirement for pAPCs in eliciting anti-VV T_{CD8+} using parent$\rightarrow$F1 mice. Following infection with an rVV expressing lymphocytic choriomeningitis virus (LCMV) nucleoprotein (NP), H-2$^b\rightarrow$H-2^{bxd} mice responded to a D^b-restricted NP determinant, but not a L^d-restricted determinant, whereas control H-2$^{dxb}\rightarrow$H-2^{dxb} mice responded to both determinants. Interestingly, H-2$^b\rightarrow$H-2^{bxd} mice responded to both determinants following LCMV infection, providing a positive control for the responsiveness of the chimeric mice to the L^d-restricted determinant (though imperfect, because more complexes may be generated on APCs in LCMV infections or more APCs may present antigen). There are two interpretations to the responsiveness of LCMV-infected H-2$^b\rightarrow$H-2^{bxd} mice to the L^d-restricted determinant: either it is presented by a non-BM-derived APC, or features of LCMV (e.g., its formidable replication in mice) enable it to selectively utilize the residual host-derived pAPCs that resist radiation ablation (estimated to be ~5% of the total number of pAPCs present).

Sigal & Rock (17) similarly used parent→F1 mice to study the requirement for BM-derived cells in priming to LCMV. They found that donor dependence of priming varied, depending on the determinant studied; D^b-restricted responses to $NP_{396-404}$ were lost in H-2^d→H-2^{bxd} mice, whereas D^b-restricted responses to GP_{33-41} were maintained in these mice. IAV priming was also examined, and once again the results varied depending on the determinants studied. H-2^d→H-2^{bxd} mice failed to respond to D^b-$NP_{366-374}$, although H-2^b→H-2^{bxd} mice were able to respond to K^d-$NP_{147-155}$. In the latter case, responses were abrogated by irradiating and reconstituting mice twice (with a 4 month interval), presumably by reducing numbers of residual host BM-derived pAPCs to ~0.25% of total pAPCs. Sigal & Rock concluded that these radiation-resistant cells were responsible for activation of $NP_{147-155}$-specific T_{CD8+} in single irradiation chimeras (and probably for the GP_{33-41} responses in H-2^d→H-2^{bxd} mice as well). It is possible, however, to explain the disparate results for individual determinants based on the degree to which the T_{CD8+} repertoire specific for the respective determinants was functionally reconstituted, that is, capable of responding to the limiting amounts of peptides presented during a virus infection. Indeed, the only result from these BM chimera experiments that can be interpreted with reasonable certainty is the failure to respond to a determinant restricted only by the recipient's haplotype. And then, only when the reconstituted T_{CD8+} repertoire demonstrates a similar dose response curve as the positive control chimera mice can we safely conclude that priming requires BM-derived APCs [although the transfer of highly purified TCR transgenic T_{CD8+} (which we term T^3_{CD8+} for the rest of this review) to reconstituted mice could ameliorate this difficulty].

Clearly, radiation chimeras have their limitations. Fortunately, there is another approach to this problem. The ablative approach pioneered by Debrick et al. (11) has been upgraded by Jung et al. (18), who ingeniously generated transgenic mice that express a diphtheria toxin receptor (DTR)–enhanced green fluorescence protein (EGFP) fusion protein under the control of the CD11c promoter. This promoter is constitutively active in nearly all conventional DC subsets (it is active in LCs only following activation; DC subsets are discussed below). Mice do not express a DTR, and consequently their cells are highly resistant to DT. Transgenic DCs express a sufficient amount of DTR-EGFP to enable their depletion by a single dose of DT. Owing to DC replenishment from precursors, depletion persists for ~2 days following treatment. Like CD11c itself, DTR-EGFP is expressed in activated T cells, a factor that potentially confounds analysis. Jung et al. neatly sidestepped this problem by transferring nontransgenic T cells prior to DT treatment and used this elegant system to demonstrate a requirement for CD11c expressing cells in T_{CD8+} responses to intracellular bacteria and parasites. The mice are now commercially available (Jax Mice, Bar Harbor, ME) and awaiting deployment in studies of viral priming and boosting of T cells.

Isolation of APCs from Virus-Infected Mice

Shortman and colleagues (19) have done yeoman's work in defining mouse DC subsets, which represent distinct lineages with unique functional profiles. DC subsets can be identified and physically separated on the basis of the differential expression of cell surface proteins. Presently there are seven defined types of mouse DC: plasmacytoid DCs (pDC) derived from blood, and six types of conventional DC, four derived from blood ($CD4^+$, $CD8^+$, $CD4^-CD8^-$, and a novel population described in 2004, discussed below), and two derived from tissues (LC, interstitial DC from dermis and tissues). All the subsets are present in lymph nodes. Only the pDC and blood-borne DCs are present in spleen, which lacks the afferent lymphatics that deliver tissue DCs to nodes. Interestingly, the $CD8^+$ DCs express the $CD8\alpha$ chain but not the $CD8\beta$ chain.

Exploring the differential roles of DC subsets in priming T_{CD8+} in virus infections has been the nearly exclusive domain of Carbone, Heath, and colleagues (20) in an elegant and comprehensive series of studies. Smith et al. (21) infected B6 mice via footpads (f.p.) with herpes simplex virus (HSV), dissociated the draining lymph nodes (DLN), and examined the abilities of isolated DLN suspensions to activate T_{CD8+} specific for the immunodominant determinant, $gB_{498-505}$. Depletion of DCs from DLN suspensions by anti-CD11c magnetic beads completely abrogated stimulation of a T_{CD8+} hybridoma, whereas depletion using antibodies specific for Mϕ, B, or T cells had no effect. $CD11c^+$ cells were then subsetted by FACS and tested for their ability to activate naive T_{CD8+} derived from a $gB_{498-505}$-specific TCR transgenic mouse. Such activity remained the exclusive province of $CD8\alpha^+$ DC in DLN harvested from 6 to 72 h post-infection (p.i.), when APC activity waned. APC activity was robust even at 6 h p.i. and peaked 6 h later. All the DC subsets contained HSV DNA, although it was not established whether DCs were infected or were simply harboring virions or subviral material.

Extending this approach to other viruses, Belz et al. (22) showed that 12, 24, or 48 h following f.p. infection with IAV or VV, $CD8\alpha^+$ DCs alone, of the 6 DLN DC populations tested, were able to activate naive T^3_{CD8+} in vitro. Similarly, following intravenous (i.v.) infection with HSV, IAV, or VV, only the $CD8\alpha^+$ population among the 4 splenic DC populations could activate naive T^3_{CD8+} in vitro. By contrast, each of the DC subsets activated T^3_{CD8+} if they were either exposed to the appropriate synthetic peptide or, most importantly, infected with each virus.

Although LCs are commonly assumed to be the principal pAPCs for pathogens entering via skin, Allan et al. (23) found that 2 days following infection with HSV via scarification, in vitro APC activity for naive T^3_{CD8+} resided exclusively with $CD8\alpha^+$ DCs among DC subsets obtained from DLNs. Histological staining for HSV antigens demonstrated that HSV gene expression was limited to the epidermis and hair follicles; infected cells were not detected in the dermis. The radiation resistance of LCs (14) made it possible to independently confirm the lack of LC involvement in HSV priming. Irradiated B6 mice were reconstituted with BM from bm1 mice (these mice possess a mutated K^b gene unable to activate $gB_{498-505}$-specific T_{CD8+}). Despite the fact that LCs remained of host origin, bm1→B6 mice (unlike B6→B6 mice) were unable to mount a primary $gB_{498-505}$ response to HSV skin infection as assessed by cytotoxicity, tetramer staining, or IFN-γ expression. Control experiments established that the bm1→B6 mice could respond to subcutaneous (s.c.) immunization with $gB_{498-505}$ synthetic peptide–sensitized DCs, but cells were pulsed with a saturating dose of peptide, leaving the possibility (as discussed above) that the chimera's T_{CD8+} were insufficiently sensitive to recognize cells presenting physiological amounts of K^b-$gB_{498-505}$ complexes.

What about other tissues? Belz et al. (24) measured the APC activities of mediastinal lymph node (MLN) populations following lung infections with IAV or HSV. In contrast to s.c. infections, APC activity was extremely low 1 day p.i., robust on day 2, peaking on day 3, and declined propitiously only after day 6. Lawrence & Braciale (25) observed a similar loss of APCs activity from MLNs between 5 and 8 days after respiratory IAV infection. Belz et al. (24) found that naive T^3_{CD8+} could be activated in vitro by $CD8\alpha^+$ DCs and a novel subset of MLN DC ($CD205^+$, $CD8^-$, $CD11b^-$) that is absent from skin draining and mesenteric LN, but present in renal and hepatic LNs. To determine the tissue origins of the DC subsets, mice were instilled with the cell staining dye CFSE (26) 6 h prior to infection with IAV. Legge & Braciale (27) had previously used this method to demonstrate that DCs in the respiratory tract demonstrated accelerated migration to MLN during the first 24 h of IAV infection, followed by decreased emigration relative to baseline. Belz et al. used this method to show that <3% of $CD8\alpha^+$ and ~50% of the $CD205^+$, $CD8^-$, $CD11b^-$ DCs in LN were stained by CFSE. Although CFSE-negative $CD8\alpha^+$ DCs could activate naive T_{CD8+} in vitro, among the $CD8\alpha^-$ DCs, only CFSE-positive cells exhibited APC activity. These findings point to $CD8\alpha^+$ DCs acquiring their antigens from either viral material that reaches the MLN or, most intriguingly, from cells that traffic to the MLN. To test the latter possibility, $TAP^{-/-}$ mice were infected with IAV and their $CD8^-$, $CD11b^-$ DCs were isolated and examined for their APC activity in vitro. $CD8^-$, $CD11b^-$ DCs alone were unable to activate naive T_{CD8+} (expected from lack of TAP activity), but activation occurred when the cells were mixed with $CD8\alpha^+$ DCs from wild-type uninfected mice, presumably caused by exchange of viral antigens and not infectious virus itself (this was not rigorously excluded, nor were the representation capacities of other DC subsets examined). On the basis of these findings, Belz et al. suggested that $CD8\alpha^+$ DCs that reside in MLN receive antigens from $CD8^-$, $CD11b^-$ DCs that emigrate from the lung and, more generally, that LN-resident $CD8\alpha^+$ DCs may regularly function to represent antigens derived from trafficking DC subsets, such as LC.

This remarkable inference represents a significant alteration in the paradigm for DC function in antigen presentation. Migrating tissue DCs could transfer antigen to multiple DLN DCs; this would provide a mechanism for amplifying T_{CD8+} responses. It will be important in future studies to determine exactly what is transferred between migratory $CD8^-$, $CD11b^-$ and resident $CD8\alpha^+$ DCs. The fact that

CD8α^+ DCs have been implicated as the principal APC in cross-priming suggests that information is transferred to CD8α^+ DCs in the form of proteins. These could have been synthesized by respiratory epithelial cells or the CD8$^-$, CD11b$^-$ DCs themselves. Alternatively, the possible transfer of infectious virus or viral genes that are translated by accepting cells needs to be carefully excluded.

Whatever the exact mechanism of information transfer, these findings are potentially important to vaccine development because they suggest that the critical target for effective T$_{CD8+}$ activation by virus-based vectors is the CD8α^+ DC population. Before banging the drum too loudly, however, we note that the available evidence is based on the APC capacities of cells in DLN suspensions, and confirmation by other methods, including in situ studies (discussed in the next section), is necessary.

Visualizing APC-T$_{CD8+}$ Interactions in Lymphoid Organs

In principle, the most direct method for determining the identity of APCs that activate T$_{CD8+}$ is to visualize interactions that lead to T$_{CD8+}$ activation. Using multiphoton confocal microscopy, researchers can now visualize these events in the lymphoid organs of living animals (termed intravital microscopy) (28, 29). Truly, cellular immunology has come full circle to its origins in Metchnikoff's eyeballing of macrophages in *flagrante delicto*. No doubt, there will be many studies to review five years hence, as intravital microscopy becomes a standard (if costly) technology in immunological research. At present, however, visualization of T$_{CD8+}$ with pAPCs in vivo is limited to a single study based exclusively on extravital microscopy.

Norbury et al. (30) used a rVV expressing IAV NP genetically conjoined to EGFP to visualize interaction with T$^3_{CD8+}$ in fixed frozen sections of the DLN of mice infected via the f.p. route. Because EGFP was targeted to the nucleus by NP, it was possible to distinguish infected cells (strong nuclear staining) from cells that acquired NP-EGFP from other cells (expected to be mostly endosomal, although such cells were not visualized). At the peak of infection (6 h), nodes contained approximately 3000 infected cells (quantitated by flow cytometry of dissociated DLN), declining fivefold 18 h later to <100 cells. On the basis of in situ staining with cell type specific mAbs, 60%–90% of infected cells were macrophages, whereas 10%–15% of infected cells were DCs. B and T cells were not detectably infected. A similar pattern was observed in spleen after i.v. infection. Many of the infected Mϕs were present in the subcapsular region and were probably infected by the bolus of virus transported via lymphatics into the LN. All the infected DCs and an equal number of Mϕs were present in cortical areas of the node, however. Because virus is probably excluded from the node interior on the basis of its size (31), these cells were likely infected either (*a*) in the subcapsular space (particularly Mϕs, which reside there in large numbers), (*b*) extranodally (particularly DCs, which are not numerous in the subcapsule), or (*c*) by virus carried in by migrating cells.

To determine which cells could activate naive T_{CD8+}, T^3_{CD8+} specific for NP-EGFP determinants were labeled ex vivo with a cell tracking dye and given i.v. to mice a day prior to rVV infection. Accumulation of T^3_{CD8+} in DLNs occurred independently of cognate antigen. By contrast, clustering of T^3_{CD8+} was antigen-dependent and did not occur following infection with a rVV expressing the same protein but with two amino acid substitutions that abrogated recognition. Approximately 80 clusters were observed per node, and ~80% of clusters occurred around infected cells. Although most infected cells in the nodes were macrophages, all the clusters formed around DCs. Norbury et al. (30) noted that NP-EGFP-negative DCs that supported cluster formation might be uninfected cells cross-presenting NP-EGFP or might have been infected but producing insufficient amounts of NP-EGFP for detection. By 24 h after infection, clusters were no longer detected, and T_{CD8+} were predominantly located in the medulla of DLNs. Similar findings were made in the spleen when mice were infected i.v.

These findings are consistent with the idea that T_{CD8+} were activated primarily by rVV-infected DCs in DLN and spleen following f.p. and i.v. infections, respectively. In support of the involvement of infected DCs in priming, Norbury et al. (30) infected splenocytes with rVVs expressing minigene products and demonstrated that these cells could activate transferred T^3_{CD8+} in $TAP^{-/-}$ mice, which were used to eliminate direct-priming via transferred virus, since these rVVs were non-immunogenic in these mice. Because, as described below, minigene-expressing cells are inactive in cross-priming (32), T_{CD8+} activation in this experiment is almost certainly due to direct-priming. Most of the immunogenicity of infected splenocytes was lost by depleting DCs.

Taken together, these findings strongly implicate infected DCs as the major source of priming in this system. Still, cluster formation cannot be equated with T_{CD8+} activation, which remains to be directly demonstrated by in situ intravital imaging. Intravital imagining should also shed light on the important issues of the duration of T_{CD8+} contact with DCs and whether T_{CD8+} are directed to DCs by some mechanism or randomly visit Mϕs and DCs and preferentially adhere to the latter.

Timing of T_{CD8+} Activation

Priming in the system used by Norbury et al. (32) appears to occur within the first 24 h p.i., on the basis of the kinetics of cluster formation and dissociation and the capacity of lymph node cells to activate T^3_{CD8+} in vitro, which was maximal at the earliest point examined (6 h) and declined by 48 h p.i. in parallel with the loss of infected cells. This differs from findings from IAV and HSV pulmonary infections, where functional APCs were detected in MLNs for up to 6 days p.i. (25, 26). In IAV infections, Legge & Braciale (27) showed that migration of DCs to MLNs occurs within 24 h p.i. and ceases afterwards. This suggests either that IAV-infected cells persist in MLNs for 5 days (this is unlikely to be due to ongoing IAV replication because IAV replicates efficiently only respiratory epithelia), or that priming is based on the persistence of cross-presented antigen. In the latter case, this would mean that class I peptide complexes are extremely long-lived on the relevant APCs or that complexes are continuously generated from viral antigens carried from the lung, which would be consistent with the findings of Belz et al. (24).

Using adoptively transferred CFSE labeled T^3_{CD8+}, Lawrence & Braciale (25) reported that T_{CD8+} division is first detected between day 3 and day 4 following IAV infection. Proliferating T_{CD8+} only appeared in the lung one day after proliferation began in the node, providing evidence that T_{CD8+} activation does not occur in the lung; these results are consistent with previous findings (33). The gap between the appearance of functionally active APCs in the node and T_{CD8+} proliferation, however, is puzzling. T^3_{CD8+} activation is detected within a few hours after s.c. infection with HSV (34), and T^3_{CD8+} proliferation is detected within a day (35). Moreover, Mempel et al. (36) visualized the interaction of adoptively transferred T^3_{CD8+} and peptide pulsed DCs in DLNs via vital microscopy and detected T_{CD8+} division within 24 h of cell transfer.

Clearly, much remains to be learned regarding the timing of T_{CD8+} activation in viral infections. It is particularly important to understand the effects of route of infection, viral tropism, and other specific viral infection features on the kinetics of activating APCs in DLNs and spleen. Further, although T^3_{CD8+} offer great experimental advantages, these results will eventually have to be squared with the properties of bona fide naive T_{CD8+}. In addition to potential intrinsic development differences between normal and transgenic T_{CD8+}, the latter are used at much higher precursor frequencies and only following adoptive transfer.

WHAT FORM OF ANTIGEN IS PRESENTED BY PAPCs TO T_{CD8+}?

Cross-Priming Versus Direct-Priming

pAPCs can present viral antigens to naive T_{CD8+} by two defined routes. Direct-priming refers to activation of naive T_{CD8+} by infected pAPCs that present peptides derived from viral gene products synthesized by their own ribosomes. The outcome of pAPC infection can range from:

1. complete virus replication cycle with the release of infectious progeny and cell death; to

2. abortive infection, in which only a limited number of viral gene products are synthesized and cells maintain viability; to

3. everything in between these extremes.

Cross-priming refers to T_{CD8+} activation by APCs presenting determinants generated from viral proteins synthesized by other cells. Because incoming virion proteins themselves can be a source of immunogenic peptides (37, 38), there is some ambiguity in defining routes of presentation when viruses are known to infect pAPCs. Indeed, though less intuitive than direct-priming, the principle of cross-priming is actually much easier to demonstrate unambiguously in experimental systems, either by immunizing animals with xenogeneic, allogeneic, or class I null cells expressing antigens from cellular genes [as in its original description (39)] or by simply injecting animals with completely noninfectious antigens (as originally described with inactivated viruses and purified proteins, and since repeated in many guises (reviewed in 40). Additionally, there is a third route (that we dub cross-dressing) in which preformed class I peptide complexes are transferred from aAPCs to pAPC (or between pAPCs). T_{CD8+} are known to obtain class I molecules from APCs via synapse formation (41), but acquisition of preformed complexes by pAPCs has not been in vivo (or even in vitro), so it remains a theory. It would, however, represent an economical means for amplifying an antigenic stimulus, as previously suggested (42).

Despite conflicting evidence from his own laboratory (43, 44), Zinkernagel has stridently argued that cross-priming is a feeble process of dubious physiological significance (45). Several studies directly refute his arguments by demonstrating that immunization of cells expressing defined antigens results in local and systemic responses easily measured ex vivo against immunodominant determinants defined by infection with viruses expressing the same antigens (ex vivo refers to measuring numbers of antigen-specific T_{CD8+} by activating immediately upon their recovery from mice, i.e., in the absence of in vitro expansion) (32, 46, 47).

Probably the most important factor in deciding the balance of cross-priming versus direct-priming in antiviral responses is the nature of the virus itself. By definition, viruses that are unable to direct expression of their genes in APCs capable of activating T_{CD8+} will be presented exclusively by cross-priming. Other important virus-specific factors include VIPR-expression, effects of infection on pAPCs, and the spectrum of cytokines induced by viral infection from infected cells and sentinel cells in the tissue (such as pDCs).

Cross-Priming Versus Direct-Priming: Virus-by-Virus

To emphasize the anticipated virus-specific differences, we have divided this section according to the virus studied.

POLIO VIRUS   Demonstrating the contribution of cross-priming in viral infections requires nimble experimental strategies to enable differentiation from direct-priming. The nimblest of all was devised by Sigal et al. (13), who used transgenic mice that express the human receptor for poliovirus (PVR). Lacking cellular receptors for poliovirus, B6 mice resist PV infection and, unlike PVR mice, fail to mount T_{CD8+} responses to PV-encoded proteins. Sigal et al. exploited this difference by generating BM chimeras in which pAPCs were of B6 origin and hence incapable of direct-priming. Although B6→PVR chimeras respond to PV-encoded antigens (including an OVA fragment inserted into the PV genome and not incorporated into virions), $TAP^{0/0}$→PVR chimeras do not, demonstrating that presentation in

B6→PVR mice is not caused by residual pAPCs resisting irradiative ablation. As described above, control experiments carefully established that these differences were extremely unlikely to be due to differences in T_{CD8+} sensitivity in the various chimeras. Thus, these experiments strongly implicated cross-priming in the generation of PV-specific T_{CD8+}.

Freigang et al. (48) recently challenged the validity of this conclusion, reporting that wild-type B6 mice are capable of responding to wild-type and recombinant PV stocks from the same source as those used by Sigal et al. Priming in B6 mice required a higher viral dose than in PVR transgenics (derived from the same breeding colony used by Sigal et al.) but could not be obtained with UV-inactivated virus. Combined with the response to OVA following immunization with recombinant PV, this demonstrated that priming could not be attributed to presentation of exogenous virion proteins. Freigang et al. argue compellingly that interpretation of the critical B6→PVR chimera experiments in Sigal et al. were clouded by the possibility that poliovirus replication in PVR mice amplified the virus dose, resulting in the infection of B6 pAPCs and therefore leading to direct-priming. In support of this contention, Freigang et al. demonstrated the presence of PV RNA in splenic DCs following infection of B6 mice (though the translation of these genes was not demonstrated in any manner) and showed that BM-derived DC cultures transfected with PV RNA could generate infectious PV (although only very small amounts).

The B6 mice used by Sigal et al. and Freigang et al. derive from different colonies, and the disparate results may be due to differences in the PV-responsiveness of the ostensibly identical mice. This does not settle the matter definitively in favor or Sigal et al., however, because Freigang et al. demonstrate the possibility that in PVR → B6 chimeras, infectious PV is transferred to pAPCs following amplification by PVR-expressing cells.

ADENOVIRUS   Prasad et al. (49) used recombinant adenoviruses (rAds) expressing IAV NP under the control of tissue-specific promoters to determine the requirement for pAPC antigen expression in priming NP-specific T_{CD8+}. The rAds used are missing a region of their genome essential for replication, and replication can only occur if gene products from this region are provided by complementing virus or transfected cells. Using rAd-NP with a universal promoter, T_{CD8+} were elicited by i.n. (intranasal), s.c., or i.v. immunization. By contrast, priming with rAd-NP with the surfactant promoter was observed following i.n. infection but not s.c. or i.v. infection. This indicates that priming requires expression of NP in cells uniquely accessed via the respiratory route, presumably the bronchiolar and alveolar cells where the promoter is active. The lack of immunogenicity via other routes provides solid evidence that NP is not expressed in pAPCs in levels sufficient to enable direct-priming. Thus, these findings strongly suggest that T_{CD8+} are activated either by infected lung cells or via cross-priming. Although the latter answer is more credible, this must be established experimentally by manipulating and characterizing pAPC populations as described in other studies and by visualizing the interactions of pAPCs with T_{CD8+} in the MLN.

VACCINIA VIRUS   rVV was the first recombinant vector used to elicit T_{CD8+} responses to inserted genes and has been the principal vector used for probing antigen processing and presentation in vitro and in vivo over the past two decades (50). Early work with VV demonstrated that the immunogenicity of inserted genes was increased if their expression was controlled by an early/late virus promoter (i.e., expressed before and after the initiation of VV DNA replication) versus a late promoter (51). This could not be explained by the quantity of antigen synthesized by infected cells because higher quantities of late antigens were present in infected mouse tissue. A possible explanation came from the finding that in cultivated mouse DCs, VV induced an abortive infection in which late genes were poorly expressed (52). Thus, if inserted gene products (which are excluded from VV virions) are generally presented via direct-priming by DCs, their poor immunogenicity when controlled by late promoters would be explained if DCs behaved similarly in vivo.

Several studies support the idea that direct-priming contributes to activation of T_{CD8+} specific for inserted rVV gene products. First, as discussed above, T^3_{CD8+} specific for inserted genes have been directly visualized interacting with infected DCs (30). Second, minigene products are highly immunogenic in VV, and as discussed below, recent evidence suggests that minigene products are extremely weak immunogens in cross-priming (32). Third, using a panel of rVVs expressing cytosolic and ER-targeted versions of minigenes, Norbury et al. (53) showed a close correlation between TAP dependence of antigenicity in vitro and immunogenicity in $TAP^{-/-}$ mice. Similarly, there was a close correlation between in vitro and in vivo TAP-dependence in the antigenicity and immunogenicity of rVVs encoding various forms of cytosolic and ER-targeted IAV NP that strongly points to direct-priming.

Norbury et al.'s study, however, noted an exception. Although in vitro presentation of rVV-expressed chicken OVA was TAP-dependent, VV-OVA infection activated T^3_{CD8+} adoptively transferred into $TAP^{-/-}$ mice. K^{bm1} splenocytes infected with VV-OVA or a rVV expressing $OVA_{257-264}$ as a cytosolic minigene product were able to activate T^3_{CD8+} in $TAP^{-/-}$ mice. Norbury et al. concluded that cross-priming of both OVA and cytosolic minigenes occurred under these conditions. This conclusion is probably valid for OVA, but later findings indicated that minigene priming could be due to expression of the minigene product in host APCs from partially UV-inactivated virus adhering to infected K^{bm1} splenocytes (C. Norbury, personal communication).

The relative contribution of direct- and cross-priming in VV infections was further examined using rVVs that express the US2 and US11 VIPRs from human cytomegalovirus (hCMV). This strategy is based on the assumption that the effect of US2 or US11 would be limited to infected cells and therefore would selectively inhibit direct-priming. Although reasonable, this assumption has not been tested, and there is clear in vitro evidence that US6, another CMV VIPR, is capable of inhibiting cross-presentation (54), although unlike US2 or US11, US6 is a soluble protein.

Basta et al. (55) used rVVs expressing US2 or US11, both able to induce the degradation of newly synthesized K^b or D^b molecules. Following intraperitoneal (i.p.) infection of B6 mice, these viruses elicited $\sim$50% of the VV-specific T_{CD8+} elicited by control rVVs. This could not be attributed to differences in viral infectivity in mice. Resolution of antigenic peptides from VV-infected cells via high performance liquid chromatography revealed that US2 selectively inhibits T_{CD8+} specific for a subset of VV peptides. T_{CD8+} responses to a similar subset of viral peptides were also reduced following immunization with VV-infected HeLa cells. Basta et al. suggested that US2 selectively interferes with peptides that were exclusively presented by direct-priming and therefore that VV antigens are presented by both cross-priming and direct-priming.

Shen et al. (56) generated their own rVV expressing US11 and found that it was far less immunogenic than control VV when given by the i.v. and particularly the i.p. routes. The effect was observed for VV antigens as well as β-galactosidase expressed by a late promoter. The latter suggests that VV late gene products can be presented by direct-priming; this may explain the residual immunogenicity of late gene products. Importantly, US2 expression had only a moderate effect on immunogenicity following intramuscular infection and no significant effects following s.c. or intradermal infection, testing either total VV-specific responses or β-galactosidase-specific T_{CD8+}. Shen et al. (56) concluded that these effects were most likely explained by route-dependent differences in the contribution of cross-priming and direct-priming to T_{CD8+} activation, but they noted that other mechanisms were possible, for example, differences in levels of cytokines induced by VV infection that could override the inhibitory effects of US11 on direct presentation.

Taken together, these findings provide moderately strong but still-inconclusive evidence that VV gene products are presented by both direct-priming and cross-priming. Although US2 had the least effect on priming via s.c. infection, Norbury et al. (30) used f.p. infection to visualize the interaction of T^3_{CD8+} with infected DCs in draining nodes. Future studies examining reasons for this discrepancy should be of interest.

IAV   Shen et al. (57) used BM chimeras generated using donor marrow derived from mice with defects in the classical cytosolic pathway ($TAP^{-/-}$) or exogenous pathway [Cathepsin S $(CatS)^{-/-}$] to examine the relative contributions of direct- and cross-priming following i.p. infection with IAV. In the same study, they provided clear evidence that CatS plays an essential role in endosomal processing of exogenous OVA delivered via phagocytosis. T_{CD8+} activation was measured in reconstituted mice by an in vivo cytotoxicity assay using target cells pulsed with either $NP_{366-374}$ or $PA_{224-232}$ peptides. Reconstitution with $CatS^{-/-}$ BM resulted in a slight reduction to $NP_{366-374}$ responses and a 50% reduction in anti-$PA_{224-232}$ activity relative to reconstitution with B6 BM. Reconstitution with $TAP^{-/-}$ BM resulted in a 75% reduction in activity to either determinant. Importantly, reconstitution with BM from $TAP^{-/-}$ $CatS^{-/-}$ mice resulted in complete inhibition in

T_{CD8+} activation to either, demonstrating that both processes contribute to priming of T_{CD8+} specific for these determinants (although with the now-familiar caveat that this conclusion is subject to potential limitations regarding the integrity of the T_{CD8+} repertoire discussed above). Because TAP is important for both direct-priming and cross-priming, the TAP dependence of priming cannot be used to distinguish these pathways. On the other hand, CatS dependence clearly implicates endosomal-dependent cross-priming as contributing to the generation of these T_{CD8+}.

MOUSE CMV   Mice have a CMV of their very own that encodes at least three VIPRs that interfere with mouse class I molecules. VIPR-deleted mCMVs have been genetically engineered and are now used to study the biological roles of VIPRs in their natural setting, including their effects on T_{CD8+} responses. Gold et al. (58) found that the m152 VIPR reduced presentation of the D^b-restricted M45$_{985-993}$ determinant to below detection limits in fibroblasts and a DC line. Despite this, deletion of m152 from CMV had no significant impact on M45$_{985-993}$ immunogenicity following virus infection. The effectiveness of the CMV VIPRs have been described to vary greatly between cell types, allomorphs, and even determinants (59, 60), but there is no evidence to suggest variability in effect of m152 on M45$_{985-993}$ presentation. Thus, in accordance with Occam's razor, it is most likely that the immunogenicity of M45$_{985-993}$ is based on cross-priming.

EBV   Epstein-Barr virus (EBV) is a herpesvirus that infects most humans, where it persists in a latent state in B cells. Maintenance of the latent state entails expression of an essential viral gene product, EBNA1. For the past decade, dogma dictated that EBNA1 avoided T_{CD8+} detection by preventing its own degradation by proteasomes (61). This story began to unravel, however, when it was found that most individuals mount a vigorous EBNA1-specific response and that EBNA1 could indeed be presented to T_{CD8+} in vitro via cross-presentation (62), making EBNA1 the poster-child for cross-priming in humans.

Alas, a new poster-child will be required as a flood of reports in the past year clearly demonstrate that multiple cells types can process and present EBNA1 determinants via the endogenous pathway (63–67). Indeed, it appears that EBNA1 avoids recognition in latently infected cells by limiting its own synthesis in a tricky and unprecedented manner (64). The EBNA1 saga provides a cautionary tale on the perils of jumping to conclusions.

A Better Mousetrap?

The findings from the various virus systems described suggest that both priming pathways contribute to antiviral T_{CD8+} responses. Although compelling, each line of evidence is limited in some nontrivial way, and resolution of the relative contributions clearly require additional experimental approaches that selectively ablate one of the pathways.

Lizée et al. (68) provide just such an approach. They generated transgenic C3H (H-2^k) mice that express wild-type K^b molecules or K^b molecules in which the Tyr residue in the exon 6 cytoplasmic domain is mutated to Phe. This Tyr is quite impressively conserved in class I molecules in vertebrates from shark to human. Using BM DCs cultured from the transgenic mice, Lizée et al. found that the Tyr→Phe substitution interferes with K^b internalization to endosomal compartments, and it interferes with the ability of cells to generate K^b-$OVA_{257-264}$ complexes from exogenous OVA. The substitution does not, however, affect the ability of cells to generate K^b-$OVA_{257-264}$ from endogenous full length or minigene products. Antigen presentation was carefully quantitated using the 25-D1.16 mAb specific for K^b-$OVA_{257-264}$ complexes (69). Most importantly, mice with mutated K^b demonstrated $\sim$ tenfold decreased T_{CD8+} responses to defined determinants following infection with either VSV or SV (Sendai virus). These findings are consistent with the idea that cross-priming plays a critical role in infections with these viruses.

Mice with mutated K^b could well be a key tool in dissecting antigen processing pathways in vivo, but it is important to note that the bête noire of BM chimera experiments also applies here: It was not established that T_{CD8+} repertoire of mice with mutated K^b are fully capable of responding to the determinants tested. It will be important to test these mice with antigens exclusively presented by direct-priming (e.g., minigene-expressing rVVs, see below) and also to use the mice in experiments using adoptively transferred T_{CD8+} to minimize uncertainties regarding T_{CD8+} responsiveness.

Influence of Cytokines on Priming Pathways

One of the most important features of the innate immune response to viruses is the release of cytokines. Type I IFNs (i.e. IFN-α/β) are of paramount importance, as their synthesis and secretion is induced by infections with nearly all types of viruses, and type I IFNs are secreted in enormous quantities by individual pDCs. Although type I IFN and other cytokines likely affect the magnitude and quality of T_{CD8+} responses significantly, little is known how cytokines modify presentation of viral antigens to T_{CD8+}. A pioneering study by Le Bon et al. (70) provides a glimpse at the possibilities, however. They found that infection with VV or LCMV greatly enhanced cross-presentation of soluble OVA injected 12 h p.i. as determined by activation of OVA-specific T_{CD8+}. Three findings linked this effect to type I interferons. First, the magnitude of the OVA-specific response was proportional to serum levels of IFN-α. Second, LCMV-induced cross-priming to OVA was not observed in type I IFN receptor$^{-/-}$ mice. Third, cross-priming was observed if IFN-α was administered to mice in the absence of virus infection. Additional evidence suggested that IFN acted by modifying DCs.

These intriguing findings suggest that type I IFNs and possibly other cytokines play an important role in controlling cross-priming in viral infections. It will be critical in future studies to determine the extent to which cross-presentation per se is enhanced by cytokines versus their induction of costimulatory molecules on cross-presenting pAPCs. In either event, these findings raise the important issue of cytokine-enhanced cross-presentation of self-antigens and how the immune system manages to avoid activation of self-specific T_{CD8+} (unless, of course, such self-specific T_{CD8+} *are* transiently induced during the course of viral infections).

How Is Information Transferred in Cross-Priming?

Immunization with molecular chaperone preparations derived from antigen-expressing cells primes T_{CD8+} responses in an antigen-specific manner (71). Several biotech startups and a small academic industry have been built around the chaperoned-peptide model of cross-priming. In this model, pAPCs acquire the peptide-based information needed to activate T_{CD8+} in the form of molecular chaperones bearing proteasome-generated peptides. Despite the unbridled optimism of venture capitalists and funding agencies, the participation of molecular chaperones in cross-priming remains uncertain. An important test of the chaperoned-peptide model is that the cross-priming capacity of cells should be related to their abilities to generate chaperone-binding peptides. Three recent studies fail to confirm this prediction, and instead point to the opposite conclusion.

Shen & Rock (72) engineered stable transfectants expressing various stable and rapidly degraded forms of OVA from transfected genes. Although the constructs generated similar amounts of K^b-$OVA_{257-264}$ complexes measured via 25-D1.16 staining of transfectants, their cross-priming capacity was related to the steady state levels of OVA. Physically disrupted cells were fractionated into soluble and insoluble fractions. Using cells expressing OVA, priming activity was limited to the soluble fraction, whereas priming activity was present in both fractions derived from cells expressing membrane-bound OVA and strongest in the membrane fraction. Importantly, the cross-priming capacity of the soluble fraction from membrane-bound OVA-expressing cells was dependent on the presence of antibody reactive forms of OVA as determined by depletion with OVA-specific polyclonal or monoclonal antibodies. Antibody depletion did not remove Hsp70, Hsp90, or gp96, the principal molecular chaperones implicated in cross-priming. Because the OVA-specific monoclonal antibodies used do not recognize fully denatured OVA, these findings indicate that the cross-priming capacity of the soluble fraction is based on transfer of antigen that maintains at least some element of native structure and not on unfolded peptide fragments free or bound to molecular chaperones.

Further evidence of the importance of proteins in cross-priming comes from Wolkers et al. (73). They generated transfected cells expressing chimeric GFP constructs consisting of determinant "A" in an NH_2-terminal ER-insertion sequence and determinant "B" at the COOH-terminus of the fusion protein and vice versa. Cells generated comparable levels of peptide-class I complexes regardless of the location of the peptide in the protein, as carefully quantitated by assaying acid-stripped peptides for activation of their cognate T_{CD8+}. Despite this, peptide location in the signal sequence was associated with greatly decreased cross-priming capacity, as determined by immunizing mice with cells unable to present the peptides owing to lack of TAP or the relevant presenting class I molecules. Rendering the signal sequence nonfunctional by removal of its hydrophobic core greatly increased the cross-priming capacity of the embedded determinant. This location-based differential immunogenicity was observed in mice unable to mount antibody responses, demonstrating that it could not be attributed to antibody-enhanced presentation of secreted GFP. (This would be highly unlikely anyway, because cross-priming should occur before sufficient amounts of antibody are secreted to influence antigen presentation, but still, it is a reassuring control). In vitro cross-presentation of the determinants from the transfected cells by a DC line paralleled their cross-priming capacity.

These findings dissociate endogenous processing and cross-priming and are therefore contrary to the chaperoned-peptide model of cross-priming. Because signal sequences, like other oligopeptides, are known to be degraded rapidly, they suggest that cross-priming is based on the transfer of proteins and not on their degradation products. Wolkers et al. (73) linked their findings to the inability of cells to cross-present a peptide present in the leader sequence of the LCMV glycoprotein, a finding used to argue against the physiological relevance of cross-priming (45) (although to be fair, another determinant in the middle of a stable LCMV protein is similarly inept at cross-priming).

Further support for protein-based cross-priming was provided by Norbury et al. (32), who found an inverse relationship between antigen stability and cross-priming. rVVs were used to express a stable or rapidly degraded form of IAV NP genetically fused to GFP. Although peptides are generated from the rapidly degraded protein at three times the rate as from the stable protein (74), cells expressing the rapidly degraded protein failed to cross-prime. This could be reversed, however, if cells were treated with lactacystin, an irreversible proteasome inhibitor. Similarly, rVV-infected cells expressing cytosolic or ER minigenes were unable to cross-prime. To prevent transfer of VV along with cells, VV-infected cells were UV-irradiated to an extent that severely compromised protein synthesis. This alone could not, however, account for the poor immunogenicity of minigene expressing cells because transiently transfected cells were also nonimmunogenic. Moreover, treating VV-infected cells with lactacystin failed to inhibit cross-priming from cells expressing stable proteins, or even enhanced it. This was also observed for IAV-infected cells, which were not irradiated (in this case virus could be neutralized by co-injecting cells with an antiviral mAb with potent virus-neutralizing activity). Norbury et al. (32) further showed that cells exposed to high concentrations of synthetic peptide were unable to cross-prime, even if the cells expressed a class I molecule able to bind the peptide but not present it T_{CD8+}.

Taken together, these three studies argue strongly that cross-priming in these systems is based on the transfer of proteins and not on peptides generated during protein maturation or via proteasomal degradation. A somewhat contrary report should be noted. Serna et al. (75) studied Mϕ-mediated cross-presentation of OVA or OVA gene fragments expressed by VV virus–infected cells, and they found that treating donor cells with proteasome inhibitors blocked ~80% of cross-presentation in vitro. Cross-presentation was also inhibited by overexpressing cytosolic oligopeptidase or aminopeptidase that presumably act by degrading proteasome products and not proteasome substrates. Cross-presentation of minigenes was not observed, providing a neat demonstration that in this system VV genes are not transferred to Mϕs and translated, but rather presentation represents bona fide cross-presentation.

On the basis of these findings, Serna et al. (75) concluded that in their system, cross-priming was based on the transfer of extended peptides generated by the proteasome that were not protected by molecular chaperones (as inferred by their sensitivity to peptidase overexpression). Whether these findings apply to cross-priming in vivo remains to be established. Serna et al. noted that the residual presentation in the presence of proteasome inhibitors could mask their effects in vivo if the threshold for T_{CD8+} activation in vivo was low. Although true, this in itself would not explain the complete lack of antigenicity of a rapidly degraded full-length protein observed by Norbury et al., the lack of immunogenicity of the signal peptide determinant observed by Wolkers et al., nor the ability of mAbs specific for native OVA to remove the cross-priming activity from the soluble fraction in Shen & Rock's study.

In any event, scientific truth is not determined by majority vote but is reached only through the application of multiple approaches in multiple systems. Additional studies to characterize the nature of the cross-priming material are clearly warranted. At the same time, there is considerable additional evidence inconsistent with the chaperoned-peptide model:

1. Molecular chaperones purified from cells are relatively poorly immunogenic and have yet to be shown capable of eliciting T_{CD8+} responses measured ex vivo, a feat attained even by boiled IAV (76).

2. It appears that many, but not all (77), of the adjuvant properties attributed to HSP70 and gp96 are due to the presence of contaminating endotoxins or lectins not eliminated in the purification process (78, 79). Some chaperones possess high-affinity binding sites for LPS (80), which greatly complicates assessing their natural role in immunity.

3. It has proven notoriously difficult to characterize peptides bound by immunogenic chaperone preparations (78). The relatively weak immunogenicity of molecular chaperones purified from cells may result from fortuitous contamination with protein antigens and mitogens.

4. Antigenic peptides can only be recovered from cells expressing a class I molecule able to protect the peptides (81), even when overexpressed as minigene products (82), suggesting that peptides are extremely short lived. Indeed, recent evidence based on peptide microinjection indicates that oligopeptides are destroyed by cells with a $t_{1/2}$ of <10 seconds (83). This is consistent with the low presentation efficiency of biosynthesized minigene products (84). Although exceptions to the rule that proteasomal products are

rapidly destroyed unless they bind to class I molecules are to be expected (it is biology, after all), the best characterized example is the protection of oligopeptides afforded by TRiC, a barrel-type molecular chaperone not implicated in cross-priming (85).

Thus, although molecular chaperones may yet prove useful for autologous tumor vaccines, where definition of target peptides is a Herculean task, or as a method of increasing the immunogenicity of defined peptides, where they show great promise (86), their physiological relevance remains uncertain.

By contrast, protein-based cross-priming is consistent with a large literature, dating back to the early 1980s, that documents the ability of proteins to induce T_{CD8+} responses (reviewed in 40). In a recent study, investigators found that given the proper protein antigen (virus-like particles in this case), the quantities of antigen required to elicit primary T_{CD8+} versus T_{CD4+} responses were similar (87). Cell debris has been shown to be immunogenic [by Zinkernagel's lab, ironically (43)], and in vitro cross-presentation based on pAPC phagocytosis of apoptotic/necrotic cells (88, 89) or nibbling of live cells (90, 91) has been clearly demonstrated. The relevance of these processes to cross-priming in vivo remains to be established, and the mechanistic basis of cross-priming will likely remain a lively research area for years to come.

How Are Cross-Priming Antigens Processed by APCs?

pAPCs can process exogenous antigens either in the endosomal/lysosomal pathway itself or in the cytosol after egress from this compartment. Readers are referred to a recent review of exogenous antigen processing for a comprehensive and thoughtful treatment of this topic (92). We limit our discussion to recent exciting developments in delineating the mechanism of cytosolic processing of phagocytosed antigens.

Gagnon et al. (93) initially described the fusion of phagosomes with the ER in macrophages, neatly dubbed the ergosome by Wilson & Villadangos (92). Houde et al. (94) extended these findings to cross-presentation by demonstrating that following macrophage internalization of OVA-beads (OVA coupled to latex beads), OVA is detected in the cytosol, and 25-D1.16-reactive K^b-OVA$_{257-264}$ complexes are generated in ER/phagosomes in a process that is TAP-dependent. Importantly, antigen presentation via this route was only partially inhibited by brefeldin A, which completely blocked presentation of endogenous antigens in the same cells. This suggests that the ergosome retains the ability of endosomes in communicating with the cell surface independently of Golgi complex-mediated transport (which is abrogated by brefeldin A treatment).

Guermonprez et al. (95) showed that the endosome-to-cytosol route previously established for DCs (96, 97) is also based on ER/phagosome fusion. Using OVA-beads, they demonstrated that 25-D1.16-reactive K^b-OVA$_{257-264}$ complexes are present in ergosomes containing OVA-beads and not other phagosomes in the same cells. In a carefully controlled series of experiments, purified phagosomes imported peptides via TAP and loaded them onto class I molecules. Because presentation was inhibited by proteasome inhibitors, Guermonprez et al. suggested a model in which antigen exits ergosomes and is processed by proteasomes associated with the same ergosome into peptides translocated back into the originating phagosome (both groups demonstrated that proteasomes were recruited to the cytosolic face of ER/phagosome membranes).

Ackerman and Cresswell (54) extended this pathway to soluble antigens by demonstrating that macropinosomes fuse with the ER in human DCs. They showed that all the cochaperones present in the class I loading complex are present in ergosomes. Further, they found that generation of cell surface K^b-$OVA_{257-264}$ complexes from soluble OVA could be blocked by co-incubating cells with a viral protein that inactivates TAP by interacting with its ER-domain; this confirms that complexes were generated in a compartment that receives internalized material. These findings are completely consistent with the Guermonprez et al. model.

Ackerman and Creswell clearly demonstrated the presence of newly synthesized class I molecules in ergosomes, and showed that ~25% of cell surface class I molecules on the DCs possess oligosaccharides typical of the ER, suggesting that they trafficked there directly from the ergosome. This finding is consistent with Gagnon's BFA results discussed above. It seems to conflict, however, with the requirement for K^b internalization in cross-presentation observed by Lizée et al. (68). This inconsistency could reflect differences between mouse and human DCs or between different class I gene products. Alternatively, mutation of the conserved Tyr in K^b may affect cross-presentation in a manner independent of its effects on internalization. Resolution of this discrepancy requires further investigation.

One attractive feature of the ergosome processing model emerging from these studies is that it could result in more efficient antigen processing than has been observed for endogenous antigen processing, which has been estimated at about 1 complex generated for every 2000 proteins degraded (74). Virus-infected pAPCs and aAPCs appear to cope with this inefficiency due to the huge flux of viral DRiPs that result from the shift from cellular protein synthesis to viral protein synthesis (98). But this low overall efficiency would seem to cripple cross-presentation, where much reduced amounts of antigen ought to be available for processing. (The word "overall" is used advisedly, because the low overall efficiency of endogenous peptide presentation may mask a high-efficiency process that operates on a fraction of DRiPs). Indeed, in the very first study to consider the efficiency of antigen processing, Pamer and colleagues (99) found that the efficiency of processing bacterial proteins released from phagosomes into the cytosol was approximately 1 complex generated for every 35 proteins degraded.

The ergosome appears to be specialized to increase the efficiency of exogenous antigen presentation. The finding that K^b-$OVA_{257-264}$ complexes are selectively generated in phagosomes containing OVA-beads (95), whereas OVA can be detected in the cytosol, provides direct evidence for the increased antigen-processing efficiency of ergosomes. This increase could result from a number of steps:

1. diversion of a set portion of incoming proteins to proteasome regardless of their structure (i.e., native versus denatured);

2. use of immunoproteasome versus standard proteasomes, as Houde et al. (94) found immunoproteasomes associated with ergosomes;

3. targeted delivery of proteasome products to TAP;

4. reducing competition from other peptides by restricting the access of ergosome associated TAP to other peptides and/or preventing degradation of cellular DRiPs by sequestering them in DALIs (100, 101); and

5. prolonging presentation of ergosome-generated peptides by reducing the internalization of ergosome-derived class I molecules, perhaps enabled by marking them with immature oligosaccharides characteristic of the ER, as suggested by Wilson & Villadangos (92).

Further use of 25-D1.16 and other TCR-like antibodies (102, 103) on different physiological substrates, including cross-presented antigens from virus-infected cells, should enable the careful comparison of the efficiencies of endogenous and exogenous processing in future studies. Also, it will be of great interest to determine whether two new proteins implicated in delivery of ER DRiPs to the cytosol (104, 105) are involved in ergosome antigen processing.

THE LONG HAUL

This review documents the tremendous progress achieved in the past five years in elucidating the pathways of presentation of viral antigens to T_{CD8+} in vivo and in vitro. The tools are now available to obtain detailed mechanistic understanding of antiviral T_{CD8+} activation in mice. There are a number of pressing questions directly relevant to vaccine design:

1. Do CD8α DCs generally play a critical role in activating anti-viral T_{CD8+}? If so, are they chosen for this role because they are simply better at it than other pAPCs or are other factors involved? In the former case, this implies that vaccines should be designed to deliver their information (polypeptides/nucleic acids) to these cells, assuming an equivalent population exists in humans.

2. What are the minimal cytokine/costimulatory signals necessary for vaccines to induce to maximize immunogenicity in cross-priming or direct-priming scenarios?

3. What is the molecular basis for cross-priming? Is it generally true that cross-priming is based on transfer of stable viral proteins? If so, are such proteins transferred with molecular chaperones or other cellular components that enhance the efficiency of cross-presentation in some manner?

4. Given this knowledge, what is the efficiency of polypeptide-vaccines based on cross-priming versus nucleic acid vaccines based on direct-priming with minigene/rapidly degraded gene products, when each vaccine is given conjunction with the optimal cytokine/costimulatory signals?

5. How does activation of memory T_{CD8+} differ from activation of naive T_{CD8+}? Precious little is known about the activation of memory T_{CD8+}, for example, their potential activation by aAPCs. This is directly relevant to boosting T_{CD8+} immunity in patients with chronic active infections with viruses such as human immunodeficiency virus, hepatitis B virus, or hepatitis C virus, or as means of increasing the memory response in patients to antigenically variable viruses such as IAV that escape existing antibody-based immunity.

Although we have come a long, long way since Metchnikoff's seminal observations of cellular immunity, rational vaccine design for inducing T_{CD8+} will require considerable additional investment of time and money. Viruses, however, are a ubiquitous, dangerous, and wily foe, and the vaccines will be well worth the effort.

The *Annual Review of Immunology* is online at
http://immunol.annualreviews.org

LITERATURE CITED

1. Metchnikoff É. 1902. Immunität bei Infektionskrankheiten. Jena, Germany: Fischer
2. Jerne NK. 1985. The generative grammar of the immune system. *Science* 229:1057–59
3. Sykulev Y, Joo M, Vturina I, Tsomides TJ, Eisen HN. 1996. Evidence that a single peptide-MHC complex on a target cell can elicit a cytolytic T cell response. *Immunity* 4:565–71
4. Davis MM, Krogsgaard M, Huppa JB, Sumen C, Purbhoo MA, et al. 2003. Dynamics of cell surface molecules during T cell recognition. *Annu. Rev. Biochem.* 72:717–42
5. Yewdell JW, Hill AB. 2002. Viral interference with antigen presentation. *Nat. Immunol.* 3:1019–25
6. Day PM, Esquivel F, Lukszo J, Bennink JR, Yewdell JW. 1995. Effect of TAP on the generation and intracellular trafficking of peptide-receptive major histocompatibility complex class I molecules. *Immunity* 2:137–47
7. Song R, Harding CV. 1996. Roles of proteosomes, transporter for antigen presentation (TAP), and b2-microglobulin in the processing of bacterial or particulate antigens via an alternate class I MHC processing pathway. *J. Immunol.* 156:4182–90
8. Bevan MJ. 2004. Helping the CD8$^+$ T-cell response. *Nat. Rev. Immunol.* 4:595–602
9. Wolkers MC, Stoetter G, Vyth-Dreese FA, Schumacher TNM. 2001. Redundancy of direct priming and cross-priming in tumor-specific CD8$^+$ T cell responses. *J. Immunol.* 167:3577–84
10. Ochsenbein AF, Sierro S, Odermatt B, Pericin M, Karrer U, et al. 2001. Roles of tumour localization, second signals and cross priming in cytotoxic T-cell induction. *Nature* 411:1058–64
11. Debrick JE, Campbell PA, Staerz UD. 1991. Macrophages as accessory cells for class I MHC-restricted immune responses. *J. Immunol.* 147:2846–51
12. Ciavarra RP, Buhrer K, van Rooijen N, Tedeschi B. 1997. T cell priming against vesicular stomatitis virus analyzed in situ: red pulp macrophages, but neither marginal metallophilic nor marginal zone macrophages, are required for priming

CD4$^+$ and CD8$^+$ T cells. *J. Immunol.* 158:1749–55

13. Sigal LJ, Crotty S, Andino R, Rock KL. 1999. Cytotoxic T-cell immunity to virus-infected non-haematopoietic cells requires presentation of exogenous antigen. *Nature* 398:77–80

14. Merad M, Manz MG, Karsunky H, Wagers A, Peters W, et al. 2002. Langerhans cells renew in the skin throughout life under steady-state conditions. *Nat. Immunol.* 3:1135–41

15. Bacik I, Cox JH, Anderson R, Yewdell JW, Bennink JR. 1994. TAP (transporter associated with antigen processing)-independent presentation of endogenously synthesized peptides is enhanced by endoplasmic reticulum insertion sequences located at the amino- but not carboxyl-terminus of the peptide. *J. Immunol.* 152:381–87

16. Lenz LL, Butz EA, Bevan MJ. 2000. Requirements for bone marrow-derived antigen-presenting cells in priming cytotoxic T cell responses to intracellular pathogens. *J. Exp. Med.* 192:1135–42

17. Sigal LJ, Rock KL. 2000. Bone marrow-derived antigen-presenting cells are required for the generation of cytotoxic T lymphocyte responses to viruses and use transporter associated with antigen presentation (TAP)-dependent and -independent pathways of antigen presentation. *J. Exp. Med.* 192:1143–50

18. Jung S, Unutmaz D, Wong P, Sano G, De los SK, et al. 2002. In vivo depletion of CD11c$^+$ dendritic cells abrogates priming of CD8$^+$ T cells by exogenous cell-associated antigens. *Immunity.* 17:211–20

19. Shortman K, Liu YJ. 2002. Mouse and human dendritic cell subtypes. *Nat. Rev. Immunol.* 2:151–61

20. Heath WR, Belz GT, Behrens GM, Smith CM, Forehan SP, et al. 2004. Cross-presentation, dendritic cell subsets, and the generation of immunity to cellular antigens. *Immunol. Rev.* 199:9–26

21. Smith CM, Belz GT, Wilson NS, Vil-

ladangos JA, Shortman K, et al. 2003. Cutting edge: conventional CD8α^+ dendritic cells are preferentially involved in CTL priming after footpad infection with herpes simplex virus-12. *J. Immunol.* 170:4437–40

22. Belz GT, Smith CM, Eichner D, Shortman K, Karupiah G, et al. 2004. Cutting edge: conventional CD8α^+ dendritic cells are generally involved in priming CTL immunity to viruses. *J. Immunol.* 172:1996–2000

23. Allan RS, Smith CM, Belz GT, van Lint AL, Wakim LM, et al. 2003. Epidermal viral immunity induced by CD8α^+ dendritic cells but not by Langerhans cells. *Science* 301:1925–28

24. Belz GT, Smith CM, Kleinert L, Reading P, Brooks A, et al. 2004. Distinct migrating and nonmigrating dendritic cell populations are involved in MHC class I-restricted antigen presentation after lung infection with virus. *Proc. Natl. Acad. Sci. USA* 101:8670–75

25. Lawrence CW, Braciale TJ. 2004. Activation, differentiation, and migration of naive virus-specific CD8$^+$ T cells during pulmonary influenza virus infection. *J. Immunol.* 173:1209–18

26. Mintern J, Li M, Davey GM, Blanas E, Kurts C, et al. 1999. The use of carboxyfluorescein diacetate succinimidyl ester to determine the site, duration and cell type responsible for antigen presentation in vivo. *Immunol. Cell Biol.* 77:539–43

27. Legge KL, Braciale TJ. 2003. Accelerated migration of respiratory dendritic cells to the regional lymph nodes is limited to the early phase of pulmonary infection. *Immunity* 18:265–77

28. Mempel TR, Scimone ML, Mora JR, Von Andrian UH. 2004. In vivo imaging of leukocyte trafficking in blood vessels and tissues. *Curr. Opin. Immunol.* 16:406–17

29. Cahalan MD, Parker I, Wei SH, Miller MJ. 2003. Real-time imaging of lymphocytes in vivo. *Curr. Opin. Immunol.* 15:372–77

30. Norbury CC, Malide D, Gibbs JS, Bennink JR, Yewdell JW. 2002. Visualizing priming of virus-specific CD8$^+$ T cells by infected dendritic cells in vivo. *Nat. Immunol.* 3:265–71

31. Gretz JE, Norbury CC, Anderson AO, Proudfoot AE, Shaw S. 2000. Lymph-borne chemokines and other low molecular weight molecules reach high endothelial venules via specialized conduits while a functional barrier limits access to the lymphocyte microenvironments in lymph node cortex. *J. Exp. Med.* 192:1425–40

32. Norbury CC, Basta S, Donohue KB, Tscharke DC, Princiotta MF, et al. 2004. CD8$^+$ T cell cross-priming via transfer of proteasome substrates. *Science* 304:1318–21

33. Doherty PC, Christensen JP. 2000. Accessing complexity: the dynamics of virus-specific T cell responses. *Annu. Rev. Immunol.* 18:561–92

34. Mueller SN, Jones CM, Chen W, Kawaoka Y, Castrucci MR, et al. 2003. The early expression of glycoprotein B from herpes simplex virus can be detected by antigen-specific CD8$^+$ T cells. *J. Virol.* 77:2445–51

35. Coles RM, Mueller SN, Heath WR, Carbone FR, Brooks AG. 2002. Progression of armed CTL from draining lymph node to spleen shortly after localized infection with herpes simplex virus 1. *J. Immunol.* 168:834–38

36. Mempel TR, Henrickson SE, Von Andrian UH. 2004. T-cell priming by dendritic cells in lymph nodes occurs in three distinct phases. *Nature* 427:154–59

37. Yewdell JW, Bennink JR, Hosaka Y. 1988. Cells process exogenous proteins for recognition by cytotoxic T lymphocytes. *Science* 239:637–40

38. Riddell SR, Rabin M, Geballe AP, Britt WJ, Greenberg PD. 1991. Class I MHC-restricted cytotoxic T lymphocyte recognition of cells infected with human cytomegalovirus does not require endoge-nous viral gene expression. *J. Immunol.* 146:2795–804

39. Bevan MJ. 1976. Cross-priming for a secondary cytotoxic response to minor H antigens with H-2 congenic cells which do not cross-react in the cytotoxic assay. *J. Exp. Med.* 143:1283–88

40. Yewdell JW, Norbury CC, Bennink JR. 1999. Mechanisms of exogenous antigen presentation by MHC class I molecules in vitro and in vivo: implications for generating CD8$^+$ T cell responses to infectious agents, tumors, transplants, and vaccines. *Adv. Immunol.* 73:1–77

41. Hudrisier D, Bongrand P. 2002. Intercellular transfer of antigen-presenting cell determinants onto T cells: molecular mechanisms and biological significance. *FASEB J.* 16:477–86

42. Smith AL, Fazekas De St. Groth B. 1999. Antigen-pulsed CD8α^+ dendritic cells generate an immune response after subcutaneous injection without homing to the draining lymph node. *J. Exp. Med.* 189:593–98

43. Bachmann MF, Kundig TM, Freer G, Li Y, Kang CY, et al. 1994. Induction of protective cytotoxic T cells with viral proteins. *Eur. J. Immunol.* 24:2228–36

44. Bachmann MF, Oxenius A, Pircher H, Hengartner H, Ashton-Richardt PA, et al. 1995. TAP1-independent loading of class I molecules by exogenous viral proteins. *Eur. J. Immunol.* 25:1739–43

45. Zinkernagel RM. 2002. On cross-priming of MHC class I-specific CTL: rule or exception? *Eur. J. Immunol.* 32:2385–92

46. Chen W, Masterman KA, Basta S, Haery-far SM, Dimopoulos N, et al. 2004. Cross-priming of CD8$^+$ T cells by viral and tumor antigens is a robust phenomenon. *Eur. J. Immunol.* 34:194–99

47. Chen W, Pang K, Masterman KG, Basta DN, Hornung F, et al. 2004. Reversal in the immunodominance hierarchy in secondary CD8$^+$ T cell responses to influenza A virus: roles for cross-presentation and

lysis-independent immunodomination. *J. Immunol.* 173:5021–27

48. Freigang S, Egger D, Bienz K, Hengartner H, Zinkernagel RM. 2003. Endogenous neosynthesis vs. cross-presentation of viral antigens for cytotoxic T cell priming. *Proc. Natl. Acad. Sci. USA* 100:13477–82

49. Prasad SA, Norbury CC, Chen W, Bennink JR, Yewdell JW. 2001. Cutting edge: recombinant adenoviruses induce CD8 T cell responses to an inserted protein whose expression is limited to nonimmune cells. *J. Immunol.* 166:4809–12

50. Bennink JR, Yewdell JW. 1990. Recombinant vaccinia viruses as vectors for studying T lymphocyte specificity and function. *Curr. Top. Microbiol. Immunol.* 163:153–84

51. Coupar BEH, Andrew ME, Both GW, Boyle DB. 1986. Temporal regulation of influenza hemagglutinin expression in vaccinia virus recombinants and effects on the immune response. *Eur. J. Immunol.* 16:1479–87

52. Bronte V, Carroll MW, Goletz TJ, Wang M, Overwijk WW, et al. 1997. Antigen expression by dendritic cells correlates with the therapeutic effectiveness of a model recombinant poxvirus tumor vaccine. *Proc. Natl. Acad. Sci. USA* 94:3183–88

53. Norbury CC, Princiotta MF, Bacik I, Brutkiewicz RR, Wood P, et al. 2001. Multiple antigen-specific processing pathways for activating naive CD8+ T cells in vivo. *J. Immunol.* 166:4355–62

54. Ackerman AL, Kyritsis C, Tampe R, Cresswell P. 2003. Early phagosomes in dendritic cells form a cellular compartment sufficient for cross presentation of exogenous antigens. *Proc. Natl. Acad. Sci. USA* 100:12889–94

55. Basta S, Chen W, Bennink JR, Yewdell JW. 2002. Inhibitory effects of cytomegalovirus proteins US2 and US11 point to contributions from direct priming and cross-priming in induction of vaccinia

virus-specific CD8+ T cells. *J. Immunol.* 168:5403–8

56. Shen X, Wong SB, Buck CB, Zhang J, Siliciano RF. 2002. Direct priming and cross-priming contribute differentially to the induction of CD8+ CTL following exposure to vaccinia virus via different route? *J. Immunol.* 169:4222–29

57. Shen L, Sigal LJ, Boes M, Rock KL. 2004. Important role of cathepsin S in generating peptides for TAP-independent MHC class I crosspresentation in vivo. *Immunity* 21:155–65

58. Gold MC, Munks MW, Wagner M, Koszinowski UH, Hill AB, Fling SP. 2002. The murine cytomegalovirus immunomodulatory gene *m152* prevents recognition of infected cells by M45-specific CTL but does not alter the immunodominance of the M45-specific CD8 T cell response in vivo. *J. Immunol.* 169:359–65

59. Holtappels R, Podlech J, Pahl-Seibert MF, Julch M, Thomas D, et al. 2004. Cytomegalovirus misleads its host by priming of CD8 T cells specific for an epitope not presented in infected tissues. *J. Exp. Med.* 199:131–36

60. Hengel H, Reusch U, Geginat G, Holtappels R, Ruppert T, et al. 2000. Macrophages escape inhibition of major histocompatibility complex class I-dependent antigen presentation by cytomegalovirus. *J. Virol.* 74:7861–68

61. Dantuma NP, Sharipo A, Masucci MG. 2002. Avoiding proteasomal processing: the case of EBNA1. *Curr. Top. Microbiol. Immunol.* 269:23–36

62. Blake N, Lee S, Redchenko I, Thomas W, Steven N, et al. 1997. Human CD8+ T cell responses to EBV EBNA1: HLA class I presentation of the (Gly-Ala)-containing protein requires exogenous processing. *Immunity* 7:791–802

63. Lee SP, Brooks JM, Al-Jarrah H, Thomas WA, Haigh TA, et al. 2004. CD8 T cell recognition of endogenously expressed Epstein-Barr virus nuclear antigen 1. *J. Exp. Med.* 199:1409–20

64. Yin Y, Manoury B, Fahraeus R. 2003. Self-inhibition of synthesis and antigen presentation by Epstein-Barr virus-encoded EBNA1. *Science* 301:1371–74

65. Tellam J, Connolly G, Green KJ, Miles JJ, Moss DJ, et al. 2004. Endogenous presentation of CD8$^+$ T cell epitopes from Epstein-Barr virus-encoded nuclear antigen 1. *J. Exp. Med.* 199:1421–31

66. Jones RJ, Smith LJ, Dawson CW, Haigh T, Blake NW, Young LS. 2003. Epstein-Barr virus nuclear antigen 1 (EBNA1) induced cytotoxicity in epithelial cells is associated with EBNA1 degradation and processing. *Virology* 313:663–76

67. Voo KS, Fu T, Wang HY, Tellam J, Heslop HE, et al. 2004. Evidence for the presentation of major histocompatibility complex class I-restricted Epstein-Barr virus nuclear antigen 1 peptides to CD8$^+$ T lymphocytes. *J. Exp. Med.* 199:459–70

68. Lizée G, Basha G, Tiong J, Julien JP, Tian M, et al. 2003. Control of dendritic cell cross-presentation by the major histocompatibility complex class I cytoplasmic domain. *Nat. Immunol.* 4:1065–73

69. Porgador A, Yewdell JW, Deng Y, Bennink JR, Germain RN. 1997. Localization, quantitation, and in situ detection of specific peptide-MHC class I complexes using a monoclonal antibody. *Immunity* 6:715–26

70. Le Bon A, Etchart N, Rossmann C, Ashton M, Hou S, et al. 2003. Cross-priming of CD8$^+$ T cells stimulated by virus-induced type I interferon. *Nat. Immunol.* 4:1009–15

71. Srivastava P. 2002. Interaction of heat shock proteins with peptides and antigen presenting cells: chaperoning of the innate and adaptive immune responses. *Annu. Rev. Immunol.* 20:395–425

72. Shen L, Rock KL. 2004. Cellular protein is the source of cross-priming antigen in vivo. *Proc. Natl. Acad. Sci. USA* 101:3035–40

73. Wolkers MC, Brouwenstijn N, Bakker AH, Toebes M, Schumacher TN. 2004. Antigen bias in T cell cross-priming. *Science* 304:1314–17

74. Princiotta MF, Finzi D, Qian SB, Gibbs J, Schuchmann S, et al. 2003. Quantitating protein synthesis, degradation, and endogenous antigen processing. *Immunity* 18:343–54

75. Serna A, Ramirez MC, Soukhanova A, Sigal LJ. 2003. Cutting edge: efficient MHC class I cross-presentation during early vaccinia infection requires the transfer of proteasomal intermediates between antigen donor and presenting cells. *J. Immunol.* 171:5668–72

76. Cho Y, Basta S, Chen W, Bennink JR, Yewdell JW. 2003. Heat-aggregated noninfectious influenza virus induces a more balanced CD8$^+$-T-lymphocyte immunodominance hierarchy than infectious virus. *J. Virol.* 77:4679–84

77. Baker-LePain JC, Sarzotti M, Fields TA, Li CY, Nicchitta CV. 2002. GRP94 (gp96) and GRP94 N-terminal geldanamycin binding domain elicit tissue nonrestricted tumor suppression. *J. Exp. Med.* 196:1447–59

78. Baker-LePain JC, Reed RC, Nicchitta CV. 2003. ISO: a critical evaluation of the role of peptides in heat shock/chaperone protein-mediated tumor rejection. *Curr. Opin. Immunol.* 15:89–94

79. Wallin RP, Lundqvist A, More SII, von Bonin A, Kiessling R, Ljunggren HG. 2002. Heat-shock proteins as activators of the innate immune system. *Trends Immunol.* 23:130–35

80. Reed RC, Berwin B, Baker JP, Nicchitta CV. 2003. GRP94/gp96 elicits ERK activation in murine macrophages: a role for endotoxin contamination in NF-κB activation and nitric oxide production. *J. Biol. Chem.* 278:31853–60

81. Falk K, Rötzschke O, Rammensee H-G. 1990. Cellular peptide composition governed by major histocompatibility complex class I molecules. *Nature* 348:248–51

82. Anton LC, Yewdell JW, Bennink JR. 1997. MHC class I-associated peptides produced from endogenous gene products with vastly different efficiencies. *J. Immunol.* 158:2535–42

83. Reits E, Griekspoor A, Neijssen J, Groothuis T, Jalink K, et al. 2003. Peptide diffusion, protection, and degradation in nuclear and cytoplasmic compartments before antigen presentation by MHC class I. *Immunity* 18:97–108

84. Fruci D, Lauvau G, Saveanu L, Amicosante M, Butler RH, et al. 2003. Quantifying recruitment of cytosolic peptides for HLA class I presentation: impact of TAP transport. *J. Immunol.* 170:2977–84

85. Kunisawa J, Shastri N. 2003. The group II chaperonin TRiC protects proteolytic intermediates from degradation in the MHC class I antigen processing pathway. *Mol. Cell* 12:565–76

86. MacAry PA, Javid B, Floto RA, Smith KG, Oehlmann W, et al. 2004. HSP70 peptide binding mutants separate antigen delivery from dendritic cell stimulation. *Immunity* 20:95–106

87. Storni T, Bachmann MF. 2004. Loading of MHC class I and II presentation pathways by exogenous antigens: a quantitative in vivo comparison. *J. Immunol.* 172:6129–35

88. Fonteneau JF, Larsson M, Bhardwaj N. 2002. Interactions between dead cells and dendritic cells in the induction of antiviral CTL responses. *Curr. Opin. Immunol.* 14:471–77

89. Albert ML. 2004. Death-defying immunity: Do apoptotic cells influence antigen processing and presentation? *Nat. Rev. Immunol.* 4:223–31

90. Harshyne LA, Zimmer MI, Watkins SC, Barratt-Boyes SM. 2003. A role for class A scavenger receptor in dendritic cell nibbling from live cells. *J. Immunol.* 170:2302–9

91. Harshyne LA, Watkins SC, Gambotto A, Barratt-Boyes SM. 2001. Dendritic cells acquire antigens from live cells for cross-presentation to CTL. *J. Immunol.* 166:3717–23

92. Wilson NS, Villadangos JA. 2004. Regulation of antigen presentation and cross-presentation in the dendritic cell network: facts, hypothesis, and immunological implications. *Adv. Immunol.* In press

93. Gagnon E, Duclos S, Rondeau C, Chevet E, Cameron PH, et al. 2002. Endoplasmic reticulum-mediated phagocytosis is a mechanism of entry into macrophages. *Cell* 110:119–31

94. Houde M, Bertholet S, Gagnon E, Brunet S, Goyette G, et al. 2003. Phagosomes are competent organelles for antigen cross-presentation. *Nature* 425:402–6

95. Guermonprez P, Saveanu L, Kleijmeer M, Davoust J, van Endert P, Amigorena S. 2003. ER-phagosome fusion defines an MHC class I cross-presentation compartment in dendritic cells. *Nature* 425:397–402

96. Rodriguez A, Regnault A, Kleijmeer M, Ricciardi-Castagnoli P, Amigorena S. 1999. Selective transport of internalized antigens to the cytosol for MHC class I presentation in dendritic cells. *Nat. Cell Biol.* 1:362–68

97. Norbury CC, Chambers BJ, Prescott AR, Ljunggren HG, Watts C. 1997. Constitutive macropinocytosis allows TAP-dependent major histocompatibility complex class I presentation of exogenous soluble antigen by bone marrow-derived dendritic cells. *Eur. J. Immunol.* 27:280–88

98. Yewdell JW, Reits E, Neefjes J. 2003. Making sense of mass destruction: quantitating MHC class I antigen presentation. *Nat. Rev. Immunol.* 3:952–61

99. Villanueva MS, Fischer P, Feen K, Pamer EG. 1994. Efficiency of MHC class I antigen processing: a quantitative analysis. *Immunity* 1:479–89

100. Lelouard H, Gatti E, Cappello F, Gresser O, Camosseto V, Pierre P. 2002.

Transient aggregation of ubiquitinated proteins during dendritic cell maturation. *Nature* 417:177–82

101. Lelouard H, Ferrand V, Marguet D, Bania J, Camosseto V, et al. 2004. Dendritic cell aggresome-like induced structures are dedicated areas for ubiquitination and storage of newly synthesized defective proteins. *J. Cell Biol.* 164:667–75

102. Cohen CJ, Denkberg G, Lev A, Epel M, Reiter Y. 2003. Recombinant antibodies with MHC-restricted, peptide-specific, T-cell receptor-like specificity: new tools to study antigen presentation and TCR-peptide-MHC interactions. *J. Mol. Recognit.* 16:324–32

103. Greten TF, Schneck JP. 2002. Development and use of multimeric major histocompatibility complex molecules. *Clin. Diagn. Lab. Immunol.* 9:216–20

104. Lilley BN, Ploegh HL. 2004. A membrane protein required for dislocation of misfolded proteins from the ER. *Nature* 429:834–40

105. Ye Y, Shibata Y, Yun C, Ron D, Rapoport TA. 2004. A membrane protein complex mediates retro-translocation from the ER lumen into the cytosol. *Nature* 429:841–47

Annu. Rev. Immunol. 2005. 23:683–747
doi: 10.1146/annurev.immunol.23.021704.115707
Copyright © 2005 by Annual Reviews. All rights reserved
First published online as a Review in Advance on January 19, 2005

IMMUNOLOGY OF MULTIPLE SCLEROSIS*

Mireia Sospedra and Roland Martin

*Cellular Immunology Section, Neuroimmunology Branch, National Institute of
Neurological Disorders and Stroke, National Institutes of Health, Bethesda, Maryland
20892-1400; email: martinr@ninds.nih.gov; sospedrm@ninds.nih.gov*

Key Words   autoimmunity, autoimmune mechanisms, neuroimmunology,
demyelinating dieseases, EAE

■ **Abstract**   Multiple sclerosis (MS) develops in young adults with a complex predisposing genetic trait and probably requires an inciting environmental insult such as
a viral infection to trigger the disease. The activation of CD4+ autoreactive T cells
and their differentiation into a Th1 phenotype are crucial events in the initial steps,
and these cells are probably also important players in the long-term evolution of the
disease. Damage of the target tissue, the central nervous system, is, however, most
likely mediated by other components of the immune system, such as antibodies, complement, CD8+ T cells, and factors produced by innate immune cells. Perturbations
in immunomodulatory networks that include Th2 cells, regulatory CD4+ T cells, NK
cells, and others may in part be responsible for the relapsing-remitting or chronic progressive nature of the disease. However, an important paradigmatic shift in the study
of MS has occurred in the past decade. It is now clear that MS is not just a disease
of the immune system, but that factors contributed by the central nervous system are
equally important and must be considered in the future.

INTRODUCTION

Multiple sclerosis (MS) is an inflammatory disease that affects the central nervous
system (CNS), i.e., the brain and spinal cord, and usually starts between 20 and
40 years of age (1, 2).[1,2] At least 350,000 individuals in the United States alone are
affected with MS. It leads to substantial disability through deficits of sensation and
of motor, autonomic, and neurocognitive function. The disease is usually not life

---

*The U.S. Government has the right to retain a nonexclusive, royalty-free license in and to
any copyright covering this paper.
[1]Owing to space restrictions, additional references for each section of this review are accessible in the Supplemental Material. Follow the Supplemental Material link from the Annual
Reviews home page at http://www.annualreviews.org.
[2]See Appendix for a full list of abbreviations used.

shortening, but its socioeconomic importance is second only to trauma in young adults (1, 2). There are two major forms of MS. Relapsing-remitting (RR)-MS is the most frequent (85%–90%) and affects women about twice as often as men. Most RR-MS patients later develop secondary progressive (SP)-MS (Figure 1). About 10%–15% of patients present with insidious disease onset and steady progression, termed primary progressive (PP)-MS. It is not clear which factors are responsible for the different courses. There is also heterogeneity in morphological alterations of the brain found by magnetic resonance imaging (MRI) (3) or histopathological evaluation (4, 5), as well as in clinical presentation, e.g., which CNS system and areas are primarily affected and whether a patient responds to treatment. The factors underlying this heterogeneity are not completely understood but include a complex genetic trait that translates into different immune abnormalities and/or increased vulnerability of CNS tissue to inflammatory insult or reduced ability to repair damage (Figure 1).

MS is still considered a $CD4^+$ Th1-mediated autoimmune disease (6, 7). This view is based on the cellular composition of brain and cerebrospinal fluid (CSF)-infiltrating cells and data from experimental allergic (autoimmune) encephalomyelitis (EAE) (8). In the EAE model, the injection of myelin components into susceptible animals leads to a $CD4^+$-mediated autoimmune disease that shares similarities with MS (6, 8) and can be adoptively transferred by encephalitogenic $CD4^+$ T cells into a naive animal (6, 8, 9). EAE cannot be transferred by antibodies, and so far it has been transferred in only two instances by $CD8^+$ T cells (10, 11), emphasizing the importance of $CD4^+$ T cells. The role of $CD4^+$ T cells in MS is supported by many parallels with EAE, but it is also supported indirectly by the fact that certain HLA class II molecules represent the strongest genetic risk factor for MS, presumably via their role as antigen-presenting molecules to pathogenic $CD4^+$ T cells.

The above considerations still apply, but research during the past decade has not only substantially increased our knowledge of the involvement of $CD4^+$ T cells in MS but also shown that the previous concepts were too simplistic and did not appropriately consider immune factors other than $CD4^+$ T cells. Another aspect might turn out to be even more important. We have for a long time almost completely ignored the contribution of the affected organ, the CNS. Pathologic and imaging studies (3, 5), as well as research of the molecular aspects of the disease in EAE and MS, now provide ample evidence that CNS-specific factors are important (12, 13). In this context, it is interesting, although historically not too surprising, that reviews on organ-specific autoimmune diseases, such as type 1 diabetes or rheumatoid arthritis, focus entirely on alterations of tolerance, specific immune cells, and other immune aspects, but rarely on the involvement of factors intrinsic to the target tissue. For MS, such an "immune-centered" view can not be upheld, and consequently in this chapter we deviate from our previous review 12 years ago (6) and consider the role of the CNS in targeting the disease process, in interactions with the immune system, and in the long-term course of MS.

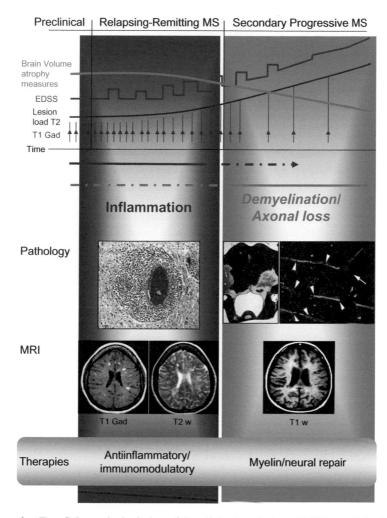

Figure 1 *Top:* Schematic depiction of the clinical evolution of MS by a clinical scale (EDSS, *red line*); the frequency of inflammatory events when studied by MRI (T1 lesions with contrast showing blood-brain barrier opening, *blue arrows*); T2 lesion load documenting all tissue damage (*blue line*); brain atrophy (*green line*). *Pathology:* Main pathological characteristics of MS. On the left, perivascular inflammation with mononuclear cells and open blood-brain barrier (courtesy of H.F. McFarland, NIB, NINDS, NIH); on the right, demyelinated areas shown in light blue and white, and, on the far right, axonal transactions (blue onion bulb-like structure) and segmental demyelination (from Reference 339, with kind permission of *N. Engl. J. Med.*). *MRI:* Typical MRI characteristics. On the left, T1-weighted image with Gadolinium contrast enhancement. White lesions indicate areas of fresh inflammation and open blood-brain barrier. T2-weighted image shows the CSF-filled ventricles in white and MS lesions in the brain parenchyma. On the right, brain atrophy with widened lateral ventricles and cortical sulci.

ETIOLOGY OF MS: IMMUNOGENETIC BACKGROUND

The etiology of MS remains unclear, but according to current data the disease develops in genetically susceptible individuals and may require additional environmental triggers. Virtually hundreds of studies in the past decades have addressed the genetic contribution, and for details the reader is referred to excellent reviews and the original articles (14, 15). Here, we try to distill from the existing literature the most relevant aspects in the context of the immunopathogenesis of MS.

The general population prevalence of MS varies between 60–200/100,000 in Northern Europe and North America, and 6–20/100,000 in low risk areas such as Japan. Population, family, and twin studies all show that the prevalence is substantially increased in family members of MS patients (14). First-degree relatives of affected individuals have an approximately 20- to 50-fold (2%–5%) higher risk to develop MS, and concordance rates in monozygotic twins vary between 20% and 35% in different studies, with the most recent studies placing it at 25% (14). Although the modest concordance rate has been viewed as a sign of environmental influences, studies of adoptees in MS families (16) and other data indicate that the genetic risk is probably higher. The search for individual susceptibility genes has so far been frustrating, despite tremendous advances. More than 20 whole genome screens have been performed in different MS populations and different geographic areas, with up to 6000 microsatellite markers and different methodologies (17). The data are strongest for one or more susceptibility genes on chromosome 6p21 in the area of the major histocompatibility complex [MHC; histocompatibility leukocyte antigen (HLA) in humans], which is thought to account for 10%–60% of the genetic risk of MS (18, 19).

THE ROLE OF THE HLA GENE COMPLEX

Similar to other T cell–mediated autoimmune diseases, in MS the specific genes that confer risk are the HLA-DR and -DQ genes, the HLA-DR15 haplotype in Caucasians (DRB1*1501, DRB5*0101, DQA1*0102, DQB1*0602) (18), but also other DRs in ethnically more distant populations. Most of the risk stems from the two DR alleles that are in very tight linkage disequilibrium, and there is also a dose effect in DR15 homozygotic MS patients (20). The contribution of DQA1*0102/-B1*0602 varies, and both additive and independent effects have been described, particularly in populations with lower overall MS prevalence (21, 22). Additional MS "risk/protective alleles" are listed in Table 1. Less information exists regarding genetic risk conferred by HLA class I alleles. Their association with MS appears to be much lower. HLA-A3 and -B7 are overrepresented in MS patients, and HLA-A201 has shown protective effects (18, 21, 23) (Table 1). With respect to associations of HLA-DR/DQ alleles with other genes, or clinical, MRI, or immunological characteristics, only limited data are available (Table 2). Genes associated with the DR15 haplotype include transforming growth factor (TGF)-β family members,

TABLE 1   Association of HLA class I and class II alleles with multiple sclerosis

MHC class I/II allele	Ethnic background/population and geographic location/country	MS subtype association	Remark
DRB1*1501[a]	Caucasians, many countries and backgrounds including Japanese, Tasmanians, and many others	All subtypes	Independent and joint with DQ; dose effect
DRB1*1503	Martinique	None	—
DRB1*1506, -1508	India	None	Joint with *1501
DRB1*15/DR3	Mexican Mestizos	None	—
DRB1*0301	Sardinia	None	—
DRB1*03/A30/B18	Central Sardinia	None	—
DRB1*0405	Sardinia	None	—
DRB1*04	Turkey/Canary Island	None	—
DRB1*04	Sweden	Progressive MS	—
DRB1*04	Russia	Higher T2 MRI load	—
DRB1*0405	Japan	OCB negativity	—
DRB1*04/DQB1*0302	Finland	None	Weak association
DRB1*0801	Ashkenazi Jews	PP-MS	—
DRB1*12	Russia	Higher T1 MRI load, higher MRI atrophy	—
DRB1*13	Northern Italy	Benign MS	—
DRB1*1303	Non-Ashkenazi Jews	None	—
DRB1*17	Germany/Sweden	None	—
DR in general	Canada	None	In DR15 negative families, independent contribution
DRB1*01/07/11	—	None	Protective
DRB1*01/DRw53	Finland	None	Protective
DRB1*01/DQB1*0501	Finland	None	Protective
DRB1*13/DQB1*0603	Finland	None	Protective
DRB1*15021	Iran	None	Protective
DQA1*0101	Colombia	None	—
DQA1*0102	Colombia	None	—
DQA1*0103	Colombia	None	Protective
DQB1*0602	Many MS populations	All subtypes	Independent and joint with DRB1*1501
DPB1*0301	Japan	Classical MS	—
DPB1*0501	Japan	Opticospinal (Asian) MS	—
A*0301	Caucasians, Russia, Sweden	Poor outcome, none	Partly independent of DR15
B*07/B*12	Caucasians, Russia	Poor outcome, none	—
A*02	Russia	More benign outcome	—
A*0201	Sweden	More benign outcome	Protective

[a]Note that wherever DRB1*1501 is mentioned in the Table, DRB5*0101 is co-expressed in this haplotype, and therefore these findings apply to DRB1*1501 and DRB5*0101.

cytotoxic T lymphocyte–associated antigen (CTLA)-4, the tumor necrosis factor (TNF) cluster, IL-1 receptor antagonist, IL-1, and estrogen receptor. Clinical factors include earlier disease onset, more often RR-MS, female gender, optic neuritis, or spinal involvement as initial event. Immunologically, higher CSF immunoglobulins, oligoclonal bands (OCB), and matrix metalloproteinase 9 (MMP-9) levels have been reported (24). $DR4^+$ patients often have a worse clinical outcome or progressive course than patients expressing $DR15^+$ (Tables 1 and 2). The above-mentioned studies on HLA associations with MS are heterogeneous with respect to sample size, methodology, ethnic background, and clinical findings. In older studies, the exact HLA class II gene has not been determined by molecular typing techniques. However, there is no doubt that HLA-DR and -DQ molecules are by far the strongest genetic risk factors in MS.

Our knowledge of how certain HLA class II genes confer risk for MS or autoimmune diseases at the molecular level is very sketchy. Several mechanisms have been considered: (*a*) Disease-associated HLA-DR and -DQ molecules have binding characteristics that lead to preferential presentation of specific sets of self peptides, e.g., myelin peptides in MS. Currently, little data support this hypothesis, and comparisons of polymorphic residues in the HLA-DR and -DQ binding pockets have not been conclusive. (*b*) As a variation of the first possibility, investigators have speculated that disease-associated HLA molecules could have binding characteristics that allow only limited sets of peptides to bind, accounting for less "complete" thymic negative selection of self-reactive T cells. Diabetes-prone NOD mice and their MHC class II ($I-A^{g7}$) have been viewed as an example for this situation (25). Given the high frequency of most autoimmune disease–associated HLA-DR and -DQ alleles in the population and the normal cellular immune function in the vast majority, we consider this mechanism unlikely in MS. (*c*) Either polymorphic residues of the T cell receptor (TCR)-exposed surfaces of the α-helical regions of DR/DQ-α and -β chains, such as the "shared motif" in rheumatoid arthritis–associated class II molecules (26) or TCR-contacting amino acids of the antigenic peptide, or both, could select an autoimmune-prone T cell repertoire. Gross abnormalities in T cell repertoires do not exist in MS patients according to current data (see below). However, we recently observed that clonally expanded T cells from the CSF of MS patients are capable of utilizing all MS-associated HLA-DR/DQ molecules in the DR15 haplotype for recognition of large sets of peptides (M. Sospedra, unpublished observation). (*d*) Gene and protein expression of one or several disease-associated DR and DQ alleles could be elevated in the CNS, enhancing antigen presentation. Comparisons of the expression of the two MS-associated DR molecules in the DR15 haplotype, DR2a (DRA1*0101 and DRB5*0101) and DR2b (DRA1*0101 and DRB1*1501), in MS patients and controls did not reveal general or tissue-specific upregulation of one DR allele (E. Prat, unpublished observation), but differential expression on B cells and monocytes. (*e*) Antigen presentation in the context of certain DR molecules could be shaped by proteases involved in antigen processing or by nonpolymorphic class II molecules such as HLA-DO and -DM that are tightly linked on chromosome 6p21.3

TABLE 2   Association of HLA-DR15 or other DR haplotypes with additional genes/chromosomal regions (part 1), or clinical/MRI/immunological criteria (part 2)

HLA-DR gene	Associated gene or clinical/MRI/immunological factor	Remark
Part 1		
DRB1*1501[a]	12p12	Gene not known
DRB1*1501	Microsatellite close to TGFB1	Gene not known
DRB1*1501	TGFB3	—
DRB1*1501	CTLA-4	—
DRB1*1501	Allele in TNF cluster	—
DRB1*1501	Area extending to DRA1* promoter	Gene not known
DRB1*1501	Allele 2 of IL-1 receptor antagonist	Association with RR-MS
DRB1*1501	Association with estrogen receptor polymorphism	—
DRB1*04/05	Association with MBP gene polymorphism in Italian and Russian MS patients	—
Part 2		
DRB1*1501	Association with relapse onset MS	—
DRB1*1501	Female gender, younger age at onset	—
DRB1*1501	Optic neuritis first sign, spinal involvement, early onset (all in a non-Japanese population)	—
DRB1*1501	Optic neuritis in children	—
DRB1*1501	Higher CSF OCB and IgG, and MMP-9	—
DRB1*1501	Higher IL-4 and TGF β levels, RR-MS	—
DRB1*1501	Anti-MOG IgA higher in asymptomatic relatives	—
DRB1*15-negative status	Worse clinical outcome	—
DRB1*04	Anti-MOG IgM elevated in patients	—
DRB1*04	Worse prognosis	—

[a]Note that wherever DRB1*1501 is mentioned in the Table, DRB5*0101 is co-expressed in this haplotype, and therefore these findings apply to DRB1*1501 and DRB5*0101.

and fulfill peptide-sorting and -loading functions. DM has been examined, but so far no association has been found in MS (27). (*f*) Engagement of HLA class II molecules leads to intracellular signaling events, e.g., anergy (28), which could be perturbed in patients with autoimmune diseases. There is currently no information on this aspect in MS.

HLA class I may act independently of class II in some patients, either via similar mechanisms or by modulation of NK cell activity. The reduced number of peptide-occupied HLA class I molecules in MS patients (29), the CD8$^+$ T cell infiltrations in the CSF and MS plaque tissue (30, 31), and the higher expression of HLA class I in the brain (32) suggest that the roles of HLA class I, CD8$^+$ T cells, and NK cells merit further study.

OTHER RISK-CONFERRING GENES

A recent review on the genetics of MS (14) pointedly remarked that the search for candidate genes has been plagued by initial positive results on specific genes in one study and subsequent negative or inconclusive data in several other reports. Polymorphisms of TCR genes, immunoglobulin loci, CCR5, and CD45 are just a few examples. Without summarizing the existing literature in depth, a few chromosomal loci have been identified in several but not all studies, and these studies used different methodologies, including the TCRβ chain locus, CTLA-4, TNF-α and -β alleles, and ICAM-1. Polymorphisms of CCR2, IL-10 receptor α, and Fas-L may confer protective effects; CCR5, IL-10, IL-4 receptor α, IL-2 receptor β, IFN-γ, vitamin D, and estrogen receptor confer risk. With respect to CNS-related genes, Notch4, a signaling molecule that is involved in both myelin development and immune function, neutral sphingomyelinase activating factor, ciliary neurotrophic factor, and the myelin basic protein (MBP) gene have been implicated. Other oligodendrocyte/CNS growth factors have been studied, but no association has been found. The role of an allele of apolipoprotein E (APOE4), which is involved in lipid metabolism and associated with the severity of Alzheimer's disease, remains controversial in MS, although an association between the APOE4 allele and higher severity/faster progression has been shown.

The above list is far from complete, and there are several reasons for the ambiguity of candidate gene searches. Methodologies and sample sizes vary; patient populations are often not stratified with respect to HLA, clinical, MRI-defined, or pathological phenotype; the ethnic background of subjects differs among studies; and the search often focuses on a few members of a gene family of interest, e.g., cytokine or TCR genes. Considering the genetic heterogeneity of the outbread human population and that almost every aspect of immune and nervous system function occurs and is regulated via highly complex interactions between multiple cell types and their soluble factors, surface receptors, signaling components, growth characteristics, and many other molecular pathways, our limited understanding is not too surprising.

GENOMICS STUDIES IN MS

The quantitative genetic trait has been difficult to dissect in MS and other complex diseases. In recent years, numerous groups have examined gene expression rather than the presence or absence of genetic polymorphisms. The development of microarray-based methods that allow the interrogation of thousands of genes in one experiment offers great advantages (33). Several investigators have employed microarrays to study gene expression patterns in MS brain tissue or peripheral blood samples. Whitney et al. (34, 35) examined plaque tissue and normal-appearing white matter in MS patients and EAE and identified four genes consistently overexpressed: the transcription factor jun-D, thrombin receptor protease-activated receptor 3, a putative ligand for IL-1 receptor-related molecule T1/ST2, and arachidonic acid 5-lipoxygenase, a molecule involved in leukotriene biosynthesis (35). Lock et al. (36) found increased transcription of MHC class II molecules; complement; T cell and B cell genes; some cytokine genes (IL-17), as well as their receptors (IL-1R, TNF p75 receptor); and glial fibrillary acidic protein (GFAP) and transcription factors. However, myelin proteins and neuronal genes were mostly underexpressed. EAE studies pointed at the relevance of G-CSF and FcRγ (36). Further studies found differential abundance of CD4, MAPKK1, nerve growth factors, HLA-DRα, and proinflammatory cytokines including osteopontin, but also some Th2 genes, α-B crystallin, and others (37–40). These studies have not been formally compared; however, immune system–related genes are prominently expressed, particularly at the acute stage of MS, and there are quantitative rather than qualitative differences between early and later stages of the disease. Examination of normal-appearing white matter, i.e., areas of the brain that appear macroscopically normal but are microscopically abnormal, demonstrated upregulation of genes involved in homeostasis and neural protection (41).

Expression studies in peripheral blood mononuclear cells (PBMC) have yielded similarly large numbers (42) of differentially expressed genes, and many are related to immune function, including MHC class II molecules; cytokines (TNF-α, IFN-γ, LTB, TNF-α receptor-associated factor 5); adhesion molecules (CD11a, CD18, CD49, integrin β7); costimulatory molecules (SLAM); T cell transcripts (TCRα, MAL); B cell or NK cell transcripts; signaling molecules (ZAP70); proteases involved in antigen processing; and many others with unknown relation to MS (42). The differential expression of only two genes from chromosome 6p21.3, i.e., heat shock protein 70 and histone family member 2, allowed investigators to separate patients and controls with 80% accuracy (43), and with the entire set of differentially expressed genes, one can accurately distinguish the two groups (43; G. Blevins, unpublished observation). Dissection of the mechanism of action of MS therapies by gene expression profiling has shown that IFN-β has not only immunomodulatory effects (e.g., increase of IL-10) but also proinflammatory effects (e.g., upregulation of CCR5 and the IL-12 receptor β2 chain) (44). Gene expression profiling also identified genes associated with partial responsiveness (e.g., IL-8 or TRAIL) to IFN-β therapy (45, 46). Although widely perceived as "fishing expeditions" and not hypothesis-driven experiments, gene expression profiling is likely to complement genetic studies and also to be instrumental in other aspects of MS research, such as identifying important functional pathways and treatment mechanisms.

ETIOLOGY OF MS: NONGENETIC FACTORS AND INFECTIOUS TRIGGERS

Nongenetic Factors in the Etiology of MS

The relatively low concordance rate of identical twins indicates a contribution of nongenetic factors to MS etiology (14, 47). This argument has to be considered with some caution because studies in congenic mice with gradually increasing numbers of lupus-associated genes have shown that the rate of disease expression can be "titrated," i.e., the fraction of animals that developed lupus was determined by the number of disease-linked genes under identical environmental influences (48). Among putative environmental factors, both infectious agents and behavioral or lifestyle influences have been proposed to induce or contribute to disease expression (49). The fact that women with the disease outnumber men with MS by 1.6–2.0:1 suggests hormonal variables as risk factors. This is supported by (a) lower relapse rates during, and disease rebound after, pregnancy (50); (b) the worsening of MS during menstruation; (c) the correlation of high estradiol and low progesterone with increased MRI disease activity; (d) gender differences in EAE susceptibility related to the protective effect of testosterone; and finally (e) the therapeutic effects of estriol in RR-MS (51). The precise mechanisms by which sex hormones may influence MS susceptibility are not known, but the stimulatory effects of estrogens on proinflammatory cytokine secretion and the reverse by androgens probably represent one mechanism.

Environmental contributions to the etiology for MS are supported by a number of factors. (a) The north to south gradient in disease prevalence on the northern hemisphere and the opposite on the southern. (b) MS distribution cannot be explained by population genetics alone. Although regions to which Northern European descendents migrated show high prevalence rates, these rates among Caucasians outside Europe are only half those in many parts of Northern Europe. (c) Migration studies show that if one migrated from an area of high prevalence of MS to an area of low prevalence before age 15–16, the low risk was acquired, whereas migration after 15–16 did not change the risk (52). One proposed causative factor is the decrease in sunlight exposure depending on the latitude. UV radiation may exert its effects either by influencing immunoregulatory cells or by the biosynthesis of vitamin D (53). The latter notion is supported by EAE data and the association of a vitamin D receptor polymorphism with MS in Japan. Melatonin secretion also depends on sunlight exposure. The lack of sunlight could induce an excess of melatonin, which enhances Th1 responses.

The geographical distribution also reflects the economic level of the country. The incidence of MS in Asia is overall low, with the highest prevalence in Japan, the most developed country in the area. Furthermore, prevalence rates have increased with the socioeconomic development in previous decades, which has been related to industrialization, urban living, pollution, occupational exposures to solvents, changes in diet and breastfeeding, smoking habits, and reduced UV light exposure. Finally, the delayed exposure to or overall reduction in childhood infections in developed countries is another factor and has led to the "hygiene hypothesis." According to this hypothesis, which is supported by findings in type 1 diabetes and EAE, there is a skewed immune responsiveness and increased propensity to develop autoimmune reactions/diseases (Th1-mediated) and allergy (Th2-mediated) in populations with delayed exposure to or overall reduction in childhood infections. However, this hypothesis is difficult to prove.

INFECTIOUS AGENTS AS TRIGGERS OF MS

Viral and bacterial infections are logical candidates as environmental triggers of MS. However, what has been stated for genetic studies also applies to research on infectious agents. Numerous reports have claimed to identify MS triggers, and almost universally these observations have later not withstood scrutiny (54, 55). Prospective studies have shown that MS relapses often follow viral infections (56). The temporal patterns and the occurrence of "MS epidemics," i.e., sudden increases in MS incidence in small, previously isolated communities, such as the one on the Faroe Islands, also point toward an infectious agent (52), although these are not uncontested. Further evidence for viral or bacterial triggers stems from EAE studies. Almost 100% of transgenic mice expressing a TCR that is specific for an encephalitogenic peptide of MBP develop EAE when the transgenic mice are housed under nonpathogen-free conditions, whereas the same animals housed in a specific-pathogen-free facility remained disease free (57).

The viral etiology of a number of human demyelinating diseases [progressive multifocal leukoencephalopathy caused by papovavirus JC; postinfectious encephalitis and subacute sclerosing panencephalitis (SSPE), both caused by measles virus; herpes simplex virus (HSV); HIV encephalopathy] explains the continued interest in viruses as triggers for MS (54, 55). Animal models of virus-induced demyelinating diseases, such as encephalitis or encephalomyelitis by Theiler's murine encephalomyelitis virus (TMEV), canine distemper virus, neurotropic strains of mouse hepatitis virus, Semliki Forest virus, Visna virus, and rat-adapted measles virus (54, 55), also support the possible involvement of a virus in MS.

Among viruses that are pathogenic in humans, those that induce persistent infection, such as herpes- or retroviruses, are suitable candidates and have been studied widely in MS. Herpesviruses are of particular interest owing to their neurotropism, ubiquitous nature, and tendency to produce latent, recurrent infections. Human herpesvirus 6 (HHV-6) and Epstein-Barr virus (EBV) are the leading candidates. The seroprevalence for both is high, i.e., >80% for HHV-6, a lymphotropic and neurotropic β-herpesvirus, and 90% for EBV, a lymphotropic γ-herpesvirus. HHV-6 can lead to meningoencephalitis, and several additional observations suggest a role in MS, including its detection in oligodendrocytes in MS plaque tissue (58) (but also in normal brains), the infection of astrocytes, and the presence of HHV-6 DNA and anti-HHV-6 IgG and IgM antibodies in serum and CSF of MS patients. However, the DNA and serological data are controversial (reviewed in 59). The existence of two different HHV-6 variants may account for some of the discrepancies. The role of HHV-6 variant A in MS is supported by its higher neurotropism, increased lymphoproliferative responses against variant A in MS patients (60), and its DNA presence in CSF from MS patients.

EBV has also been linked with MS. Anti-EBV antibodies are elevated in patients with MS, i.e., the seropositivity rate of MS patients is 100% versus approximately 90% in the general population, and MS patients reactivate latent EBV infections more often, correlating with relapses (61). Serum anti-EBV IgG levels prior to onset of MS have been reported as a strong disease predictor, a history of infectious mononucleosis is more common in MS patients, and the risk of developing MS is higher for individuals who suffered from infectious mononucleosis at a young age (62). Furthermore, some patients with neurological sequelae of primary EBV infection develop MS.

Human herpesvirus 1 (HSV-1) and varicella zoster virus (VZV or HSV-3) have also been considered as MS-triggering agents on the basis either of CSF antibody studies, casuistic observations, or the finding that VZV encephalitis is characterized by demyelination. Finally, MS-associated retroviruses have been linked with disease on the basis of the detection of extracellular virions in plasma and CSF of MS patients; however, their role is currently not clear.

Among bacteria, *Chlamydia pneumoniae* (Cpn) has been implicated in MS. Cpn is a Gram-negative intracellular bacterium and common pathogen of the respiratory system. Following an initial report (63), many studies examined an association between Cpn and MS. Current data are contradictory. Whereas one study reported the presence of Cpn in the CSF of a large percentage of MS patients compared with controls (64), other studies failed to observe an association between Cpn and MS (65).

The difficulty in identifying a single microorganism as the cause of MS probably indicates that Koch's paradigm "one organism, one disease" does not apply to this complex disease. Current data suggest that MS could be induced and/or exacerbated by many different microbial infections, and the responsible agents are most likely ubiquitous pathogens that are highly prevalent in the general population.

MECHANISMS: HOW INFECTIOUS AGENTS MAY INDUCE MS

Two main mechanisms have been proposed to explain how infections could induce MS: (*a*) molecular mimicry, i.e., the activation of autoreactive cells by cross reactivity between self-antigens and foreign agents; and (*b*) bystander activation, which assumes that autoreactive cells are activated because of nonspecific inflammatory events that occur during infections. A third proposal is that infections induce MS through a combination of these two mechanisms.

Molecular Mimicry

Molecular mimicry involves reactivity of T and B cells with either peptides or antigenic determinants shared by infectious and self-antigens. The recognition of self-antigens at intermediate levels of affinity by T cells during thymic selection leads to positive selection and export of these T cells to the periphery. Cross-reactivity of these potentially self-reactive T cells with foreign antigens can lead to activation during infection, migration across the blood-brain barrier (BBB), CNS infiltration, and, if they recognize antigens expressed in the brain, tissue damage and potentially an autoimmune disease like MS (Figure 2).

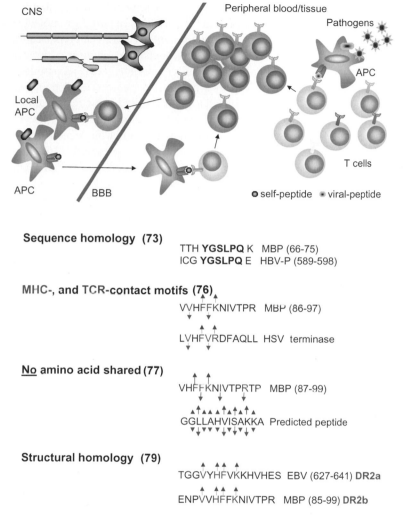

Figure 2   The evolution of the molecular mimicry concept and activation of autoreactive T cells via cross-reactivity with foreign antigens (for details, see text).

For example, MBP is a candidate autoantigen in MS on the basis of numerous pieces of evidence (6). MBP-specific T cells can be isolated from MS patients and controls (66–72). However, their activation state in MS patients, proinflammatory phenotype, higher antigen avidity, and preferential memory origin suggest that they had been activated in vivo, e.g., by cross-reactive infectious antigens during infections. Many studies have looked for cross-reactive antigens between MBP and foreign agents. Initially, the search was guided by the concept that humoral and cellular immune reactivity is exquisitely specific and that complete homology between foreign proteins and MBP is required for molecular mimicry. Although examples of such stringent homology have been reported for MBP and viruses (73, 74) (Figure 2), complete sequence matching is a rare event. Subsequent research of the molecular requirements for T cell recognition found that certain amino acid positions in a peptide are more critical than others for the interactions within the trimolecular complex, and most residues, except for the primary TCR contact, allowed for some degree of variation (75). On the basis of these observations, a search algorithm assumed that molecular mimicry can occur as long as a MHC and TCR contact motif is preserved (76) (Figure 2). The activation of MBP-specific T cell clones (TCC) derived from MS patients by viral and bacterial peptides sharing this motif with MBP confirmed the prediction that sequence homology was not required for cross-recognition (76) (Figure 2). Subsequently, the recognition by a $MBP_{(83-99)}$-specific TCC was systematically dissected using single amino acid substitutions in each position of the peptide sequence (77). These data demonstrate that cross-reactivity can occur with peptides that share no amino acid in their sequence and that each amino acid in the peptide contributes independently to TCR recognition (78) (Figure 2). Recently, the concept evolved even further; Lang et al. (79) showed that different peptides bound to different class II molecules can lead to cross-reactivity by the same TCR as long as the complexes share similarity in charge distribution and overall shape (Figure 2). Together, these observations offer new perspectives on the concept of molecular mimicry and indicate that cross-reactivity occurs frequently. Additional evidence for molecular mimicry stems from animal experiments showing that mice expressing viral proteins as tissue-specific transgenes develop autoimmune diseases after viral infection (80, 81). Recently, a model for virus infection that leads to molecular mimicry has been developed, in which an encephalitogenic virus (TEMV) encodes a mimic peptide for an encephalitogenic myelin proteolipid protein (PLP) that is naturally expressed by *Haemophilus influenzae*. The infection with this recombinant virus induces early onset of disease, which indicates that CNS infection with a pathogen containing a mimic epitope for a self-myelin antigen can induce a cross-reactive T cell response, resulting in autoimmune demyelinating disease (82). Although all these findings demonstrate that molecular mimicry is a viable hypothesis that can explain the link between infection and MS, evidence for this phenomenon in human autoimmune diseases is still scarce.

Bystander Activation

Bystander activation mechanisms can be classified into two categories. The first category encompasses TCR-independent bystander activation of autoreactive T cells by inflammatory cytokines, superantigens, and molecular pattern recognition, e.g., Toll-like receptor (TLR) activation. The second category involves the unveiling of host antigens and the adjuvant effect of infectious agents on antigen-presenting cells (APCs). Several proinflammatory cytokines and chemokines are produced during infection, and these molecules have long been considered the main activators of virus-specific CD8$^+$ T cells and inducers of the autoimmune process (83). Most of the activated CD8$^+$ T cells are specific for viral antigens, however, and cytokines alone are unlikely to cause the activation and differentiation of T cells in the absence of a specific antigen (84), which suggests that bystander activation requires the cooperation of several mechanisms to induce autoimmunity. Although the administration of cytokines can induce disease relapses in EAE, there are few examples in which the local overexpression of inflammatory cytokines/chemokines alone can break tolerance in healthy animals. The local expression of IL-2, IL-12, and IFN-γ-inducible protein (IP)-10 in diabetes can lead to inflammation but not to clinical disease, and only the overexpression of IFN-γ in pancreatic β cells disrupts tolerance to autoantigens, probably owing to enhanced presentation of self-antigens.

Superantigen exposure has also been proposed as a bystander activation mechanism. These toxins can induce relapses in the EAE model via interactions with MBP-specific TCC that express certain TCR Vβ chains (85).

Bystander activation via another group of infectious agent–derived and proinflammatory factors, such as TLRs, has also been described (86). One of them, lipopolysaccharide (LPS), binds to TLR4 and initiates innate immune responses to common Gram-negative bacteria such as Cpn. TLR4 activation by LPS increases the expression of cytokines as well as of reactive oxygen species. TLR4 in the CNS is mainly expressed on microglia but not on astrocytes or oligodendrocytes. LPS-TLR4 interactions may occur in MS during an infection with bacteria such as Cpn and induce the activation of monocytes and microglia, i.e., the adjuvant effect on APCs. Alternatively, LPS-TLR4 interactions may activate autoreactive T cells in the periphery. Bacteria injected into the brain parenchyma are able to induce inflammatory responses only after peripheral sensitization.

Another mechanism of bystander activation that depends on specific TCR recognition is the unveiling of host antigens as a consequence of viral tissue damage. Activated virus-specific T cells traffic to the infected tissue, where they recognize viral epitopes and kill infected cells, resulting in the destruction of self-tissue and the release of autoantigens. The presentation of autoantigens together with the adjuvant effect of infectious agents can then result in the de novo activation of autoreactive T cells and later to epitope spreading. This process occurs in the TMEV mouse model for MS, in which an initial virus-specific T cell response broadens or spreads to myelin proteins during persistent infection of the CNS (87). Spreading of the T cell response can include the presentation of cryptic epitopes that are usually not processed or presented as immunodominant epitopes but that can be presented during specific conditions associated with viral infection (88). During viral infection, the expression of self-proteins in the infected tissue is often upregulated (89), tissue-specific APCs are activated, and the expression pattern of proteases in these APCs can be altered, which leads to processing of cryptic epitopes that are not generated during "normal" processing (90). The recognition of such cryptic epitopes is probably more important during progression and perpetuation of the autoimmune response.

Recently, Pender (91) suggested that MS, like other chronic autoimmune diseases, could be based on infection of autoreactive B lymphocytes by EBV. In this scenario, autoreactive B cells are infected by EBV, proliferate, and turn into latently infected B cells that are resistant to apoptosis because they express virus-encoded antiapoptotic molecules. The presence of infected B cells in the target tissue can result in costimulation of autoreactive T cells, which prevents these cells from undergoing activation-induced apoptosis.

THE "MAJOR PLAYERS"

$CD4^+$ T Cells

EVIDENCE FOR INVOLVEMENT OF $CD4^+$ T CELLS IN MS   Following the description of MS by Charcot in 1868 (92), and the observation by Pasteur at the turn to the twentieth century (93) of acute postvaccinal encephalomyelitis in rabies vaccinees, Rivers showed in 1933 (94) that the injection of spinal cord or brain homogenates into healthy primates caused a disease similar to MS, leading to the hypothesis that MS is an autoimmune disease. Several decades later, investigators began to study systematically the experimental disease in rodents and made the seminal observations that still dominate our thinking about the pathogenesis of MS (8, 9, 95). They showed that the injection of defined protein components of the myelin sheath together with an adjuvant into naive susceptible animals caused either an acute, chronic, or relapsing-remitting encephalomyelitis, which is now referred to as EAE. The observation that EAE could be transferred by in vitro reactivated myelin-specific $CD4^+$ T cells (passive or adoptive transfer EAE) (8, 9) convincingly documented that EAE can be directly induced with autoreactive T cells in naive animals. Unlike myasthenia gravis, which is also an autoimmune disease affecting striated muscle, EAE cannot be transferred by antibodies. This fact led investigators to conclude that MS is likely a T cell–mediated autoimmune disease. As we discuss below, this view is too simplistic. However, current evidence on the induction and perpetuation of MS still favors $CD4^+$ autoreactive T cells as a central factor for the autoimmune pathogenesis of MS by the following arguments: (a) $CD4^+$ T cells contribute to the CNS- and CSF-infiltrating inflammatory cells in MS; (b) genetic risk is to a substantial degree conferred by HLA-DR and -DQ molecules; (c) humanized transgenic mice expressing either HLA-DR or -DQ molecules are susceptible to EAE (96–98), and mice expressing both MS-associated HLA-DR molecules and MS patient–derived MBP-specific TCR develop spontaneous or induced EAE (99, 100); (d) a therapeutic trial with an altered peptide ligand (APL) of $MBP_{(83-99)}$ induced cross-reactive $CD4^+$ T cells with Th1 phenotype that led to disease exacerbations of MS patients (101); (e) antibody production, $CD8^+$ maturation, and many other steps of adaptive and innate immune function are at least in part controlled by CD4$^+$ helper T cells. Unlike our previous review of this subject (6), we do not describe EAE data in detail here, but rather refer the reader to the original literature and reviews (8, 102, 103). We focus instead on MS.

One of the first striking observations in the early investigations of the involvement of CD4$^+$ T cells in MS was that MBP-specific T cells were readily found in both MS patients and healthy controls (66), indicating that previous concepts about the efficiency of central tolerance mechanisms and the elimination of autoreactive T cells were probably not correct (68–71). The fact that such autoreactive T cells from the normal T cell repertoire of Lewis rats can induce EAE (104) suggested to investigators that their equivalent in humans might also be relevant for MS. During the subsequent two decades, every aspect of CD4$^+$ T cells in MS has been the subject of exhaustive research. We are not able to cover all these data in detail, but we summarize the main findings.

FREQUENCY OF CD4$^+$ AUTOREACTIVE T CELLS   Frequencies of autoreactive T cells in MS patients and healthy controls vary greatly depending on the methodology (71, 72, 105–109). Whereas tissue culture–based techniques have shown frequencies of about 1 MBP-specific cell per 10^6-10^7 PBMC (71, 105), approximately 1–2 orders of magnitude higher numbers were observed with enzyme-linked immunospot (ELISPOT) assays, which detect IFN-γ-secreting cells (72). Newer methods, which employ quantitative polymerase chain reaction to follow individual TCC via their specific TCR CDR3 regions, observe frequencies of $1/10^4$ or even higher (107, 109). Flow cytometry–based techniques that follow the proliferating cell fraction upon stimulation with a myelin antigen observe frequencies in a similar range (110). Tetramer-based assays currently do not work for autoreactive HLA class II–restricted T cells, probably owing to low-affinity TCR recognition of autoantigens. Most studies comparing MBP- or PLP-specific T cells in MS patients and controls observe elevations in precursor frequencies in MS patients (111). Furthermore, the number of myelin-specific T cells with mutations of the hypoxanthine phosphoribosyl transferase gene, which occur in the proliferating T cell pool, is elevated in MS (112, 113). Up to 2000-fold expansions of MBP$_{(83–99)}$-specific T cells have been described during exacerbation of patients in a treatment trial with an APL based on the immunodominant MBP$_{(83–99)}$ peptide (101). Most APL-specific T cells cross-reacted with MBP$_{(83–99)}$, and these cells were also found in the CSF and exhibited a Th1 phenotype, all supporting their involvement in disease exacerbation (101). Finally, TCR CDR3-based molecular tracking of individual clones showed that MBP- and APL-specific T cells had preexisted in the patient's peripheral blood long before APL therapy but were markedly expanded during disease exacerbation (107). Most studies of autoreactive T cells in MS used relatively high concentrations (10–50 μg/ml) of either whole native or recombinant proteins or peptides. Under normal conditions, and even under disease conditions such as stroke, such high concentrations of myelin antigens are probably rarely reached, and T cell activation by autoantigens will only result if other factors, such as strong activation of innate immune mechanisms, upregulation of MHC and costimulatory molecules, and proinflammatory cytokines, occur. However, high-avidity T cells that respond at low antigen concentrations to myelin proteins/peptides and that are likely more relevant to disease are clearly also increased in MS patients and mostly express a proinflammatory phenotype (108).

Antigen Specificity of Myelin-Specific CD4$^+$ T Cells

MYELIN BASIC PROTEIN (MBP)   MBP is the best-studied myelin protein in MS. It is the second most abundant myelin protein (approximately 30%–40%) after PLP, is relatively easy to isolate owing to its physicochemical characteristics, and was the first that was used extensively in EAE. There are five MBP isoforms with 14.0–21.5 kDa molecular weights in mammals that result from differential splicing of eleven axons within the Golli-MBP locus (114). The highly basic MBP is positioned at the intracellular surface of myelin membranes, and via interactions with acidic lipid moieties it is involved in maintaining the structure of compact myelin. The most abundant 18.5 kDa isoform (170 amino acid length) has been used in most immunological studies. Unlike myelin oligodendrocyte glycoprotein (MOG) and PLP, MBP is found in significant quantities in both central and peripheral myelin, and MBP transcripts have also been demonstrated in peripheral lymphoid organs (115). EAE can be induced with MBP in several mouse and rat strains, guinea pigs, and nonhuman primates (103). The most important encephalitogenic areas are depicted in Figure 3. An important parallel between rodent and primate EAE models and MBP-specific immune responses in humans is the striking overlap between epitopes that are encephalitogenic in the context of EAE-associated MHC class II alleles and MBP regions that are immunodominant in the context of MS-associated HLA-DR alleles, i.e., HLA-DR2a (DRB5*0101), -DRb (DRB1*1501), and -DRB1*0401/0404/0405 (69–71, 116, 117) (Figure 3). This applies to the immunodominant MBP$_{(83–99)}$ or MBP$_{(84–102)}$ epitope, a promiscuous binder to all the above MS-associated HLA-DR molecules (118–120), as well as to the immunodominant MBP$_{(111–129)}$ epitope in the context of DRB1*0401 (121) and the region of MBP that is immunodominant with DR2a (71, 122) and other DR alleles (123). For high-avidity myelin-specific T cells, MBP$_{(83–99)}$ is not immunodominant, but MBP$_{(13–32)}$, MBP$_{(111–129)}$, and MBP$_{(146–170)}$ are (108). Most of these peptides are promiscuous HLA-DR binders; however, the predicted affinity to HLA-DR2a, -DR2b, -DR4, and other DR alleles is low, indicating that deletion of T cells with high functional avidity for these MBP epitopes in the thymus is incomplete. This situation is similar to MBP Ac1-11 epitope in PL/J mice (114, 124). The poor binding affinity of the latter MBP epitope to IA^u supports the view that complexes of MBP Ac1-11 with IA^u are unstable and therefore inefficient in negative selection (125). MBP Ac1-11-specific TCR transgenic mice develop EAE depending on the level of microbial exposure or after induction with pertussis (57, 126). The encephalitogenic potential of a MS patient–derived T cell was demonstrated in a transgenic mouse expressing a MBP$_{(84–104)}$-specific TCR and HLA-DR15 (99).

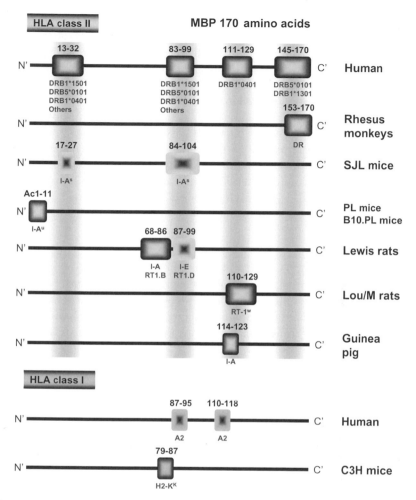

Figure 3   Immunodominant regions of MBP in humans and various EAE models in different species. MHC class II–restricted epitopes are shown on top (*green*), those that are recognized in the context of MHC class I and/or encephalitogenic in EAE at the bottom (*blue*).

EAE could readily be induced, and about 4% of these animals developed spontaneous disease. Furthermore, the same TCR cross-reacts with an EBV-derived peptide in the context of DR2a, supporting molecular mimicry (79). The complex of HLA-DR2b and MBP$_{(84-102)}$ was also detected in the brains of MS patients via staining with a monoclonal antibody, which supports the notion that the immunodominant autoantigenic peptide is presented locally (127). A recent humanized transgenic mouse model that combines another MS patient–derived MBP$_{(83-99)}$-specific TCR and DR2a also readily develops active and passive EAE, although we do not know yet whether spontaneous disease will occur (J. Shukaliak-Quandt, unpublished observation). $MBP_{(83-99)}$ has received the most attention; however, EAE can also be induced in humanized transgenic mice expressing a $MBP_{(111-129)}$-specific MS patient–derived TCR together with the restriction element DRB1*0401 (100). Interestingly, only adoptive transfer EAE was inducible in this model, and some animals not only develop signs of conventional EAE, i.e., limp tail, flaccid hind limb paresis, or paralysis, but also show signs of involvement of caudal cranial nerves with swallowing difficulties and ataxia, which indicate that clinical/phenotypic heterogeneity is related to the inducing myelin peptide (102).

Additional evidence supporting a role for MBP in MS includes cross-reactivity between $MBP_{(84-102)}$-specific Th1 cells and an identical sequence in the U24 antigen of HHV-6 (74), broader responses to MBP, and intra- and interindividual fluctuations of the specificities over time, without clear relation to inflammatory MRI activity.

PROTEOLIPID PROTEIN (PLP) PLP is the most abundant CNS myelin protein (about 50%), highly hydrophobic and evolutionarily conserved across species. In mice, there are two main transcripts, the full-length 276 amino acid isoform; and DM-20, an isoform that lacks 35 amino acids and is mainly expressed in brain and spinal cord prior to myelination but also in peripheral lymphoid organs, where full-length PLP is barely found (114, 115, 128). The differential peripheral expression is relevant for one major encephalitogenic and immunodominant $PLP_{(139-154)}$ peptide that is contained in full-length PLP, but is not contained in DM-20 (115, 128) and therefore is not available for thymic negative selection. Consequently, high frequencies of $PLP_{(139-154)}$-specific T cells have been observed even in naive unprimed animals (128, 129). PLP is a stronger encephalitogen compared with MBP, at least in some EAE models, particularly in SJL/J mice, in which $PLP_{(139-151)}$ is dominant (130, 131). PLP TCR transgenic mice on the SJL/J background develop spontaneous EAE with very high frequency (129). Upon EAE induction with whole spinal cord homogenate in SJL/J mice, the dominant T cell response is directed against $PLP_{(139-151)}$, and during disease relapses predictable epitope spreading occurs to $PLP_{(178-191)}$ and later to $MBP_{(89-101)}$ (130, 131). If EAE in SJL/J mice is induced with either the secondary $PLP_{(178-191)}$ epitope or with $MBP_{(89-101)}$, further waves of the disease always involve reactivity to $PLP_{(139-151)}$ (130, 131). Numerous other PLP peptides are encephalitogenic, including $PLP_{(178-191)}$, $PLP_{(43-64)}$, $PLP_{(56-70)}$, and $PLP_{(104-117)}$ in SJL/J mice, $PLP_{(217-233)}$ in Lewis rats, and $PLP_{(56-70)}$ in Biozzi mice. Although examined less extensively for PLP, the above parallels between encephalitogenic MBP epitopes in EAE and immunodominant peptides in humans are also observed. $PLP_{(104-117)}$, $PLP_{(142-153)}$, $PLP_{(184-199)}$, and $PLP_{(190-209)}$ peptides are immunodominant in the context of the MS-associated DR2 alleles, but these peptides also bind to other HLA-DR alleles (132, 133). Further immunodominant epitopes are $PLP_{(30-49)}$, $PLP_{(40-60)}$, $PLP_{(89-106)}$, and $PLP_{(95-116)}$ (97, 134–136). As is the case in the mouse, the human thymus does not express $PLP_{(139-151)}$, which at least in part explains the immunodominance in humans. The frequencies and skew toward a Th1 phenotype of PLP-specific T cells are increased in MS, but not in every study. $PLP_{(139-151)}$ and $PLP_{(178-191)}$ are main targets of high-avidity T cells and are clearly elevated in MS patients (108).

MYELIN OLIGODENDROCYTE GLYCOPROTEIN (MOG)   MOG, a 218 amino acid transmembrane glycoprotein of the Ig superfamily, is much less abundant than the major myelin proteins (0.01%–0.05%), and it is not located in compact myelin but rather on the outer surface of the oligodendrocyte membrane. Owing to this "strategic" location, it is directly accessible to antibodies and believed to be relevant as a target for both cellular and humoral immune responses in MS. MOG is expressed late in myelination and is only found in the brain/spinal cord and the retina, not in peripheral nerve. Furthermore, MOG expression is either completely or almost completely lacking in peripheral lymphoid tissues (114, 115). MOG-induced EAE is best examined in C57/BL6 mice, in which the $MOG_{(35-55)}$ peptide induces a chronic, nonrelapsing EAE (137). A recent MOG TCR transgenic mouse model on the B6 background showed spontaneous EAE with inflammation, demyelination, and axonal damage in brain and spinal cord in a small fraction of animals, while 35% developed spontaneous optic neuritis (138). Optic neuritis is also seen in MOG-induced EAE in DA rats (102), and the relatively higher expression of MOG in the optic nerve has been proposed as one explanation for the involvement of the optic nerve (138). Differences in lesion location, as well as in the involvement of antibodies versus T cells in different EAE models support the notion that the inducing antigens and immunogenetic background contribute to disease phenotype (102, 139).

Overall, much less information is available on the fine specificity of human MOG-reactive T cells when compared with MBP and PLP. Immunodominant epitopes have been located in the Ig-like extracellular domain of $MOG_{(1-22)}$, $MOG_{(11-30)}$, $MOG_{(21-40)}$, $MOG_{(31-50)}$, $MOG_{(34-56)}$, $MOG_{(63-87)}$, $MOG_{(64-96)}$, $MOG_{(71-90)}$ (140–142), which also harbor several encephalitogenic epitopes (143), but immunodominant areas have also been found in the intracellular parts of MOG. $MOG_{(146-154)}$ is immunodominant with both DR15 (DRB1*1501) and DR4 (DRB1*0401) (144). Weissert et al. (144) reported stronger responses toward intracellular portions of MOG and to different MOG peptides in MS patients, whereas the reverse was observed by Lindert et al. (145). $MOG_{(1-20)}$ and $MOG_{(35-55)}$ peptides are among the 6/15 myelin peptides from MBP, PLP, MOG, and CNPase that account for clearly elevated high-avidity myelin-specific T cell responses in MS patients, which supports the importance of MOG (108).

Other Myelin and Nonmyelin Antigens as Targets for CD4$^+$ T Cells

Investigators have examined the role of a few other myelin components and nonmyelin proteins and glycolipids as antigens for CD4$^+$ T cells. The order in which they are mentioned here does not reflect their importance, which is not yet known.

MYELIN-ASSOCIATED GLYCOPROTEIN (MAG)   MAG is a large (approximately 100 kDa) myelin glycoprotein located at the inner surface of the myelin sheath opposing the axon surface. It accounts for less than 1% of total myelin protein in the CNS and is even less abundant in the peripheral nervous system (PNS). The pathogenetic relevance of MAG has been documented for polyneuropathies by anti-MAG IgM (146). MAG$_{(97-112)}$ is encephalitogenic in ABH (H-2A^{g7}) mice (147), and elevated MAG-specific T and B cell responses have been observed in the CSF of MS patients by ELISPOT assays (148). Among the few MAG peptides that have been examined, C-terminal areas, i.e., MAG$_{(596-612)}$ and MAG$_{(609-626)}$, are relatively immunodominant (148). The preferential location of CNS lesions in cerebellum, centrum semiovale, and forebrain in MAG-induced EAE in Lewis rats supports the notion that the antigen specificity is related to lesion location (102).

2′,3′-CYCLIC NUCLEOTIDE 3′ PHOSPHODIESTERASE (CNPase)   CNPase exists in two splice variants (CNPase I and II, 46 kDa and 48 kDa) and makes up 3%–4% of total myelin protein. It is located in oligodendrocytes, mainly around the nucleus and in the paranodal loops, but it is also expressed in peripheral Schwann cells and, although much less, in lymphoid tissues. Its exact role is not clear. Encephalito-genicity could not be demonstrated so far (147); however, immunization of Lewis rats with a CNPase peptide with homology with mycobacterial HSP65 resulted in protection from EAE (149). CNPase is immunogenic both in rodents and in humans, and studies of the reactivity to either recombinant or native CNPase and to overlapping CNPase peptides have located a number of areas with promiscuous binding to several HLA-DR alleles, including the MS-associated DR15 molecules (150, 151). A C-terminal area [CNPase$_{(343-373)}$] is one of the immunodominant epitopes that is recognized preferentially by high-avidity myelin-specific T cells of MS patients (108).

MYELIN-ASSOCIATED OLIGODENDROCYTIC BASIC PROTEIN (MOBP)   MOBP was discovered recently. Several splice variants exist, and the 81 amino acid isoform is most abundant in rodent and human myelin. MOBP is exclusively expressed in oligodendrocytes, appears late in myelination, and is located in the major dense line of compact myelin. MOBP is encephalitogenic in SJL/J mice, and the encephalito-genic epitope is located within amino acids 37–60 (152, 153). Preliminary studies of cellular anti-MOBP responses in MS patients and controls identified one im-munodominant region, MOBP$_{(21-39)}$ (152), and the reactivity of MOBP-specific T cells cofluctuated with inflammatory MRI activity (154).

OLIGODENDROCYTE-SPECIFIC GLYCOPROTEIN (OSP)   OSP is the third most abun-dant myelin protein (7%), is expressed in the CNS and testis, and is located in tight junctions. These characteristics led it to be grouped in the family of tight junction proteins and to be renamed as OSP/Claudin-11. Several OSP peptides induce EAE in SJL/J mice, and OSP-specific antibodies are found in the CSF of RR-MS patients (155). By testing PBMC from RR-MS and SP-MS patients with overlapping OSP peptides, investigators identified a number of immunogenic areas and observed overall strong responses in both healthy controls and RR-MS patients but decreased reactivity in SP-MS (156).

α-B CRYSTALLIN (αB-C)   Unlike the myelin proteins discussed above, αB-C was identified as a candidate target in MS patients and not in EAE models. Van Noort and colleagues (157) fractionated MS brain–derived proteins and then tested the proliferation of PBMC from MS patients and healthy controls against brain protein fractions. They observed prominent reactivity in one of the fractions and identified the small heat shock protein αB-C as the relevant antigen (157). αB-C is a major constituent of the eye lens, but it is also expressed in astrocytes and oligodendrocytes in active MS lesions. A cryptic epitope of α-B crystallin, αB-C$_{(1-16)}$, is weakly encephalitogenic in Biozzi ABH mice. In addition to the demonstration of strong responses to αB-C-containing MS brain–derived protein fractions, DRB1*1501-restricted CD4$^+$ Th1 T cells in MS patients responded to peptides αB-C$_{(21-40)}$ and αB-C$_{(41-60)}$, although less to αB-C$_{(131-150)}$ (158). Other investigators documented comparable T cell responses to αB-C in MS patients and healthy controls (159).

S100β PROTEIN   Linington and colleagues (160) examined the astrocyte-derived calcium-binding protein S100 in Lewis rats and observed a strong immune response against the S100β epitope (amino acids 76–91). Unlike myelin antigens, S100 immunization or adoptive transfer of S100-specific T cells led to a panencephalitis and uveoretinitis. However, disease induction with S100 led to little if any clinical deficit (160). The lack of clinical disease was related to the decreased macrophage recruitment, despite massive T cell infiltrates (160). Also, unlike MBP-specific T cell lines, S100-specific T cells did not show cytotoxic activity. These observations parallel data from MS patients. Both CD4$^+$ and CD8$^+$ T cells specific for S100β can be isolated with no differences among the groups (159, 161). S100-specific CD4$^+$ T cells exhibited cytotoxic activity less often compared with MBP-specific T cells from the same donors (161).

TRANSALDOLASE-H (Tal-H)   Tal-H was discovered on the basis of homologies with the gag p17 protein of human T lymphotropic virus type I (162). Tal-H is a key enzyme of the pentose phosphate pathway and is expressed in oligodendrocytes, Schwann cells, and lymphoid tissues. High-affinity antibodies against Tal-H have been found in the serum and CSF of MS patients, and Tal-H also stimulates proliferation of MS PBMC (163).

IMMUNOGLOBULINS AS T CELL ANTIGENS   Vartdal and colleagues (164) examined the interesting hypothesis that the intrathecal Ig synthesis is involved in perpetuating the CD4$^+$ T cell response. They found proliferative reactivity of T cells to CSF Ig in 14 out of 21 MS patients and 4 out of 17 other neurological controls, and preliminary studies indicate that CD4$^+$ T cells responded in a DR-restricted fashion (164). We have recently identified an IgG peptide as one target of a CD4$^+$ TCC (MN36) that was clonally expanded in the CSF of a MS patient during exacerbation (M. Sospedra, unpublished observation). The specificity of the TCC was identified with an unbiased technique, i.e., positional scanning combinatorial peptide libraries, and it supports the above hypothesis (164, 165) that CSF-derived Ig may serve as an autoantigen that perpetuates the autoreactive T cell response.

LIPID COMPONENTS AS ANTIGENS FOR CD4$^+$ T CELLS IN MS   Paralleling the observation of elevated antiganglioside antibodies, particularly in the chronic progressive form of MS (166), Pender and colleagues (167) found enhanced T cell reactivity against gangliosides GM3 and GQ1b in PP-MS patients only. These findings suggest that ganglioside-specific T cells can contribute to axonal damage in PP-MS, although further studies are required, particularly with respect to which cell types and molecular mechanisms are involved in lipid recognition in MS.

ANTIGEN AVIDITY: CROSS-REACTIVITY AND DEGENERACY OF CD4$^+$ T CELL RECOGNITION   Despite long-held views that cellular immune responses are highly specific, it is now firmly established that the ability of T cells for cross-reactivity or degeneracy is a normal phenomenon. Degenerate T cell recognition is not only required for thymic positive selection on thymic self peptides but also for host protection against potential antigens that outnumber the available T cells/TCRs by several orders of magnitude. For self-antigens expressed in the thymus (e.g., MBP), only T cells recognizing these antigens with low functional avidity are positively selected. In agreement, most MBP-specific T cell lines respond to antigen at relatively high concentrations in the micromolar range (69–71, 168), and pathogen-derived peptides have been identified that activate MBP-specific TCC at several orders of magnitude lower concentrations (169). However, high-avidity myelin-reactive TCC also exist in the periphery, and they are elevated in MS patients compared with controls (108). Furthermore, during a trial with an APL peptide derived from MBP$_{(83-99)}$, we identified TCC responding to both the APL peptide and MBP$_{(83-99)}$ at subnanomolar concentrations (101), and one of these TCC was already present in the peripheral blood seven years before the APL trial (107). It is not clear whether changes in functional avidity occur during the disease process in the periphery, either by changes in the requirements for costimulation or the TCR-associated signaling machinery, or whether high-avidity T cells pass "thymic inspection" because central tolerance is less stringent in MS. With respect to self-antigens that are not or are barely expressed in the thymus, such as MOG or the full length PLP isoform, it is expected that autoreactive T cells are deleted less efficiently in the thymus. This has been confirmed for PLP$_{(139-154)}$-specific T cells in SJL/J mice. Furthermore, the six myelin peptides (three MBP, one PLP, and two MOG peptides) that are immunodominant for high-avidity T cells are either derived from proteins that are not expressed in the thymus ($PLP_{(139-154)}$ and the two MOG peptides) or that reside in areas that poorly bind to the MS-associated HLA-DR (108).

Recent observations suggest that the extent of cross-reactivity increases either during the disease process, upon entering of the CNS/CSF, or during long-term antigen stimulation within the CNS. CSF-derived and clonally expanded TCC during disease exacerbation show a considerably higher degree of cross-reactivity/degeneracy than previously studied peripheral blood-derived TCC (M. Sospedra, unpublished observation; 169, 170). Some of these TCC further demonstrate a high degree of promiscuity in HLA restriction, i.e., restriction by both MS-associated DR and DQ molecules (M. Sospedra, unpublished observation).

HLA-RESTRICTION AND FUNCTIONAL CHARACTERISTICS OF AUTOREACTIVE $CD4^+$ T CELLS   Most myelin-specific $CD4^+$ T cells are restricted by HLA-DR molecules (68, 69, 71, 116–118, 121, 168, 171). MBP-specific T cell lines are mainly restricted by MS-associated DR alleles (Figure 3), and the immunodominant peptides are either promiscuous binders to all of them [$MBP_{(83-99)}$] or are recognized with one HLA molecule, e.g., $MBP_{(111-129)}$ with DRB1*0401 (121). Investigators do not currently know what accounts for these parallels, but the peptide binding characteristics of the disease-associated class II alleles, as well as the preferential generation of certain protein fragments by the processing machinery, are probably important. A few myelin-specific T cell lines have been restricted by DQ or DP molecules (68, 71), although the reasons are not clear. Nonetheless, the observation that myelin-specific T cells in Japanese patients with Asian-type (optico-spinal) MS were in part HLA-DP5-restricted supports the notion that important interactions occur among specific HLA class II molecules, T cell response, and disease characteristics, because HLA-DP5 is associated with Asian-type MS (172). Another study suggests that HLA-DP can be relevant for epitope spreading in MS (173).

With respect to function, the aggregate data support the idea that myelin-specific T cells are skewed toward a Th1 phenotype (72, 108, 111, 132, 174). It is important to consider the methodology of the respective study and the patients' disease state and subtype. Fluctuations of cytokine secretion have, for example, been linked to the MRI-documented inflammatory activity, and elevated expression of IFN-γ and TNF-α and reduced IL-10 have correlated with disease activity (175). Even though inflammation decreases during SP-MS (Figure 1), the secretion of proinflammatory cytokines IL-12, IL-18, and IFN-γ are elevated during later stages (176, 177), the activation of Th1 cells is less strictly controlled, and Th1 markers CCR5 and TIM-3 are upregulated (178, 179). When the specificity and cytokine expression of high-avidity T cells has been linked to MRI characteristics in MS patients, correlations have been observed between MOG-specific Th0/2 cells and less inflammation, as well as between MBP-specific Th1 cells and a more destructive disease process (108).

The cytotoxic activity of $CD4^+$ T cells is relatively poorly understood compared with that of $CD8^+$ T cells. MBP-specific $CD4^+$ T cells mediate both perforin- and

Fas/Fas-L-mediated cytotoxicity of MBP or MBP peptide–pulsed targets. When comparing MBP-specific T cells restricted by either DR2a or DR2b, only the former employ perforin-mediated killing or are noncytotoxic, whereas DR2b-restricted T cells exclusively exhibit Fas/Fas-L-mediated cytolysis (122, 171, 180, 181). Currently, it is not known how this relates to the pathogenesis of MS. It is unlikely that direct lysis of oligodendrocytes, and even fewer neurons, involves CD4$^+$ T cells because neither type of CNS cells express HLA class II. A subtype of MBP-specific CD4$^+$ TCR$\alpha\beta^+$ T cells expresses the neural cell adhesion molecule family member CD56 (also a marker for NK cells) and is capable of lysing CD56$^+$ target cells via homotypic CD56-CD56 interactions independent of HLA restriction (180). A number of CNS cells, including oligodendrocytes, express CD56, and CD4$^+$ CD56$^+$ T cells can indeed lyse oligodendrocytes in an HLA-unrestricted fashion (182).

Furthermore, the requirement for costimulation, i.e., the interaction of CD80/86 on APCs with CD28 on T cells, as well as the control via the negative costimulator CTLA-4, is perturbed in CD4$^+$ T cells in MS. CD4$^+$ myelin-specific T cells, as well as T cells with specificity for other antigens, are less dependent or independent of costimulation (183–186), and they do not respond, or respond less, to CTLA-4 (185, 187). The latter is due to the absence of CTLA-4 upon activation on CD4$^+$ CD28$^-$ T cells. Furthermore, this cell population is characterized by a clear Th1 skew, seemingly increased proliferative capacity, and relative enrichment for autoreactive T cells (185). The susceptibility to activation-induced cell death via Fas/Fas-L interactions is not generally impaired. However, data—including the increased expression of the antiapoptotic molecules survivin, bcl-2, and inhibitor of apoptosis (IAP) family members IAP, IAP-2 and X-IAP in MS T cells, their heightened expression during disease exacerbations, and downregulation by IFN-β—all suggest that the regulation of apoptosis is perturbed in MS, although some aspects are not different from controls.

CD4$^+$ immunoregulatory T cells (Tregs) are characterized by CD25^{high} expression and the transcription factor Fox-P3 (188, 189). CD4$^+$CD25$^+$ Tregs suppress T cell proliferation by both cell-cell contact and cytokine-mediated mechanisms. The number and function of CD4$^+$CD25$^+$ Tregs appear reduced in MS patients (190). CD4$^+$ Th2/3 cells and their cytokines IL-4, IL-10, and TGF-β are probably largely beneficial in MS (191); however, under certain circumstances Th2 cells can induce EAE (192), and Th2-controlled cell populations, e.g., mast cells, can contribute to tissue damage in MS.

TCR REPERTOIRE   Early EAE studies have demonstrated a restricted TCR repertoire in some models. Initial data in MS patients appeared to confirm these data, and a restricted expression of Vβ17 was described (193); however, this particular report was heavily influenced by data from one individual. Subsequent research has described a restricted TCR repertoire either within single MS patients, but not interindividually (194), or across the entire MS populations (195), or not (196). Among the most often found Vβ chains are Vβ5.2, Vβ5.3, and Vβ6.2

(117, 195, 197), or in PLP-specific T cells Vβ2 (136). Subsequent studies have examined CDR3 spectratypes or oligoclonality by single-strand conformational polymorphism typing and sequencing (136, 197–201). They described (*a*) an association of oligoclonal TCR CDR3 spectratypes, particularly in Vβ5.2 T cells (200); (*b*) prevalence of TCR Vβ13-associated junctional sequences at disease onset (198); (*c*) increased MBP reactivity and IFN-γ and IL-2 secretion in CD4$^+$ and CD8$^+$ T cells with altered CDR3 length distributions (199); (*d*) an oligoclonal expansion of T cells with distinct TCRs in the CSF (201; M. Sospedra, unpublished observation); and (*e*) the observation of Vβ5.2-associated junctional sequences from MS brain–derived TCRs similar to an MBP TCC (117, 197), as well as CDR3 motifs in PLP-specific T cells that showed homologies with TCRs from MS brains (136). Finally, the comparison of the TCR Vα chain usage in monozygous concordant and discordant twins showed that the overall TCR Vα chain repertoire in discordant twins is different, and not only in MBP-specific but also in tetanus-specific T cells (202). A recent study that focused on the CDR3 spectratypes in naive T cells of discordant monozygous twins found similar distortions in both the healthy and diseased twins (203). Such repertoire shifts in naive T cells may predispose one to MS development, but they are probably not sufficient.

CD8$^+$ T Cells

Much less is known about CD8$^+$ T cells than CD4$^+$ T cells, not only in MS but in other human autoimmune diseases as well. Technical difficulties in growing and characterizing CD8$^+$ TCC have probably contributed to this temporary neglect. In the context of effector functions, however, CD8$^+$ T cells are much better suited than CD4$^+$ T cells to mediate CNS damage for the following reasons: (*a*) Except for microglia, none of the resident CNS cells express MHC class II; it can be induced on astrocytes by IFN-γ (32), but not on oligodendrocytes or neurons, and therefore the latter can only be recognized by CD8$^+$ T cells (204, 205); (*b*) prominent oligoclonal expansions of CD8$^+$ memory T cells have been found in the CSF (31) and in MS brain tissue (206), and a persistence of CD8$^+$ TCC in CSF and blood (206); (*c*) CD8$^+$ T cells are more prevalent in MS brain tissue than are CD4$^+$ T cells (207); (*d*) MHC class I can be induced on neurons that are functionally compromised (208), and CD8$^+$ virus-specific T cells can directly lyse neurons via Fas/Fas-L-mediated cytolysis (205); (*e*) a number of HLA class I–restricted myelin epitopes have been described for MBP, PLP, MAG, and others (110, 209–211), and the CD8$^+$ cytotoxic T cell response to MBP is increased in MS patients (211); (*f*) CD8$^+$ myelin-specific T cells secrete chemoattractants (IL-16 and IP-10) for CD4$^+$ myelin-specific T cells (212); and (*g*) the MBP$_{(79-87)}$-specific CD8$^+$ TCC from wild-type C3H mice are encephalitogenic and induce a disease phenotype that resembles MS more closely with respect to the presence of ataxia and spasticity than some of the CD4$^+$ T cell–mediated EAE models (10) (Figure 2). Further data supporting a role for CD8$^+$ T cells in MS are the increased production of lymphotoxin (LT) in SP-MS patients, their increased adhesion to brain venules, an increased frequency of $CD8^+$ T cells against EBV epitopes in MS patients, and a correlation between cytokine production by $CD8^+$ T cells and MRI-documented tissue destruction (213). Taken together, there is little doubt that both $CD4^+$ and $CD8^+$ T cell responses contribute to MS pathogenesis, albeit at different steps and with different roles.

B Cells and Antibodies in MS

The observation that Igs are elevated in the CSF of MS patients (214) has been the most important and earliest evidence suggesting a role for B cells and antibodies in the pathology of MS. The correlations between increased CSF Ig with episodes of worsening and the absence of OCB in some patients with benign MS also suggest the involvement of humoral responses.

B cells do not cross the intact BBB; however, once inflammation has started, B cells, antibodies, and complement can enter the CNS. The observation of increased Igs in the CSF in MS patients (214), but not in the serum, indicates local production. B cell activation can occur because of stimulation with antigen from either self or foreign proteins, through a random bystander effect during inflammation in MS lesions, or by superantigen stimulation. Sequence analysis of the Ig variable regions have shown a high frequency of clonally expanded memory B cells that express variable heavy chain-4 type in MS CSF (215) and also in lesions (216, 217), which suggests selection by a specific antigen. In addition, CSF Igs of MS patients show an oligoclonal distribution, i.e., only a limited number of B cell clones contributes to the increased CSF Igs (218, 219). B cells and antibodies can contribute to MS disease pathogenesis in various ways. (*a*) B cells can serve as APCs for autoreactive T cells. Supporting this mechanism is the observation that the epitope specificity of the antibodies generated during EAE, the encephalitogenic T cell epitopes, and the immunodominant T and B cell epitopes in humans often overlap (220, 221). (*b*) B cells provide costimulation to autoreactive T cells. (*c*) B cells and tissue-bound Ig can recruit autoreactive T cells to the CNS (222). (*d*) Idiotope-specific T cells may be activated by CSF Igs, and these T cells sustain B cells that produce such idiotopes (164). (*e*) The production of myelin-specific antibodies and the destruction of myelin within plaques appear to be the most important way that B cells contribute to pathogenesis.

In 1959, investigators demonstrated that humoral factors may have a role in inflammatory demyelination by the in vitro demyelinating activity of a serum factor (223), which was later identified as myelin-specific Igs. Further support came from histopathological studies of CNS tissue and the analysis of CSF. B cells, plasma cells, and myelin-specific antibodies are detected in MS plaques and in areas of active demyelination in MS patients (224–226). Antibodies can cause demyelination by opsonization of myelin for phagocytosis (227–229). Another antibody-mediated mechanism of demyelination acts via complement activation, leading to membrane attack complex (MAC) deposition and complement-mediated cytolysis (230). Studies of MS lesions found complement in areas of active demyelination

(5, 231), and neurological disability and terminal complement concentrations in CSF correlate in MS (232). MAC-enriched vesicles in MS CSF support this mechanism (233). The demyelinating potential of antibody in EAE has been correlated with complement fixation, and soluble complement receptor inhibits EAE severity.

The antigen specificity or specificities of CSF antibodies in MS have yet to be established. Most of the CSF OCB are not directed against the major myelin components (234), but sometimes against infectious agents (235). Several comprehensive reviews have been published on this subject (236–238), and below we emphasize recent data. Assuming a pathogenic role of autoantibodies in MS, the search for autoantigens has focused on myelin proteins and other CNS components. A pathogenic contribution of MBP-specific antibodies in EAE has not been established and is controversial in MS. Although some studies emphasize the relevance of MBP-specific antibodies (239, 240), others fail to confirm these data. Unbiased screenings of antigen libraries with CSF Igs did not identify MBP epitopes (241). Technical considerations, as well as the low-affinity interactions of these antibodies (242), contribute to the controversial results. Increased numbers of anti-PLP-secreting B cells have been detected in the CSF of MS patients (243), and those with a prominent anti-PLP response are distinct from patients with anti-MBP antibodies (244). Igs against minor myelin components have also been shown. MOG is the most interesting candidate B cell autoantigen in MS. Anti-MOG antibodies are able to cause myelin destruction in EAE (245–248), in contrast to anti-MBP or -PLP antibodies (249). Anti-MOG antibodies have also been found in human MS lesions (226). The B cell response to MOG is enhanced in MS (145, 250). Serum anti-MOG antibodies in patients with first CNS symptoms of MS and MRI lesions are predictive of subsequent exacerbations and the diagnosis of definitive MS (251); however, because anti-MOG antibodies are also frequent in controls, important questions remain.

Antibodies with specificity against minor myelin components, other autoantigens, lipids, and DNA are summarized in Table 3. The observation that autoantibodies against ubiquitous antigens are present in MS suggests that less biased search approaches should be applied. A recent flow cytometry study compared antibody binding to human cell lines between patients with MS and patients with other inflammatory CNS diseases (252). The study observed antibodies to oligodendrocyte precursors without differences between RR-MS and SP-MS. Binding to a neuronal cell line was increased in SP-MS. Although the antigens targeted by these antibodies have to be elucidated, this approach to identifying accessible cell surface autoantigens that could mediate demyelination or neuronal damage appears promising. Another unbiased method employs array-based or proteomics technologies to characterize autoantibodies directed against candidate antigens in cohorts of autoimmune and control patients, as well as in experimental autoimmune conditions (253).

Interestingly, antibodies may also play beneficial roles in two ways. First, they may skew the cytokine pattern toward Th2. Rats treated with an encephalitogenic

TABLE 3   Antibody specificities against CNS components other than MOG and MBP

Target antigen	Remarks
Myelin-associated glycoprotein (MAG)	Low titers in MS; possible involvement in progression
Oligodendrocyte-specific protein (OSP)	Minor myelin component
2'3'cyclic nucleotide 3'-phosphodiesterase (CNPase)	—
Transaldolase-H	Oligodendrocyte component
Glyco-shingolipids	Lipid component of myelin
Sulfatides	Lipid component of myelin
GD1a and GM3 (ganglioside)	Lipid component of myelin
Galactocerebroside (Gal-C)	Major myelin lipid; anti-Gal-C has demyelinating activity in vitro; anti-Gal-C antibodies exacerbate EAE
α-B crystallin (small heat shock protein)	Detected in MS sera; isotype prevalence controversial
Neurofilament-L (NF-L)	Elevated in MS CSF, suggested as indicator of axonal damage; elevated in the CSF in progressive MS
AN2 (oligodendrocyte surface glycoprotein)	Expression of AN2 on oligodendrocyte precursor cells suggests involvement in suppression of remyelination
Nogo-A (neurite outgrowth inhibitor)	Anti-Nogo antibodies are frequent in serum and CSF of MS patients, but also in controls
Proteasome (protein complex involved in processing and chaperone function)	Anti-proteasome antibodies found in serum and CSF in MS
DNA	High-affinity antibodies found in MS CSF; from the role of anti-DNA antibodies in CNS lupus, it is speculated that they might bind to neurons and oligodendrocytes

peptide of MBP coupled to monoclonal anti-IgD are resistant to induction of EAE after sequent challenge with MBP in CFA (254). Second, antibodies against CNS components, e.g., Nogo-A, can foster myelin repair. IgM antibodies against certain CNS antigens enhance remyelination in different animal models of MS (255). Further evidence for a beneficial role of antibodies stems from the use of pooled intravenous Ig in the therapy of MS (256), which acts through a number of mechanisms, including Fc-receptor blockade, inactivation of cytokines, complement inhibition, blocking of CD4 and MHC, and modulation of apoptosis (257).

INNATE IMMUNE MECHANISMS IN MS

Innate immune responses involve (*a*) recognition of conserved molecular structures produced by microbial pathogens via TLRs, cells such as macrophages, neutrophils, and mast cells, and effector mechanisms such as the production of lysozyme, lactoferrin, phagocyte oxidase, and nitric oxide; and (*b*) the recognition of molecular structures expressed only on normal, uninfected host cells that serve as indicators of "normality" and inhibit immune activation [NK cells, complement, and receptors of the C-type lectin family (258)]. Although the innate immune system's main role is self-protection and maintenance of homeostasis, innate immune mechanisms can in some circumstances result in destructive autoimmunity. We summarize important findings and include observations that suggest a role for NKT cells and $\gamma\delta$ T cells in the pathogenesis of MS.

Toll-Like Receptors (TLR)

TLR function as sentinels by recognizing conserved pathogen-associated molecular patterns and generating proinflammatory signals that initiate adaptive immune responses. They are expressed by a wide array of immune and nonimmune cells. Inappropriate TLR signaling may contribute to diseases such as MS. TLR engagement on dendritic cells (DCs) inhibits immunosuppressive effects of $CD4^+CD25^+$ regulatory cells on effector T cells via IL-6 (259), and mice deficient in IL-6 are more resistant to induction of autoimmune diseases (260). TLRs could further play a role by breaking peripheral tolerance to self-antigens during chronic infections. Assuming that autoreactive T cells are part of the normal T cell population and tightly regulated, it has been hypothesized that tolerance is maintained in a similar manner to mature T cells after recognition of antigen presented by resting or inactivated DCs (261). Under normal conditions, APCs remain in their resting state and induce tolerance in autoreactive T cells, whereas danger signals activate APCs and may convert tolerized autoreactive T cells into effector cells. The increase of MS exacerbations around viral infections supports this concept (56), and pretreatment of mice with bacterially derived DNA exacerbates EAE (262). In a recent EAE study, the stimulation of TLR9 with CpG oligonucleotides breaks tolerance and renders lymph node cells reactive against a self-antigen to which they were previously unresponsive (86, 263).

Mast Cells

Mast cells are activated during allergic reactions through crosslinking of surface IgE receptors, which leads to degranulation of multiple mediators. Mast cells are ubiquitously distributed among tissues including the brain, but their numbers in the CNS are low and their role unclear. Investigators have suggested several effects of mast cells in MS (264). Elevated numbers in MS plaques were originally shown in 1890 (265) and later confirmed by others (266). They are attracted to MS lesions via chemokines. RANTES, a potent attractant for mast cells, is elevated in

MS lesions (39). Interestingly, mast cell–released mediators such as tryptase and histamine are increased in the CSF of MS patients. Gene expression profiling of MS plaques also demonstrated elevated expression of mast cell mediators in acute lesions (36). Mast cells and their mediators can act in MS during BBB opening and augment CNS infiltration via increased recruitment, adhesion, rolling, and extravasation of leukocytes through the chemokines/cytokines lymphotactin and IL-16, through TNF-α and IL-1-mediated induction of ICAM-1 and VCAM-1 expression, and through the effects of histamine and tryptase on leukocyte rolling. Mast cell proteases such as tryptase and chymase activate matrix metalloproteinase (MMP) precursors, and mast cells can also synthesize MMP-2 and MMP-9 directly. It has been suggested that mast cells may act as APCs and influence MS by shaping Th1/Th2 responses, but a clear demonstration of this role is lacking. Finally, mast cell degranulation in response to MBP can lead to demyelination in vitro via proteolytic enzymes. Mast cell mediators can participate in the destruction of oligodendrocytes and neurons. With respect to the gender bias of MS and the elevated inflammatory activity in women, it is interesting to note that mast cells express estrogen receptors.

Nitric Oxide Synthase

Phagocytes (granulocytes and macrophages) are equipped with the enzymatic machinery to generate highly toxic reactive oxygen and nitrogen intermediates, which exert potent antimicrobial activities. The enzyme inducible nitric oxide synthase (iNOS) generates large amounts of nitric oxide (NO), a short-lived and bioactive free radical that is toxic to bacteria. NOS has been found in MS lesions, suggesting a role in MS pathology (267). Although initial studies have shown that NO can mediate microglia-induced cytotoxicity (268) and also necrosis of rodent oligodendrocytes (269), the actual role of NOS in CNS injury in MS is not clear. Results from blocking NOS in EAE are not conclusive, and additional data suggest that NO may even have an antiapoptotic effect or modulate immune responses in a beneficial way.

NK Cells

An association between decreased NK cell activity and MS was first reported in 1980 (270), and later studies expanded this knowledge (271), although findings remain controversial. Potential explanations are disease heterogeneity among patient groups and fluctuations of NK activity and number during the disease course. NK lysis is reduced prior to and during acute exacerbations compared with chronic disease (271, 272) and normal during stable phases. Multi-parameter flow cytometry demonstrated that NK cells are significantly reduced in MS (273). Furthermore, NK deficiencies exist in peripheral blood, placques, and CSF of MS patients (274). Furthermore, NK cell depletion in two different EAE models exacerbate disease (275, 276), whereas the transfer of in vitro generated NK cells decrease autoimmunity (277). NK cells could suppress autoimmunity by cytokine production (IL-5,

IL-13, TGF-β) or by the induction of target lysis via perforin- and/or TRAIL-dependent mechanisms. Supporting data come from perforin-deficient lpr mice that developed severe autoimmunity (278) and blockage of TRAIL-exacerbated EAE (279). In a recent phase II clinical trial with a humanized monoclonal antibody against the IL-2 receptor α chain in MS (280), we observed marginal effects on CD4$^+$ T cells but an expansion of CD56^{bright} immunoregulatory NK cells. The relative and absolute expansion of the latter NK cell population and their increased perforin expression correlate highly with the reduction of the inflammatory activity, and in vitro experiments demonstrated direct lysis of activated CD4$^+$ T cells via perforin (B. Bielekova, unpublished observation). These observations indicate that NK cells may exert important immunoregulatory functions in MS.

Complement

Complement serves as an auxiliary system in antimicrobial defenses. The human brain is considered an immunoprivileged site and separated from the periphery via the BBB. Nevertheless, all major CNS cells produce most of the complement proteins. Astrocytes are the main CNS complement source, thus providing immune defense against pathogens, and also contributing to damage in some diseases. Demyelination not only results from an autoimmune response against myelin via the classical pathway, but also from direct complement activation after binding of complement to myelin. Purified CNS myelin, but not PNS myelin, can activate the classical pathway (281). Furthermore, mature rat oligodendrocytes are lysed in vitro by complement in the absence of antimyelin antibodies (282). MOG may be capable of binding and activating the C1q component of complement (283) because it harbors a domain similar to the C1q-binding sequence of antibodies. Complement activation results in oligodendrocyte lysis and chemoattraction of macrophages. Susceptibility of oligodendrocytes to complement injury could be facilitated by the lack of the protective and ubiquitously distributed complement inhibitors. CR1 (CD35), membrane cofactor protein (CD46), and homologous restriction factor were not expressed on oligodendrocytes, whereas CD59 showed substantial heterogeneity (283, 284).

NKT Cells

NKT cells share characteristics with T and NK cells and play a regulatory role in autoimmunity as well as in immune responses to tumors and infections via secretion of high levels of IL-4 and IFN-γ. Both CD4$^-$ and CD4$^+$ cells contain NKT cells, and in humans CD4$^-$ and CD4$^+$ cells express a conserved canonical TCRα chain, Vα24JαQ, paired with a selected Vβ11 segment. NKT cells recognize glycolipids presented by the nonclassical class I–like CD1d molecule (285). A considerable reduction of Vα24JαQ$^+$ cells among Vα24$^+$ cells has been observed in MS blood (286) and confirmed by another group that also showed reduced Vα24 Vβ11$^+$ NKT cells (287). A further study failed to detect decreased NKT cells within Vα24$^+$ cells, but did detect reduced production of IL-4 by Vα24JαQ TCC (288). A role for NKT cells in MS is supported by EAE data. An analog of α-galactosylceramide (GalCer), a synthetic glycolipid that binds CD1d and stimulates mouse and human NKT cells, suppresses EAE by selective IL-4 induction (289). CD4$^+$ NKT cells are probably the main NKT regulatory population.

$\gamma\delta$ T Cells

$\gamma\delta$ T cells represent another distinct lymphocyte population that mediates host defense and immunoregulatory functions. The expression of NK cell inhibitory receptors on human $\gamma\delta$ T cells indicates a role for $\gamma\delta$ T cells in tumor immunity and autoimmunity. Two main fractions of $\gamma\delta$ T cells have been described. One fraction of $\gamma\delta$ T cells expresses Vγ1 within epithelial tissues, where it may provide a first line of defense against infections and cancer. The second fraction that expresses Vγ2 represents the majority of peripheral blood $\gamma\delta$ T cells. This fraction infiltrates chronic lesions and is detected in the CSF of MS patients (290, 291). Interestingly, oligodendrocytes selectively stimulate the expansion of the Vγ2 subtype of $\gamma\delta$ T cells (292). Limited TCR heterogeneity of CSF-infiltrating $\gamma\delta$ T cells in MS suggests a common antigen reactivity (293, 294). Human $\gamma\delta$ T cells can lyse oligodendrocytes via perforin without the need for APCs, possibly through recognition of heat shock proteins (291, 295), αB crystallin, or even non-peptide antigens (296). These findings, together with EAE studies in which $\gamma\delta$ T cells appear to be important early mediators of damage (297), support a role for $\gamma\delta$ T cells in MS pathogenesis.

CYTOKINES AND CHEMOKINES IN MS

Cytokines

Cytokines orchestrate all phases of immune responses, act in highly complex, dynamic networks in paracrine and/or autocrine fashion, and often exert overlapping and in part redundant functions via multi-component receptor molecules that may be shared by different cell types. To maintain homeostasis, a dynamic balance between pro- and anti-inflammatory cytokines is required. Proinflammatory cytokines are thought to play a role in the pathogenesis of MS via immune system activation in the periphery and/or by directly damaging the oligodendrocyte/myelin unit. Anti-inflammatory cytokines, e.g., IL-4, have been considered beneficial. We summarize the main findings about proinflammatory cytokines (IFN-γ, TNF-α, IL-12, IL-17, and IL-23), anti-inflammatory cytokines (IL-4, IL-10), and others exerting both effects (IL-6) in MS (298). Proinflammatory cytokines can participate in the pathogenesis of MS at different points. Elevated numbers of blood cells expressing TNF-α mRNA (299), serum TNF-α concentrations (300), and PBMC secreting TNF-α (301) have been reported in MS patients. Nevertheless, therapy with a soluble TNF-α receptor Ig fusion protein or anti-TNF-α leads to increased and prolonged MS exacerbations (302). Results about IFN-γ in the blood of MS patients are conflicting. Although higher numbers of PBMC expressing IFN-γ mRNA and serum levels (300) have been found in MS, other studies found no differences (303). A therapeutic trial with IFN-γ in MS resulted in disease exacerbation (304). The role of IFN-γ in EAE is also not clear. The prevailing perception is that IFN-γ-secreting T cells are encephalitogenic, but IFN-γ-knockout animals develop much worse or even lethal EAE compared with wild-type littermates. IL-12, a main stimulator of IFN-γ has been implicated as a proinflammatory cytokine (305), but recent data indicate that IL-23, a cytokine that shares the p40 chain with IL-12, is the main mediator of these effects (306). In MS, some studies have reported higher numbers of PBMC expressing IL-12 p40 mRNA (307), but other studies found no differences (308).

Data about anti-inflammatory cytokines in MS are similarly contradictory. Decreased numbers of PBMC secreting IL-10 and lower serum levels of IL-10 in MS have been reported (309). Moreover, investigators have described decreases in IL-10 expression but elevated numbers of PBMC expressing IL-10 mRNA before clinical relapses (310). Therefore, the role of IL-10 in MS is currently not clear. Increased levels of IL-6, a cytokine with pro- and anti-inflammatory capacities, have been shown in MS patient serum (301). Within the CSF and brain, proinflammatory cytokines can damage the oligodendrocyte/myelin unit. Higher numbers of mononuclear CSF cells expressing TNF-α and IFN-γ have been detected in MS patients. TNF-α has proinflammatory functions but is also involved in tissue repair in the brain. Proinflammatory cytokines have also been found in active MS lesions (311, 312). The expression of TNF-α is elevated in active demyelinating lesions compared with inactive/remyelinating lesions (313), and transgenic mice overexpressing TNF-α and IFN-γ driven by the astrocyte-specific GFAP promoter induced demyelination (314). Investigators have proposed different mechanisms for this demyelination: (a) TNF-α and IFN-γ may be toxic for oligodendrocytes; (b) cytokines may activate macrophages and microglia, which then phagocytose myelin; and (c) proinflammatory cytokines may be involved in apoptosis induction/execution and subsequent demyelination. The addition of IFN-γ to cultured oligodendrocytes renders them susceptible to Fas ligand–mediated apoptosis by inducing Fas expression on their surface (315). The proinflammatory cytokines IL-12 and IL-17 are also elevated in CSF and brain lesion of MS patients (36).

Unexpectedly high numbers of cells expressing IL-4 mRNA have been observed in MS CSF lesions (316). Studies on IL-10 and IL-6 have been contradictory. Assuming a beneficial role of the Th2 cytokines, at least two interpretations can be proposed: (a) These cytokines, mainly IL-10, could be involved in MS pathogenesis by augmenting B cell proliferation, differentiation, and antibody production. In line with this hypothesis, a correlation between IL-10 levels and IgG in the CSF of MS patients has been reported (317). (b) The presence of IL-4, IL-10, and TGF-β in CSF or MS brain parenchyma could reflect ongoing immunoregulatory mechanisms that are initiated after disease exacerbations and are important for disease resolution/prevention in EAE (318).

Chemokines

Chemokines and their receptors play a central role in the inflammatory recruitment of leukocytes and other cell types. Trafficking of inflammatory T cells into the CNS is a crucial step in MS and begins with weak adhesion and rolling on the endothelium of the BBB, followed by firm arrest on the luminal side of the endothelium and subsequent diapedesis across the BBB. Chemokines induce and activate leukocyte adhesion molecules that mediate firm adhesion to the endothelium and establish a chemotactic concentration gradient that results in recruitment across the endothelial monolayer. The induction of proteolytic enzymes facilitates BBB opening (319), and subsequently chemokines mediate retention of leukocytes in the CNS. Numerous reports analyze the roles of chemokines and their receptors in intrathecal accumulation of T cells in MS (320). Among the various chemokine receptors, CCR5 and CXCR3 have received attention as key receptors on Th1 cells, as have CCR3 and CCR4 on Th2 cells. Furthermore, CCR7, an important marker for the capacity of mononuclear cells to migrate to secondary lymphoid organs, is also of interest. This section summarizes the main findings on chemokines in the blood, CSF, and lesions in MS.

BLOOD   CCR5 expression is increased on circulating T cells in MS patients (321, 322) and during disease relapse, suggesting a pathogenic role of CCR5$^+$ T cells (323). Increased CXCR3 expression on circulating T cells has been shown in some but not all studies (322). T cells expressing CCR5 and CXCR3 in MS produce high quantities of IFN-γ and TNF-α (324), and MBP-specific Th1 cells express high levels of CXCR3 and CXCR6 (325). The effects of IFN-β treatment on chemokine and chemokine receptor expression are controversial.

CSF   CCL5 (RANTES) and CXCL10 (IP-10) are elevated in MS CSF, whereas CCL2 (MCP-1) is significantly decreased (326). The increase of CXCL10 (IP-10) and decrease of CCL2 (MCP-1) has been confirmed to take place during MS exacerbations and not to occur during remissions (327). CCL2 (MCP-1) decreases correlate with active MRI, i.e., presence of inflammation and gadolinium-enhancing lesions in the brain (328), suggesting a Th1 polarization in active MS. CCL3 (MIP-1α) has been found in the CSF of MS patients, as well as in other neuroinflammatory diseases. The source of these chemokines in the CSF remains to be elucidated.

With respect to chemokine receptors, initial studies document a higher proportion of CSF T cells that express CXCR3 and CCR5 (326) compared with PBMC. Because CSF T cells are enriched for the CD4$^+$/CD45RO$^+$ subset, corrections for this bias have shown that only CXCR3, but not other receptors (CCR1-3, CCR5, and CCR6), is relatively increased on CSF (329). Interestingly, the same has been observed in controls and interpreted such that the presence of CXCR3$^+$ cells in the CSF is independent of CNS inflammation (326). CXCR3 expression probably facilitates the entry of T cells into the CSF, and CXCL10 (IP-10) mediates the retention in the inflamed CNS. CCR5$^+$ and CXCR3$^+$ Th1 cells in the CSF also express CCR7 (330), and CSF-infiltrating monocytes express higher CCR1 and CCR5 levels (331). But similar results were obtained in controls, suggesting that the presence of CCR1$^+$/CCR5$^+$ monocytes in the CSF is independent of CNS inflammation.

BRAIN LESIONS   A number of chemokines and the corresponding receptors have been detected in MS brain lesions, indicating that they might evolve into interesting therapeutic targets. CCL3 (MIP-1α), CCL4 (MIP-1β), and CCL5 (RANTES) are expressed within MS lesions, CCL4 in parenchymal inflammatory cells (macrophages and microglia), CCL3 also in parenchymal inflammatory cells and activated neuroglia (332), and CCL5 in perivascular inflammatory cells and (though less so) in astrocytes (39, 332, 333). Other chemokines in active MS lesions include CCL2 (MCP-1), CCL7 (MCP-3), CCL8 (MCP-2), and CXCL10 (IP-10). CXCR3 is expressed on the majority of perivascular T cells in MS brain lesions, and CCR5 on a subset of these cells. CCR1 has been found on newly infiltrating monocytes (331), CCR2 and CCR3 on macrophages (333), and CCR5 on infiltrating monocytes and activated microglia cells (324, 326, 333).

A role for chemokines and their receptors in MS is supported by EAE data. Increased expression of CCL2, CCL3, CCL5, and CXCL10 in EAE is associated with disease progression, and in vivo depletion improves EAE (334). Mice deficient in CCR2 (335), and to a lesser extent in CCR1 (336), fail to exhibit EAE symptoms. In contrast, CCR5-deficient mice showed disease severity similar to controls (337), which suggests that T cell accumulation in the CNS during EAE does not function through CCR5.

Polymorphisms in genes for chemokines and their receptors have been proposed to confer susceptibility or protection in MS, although definitive evidence is still lacking. The CCR5 Δ32 mutation leads to a nonfunctional receptor that has been associated with decreased severity of MS. Although homozygous individuals for CCR5 Δ32 were not protected from MS, heterozygosity for Δ32 has been linked to prolonged disease-free intervals and a delay in MS onset. Microsatellite polymorphisms in CCL7 (MCP-3) have also been associated with disease resistance to MS.

PATHOGENETIC STAGES IN THE DISEASE PROCESS IN MS: LESION PATHOLOGY

Figure 4 summarizes the most important events in MS. Potentially autoreactive CD4$^+$ T cells are activated in the periphery by recognizing, for example, a viral peptide in the context of costimulatory and other less-defined signals (step 1). Factors that contribute to a proinflammatory environment include a number of cytokines from both T cells and APCs (e.g., IL-12, IFN-γ), the strength of activation, and the infectious context ("danger"). Activated autoreactive T cells

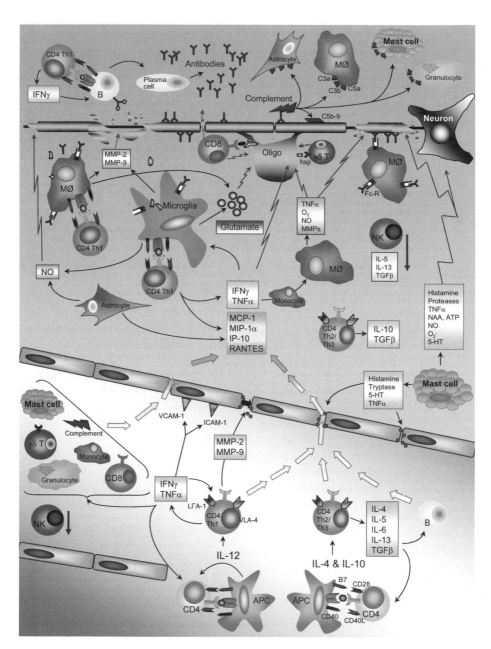

Figure 4 Schematic diagram depicting the pathogenetic steps and contributing factors that lead to tissue damage in MS (see text for details).

adhere to the BBB endothelium via adhesion molecules (LFA-1 and VLA-4), and transmigrate into the brain parenchyma through cerebrovascular endothelial cells (step 2). Several mechanisms are still unclear, including what guides autoreactive $CD4^+$ T cells to the CNS; whether antigen presentation is required in deep cervical lymph nodes, a putative draining site for brain-derived antigen; and whether a chemokine gradient from inside the brain parenchyma to the blood exists during the initial event. However, experiments in EAE have shown that adoptively transferred encephalitogenic T cells are transiently found in deep cervical lymph nodes and then locally reactivated in the CNS, as shown by downmodulation of their TCR (338). Subsequently, proinflammatory cytokines (IFN-γ, IL-23, TNF-α, LT) and chemokines (RANTES, IP-10, IL-8, and others) (*a*) activate resident cells, such as microglia and astrocytes; (*b*) recruit other immune cells, including monocytes, $CD8^+$ T cells, B cells, and mast cells, from the peripheral blood; and (*c*) orchestrate the formation of the inflammatory lesion (step 3) . The formation of the inflammatory lesion is characterized by an open BBB with tissue edema after mediator/protease release from mast cells, monocytes, and T cells, as well as by a host of proinflammatory molecules and oxygen and nitrogen radicals. Damage of CNS tissue, i.e., the myelin sheath, oligodendrocytes, and axons, occurs already at this early inflammatory stage (step 4). During the above steps, $CD4^+$ autoreactive T cells are likely driving the process, whereas their role in the effector phase is probably secondary. Numerous processes may lead to myelin/oligodendrocyte and axonal damage, including radicals, TNF-α, LT, and direct complement deposition, as well as antibody-mediated complement activation and antibody-dependent cellular cytotoxicity via Fc-receptors, myelin phagocytosis, direct lysis of axons by $CD8^+$ cytotoxic T lymphocytes, the secretion of proteases, and apoptosis of oligodendrocytes. Furthermore, the increased production and decreased degradation or reuptake of the excitatory neurotransmitter glutamate by astrocytes leads to glutamate-mediated excitotoxicity of oligodendrocytes via glutamate receptor-mediated calcium influx (12). The inflammatory event lasts from a few days to two weeks. The "aftermath" is characterized by stretches of demyelinated axons, apoptotic oligodendrocytes and T cells, axon transsections with onion bulb-like protrusions owing to interrupted axonal transport (339) (Figure 1), macrophages loaded with phagocytosed myelin lipids, and the activation and beginning proliferation of astrocytes. Besides clearing debris, lesion resolution (step 5) further includes a relative dominance of Th2/Th3 cytokines, such as IL-10 and TGF-β, and the secretion of various growth factors (brain-derived neurotrophic factor, platelet-derived growth factor, ciliary neurotrophy factor, and fibroblast growth factors) by both resident cells and T cells. Oligodendrocyte precursors that are still present in the adult CNS are also activated, and surviving oligodendrocytes begin to re-myelinate denuded internode areas, although the original thickness of the compact myelin is not reached again and hence nerve conduction velocity is slower in these "repaired" areas, despite some compensatory redistribution of sodium channels. Inhibitory signals between axonal and myelin structures, including Nogo, MAG, and OMgp, all of which interact with Nogo receptors and are physiologically relevant during shaping and maintenance of the intricate cytoarchitecture in the CNS, impede the repair process (340). "Repaired" myelin differs from mature adult myelin in its relative composition of myelin protein isoforms and/or post-translational modifications. The relative abundance of citrullinated C8-MBP is one example. C8-MBP is less basic than mature MBP owing to modification of six arginines into citrullines (341). C8-MBP increases during the course of MS and probably results in functionally impaired myelin, as well as in increased vulnerability to further damage (342). C8-specific T cells have been found in MS patients. During the months and years following an inflammatory event, the cellular composition of the plaque changes dramatically. Chronic plaques may show smoldering inflammation, but they are often devoid of inflammatory cells and characterized by loss of myelin and axons, relative increases in astrocytes (but overall lower cellularity), and deposition of scar tissue.

The cellular composition and involved molecular pathways vary among patients (5). Besides the recognition of pathological heterogeneity, other "forgotten" aspects, such as axonal injury, have received new attention (339). Investigators have identified four pathologic MS subtypes on the basis of the relative contribution of different immune cells, antibody and complement deposition, myelin loss, and oligodendrocyte death (5). Interestingly, patterns differ interindividually, but not intraindividually. The following pathologic subtypes are described by Brück and colleagues (343):

Pattern I. This pattern is predominated by T cells and macrophages, and candidate effector molecules include TNF-α, IFN-γ, and radical species.

Pattern II. In this pattern, antibody and complement deposition predominate, and both MOG- and MBP-specific antibodies are involved. The mechanism of tissue destruction shares similarities with those observed in Guillain Barré syndrome, an acute inflammatory demyelinating disease of the PNS.

Pattern III. Lesions impress by preferential loss of MAG and oligodendrogliopathy, and a vasculitic mechanism is suspected on the basis of parallels with focal cerebral ischemia. Furthermore, the vulnerability of oligodendrocytes may be increased by immune responses against heat shock proteins in this pattern.

Pattern IV. This pattern, marked by nonapoptotic oligodendrocyte degeneration, is the least common and occurs primarily in PP-MS (343). The overall extent of inflammation is highest in RR-MS and declines over time, with the evolution into SP-MS (Figure 1).

Further pathologic observations that deserve mention include the axonal loss, which was originally described by Charcot (92) and others in the mid-nineteenth century. Substantial axonal loss may occur during the earliest stages of disease. It is closely related to neurological disability, and, as mentioned above, several effector mechanisms, including antiganglioside antibodies and CD8[+] CTL, are probably involved. Finally, a number of findings indicate that contributors to tissue vulnerability and aberrant repair include the vulnerability of CNS tissue, the local dysregulation of apoptosis mechanisms such as higher expression of bcl-2 on oligodendrocytes during RR-MS, glutamate-mediated excitotoxicity (12, 344), and the reexpression of developmentally important recognition molecules (Jagged1/Notch) (13).

LESSONS FROM THERAPIES

The concept of MS as an autoimmune inflammatory disease is supported by the response to immunomodulatory and suppressive treatments. Glucocorticoids, applied intravenously and at high doses during acute clinical exacerbations of MS, act broadly as anti-inflammatory agents by reducing edema and arachidonic acid metabolites and by decreasing and modulating IL-1, IL-2, IL-4, IL-5, IL-6, IFN-γ, TNF-$\alpha\beta$, fibrin deposition, and other mechanisms.

A number of chemotherapeutic agents with similarly broad activities but long-term immunosuppressive effects are used at more advanced stages of the disease, i.e., the transition from RR-MS to SP-MS, or in patients with aggressive disease who do not respond or who incompletely respond to the approved agents. Immunosuppressants include mitoxantrone, cyclophosphamide, methotrexate, azathioprine, cladribin, and mycophenolate. Interestingly, their mechanism of action in autoimmune diseases is relatively poorly understood; however, we do know that cyclophosphamide not only has apoptosis-inducing activities but also induces Th2 cells in MS.

IFN-β is approved for treatment of RR-MS and is currently the agent that is most broadly used. It was originally explored as an antiviral agent, but in recent years it has been shown that it has immunomodulatory activities. These immunomodulatory activities include the upregulation and increased shedding of adhesion molecules, induction of IL-10 and neurotrophic factors, blocking of BBB opening via inhibition of MMP-2 and -9, and reduction of cell adhesion to the BBB. IFN-β reduces disease exacerbations by only about 30% and has a modest impact on disease progression. IFN-β is a clear step forward in MS therapy, but the frequency of subcutaneous injections of IFN-β, the flu-like symptoms that occur at the beginning of therapy, the modest activity required of patients, and the treatment failures are all reasons to search for better agents.

Glatiramer-acetate (GA, copolymer-1, Cop-1) is another approved therapy for RR-MS, with similar or slightly lower efficacy than IFN-β at high doses. However, GA has a more favorable side-effect profile than IFN-β (345). GA is a random copolymer of the four amino acids Ala, Lys, Glu, and Tyr, with various lengths and fixed molar ratios of 4.5:3.6:1.5:1 (346). It was originally developed as a mimic of MBP and to induce EAE (346). Fortuitously, GA blocks the experimental disease (346). Initially, it was assumed that it acts primarily by displacing autoantigenic peptides from HLA class II binding grooves, i.e., via competition for binding. Later, a host of other activities were shown, including polyclonal T cell stimulation, partial agonist effects, Th2 activation and cross-reactivity with myelin peptides, shift of the antibody response toward IgG4, interference with DC differentiation, and induction of brain-derived neurotrophic factors (347, 348). The most important effect of GA is most likely the relative skew toward Th2 reactivity. When inflammatory activity is monitored via MRI, IFN-β reduces BBB opening almost immediately, but it takes much longer until an effect of GA is observed. Currently, attempts are ongoing to develop better defined and more active peptidic compounds.

Other promising therapeutic strategies include humanized monoclonal antibodies against VLA-4 (natalizumab), which blocks BBB migration of T cells and their activation and reduces brain inflammation (349), and against the IL-2 receptor α chain (daclizumab), which activates and expands immunoregulatory NK cells (280). Daclizumab reduces brain inflammation by almost 80% in patients with high disease activity who have failed IFN-β treatment (280), but daclizumab is also effective as monotherapy (J. Rose, personal communication). Anti-CD52 leads to long-lasting lymphopenia and also reduces inflammatory activity in MS (350). Numerous other monoclonal antibodies (e.g., against CD20$^+$ B cells and CD40L) are either in preclinical or clinical testing. Promising results have also been observed with estriols (51) and the cholesterin-lowering statins (351, 352).

Further strategies include modulators of cAMP levels, e.g., phosphodiesterase type 4 inhibitor, pentoxifylline (353), and β-adrenergic agents, inhibitors of chemokine receptors (CCR2 antagonists), blocking agents of CD4, retinoic acid, vitamin A and D derivatives, peroxisome proliferator-activated receptoragonists, DNA vaccination, and numerous others. Many of these agents have appeared promising in EAE but later not shown activity in MS. For example, the phosphodiesterase type 4 inhibitor Rolipram had shown prophylactic and therapeutic activity in EAE, but in a recent clinical trial in MS showed no disease reduction (B. Bielekova, unpublished observation). Paradoxic effects have been observed with therapies aimed at TNF or TNF-receptors (see above). Furthermore, in rheumatoid arthritis, where TNF-blocking agents have become standard therapy, a number of cases developed acute inflammatory demyelination or MS. Caution must therefore be used both in extrapolating animal data to humans or information from one autoimmune disease to another.

REESTABLISHING TOLERANCE

Reestablishing tolerance to autoantigens and specific and subtle therapeutic interventions remain important goals. The question is whether they can be achieved in complex and heterogeneous diseases such as MS. Currently, investigators are pursuing two main lines. The first is modulation of antigen-specific T cell responses via induction of anergy or activation-induced cell death. The latter is achieved through intravenous immunization with either autoantigenic peptides, proteins/fusion proteins, or DNAs that code for these proteins with and without covaccination with DNAs coding for anti-inflammatory cytokines, or by APL peptides. The second investigative line is methods to induce anti-idiotypic T cells directed either at TCR CDR2 or CDR3 regions of autoantigen-specific TCR chains, or vaccination with whole, inactivated, autoreactive T cells.

Currently, it is not clear whether either of these approaches can be successful. We have already mentioned the negative experience with a high dose of APL peptide, which not only led to hypersensitivity reactions but also to disease exacerbations (101). Lower doses appeared to induce a Th2 bias, and a currently ongoing trial with the same APL will hopefully solve whether APL therapy is viable. T cell vaccination (354) or immunization with CDR2 peptides have been well tolerated (355). With respect to their mechanisms, the induction of CDR2-specific T cells that secreted IL-10 has been shown (355). T cell vaccination has led to the reduction of MBP-specific T cells, apparently via CD8$^+$ cytolytic T cells, and treatment with anti-Vβ5.2/5.3 led to the reduction of Vβ5.2/5.3-expressing T cells; however, the effect on reducing MRI activity was below expectations (356). In summary, our incomplete understanding of antigen-specific T cell responses in MS, the disease heterogeneity, and its complex pathogenesis are among the factors that render specific immune intervention very challenging.

A more drastic approach toward reestablishing tolerance is hematopoietic stem cell transplantation (HSCT) via abrogation of the hematopoietic or lymphopoietic system by chemotherapy/irradiation, or optionally via lymphocyte-depleting steps such as antilymphocyte antibodies and subsequent infusion of autologous hematopoietic (CD34$^+$) stem cells. Although still considered a high-risk procedure, HSCT offers the prospect of stopping the autoimmune process and curing at least the inflammatory aspects. Recent trials revealed that (*a*) inflammatory disease activity is completely halted in the majority of patients (357); (*b*) progression of clinical disability continues in patients with advanced disease (358, 359) and therefore HSCT probably must be applied earlier when neurological deficit is limited but the patient clearly has aggressive disease; (*c*) low-risk protocols have to be explored and improved, and such studies are currently ongoing; and (*d*) long-term follow-up is necessary, and we need to understand the mechanism of action. With respect to the latter point, HSCT indeed leads to rejuvenation of the immune system, with increased recent thymic emigrants, reactivation of the thymus, a net increase of naive CD4$^+$ T cells, and the reestablishment of a more diverse TCR repertoire. Transiently after HSCT, there is also increased apoptosis of T cells and a relative increase of CD4$^+$CD25$^+$ regulatory T cells (P.A. Muraro, unpublished observation).

New approaches toward specific immune intervention clearly need to be defined, but recent progress in immunomodulation has been very promising. We believe that future therapies toward tissue repair and neuroprotection are only meaningful if the inflammatory components of MS can be contained or completely stopped.

CONCLUDING REMARKS

Exciting progress has been made in understanding MS pathogenesis in the past decade. Every aspect has become more complicated, and our previous concept of MS as "simply" a CD4$^+$ Th1 cell–mediated autoimmune disease must be revisited. We now recognize that the complex genetic background in concert with environmental triggers—most likely common viral infections, but mitigated by many other factors—is responsible for the heterogeneity of every aspect of the disease, including pathologic mechanisms, clinical and MRI presentation, and response to treatments. Many components of the innate and adaptive immune systems, and in the latter CD4$^+$ T cells, CD8$^+$ T cells, and antibodies, all contribute to different aspects of the disease process. In addition, factors other than the autoimmune response clearly shape the disease. The vulnerability of the CNS to inflammatory insult and/or its inability to repair tissue is equally heterogeneous among different patients, and we will only understand the full scope of disease etiology and pathogenesis if we consider both immune system and nervous system and their mutual interactions in MS. The latter point is particularly relevant when we try to block the disease process or even repair already inflicted damage and prevent it in the future through single agent, cell-based, or combination therapies. These treatments will likely become much more complex than those currently applied.

APPENDIX

Abbreviations used: αB-C, α-B crystallin; ADCC, antibody-dependent cellular cytotoxicity; APC, antigen-presenting cell; APL, altered peptide ligand; APOE, apolipoprotein E; BBB, blood-brain barrier; CNPase, 2′,3′-cyclic nucleotide 3′ phosphodiesterase; CNS, central nervous system; Cpn, *Chlamydia pneumoniae;* CTLA, cytotoxic T lymphocyte–associated antigen; DC, dendritic cell; EAE, experimental allergic encephalomyelitis; EBV, Epstein-Barr virus; ELISPOT, enzyme-linked immunospot; GA, glatiramer-acetate; G-CSF, granulocyte colony-stimulating factor; GFAP, glial fibrillary acidic protein; HHV, human herpesvirus; HLA, histocompatibility leukocyte antigen; HSCT, hematopoietic stem cell transplantation; HSV, herpes simplex virus; IAP, inhibitor of apoptosis; IFN, interferon; IP, IFN-γ-inducible protein; LT, lymphotoxin; MAC, membrane attack complex; MAG, myelin-associated glycoprotein; MBP, myelin basic protein; MCP, monocyte chemoattractant protein; MHC, major histocompatibility complex; MRI, magnetic resonance imaging; MMP, matrix metalloproteinase; MOBP, myelin-associated oligodendrocytic basic protein; MOG, myelin oligodendrocyte glycoprotein; MS, multiple sclerosis; NO, nitric oxide; NOS, nitric oxide synthase; OCB, oligoclonal bands; OSP, oligodendrocyte-specific glycoprotein; PBMC, peripheral blood mononuclear cells; PLP, proteolipid protein; PNS, peripheral nervous system; PP-MS, primary progressive MS; RR-MS, relapsing-remitting MS; SP-MS, secondary progressive MS; TCC, T cell clones; TCR, T cell receptor; TGF, transforming growth factor, TLR, Toll-like receptor; TNF, tumor necrosis factor; TRAIL, TNF-related apoptosis-inducing ligand; Treg, immunoregulatory T cell; VZV, varicella zoster virus.

ACKNOWLEDGMENTS

We realize that many studies could not be considered, and we apologize to the authors of these works. Our summary views try, however, to take them into account.

I (R.M.) thank Hans-Wolfgang Kreth, MD, Department of Pediatrics, University of Würzburg, Germany, my first teacher in immunology, and Henry F. McFarland, MD, Neuroimmunology Branch, NINDS, NIH, Bethesda, my long-term mentor, for his advice and support. Further, we acknowledge the work of our coworkers and prior investigators at the Cellular Immunology Section and Neuroimmunology Branch, NINDS, NIH, whose research during recent years has contributed to this review.

The *Annual Review of Immunology* is online at
http://immunol.annualreviews.org

LITERATURE CITED

1. McFarlin DE, McFarland HF. 1982. Multiple sclerosis (first of two parts). *N. Engl. J. Med.* 307:1183–88
2. McFarlin DE, McFarland HF. 1982. Multiple sclerosis (second of two parts). *N. Engl. J. Med.* 307:1246–51
3. McFarland HF. 1999. Correlation between MR and clinical findings of disease activity in multiple sclerosis. *Am. J. Neuroradiol.* 20:1777–78
4. Raine CS, Scheinberg LC. 1988. On the immunopathology of plaque development and repair in multiple sclerosis. *J. Neuroimmunol.* 20:189–201
5. Lucchinetti C, Bruck W, Parisi J, Scheithauer B, Rodriguez M, Lassmann H. 2000. Heterogeneity of multiple sclerosis lesions: implications for the pathogenesis of demyelination. *Ann. Neurol.* 47:707–17
6. Martin R, McFarland HF, McFarlin DE. 1992. Immunological aspects of demyelinating diseases. *Annu. Rev. Immunol.* 10:153–87
7. Hafler DA. 2004. Multiple sclerosis. *J. Clin. Invest.* 113:788–94
8. Zamvil SS, Steinman L. 1990. The T lymphocyte in experimental allergic encephalomyelitis. *Annu. Rev. Immunol.* 8:579–621
9. Pettinelli CB, McFarlin DE. 1981. Adoptive transfer of experimental allergic encephalomyelitis in SJL/J mice after in vitro activation of lymph node cells by myelin basic protein: requirement for Lyt 1+ 2-T lymphocytes. *J. Immunol.* 127:1420–23
10. Huseby ES, Liggitt D, Brabb T, Schnabel B, Ohlen C, Goverman J. 2001. A pathogenic role for myelin-specific CD8+ T cells in a model for multiple sclerosis. *J. Exp. Med.* 194:669–76
11. Sun DM, Whitaker JN, Huang ZG, Liu D, Coleclough C, et al. 2001. Myelin antigen-specific CD8+ T cells are encephalitogenic and produce severe disease in C57BL/6 mice. *J. Immunol.* 166:7579–87
12. Pitt D, Werner P, Raine CS. 2000. Glutamate excitotoxicity in a model of multiple sclerosis. *Nat. Med.* 6:67–70
13. John GR, Shankar SL, Shafit-Zagardo B, Massimi A, Lee SC, et al. 2002. Multiple sclerosis: re-expression of a developmental pathway that restricts oligodendrocyte maturation. *Nat. Med.* 8:1115–21
14. Dyment DA, Ebers GC, Sadovnick AD. 2004. Genetics of multiple sclerosis. *Lancet Neurol.* 3:104–10
15. Haines JL, Bradford Y, Garcia ME, Reed AD, Neumeister E, et al. 2002. Multiple susceptibility loci for multiple sclerosis. *Hum. Mol. Genet.* 11:2251–56
16. Ebers GC, Sadovnick AD, Risch NJ. 1995. A genetic basis for familial aggregation in multiple sclerosis. Canadian Collaborative Study Group. *Nature* 377:150–51

17. GAMES, Transatlantic Multiple Sclerosis Genetics Cooperative. 2003. A meta-analysis of whole genome linkage screens in multiple sclerosis. *J. Neuroimmunol.* 143:39–46

18. Hillert J, Olerup O. 1993. HLA and MS. *Neurology* 43:2426–27

19. Haines JL, Terwedow HA, Burgess K, Pericak-Vance MA, Rimmler JB, et al. 1998. Linkage of the MHC to familial multiple sclerosis suggests genetic heterogeneity. *Hum. Mol. Genet.* 7:1229–34

20. Barcellos LF, Oksenberg JR, Begovich AB, Martin ER, Schmidt S, et al. 2003. HLA-DR2 dose effect on susceptibility to multiple sclerosis and influence on disease course. *Am. J. Hum. Genet.* 72:710–16

21. Fogdell-Hahn A, Ligers A, Gronning M, Hillert J, Olerup O. 2000. Multiple sclerosis: a modifying influence of HLA class I genes in an HLA class II associated autoimmune disease. *Tissue Antigens* 55:140–48

22. Fernandez O, Fernandez V, Alonso A, Caballero A, Luque G, et al. 2004. DQB1*0602 allele shows a strong association with multiple sclerosis in patients in Malaga, Spain. *J. Neurol.* 251:440–44

23. Bertram J, Kuwert E. 1982. HLA antigen frequencies in multiple sclerosis. *Eur. J. Neurol.* 7:74–79

24. Sellebjerg F, Jensen J, Madsen HO, Svejgaard A. 2000. HLA DRB1*1501 and intrathecal inflammation in multiple sclerosis. *Tissue Antigens* 55:312–18

25. Ridgway WM, Ito H, Fasso M, Yu C, Fathman CG. 1998. Analysis of the role of variation of major histocompatibility complex class II expression on nonobese diabetic (NOD) peripheral T cell response. *J. Exp. Med.* 188:2267–75

26. Merryman PF, Crapper RM, Lee S, Gregersen PK, Winchester RJ. 1989. Class II major histocompatibility complex gene sequences in rheumatoid arthritis. The third diversity regions of both DRβ1 genes in two DR1, DRw10-positive individuals specify the same inferred amino acid sequence as the DRβ1 and DRβ2 genes of a DR4 (Dw14) haplotype. *Arthritis Rheum.* 32:251–58

27. Ristori G, Carcassi C, Lai S, Fiori P, Cacciani A, et al. 1997. HLA-DM polymorphisms do not associate with multiple sclerosis: an association study with analysis of myelin basic protein T cell specificity. *J. Neuroimmunol.* 77:181–84

28. Matsuoka T, Tabata H, Matsushita S. 2001. Monocytes are differentially activated through HLA-DR, -DQ, and -DP molecules via mitogen-activated protein kinases. *J. Immunol.* 166:2202–8

29. Li F, Linan MJ, Stein MC, Faustman DL. 1995. Reduced expression of peptide-loaded HLA class I molecules on multiple sclerosis lymphocytes. *Ann. Neurol.* 38:147–54

30. Babbe H, Roers A, Waisman A, Lassmann H, Goebels N, et al. 2000. Clonal expansions of CD8$^+$ T cells dominate the T cell infiltrate in active multiple sclerosis lesions as shown by micromanipulation and single cell polymerase chain reaction. *J. Exp. Med.* 192:393–404

31. Jacobsen M, Cepok S, Quak E, Happel M, Gaber R, et al. 2002. Oligoclonal expansion of memory CD8$^+$ T cells in cerebrospinal fluid from multiple sclerosis patients. *Brain* 125:538–50

32. Head JR, Griffin WST. 1985. Functional capacity of solid tissue transplants in brain: evidence for immonological privilege. *Proc. R. Soc. London Ser. B* 224:375–87

33. DeRisi J, Penland L, Brown PO, Bittner ML, Meltzer PS, et al. 1996. Use of a cDNA microarray to analyse gene expression patterns in human cancer. *Nat. Genet.* 14:457–60

34. Whitney LW, Becker KG, Tresser NJ, Caballero-Ramos CI, Munson PJ, et al. 1999. Analysis of gene expression in mutiple sclerosis lesions using cDNA microarrays. *Ann. Neurol.* 46:425–28

35. Whitney LW, Ludwin SK, McFarland HF,

Biddison WE. 2001. Microarray analysis of gene expression in multiple sclerosis and EAE identifies 5-lipoxygenase as a component of inflammatory lesions. *J. Neuroimmunol.* 121:40–48

36. Lock C, Hermans G, Pedotti R, Brendolan A, Schadt E, et al. 2002. Gene-microarray analysis of multiple sclerosis lesions yields new targets validated in autoimmune encephalomyelitis. *Nat. Med.* 8:500–8

37. Tajouri L, Mellick AS, Ashton KJ, Tannenberg AE, Nagra RM, et al. 2003. Quantitative and qualitative changes in gene expression patterns characterize the activity of plaques in multiple sclerosis. *Brain Res. Mol. Brain Res.* 119:170–83

38. Mycko MP, Papoian R, Boschert U, Raine CS, Selmaj KW. 2004. Microarray gene expression profiling of chronic active and inactive lesions in multiple sclerosis. *Clin. Neurol. Neurosurg.* 106:223–29

39. Baranzini SE, Elfstrom C, Chang SY, Butunoi C, Murray R, et al. 2000. Transcriptional analysis of multiple sclerosis brain lesions reveals a complex pattern of cytokine expression. *J. Immunol.* 165:6576–82

40. Chabas D, Baranzini SE, Mitchell D, Bernard CC, Rittling SR, et al. 2001. The influence of the proinflammatory cytokine, osteopontin, on autoimmune demyelinating disease. *Science* 294:1731–35

41. Graumann U, Reynolds R, Steck AJ, Schaeren-Wiemers N. 2003. Molecular changes in normal appearing white matter in multiple sclerosis are characteristic of neuroprotective mechanisms against hypoxic insult. *Brain Pathol.* 13:554–73

42. Achiron A, Gurevich M, Friedman N, Kaminski N, Mandel M. 2004. Blood transcriptional signatures of multiple sclerosis: unique gene expression of disease activity. *Ann. Neurol.* 55:410–17

43. Bomprezzi R, Ringner M, Kim S, Bittner ML, Khan J, et al. 2003. Gene expression profile in multiple sclerosis patients and healthy controls: identifying pathways relevant to disease. *Hum. Mol. Genet.* 12:2191–99

44. Wandinger KP, Sturzebecher CS, Bielekova B, Detore G, Rosenwald A, et al. 2001. Complex immunomodulatory effects of interferon-β in multiple sclerosis include the upregulation of T helper 1-associated marker genes. *Ann. Neurol.* 50:349–57

45. Sturzebecher S, Wandinger KP, Rosenwald A, Sathyamoorthy M, Tzou A, et al. 2003. Expression profiling identifies responder and non-responder phenotypes to interferon-β in multiple sclerosis. *Brain* 126:1419–29

46. Wandinger KP, Lunemann JD, Wengert O, Bellmann-Strobl J, Aktas O, et al. 2003. TNF-related apoptosis inducing ligand (TRAIL) as a potential response marker for interferon-β treatment in multiple sclerosis. *Lancet* 361:2036–43

47. McFarland HF. 1992. Twin studies and multiple sclerosis. *Ann. Neurol.* 32:722–23

48. Wakeland EK, Liu K, Graham RR, Behrens TW. 2001. Delineating the genetic basis of systemic lupus erythematosus. *Immunity* 15:397–408

49. Coo H, Aronson KJ. 2004. A systematic review of several potential non-genetic risk factors for multiple sclerosis. *Neuroepidemiology* 23:1–12

50. Runmarker B, Andersen O. 1995. Pregnancy is associated with a lower risk of onset and a better prognosis in multiple sclerosis. *Brain* 118(Part 1):253–61

51. Sicotte NL, Liva SM, Klutch R, Pfeiffer P, Bouvier S, et al. 2002. Treatment of multiple sclerosis with the pregnancy hormone estriol. *Ann. Neurol.* 52:421–28

52. Kurtzke JF. 1983. Epidemiology of multiple sclerosis. In *Multiple Sclerosis*, ed. JF Hallpike, CWM Adams, WW Tourtelotte, pp. 49–95. Baltimore, MD: Williams & Wilkins

53. Hayes CE. 2000. Vitamin D: a natural

inhibitor of multiple sclerosis. *Proc. Nutr. Soc.* 59:531–35

54. Johnson RT. 1994. The virology of demyelinating diseases. *Ann. Neurol.* 36(Suppl.):S54–60

55. Soldan SS, Jacobson S. 2001. Role of viruses in etiology and pathogenesis of multiple sclerosis. *Adv. Virus Res.* 56: 517–55

56. Sibley WA, Bamford CR, Clark K. 1985. Clinical viral infections and multiple sclerosis. *Lancet* 1:1313–15

57. Goverman J, Woods A, Larson L, Weiner LP, Hood L, Zaller DM. 1993. Transgenic mice that express a myelin basic protein-specific T cell receptor develop spontaneous autoimmunity. *Cell* 72:551–60

58. Challoner PB, Smith KT, Parker JD, MacLeod DL, Coulter SN, et al. 1995. Plaque-associated expression of human herpesvirus 6 in multiple sclerosis. *Proc. Natl. Acad. Sci. USA* 92:7440–44

59. Moore FG, Wolfson C. 2002. Human herpes virus 6 and multiple sclerosis. *Acta Neurol. Scand.* 106:63–83

60. Soldan SS, Leist TP, Juhng KN, McFarland HF, Jacobson S. 2000. Increased lymphoproliferative response to human herpesvirus type 6A variant in multiple sclerosis patients. *Ann. Neurol.* 47:306–13

61. Wandinger KP, Jabs W, Siekhaus A, Bubel S, Trillenberg P, et al. 2000. Association between clinical disease activity and Epstein-Barr virus reactivation in MS. *Neurology* 55:178–84

62. Martyn CN, Cruddas M, Compston DA. 1993. Symptomatic Epstein-Barr virus infection and multiple sclerosis. *J. Neurol. Neurosurg. Psychiatry* 56:167–68

63. Sriram S, Mitchell W, Stratton C. 1998. Multiple sclerosis associated with *Chlamydia pneumoniae* infection of the CNS. *Neurology* 50:571–72

64. Sriram S, Stratton CW, Yao S, Tharp A, Ding L, et al. 1999. *Chlamydia pneumoniae* infection of the central nervous sys-

tem in multiple sclerosis. *Ann. Neurol.* 46:6–14

65. Pucci E, Taus C, Cartechini E, Morelli M, Giuliani G, et al. 2000. Lack of Chlamydia infection of the central nervous system in multiple sclerosis. *Ann. Neurol.* 48:399–400

66. Burns J, Rosenzweig A, Zweiman B, Lisak RP. 1983. Isolation of myelin basic protein-reactive T-cell lines from normal human blood. *Cell Immunol.* 81:435–40

67. Richert JR, McFarlin DE, Rose JW, McFarland HF, Greenstein JI. 1983. Expansion of antigen-specific T cells from cerebrospinal fluid of patients with multiple sclerosis. *J. Neuroimmunol.* 5:317–24

68. Chou YK, Vainiene M, Whitham R, Bourdette D, Chou CH, et al. 1989. Response of human T lymphocyte lines to myelin basic protein: association of dominant epitopes with HLA class II restriction molecules. *J. Neurosci. Res.* 23:207–16

69. Martin R, Jaraquemada D, Flerlage M, Richert J, Whitaker J, et al. 1990. Fine specificity and HLA restriction of myelin basic protein-specific cytotoxic T cell lines from multiple sclerosis patients and healthy individuals. *J. Immunol.* 145:540–48

70. Pette M, Fujita K, Kitze B, Whitaker JN, Albert E, et al. 1990. Myelin basic protein-specific T lymphocyte lines from MS patients and healthy individuals. *Neurology* 40:1770–76

71. Ota K, Matsui M, Milford EL, Mackin GA, Weiner HL, Hafler DA. 1990. T-cell recognition of an immunodominant myelin basic protein epitope in multiple sclerosis. *Nature* 346:183–87

72. Olsson T, Zhi WW, Hojeberg B, Kostulas V, Jiang YP, et al. 1990. Autoreactive T lymphocytes in multiple sclerosis determined by antigen-induced secretion of interferon-γ. *J. Clin. Invest.* 86:981–85

73. Fujinami RS, Oldstone MB. 1985. Amino acid homology between the encephalitogenic site of myelin basic protein and

virus: mechanism for autoimmunity. *Science* 230:1043–45

74. Tejada-Simon MV, Zang YCQ, Hong J, Rivera VM, Zhang JWZ. 2003. Cross-reactivity with myelin basic protein and human herpesvirus-6 in multiple sclerosis. *Ann. Neurol.* 53:189–97

75. Evavold BD, Sloan-Lancaster J, Hsu BL, Allen PM. 1993. Separation of T helper 1 clone cytolysis from proliferation and lymphokine production using analog peptides. *J. Immunol.* 150:3131–40

76. Wucherpfennig KW, Strominger JL. 1995. Molecular mimicry in T cell-mediated autoimmunity: viral peptides activate human T cell clones specific for myelin basic protein. *Cell* 80:695–705

77. Hemmer B, Vergelli M, Gran B, Ling N, Conlon P, et al. 1998. Predictable TCR antigen recognition based on peptide scans leads to the identification of agonist ligands with no sequence homology. *J. Immunol.* 160:3631–36

78. Hemmer B, Pinilla C, Gran B, Vergelli M, Ling N, et al. 2000. Contribution of individual amino acids within MHC molecule or antigenic peptide to TCR ligand potency. *J. Immunol.* 164:861–71

79. Lang HL, Jacobsen H, Ikemizu S, Andersson C, Harlos K, et al. 2002. A functional and structural basis for TCR cross-reactivity in multiple sclerosis. *Nat. Immunol.* 3:940–43

80. Ohashi PS, Oehen S, Buerki K, Pircher II, Ohashi CT, et al. 1991. Ablation of "tolerance" and induction of diabetes by virus infection in viral antigen transgenic mice. *Cell* 65:305–17

81. Oldstone MB, Nerenberg M, Southern P, Price J, Lewicki H. 1991. Virus infection triggers insulin-dependent diabetes mellitus in a transgenic model: role of anti-self (virus) immune response. *Cell* 65:319–31

82. Olson JK, Croxford JL, Miller SD. 2004. Innate and adaptive immune requirements for induction of autoimmune demyelinating disease by molecular mimicry. *Mol. Immunol.* 40:1103–8

83. Tough DF, Sprent J. 1996. Viruses and T cell turnover: evidence for bystander proliferation. *Immunol. Rev.* 150:129–42

84. Murali-Krishna K, Altman JD, Suresh M, Sourdive DJ, Zajac AJ, et al. 1998. Counting antigen-specific CD8 T cells: a reevaluation of bystander activation during viral infection. *Immunity* 8:177–87

85. Brocke S, Gaur A, Piercy C, Gautam A, Gijbels K, et al. 1993. Induction of relapsing paralysis in experimental autoimmune encephalomyelitis by bacterial superantigen. *Nature* 365:642–44

86. Waldner H, Collins M, Kuchroo VK. 2004. Activation of antigen-presenting cells by microbial products breaks self tolerance and induces autoimmune disease. *J. Clin. Invest.* 113:990–97

87. Miller SD, Vanderlugt CL, Begolka WS, Pao W, Yauch RL, et al. 1997. Persistent infection with Theiler's virus leads to CNS autoimmunity via epitope spreading. *Nat. Med.* 3:1133–36

88. Horwitz MS, Bradley LM, Harbertson J, Krahl T, Lee J, Sarvetnick N. 1998. Diabetes induced by Coxsackie virus: initiation by bystander damage and not molecular mimicry. *Nat. Med.* 4:781–85

89. Barnaba V. 1996. Viruses, hidden self-epitopes and autoimmunity. *Immunol. Rev.* 152:47–66

90. Opdenakker G, Van Damme J. 1994. Cytokine-regulated proteases in autoimmune diseases. *Immunol. Today* 15:103–7

91. Pender MP. 2003. Infection of autoreactive B lymphocytes with EBV, causing chronic autoimmune diseases. *Trends Immunol.* 24:584–88

92. Charcot J. 1868. Histologie de la sclerose en plaque. *Gaz. Hopitaux* 41:554–66

93. Remlinger J. 1905. Accidents paralytiques au cours du traitment antirabique. *Ann. Inst. Pasteur* 19:625–46

94. Rivers TM, Sprunt DH, Berry GP. 1933. Observations on attempts to produce acute disseminated encephalomyelitis in monkeys. *J. Exp. Med.* 58:39–53

95. Ben-Nun A, Cohen IR. 1982. Experimental autoimmune encephalomyelitis (EAE) mediated by T cell lines: process of selection of lines and characterization of the cells. *J. Immunol.* 129:303–8

96. Das P, Drescher KM, Geluk A, Bradley DS, Rodriguez M, David CS. 2000. Complementation between specific HLA-DR and HLA-DQ genes in transgenic mice determines susceptibility to experimental autoimmune encephalomyelitis. *Hum. Immunol.* 61:279–89

97. Kawamura K, Yamamura T, Yokoyama K, Chui DH, Fukui Y, et al. 2000. HLA-DR2-restricted responses to proteolipid protein 95–116 peptide cause autoimmune encephalitis in transgenic mice. *J. Clin. Invest.* 105:977–84

98. Forsthuber TG, Shive CL, Wienhold W, deGraaf K, Spack EG, et al. 2001. T cell epitopes of human myelin oligodendrocyte glycoprotein identified in HLA-DR4 (DRB1*0401) transgenic mice are encephalitogenic and are presented by human B cells. *J. Immunol.* 167:7119–25

99. Madsen LS, Andersson EC, Jansson L, Krogsgaard M, Andersen CB, et al. 1999. A humanized model for multiple sclerosis using HLA-DR2 and a human T-cell receptor. *Nat. Genet.* 23:343–47

100. Quandt JA, Baig M, Yao K, Kawamura K, Huh J, et al. 2004. Unique clinical and pathological features in HLA-DRB1*0401-restricted MBP 111–129–specific humanized transgenic mice. *J. Exp. Med.* 200:223–34

101. Bielekova B, Goodwin B, Richert N, Cortese I, Kondo T, et al. 2000. Encephalitogenic potential of the myelin basic protein peptide (amino acids 83–99) in multiple sclerosis: results of a phase II clinical trial with an altered peptide ligand. *Nat. Med.* 6:1167–75

102. Berger T, Weerth S, Kojima K, Linington C, Wekerle H, Lassmann H. 1997. Experimental autoimmune encephalomyelitis: the antigen specificity of T lymphocytes determines the topography of lesions in the central and peripheral nervous system. *Lab. Invest.* 76:355–64

103. Wekerle H, Kojima K, Lannes-Vieira J, Lassmann H, Linington C. 1994. Animal models. *Ann. Neurol.* 36:S47–53

104. Schluesener HJ, Wekerle H. 1985. Autoaggressive T lymphocyte lines recognizing the encephalitogenic region of myelin basic protein: in vitro selection from unprimed rat T lymphocyte populations. *J. Immunol.* 135:3128–33

105. Martin R, Voskuhl R, Flerlage M, McFarlin DE, McFarland HF. 1993. Myelin basic protein-specific T-cell responses in identical twins discordant or concordant for multiple sclerosis. *Ann. Neurol.* 34:524–35

106. Bieganowska KD, Ausubel LJ, Modabber Y, Slovik E, Messersmith W, Hafler DA. 1997. Direct ex vivo analysis of activated, Fas-sensitive autoreactive T cells in human autoimmune disease. *J. Exp. Med.* 185:1585–94

107. Muraro PA, Wandinger KP, Bielekova B, Gran B, Marques A, et al. 2003. Molecular tracking of antigen-specific T cell clones in neurological immune-mediated disorders. *Brain* 126:20–31

108. Bielekova B, Sung MH, Kadom N, Simon R, McFarland H, Martin R. 2004. Expansion and functional relevance of high-avidity myelin-specific CD4+ T cells in multiple sclerosis. *J. Immunol.* 172:3893–904

109. Hong J, Zang YCQ, Li SF, Rivera VM, Zhang JWZ. 2004. Ex vivo detection of myelin basic protein-reactive T cells in multiple sclerosis and controls using specific TCR oligonucleotide probes. *Eur. J. Immunol.* 34:870–81

110. Crawford MP, Yan SX, Ortega SB, Mehta RS, Hewitt RE, et al. 2004. High prevalence of autoreactive, neuroantigen-specific CD8+ T cells in multiple sclerosis revealed by novel flow cytometric assay. *Blood* 103:4222–31

111. Olsson T, Sun J, Hillert J, Hojeberg B, Ekre HP, et al. 1992. Increased numbers

of T cells recognizing multiple myelin basic protein epitopes in multiple sclerosis. *Eur. J. Immunol.* 22:1083–87

112. Allegretta M, Nicklas JA, Sriram S, Albertini RJ. 1990. T cells responsive to myelin basic protein in patients with multiple sclerosis. *Science* 247:718–21

113. Trotter JL, Damico CA, Cross AH, Pelfrey CM, Karr RW, et al. 1997. HPRT mutant T-cell lines from multiple sclerosis patients recognize myelin proteolipid protein peptides. *J. Neuroimmunol.* 75:95–103

114. Seamons A, Perchellet A, Goverman J. 2003. Immune tolerance to myelin proteins. *Immunol. Res.* 28:201–21

115. Bruno R, Sabater L, Sospedra M, Ferrer-Francesch X, Escudero D, et al. 2002. Multiple sclerosis candidate autoantigens except myelin oligodendrocyte glycoprotein are transcribed in human thymus. *Eur. J. Immunol.* 32:2737–47

116. Pette M, Fujita K, Wilkinson D, Altmann DM, Trowsdale J, et al. 1990. Myelin autoreactivity in multiple sclerosis: recognition of myelin basic protein in the context of HLA-DR2 products by T lymphocytes of multiple sclerosis patients and healthy donors. *Proc. Natl. Acad. Sci. USA* 87:7968–72

117. Martin R, Howell MD, Jaraquemada D, Flerlage M, Richert J, et al. 1991. A myelin basic protein peptide is recognized by cytotoxic T cells in the context of four HLA-DR types associated with multiple sclerosis. *J. Exp. Med.* 173:19–24

118. Valli A, Sette A, Kappos L, Oseroff C, Sidney J, et al. 1993. Binding of myelin basic protein peptides to human histocompatibility leukocyte antigen class II molecules and their recognition by T cells from multiple sclerosis patients. *J. Clin. Invest.* 91:616–28

119. Wucherpfennig KW, Sette A, Southwood S, Oseroff C, Matsui M, et al. 1994. Structural requirements for binding of an immunodominant myelin basic protein peptide to DR2 isotypes and for its recognition by human T cell clones. *J. Exp. Med.* 179:279–90

120. Vogt AB, Kropshofer H, Kalbacher H, Kalbus M, Rammensee HG, et al. 1994. Ligand motifs of HLA-DRB5*0101 and DRB1*1501 molecules delineated from self-peptides. *J. Immunol.* 153:1665–73

121. Muraro PA, Vergelli M, Kalbus M, Banks DE, Nagle JW, et al. 1997. Immunodominance of a low-affinity major histocompatibility complex-binding myelin basic protein epitope (residues 111–129) in HLA-DR4 (B1*0401) subjects is associated with a restricted T cell receptor repertoire. *J. Clin. Invest.* 100:339–49

122. Vergelli M, Kalbus M, Rojo SC, Hemmer B, Kalbacher H, et al. 1997. T cell response to myelin basic protein in the context of the multiple sclerosis-associated HLA-DR15 haplotype: peptide binding, immunodominance and effector functions of T cells. *J. Neuroimmunol.* 77:195–203

123. Richert JR, Robinson ED, Deibler GE, Martenson RE, Dragovic LJ, Kies MW. 1989. Human cytotoxic T-cell recognition of a synthetic peptide of myelin basic protein. *Ann. Neurol.* 26:342–46

124. Wraith DC, Smilek DE, Mitchell DJ, Steinman L, McDevitt HO. 1989. Antigen recognition in autoimmune encephalomyelitis and the potential for peptide-mediated immunotherapy. *Cell* 59:247–55

125. Fairchild PJ, Wraith DC. 1992. Peptide-MHC interaction in autoimmunity. *Curr. Opin. Immunol.* 4:748–53

126. Lafaille JJ, Nagashima K, Katsuki M, Tonegawa S. 1994. High incidence of spontaneous autoimmune encephalomyelitis in immunodeficient anti-myelin basic protein T cell receptor transgenic mice. *Cell* 78:399–408

127. Krogsgaard M, Wucherpfennig KW, Cannella B, Hansen BE, Svejgaard A, et al. 2000. Visualization of myelin basic protein (MBP) T cell epitopes in multiple sclerosis lesions using a monoclonal

antibody specific for the human histocompatibility leukocyte antigen (HLA)-DR2-MBP 85–99 complex. *J. Exp. Med.* 191: 1395–412

128. Klein L, Klugmann M, Nave K-A, Tuohy VK, Kyewski B. 2000. Shaping of the autoreactive T-cell repertoire by a splice variant of self protein expressed in thymic epithelial cells. *Nat. Med.* 6:56–62

129. Waldner H, Whitters MJ, Sobel RA, Collins M, Kuchroo VK. 2000. Fulminant spontaneous autoimmunity of the central nervous system in mice transgenic for the myelin proteolipid protein-specific T cell receptor. *Proc. Natl. Acad. Sci. USA* 97:3412–17

130. Kennedy MK, Tan LJ, Dal Canto MC, Tuohy VK, Lu ZJ, et al. 1990. Inhibition of murine relapsing experimental autoimmune encephalomyelitis by immune tolerance to proteolipid protein and its encephalitogenic peptides. *J. Immunol.* 144: 909–15

131. Vanderlugt CL, Miller SD. 2002. Epitope spreading in immune-mediated diseases: implications for immunotherapy. *Nat. Rev. Immunol.* 2:85–95

132. Correale J, McMillan M, McCarthy K, Le T, Weiner LP. 1995. Isolation and characterization of autoreactive proteolipid protein-peptide specific T-cell clones from multiple sclerosis patients. *Neurology* 45:1370–78

133. Greer JM, Csurhes PA, Cameron KD, McCombe PA, Good MF, Pender MP. 1997. Increased immunoreactivity to two overlapping peptides of myelin proteolipid protein in multiple sclerosis. *Brain* 120(Part 8):1447–60

134. Pelfrey CM, Trotter JL, Tranquill LR, McFarland HF. 1993. Identification of a novel T cell epitope of human proteolipid protein (residues 40–60) recognized by proliferative and cytolytic CD4$^+$ T cells from multiple sclerosis patients. *J. Neuroimmunol.* 46:33–42

135. Pelfrey CM, Trotter JL, Tranquill LR, McFarland HF. 1994. Identification of a second T cell epitope of human proteolipid protein (residues 89–106) recognized by proliferative and cytolytic CD4$^+$ T cells from multiple sclerosis patients. *J. Neuroimmunol.* 53:153–61

136. Kondo T, Yamamura T, Inobe J, Ohashi T, Takahashi K, Tabira T. 1996. TCR repertoire to proteolipid protein (PLP) in multiple sclerosis (MS): homologies between PLP-specific T cells and MS-associated T cells in TCR junctional sequences. *Int. Immunol.* 8:123–30

137. Mendel I, Kerlero de Rosbo N, Ben-Nun A. 1995. A myelin oligodendrocyte glycoprotein peptide induces typical chronic experimental autoimmune encephalomyelitis in H-2b mice: fine specificity and T cell receptor Vβ expression of encephalitogenic T cells. *Eur. J. Immunol.* 25:1951–59

138. Bettelli E, Pagany M, Weiner HL, Linington C, Sobel RA, Kuchroo VK. 2003. Myelin oligodendrocyte glycoprotein-specific T cell receptor transgenic mice develop spontaneous autoimmune optic neuritis. *J. Exp. Med.* 197:1073–81

139. Tsunoda I, Kuang LQ, Theil DJ, Fujinami RS. 2000. Antibody association with a novel model for primary progressive multiple sclerosis: induction of relapsing-remitting and progressive forms of EAE in H2s mouse strains. *Brain Pathol.* 10:402–18

140. Kerlero de Rosbo N, Hoffman M, Mendel I, Yust I, Kaye J, et al. 1997. Predominance of the autoimmune response to myelin oligodendrocyte glycoprotein (MOG) in multiple sclerosis: reactivity to the extracellular domain of MOG is directed against three main regions. *Eur. J. Immunol.* 27:3059–69

141. Wallstrom E, Khademi M, Andersson M, Weissert R, Linington C, Olsson T. 1998. Increased reactivity to myelin oligodendrocyte glycoprotein peptides and epitope mapping in HLA DR2(15)$^+$ multiple sclerosis. *Eur. J. Immunol.* 28:3329–35

142. Koehler NK, Genain CP, Giesser B,

Hauser SL. 2002. The human T cell response to myelin oligodendrocyte glycoprotein: a multiple sclerosis family-based study. *J. Immunol.* 168:5920–27

143. Iglesias A, Bauer J, Litzenburger T, Schubart A, Linington C. 2001. T- and B-cell responses to myelin oligodendrocyte glycoprotein in experimental autoimmune encephalomyelitis and multiple sclerosis. *Glia* 36:220–34

144. Weissert R, Kuhle J, de Graaf KL, Wienhold W, Herrmann MM, et al. 2002. High immunogenicity of intracellular myelin oligodendrocyte glycoprotein epitopes. *J. Immunol.* 169:548–56

145. Lindert RB, Haase CG, Brehm U, Linington C, Wekerle H, Hohlfeld R. 1999. Multiple sclerosis: B- and T-cell responses to the extracellular domain of the myelin oligodendrocyte glycoprotein. *Brain* 122(Part 11):2089–100

146. Steck AJ, Murray N, Meier C, Page N, Perruisseau G. 1983. Demyelinating neuropathy and monoclonal IgM antibody to myelin-associated glycoprotein. *Neurology* 33:19–23

147. Morris-Downes MM, McCormack K, Baker D, Sivaprasad D, Natkunarajah J, Amor S. 2002. Encephalitogenic and immunogenic potential of myelin-associated glycoprotein (MAG), oligodendrocyte-specific glycoprotein (OSP) and 2′,3′-cyclic nucleotide 3′-phosphodiesterase (CNPase) in ABH and SJL mice. *J. Neuroimmunol.* 122:20–33

148. Andersson M, Yu M, Soderstrom M, Weerth S, Baig S, et al. 2002. Multiple MAG peptides are recognized by circulating T and B lymphocytes in polyneuropathy and multiple sclerosis. *Eur. J. Neurol.* 9:243–51

149. Birnbaum G, Kotilinek L, Schlievert P, Clark HB, Trotter J, et al. 1996. Heat shock proteins and experimental autoimmune encephalomyelitis (EAE): I. Immunization with a peptide of the myelin protein 2′,3′ cyclic nucleotide 3′ phosphodiesterase that is cross-reactive with a heat shock protein alters the course of EAE. *J. Neurosci. Res.* 44:381–96

150. Rosener M, Muraro PA, Riethmuller A, Kalbus M, Sappler G, et al. 1997. 2′,3′-cyclic nucleotide 3′-phosphodiesterase: a novel candidate autoantigen in demyelinating diseases. *J. Neuroimmunol.* 75:28–34

151. Muraro PA, Kalbus M, Afshar G, McFarland HF, Martin R. 2002. T cell response to 2′,3′-cyclic nucleotide 3′-phosphodiesterase (CNPase) in multiple sclerosis patients. *J. Neuroimmunol.* 130:233–42

152. Holz A, Bielekova B, Martin R, Oldstone MB. 2000. Myelin-associated oligodendrocytic basic protein: identification of an encephalitogenic epitope and association with multiple sclerosis. *J. Immunol.* 164:1103–9

153. Kaye JF, Kerlero de Rosbo N, Mendel I, Flechter S, Hoffman M, et al. 2000. The central nervous sytem-specific myelin oligodendrocytic basic protein (MOBP) is encephalitogenic and a potential target antigen in multiple sclerosis (MS). *J. Neuroimmunol.* 102:189–98

154. Arbour N, Holz A, Sipe JC, Naniche D, Romine JS, et al. 2003. A new approach for evaluating antigen-specific T cell responses to myelin antigens during the course of multiple sclerosis. *J. Neuroimmunol.* 137:197–209

155. Bronstein JM, Lallone RL, Seitz RS, Ellison GW, Myers LW. 1999. A humoral response to oligodendrocyte-specific protein in MS: a potential molecular mimic. *Neurology* 53:154–61

156. Vu T, Myers LW, Ellison GW, Mendoza F, Bronstein JM. 2001. T-cell responses to oligodendrocyte-specific protein in multiple sclerosis. *J. Neurosci. Res.* 66:506–9

157. van Noort JM, van Sechel AC, Bajramovic JJ, el Ouagmiri M, Polman CH, et al. 1995. The small heat-shock protein αB-crystallin as candidate autoantigen in multiple sclerosis. *Nature* 375:798–801

158. Chou YK, Burrows GG, LaTocha D,

Wang C, Subramanian S, et al. 2004. CD4 T-cell epitopes of human αB-crystallin. *J. Neurosci. Res.* 75:516–23

159. Saez-Torres I, Brieva L, Espejo C, Barrau MA, Montalban X, Martinez-Caceres EM. 2002. Specific proliferation towards myelin antigens in patients with multiple sclerosis during a relapse. *Autoimmunity* 35:45–50

160. Kojima K, Berger T, Lassmann H, Hinze-Selch D, Zhang Y, et al. 1994. Experimental autoimmune panencephalitis and uveoretinitis transferred to the Lewis rat by T lymphocytes specific for the S100β molecule, a calcium binding protein of astroglia. *J. Exp. Med.* 180:817–29

161. Schmidt S, Linington C, Zipp F, Sotgiu S, de Waal Malefyt R, et al. 1997. Multiple sclerosis: comparison of the human T-cell response to S100β and myelin basic protein reveals parallels to rat experimental autoimmune panencephalitis. *Brain* 120(Part 8):1437–45

162. Banki K, Colombo E, Sia F, Halladay D, Mattson DH, et al. 1994. Oligodendrocyte-specific expression and autoantigenicity of transaldolase in multiple sclerosis. *J. Exp. Med.* 180:1649–63

163. Colombo E, Banki K, Tatum AH, Daucher J, Ferrante P, et al. 1997. Comparative analysis of antibody and cell-mediated autoimmunity to transaldolase and myelin basic protein in patients with multiple sclerosis. *J. Clin. Invest.* 99:1238–50

164. Holmoy T, Vandvik B, Vartdal F. 2003. T cells from multiple sclerosis patients recognize immunoglobulin G from cerebrospinal fluid. *Mult. Scler.* 9:228–34

165. Holmoy T, Vartdal F. 2004. Cerebrospinal fluid T cells from multiple sclerosis patients recognize autologous Epstein-Barr virus-transformed B cells. *J. Neurovirol.* 10:52–56

166. Sadatipour BT, Greer JM, Pender MP. 1998. Increased circulating antiganglioside antibodies in primary and secondary progressive multiple sclerosis. *Ann. Neurol.* 44:980–83

167. Pender MP, Csurhes PA, Wolfe NP, Hooper KD, Good MF, et al. 2003. Increased circulating T cell reactivity to GM3 and GQ1b gangliosides in primary progressive multiple sclerosis. *J. Clin. Neurosci.* 10:63–66

168. Meinl E, Weber F, Drexler K, Morelle C, Ott M, et al. 1993. Myelin basic protein-specific T lymphocyte repertoire in multiple sclerosis. Complexity of the response and dominance of nested epitopes due to recruitment of multiple T cell clones. *J. Clin. Invest.* 92:2633–43

169. Hemmer B, Fleckenstein BT, Vergelli M, Jung G, McFarland H, et al. 1997. Identification of high potency microbial and self ligands for a human autoreactive class II-restricted T cell clone. *J. Exp. Med.* 185:1651–59

170. Zhao Y, Gran B, Pinilla C, Markovic-Plese S, Hemmer B, et al. 2001. Combinatorial peptide libraries and biometric score matrices permit the quantitative analysis of specific and degenerate interactions between clonotypic TCR and MHC peptide ligands. *J. Immunol.* 167:2130–41

171. Jaraquemada D, Martin R, Rosen-Bronson S, Flerlage M, McFarland HF, Long EO. 1990. HLA-DR2a is the dominant restriction molecule for the cytotoxic T cell response to myelin basic protein in DR2Dw2 individuals. *J. Immunol.* 145:2880–85

172. Minohara M, Ochi H, Matsushita S, Irie A, Nishimura Y, Kira J. 2001. Differences between T-cell reactivities to major myelin protein-derived peptides in opticospinal and conventional forms of multiple sclerosis and healthy controls. *Tissue Antigens* 57:447–56

173. Yu M, Kinkel RP, Weinstock-Guttman B, Cook DJ, Tuohy VK. 1998. HLA-DP: a class II restriction molecule involved in epitope spreading during the development of multiple sclerosis. *Hum. Immunol.* 59:15–24

174. Hemmer B, Vergelli M, Calabresi P, Huang T, McFarland HF, Martin R. 1996.

Cytokine phenotype of human autoreactive T cell clones specific for the immunodominant myelin basic protein peptide (83–99). *J. Neurosci. Res.* 45:852–62

175. Correale J, Gilmore W, McMillan M, Li S, McCarthy K, et al. 1995. Patterns of cytokine secretion by autoreactive proteolipid protein-specific T cell clones during the course of multiple sclerosis. *J. Immunol.* 154:2959–68

176. Balashov KE, Smith DR, Khoury SJ, Hafler DA, Weiner HL. 1997. Increased interleukin 12 production in progressive multiple sclerosis: induction by activated CD4$^+$ T cells via CD40 ligand. *Proc. Natl. Acad. Sci. USA* 94:599–603

177. Karni A, Koldzic DN, Bharanidharan P, Khoury SJ, Weiner HL. 2002. IL-18 is linked to raised IFN-γ in multiple sclerosis and is induced by activated CD4$^+$ T cells via CD40-CD40 ligand interactions. *J. Neuroimmunol.* 125:134–40

178. Monney L, Sabatos CA, Gaglia JL, Ryu A, Waldner H, et al. 2002. Th1-specific cell surface protein Tim-3 regulates macrophage activation and severity of an autoimmune disease. *Nature* 415:536–41

179. Khademi M, Illes Z, Gielen AW, Marta M, Takazawa N, et al. 2004. T Cell Ig- and mucin-domain-containing molecule-3 (TIM-3) and TIM-1 molecules are differentially expressed on human Th1 and Th2 cells and in cerebrospinal fluid-derived mononuclear cells in multiple sclerosis. *J. Immunol.* 172:7169–76

180. Vergelli M, Le H, van Noort JM, Dhib-Jalbut S, McFarland H, Martin R. 1996. A novel population of CD4$^+$CD56$^+$ myelin-reactive T cells lyses target cells expressing CD56/neural cell adhesion molecule. *J. Immunol.* 157:679–88

181. Vergelli M, Hemmer B, Muraro PA, Tranquill L, Biddison WE, et al. 1997. Human autoreactive CD4$^+$ T cell clones use perforin- or Fas/Fas ligand-mediated pathways for target cell lysis. *J. Immunol.* 158:2756–61

182. Antel JP, McCrea E, Ladiwala U, Qin YF, Becher B. 1998. Non-MHC-restricted cell-mediated lysis of human oligodendrocytes in vitro: relation with CD56 expression. *J. Immunol.* 160:1606–11

183. Scholz C, Patton KT, Anderson DE, Freeman GJ, Hafler DA. 1998. Expansion of autoreactive T cells in multiple sclerosis is independent of exogenous B7 costimulation. *J. Immunol.* 160:1532–38

184. Lovett-Racke AE, Trotter JL, Lauber J, Perrin PJ, June CH, Racke MK. 1998. Decreased dependence of myelin basic protein-reactive T cells on CD28-mediated costimulation in multiple sclerosis patients. A marker of activated/memory T cells. *J. Clin. Invest.* 101:725–30

185. Markovic-Plese S, Cortese I, Wandinger KP, McFarland HF, Martin R. 2001. CD4$^+$CD28$^-$ costimulation-independent T cells in multiple sclerosis. *J. Clin. Invest.* 108:1185–94

186. Chitnis T, Khoury SJ. 2003. Role of costimulatory pathways in the pathogenesis of multiple sclerosis and experimental autoimmune encephalomyelitis. *J. Allergy Clin. Immunol.* 112:837–50

187. Oliveira EM, Bar-Or A, Waliszewska AI, Cai G, Anderson DE, et al. 2003. CTLA-4 dysregulation in the activation of myelin basic protein reactive T cells may distinguish patients with multiple sclerosis from healthy controls. *J. Autoimmun.* 20:71–81

188. Hori S, Nomura T, Sakaguchi S. 2003. Control of regulatory T cell development by the transcription factor Foxp3. *Science* 299:1057–61

189. Zhang X, Koldzic DN, Izikson L, Reddy J, Nazareno RF, et al. 2004. IL-10 is involved in the suppression of experimental autoimmune encephalomyelitis by CD25$^+$CD4$^+$ regulatory T cells. *Int. Immunol.* 16:249–56

190. Viglietta V, Baecher-Allan C, Weiner HL, Hafler DA. 2004. Loss of functional suppression by CD4$^+$CD25$^+$ regulatory

T cells in patients with multiple sclerosis. *J. Exp. Med.* 199:971–79

191. Weiner HL, Friedman A, Miller A, Khoury SJ, Al-Sabbagh A, et al. 1994. Oral tolerance: immunologic mechanisms and treatment of animal and human organ-specific autoimmune diseases by oral administration of autoantigens. *Annu. Rev. Immunol.* 12:809–37

192. Lafaille JJ, Keere FV, Hsu AL, Baron JL, Haas W, et al. 1997. Myelin basic protein-specific T helper 2 (Th2) cells cause experimental autoimmune encephalomyelitis in immunodeficient hosts rather than protect them from the disease. *J. Exp. Med.* 186:307–12

193. Wucherpfennig KW, Ota K, Endo N, Seidman JG, Rosenzweig A, et al. 1990. Shared human T cell receptor Vβ usage to immunodominant regions of myelin basic protein. *Science* 248:1016–19

194. Ben-Nun A, Liblau RS, Cohen L, Lehmann D, Tournier-Lasserve E, et al. 1991. Restricted T-cell receptor Vβ gene usage by myelin basic protein-specific T-cell clones in multiple sclerosis: predominant genes vary in individuals. *Proc. Natl. Acad. Sci. USA* 88:2466–70

195. Kotzin BL, Karuturi S, Chou YK, Lafferty J, Forrester M, et al. 1991. Preferential T-cell receptor β-chain variable gene use in myelin basic protein-reactive T-cell clones from patients with multiple sclerosis. *Proc. Natl. Acad. Sci. USA* 88:9161–65

196. Afshar G, Muraro PA, McFarland HF, Martin R. 1998. Lack of over-expression of T cell receptor Vβ5.2 in myelin basic protein-specific T cell lines derived from HLA-DR2 positive multiple sclerosis patients and controls. *J. Neuroimmunol.* 84:7–13

197. Oksenberg JR, Stuart S, Begovich AB, Bell RB, Erlich HA, et al. 1990. Limited heterogeneity of rearranged T-cell receptor V α transcripts in brains of multiple sclerosis patients. *Nature* 345:344–46

198. Demoulins T, Mouthon F, Clayette P, Be-quet D, Gachelin G, Dormont D. 2003. The same TCR (N)Dβ(N)Jβ junctional region is associated with several different vβ13 subtypes in a multiple sclerosis patient at the onset of the disease. *Neurobiol. Dis.* 14:470–82

199. Laplaud DA, Ruiz C, Wiertlewski S, Brouard S, Berthelot L, et al. 2004. Blood T-cell receptor β chain transcriptome in multiple sclerosis. Characterization of the T cells with altered CDR3 length distribution. *Brain* 127:981–95

200. Matsumoto Y, Yoon WK, Jee Y, Fujihara K, Misu T, et al. 2003. Complementarity-determining region 3 spectratyping analysis of the TCR repertoire in multiple sclerosis. *J. Immunol.* 170:4846–53

201. Gestri D, Baldacci L, Taiuti R, Galli E, Maggi E, et al. 2001. Oligoclonal T cell repertoire in cerebrospinal fluid of patients with inflammatory diseases of the nervous system. *J. Neurol. Neurosurg. Psychiatry* 70:767–72

202. Utz U, Biddison WE, McFarland HF, McFarlin DE, Flerlage M, Martin R. 1993. Skewed T-cell receptor repertoire in genetically identical twins correlates with multiple sclerosis. *Nature* 364:243–47

203. Haegert DG, Galutira D, Murray TJ, O'Connor P, Gadag V. 2003. Identical twins discordant for multiple sclerosis have a shift in their T-cell receptor repertoires. *Clin. Exp. Immunol.* 134:532–37

204. Jurewicz A, Biddison WE, Antel JP. 1998. MHC class I-restricted lysis of human oligodendrocytes by myelin basic protein peptide-specific CD8 T lymphocytes. *J. Immunol.* 160:3056–59

205. Medana IM, Gallimore A, Oxenius A, Martinic MM, Wekerle H, Neumann H. 2000. MHC class I-restricted killing of neurons by virus-specific CD8+ T lymphocytes is effected through the Fas/FasL, but not the perforin pathway. *Eur. J. Immunol.* 30:3623–33

206. Skulina C, Schmidt S, Dornmair K, Babbe H, Roers A, et al. 2004. Multiple sclerosis: brain-infiltrating CD8+ T cells persist

as clonal expansions in the cerebrospinal fluid and blood. *Proc. Natl. Acad. Sci. USA* 101:2428–33

207. Cabarrocas J, Bauer J, Piaggio E, Liblau R, Lassmann H. 2003. Effective and selective immune surveillance of the brain by MHC class I-restricted cytotoxic T lymphocytes. *Eur. J. Immunol.* 33:1174–82

208. Neumann H. 2003. Molecular mechanisms of axonal damage in inflammatory central nervous system diseases. *Curr. Opin. Neurol.* 16:267–73

209. Tsuchida T, Parker KC, Turner RV, McFarland HF, Coligan JE, Biddison WE. 1994. Autoreactive CD8$^+$ T-cell responses to human myelin protein-derived peptides. *Proc. Natl. Acad. Sci. USA* 91: 10859–63

210. Honma K, Parker KC, Becker KG, McFarland HF, Coligan JE, Biddison WE. 1997. Identification of an epitope derived from human proteolipid protein that can induce autoreactive CD8$^+$ cytotoxic T lymphocytes restricted by HLA-A3: evidence for cross-reactivity with an environmental microorganism. *J. Neuroimmunol.* 73:7–14

211. Zang YCQ, Li SF, Rivera VM, Hong J, Robinson RR, et al. 2004. Increased CD8$^+$ cytotoxic T cell responses to myelin basic protein in multiple sclerosis. *J. Immunol.* 172:5120–27

212. Biddison WE, Cruikshank WW, Center DM, Pelfrey CM, Taub DD, Turner RV. 1998. CD8$^+$ myelin peptide-specific T cells can chemoattract CD4$^+$ myelin peptide-specific T cells: importance of IFN-inducible protein 10. *J. Immunol.* 160:444–48

213. Killestein J, Eikelenboom MJ, Izeboud T, Kalkers NF, Ader HJ, et al. 2003. Cytokine producing CD8$^+$ T cells are correlated to MRI features of tissue destruction in MS. *J. Neuroimmunol.* 142:141–48

214. Kabat EA, Freedman DA, Murray JP, Knaub V. 1950. A study of the cristalline albumin, gamma globulin and total protein in the cerebrospinal fluid of one hundred cases of multiple sclerosis and in other diseases. *Am. J. Med. Sci.* 219:55–64

215. Qin Y, Duquette P, Zhang Y, Talbot P, Poole R, Antel J. 1998. Clonal expansion and somatic hypermutation of V$_H$ genes of B cells from cerebrospinal fluid in multiple sclerosis. *J. Clin. Invest.* 102:1045–50

216. Owens GP, Kraus H, Burgoon MP, Smith-Jensen T, Devlin ME, Gilden DH. 1998. Restricted use of VH4 germline segments in an acute multiple sclerosis brain. *Ann. Neurol.* 43:236–43

217. Baranzini SE, Jeong MC, Butunoi C, Murray RS, Bernard CC, Oksenberg JR. 1999. B cell repertoire diversity and clonal expansion in multiple sclerosis brain lesions. *J. Immunol.* 163:5133–44

218. Walsh MJ, Tourtellotte WW. 1986. Temporal invariance and clonal uniformity of brain and cerebrospinal IgG, IgA, and IgM in multiple sclerosis. *J. Exp. Med.* 163:41–53

219. Sharief MK, Thompson EJ. 1991. Intrathecal immunoglobulin M synthesis in multiple sclerosis. Relationship with clinical and cerebrospinal fluid parameters. *Brain* 114(Part 1A):181–95

220. Wang LY, Fujinami RS. 1997. Enhancement of EAE and induction of autoantibodies to T-cell epitopes in mice infected with a recombinant vaccinia virus encoding myelin proteolipid protein. *J. Neuroimmunol.* 75:75–83

221. Wucherpfennig KW, Catz I, Hausmann S, Strominger JL, Steinman L, Warren KG. 1997. Recognition of the immunodominant myelin basic protein peptide by autoantibodies and HLA-DR2-restricted T cell clones from multiple sclerosis patients. Identity of key contact residues in the B-cell and T-cell epitopes. *J. Clin. Invest.* 100:1114–22

222. Lou YH, Park KK, Agersborg S, Alard P, Tung KS. 2000. Retargeting T cell-mediated inflammation: a new perspective on autoantibody action. *J. Immunol.* 164: 5251–57

223. Bornstein MB, Appel SH. 1959. Demyelination in cultures of rat cerebellum produced by experimental allergic encephalomyelitic serum. *Trans. Am. Neurol. Assoc.* 84:165–66

224. Esiri MM. 1977. Immunoglobulin-containing cells in multiple-sclerosis plaques. *Lancet* 2:478

225. Mattson DH, Roos RP, Arnason BG. 1980. Isoelectric focusing of IgG eluted from multiple sclerosis and subacute sclerosing panencephalitis brains. *Nature* 287:335–37

226. Genain CP, Cannella B, Hauser SL, Raine CS. 1999. Identification of autoantibodies associated with myelin damage in multiple sclerosis. *Nat. Med.* 5:170–75

227. Trotter J, DeJong LJ, Smith ME. 1986. Opsonization with antimyelin antibody increases the uptake and intracellular metabolism of myelin in inflammatory macrophages. *J. Neurochem.* 47:779–89

228. Goldenberg PZ, Kwon EE, Benjamins JA, Whitaker JN, Quarles RH, Prineas JW. 1989. Opsonization of normal myelin by anti-myelin antibodies and normal serum. *J. Neuroimmunol.* 23:157–66

229. van der Laan LJ, Ruuls SR, Weber KS, Lodder IJ, Dopp EA, Dijkstra CD. 1996. Macrophage phagocytosis of myelin in vitro determined by flow cytometry: Phagocytosis is mediated by CR3 and induces production of tumor necrosis factor-α and nitric oxide. *J. Neuroimmunol.* 70: 145–52

230. Mead RJ, Singhrao SK, Neal JW, Lassmann H, Morgan BP. 2002. The membrane attack complex of complement causes severe demyelination associated with acute axonal injury. *J. Immunol.* 168: 458–65

231. Storch MK, Piddlesden S, Haltia M, Iivanainen M, Morgan P, Lassmann H. 1998. Multiple sclerosis: in situ evidence for antibody- and complement-mediated demyelination. *Ann. Neurol.* 43:465–71

232. Sellebjerg F, Jaliashvili I, Christiansen M, Garred P. 1998. Intrathecal activation of the complement system and disability in multiple sclerosis. *J. Neurol. Sci.* 157: 168–74

233. Scolding NJ, Morgan BP, Houston WA, Linington C, Campbell AK, Compston DA. 1989. Vesicular removal by oligodendrocytes of membrane attack complexes formed by activated complement. *Nature* 339:620–22

234. Trotter JL, Rust RS. 1989. *Human Cerebrospinal Fluid Immunology*, ed. RM Herndon, RA Brumback, pp. 179–226. Amsterdam: Martinus Nyhoff

235. Sindic CJ, Monteyne P, Laterre EC. 1994. The intrathecal synthesis of virus-specific oligoclonal IgG in multiple sclerosis. *J. Neuroimmunol.* 54:75–80

236. Archelos JJ, Storch MK, Hartung HP. 2000. The role of B cells and autoantibodies in multiple sclerosis. *Ann. Neurol.* 47: 694–706

237. Cross AH, Trotter JL, Lyons J. 2001. B cells and antibodies in CNS demyelinating disease. *J. Neuroimmunol.* 112:1–14

238. Dharmasaroja P. 2003. Specificity of autoantibodies to epitopes of myelin proteins in multiple sclerosis. *J. Neurol. Sci.* 206:7–16

239. Warren KG, Catz I. 1993. Increased synthetic peptide specificity of tissue-CSF bound anti-MBP in multiple sclerosis. *J. Neuroimmunol.* 43:87–96

240. Reindl M, Linington C, Brehm U, Egg R, Dilitz E, et al. 1999. Antibodies against the myelin oligodendrocyte glycoprotein and the myelin basic protein in multiple sclerosis and other neurological diseases: a comparative study. *Brain* 122(Part 11):2047–56

241. Cortese I, Tafi R, Grimaldi LM, Martino G, Nicosia A, Cortese R. 1996. Identification of peptides specific for cerebrospinal fluid antibodies in multiple sclerosis by using phage libraries. *Proc. Natl. Acad. Sci. USA* 93:11063–67

242. O'Connor KC, Chitnis T, Griffin DE, Piyasirisilp S, Bar-Or A, et al. 2003.

Myelin basic protein-reactive autoantibodies in the serum and cerebrospinal fluid of multiple sclerosis patients are characterized by low-affinity interactions. *J. Neuroimmunol.* 136:140–48

243. Sun JB, Olsson T, Wang WZ, Xiao BG, Kostulas V, et al. 1991. Autoreactive T and B cells responding to myelin proteolipid protein in multiple sclerosis and controls. *Eur. J. Immunol.* 21:1461–68

244. Warren KG, Catz I, Johnson E, Mielke B. 1994. Anti-myelin basic protein and anti-proteolipid protein specific forms of multiple sclerosis. *Ann. Neurol.* 35:280–89

245. Schluesener HJ, Sobel RA, Linington C, Weiner HL. 1987. A monoclonal antibody against a myelin oligodendrocyte glycoprotein induces relapses and demyelination in central nervous system autoimmune disease. *J. Immunol.* 139:4016–21

246. Linington C, Bradl M, Lassmann H, Brunner C, Vass K. 1988. Augmentation of demyelination in rat acute allergic encephalomyelitis by circulating mouse monoclonal antibodies directed against a myelin/oligodendrocyte glycoprotein. *Am. J. Pathol.* 130:443–54

247. Storch MK, Stefferl A, Brehm U, Weissert R, Wallstrom E, et al. 1998. Autoimmunity to myelin oligodendrocyte glycoprotein in rats mimics the spectrum of multiple sclerosis pathology. *Brain Pathol.* 8:681–94

248. Litzenburger T, Fassler R, Bauer J, Lassmann H, Linington C, et al. 1998. B lymphocytes producing demyelinating autoantibodies: development and function in gene-targeted transgenic mice. *J. Exp. Med.* 188:169–80

249. Genain CP, Nguyen MH, Letvin NL, Pearl R, Davis RL, et al. 1995. Antibody facilitation of multiple sclerosis-like lesions in a nonhuman primate. *J. Clin. Invest.* 96:2966–74

250. Sun J, Link H, Olsson T, Xiao BG, Andersson G, et al. 1991. T and B cell responses to myelin-oligodendrocyte glycoprotein in multiple sclerosis. *J. Immunol.* 146:1490–95

251. Berger T, Rubner P, Schautzer F, Egg R, Ulmer H, et al. 2003. Antimyelin antibodies as a predictor of clinically definite multiple sclerosis after a first demyelinating event. *N. Engl. J. Med.* 349:139–45

252. Lily O, Palace J, Vincent A. 2004. Serum autoantibodies to cell surface determinants in multiple sclerosis: a flow cytometric study. *Brain* 127:269–79

253. Robinson WH, Fontoura P, Lee BJ, de Vegvar HE, Tom J, et al. 2003. Protein microarrays guide tolerizing DNA vaccine treatment of autoimmune encephalomyelitis. *Nat. Biotechnol.* 21:1033–39

254. Saoudi A, Simmonds S, Huitinga I, Mason D. 1995. Prevention of experimental allergic encephalomyelitis in rats by targeting autoantigen to B cells: evidence that the protective mechanism depends on changes in the cytokine response and migratory properties of the autoantigen-specific T cells. *J. Exp. Med.* 182:335–44

255. Rodriguez M, Lennon VA. 1990. Immunoglobulins promote remyelination in the central nervous system. *Ann. Neurol.* 27:12–17

256. Achiron A, Gabbay U, Gilad R, Hassin-Baer S, Barak Y, et al. 1998. Intravenous immunoglobulin treatment in multiple sclerosis. Effect on relapses. *Neurology* 50:398–402

257. Sewell WA, Jolles S. 2002. Immunomodulatory action of intravenous immunoglobulin. *Immunology* 107:387–93

258. van Kooyk Y, Geijtenbeek TB. 2002. A novel adhesion pathway that regulates dendritic cell trafficking and T cell interactions. *Immunol. Rev.* 186:47–56

259. Pasare C, Medzhitov R. 2003. Toll pathway-dependent blockade of CD4+ CD25+ T cell-mediated suppression by dendritic cells. *Science* 299:1033–36

260. Ohshima S, Saeki Y, Mima T, Sasai M, Nishioka K, et al. 1998. Interleukin

6 plays a key role in the development of antigen-induced arthritis. *Proc. Natl. Acad. Sci. USA* 95:8222–26

261. Hawiger D, Inaba K, Dorsett Y, Guo M, Mahnke K, et al. 2001. Dendritic cells induce peripheral T cell unresponsiveness under steady state conditions in vivo. *J. Exp. Med.* 194:769–79

262. Tsunoda I, Tolley ND, Theil DJ, Whitton JL, Kobayashi H, Fujinami RS. 1999. Exacerbation of viral and autoimmune animal models for multiple sclerosis by bacterial DNA. *Brain Pathol.* 9:481–93

263. Ichikawa HT, Williams LP, Segal BM. 2002. Activation of APCs through CD40 or Toll-like receptor 9 overcomes tolerance and precipitates autoimmune disease. *J. Immunol.* 169:2781–87

264. Zappulla JP, Arock M, Mars LT, Liblau RS. 2002. Mast cells: new targets for multiple sclerosis therapy? *J. Neuroimmunol.* 131:5–20

265. Neumann J. 1890. Über das Vorkommen der sogenannten "Mastzellen" bei pathologischen Veränderungen des Gehirns. *Virchow's Arch. Pathol. Anat.* 122:378–80

266. Kruger PG. 2001. Mast cells and multiple sclerosis: a quantitative analysis. *Neuropathol. Appl. Neurobiol.* 27:275–80

267. Bo L, Dawson TM, Wesselingh S, Mork S, Choi S, et al. 1994. Induction of nitric oxide synthase in demyelinating regions of multiple sclerosis brains. *Ann. Neurol.* 36:778–86

268. Merrill JE, Ignarro LJ, Sherman MP, Melinek J, Lane TE. 1993. Microglial cell cytotoxicity of oligodendrocytes is mediated through nitric oxide. *J. Immunol.* 151:2132–41

269. Mitrovic B, Ignarro LJ, Vinters HV, Akers MA, Schmid I, et al. 1995. Nitric oxide induces necrotic but not apoptotic cell death in oligodendrocytes. *Neuroscience* 65:531–39

270. Benczur M, Petranyi GG, Palffy G, Varga M, Talas M, et al. 1980. Dysfunction of natural killer cells in multiple sclerosis: a possible pathogenetic factor. *Clin. Exp. Immunol.* 39:657–62

271. Kastrukoff LF, Morgan NG, Zecchini D, White R, Petkau AJ, et al. 1998. A role for natural killer cells in the immunopathogenesis of multiple sclerosis. *J. Neuroimmunol.* 86:123–33

272. Kastrukoff LF, Lau A, Wee R, Zecchini D, White R, Paty DW. 2003. Clinical relapses of multiple sclerosis are associated with 'novel' valleys in natural killer cell functional activity. *J. Neuroimmunol.* 145:103–14

273. Munschauer FE, Hartrich LA, Stewart CC, Jacobs L. 1995. Circulating natural killer cells but not cytotoxic T lymphocytes are reduced in patients with active relapsing multiple sclerosis and little clinical disability as compared to controls. *J. Neuroimmunol.* 62:177–81

274. Weber WE, Buurman WA, Vandermeeren MM, Medaer RH, Raus JC. 1987. Fine analysis of cytolytic and natural killer T lymphocytes in the CSF in multiple sclerosis and other neurologic diseases. *Neurology* 37:419–25

275. Zhang B, Yamamura T, Kondo T, Fujiwara M, Tabira T. 1997. Regulation of experimental autoimmune encephalomyelitis by natural killer (NK) cells. *J. Exp. Med.* 186:1677–87

276. Matsumoto Y, Kohyama K, Aikawa Y, Shin T, Kawazoe Y, et al. 1998. Role of natural killer cells and TCR $\gamma\delta$ T cells in acute autoimmune encephalomyelitis. *Eur. J. Immunol.* 28:1681–88

277. Smeltz RB, Wolf NA, Swanborg RH. 1999. Inhibition of autoimmune T cell responses in the DA rat by bone marrow-derived NK cells in vitro: implications for autoimmunity. *J. Immunol.* 163:1390–97

278. Peng SL, Moslehi J, Robert ME, Craft J. 1998. Perforin protects against autoimmunity in lupus-prone mice. *J. Immunol.* 160:652–60

279. Hilliard B, Wilmen A, Seidel C, Liu TS, Goke R, Chen Y. 2001. Roles of TNF-related apoptosis-inducing ligand in

experimental autoimmune encphalomyelitis. *J. Immunol.* 166:1314–19

280. Bielekova B, Richert N, Howard T, Blevins G, Markovic-Plese S, et al. 2004. Humanized anti-CD25 (daclizumab) inhibits disease activity in multiple sclerosis patients failing to respond to interferon β. *Proc. Natl. Acad. Sci. USA* 101:8705–8

281. Vanguri P, Shin ML. 1986. Activation of complement by myelin: identification of C1-binding proteins of human myelin from central nervous tissue. *J. Neurochem.* 46:1535–41

282. Scolding NJ, Morgan BP, Houston A, Campbell AK, Linington C, Compston DA. 1989. Normal rat serum cytotoxicity against syngeneic oligodendrocytes. Complement activation and attack in the absence of anti-myelin antibodies. *J. Neurol. Sci.* 89:289–300

283. Johns TG, Bernard CC. 1997. Binding of complement component C1q to myelin oligodendrocyte glycoprotein: a novel mechanism for regulating CNS inflammation. *Mol. Immunol.* 34:33–38

284. Piddlesden SJ, Morgan BP. 1993. Killing of rat glial cells by complement: deficiency of the rat analogue of CD59 is the cause of oligodendrocyte susceptibility to lysis. *J. Neuroimmunol.* 48:169–75

285. Park SH, Bendelac A. 2000. CD1-restricted T-cell responses and microbial infection. *Nature* 406:788–92

286. Illes Z, Kondo T, Newcombe J, Oka N, Tabira T, Yamamura T. 2000. Differential expression of NK T cell $V\alpha24J\alpha Q$ invariant TCR chain in the lesions of multiple sclerosis and chronic inflammatory demyelinating polyneuropathy. *J. Immunol.* 164:4375–81

287. van der Vliet HJ, von Blomberg BM, Nishi N, Reijm M, Voskuyl AE, et al. 2001. Circulating $V\alpha24^+V\beta11^+$ NKT cell numbers are decreased in a wide variety of diseases that are characterized by autoreactive tissue damage. *Clin. Immunol.* 100:144–48

288. Gausling R, Trollmo C, Hafler DA.

2001. Decreases in interleukin-4 secretion by invariant CD4$^-$CD8$^-$ $V\alpha24J\alpha Q$ T cells in peripheral blood of patients with relapsing-remitting multiple sclerosis. *Clin. Immunol.* 98:11–17

289. Miyamoto K, Miyake S, Yamamura T. 2001. A synthetic glycolipid prevents autoimmune encephalomyelitis by inducing TH2 bias of natural killer T cells. *Nature* 413:531–34

290. Triebel F, Hercend T. 1989. Subpopulations of human peripheral T $\gamma\delta$ lymphocytes. *Immunol. Today* 10:186–88

291. Battistini L, Salvetti M, Ristori G, Falcone M, Raine CS, Brosnan CF. 1995. $\gamma\delta$ T cell receptor analysis supports a role for HSP 70 selection of lymphocytes in multiple sclerosis lesions. *Mol. Med.* 1:554–62

292. Freedman MS, Bitar R, Antel JP. 1997. $\gamma\delta$ T-cell-human glial cell interactions. II. Relationship between heat shock protein expression and susceptibility to cytolysis. *J. Neuroimmunol.* 74:143–48

293. Nick S, Pileri P, Tongiani S, Uematsu Y, Kappos L, De Libero G. 1995. T cell receptor $\gamma\delta$ repertoire is skewed in cerebrospinal fluid of multiple sclerosis patients: molecular and functional analyses of antigen-reactive $\gamma\delta$ clones. *Eur. J. Immunol.* 25:355–63

294. Stinissen P, Vandevyver C, Medaer R, Vandegaer L, Nies J, et al. 1995. Increased frequency of $\gamma\delta$ T cells in cerebrospinal fluid and peripheral blood of patients with multiple sclerosis. Reactivity, cytotoxicity, and T cell receptor V gene rearrangements. *J. Immunol.* 154:4883–94

295. Birnbaum G, Kotilinek L, Albrecht L. 1993. Spinal fluid lymphocytes from a subgroup of multiple sclerosis patients respond to mycobacterial antigens. *Ann. Neurol.* 34:18–24

296. Constant P, Davodeau F, Peyrat MA, Poquet Y, Puzo G, et al. 1994. Stimulation of human $\gamma\delta$ T cells by nonpeptidic mycobacterial ligands. *Science* 264:267–70

297. Rajan AJ, Gao YL, Raine CS, Brosnan CF. 1996. A pathogenic role for $\gamma\delta$ T cells

in relapsing-remitting experimental allergic encephalomyelitis in the SJL mouse. *J. Immunol.* 157:941–49

298. Bielekova B, Martin R. 2004. Development of biomarkers in multiple sclerosis. *Brain* 127:1463–78

299. Navikas V, He B, Link J, Haglund M, Soderstrom M, et al. 1996. Augmented expression of tumour necrosis factor-α and lymphotoxin in mononuclear cells in multiple sclerosis and optic neuritis. *Brain* 119(Part 1):213–23

300. Hohnoki K, Inoue A, Koh CS. 1998. Elevated serum levels of IFN-γ, IL-4 and TNF-α/unelevated serum levels of IL-10 in patients with demyelinating diseases during the acute stage. *J. Neuroimmunol.* 87:27–32

301. Ozenci V, Kouwenhoven M, Huang YM, Kivisakk P, Link H. 2000. Multiple sclerosis is associated with an imbalance between tumour necrosis factor-α (TNF-α)- and IL-10-secreting blood cells that is corrected by interferon-β (IFN-β) treatment. *Clin. Exp. Immunol.* 120:147–53

302. The Lenercept Multiple Sclerosis Study Group and The University of British Columbia MS/MRI Analysis Group. 1999. TNF neutralization in MS: results of a randomized, placebo-controlled multicenter study. *Neurology* 53:457–65

303. Nguyen LT, Ramanathan M, Munschauer F, Brownscheidle C, Krantz S, et al. 1999. Flow cytometric analysis of in vitro proinflammatory cytokine secretion in peripheral blood from multiple sclerosis patients. *J. Clin. Immunol.* 19:179–85

304. Panitch HS, Hirsch RL, Schindler J, Johnson KP. 1987. Treatment of multiple sclerosis with γ interferon: exacerbations associated with activation of the immune system. *Neurology* 37:1097–102

305. Segal BM, Dwyer BK, Shevach EM. 1998. An interleukin (IL)-10/IL-12 immunoregulatory circuit controls susceptibility to autoimmune disease. *J. Exp. Med.* 187:537–46

306. Cua DJ, Sherlock J, Chen Y, Murphy CA, Joyce B, et al. 2003. Interleukin-23 rather than interleukin-12 is the critical cytokine for autoimmune inflammation of the brain. *Nature* 421:744–48

307. Matusevicius D, Kivisakk P, Navikas V, Soderstrom M, Fredrikson S, Link H. 1998. Interleukin-12 and perforin mRNA expression is augmented in blood mononuclear cells in multiple sclerosis. *Scand. J. Immunol.* 47:582–90

308. Heesen C, Sieverding F, Schoser BG, Hadji B, Kunze K. 1999. Interleukin-12 is detectable in sera of patients with multiple sclerosis—association with chronic progressive disease course? *Eur. J. Neurol.* 6:591–96

309. Huang WX, Huang P, Link H, Hillert J. 1999. Cytokine analysis in multiple sclerosis by competitive RT—PCR: a decreased expression of IL-10 and an increased expression of TNF-α in chronic progression. *Mult. Scler.* 5:342–48

310. Navikas V, Link J, Palasik W, Soderstrom M, Fredrikson S, et al. 1995. Increased mRNA expression of IL-10 in mononuclear cells in multiple sclerosis and optic neuritis. *Scand. J. Immunol.* 41:171–78

311. Windhagen A, Newcombe J, Dangond F, Strand C, Woodroofe MN, et al. 1995. Expression of costimulatory molecules B7-1 (CD80), B7-2 (CD86), and interleukin 12 cytokine in multiple sclerosis lesions. *J. Exp. Med.* 182:1985–96

312. Cannella B, Raine CS. 1995. The adhesion molecule and cytokine profile of multiple sclerosis lesions. *Ann. Neurol.* 37:424–35

313. Bitsch A, Kuhlmann T, Da Costa C, Bunkowski S, Polak T, Bruck W. 2000. Tumour necrosis factor α mRNA expression in early multiple sclerosis lesions: correlation with demyelinating activity and oligodendrocyte pathology. *Glia* 29:366–75

314. Owens T, Wekerle H, Antel J. 2001. Genetic models for CNS inflammation. *Nat. Med.* 7:161–66

315. Pouly S, Becher B, Blain M, Antel JP. 2000. Interferon-γ modulates human

oligodendrocyte susceptibility to Fas-mediated apoptosis. *J. Neuropathol. Exp. Neurol.* 59:280–86

316. Link J, Soderstrom M, Olsson T, Hojeberg B, Ljungdahl A, Link H. 1994. Increased transforming growth factor-β, interleukin-4, and interferon-γ in multiple sclerosis. *Ann. Neurol.* 36:379–86

317. Nakashima I, Fujihara K, Misu T, Okita N, Takase S, Itoyama Y. 2000. Significant correlation between IL-10 levels and IgG indices in the cerebrospinal fluid of patients with multiple sclerosis. *J. Neuroimmunol.* 111:64–67

318. Issazadeh S, Mustafa M, Ljungdahl Å, Höjeberg B, Dagerlind Å, et al. 1995. Interferon-γ, interleukin-4 and transforming growth factor β in experimental autoimmune encephalomyelitis in Lewis rats: dynamics of cellular mRNA expression in the central nervous system and lymphoid cells. *J. Neurosci. Res.* 40:579–90

319. Sindern E. 2004. Role of chemokines and their receptors in the pathogenesis of multiple sclerosis. *Front Biosci.* 9:457–63

320. Trebst C, Ransohoff RM. 2001. Investigating chemokines and chemokine receptors in patients with multiple sclerosis: opportunities and challenges. *Arch. Neurol.* 58:1975–80

321. Calabresi PA, Martin R, Jacobson S. 1999. Chemokines in chronic progressive neurological diseases: HTLV-1 associated myelopathy and multiple sclerosis. *J. Neurovirol.* 5:102–8

322. Strunk T, Bubel S, Mascher B, Schlenke P, Kirchner H, Wandinger KP. 2000. Increased numbers of CCR5$^+$ interferon-γ- and tumor necrosis factor-α-secreting T lymphocytes in multiple sclerosis patients. *Ann. Neurol.* 47:269–73

323. Misu T, Onodera H, Fujihara K, Matsushima K, Yoshie O, et al. 2001. Chemokine receptor expression on T cells in blood and cerebrospinal fluid at relapse and remission of multiple sclerosis: imbalance of Th1/Th2-associated

chemokine signaling. *J. Neuroimmunol.* 114:207–12

324. Balashov KE, Rottman JB, Weiner HL, Hancock WW. 1999. CCR5$^+$ and CXCR3$^+$ T cells are increased in multiple sclerosis and their ligands MIP-1α and IP-10 are expressed in demyelinating brain lesions. *Proc. Natl. Acad. Sci. USA* 96:6873–78

325. Calabresi PA, Yun SH, Allie R, Whartenby KA. 2002. Chemokine receptor expression on MBP-reactive T cells: CXCR6 is a marker of IFNγ-producing effector cells. *J. Neuroimmunol.* 127:96–105

326. Sorensen TL, Tani M, Jensen J, Pierce V, Lucchinetti C, et al. 1999. Expression of specific chemokines and chemokine receptors in the central nervous system of multiple sclerosis patients. *J. Clin. Invest.* 103:807–15

327. Sorensen TL, Sellebjerg F, Jensen CV, Strieter RM, Ransohoff RM. 2001. Chemokines CXCL10 and CCL2: differential involvement in intrathecal inflammation in multiple sclerosis. *Eur. J. Neurol.* 8:665–72

328. Sindern E, Niederkinkhaus Y, Henschel M, Ossege LM, Patzold T, Malin JP. 2001. Differential release of β-chemokines in serum and CSF of patients with relapsing-remitting multiple sclerosis. *Acta Neurol. Scand.* 104:88–91

329. Kivisakk P, Trebst C, Liu Z, Tucky BH, Sorensen TL, et al. 2002. T-cells in the cerebrospinal fluid express a similar repertoire of inflammatory chemokine receptors in the absence or presence of CNS inflammation: implications for CNS trafficking. *Clin. Exp. Immunol.* 129:510–18

330. Giunti D, Borsellino G, Benelli R, Marchese M, Capello E, et al. 2003. Phenotypic and functional analysis of T cells homing into the CSF of subjects with inflammatory diseases of the CNS. *J. Leukoc. Biol.* 73:584–90

331. Trebst C, Sorensen TL, Kivisakk P, Cathcart MK, Hesselgesser J, et al. 2001.

CCR1$^+$/CCR5$^+$ mononuclear phagocytes accumulate in the central nervous system of patients with multiple sclerosis. *Am. J. Pathol.* 159:1701–10

332. Boven LA, Montagne L, Nottet HS, De Groot CJ. 2000. Macrophage inflammatory protein-1α (MIP-1α), MIP-1β, and RANTES mRNA semiquantification and protein expression in active demyelinating multiple sclerosis (MS) lesions. *Clin. Exp. Immunol.* 122:257–63

333. Simpson J, Rezaie P, Newcombe J, Cuzner ML, Male D, Woodroofe MN. 2000. Expression of the β-chemokine receptors CCR2, CCR3 and CCR5 in multiple sclerosis central nervous system tissue. *J. Neuroimmunol.* 108:192–200

334. Elhofy A, Kennedy KJ, Fife BT, Karpus WJ. 2002. Regulation of experimental autoimmune encephalomyelitis by chemokines and chemokine receptors. *Immunol. Res.* 25:167–75

335. Fife BT, Huffnagle GB, Kuziel WA, Karpus WJ. 2000. CC chemokine receptor 2 is critical for induction of experimental autoimmune encephalomyelitis. *J. Exp. Med.* 192:899–905

336. Rottman JB, Slavin AJ, Silva R, Weiner HL, Gerard CG, Hancock WW. 2000. Leukocyte recruitment during onset of experimental allergic encephalomyelitis is CCR1 dependent. *Eur. J. Immunol.* 30:2372–77

337. Tran EH, Kuziel WA, Owens T. 2000. Induction of experimental autoimmune encephalomyelitis in C57BL/6 mice deficient in either the chemokine macrophage inflammatory protein-1α or its CCR5 receptor. *Eur. J. Immunol.* 30:1410–15

338. Flugel A, Berkowicz T, Ritter T, Labeur M, Jenne DE, et al. 2001. Migratory activity and functional changes of green fluorescent effector cells before and during experimental autoimmune encephalomyelitis. *Immunity* 14:547–60

339. Trapp BD, Peterson J, Ransohoff RM, Rudick R, Mork S, Bo L. 1998. Axonal transection in the lesions of multiple sclerosis. *N. Engl. J. Med.* 338:278–85

340. Karnezis T, Mandemakers W, McQualter JL, Zheng B, Ho PP, et al. 2004. The neurite outgrowth inhibitor Nogo A is involved in autoimmune-mediated demyelination. *Nat. Neurosci.* 7:736–44

341. Whitaker JN, Kirk KA, Herman PK, Zhou SR, Goodin RR, et al. 1992. An immunochemical comparison of human myelin basic protein and its modified, citrullinated form, C8. *J. Neuroimmunol.* 36:135–46

342. Wood DD, Bilbao JM, O'Connors P, Moscarello MA. 1996. Acute multiple sclerosis (Marburg type) is associated with developmentally immature myelin basic protein. *Ann. Neurol.* 40:18–24

343. Bruck W, Lucchinetti C, Lassmann H. 2002. The pathology of primary progressive multiple sclerosis. *Mult. Scler.* 8:93–97

344. Werner P, Pitt D, Raine CS. 2001. Multiple sclerosis: altered glutamate homeostasis in lesions correlates with oligodendrocyte and axonal damage. *Ann. Neurol.* 50:169–80

345. Johnson KP, Brooks BR, Cohen JA, Ford CC, Goldstein J, et al. 1995. Copolymer 1 reduces relapse rate and improves disability in relapsing-remitting multiple sclerosis: results of a phase III multicenter, double-blind placebo-controlled trial. *Neurology* 45:1268–76

346. Arnon R. 1996. The development of Cop1 (Copaxone), an innovative drug for the treatment of multiple sclerosis: personal reflections. *Immunol. Lett.* 50:1–15

347. Ziemssen T, Kumpfel T, Klinkert WE, Neuhaus O, Hohlfeld R. 2002. Glatiramer acetate-specific T-helper 1- and 2-type cell lines produce BDNF: implications for multiple sclerosis therapy. Brain-derived neurotrophic factor. *Brain* 125:2381–91

348. Chen M, Valenzuela RM, Dhib-Jalbut S. 2003. Glatiramer acetate-reactive T cells

produce brain-derived neurotrophic factor. *J. Neurol. Sci.* 215:37–44

349. Miller DH, Khan OA, Sheremata WA, Blumhardt LD, Rice GP, et al. 2003. A controlled trial of natalizumab for relapsing multiple sclerosis. *N. Engl. J. Med.* 348:15–23

350. Coles AJ, Wing MG, Molyneux P, Paolillo A, Davie CM, et al. 1999. Monoclonal antibody treatment exposes three mechanisms underlying the clinical course of multiple sclerosis. *Ann. Neurol.* 46:296–304

351. Youssef S, Stuve O, Patarroyo JC, Ruiz PJ, Radosevich JL, et al. 2002. The HMG-CoA reductase inhibitor, atorvastatin, promotes a Th2 bias and reverses paralysis in central nervous system autoimmune disease. *Nature* 420:78–84

352. Vollmer T, Key L, Durkalski V, Tyor W, Corboy J, et al. 2004. Oral simvastatin treatment in relapsing-remitting multiple sclerosis. *Lancet* 363:1607–8

353. Weber F, Polak T, Gunther A, Kubuschok B, Janovskaja J, et al. 1998. Synergistic immunomodulatory effects of interferon-β1b and the phosphodiesterase inhibitor pentoxifylline in patients with relapsing-remitting multiple sclerosis. *Ann. Neurol.* 44:27–34

354. Zhang JZ, Rivera VM, Tejada-Simon MV, Yang DY, Hong J, et al. 2002. T cell vaccination in multiple sclerosis: results of a preliminary study. *J. Neurol.* 249:212–18

355. Vandenbark AA, Chou YK, Whitham R, Mass M, Buenafe A, et al. 1996. Treatment of multiple sclerosis with T-cell receptor peptides: results of a double-blind pilot trial. *Nat. Med.* 2:1109–15

356. Killestein J, Olsson T, Wallstrom E, Svenningsson A, Khademi M, et al. 2002. Antibody-mediated suppression of $V\beta5.2/5.3^+$ T cells in multiple sclerosis: results from an MRI-monitored phase II clinical trial. *Ann. Neurol.* 51:467–74

357. Mancardi GL, Saccardi R, Filippi M, Gualandi F, Murialdo A, et al. 2001. Autologous hematopoietic stem cell transplantation suppresses Gd-enhanced MRI activity in MS. *Neurology* 57:62–68

358. Burt RK, Cohen BA, Russell E, Spero K, Joshi A, et al. 2003. Hematopoietic stem cell transplantation for progressive multiple sclerosis: failure of a total body irradiation-based conditioning regimen to prevent disease progression in patients with high disability scores. *Blood* 102:2373–78

359. Nash RA, Bowen JD, McSweeney PA, Pavletic SZ, Maravilla KR, et al. 2003. High-dose immunosuppressive therapy and autologous peripheral blood stem cell transplantation for severe multiple sclerosis. *Blood* 102:2364–72

Annu. Rev. Immunol. 2005. 23:749–86
doi: 10.1146/annurev.immunol.21.120601.141025
Copyright © 2005 by Annual Reviews. All rights reserved
First published online as a Review in Advance on January 7, 2005

Mast Cells as "Tunable" Effector and Immunoregulatory Cells: Recent Advances

Stephen J. Galli, Janet Kalesnikoff,
Michele A. Grimbaldeston, Adrian M. Piliponsky,
Cara M.M. Williams, and Mindy Tsai

*Department of Pathology, Stanford University School of Medicine, Stanford,
California 94305; email: sgalli@stanford.edu*

Key Words acquired immunity, allergy, basophils, cytokines, inflammation, innate immunity, signaling, tissue remodeling

■ **Abstract** This review focuses on recent progress in our understanding of how mast cells can contribute to the initiation, development, expression, and regulation of acquired immune responses, both those associated with IgE and those that are apparently expressed independently of this class of Ig. We emphasize findings derived from in vivo studies in mice, particularly those employing genetic approaches to influence mast cell numbers and/or to alter or delete components of pathways that can regulate mast cell development, signaling, or function. We advance the hypothesis that mast cells not only can function as proinflammatory effector cells and drivers of tissue remodeling in established acquired immune responses, but also may contribute to the initiation and regulation of such responses. That is, we propose that mast cells can also function as immunoregulatory cells. Finally, we show that the notion that mast cells have primarily two functional configurations, off (or resting) or on (or activated for extensive mediator release), markedly oversimplifies reality. Instead, we propose that mast cells are "tunable," by both genetic and environmental factors, such that, depending on the circumstances, the cell can be positioned phenotypically to express a wide spectrum of variation in the types, kinetics, and/or magnitude of its secretory functions.

INTRODUCTION

Mast cells are derivatives of hematopoietic progenitor cells that migrate into virtually all vascularized tissues, where they complete their maturation (1–6).[1] Mature mast cells normally reside close to epithelia, blood vessels, nerves, and, in the airways and gastrointestinal tract, near smooth muscle cells and mucus-producing glands (1–6). In certain circumstances, morphologically identifiable mast cells can

---

[1] See Appendix for a full list of abbreviations used in this review.

0732-0582/05/0423-0749$14.00

migrate locally in the tissues, including into epithelia (1–4). In some species, including murine rodents, mast cells also occur within mesothelium-lined cavities, such as the peritoneal cavity (1–6).

Mast cells are not to be confused with basophils, which share some phenotypic and functional properties with mast cells but that differ from mast cells in important aspects of natural history, mediator content, and function (5, 6). In contrast to mast cells, basophils are circulating granulocytes that typically mature in the bone marrow, circulate in the blood as mature cells, and can be recruited into tissues at sites of immunological or inflammatory responses (5, 6). Whereas tissue and peritoneal mast cells can be long-lived and can reenter the cell cycle to undergo proliferation locally, mature basophils, like other granulocytes, appear to lack the potential to proliferate and are thought to undergo apoptosis in the tissues after participating in the biological process that elicited their entry into the tissues (4–6).

Upon appropriate activation (e.g., via aggregation of the FcεRI), both mast cells and basophils can produce a similar, but not identical, spectrum of proinflammatory mediators, as well as certain cytokines and chemokines (2, 5–11) (Table 1). Notably, several lines of evidence, particularly those derived from studies in mice, indicate that the mediator content of particular mast cell populations, as well as other aspects of their phenotype such as the ability of the cell to respond to particular stimuli (or pharmacological inhibitors) of activation, can be modulated, in at least some cases reversibly, by cytokines, growth factors, and other microenvironmental signals (1, 2, 4, 12–15).

This "plasticity" of multiple aspects of the mast cell's phenotype, resulting in the development of phenotypically distinct populations of mast cells in different anatomical sites, as well as in different animal species, is called "mast cell heterogeneity" (1, 2, 4, 12–15). In our view, the most compelling hypothesis to account for such heterogeneity in mast cell phenotypes is the most obvious one: The ability of the lineage to generate individual mast cell populations that exhibit differences in biochemical and functional properties (depending on the anatomical site in which the cells reside and/or the biological processes in which they participate) allows greater flexibility and diversity of mast cell responsiveness to meet the requirements of the physiological, immunological, inflammatory, or other biological responses in which this cell can be involved.

In IgE-associated biological responses, the crosslinking of FcεRI-bound IgE with multivalent antigen (Ag) initiates the activation of mast cells or basophils by promoting aggregation of FcεRI (16–24). This FcεRI-dependent cell activation process results in downstream events that lead to the secretion of three classes of mediators: (*a*) the extracellular release of preformed mediators stored in the cells' cytoplasmic granules, e.g., vasoactive amines, neutral proteases, proteoglycans, and some cytokines and growth factors, by a process called degranulation [or, to distinguish it from "piecemeal" degranulation (25–27), it also can be called anaphylactic degranulation or compound exocytosis], which involves the fusion of the cytoplasmic granule membranes with the cell's plasma membrane; (*b*) the de novo synthesis of proinflammatory lipid mediators, such as prostaglandins and

TABLE 1   Secreted products of mast cells and basophils[a]

	Basophils	Mast Cells
Major mediators stored preformed in cytoplasmic granules	Histamine, chondroitin sulfates, neutral protease with bradykinin-generating activity, β-glucuronidase, elastase, cathepsin G-like enzyme, major basic protein, Charcot-Leyden crystal protein, peroxidase, carboxypeptidase A[b]	Histamine, serotonin (in murine rodents), heparin and/or chondroitin sulfates, neutral proteases (chymases and/or tryptases[b]), major basic protein, many acid hydrolases, cathepsin, carboxypeptidases, peroxidase
Major lipid mediators produced on appropriate activation	LTC$_4$	PGE$_2$, PGD$_2$, LTB$_4$, and LTC$_4$, platelet-activating factor
Cytokines released on appropriate activation[c]	IL-4, IL-13, and probably several chemokines (in mice)[c]	TNF[d], TGF-β, MIP-1α, VPF/VEGF[d], FGF-2[d], LIF, IFN-α, IFN-β, IFN-γ, GM-CSF, MCP-1, IL-1α, IL-1β, IL-3, IL-4, IL-5, IL-6, IL-8, IL-10, IL-9, IL-11, IL-12, IL-13, IL-15, IL-16, IL-18, IL-25 (and probably many more)
Anti-microbial peptides	?	Cathelicidin (human mast cells: LL-37; murine mast cells: CRAMP[e])

[a]Table adapted from Reference 204.

[b]Under certain conditions, tryptase+, chymase+, carboxypeptidase A+ and c-Kit+ granulated cells, that appear to be basophils by morphology and are reactive with an antibody against BSP-1 (which stains basophils but not mast cells), can be observed in the peripheral blood. Adapted from Li et al. (202).

[c]Based on microarray data (11).

[d]Several lines of evidence indicate that certain cytokines produced by mast cells, such as tumor necrosis factor (TNF), fibroblast growth factor (FGF)-2 and vascular permeability factor (VPF)/vascular endothelial growth factor (VEGF), are released in part from preformed stores, some of which may be physically associated with the cells' cytoplasmic granules.

[e]CRAMP: cathelin-related antimicrobial peptide (203).

leukotrienes; and (c) the synthesis and secretion of many growth factors, cytokines, and chemokines (2, 7–10, 16–18, 21–24).

Because they can release potent biologically active mediators in response to challenge with IgE and specific Ag, mast cells and basophils have long been regarded as key effector cells in IgE-associated immediate hypersensitivity and allergic disorders, as well as in certain protective immune responses to parasites (2, 3, 5, 10, 16, 17, 21, 28). The IgE-dependent release of mediators can begin within minutes of Ag challenge, and the critical role of mast cells and basophils in certain acute allergic reactions (such as anaphylaxis and acute attacks of "atopic" asthma) is now widely accepted. By contrast, the importance of these cells (as opposed to other potential effector cells) in the chronic inflammation and other long-term tissue changes observed in some IgE-associated disorders, including asthma, has been debated for some time (7, 17, 29, 30).

The same is true of the proposed importance of mast cells in certain T cell–dependent immune responses, such as contact hypersensitivity (CHS): Some studies have strongly implicated mast cells as important contributors to the responses (31–33), whereas others have detected no such role (34–38). Although the mechanisms that account for mast cell activation during CHS remain to be fully understood (as discussed below), there is no doubt that mast cells (or basophils) can be activated to express effector function by many mechanisms that are independent of the FcεRI, and these cells are now thought to participate in a wide variety of physiological or pathological processes independently of IgE (2, 3, 5, 7, 17, 39–51). For example, mast cells are essential for the full expression of certain innate immune responses in mice (40, 43, 49, 52) and have been implicated as potentially critical participants in many other settings (such as angiogenesis, host responses to neoplasia, and certain autoimmune disorders) (2, 3, 5, 7, 39, 41, 42, 46–48, 50, 51).

In this review, we briefly summarize the current understanding of the positive and negative regulation of signaling in mast cells via the FcεRI, including recent work indicating that the cell's functional properties can be modified (or "tuned") by actions of IgE in the absence of known Ag. We then describe a model system in which many proposed mast cell functions can be analyzed in vivo by comparing the expression of biological responses in (*a*) wild-type mice, (*b*) mice that essentially lack mast cells (but also express other phenotypic abnormalities) because of defective expression and/or function of the c-kit receptor, and (*c*) c-*kit* mutant, genetically mast cell–deficient mice that have been selectively repaired of their mast cell deficiency, so-called "mast cell knockin mice." Finally, we illustrate how mast cell knockin mice have been used to identify and characterize the potentially diverse contributions of mast cells to the induction, expression, and regulation of IgE-associated and other acquired immune responses.

MAST CELL SIGNALING

FcεRI Signaling Events

Mast cells express an array of immunoreceptors and other surface receptors that allow these cells to respond to many different stimuli, such as stem cell factor (SCF), interleukin-3 (IL-3), lipopolysaccharide (LPS), certain products of complement activation, and some neuropeptides, and to participate in a wide variety of physiological and pathological processes (1–6). However, the best-studied mechanism for the activation of mast cells for immunologically specific function is the interaction of specific Ag with IgE bound to its high-affinity receptor, FcεRI, on the cell surface, resulting in the aggregation of the receptors and the initiation of intracellular signaling (16–24). Because a number of excellent reviews on mast cell signaling via the FcεRI have been published recently (17–24), this section focuses primarily on some new developments that employ genetically altered mice to elucidate aspects of the positive or negative regulation of signaling initiated by this receptor.

In both humans and rodents, FcεRI is expressed on the surface of mast cells (and basophils) as a heterotetrameric receptor composed of an IgE-binding α subunit, a four transmembrane-spanning β subunit, and two identical disulphide linked γ subunits (17, 18, 20, 21). The γ subunits are important for initiating signaling events downstream of this receptor because they each contain one immunoreceptor tyrosine-based activation motif (ITAM), and the β subunit serves as an important amplifier of IgE- and Ag-induced signaling events (17, 20). Monomeric IgE binds to FcεRI at a very high affinity (1×10^{10} M^{-1}), and this interaction has a slow rate of dissociation (17, 18); thus, FcεRI binds IgE and retains it for long periods, setting the stage for an immediate allergic or inflammatory response upon exposure to Ag.

Like all immunoreceptor family members, FcεRI lacks intrinsic tyrosine kinase activity (2, 17–19). IgE- and Ag-induced crosslinking of FcεRI initiates a complex series of phosphate transfer events via the activation of Src, Syk, and Tec family protein tyrosine kinases (17, 19, 21–23) (Figure 1). These early phosphorylation events lead to the recruitment of adaptor molecules [e.g., LAT (linker for activation of T cells), SLP-76 (SH2-containing leukocyte protein of 76 kDa), and NTAL (non–T cell activation linker) (22, 23, 53)] and the activation of enzymes, such as PLCγ (phospholipase Cγ), which regulates intracellular calcium release and PKC (protein kinase C) activity by hydrolyzing the membrane phospholipid PI-4,5-P$_2$(phosphatidyl inositol 4,5,-bisphosphate) to form soluble IP$_3$(inositol 1,4,5-trisphosphate) and membrane bound DAG (diacylglycerol). Recruitment and activation of SLP-76, Vav, Shc, Grb2, and Sos culminate in the activation of the small GTPases, Ras, Rac, and Rho. These GTPases regulate activation of the MAPK (mitogen-activated protein kinase) family members, ERK (extracellular signal-regulated kinase), JNK (c-Jun N-terminal kinase), and p38, which regulate the activity of numerous transcription factors important for cytokine production and the activity of PLA$_2$ (phospholipase A$_2$) to generate arachidonic acid metabolites. A mast cell–specific Ras guanine nucleotide releasing protein, RasGRP4, has recently been identified (54). RasGRP4 contributes to mast cell granule formation (54) and ionophore-induced PGD$_2$ (prostaglandin D$_2$) expression (55). However, it has not yet been reported whether RasGRP4 has any role in FcεRI-dependent mast cell activation.

Another primary target of FcεRI signaling is PI3K (Figure 1). The SH2 domain-containing p85 regulatory subunit of PI3K mediates its recruitment to the membrane, which allows the associated p110 catalytic subunit to phosphorylate PI-4,5-P$_2$ and generate the important second messenger, PI-3,4,5-P$_3$. Our understanding of FcεRI-induced activation of PI3K has increased dramatically over the past three years. The adaptor protein Gab2, which quickly becomes tyrosine phosphorylated after FcεRI aggregation, was recently reported to link the IgE receptor with PI3K activation by binding to the p85 regulatory subunit (22, 23). In addition, the Src family kinase Fyn was newly identified as the principal kinase that positively regulates Gab2 phosphorylation (independent of Lyn, Syk, or LAT) (22, 56). Similar to Lyn, Fyn appears to associate with the FcεRI β subunit in mast cells, and this interaction is enhanced by FcεRI aggregation; the recruitment of two Src family kinases to the FcεRI is reminiscent of early signaling events downstream of the T cell (Lck and Fyn) and B cell (Lyn and Fyn) receptors (22, 23). The signaling

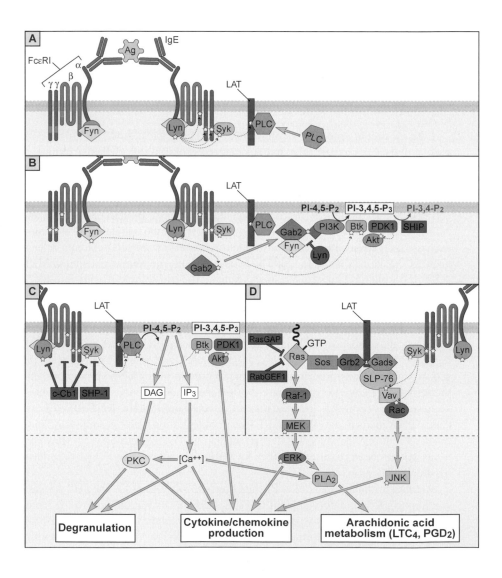

pathways outlined above and their contributions toward mast cell activation are illustrated in Figure 1; however, their compartmentalization is reviewed elsewhere (21–23).

Negative Regulation of FcεRI Signaling

Several negative intracellular regulators modulate the signaling events initiated by FcεRI and other "activating" receptors on mast cells [e.g., c-kit, IL-3R, Toll-like

---

Figure 1   FcεRI-mediated signaling events. (*A*) Ag-induced crosslinking of FcεRI activates Lyn, which is associated with the β chain, to phosphorylate (*star symbol*) the β and γ chain ITAMs. Once phosphorylated, the β chain ITAM binds to the SH2 domain of additional Lyn molecules, while the γ chain ITAM recruits Syk to the receptor complex, where it is phosphorylated and activated by Lyn. Lyn and Syk phosphorylate many adaptors and enzymes (indicated by - - ≫). Syk phosphorylates LAT, which then recruits the SH2 domain of PLCγ. (*C*) At the membrane, PLCγ is phosphorylated by both Syk and Btk. These phosphorylation events activate PLCγ to hydrolyze the membrane bound lipid, PI-4,5-P_2, to IP_3 and DAG, which positively regulate calcium (Ca^{2+}) flux and PKC activity, respectively. (*B*) FcεRI aggregation also activates Fyn, which is associated with the β chain, to phosphorylate Gab2. Phosphorylated Gab2 serves as a docking site for additional Fyn molecules and binds to the SH2 domain of the p85 subunit of PI3K (phosphoinositide 3-kinase), recruiting the p110 catalytic subunit to the membrane, where it phosphorylates PI-4,5-P_2 to generate PI-3,4,5-P_3. PI-3,4,5-P_3 recruits a number of PH domain–containing proteins, including Btk (which is then phosphorylated by Lyn and autophosphorylates for full activation), PLCγ, PDK1 (3-phosphoinositide-dependent kinase 1, which phosphorylates Akt), and Akt (which enhances cell survival and cytokine production). (*D*) Phosphorylated LAT also recruits the adaptor molecules Grb2, Gads, and SLP-76. At the membrane, the Grb2-associated effector molecule, Sos, which is a guanine nucleotide exchange factor, activates Ras. SLP-76 is phosphorylated by Syk, then recruits the SH2 domain of the guanine nucleotide exchange factor, Vav, which is also phosphorylated by Syk prior to its activation of Rac. Vav has recently been shown to regulate PLCγ phosphorylation as well. Arrows indicate the contributions of these signaling pathways toward mast cell degranulation, arachidonic acid metabolism, and cytokine/chemokine production. As indicated in the text, FcεRI aggregation activates a number of proteins that negatively regulate these positive signaling pathways (indicated by ⊣ in *red*). Lyn, which initiates both activating and inhibitory signals, negatively regulates Gab2 phosphorylation events. Other negative regulators include c-Cbl (which facilitates the ubiquitination of FcεRI, Lyn, and Syk), the tyrosine phosphatase SHP-1 (which dephosphorylates Syk), the lipid phosphatase SHIP (which catalyzes the hydrolysis of PI-3,4,5-P_3), RasGAP (which enhances the intrinsic GTPase activity of Ras), and RabGEF1 (which binds to GTP-bound Ras and negatively regulates activation of the Ras/Raf/ERK pathway). (Figure adapted from References 21–23.)

receptors (TLRs), etc.]. Important negative regulators of mast cell signaling events include the tyrosine phosphatase SHP-1 (SH2-containing protein tyrosine phosphatase-1) (57, 58), the lipid phosphatases SHIP (SH2-containing inositol 5' phosphatase) and SHIP2 (57, 59), and the E3 ubiquitin ligase c-Cbl (60, 61) (Figure 1). Interestingly, some signaling molecules initiate both activating and inhibitory signals; for example, Lyn phosphorylation of FcεRI ITAMs initiates signaling events downstream of this receptor, whereas its phosphorylation of immunoreceptor tyrosine-based inhibitory motifs (ITIMs; outlined below) leads to the recruitment of inhibitory signaling molecules such as SHIP, and Lyn also appears to negatively regulate Gab2 phosphorylation events (22, 56). Furthermore, Lyn knockout mast cells and mice are hyperresponsive to IgE and Ag stimulation, highlighting Lyn's important role as a negative regulator of the allergic response (22, 23, 62).

Multiple functionally distinct effectors of Ras have recently been identified, and these proteins are thought to mediate the many biological actions of Ras (63). Using functional genomics approaches, our group has recently identified Rab guanine nucleotide exchange factor 1 (RabGEF1) as a novel negative regulator of IgE- and Ag-induced mast cell activation (64) (Figure 1). RabGEF1 binds to Ras and negatively regulates the Ras/Raf/ERK signaling cascade. Mast cells derived from RabGEF1 knockout mice exhibit enhanced degranulation and increased release of cytokines and lipid mediators in response to IgE and Ag stimulation. Mice lacking RabGEF1 have increased perinatal mortality and develop severe inflammation of the skin (64). Because RabGEF1 is expressed in many different tissues and RabGEF1 knockout mice exhibit many distinct phenotypic abnormalities, it is likely that multiple cell lineages expressing RabGEF1 contribute to the complex phenotype of these mice.

In addition to the negative intracellular regulators highlighted above, signaling events initiated by FcεRI and other ITAM-containing immunoreceptors are negatively regulated by coaggregation with ITIM-containing receptors (19, 21, 65, 66). These receptors traverse the plasma membrane once, and their N-terminal extracellular domains consist of either C-type lectin domains [e.g., Ly49 and MAFA (mast cell function–associated antigen)] or Ig-like domains [e.g., FcγRIIB, KIR (killer inhibitory receptor), gp49B1, PIR-B (paired Ig-like receptor-B), and SIRP (signal regulatory protein)] domains (19, 66). Each of these receptors contains at least one cytoplasmic ITIM (I/VxYxxL) that becomes phosphorylated after coaggregation with FcεRI and attenuates immunoreceptor-induced signaling events through the recruitment of specific SH2-containing phosphatases (i.e., SHP-1, SHP-2, SHIP or SHIP2) (19, 21, 65, 66).

The low-affinity IgG receptor, FcγRIIB, was the first identified ITIM-containing receptor; FcγRIIB has been shown to inhibit signaling events when coaggregated with FcεRI and the SCF receptor, c-kit, on mast cells (19, 21, 66–68) (Figure 2). Moreover, FcγRII$^{-/-}$ mice exhibited enhanced passive cutaneous anaphylaxis in vivo (69). To date, FcγRIIB is the only inhibitory receptor shown to recruit SHIP and coaggregate with FcεRI in vivo, making it a desirable therapeutic target (70). Another ITIM-containing receptor, gp49B1, is preferentially expressed on mast cells, macrophages, and activated natural killer (NK) cells. This inhibitory receptor contains two ITIMs, which bind to SHP-1 following antibody-induced coaggregation of gp49B1 with FcεRI, thus inhibiting IgE- and Ag-induced degranulation and LTC_4 synthesis; moreover, gp49B1 knockout mice display increased sensitivity to IgE- and Ag-induced passive cutaneous anaphylaxis (19, 21, 67, 71). The integrin $\alpha_v\beta_3$ was recently reported to be a ligand for mouse gp49B1; thus, gp49B1 may represent an innate pathway for the downregulation of IgE- and Ag-induced mast cell activation (67, 71).

Other inhibitory receptors expressed on mast cells include MAFA (19, 23, 65, 72), PIR-B (19, 67), and SIRPα (19, 67). PIR-B and SIRPα both contain four ITIMs that interact with SHP-1 and SHP-2 to downregulate IgE- and Ag-induced signaling events, including degranulation, when they are expressed as chimeric receptors containing the extracellular domain of FcγRIIB and are then coaggregated with FcεRI (19, 67). Although the ligand for PIR-B remains elusive, IAP (integrin-associated protein)/CD47, a ubiquitously expressed cell surface glycoprotein that regulates adhesion, was recently identified as a ligand for SIRPα (19).

An interesting area for future study is the extent to which the various ITIM-containing surface structures or other (intracellular) molecules that can negatively regulate FcεRI-dependent signaling actually come into play during naturally occurring adaptive or pathological responses involving IgE in vivo. Clearly, such work may have important therapeutic implications.

Factors Affecting (or "Tuning") the Mast Cell's Functional "Secretory Phenotype"

Although it has been traditional to think of mast cells, at least from the perspective of mediator secretion, as being either off (or resting) or on (or activated for extensive mediator release), both older and more recent evidence suggests that this view significantly oversimplifies reality. On the basis of ultrastructural evidence, A. Dvorak et al. (25–27) proposed that basophils and mast cells can release cytoplasmic granule-associated mediators by a process called "piecemeal degranulation," in which small vehicles carry granule contents from the cytoplasmic granules to the plasma membrane. Evidence for this proposed mechanism has recently been reported in eosinophils as well (73, 74). Moreover, mast cells can express "differential" release of mediators under certain circumstances (e.g., serotonin rather than histamine in response to challenge with Compound 48/80 or IgE and Ag when the cells are stimulated in the presence of amitriptyline; Reference 75) or certain cytokines rather than preformed granule-associated mediators in response to LPS (76). In such cases, mast cells are thought to exhibit a pattern of stimulus-dependent mediator release that can differ from that associated with classical IgE- and Ag-induced "anaphylactic degranulation," both in kinetics and in amounts and/or spectrum of secreted mediators.

More recently, evidence has been presented that mast cells can exhibit variation in their intrinsic responsiveness to various activating stimuli, and in some cases may actually secrete products in the absence of known mast cell stimuli. For example,

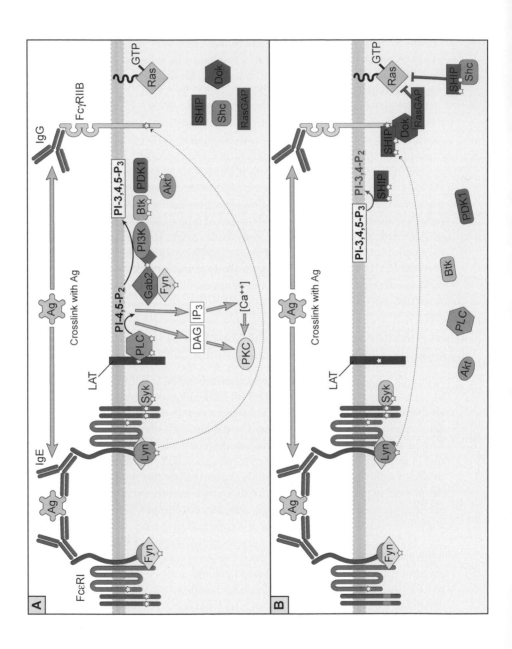

mast cells derived from mice lacking certain proteins that negatively regulate mast cell activation (e.g., SHIP, RabGEF1, etc.), exhibit increased sensitivity to activating stimuli, and/or release substantially larger amounts of mediators once stimulated; in some cases, such cells exhibit evidence of activation even in the absence of known stimuli (59, 64, 77).

These findings suggest that naturally occurring variations in levels of expression of such proteins (and/or of proteins that positively regulate secretion) within the population, or genetic variation in the structure and function of such proteins, also may contribute to variation in the secretory phenotype of mast cells in different individuals and thereby influence their susceptibility to the development (and/or the severity) of allergic inflammation or other mast cell–associated responses. Indeed, deficiencies in a positive signaling molecule downstream of $Fc\varepsilon RI$ (i.e., Syk) have been reported in "nonreleaser" basophils (that do not degranulate in response to $Fc\varepsilon RI$ crosslinking) (78), whereas deficiencies in a negative signaling molecule (i.e., SHIP) have been reported in "hyper-releasable" basophils derived from highly allergic donors (79). Finally, defective variants of RasGRP4 that contribute to mast cell granule formation (54) and ionophore-induced PGD_2 expression (55) have been reported in subjects with asthma, mastocytosis, or mast cell leukemia (54).

Making matters more complicated (and interesting), it was recently found that IgE alone, in the absence of known Ag, not only can result in enhanced surface expression of the $Fc\varepsilon RI$ (80–87) but also can induce signaling events that enhance mouse mast cell survival in vitro and in vivo (21, 88, 89). And some IgEs can enhance mast cell histamine content (89, 90) and/or induce secretion of mast cell mediators (21, 88, 89, 91), at least in vitro. Moreover, different mouse monoclonal IgE molecules vary in their ability to induce signaling events in mouse mast cells (89). Although the mechanisms underlying such effects are not fully understood, the signaling and biological consequences of exposure of mast cells to such IgEs, in the absence of known Ag, closely resemble those induced by IgE- and Ag-dependent aggregation of the $Fc\varepsilon RI$ (89).

How can these effects of IgE be explained? One clue comes from the recent findings concerning the mouse monoclonal anti-DNP IgE, SPE-7 (Sigma) (88, 89, 92). Of the IgE monoclonal antibodies reported so far, SPE-7 displays the strongest signaling potential in mast cells (88, 89). Moreover, SPE-7 has an antigen-binding site that can exist in at least two isomeric conformations, which permit it to bind to

---

←

Figure 2 $Fc\gamma RIIB$-mediated inhibition of $Fc\varepsilon RI$ signaling pathways. (*A*) Ag-induced coaggregation of $Fc\varepsilon RI$ with $Fc\gamma RIIB$ induces Lyn, which is associated with the $Fc\varepsilon RI$ β chain, to phosphorylate (*star symbol*) the ITIM of $Fc\gamma RIIB$. (*B*) This phosphorylation event leads to the recruitment of SHIP, which catalyzes the hydrolysis of $PI\text{-}3,4,5\text{-}P_3$ to $PI\text{-}3,4\text{-}P_2$ and inhibits $Fc\varepsilon RI$-induced membrane recruitment of Btk, $PLC\gamma$, PDK-1, and Akt. $Fc\gamma RIIB$ coaggregation also induces the phosphorylation of SHIP, which leads to the subsequent inhibition of Ras activation as indicated. (Figure adapted from Reference 21.)

two chemically and structurally distinct Ags (92). These findings suggest that, in addition to serum IgE levels per se [which can regulate levels of surface expression of the FcεRI on mast cells (80–87)], the Ag "multispecificity" of particular IgE molecules in individual subjects also may contribute to the range of allergic inflammation and disease observed across the population. Indeed, extrapolating broadly from the findings with SPE-7 (92), one at least has to consider the possibility that all IgE antibodies might be able to recognize not only the Ag to which they are known to have specificity (such as those that are routinely included in panels of allergens for clinical testing), but also at least one "unknown" Ag. Moreover, in theory, such unknown Ags could include those contained either in exogenous or endogenous molecules.

Adding another layer of complexity to the regulation of mast cell activation levels in vivo is the observation that activated mast cells can respond to, and in some cases produce, a myriad of mediators that may serve to amplify responses to other specific activation signals. For example, adenosine represents a potentially important autocrine signal for the activation of mast cells (93–96). Laffargue et al. (95) provided evidence that IgE- and Ag-mediated mast cell activation induces the release of adenosine, which activates PI3Kγ, through the A(3) adenosine receptor expressed on mast cells (97), and leads to a transient increase in PI-3,4,5-P$_3$ levels that can initiate a sustained calcium influx and mast cell degranulation. Signaling via PI3Kγ is also required for optimal enhancement of cutaneous vascular permeability during IgE- and Ag-dependent passive systemic anaphylaxis in vivo. However, this signaling requirement may reflect the PI3Kγ-dependent signaling from G protein–coupled receptors (GPCRs), which are activated by ligands other than adenosine and are released during this immune response (95, 97). Thus, in addition to effects of IgE, autocrine or paracrine stimulation of mast cells via GPCRs may also contribute to the modulation of mast cell activation levels. Finally, it is likely that signaling via other classes of molecules expressed on the mast cell surface, such as TLRs (98) or members of the transient receptor potential (vanilloid) (TRPV) family (99), may also have effects that can alter mast cell responsiveness to signaling via the FcεRI or other receptors through which these cells express immunologically specific function.

Taken together, such findings suggest that, depending on the intrinsic (i.e., genetic) secretory phenotype of one's mast cells, and one's personal exposure to various species and levels of IgE (and/or other stimuli of mast cell activation), one's mast cells may exhibit a wide spectrum of functional "activation levels" in vivo. These may range from truly resting (in which essentially no mediators are released and no secretory function is expressed) to low levels of activation that include the secretion of small quantities of some mediators, such as immunomodulatory cytokines (21, 24, 88, 89, 91, 100), to the highly activated states associated with the release of large amounts of all classes of mediators that characterize mast cells participating in acute allergic reactions. Moreover, Bryce et al. (33) recently provided evidence that even "physiological" levels of IgE, through effects mediated via the FcRγ chain of FcεRI, can prime mouse mast cells to exhibit enhanced levels of mRNA for certain mast cell mediators, including cytokines and a chemokine that can have a variety of proinflammatory and/or immunoregulatory effects, upon exposure of the skin to a sensitizing hapten in vivo. Thus, IgE appears to be able to adjust the mast cell's potential to produce cytokines and chemokines in response to signals initiated by the animal's first exposure to a sensitizing hapten.

The term "tuning" can be used to describe the adjustment of a radio receiver or laser to receive or transmit signals at one specific point along a potentially broad spectrum of frequencies, or to refer to adjusting an apparatus for optimal performance. We use the term "tuning" to describe how a constellation of genetic and/or environmental factors (including IgE itself) can position, or "tune," mast cells within a broad spectrum of functional responsiveness. At one extreme (e.g., in the absence of IgE), mast cells may be tuned to be highly resistant to some or all stimuli of activation; at the other extreme (e.g., in the absence of critical negative regulators of signaling via the FcεRI, such as SHIP or RabGEF1), the cell may actually secrete mediators in the absence of known stimuli of activation, and may produce much larger quantities of mediators when stimulated with IgE and Ag (64, 77).

Mast Cell Knockin Mice as a Model for Studying Mast Cell Function In Vivo

Normal mast cell development and survival, and therefore mast cell function, are disrupted in c-kit/W mutant animals that either lack expression of the c-kit receptor or express c-kit with significantly reduced tyrosine kinase activity. Several mast cell–deficient rodents, such as Kit^W/Kit^{W-v}, Kit^{W-41}/Kit^{W-41}, and Kit^{W-f}/Kit^{W-f} mice, as well as Kit^{W-s}/Kit^{W-s} rats, have been used to investigate mast cell biology in vivo (1, 4, 101). Among these, WBB6F1-Kit^W/Kit^{W-v} mice are the most commonly used. Adult Kit^W/Kit^{W-v} mice ordinarily have <1% the wild-type levels of skin mast cells, and usually no detectable mast cells in the peritoneal cavity, respiratory system, gastrointestinal tract, or other sites (102). However, these mice also have other abnormalities owing to the lack of normal c-kit function, including a virtually complete lack of germ cells, interstitial cells of Cajal, and cutaneous melanocytes, a moderate anemia, and other more subtle abnormalities (1, 4, 101).

Although the lack of tissue mast cells in Kit^{W-sh}/Kit^{W-sh} mice was documented long ago (103), these mice are now being characterized in more detail as a model for the study of mast cell function in vivo (104, 105). Unlike other c-kit/W mutations that affect multiple cell lineages as a result of an altered c-kit coding region, the "W-$sash$" (W^{sh}) mutation, an inversion mutation upstream of the c-kit transcriptional site on mouse chromosome 5 (106), has been reported to impair primarily the development of mast cells and melanocytes (107, 108). In vitro–derived mast cells generated from Kit^{W-sh}/Kit^{W-sh} mice do not express c-kit mRNA (107, 108).

Like WBB6F1-Kit^W/Kit^{W-v} mice, C57BL/6-Kit^{W-sh}/Kit^{W-sh} mice are profoundly mast cell–deficient (103–105, 107, 108) and can accept mast cell transplantation by adoptive transfer into the peritoneal cavity (104, 105) or via the intradermal or intravenous routes (105). However, compared with Kit^W/Kit^{W-v} mice, Kit^{W-sh}/Kit^{W-sh} mice exhibit fewer other phenotypic abnormalities; for example, Kit^{W-sh}/Kit^{W-sh} mice are neither anemic nor sterile. As a result, Kit^{W-sh}/Kit^{W-sh} mice may offer some advantages over Kit^W/Kit^{W-v} mice as a model for analyzing certain mast cell functions in vivo. Certainly, the fertility of the Kit^{W-sh}/Kit^{W-sh} mice is advantageous when one wishes to produce mast cell–deficient mice that also have other defined genetic abnormalities; in the case of the sterile Kit^W/Kit^{W-v} mice, more complex and expensive breeding strategies must be employed for this purpose (109, 110).

The mast cell activity in genetically mast cell–deficient c-*kit* mutant mice can be selectively reconstituted (i.e., mast cell reconstitution can be achieved without replacing the recipient's other hematopoietic cells with those of donor origin) by the adoptive transfer of genetically compatible, in vitro–derived mast cells (111). Such mast cells can be derived from the bone marrow cells of either the congenic wild-type mice or various transgenic or knockout mice [bone marrow–derived, cultured mast cells (BMCMCs)] (111), from other sources of hematopoietic cells, or directly from embryonic stem cells [embryonic stem cell–derived cultured mast cells (ESCMCs)] (112). With BMCMCs, the mast cells can be administered by intravenous, intraperitoneal, or intradermal injection (1, 4, 111) or by direct injection into the anterior wall of the stomach (113), thus producing the so-called mast cell knockin mice.

Notably, depending on the anatomical site in which they reside, such adoptively transferred BMCMCs gradually acquire multiple phenotypic characteristics of the corresponding native mast cell populations found in the congenic wild-type mice (111). And in certain anatomical sites, such as the skin and peritoneal cavity, the locally injected BMCMCs can acquire a tissue distribution, and numbers, that closely resemble those of the corresponding mast cell populations in wild-type mice (1, 4, 111, 114). However, certain aspects of the phenotype of such adoptively transferred mast cells may not be identical to those of the native populations of mast cells in the corresponding sites in the wild-type mice. For example, because the content of stored mediators in mast cells increases with age, the adoptively transferred mast cells may have lower levels of these mediators than the corresponding native mast cell populations in the wild-type mice (111).

Moreover, in some anatomical sites, the distribution and numbers of mast cells in mast cell knockin mice may not be identical to those of the corresponding native mast cell populations in the normal mice. For example, intravenous injection of WBB6F1-Kit^W/Kit^{W-v} mice with $Kit^{+/+}$ (wild-type) BMCMCs results in a pattern of mast cell distribution in the respiratory tract of the mast cell knockin mice that differs from that in the wild-type mice, with fewer in the trachea but more in the lung periphery than in the wild-type mice (115, 116). Intravenous administration of BMCMCs also failed to reconstitute mast cells in the central nervous system, lymph nodes, or hearts of WBB6F1-Kit^W/Kit^{W-v} mice, and resulted in higher than normal numbers of mast cells in the spleen (117). Finally, upon transfer to a new anatomical site, certain adoptively transferred mast cell populations (such as mature peritoneal mast cells) may retain aspects of their phenotype (such as a pattern of mast cell protease expression) that are not fully "appropriate" for the new anatomical site in which they reside (118, 119).

These observations emphasize the importance of characterizing how much reconstitution of mast cell populations in mast cell–deficient mice has been achieved in the particular model system under investigation. At a minimum, investigators should quantify the numbers of mast cells in the mast cell knockin mice and assess their tissue distribution compared with the corresponding features of the native mast cell populations in the congenic wild-type mice. In some types of experiments, researchers may need to evaluate certain aspects of the phenotype of the cells as well. Because the time required for the appearance of morphologically identifiable mast cells in different anatomical sites after the adoptive transfer of bone marrow cells (102, 120) or BMCMCs (117) can vary, one must select the interval between injecting the mast cells and performing the experiments in the mast cell–reconstituted mice on the basis of published experience with these model systems or one's own data regarding the specific model under investigation. For example, the success of mast cell reconstitution in restoring wild-type levels of resistance to lethality after cecal ligation and puncture in mast cell–deficient mice appears to require not only the presence of mast cells within the peritoneal cavity, but also the infiltration of the adoptively transferred mast cells into the mesentery of the recipient mice (121).

Interestingly, depending on the model system under investigation, mast cell knockin mice may exhibit mast cell–dependent biological responses which, in terms of the magnitude of the features examined, are statistically indistinguishable from those in the wild-type mice, despite documented differences in the numbers and/or anatomical distribution of mast cells in the wild-type versus mast cell knockin mice (116). One likely explanation for such observations is that the numbers and distribution of adoptively transferred mast cells in the mast cell knockin mice are sufficient to produce the types, amounts, and tissue distribution of biologically active mediators critical for the normal expression of the particular aspect of the response under investigation. This conclusion is supported by studies showing that rather modest levels of mast cell activation induced by the direct injection of SCF into the skin of mice resulted in maximal levels of local tissue swelling, but only suboptimal levels of local deposition of cross-linked fibrin (122). Thus, submaximal levels of mast cell activation may be sufficient for the full expression of certain aspects of the biological response under investigation (in the example given, the associated tissue swelling), whereas the optimal expression of other aspects of the same response (e.g., fibrin deposition) may require higher levels of local mast cell activation.

One also can employ mouse ESCMCs to analyze the effects of specific genetic manipulations on mast cell development, survival, and/or function in vivo (101, 112) as well as in vitro (101, 112, 123). As genetic modifications of ES cells can be readily performed, and large quantities of highly purified mast cells can be generated from mouse ES cells by in vitro differentiation, one can generate mouse

ESCMCs from wild-type or genetically altered ES cells to assess the effects of these constitutive or inducible genetic alterations on the differentiation, lineage commitment, and maturation of mast cells in vitro.

We have used this model system to assess the function of wild-type or genetically altered ESCMCs of 129Sv origin after their transfer into the skin (112) or peritoneal cavity (124) of WBB6F1- Kit^W/Kit^{W-v} mice. However, even though strains 129Sv and C57BL/6 (one of the parental strains of WBB6F1 mice) are MHC identical (H-2^b), there are differences between 129Sv and C57BL/6 strains at minor histocompatibility loci. Perhaps for this reason, we have found that intravenous injection of 129Sv ESCMCs does not result in long-term systemic repair of the mast cell deficiency of WBB6F1- Kit^W/Kit^{W-v} mice. Therefore, it will be of interest to compare the abilities of C57BL/6 or WBB6F1 ESCMCs (64), as opposed to 129Sv ESCMCs, to achieve long-term local or systemic selective reconstitution of mast cell populations in either C57BL/6-Kit^{W-sh}/Kit^{W-sh} or WBB6F1-Kit^W/Kit^{W-v} mast cell–deficient mice, respectively.

In conclusion, genetically mast cell–deficient mice and mast cell knockin mice provide a useful approach for directly assessing the expression of biological responses in vivo in the presence or virtual absence of wild-type mast cells or mast cells with certain genetic alterations [including embryonic or perinatal lethal mutations (112, 124)] that affect mast cell phenotype or function. As with any animal model system, one must always interpret the results obtained in specific experiments in the context of the important features of the model. In the case of mast cell knockin mice, these include the numbers, tissue distribution, and phenotype of the adoptively transferred mast cell populations compared with those of the corresponding native mast cell populations in the congenic wild-type mice. One must also assess directly whether the biological response under examination can actually induce the development of mast cells in the genetically mast cell–deficient mice studied. Although this has been reported in only a few special circumstances (109, 125–130), and represents evidence of the activation of largely c-kit-independent pathways of mast cell development and survival, one must always appropriately examine the mast cell–deficient mice at the end of the experiment to address this possibility. The general approach for using mast cell knockin mice for analyzing the roles of mast cells in biological responses in vivo is shown in Figure 3.

ROLES OF MAST CELLS IN ACQUIRED IMMUNE RESPONSES

Mast Cells in IgE-Dependent Immune Responses

In the mouse, studies of IgE-dependent biological responses that have been conducted by passively transferring IgE antibodies (or injecting anti-IgE antibodies) into wild-type mice, genetically mast cell–deficient mice and, in some cases, mast cell knockin mice indicate that essentially all measured aspects of the responses are entirely mast cell–dependent. These include the associated acute tissue swelling

(131, 132) and local fibrin disposition (131), the acutely enhanced airway hyper-reactivity (AHR) to methacholine (133), the local recruitment of leukocytes to the skin (132) or stomach wall (113), and the cardiopulmonary changes and death secondary to anti-IgE-induced anaphylaxis (133–135).

Indeed, except for one model system in which the immune response to a penicillin Ag was reported to elicit an IgE-associated specific antibody response in the absence of associated Ag-specific IgG1 antibodies (136, 137), all other published evidence indicates that there is no substitute for mast cells in the elicitation of wholly IgE-dependent biological responses in mice in vivo. However, further studies may reveal at least some IgE-dependent biological responses in which partial or even full immunological function can be conferred by basophils rather than (or in addition to) mast cells.

Mast Cells in IgG1-Dependent Immune Responses

Acquired immune responses in the mouse that are associated with Ag-specific IgE are usually also associated with Ag-specific IgG1 (reviewed in 134, 138), and mast cells can be activated for Ag-specific mediator release by IgG1-dependent (139), in addition to IgE-independent, mechanisms. Accordingly, many immune responses to parasites or experimental Ags that elicit Th2 cell–associated immune responses involve the elicitation of immunologically specific mast cell function by both IgE/FcεRI- and IgG1/FcγRIII-dependent mechanisms.

In models of active or passive systemic anaphylaxis, the relative importance of mast cells, IgE antibodies, or IgG1 antibodies in eliciting the biological features of the response can be assessed using mice deficient in mast cells, or in the ability to respond to signaling via FcεRI versus FcγRIII (reviewed in 134, 138). Such work has shown that both IgE and IgG1 antibodies can contribute to the features of active systemic anaphylaxis in the mouse, with the IgE-dependent components being largely mast cell–dependent but the IgG1-dependent components involving the participation of cell types in addition to the mast cells (reviewed in 134, 138).

Mast Cells in Mouse Models of Asthma

Relatively few studies of asthma models have been conducted using mast cell knockin mice. However, all such studies published so far have revealed that mast cells can directly or indirectly enhance the magnitude of multiple features of the response, including (a) AHR to cholinergic stimulation (116, 140, 141), (b) infiltration of eosinophils (116, 141, 142) and other leukocytes (142) into the airways and/or bronchoalveolar lavage fluid, (c) numbers of proliferating cells in the airway epithelium (116), (d) lung collagen deposition (142, 143), (e) airway mucus production, and (f) the local enhancement of the expression of genes associated with inflammation and tissue remodeling (142). Notably, these roles of mast cells have been revealed in mouse models of asthma that either omitted artificial adjuvants at the time of Ag sensitization (116, 142) or employed relatively low doses of Ag for sensitization or challenge (140, 141). This work, and other lines of evidence, indicate that a key role of mast cells in IgE-associated immune responses (and probably many other settings) is to amplify the local expression of both acute and long-term tissue responses to otherwise relatively weak biological signals (7, 142).

In a model of nonatopic asthma induced by epicutaneous sensitization and intranasal challenge with dinitoflourobenze (DNFB), mast cells were required for the acute changes in vascular permeability and acute bronchoconstriction induced by DNFB challenge, as well as for the tracheal hyperreactivity detected 24 or 48 h after challenge (144). Although the mechanisms responsible for mast cell activation in this model were not described, it has been reported, on the basis of work using mast cell knockin mice, that hapten-specific mast cell activation in the skin can be mediated by immunoglobulin light chains (145). In other settings, including many standard protocols for inducing allergic inflammation of the airways in mice that employ artificial adjuvants and relatively high doses of Ag for sensitization and challenge, no contributions of mast cells were detected to such features of the responses as eosinophil infiltration or AHR (116, 146–149).

Mast Cells in Other Models of Host Defense or Disease Associated with IgE and IgG1 Antibody Responses

Approaches similar to those used for studies of asthma models can be used to examine the relative importance of IgE (whose FcεRI-dependent effects in normal mice can only reflect actions on mast cells and/or basophils) as opposed to IgG1 (that can elicit Ag-dependent functional responses in macrophages and other cell types, in addition to mast cells) in other complex biological responses, such as those elicited by parasite infection (109, 150–153) or in models of autoimmune disorders (39, 41, 46). An example of the latter is a mouse model of destructive

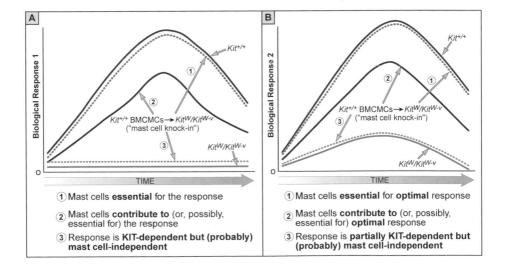

arthritis, which can be elicited in mice that have received passive transfer of anti-bodies, including IgG1 antibodies, with specificity for an autoantigen; in this model system, mast cells and $Fc\gamma$ RIII are required for maximal development of the joint pathology (46). Mast cells can also promote disease incidence and severity in a mouse model of experimental allergic encephalomyelitis (EAE) (39). Moreover, it was recently reported that Kit^W/Kit^{W-v} mice selectively repaired with BMCMCs derived from $Fc\gamma$ RIIB$^{-/-}$ mice exhibited more severe EAE than the wild-type control mice affected with the same disease (154). This finding suggests that

---

Figure 3   Interpretation of possible findings in experiments using mast cell knockin mice. (A) For the biological response illustrated, the feature measured is not expressed at all in the mast cell–deficient mice. Various possible results are shown for the expression of that feature of the response in the mast cell knockin mice (i.e., $Kit^{+/+}$ BMCMCs $\rightarrow$ Kit^W/Kit^{W-v} mice). In scenario 2, mast cells might still be essential for the expression of the response if the lower-than-wild-type response illustrated reflected the fact that, in the organ or anatomical site analyzed, there were significantly fewer mast cells in the mast cell knockin mouse than in the wild-type mouse and/or if the adoptively transferred and native mast cell populations in the respective groups exhibited significant differences in some key aspects of phenotype. In scenario 3, mast cells might still be involved in the expression of the response illustrated if, in the mast cell knockin mice, adoptive transfer of mast cells failed to achieve reconstitution of the mast cell population at the anatomical site of interest. (B) For this biological response, the feature measured is expressed in the mast cell–deficient mice, but to a lesser extent than in the wild-type mice. In examples of this type, the experiments evaluate the extent that mast cells might contribute to optimal (i.e., wild-type levels) expression of the feature of the response analyzed. In individual biological responses, particularly complex responses such as those that occur in response to pathogens or in subjects actively immunized to an Ag, some features of the response may have patterns of mast cell involvement like those shown in (A), whereas other features of the same response may have patterns like those illustrated in (B). In some biological responses, no differences can be observed between the features of the responses of the wild-type and mast cell–deficient mice. Although this result does not formally rule out any contribution of mast cells to the features of the response analyzed, it indicates that at least one other element (present in both the wild-type and mast cell–deficient mice) must contribute to the expression of the feature analyzed in a way that is similar to or overlapping with any contribution of the mast cell. Note that whereas responses evaluated in WBB6F1–$Kit^{+/+}$ versus Kit^W/Kit^{W-v} mice are illustrated in (A) and (B), the same principles apply for responses evaluated in C57BL/6–$Kit^{+/+}$ versus Kit^{W-sh}/Kit^{W-sh} mice. Also, one may substitute for the wild-type BMCMCs shown in the figure genetically compatible BMCMCs or ESCMCs that express defined, genetically determined modifications affecting mast cell phenotype and/or function. Using this approach, one can analyze mechanistically how mast cells express their function in those biological responses that exhibit mast cell–dependent components.

signals transmitted via the mast cell's $Fc\gamma RIIB$ can diminish those mast cell functions that promote disease in this model system.

In parasite infections, passive transfer studies have shown that mast cells and IgE are required for the expression of acquired host resistance to the feeding of larval *Haemaphysalis longicornis* ticks (152). However, in other models examining active immunity to the feeding of larval ticks, morphological evidence in mice (155) and antibody inhibition studies in guinea pigs (156) suggest that basophils may have a more important role. In one model of infection with *Leishmania major*, mast cells contributed to the intensity of the pathology associated with the cutaneous infection but did not detectably influence the success of the infection; however, the approach used for quantifying viable organisms in that study was not very sensitive for detecting differences in the numbers of *L. major* present in these mice (153).

It has been difficult to prove that mast cells have a critical role in the expression of acquired immunity to enteric parasites, such as nematodes. Although there is much evidence that is consistent with this possibility (reviewed in 28, 109, 157), such a role has not so far been confirmed using mast cell knockin mice, perhaps because of a failure of adoptively transferred BMCMCs (151) [as opposed to mast cells derived from adoptively transferred bone marrow cells (150)] to populate the intestinal epithelium of the recipient c-*kit* mutant mice. Moreover, two studies have suggested that mast cells might actually contribute to the fecundity of some nematodes during the primary infections (158, 159), perhaps by promoting inflammation and enhanced vascular permeability at the site of infection.

Mast Cells in Contact Hypersensitivity (CHS) and Other T Cell–Mediated Immune Responses

The interactions between mast cells and T cells that occur during the initiation, development, and expression of CHS and other T cell–associated immune responses are likely to be quite complex. Morphologic studies demonstrate that mast cells reside in close physical proximity to infiltrating T cells in inflamed allergic tissues and at sites of helminth infections (160, 161) as well as in CHS responses (162). This juxtaposition of mast cells and T cells may facilitate bidirectional signaling between these two cell types. Indeed, in vitro and in vivo studies indicate that T cell–derived IL-3 (109, 163) and the β-chemokines macrophage inflammatory protein-1α (MIP-1α) and monocyte chemoattractant protein-1 (MCP-1) (164, 165) can contribute to mast cell proliferation and activation, respectively.

On the basis of in vitro evidence, investigators have reported that activated mast cells can influence T cell–dependent inflammation via the following mechanisms: (*a*) Ag presentation by mast cells to T cells through either an MHC class I– or class II–restricted and costimulatory molecule-dependent mechanism in both humans and rodents (166–173); (*b*) promotion of T cell migration to inflammatory sites directly, either by mast cell–derived chemotactic factors, such as lymphotactin and IL-16 (which are preferentially chemotactic for $CD8^+$ or $CD4^+$ T cells, respectively) (174) or by leukotriene B_4 (LTB_4) (175), or indirectly, by mast cell–mediated upregulation of cell surface adhesion molecule expression, such as E-selectin, intercellular adhesion molecule (ICAM)-1, and vascular cell adhesion molecule (VCAM)-1, on endothelial cells (176, 177); and (c) effects on T cell polarization whereby mediators potentially derived from mast cells, such as IL-4 and histamine, can polarize T cells to preferentially differentiate toward the Th2-like phenotype (44, 178).

In addition, direct contact with PMA-activated T lymphocytes, but not with resting T cells, induced murine BMCMCs or human mast cells to release histamine, TNF, and matrix metalloproteinase-9 (MMP-9) (179–181). In this system, mast cell activation was augmented by leukocyte function–associated antigen (LFA)-1/ICAM-1-mediated heterotypic aggregation with activated T cells. In vitro data also suggest that regulation of mast cell–derived MMP-9, an enzyme that participates in extracellular matrix remodeling and thereby facilitates leukocyte trafficking into an inflamed site (182), may be promoted in an autocrine manner by the release of mast cell TNF (181). These studies clearly support the concept of functionally important mast cell–T cell interactions, but the difficult challenge remains of verifying the occurrence and biological importance of these cell-cell interactions using appropriate in vivo genetic approaches.

Experimental models of CHS responses to chemical haptens have been widely used to investigate mechanisms of immune sensitization (183). The generation of CHS requires both an effective sensitization phase, which occurs after the initial exposure to the hapten, followed by an elicitation phase that is characterized by edema and leukocyte recruitment upon reexposure to the same hapten. The migration of hapten-bearing antigen-presenting cells from the affected site to draining lymph nodes during the initial sensitization phase is crucial for Ag-specific T cell memory responses to subsequent exposures (184, 185).

Disparate findings in studies using genetically mast cell–deficient mice to investigate the roles of mast cells in CHS responses have resulted in some confusion in the literature (31–38). And, in a study employing BMCMC-reconstituted Kit^{W-f}/Kit^{W-f} mice, Villa et al. (186) reported that mast cells contributed to the tissue swelling associated with a delayed-type hypersensitivity response to subcutaneous challenge with ovalbumin.

However, it now appears that mast cells may either have important roles in augmenting certain features of the CHS responses or make no detectable contribution to these reactions, depending on the conditions of the experiment (33). Factors that may influence the importance of the mast cell's role in CHS responses include the type and concentration of hapten and the choice of vehicle to apply the hapten during the sensitization and elicitation phases of the response (33).

The variability in the importance of the mast cell's role in the expression of features of CHS responses, depending on the particular conditions of the experimental model tested, is reminiscent of findings in mouse models of asthma (as discussed above). In these, and probably many other settings, whether the mast cell has an important or entirely redundant role in a particular example of an immune response may reflect the specific features of the protocol examined; the role of the mast cell is likely to be most evident when its ability to amplify aspects of the response that otherwise would only weakly be expressed is most important.

Recently, Bryce et al. (33) demonstrated that IgE antibodies are required for optimal immune sensitization to chemical haptens in certain models of CHS. In that study, $IgE^{-/-}$, $FcR\gamma^{-/-}$, and Kit^W/Kit^{W-v} mice all exhibited attenuated CHS responses to oxazolone (Ox) when the hapten was administered in 100% ethanol at a concentration of 2% for sensitization and the mice were challenged five days later with 1.0% Ox (33). In this model, $IgE^{-/-}$ or Kit^W/Kit^{W-v} mice exhibited significant impairment in the reduction in the numbers of dendritic cells (DCs) in the epidermis in response to initial exposure to hapten. Bryce et al. (33) presented evidence that (in the absence of known Ag but presumably signaling via the $FcR\gamma$ chain on mast cells) IgE was necessary for optimal cutaneous expression of several mast cell–associated mRNAs 1 h after initial application of Ox to the skin in the sensitization phase of CHS. These mRNAs included those for the mast cell–associated protease, mouse mast cell protease-6 (MMCP-6), as well as several cytokines (IL-1β, IL-6, and TNF) and a chemokine (MCP-1) known to have effects on DC migration, maturation, and function. Accordingly, Bryce et al. (33) speculated that "physiological" levels of IgE can be required for optimal immune sensitization in certain models of CHS because such IgE sustains Ag-independent, but FcεRI-dependent, "priming" effects on dermal mast cells. Under some circumstances, IgE- and Ag-dependent activation of mast cells may also contribute to the elicitation phase of CHS to unrelated haptens (187) or promote the migration of skin Langerhans cells to draining lymph nodes (187a).

Potential Anti-Inflammatory or Immunosuppressive Roles of Mast Cells

If one analyzes the known biological effects of the many mediators that can be produced by mast cells (Table 1), one finds that several of these products, including TGF-β_1, IL-4, and histamine, can have effects that are anti-inflammatory and/or that might negatively regulate aspects of acquired immune responses. However, to date, only one of the many potential anti-inflammatory activities of mast cells has been verified using genetic approaches in vivo: the ability of mast cells, through effects mediated at least in part by histamine, to contribute to the immunosuppressive actions of ultraviolet-B irradiation on the expression of CHS responses in mice (188).

In addition to secreting products that can themselves exert anti-inflammatory or immunosuppressive effects, mast cells also can release mediators that degrade proinflammatory molecules. For example, mast cell tryptase efficiently cleaves the neuropeptide, calcitonin gene-related peptide (CGRP), to an inactive form, thereby abolishing the potent and long-acting vasodilator actions observed when CGRP is injected into skin in vivo (189). By contrast, increased secretion of mast cell tryptase in certain disorders, such as bronchial asthma, may have other effects that augment neurogenic inflammation (190). Accordingly, in the context of a complex biological response such as experimental or naturally occurring asthma, it may be very difficult to predict whether, and under what circumstances, mast cell activation resulting in the release of tryptase (and/or other mediators that can have some effects that promote and others that suppress inflammation) might have net anti-inflammatory as opposed to proinflammatory effects. Indeed, the mast cell might express both functions in some biological processes, but at different stages in the development or resolution of the response.

CONCLUSIONS: MAST CELLS AS "TUNABLE" INITIATORS, AMPLIFIERS, AND REGULATORS OF ACQUIRED IMMUNE RESPONSES

As summarized in Table 2, mast cells are very well suited to influence the initiation, development, expression, and regulation of acquired immune responses. Their role as effector cells in the development of the inflammation associated with certain acquired immune responses (especially those associated with IgE)

TABLE 2   Properties of mast cells that facilitate their effector and immunoregulatory roles in acquired immunity

---

Wide tissue distribution, including near epithelial surfaces, blood vessels, smooth muscle, and nerves

Long-lived and can re-enter cell cycle and proliferate locally

Populations can expand in numbers (via recruitment and maturation of precursors and/or by proliferation of mature mast cells) and/or change their tissue distribution or aspects of phenotype (e.g., content of stored mediators) during immune responses

Source of many mediators, cytokines, and chemokines with potential proinflammatory, anti-inflammatory, and/or immunoregulatory effects

Can be activated to release such mediators by many different stimuli, acting via several signaling pathways, during innate or acquired immune responses

Depending on the type and concentration of the particular stimulus of activation, "activated" mast cells can release either all classes of mediators at high levels or may release certain mediators more selectively

Secretory function is subject to complex positive and negative regulation, by factors acting at the cell surface or intracellularly (note: naturally occurring genetic alterations in elements of these regulatory pathways, that result in altered cell function, already have been described)

Are "rechargeable" (can participate in multiple cycles of activation for mediator release)

Can functionally interact with other cell types (including T cells, B cells, and DCs) both by releasing mediators and by cell-cell interactions

Can be functionally "tuned," by genetic and/or environmental factors, to acquire more "proinflammatory" and/or "immunoregulatory" phenotypes [e.g., by Ag-independent actions of IgE that can influence (a) surface expression of $Fc\varepsilon RI$; (b) synthesis and/or storage of secreted products, cytokines, and chemokines; and (c) secretory function; by certain cytokines, including SCF, etc.; and by stimuli acting on the cells' surface receptors other than $Fc\varepsilon RI$, such as GPCRs, TLRs, etc.]

---

is well known and reflects the ability of mast cells to secrete many biologically active molecules that can initiate and/or promote acute and long-lasting aspects of inflammation. However, their products also can regulate tissue remodeling by mechanisms that are likely to include direct effects on resident target cells, as well as indirect effects such as the promotion of inflammatory responses (5, 7, 46, 110, 116, 142, 143, 191, 192). Through such functions, mast cells either can be essential for the expression of immune responses in sensitized individuals (e.g., in the case of certain IgE-dependent responses), or can significantly contribute to the expression or magnitude of such reactions (e.g., in the case of certain T cell–dependent responses).

However, if one considers the diverse potential biological effects of mast cell mediators, as well as some of the cellular functions of this lineage that have been demonstrated in vitro, one can propose several mechanisms by which mast cells that have been activated during an innate immune response might contribute significantly to the generation, magnitude, or time course of the subsequent acquired immune response to the inciting agent. Such potential roles include the ability to act as Ag-processing and presenting cells, although this function so far has been demonstrated primarily in vitro (166, 167, 172, 193) or by the adoptive transfer of Ag-treated mast cells in vivo (186). Mast cells also have the potential to influence the migration, maturation, and/or function of DCs (194–197) and to influence the biology of other cell types that contribute to these responses, including T cells and B cells (8–10, 198). Thus, in such settings, mast cells have the potential to function as immunoregulatory cells. Moreover, in certain circumstances, the mast cell's immunoregulatory functions not only can influence the magnitude or time course of the acquired immune response, but may even be essential for its occurrence. Although the potential for mast cells to influence significantly the development or characteristics of acquired immune responses has been much discussed recently (43, 170, 192, 198, 199), only a few studies provide compelling evidence, derived from studies in mast cell knockin mice, that the mast cell actually can express such roles in vivo (33, 186, 191). This represents an important area for future work.

It should be emphasized that several of the mast cell's characteristics that are important to its roles as an effector and/or immunoregulatory cell can be influenced significantly by genetic alterations that affect key molecules in those pathways that positively or negatively regulate mast cell function. In the case of signaling via the FcεRI, spontaneous or induced genetic alterations in such molecules can result in enhanced (59, 64, 77, 88) or diminished (78) mast cell (and/or, in some cases, basophil) secretory function. And it has been proposed that genetic factors influencing the structure or expression of the FcεRI β chain, itself a key amplifier of signaling via this receptor, also may account for variation in the secretory responsiveness of mast cells and basophils (17, 18). Thus, depending on the genotype, an individual's mast cells might be either hyper- or hyporesponsive to signaling initiated at the FcεRI, or via other receptors. These observations have obvious implications with respect to the pathogenesis, the expression and, potentially, the treatment of disorders in which mast cells (and/or basophils) have important roles.

Finally, even with genetically normal mast cells, a number of environmental factors can contribute to the stimulus threshold required for activation of the cells' secretory function, and/or to the regulation of the type, magnitude, or duration of the cells' secretory responses. The most straightforward of these are the local concentrations of IgE, and the specific Ag(s) recognized by such antibodies. Others include the concentration of IgE (and the structure of the IgE) to which the cells are exposed in the absence of known Ag, the types and concentrations of other factors that can either activate the cells directly or modulate their responsiveness to IgE and Ag or other signals, the presence of other cell types that can modulate the function of the mast cell via contact-dependent or other mechanisms, and so forth.

In this context, it is important to emphasize that individual stimuli of mast cell secretion can elicit distinct, though sometimes overlapping, patterns of mediator secretion. For example, although IgE and specific Ag can induce the cells to release large quantities of all classes of mediators, Church et al. (200) have reported that neuropeptides favor the release of preformed mediators, whereas LPS and other stimuli that are identified by mast cell TLRs favor the release of certain cytokines (and may induce little or no release of preformed mediators) (10, 76, 201). Furthermore, even the same class of stimulus can, depending on the circumstances, induce patterns of mediator release that differ in their kinetics or spectrum of secreted products. For example, in vitro evidence indicates that certain monomeric IgEs can induce mouse mast cells to release all classes of mediators, but with a slower time course than is observed with IgE and specific Ag (89), and low levels of FcεRI aggregation with IgE and Ag result in the release of larger amounts of certain cytokines and chemokines than other cytokines or preformed mediators (100). Moreover, morphological and immunoelectron microscopic evidence indicates that mast cells and basophils can release mediators by a process of "piecemeal" degranulation, as well as by classical "anaphylactic-type" degranulation (25–27). Much work will likely be required to understand the regulation and biological importance of piecemeal degranulation. Yet the data already in hand suggest that this potential mechanism of mediator secretion offers the mast cell yet another option for modulating its function, in terms of the kinetics and magnitude of its mediator secretion, and perhaps in terms of the specific types of products released, in response to the requirements of the particular biological process in which the cell participates.

During a complex biological response (such as an immune response to foreign Ags or pathogens), many of the different factors that can influence the threshold for mast cell activation, the type, kinetics, and/or magnitude of the secretory response, and the pattern of secreted products the cells release upon appropriate stimulation may be present simultaneously and/or at different times during the evolution of the response. Accordingly, one can envision that the type, intensity, kinetics, and pattern of mast cell secretory responsiveness can be "tuned," not only genetically but also environmentally, over a very wide range. This realization has substantial biological, and perhaps clinical, significance. It is becoming increasingly evident that, depending on the context, mast cell function can contribute either to health (e.g., in some examples of host defense) or disease (e.g., in certain allergic or autoimmune disorders, and in other settings). Therefore, elucidating how mast cell phenotype and function are regulated, and how the cells' secretory repertoire is "tuned," not only represent opportunities to understand better the many important biological responses in which this cell participates, but may provide new insights into how mast cells might be manipulated to achieve therapeutic ends.

APPENDIX

Abbreviations used: AHR, airway hyperreactivity; BMCMC, bone marrow–derived, cultured mast cell; CGRP, calcitonin gene-related peptide; CHS, contact hypersensitivity; CRAMP, cathelin-related antimicrobial peptide; DAG, diacyl-glycerol; DC, dendritic cell; DNFB, dinitoflourobenze; EAE, experimental allergic encephalomyelitis; ERK, extracellular signal-regulated kinase; ES, embryonic stem cell; ESCMC, embryonic stem cell–derived cultured mast cell; FGF, fibroblast growth factor; GPCRs, G protein–coupled receptors; IAP, integrin-associated protein; ICAM, intercellular adhesion molecule; IL, interleukin; IP_3, inositol 1,4,5-trisphosphate; ITAM, immunoreceptor tyrosine-based activation motif; ITIM, immunoreceptor tyrosine-based inhibitory motif; JNK, c-Jun N-terminal kinase; KIR, killer inhibitory receptor; LAT, linker for activation of T cells; LFA, leukocyte function–associated antigen; LPS, lipopolysaccharide; LTB_4, leukotriene B_4; MAFA, mast cell function–associated antigen; MAPK, mitogen-activated protein kinase; MCP-1, monocyte chemoattractant protein-1; MIP-1α, macrophage inflammatory protein-1α; MMP-9, matrix metalloproteinase-9; NK, natural killer; NTAL, non–T cell activation linker; Ox, oxazolone; PDK1, 3-phosphoinositide-dependent kinase 1; PGD_2, prostaglandin D_2; PI3K, phosphoinositide 3-kinase; PI-4,5-P_2, phosphatidyl inositol 4,5,-bisphosphate; PIR-B, paired Ig-like receptor-B; PKC, protein kinase C; PLA_2, phospholipase A_2; PLCγ, phospholipase Cγ; RabGEF1, Rab guanine nucleotide exchange factor 1; RasGRP, Ras guanine nucleotide releasing protein; SCF, stem cell factor; SHIP, SH2-containing inositol 5' phosphatase; SHP-1, SH2-containing protein tyrosine phosphatase-1; SIRP, signal regulatory protein; SLP-76, SH2-containing leukocyte protein of 76 kDa; TLR, Toll-like receptors; TNF, tumor necrosis factor; TRPV, transient receptor potential (vanilloid); VCAM, vascular cell adhesion molecule; VEGF, vascular endothelial growth factor; VPF, vascular permeability factor.

ACKNOWLEDGMENTS

Our work is supported by NIH grants (AI-23990, CA-72074, and HL-67674, to S.J.G.), and postdoctoral fellowships from the Natural Sciences and Engineering Research Council of Canada (NSERC) (to J.K.) and the National Health and Medical Research Council of Australia C. J. Martin Fellowship (to M.A.G.). We thank our many colleagues and collaborators for helpful discussions.

**The *Annual Review of Immunology* is online at
http://immunol.annualreviews.org**

LITERATURE CITED

1. Kitamura Y. 1989. Heterogeneity of mast cells and phenotypic change between subpopulations. *Annu. Rev. Immunol.* 7:59–76

2. Metcalfe DD, Baram D, Mekori YA. 1997. Mast cells. *Physiol. Rev.* 77(4): 1033–79

3. Galli SJ, Lantz CS. 1999. Allergy. In *Fundamental Immunology*, ed. WE Paul, pp. 1137–84. Philadelphia, PA: Lippincott-Raven

4. Galli SJ, Zsebo KM Geissler EN. 1994. The kit ligand, stem cell factor. *Adv. Immunol.* 55:1–96

5. Galli SJ, Metcalfe DD, Arber DA, Dvorak AM. 2005. Basophils and mast cells and their disorders. In *Williams Hematology*, ed. E Beutler, MA Lichtman, BS Coller, TJ Kipps, U Seligsohn. New York: McGraw-Hill. In press

6. Galli SJ. 2000. Mast cells and basophils. *Curr. Opin. Hematol.* 7(1):32–39

7. Williams CMM, Galli SJ. 2000. The diverse potential effector and immunoregulatory roles of mast cells in allergic disease. *J. Allergy Clin. Immunol.* 105(5): 847–59

8. Sayama K, Diehn M, Matsuda K, Lunderius C, Tsai M, et al. 2002. Transcriptional response of human mast cells stimulated via the FcεRI and identification of mast cells as a source of IL-11. *BMC Immunol.* 3(1):5

9. Nakajima T, Inagaki N, Tanaka H, Tanaka A, Yoshikawa M, et al. 2002. Marked increase in CC chemokine gene expression in both human and mouse mast cell transcriptomes following Fcε receptor I cross-linking: an interspecies comparison. *Blood* 100(12):3861–68

10. Okumura S, Kashiwakura J, Tomita H, Matsumoto K, Nakajima T, et al. 2003. Identification of specific gene expression profiles in human mast cells mediated by Toll-like receptor 4 and FcεRI. *Blood* 102(7):2547–54

11. Voehringer D, Shinkai K, Locksley RM. 2004. Type 2 immunity reflects orchestrated recruitment of cells committed to IL-4 production. *Immunity* 20(3):267–77

12. Enerback L, Lowhagen GB. 1979. Long term increase of mucosal mast cells in the rat induced by administration of compound 48/80. *Cell Tissue Res.* 198(2):209–15

13. Bienenstock J, Befus D, Denburg J, Goto T, Lee T, et al. 1985. Comparative aspects of mast cell heterogeneity in different species and sites. *Int. Arch. Allergy Appl. Immunol.* 77(1–2):126–29

14. Galli SJ. 1990. New insights into "the riddle of the mast cells": microenvironmental regulation of mast cell development and phenotypic heterogeneity. *Lab. Invest.* 62(1):5–33

15. Huang C, Sali A, Stevens RL. 1998. Regulation and function of mast cell proteases in inflammation. *J. Clin. Immunol.* 18(3):169–83

16. Metzger H. 1992. The receptor with high affinity for IgE. *Immunol. Rev.* 125:37–48

17. Turner H, Kinet JP. 1999. Signalling through the high-affinity IgE receptor FcεRI. *Nature* 402(Suppl.):B24-30

18. Kinet JP. 1999. The high-affinity IgE receptor (FcεRI): from physiology to pathology. *Annu. Rev. Immunol.* 17:931–72

19. Ott VL, Cambier JC. 2000. Activating and inhibitory signaling in mast cells: new opportunities for therapeutic intervention? *J. Allergy Clin. Immunol.* 106(3):429–40

20. Nadler MJ, Matthews SA, Turner H, Kinet JP, et al. 2000. Signal transduction by the high-affinity immunoglobulin E receptor FcεRI: coupling form to function. *Adv. Immunol.* 76:325–55

21. Kawakami T, Galli SJ. 2002. Regulation of mast-cell and basophil function and survival by IgE. *Nat. Rev. Immunol.* 2(10):773–86

22. Rivera J. 2002. Molecular adapters in FcεRI signaling and the allergic response. *Curr. Opin. Immunol.* 14(6): 688–93

23. Siraganian RP. 2003. Mast cell signal transduction from the high-affinity IgE receptor. *Curr. Opin. Immunol.* 15(6): 639–46

24. Blank U, Rivera J. 2004. The ins and outs of IgE-dependent mast-cell exocytosis. *Trends Immunol.* 25(5):266–73

25. Dvorak AM, Dvorak HF, Karnovsky MJ. 1972. Uptake of horseradish peroxidase by guinea pig basophilic leukocytes. *Lab. Invest.* 26(1):27–39

26. Dvorak AM. 1992. Basophils and mast cells: piecemeal degranulation in situ and ex vivo: a possible mechanism for cytokine-induced function in disease. *Immunol. Ser.* 57:169–271

27. Dvorak AM, Tepper RI, Weller PF, Morgan ES, Estrella P, et al. 1994. Piecemeal degranulation of mast cells in the inflammatory eyelid lesions of interleukin-4 transgenic mice. Evidence of mast cell histamine release in vivo by diamine oxidase-gold enzyme-affinity ultrastructural cytochemistry. *Blood* 83(12):3600–12

28. Miller HR. 1996. Mucosal mast cells and the allergic response against nematode parasites. *Vet. Immunol. Immunopathol.* 54(1–4):331–36

29. Wedemeyer J, Tsai M, Galli SJ. 2000. Roles of mast cells and basophils in innate and acquired immunity. *Curr. Opin. Immunol.* 12(6):624–31

30. Galli SJ. 1997. Complexity and redundancy in the pathogenesis of asthma: reassessing the roles of mast cells and T cells. *J. Exp. Med.* 186(3):343–47

31. Askenase PW, Van Loveren H, Kraeuter-Kops S, Ron Y, Meade R, et al. 1983. Defective elicitation of delayed-type hypersensitivity in W/W^v and Sl/Sl^d mast cell-deficient mice. *J. Immunol.* 131(6): 2687–94

32. Biedermann T, Kneilling M, Mailhammer R, Maier K, Sander CA, et al. 2000. Mast cells control neutrophil recruitment during T cell-mediated delayed-type hypersensitivity reactions through tumor necrosis factor and macrophage inflammatory protein 2. *J. Exp. Med.* 192(10): 1441–52

33. Bryce PJ, Miller ML, Miyajima I, Tsai M, Galli SJ, et al. 2004. Immune sensitization in the skin is enhanced by antigen-independent effects of IgE. *Immunity* 20(4):381–92

34. Thomas WR, Schrader JW. 1983. Delayed hypersensitivity in mast-cell-deficient mice. *J. Immunol.* 130(6): 2565–67

35. Galli SJ, Hammel I. 1984. Unequivocal delayed hypersensitivity in mast cell-deficient and beige mice. *Science* 226(4675):710–13

36. Mekori YA, Galli SJ. 1985. Undiminished immunologic tolerance to contact sensitivity in mast cell-deficient W/W^v and Sl/Sl^d mice. *J. Immunol.* 135(2):879–85

37. Mekori YA, Weitzman GL, Galli SJ. 1985. Reevaluation of reserpine-induced suppression of contact sensitivity. Evidence that reserpine interferes with T lymphocyte function independently of an effect on mast cells. *J. Exp. Med.* 162(6):1935–53

38. Ha TY, Reed ND, Crowle PK. 1986. Immune response potential of mast cell-deficient W/W^v mice. *Int. Arch. Allergy Appl. Immunol.* 80(1):85–94

39. Secor VH, Secor WE, Gutekunst CA, Brown MA. 2000. Mast cells are essential for early onset and severe disease in

a murine model of multiple sclerosis. *J. Exp. Med.* 191(5):813–22

40. Mekori YA, Metcalfe DD. 2000. Mast cells in innate immunity. *Immunol. Rev.* 173:131–40

41. Chen R, Ning G, Zhao ML, Fleming MG, Diaz LA, et al. 2001. Mast cells play a key role in neutrophil recruitment in experimental bullous pemphigoid. *J. Clin. Invest.* 108(8):1151–58

42. Gurish MF, Austen KF. 2001. The diverse roles of mast cells. *J. Exp. Med.* 194(1):F1–5

43. Malaviya R, Abraham SN. 2001. Mast cell modulation of immune responses to bacteria. *Immunol. Rev.* 179:16–24

44. Jutel M, Watanabe T, Klunker S, Akdis M, Thomet OA, et al. 2001. Histamine regulates T-cell and antibody responses by differential expression of H1 and H2 receptors. *Nature* 413(6854):420–25

45. Benoist C, Mathis D. 2002. Mast cells in autoimmune disease. *Nature* 420(6917): 875–78

46. Lee DM, Friend DS, Gurish MF, Benoist C, Mathis D, et al. 2002. Mast cells: a cellular link between autoantibodies and inflammatory arthritis. *Science* 297(5587):1689–92

47. Pedotti R, De Voss JJ, Steinman L, Galli SJ. 2003. Involvement of both "allergic" and "autoimmune" mechanisms in EAE, MS and other autoimmune diseases. *Trends Immunol.* 24(9):479–84

48. Maurer M, Theoharides T, Granstein RD, Bischoff SC, Bienenstock J, et al. 2003. What is the physiological function of mast cells? *Exp. Dermatol.* 12(6):886–910

49. Galli SJ, Chatterjea D, Tsai M. 2004. Roles of mast cells and basophils in innate immunity. In *The Innate Immune Response to Infection*, ed. SHE Kaufman, R Medzhitov, S Gordon, pp. 111–32. Berlin: ASM Press

50. Theoharides TC, Conti P. 2004. Mast cells: the JEKYLL and HYDE of tumor growth. *Trends Immunol.* 25(5):235–41

51. Theoharides TC, Cochrane DE. 2004. Critical role of mast cells in inflammatory diseases and the effect of acute stress. *J. Neuroimmunol.* 146(1–2):1–12

52. Galli SJ, Maurer M, Lantz CS. 1999. Mast cells as sentinels of innate immunity. *Curr. Opin. Immunol.* 11(1):53–59

53. Wu JN, Jordan MS, Silverman MA, Peterson EJ, Koretzky GA. 2004. Differential requirement for adapter proteins Src homology 2 domain-containing leukocyte phosphoprotein of 76 kDa and adhesion- and degranulation-promoting adapter protein in FcεRI signaling and mast cell function. *J. Immunol.* 172(11): 6768–74

54. Yang Y, Li L, Wong GW, Krilis SA, Madhusudhan MS, et al. 2002. RasGRP4, a new mast cell-restricted Ras guanine nucleotide-releasing protein with calcium- and diacylglycerol-binding motifs. Identification of defective variants of this signaling protein in asthma, mastocytosis, and mast cell leukemia patients and demonstration of the importance of RasGRP4 in mast cell development and function. *J. Biol. Chem.* 277(28):25756–74

55. Li L, Yang Y, Stevens RL. 2003. RasGRP4 regulates the expression of prostaglandin D2 in human and rat mast cell lines. *J. Biol. Chem.* 278(7):4725–29

56. Nadler MJ, Kinet JP. 2002. Uncovering new complexities in mast cell signaling. *Nat. Immunol.* 3(8):707–8

57. Heneberg P, Draber P. 2002. Nonreceptor protein tyrosine and lipid phosphatases in type I Fcε receptor-mediated activation of mast cells and basophils. *Int. Arch. Allergy Immunol.* 128(4):253–63

58. Kamata T, Yamashita M, Kimura M, Murata K, Inami M, et al. 2003. Src homology 2 domain-containing tyrosine phosphatase SHP-1 controls the development of allergic airway inflammation. *J. Clin. Invest.* 111(1):109–19

59. Rauh MJ, Kalesnikoff J, Hughes M,

Sly L, Lam V, et al. 2003. Role of Src homology 2-containing-inositol 5′-phosphatase (SHIP) in mast cells and macrophages. *Biochem. Soc. Trans.* 31:286–91

60. Qu X, Sada K, Kyo S, Maeno K, Miah SM, et al. 2004. Negative regulation of FcεRI-mediated mast cell activation by a ubiquitin-protein ligase Cbl-b. *Blood* 103(5):1779–86

61. Ota Y, Samelson LE. 1997. The product of the proto-oncogene c-cbl: a negative regulator of the Syk tyrosine kinase. *Science* 276(5311):418–20

62. Odom S, Gomez G, Kovarova M, Furumoto Y, Ryan JJ, et al. 2004. Negative regulation of immunoglobulin E-dependent allergic responses by Lyn kinase. *J. Exp. Med.* 199(11):1491–502

63. Shields JM, Pruitt K, McFall A, Shaub A, Der CJ. 2000. Understanding Ras: "It ain't over 'til it's over." *Trends Cell Biol.* 10(4):147–54

64. Tam S-Y, Tsai M, Snouwaert JN, Kalesnikoff J, Scherrer D, et al. 2004. RabGEF1 is a negative regulator of mast cell activation and skin inflammation. *Nat. Immunol.* 5:844–52

65. Gergely J, Pecht I, Sarmay G. 1999. Immunoreceptor tyrosine-based inhibition motif-bearing receptors regulate the immunoreceptor tyrosine-based activation motif-induced activation of immune competent cells. *Immunol. Lett.* 68(1):3–15

66. Scharenberg AM. 1999. The inhibitory receptor superfamily: potential relevance to atopy. *Curr. Opin. Immunol.* 11(6):621–25

67. Katz HR. 2002. Inhibitory receptors and allergy. *Curr. Opin. Immunol.* 14(6):698–704

68. Abramson J, Rozenblum G, Pecht I. 2003. Dok protein family members are involved in signaling mediated by the type 1 Fcε receptor. *Eur. J. Immunol.* 33(1):85–91

69. Takai T, Ono M, Hikida M, Ohmori H, Ravetch JV. 1996. Augmented humoral and anaphylactic responses in FcγRII-deficient mice. *Nature* 379(6563):346–49

70. Zhu D, Kepley CL, Zhang M, Zhang K, Saxon A. 2002. A novel human immunoglobulin Fcγ Fcε bifunctional fusion protein inhibits FcεRI-mediated degranulation. *Nat. Med.* 8(5):518–21

71. Katz HR. 2002. Inhibition of anaphylactic inflammation by the gp49B1 receptor on mast cells. *Mol. Immunol.* 38(16–18):1301–5

72. Song J, Hagen G, Smith SM, Roess DA, Pecht I, et al. 2002. Interactions of the mast cell function-associated antigen with the type I Fcε receptor. *Mol. Immunol.* 38(16–18):1315–21

73. Lacy P, Logan MR, Bablitz B, Moqbel R. 2001 Fusion protein vesicle-associated membrane protein 2 is implicated in IFN-γ-induced piecemeal degranulation in human eosinophils from atopic individuals. *J. Allergy Clin. Immunol.* 107(4):671–78

74. Bandeira-Melo C, Woods LJ, Phoofolo M, Weller PF. 2002. Intracrine cysteinyl leukotriene receptor-mediated signaling of eosinophil vesicular transport-mediated interleukin-4 secretion. *J. Exp. Med.* 196(6):841–50

75. Theoharides TC, Bondy PK, Tsakalos ND, Askenase PW. 1982. Differential release of serotonin and histamine from mast cells. *Nature* 297(5863):229–31

76. Leal-Berumen I, Conlon P, Marshall JS. 1994. IL-6 production by rat peritoneal mast cells is not necessarily preceded by histamine release and can be induced by bacterial lipopolysaccharide. *J. Immunol.* 152(11):5468–76

77. Huber M, Helgason CD, Damen JE, Liu L, Humphries RK, Krystal G. 1998. The src homology 2-containing inositol phosphatase (SHIP) is the gatekeeper of mast cell degranulation. *Proc. Natl. Acad. Sci. USA* 95(19):11330–35

78. Kepley CL, Youssef L, Andrews RP, Wilson BS, Oliver JM. 1999. Syk deficiency in nonreleaser basophils. *J. Allergy Clin. Immunol.* 104:279–84

79. Vonakis BM, Gibbons S Jr, Sora R, Langdon JM, MacDonald SM. 2001. Src homology 2 domain-containing inositol 5′ phosphatase is negatively associated with histamine release to human recombinant histamine-releasing factor in human basophils. *J. Allergy Clin. Immunol.* 108(5):822–31

80. Hsu C, MacGlashan D Jr. 1996. IgE antibody up-regulates high affinity IgE binding on murine bone marrow-derived mast cells. *Immunol. Lett.* 52(2–3):129–34

81. Yamaguchi M, Lantz CS, Oettgen HC, Katona IM, Fleming T, et al. 1997. IgE enhances mouse mast cell FcεRI expression in vitro and in vivo: evidence for a novel amplification mechanism in IgE-dependent reactions. *J. Exp. Med.* 185(4):663–72

82. Lantz CS, Yamaguchi M, Oettgen HC, Katona IM, Mijama I, et al. 1997. IgE regulates mouse basophil FcεRI expression in vivo. *J. Immunol.* 158(6):2517–21

83. Yamaguchi M, Sayama K, Yano K, Lantz CS, Noben-Trauth N, et al. 1999. IgE enhances Fcε receptor I expression and IgE-dependent release of histamine and lipid mediators from human umbilical cord blood-derived mast cells: synergistic effect of IL-4 and IgE on human mast cell Fcε receptor I expression and mediator release. *J. Immunol.* 162(9):5455–65

84. MacGlashan D Jr, Xia HZ, Schwartz LB, Gong J. 2001. IgE-regulated loss, not IgE-regulated synthesis, controls expression of FcεRI in human basophils. *J. Leukoc. Biol.* 70(2):207–18

85. Kubo S, Matsuoka K, Taya C, Kitamura F, Takai T, et al. 2001. Drastic upregulation of FcεRI on mast cells is induced by IgE binding through stabilization and accumulation of FcεRI on the

cell surface. *J. Immunol.* 167(6):3427–34

86. Borkowski TA, Jouvin MH, Lin SY, Kinet JP. 2001. Minimal requirements for IgE-mediated regulation of surface FcεRI. *J. Immunol.* 167(3):1290–96

87. Saini SS, MacGlashan D. 2002. How IgE upregulates the allergic response. *Curr. Opin. Immunol.* 14(6):694–97

88. Kalesnikoff J, Huber M, Lam V, Damen JE, Zhang J, et al. 2001. Monomeric IgE stimulates signaling pathways in mast cells that lead to cytokine production and cell survival. *Immunity* 14(6):801–11

89. Kitaura J, Song J, Tsai M, Asai K, Maeda-Yamamoto M, et al. 2003. Evidence that IgE molecules mediate a spectrum of effects on mast cell survival and activation via aggregation of the FcεRI. *Proc. Natl. Acad. Sci. USA* 100(22):12911–16

90. Tanaka S, Takasu Y, Mikura S, Satoh N, Ichikawa A. 2002. Antigen-independent induction of histamine synthesis by immunoglobulin E in mouse bone marrow-derived mast cells. *J. Exp. Med.* 196(2):229–35

91. Asai K, Kitaura J, Kawakami Y, Yamagata N, Tsai M, et al. 2001. Regulation of mast cell survival by IgE. *Immunity* 14(6):791–800

92. James LC, Roversi P, Tawfik DS. 2003. Antibody multispecificity mediated by conformational diversity. *Science* 299(5611):1362–67

93. Marquardt DL, Parker CW, Sullivan TJ. 1978. Potentiation of mast cell mediator release by adenosine. *J. Immunol.* 120:871–88

94. Marquardt DL, Walker LL, Wasserman SI. 1986. Cromolyn inhibition of mediator release in mast cells derived from mouse bone marrow. *Am. Rev. Respir. Dis.* 113:1105–19

95. Laffargue M, Calvez R, Finan P, Trifillieff A, Barbier M, et al. 2002. Phosphoinositide 3-kinase γ is an essential

amplifier of mast cell function. *Immunity* 16:441–51

96. Wymann MP, Bjorklof K, Calvez R, Finan P, Thomast M, et al. 2003. Phosphoinositide 3-kinase γ: a key modulator in inflammation and allergy. *Biochem. Soc. Trans.* 31(Pt. 1):275–80

97. Tilley SL, Wagoner VA, Salvatore CA, Jacobson MA, Koller BH. 2000. Adenosine and inosine increase cutaneous vasopermeability by activating A(3) receptors on mast cells. *J. Clin. Invest.* 105:361–67

98. Okumura S, Kashiwakura J, Tomita H, Matsumoto K, Nakajima T, et al. 2003. Identification of specific gene expression profiles in human mast cells mediated by Toll-like receptor 4 and FcεRI. *Blood* 102:2547–54

99. Stokes AJ, Shimoda LM, Koblan-Huberson M, Adra CN, Turner H. 2004. A TRPV2-PKA signaling module for transduction of physical stimuli in mast cells. *J. Exp. Med.* 200(2):137–47

100. Gonzalez-Espinosa C, Odom S, Olivera A, Hobson JP, Martinez ME, et al. 2003. Preferential signaling and induction of allergy-promoting lymphokines upon weak stimulation of the high affinity IgE receptor on mast cells. *J. Exp. Med.* 197(11):1453–65

101. Tsai M, Tam SY, Wedemeyer J, Galli SJ. 2002. Mast cells derived from embryonic stem cells: a model system for studying the effects of genetic manipulations on mast cell development, phenotype, and function in vitro and in vivo. *Int. J. Hematol.* 75(4):345–49

102. Kitamura Y, Go S, Hatanaka K. 1978. Decrease of mast cells in W/W^v mice and their increase by bone marrow transplantation. *Blood* 52(2):447–52

103. Stevens J, Loutit JF. 1982. Mast cells in spotted mutant mice (*W Ph mi*). *Proc. R. Soc. London B Biol. Sci.* 215(1200):405–9

104. Mallen-St Clair J, Pham CT, Villalta SA, Caughey GH, Wolters PJ. 2004.

Mast cell dipeptidyl peptidase I mediates survival from sepsis. *J. Clin. Invest.* 113(4):628–34

105. Grimbaldeston MA, Chen C-C, Tam S-Y, Tsai M, Galli SJ. 2005. Mast cell deficient *W-sash* c-*kit* mutant Kit^{W-sh}/Kit^{W-sh} mice as a model for investigating mast cell biology in vivo. *FASEB J.* (Abstr.) In press

106. Berrozpe G, Timokhina I, Yukl S, Tajima Y, Ono M, et al. 1999. The *W(sh)*, *W(57)*, and *Ph* Kit expression mutations define tissue-specific control elements located between -23 and -154 kb upstream of *Kit*. *Blood* 94(8):2658–66

107. Duttlinger R, Manova K, Chu TY, Gyssler C, Zelenetz AD, et al. 1993. *W-sash* affects positive and negative elements controlling c-*kit* expression: ectopic c-*kit* expression at sites of kit-ligand expression affects melanogenesis. *Development* 118(3):705–17

108. Yamazaki M, Tsujimura T, Morii E, Isozaki K, Onoue H, et al. 1994. C-*kit* gene is expressed by skin mast cells in embryos but not in puppies of W^{sh}/W^{sh} mice: age-dependent abolishment of c-*kit* gene expression. *Blood* 83(12):3509–16

109. Lantz CS, Boesiger J, Song CH, Mach N, Kobayashi T, et al. 1998. Role for interleukin-3 in mast-cell and basophil development and in immunity to parasites. *Nature* 392(6671):90–93

110. Coussens LM, Raymond WW, Bergers G, Laig-Webster M, Behrendtsen O, et al. 1999. Inflammatory mast cells up-regulate angiogenesis during squamous epithelial carcinogenesis. *Genes Dev.* 13(11):1382–97

111. Nakano T, Sonoda T, Hayashi C, Yamatodani A, Kanayama Y, et al. 1985. Fate of bone marrow-derived cultured mast cells after intracutaneous, intraperitoneal, and intravenous transfer into genetically mast cell-deficient W/W^v mice. Evidence that cultured mast cells can give rise to both connective tissue type

and mucosal mast cells. *J. Exp. Med.* 162(3):1025–43

112. Tsai M, Wedemeyer J, Ganiatsas S, Tam SY, Zon LI, et al. 2000. In vivo immunological function of mast cells derived from embryonic stem cells: an approach for the rapid analysis of even embryonic lethal mutations in adult mice in vivo. *Proc. Natl. Acad. Sci. USA* 97(16):9186–90

113. Wershil BK, Furuta GT, Wang ZS, Galli SJ. 1996. Mast cell-dependent neutrophil and mononuclear cell recruitment in immunoglobulin E-induced gastric reactions in mice. *Gastroenterology* 110(5):1482–90

114. Otsu K, Nakano T, Kanakura Y, Asai H, Katz HR, et al. 1987. Phenotypic changes of bone marrow-derived mast cells after intraperitoneal transfer into W/W^v mice that are genetically deficient in mast cells. *J. Exp. Med.* 165(3):615–27

115. Martin TR, Takeishi T, Katz HR, Austen KF, Drazen JM, et al. 1993. Mast cell activation enhances airway responsiveness to methacholine in the mouse. *J. Clin. Invest.* 91(3):1176–82

116. Williams CMM, Galli SJ. 2000. Mast cells can amplify airway reactivity and features of chronic inflammation in an asthma model in mice. *J. Exp. Med.* 192(3):455–62

117. Tanzola MB, Robbie-Ryan M, Gutekunst CA, Brown MA. 2003. Mast cells exert effects outside the central nervous system to influence experimental allergic encephalomyelitis disease course. *J. Immunol.* 171(8):4385–91

118. Lee YM, Jippo T, Kim DK, Katsu Y, Tsujino K, et al. 1998. Alteration of protease expression phenotype of mouse peritoneal mast cells by changing the microenvironment as demonstrated by in situ hybridization histochemistry. *Am. J. Pathol.* 153(3):931–36

119. Jippo T, Lee YM, Ge Y, Kim DK, Okabe

M, et al. 2001. Tissue-dependent alteration of protease expression phenotype in murine peritoneal mast cells that were genetically labeled with green fluorescent protein. *Am. J. Pathol.* 158(5):1695–701

120. Du T, Friend DS, Austen KF, Katz HR. 1996. Tissue-dependent differences in the asynchronous appearance of mast cells in normal mice and in congenic mast cell-deficient mice after infusion of normal bone marrow cells. *Clin. Exp. Immunol.* 103(2):316–21

121. Jippo T, Morii E, Ito A, Kitamura Y. 2003. Effect of anatomical distribution of mast cells on their defense function against bacterial infections: demonstration using partially mast cell-deficient *tg/tg* mice. *J. Exp. Med.* 197(11):1417–25

122. Wershil BK, Tsai M, Geissler EN, Zsebo KM, Galli SJ. 1992. The rat c-kit ligand, stem cell factor, induces c-kit receptor-dependent mouse mast cell activation in vivo. Evidence that signaling through the c-kit receptor can induce expression of cellular function. *J. Exp. Med.* 175(1): 245–55

123. Garrington TP, Ishizuka T, Papst PJ, Chayama K, Webb S, et al. 2000. MEKK2 gene disruption causes loss of cytokine production in response to IgE and c-Kit ligand stimulation of ES cell-derived mast cells. *EMBO J.* 19(20): 5387–95

124. Maurer M, Wedemeyer J, Metz M, Piliponsky AM, Weller K, et al. 2004. Mast cells promote homeostasis by limiting endothelin-1 induced toxicity. *Nature.* 432:512–16

125. Alizadeh H, Murrell KD. 1984. The intestinal mast cell response to *Trichinella spiralis* infection in mast cell-deficient W/W^v mice. *J. Parasitol.* 70(5):767–73

126. Galli SJ, Arizono N, Murakami T, Dvorak AM, Fox JG. 1987. Development of large numbers of mast cells at sites of

idiopathic chronic dermatitis in genetically mast cell-deficient WBB6F1-*W/W^v* mice. *Blood* 69(6):1661–66

127. Gordon JR, Galli SJ. 1990. Phorbol 12-myristate 13-acetate-induced development of functionally active mast cells in *W/W^v* but not *Sl/Sl^d* genetically mast cell-deficient mice. *Blood* 75(8):1637–45

128. Ody C, Kindler V, Vassalli P. 1990. Interleukin 3 perfusion in *W/W^v* mice allows the development of macroscopic hematopoietic spleen colonies and restores cutaneous mast cell number. *J. Exp. Med.* 172(1):403–6

129. Khan AI, Horii Y, Tiuria R, Sato Y, Nawa Y. 1993. Mucosal mast cells and the expulsive mechanisms of mice against *Strongyloides venezuelensis*. *Int. J. Parasitol.* 23(5):551–55

130. Theoharides TC, el-Mansoury M, Letourneau R, Boucher W, Rozniecki JJ. 1993. Dermatitis characterized by mastocytosis at immunization sites in mast-cell-deficient *W/W^v* mice. *Int. Arch. Allergy Immunol.* 102(4):352–61

131. Wershil BK, Mekori YA, Murakami T, Galli SJ. 1987. 125I-fibrin deposition in IgE-dependent immediate hypersensitivity reactions in mouse skin. Demonstration of the role of mast cells using genetically mast cell-deficient mice locally reconstituted with cultured mast cells. *J. Immunol.* 139(8):2605–14

132. Wershil BK, Wang ZS, Gordon JR, Galli SJ. 1991. Recruitment of neutrophils during IgE-dependent cutaneous late phase reactions in the mouse is mast cell-dependent. Partial inhibition of the reaction with antiserum against tumor necrosis factor-alpha. *J. Clin. Invest.* 87(2):446–53

133. Martin TR, Galli SJ, Katona IM, Drazen JM. 1989. Role of mast cells in anaphylaxis. Evidence for the importance of mast cells in the cardiopulmonary alterations and death induced by anti-IgE in mice. *J. Clin. Invest.* 83(4):1375–83

134. Miyajima I, Dombrowicz D, Martin TR, Ravetch JV, Kinet JP, et al. 1997. Systemic anaphylaxis in the mouse can be mediated largely through IgG1 and FcγRIII. Assessment of the cardiopulmonary changes, mast cell degranulation, and death associated with active or IgE- or IgG1-dependent passive anaphylaxis. *J. Clin. Invest.* 99(5):901–14

135. Takeishi T, Martin TR, Katona IM, Finkelman FD, Galli SJ. 1991. Differences in the expression of the cardiopulmonary alterations associated with anti-immunoglobulin E-induced or active anaphylaxis in mast cell-deficient and normal mice. Mast cells are not required for the cardiopulmonary changes associated with certain fatal anaphylactic responses. *J. Clin. Invest.* 88(2):598–608

136. Choi IH, Shin YM, Park JS, Lee MS, Han EH, et al. 1998. Immunoglobulin E-dependent active fatal anaphylaxis in mast cell-deficient mice. *J. Exp. Med.* 188(9):1587–92

137. Choi IW, Kim YS, Kim DK, Choi JH, Seo KH, et al. 2003. Platelet-activating factor-mediated NF-κB dependency of a late anaphylactic reaction. *J. Exp. Med.* 198(1):145–51

138. Strait RT, Morris SC, Yang M, Qu XW, Finkelman FD. 2002. Pathways of anaphylaxis in the mouse. *J. Allergy Clin. Immunol.* 109(4):658–68

139. Latour S, Bonnerot C, Fridman WH, Daeron M. 1992. Induction of tumor necrosis factor-α production by mast cells via FcγR. Role of the FcγRIII γ subunit. *J. Immunol.* 149(6):2155–62

140. Kobayashi T, Miura T, Haba T, Sato M, Serizawa I, et al. 2000. An essential role of mast cells in the development of airway hyperresponsiveness in a murine asthma model. *J. Immunol.* 164(7):3855–61

141. Kung TT, Stelts D, Zurcher JA, Jones H, Umland SP, et al. 1995. Mast cells modulate allergic pulmonary eosinophilia in

mice. *Am. J. Respir. Cell Mol. Biol.* 12(4):404–9

142. Yu M, Tsai M, Tam S-Y, Galli SJ. 2005. Mast cells mediate multiple features of asthmatic responses in a mouse model of chronic asthma. *J. Allergy Clin. Immunol.* (Abstr.) In press

143. Masuda T, Tanaka H, Komai M, Nagao K, Ishizaki M, et al. 2003. Mast cells play a partial role in allergen-induced subepithelial fibrosis in a murine model of allergic asthma. *Clin. Exp. Allergy* 33(5):705–13

144. Kraneveld AD, van der Kleij HP, Kool M, van Houwelingen AH, Weitenberg AC, et al. 2002. Key role for mast cells in nonatopic asthma. *J. Immunol.* 169(4): 2044–53

145. Redegeld FA, van der Heijden MW, Kool M, Heijdra BM, Garssen J, et al. 2002. Immunoglobulin-free light chains elicit immediate hypersensitivity-like responses. *Nat. Med.* 8(7):694–701

146. Nogami M, Suko M, Okudaira H, Miyamoto T, Shiga J, et al. 1990. Experimental pulmonary eosinophilia in mice by Ascaris suum extract. *Am. Rev. Respir. Dis.* 141:1289–95

147. Okudaira H, Nogami M, Matsuzaki G, Dohi M, Suko M, et al. 1991. T-cell-dependent accumulation of eosinophils in the lung and its inhibition by monoclonal anti-interleukin-5. *Int. Arch. Allergy Appl. Immunol.* 94(1–4):171–73

148. Brusselle GG, Kips JC, Tavernier JH, van der Heyden JG, Cuvelier CA, et al. 1994. Attenuation of allergic airway inflammation in IL-4 deficient mice. *Clin. Exp. Allergy* 24(1):73–80

149. Takeda K, Hamelmann E, Joetham A, Shultz LD, Larsen GL, et al. 1997. Development of eosinophilic airway inflammation and airway hyperresponsiveness in mast cell-deficient mice. *J. Exp. Med.* 186(3):449–54

150. Nawa Y, Kiyota M, Korenaga M, Kotani M. 1985. Defective protective capacity of *W/W^v* mice against *Strongyloides ratti*

infection and its reconstitution with bone marrow cells. *Parasite Immunol.* 7(4): 429–38

151. Abe T, Nawa Y. 1987. Reconstitution of mucosal mast cells in *W/W^v* mice by adoptive transfer of bone marrow-derived cultured mast cells and its effects on the protective capacity to *Strongyloides ratti*-infection. *Parasite Immunol.* 9(1):31–38

152. Matsuda H, Watanabe N, Kiso Y, Hirota S, Ushio H, et al. 1990. Necessity of IgE antibodies and mast cells for manifestation of resistance against larval *Haemaphysalis longicornis* ticks in mice. *J. Immunol.* 144(1):259–62

153. Wershil BK, Theodos CM, Galli SJ, Titus RG. 1994. Mast cells augment lesion size and persistence during experimental *Leishmania major* infection in the mouse. *J. Immunol.* 152(9):4563–71

154. Robbie-Ryan M, Tanzola MB, Secor VH, Brown MA. 2003. Cutting edge: Both activating and inhibitory Fc receptors expressed on mast cells regulate experimental allergic encephalomyelitis disease severity. *J. Immunol.* 170(4):1630–34

155. Steeves EB, Allen JR. 1991. Tick resistance in mast cell-deficient mice: histological studies. *Int. J. Parasitol.* 21(2):265–68

156. Brown SJ, Galli SJ, Gleich GJ, Askenase PW. 1982. Ablation of immunity to *Amblyomma americanum* by anti-basophil serum: cooperation between basophils and eosinophils in expression of immunity to ectoparasites (ticks) in guinea pigs. *J. Immunol.* 129(2):790–96

157. Galli SJ, Askenase PW. 1986. Cutaneous basophil hypersensitivity. In *The Reticuloendothelial System: A Comprehensive Treatise.* Vol. IX: *Hypersensitivity*, ed. P Abramoff, SM Phillips, MR Escobar, pp. 321–69. New York: Plenum

158. Arizono N, Kasugai T, Yamada M, Okada M, Morimoto M, et al. 1993.

Infection of *Nippostrongylus brasiliensis* induces development of mucosal-type but not connective tissue-type mast cells in genetically mast cell-deficient *Ws/Ws* rats. *Blood* 81(10):2572–78

159. Newlands GF, Miller HR, MacKellar A, Galli SJ. 1995. Stem cell factor contributes to intestinal mucosal mast cell hyperplasia in rats infected with *Nippostrongylus brasiliensis* or *Trichinella spiralis*, but anti-stem cell factor treatment decreases parasite egg production during *N. brasiliensis* infection. *Blood* 86(5):1968–76

160. Friedman MM, Kaliner MA. 1987. Human mast cells and asthma. *Am. Rev. Respir. Dis.* 135(5):1157–64

161. Smith TJ, Weis JH. 1996. Mucosal T cells and mast cells share common adhesion receptors. *Immunol. Today* 17(2):60–63

162. Dvorak HF, Mihm MC Jr, Dvorak AM. 1976. Morphology of delayed-type hypersensitivity reactions in man. *J. Invest. Dermatol.* 67:391–401

163. Razin E, Ihle JN, Seldin D, Mencia-Huerta JM, Katz HR, et al. 1984. Interleukin 3: a differentiation and growth factor for the mouse mast cell that contains chondroitin sulfate E proteoglycan. *J. Immunol.* 132(3):1479–86

164. Alam R, Kumar D, Anderson-Walters D, Forsythe PA. 1994. Macrophage inflammatory protein-1α and monocyte chemoattractant peptide-1 elicit immediate and late cutaneous reactions and activate murine mast cells in vivo. *J. Immunol.* 152(3):1298–303

165. Wang HW, Tedla N, Lloyd AR, Wakefield D, McNeil PH. 1998. Mast cell activation and migration to lymph nodes during induction of an immune response in mice. *J. Clin. Invest.* 102(8):1617–26

166. Frandji P, Oskeritzian C, Cacaraci F, Lapeyre J, Peronet R, et al. 1993. Antigen-dependent stimulation by bone marrow-derived mast cells of MHC class II-restricted T cell hybridoma. *J. Immunol.* 151(11):6318–28

167. Fox CC, Jewell SD, Whitacre CC. 1994. Rat peritoneal mast cells present antigen to a PPD-specific T cell line. *Cell Immunol.* 158(1):253–64

168. Malaviya R, Ross EA, MacGregor JI, Ikeda T, Little JR, et al. 1994. Mast cell phagocytosis of FimH-expressing enterobacteria. *J. Immunol.* 152(4):1907–14

169. Malaviya R, Twesten NJ, Ross EA, Abraham SN, Pfeifer JD. 1996. Mast cells process bacterial Ags through a phagocytic route for class I MHC presentation to T cells. *J. Immunol.* 156(4):1490–96

170. Mecheri S, David B. 1997. Unravelling the mast cell dilemma: Culprit or victim of its generosity? *Immunol. Today* 18(5):212–15

171. Grabbe J, Karau L, Welker P, Ziegler A, Henz BM. 1997. Induction of MHC class II antigen expression on human HMC-1 mast cells. *J. Dermatol. Sci.* 16(1):67–73

172. Frandji P, Mourad W, Tkaczyk C, Singer M, David B, et al. 1998. IL-4 mRNA transcription is induced in mouse bone marrow-derived mast cells through an MHC class II-dependent signaling pathway. *Eur. J. Immunol.* 28(3):844–54

173. Dimitriadou V, Mecheri S, Koutsilieris M, Fraser W, Al-Daccak R, et al. 1998. Expression of functional major histocompatibility complex class II molecules on HMC-1 human mast cells. *J. Leukoc. Biol.* 64(6):791–99

174. Rumsaeng V, Cruikshank WW, Foster B, Prussin C, Kirshenbaum AS, et al. 1997. Human mast cells produce the CD4$^+$ T lymphocyte chemoattractant factor, IL-16. *J. Immunol.* 159(6):2904–10

175. Ott VL, Cambier JC, Kappler J, Marrack P, Swanson BJ. 2003. Mast cell-dependent migration of effector CD8$^+$ T cells through production of leukotriene B$_4$. *Nat. Immunol.* 4(10):974–81

176. Walsh LJ, Trinchieri G, Waldorf HA, Whitaker D, Murphy GF. 1991. Human dermal mast cells contain and release tumor necrosis factor α, which induces endothelial leukocyte adhesion molecule 1. *Proc. Natl. Acad. Sci. USA* 88(10):4220–24

177. Meng H, Marchese MJ, Garlick JA, Jelaska A, Korn JH, et al. 1995. Mast cells induce T-cell adhesion to human fibroblasts by regulating intercellular adhesion molecule-1 and vascular cell adhesion molecule-1 expression. *J. Invest. Dermatol.* 105(6):789–96

178. Jutel M, Watanabe T, Akdis M, Blaser K, Akdis CA. 2002. Immune regulation by histamine. *Curr. Opin. Immunol.* 14(6):735–40

179. Inamura N, Mekori YA, Bhattacharyya SP, Bianchine PJ, Metcalfe DD. 1998. Induction and enhancement of FcεRI-dependent mast cell degranulation following coculture with activated T cells: dependency on ICAM-1- and leukocyte function-associated antigen (LFA)-1-mediated heterotypic aggregation. *J. Immunol.* 160(8):4026–33

180. Bhattacharyya SP, Drucker I, Reshef T, Kirshenbaum AS, Metcalfe DD, et al. 1998. Activated T lymphocytes induce degranulation and cytokine production by human mast cells following cell-to-cell contact. *J. Leukoc. Biol.* 63(3):337–41

181. Baram D, Vaday GG, Salamon P, Drucker I, Hershkoviz R, et al. 2001. Human mast cells release metalloproteinase-9 on contact with activated T cells: juxtacrine regulation by TNF-α. *J. Immunol.* 167(7):4008–16

182. Sitia G, Isogawa M, Iannacone M, Campbell IL, Chisari FV, et al. 2004. MMPs are required for recruitment of antigen-nonspecific mononuclear cells into the liver by CTLs. *J. Clin. Invest.* 113(8):1158–67

183. Grabbe S, Schwarz T. 1998. Immunoregulatory mechanisms involved in elicitation of allergic contact hypersensitivity. *Immunol. Today* 19(1):37–44

184. Macatonia SE, Knight SC, Edwards AJ, Griffiths S, Fryer P. 1987. Localization of antigen on lymph node dendritic cells after exposure to the contact sensitizer fluorescein isothiocyanate. Functional and morphological studies. *J. Exp. Med.* 166(6):1654–67

185. Steinman RM, Pack M, Inaba K. 1997. Dendritic cells in the T-cell areas of lymphoid organs. *Immunol. Rev.* 156:25–37

186. Villa I, Skokos D, Tkaczyk C, Peronet R, David B, et al. 2001. Capacity of mouse mast cells to prime T cells and to induce specific antibody responses in vivo. *Immunology* 102(2):165–72

187. Ptak W, Geba GP, Askenase PW. 1991. Initiation of delayed-type hypersensitivity by low doses of monoclonal IgE antibody. Mediation by serotonin and inhibition by histamine. *J. Immunol.* 146(11):3929–36

187a. Jawat DM, Albert EJ, Rowden G, Haidl ID, Marshall JS. 2004. IgE-mediated mast cell activation induces Langerhans cell migration in vivo. *J. Immunol.* 173(8):5275–82

188. Hart PH, Grimbaldeston MA, Swift GJ, Jaksic A, Noonan FP, et al. 1998. Dermal mast cells determine susceptibility to ultraviolet B-induced systemic suppression of contact hypersensitivity responses in mice. *J. Exp. Med.* 187(12):2045–53

189. Brain SD, Williams TJ. 1988. Substance P regulates the vasodilator activity of calcitonin gene-related peptide. *Nature* 335(6185):73–75

190. Berger P, Perng DW, Thabrew H, Compton SJ, Cairns JA, et al. 2001. Tryptase and agonists of PAR-2 induce the proliferation of human airway smooth muscle cells. *J. Appl. Physiol.* 91(3):1372–79

191. McLachlan JB, Hart JP, Pizzo SV, Shelburne CP, Staats HF, et al. 2003. Mast cell-derived tumor necrosis factor induces hypertrophy of draining lymph

nodes during infection. *Nat. Immunol.* 4(12):1199–205

192. Galli SJ, Nakae S. 2003. Mast cells to the defense. *Nat. Immunol.* 4(12):1160–62

193. Eager KB, Hackett CJ, Gerhard WU, Bennink J, Eisenlohr LC, et al. 1989. Murine cell lines stably expressing the influenza virus hemagglutinin gene introduced by a recombinant retrovirus vector are constitutive targets for MHC class I- and class II-restricted T lymphocytes. *J. Immunol.* 143(7):2328–35

194. Caron G, Delneste Y, Roelandts E, Duez C, Bonnefoy JY, et al. 2001. Histamine polarizes human dendritic cells into Th2 cell-promoting effector dendritic cells. *J. Immunol.* 167(7):3682–86

195. Stoitzner P, Ratzinger G, Koch F, Janke K, Scholler T, et al. 2001. Interleukin-16 supports the migration of Langerhans cells, partly in a CD4-independent way. *J. Invest. Dermatol.* 116(5):641–49

196. Cumberbatch M, Dearman RJ, Antonopoulos C, Groves RW, Kimber I. 2001. Interleukin (IL)-18 induces Langerhans cell migration by a tumour necrosis factor-α- and IL-1β-dependent mechanism. *Immunology* 102(3):323–30

197. Kabashima K, Sakata D, Nagamachi M, Miyachi Y, Inaba K, et al. 2003. Prostaglandin E2-EP4 signaling initiates skin immune responses by promoting migration and maturation of Langerhans cells. *Nat. Med.* 9(6):744–49

198. Mekori YA, Metcalfe DD. 1999. Mast cell-T cell interactions. *J. Allergy Clin. Immunol.* 104:517–23

199. Brown MA, Tanzola MB, Robbie-Ryan M. 2002. Mechanisms underlying mast cell influence on EAE disease course. *Mol. Immunol.* 38(16–18):1373–78

200. Church MK, el-Lati S, Caulfield JP. 1991. Neuropeptide-induced secretion from human skin mast cells. *Int. Arch. Allergy Appl. Immunol.* 94(1–4):310–18

201. Varadaradjalou S, Feger F, Thieblemont N, Hamouda NB, Pleau JM, et al. 2003. Toll-like receptor 2 (TLR2) and TLR4 differentially activate human mast cells. *Eur. J. Immunol.* 33(4):899–906

202. Li L, Li Y, Reddel SW, Cherrian M, Friend DS, et al. 1998. Identification of basophilic cells that express mast cell granule proteases in the peripheral blood of asthma, allergy, and drug-reactive patients. *J. Immunol.* 161(9):5079–86

203. Di Nardo A, Vitiello A, Gallo RL. 2003. Cutting edge: mast cell antimicrobial activity is mediated by expression of cathelicidin antimicrobial peptide. *J. Immunol.* 170(5):2274–78

204. Weller PF, Tsai M, Galli SJ. 2003. Eosinophils, basophils, and mast cells. In *Blood: Principles and Practice of Hematology*, ed. RI Handin, SE Lux, TP Stossel TP, pp. 569–88. Philadelphia, PA: JB Lippincott. 2nd ed.

Annu. Rev. Immunol. 2005. 23:787–819
doi: 10.1146/annurev.immunol.23.021704.115719
Copyright © 2005 by Annual Reviews. All rights reserved
First published online as a Review in Advance on December 16, 2004

NETWORK COMMUNICATIONS: Lymphotoxins, LIGHT, and TNF

Carl F. Ware

*Division of Molecular Immunology, La Jolla Institute for Allergy and Immunology,
San Diego, California 92121; email: cware@liai.org*

Key Words   autoimmunity, chemokine, infectious disease, interferon, lymphoid
organs

■ **Abstract**   Lymphotoxins (LT) provide essential communication links between
lymphocytes and the surrounding stromal and parenchymal cells and together with
the two related cytokines, tumor necrosis factor (TNF) and LIGHT (LT-related inducible ligand that competes for glycoprotein D binding to herpesvirus entry mediator
on T cells), form an integrated signaling network necessary for efficient innate and
adaptive immune responses. Recent studies have identified signaling pathways that
regulate several genes, including chemokines and interferons, which participate in the
development and function of microenvironments in lymphoid tissue and host defense.
Disruption of the LT/TNF/LIGHT network alleviates inflammation in certain autoimmune disease models, but decreases resistance to selected pathogens. Pharmacological
disruption of this network in human autoimmune diseases such as rheumatoid arthritis
alleviates inflammation in a significant number of patients, but not in other diseases,
a finding that challenges our molecular paradigms of autoimmunity and perhaps will
reveal novel roles for this network in pathogenesis.

INTRODUCTION

Cytokines provide essential communication signals for the highly motile cells of
the immune system. Positional location within the different organs and subsequent
differentiation to acquire effector function require that lymphocytes communicate
with the surrounding tissue, with the role of communicator often played by tumor
necrosis factor (TNF) and lymphotoxin (LT)-related cytokines.[1] Lymphotoxins are
part of a complex communication system linking lymphocytes and surrounding
parenchymal and stromal cells that can act locally or at distant sites. Two distinct
structural forms of LT are recognized, LTα and LTβ, each localizing to distinct
physical compartments (secreted or membrane restricted). Alone or in combination, LTα and LTβ form trimeric molecules that engage different cellular receptors
and account, in part, for the specificity in eliciting distinct cellular responses. The

---

[1]See Appendix for a full list of abbreviations used.

extent to which the biological processes are regulated by LTαβ is now being elucidated, although the clinical importance of LT has yet to be fully realized, especially
when compared with its close structural homologue, TNF.

Lymphotoxin-α (formerly known as TNFβ) and TNF were once considered
redundant forms. However, as a complex with LTβ, LTα has emerged with roles
in the immune system quite distinct from that of TNF, a theme repeatedly corroborated at the molecular and cellular levels. Recent evidence indicates that for
some physiological processes TNF and LTαβ work together as components of an
integrated signaling network. This signaling network is defined in part by commu-
nal sharing of receptors and ligands: LTα, LTβ, TNF, and LIGHT are linked into
a common signaling network involving five distinct receptors (Figure 1). Moreover, the LT/TNF network is connected to specific chemokines, interferons, and
other TNF family ligands in larger arrays of signaling networks. The concept of
integrated signaling networks has important implications for the use of therapies
targeted at these cytokines.

In the clinic, TNF/LTα have proven to be important targets for suppressing inflammation in certain autoimmune diseases, including rheumatoid arthritis (RA)
and inflammatory bowel syndrome, but not others, such as multiple sclerosis (MS).

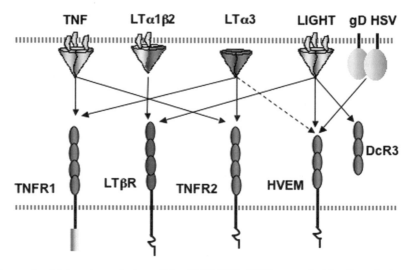

Figure 1   Molecular switches of the LT/TNF/LIGHT network. The ligands (*upper
portion*) are depicted as membrane-anchored or secreted trimers, with the solid lines
indicating their respective high-affinity receptors (*lower portion*); dashed line indicates
relatively low-affinity binding. Cysteine-rich domains in the various receptors are depicted in blue; the yellow box in the cytosolic region indicates presence of a death
domain and black squiggle line a TRAF binding motif. Decoy receptor 3 (DcR3) lacks
a transmembrane domain. Glycoprotein D (gD) is an envelope protein of the HSV
virion and is expressed on the surface of infected cells.

Moreover, side effects of TNF inhibitors include increased susceptibility to certain infectious diseases. Recent advances in identifying the molecular mechanisms in LT/TNF signaling may help clarify seemingly contradictory results in human patients treated with TNF/LT inhibitors. Here we review the structural and functional features of the LT/TNF/LIGHT signaling systems, in the context of the larger signaling networks. Although LT are well defined as key elements required for lymphoid organogenesis and organization, the effector genes activated by LT signaling pathways are just now beginning to emerge. Clinical results using LT/TNF inhibitors in various human autoimmune diseases suggest that the mechanisms controlling inflammation are much more complex than current models predict.

COMPONENTS OF THE NETWORK

Lymphotoxins and TNF are members of the TNF superfamily, a diversified family of ligands and corresponding family of receptors defined by a cysteine-rich ectodomain that control signaling pathways that initiate cell death, survival, and cellular differentiation. More than 20 distinct ligand-receptor systems now recognized in the TNF superfamily are involved in regulating the development and function of bone, neuronal, ectodermal, and lymphoid organs (reviewed in 1–3). The genes encoding LTβ, TNF, and LTα reside in a tightly linked loci within the major histocompatibility complex on Chromosome (Chr) 6 in humans (Chr 17 in the mouse). The receptors TNFR1, CD27, and LTβR are linked on Chr 12 (mouse Chr 6). Three other MHC paralogus genomic regions contain the related family members (Chr 19 LIGHT, CD27L, 41BBL; Chr 1 FasL, GITRL, Ox40L; Chr 9 CD30, TL1A) revealed by their conserved gene structure, transcriptional orientation, and function (4, 5). The receptors for these ligands (except FasL) are linked on Chr 1p36.

Molecular Switches: Ligands and Receptors

The signaling network in which lymphotoxins act is complex, comprising unique and shared ligand-receptor systems (Figure 1). LTα and LTβ form three distinct ligands. LTα can exist as a homotrimer (LTα3) that is exclusively secreted owing to cleavage of its traditional signal peptide, a unique feature in the TNF superfamily. LTα3, like TNF, binds two receptors, TNFR1 and TNFR2. Two membrane-anchored heterotrimers can be formed by LTβ and LTα during biosynthesis: LTα1β2 (the predominant form) and LTα2β1. LTβ, like other TNF superfamily ligands, is a type II transmembrane protein but lacks a traditional signal peptide cleavage site anchoring the bound LTα subunit to the cell surface. The LTβ subunit in the LTα1β2 heterotrimer changes the receptor binding specificity to engage with high affinity the LTβ receptor (LTβR). Although the LTα2β1 binds TNFR1, 2, and LTβR (with low avidity, mid-nM range), it is a minor form expressed by T cells (<2%) and thus has no defined role. The LTβ-related ligand LIGHT, the most recently defined member of the network, binds to the herpesvirus entry mediator

(HVEM), which was discovered as an entry route for herpes simplex virus (HSV) (6). Glycoprotein D of HSV is a virokine encoded by HSV that blocks LIGHT binding to HVEM (7). LTβR is a second receptor for LIGHT (7–9). HVEM may also serve as a third receptor for LTα, although binding is relatively weak (7). DcR3 is a secreted receptor for LIGHT, Fas ligand, and TL1A (10), demonstrating a broader functionally conserved relationship among these ligands.

Targeted deletion of the LT/TNF ligands and receptors in mice has aided significantly in defining unique and complementary physiological roles associated with each cytokine system (reviewed in 11, 12). The phenotypes of mice deficient in the LT system are complex and affect multiple aspects of the immune system, including lymphoid organ development and organization and host defense systems (see Table 1). As expected for a simple signaling system, genetic deletion of the ligand or receptor is expected to give identical phenotypes, which was partially true for the LT/TNF systems. For instance, with the lymph node–deficient phenotype, LT$\alpha^{-/-}$ and LTβR$^{-/-}$ are replicas, whereas the TNF$^{-/-}$ and TNFR$^{-/-}$ mice have a full complement of LN, which clearly separated the biological processes signaled by these two systems. However, LT$\beta^{-/-}$ mice lacked most LN but retained some mesenteric LN, implying there must be another ligand for LTβR. However, LIGHT$^{-/-}$ mice had a full complement of LN, although LIGHT can

TABLE 1   Genetic deficiencies in LT$\alpha\beta$/TNF/LIGHT

Gene deletion	Phenotypes					
	LN[a]	PP[b]	Architecture[c]	NK[d]	NKT[e]	DC[f]
LTα	−	−	Disrupted	Impaired	Impaired	Migration
LTβ	−	−	Disrupted	Impaired	Impaired	Migration
LIGHT	+	+	+	+	+	+
LTβ-B[g]	+	+	Disrupted	Nr	Nr	Nr
LTβ-T[g]	+	+	+	Nr	Nr	Nr
TNF	+	−	Disrupted MZ	+	+	Maturation
LTβR	−	−	Disrupted	−	−	Migration
TNFR1	+	−	Disrupted MZ	+	+	Maturation
TNFR2	+	+	+	+	+	+

[a]Lymph nodes; LT$\beta^{-/-}$ mice have ~75% of mesenteric LN.

[b]Peyer's patches.

[c]Architecture of the splenic white pulp includes T- and B-zone segregation; marginal zone (MZ); germinal center; follicular dendritic cell network.

[d]Natural killer (NK) cell deficiency includes reduced cell numbers and enhanced tumor susceptibility.

[e]NKT cells Vα14 subset.

[f]Dendritic cells phenotype includes impairment of migration to spleen or maturation in bone marrow.

[g]LTβ conditionally deleted in B cells or T cells. LTβ-B showed partial disruption in architecture; normal for LTβ-T, but combined knockout in both B and T cells was worse than LTβ-B.

Absent, −; normal, +; not reported, Nr.

contribute to LN development, as revealed by LIGHT$^{-/-}$ LT$\beta^{-/-}$ double knockout mice. A common phenotype linking LT and TNF pathways is seen in the formation of Peyer's patches (PP), which are poorly developed or missing in some TNF/TNFR1-deficient mice as well as in LT$\alpha^{-/-}$, LT$\beta^{-/-}$, and LTβR$^{-/-}$ mice. Some collateral damage to neighboring genes may indeed have occurred by the targeting vector imposed by the tight genetic linkage of the LTα/LTβ/TNF loci. However, a comparison of mice deficient in all three ligands (TNF, LTα, and LTβ) with individually gene-deficient mice indicated that LT and TNF systems functioned largely independently but overlapped in organizing the microarchitecture of the spleen, particularly in the compartmentalization of T and B cells (13). More recent results using mice conditionally deleted for LT or TNF in T or B lymphocytes are challenging some previous assumptions, particularly in distinguishing between the roles played by LT during lymphoid organ development, homeostasis and maturation (14, 15).

The TNF-TNFR1 system provides a key element as a sentinel cytokine produced by innate recognition pathways that are involved in promoting inflammatory processes, whereas LT$\alpha\beta$ signaling is centered more in the realm of development and homeostasis of lymphoid tissue, although LTα signaling can promote the formation of tertiary lymphoid tissues at sites of chronic inflammation (16). The biology of LIGHT at present seems more prominent in regulating T cell–based inflammatory reactions, particularly in the mucosal tissue. At the same time, the evidence points to significant overlap in biological responses among these cytokines. Attempts to understand the mechanisms underlying this network at the level of signaling cascades have focused on the NF-κB family of transcription factors, which in gene-deficient mice share common phenotypes with the LT/TNF system.

SIGNAL TRANSMISSION

Receptor signaling is initiated by ligand-induced clustering of cell surface receptors. Trivalent ligands or bivalent receptor-specific antibodies function as agonists for TNFR or LTβR. The receptor aggregation model seems to apply for all members of the TNF superfamily, although for apoptosis induction by Fas ligand and TRAIL higher ordered aggregation of receptors may be required (17).

A basic framework has been assembled for TNFR1 and LTβR pathways that lead to cell death and activation of the NF-κB transcription factor family, although the mechanisms governing signaling specificity, signal relay, and kinetics of activation remain active research areas (Figure 2). The coupling of activated TNF receptors to various adaptor proteins that link to intracellular signaling pathways is a complex process. TNFR1 as a death domain (DD)–containing receptor can couple to the apoptotic cascade via TNFR-associated DD (TRADD). LTβR, TNFR2, and HVEM utilize TNFR receptor-associated factors (TRAFs), a family of zinc RING finger proteins, to connect to intracellular signaling pathways. However, TNFR1 also engages TRAF2 via TRADD, coupling it to NF-κB activation, a crucial regulatory point in cellular resistance to apoptosis. Recent experiments by Micheau

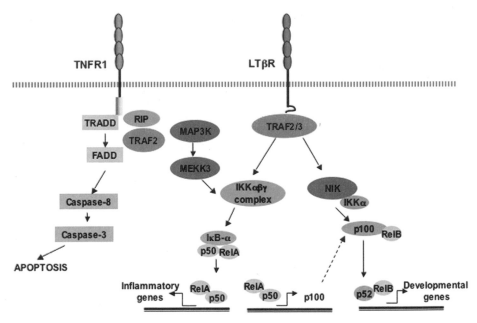

Figure 2   TNFR1 and LTβR signal transmission pathways for cell death and NF-κB activation. The death domain recruits TRADD/FADD leading to Caspase 8 activation linking TNF to the apoptotic pathway. TNFR1 can also engage TRAF2 to activate the canonical NF-κB pathway (p50/p65) via IκB degradation. This pathway controls many inflammatory genes and p100 synthesis. The LTβR induces both the canonical and the NF-κB2 pathway via the processing of p100 and formation of p52/RelB target genes.

et al. (18) have determined the importance of the FLICE inhibitory protein (FLIP) in resistance to apoptosis signaling. FLIP functions as an attenuating switch for apoptosis by displacing the FADD-Caspase 8 complex. However, FLIP expression is dependent on activation of NF-κB1/relA and transcription/translation, which are often compromised in pathogen-infected cells. Thus, the apoptotic pathway becomes the dominant default pathway in cells that are biosynthetically compromised.

The TRAF family includes six members that are related to a larger number of proteins (19), defined by a common C-terminal domain folded as a beta sandwich that form trimers. TRAFs can also contain RING finger and multiple zinc fingers typically at the N terminus, which can contribute to ubiquitinylation of substrates (20), and a coiled coil domain that acts to stabilize the trimeric structure (21). The TRAF interacting region in LTβR and other TNFR are short peptide motifs (22). The crystal structure of the TRAF domain of TRAF3 and TRAF2 provided key insight into the mechanism of receptor binding. The mushroom-shaped TRAF domain contains a peptide-binding crevice in each subunit that allows accommodation of a surprisingly large variety of sequences and conformations contained within the myriad of receptors and regulators that bind TRAF (22). The TRAF-binding crevice may have evolved this plasticity to accommodate the large expansion of the TNFR superfamily, thereby providing a greater capacity to link to various signaling pathways. The zinc RING finger moiety appears to function as part of a ubiquitin ligase complex leading to proteosome degradation, a feature common to the activation or turnover of many components in these signaling pathways. Currently, biochemical evidence indicates that TRAF2 and 3 are important in enabling lymphotoxins to activate NF-κB. However, an unresolved conundrum remains in that genetic deletions of TRAF2 or 3 in mice do not phenocopy LT deficiency. The other TRAF members, such as TRAF5, are important for signaling by Ox40 (23), whereas TRAF6 is necessary for signaling by IL-1 receptor and Toll-like receptors (24, 25), as well as some other TNFR superfamily members including RANK and CD40 (26). In each case, NF-κB is an important target of the signaling pathway.

NF-κB is a major control point for the expression of inducible genes regulating inflammation that underlie innate and adaptive defenses. Recent results showing that distinct forms of the NF-κB family of transcription factors are activated by TNF-TNFR1 and LT$\alpha\beta$-LTβR systems have provided new insight into the differential actions of these cytokines. Moreover, these results provide evidence of a plausible mechanism for overlapping phenotypes in mice deficient in LT and NF-κB. The NF-κB family comprises five members: RelA (p65), RelB, c-Rel, NF-κB1 (p50 and its precursor p105), and NF-κB2 (p52 and its precursor p100). These proteins form a collection of homodimers and heterodimers that can function as transcriptional activators or inhibitors. The NF-κB family of transcription factors regulates hundreds of genes crucial to the development of cells and organs of the innate and adaptive immune responses (27–30). NF-κB1/RelA is most closely associated with activation by inflammatory stimuli. NF-κB1 complex is held in a latent form in the cytosol by the Inhibitors of κB (IκB), requiring the IκB kinase complex (IKK) to phosphorylate IκB, inducing ubiquitination and degradation by the proteosome and releasing the NF-κB1/relA dimer for transport into the nucleus. The IKK complex is composed of two catalytic subunits (IKKα and IKKβ) and a regulatory subunit (IKKγ, also called NEMO) and is the point of convergence of varied stimuli.

LTβR, unlike TNFR1, activates NF-κB2 by a mechanism distinct from that of NF-κB1 (31–35). The NF-κB2 pathway, which mediates the processing of p100 to p52, is dependent on the NF-κB-inducing kinase (NIK) and IKKα, but is independent of IKKβ and γ (33, 35–37). Activation of the p52/RelB pathway by LTβR signaling results in the translocation of the NF-κB2/relB dimers to the nucleus, leading to gene transcription involved in the development of lymphoid organs and maintenance of architecture in secondary lymphoid organs. Like LTβR$^{-/-}$ mice, alymphoplasia (*aly*) mice, which contain a point mutation in the TRAF-binding region of NIK required to activate the IKKα complex, and NIK$^{-/-}$ mice lack secondary lymphoid organs and have disrupted splenic microarchitecture (37, 38).

The capacity of TNFR1 to activate proinflammatory genes is relative strong when compared with LTβR (39). In part, this may be due to the ability of LTβR to activate the IKKα-dependent NF-κB2 pathway, which can attenuate gene expression turned on by NF-κB1/relA (33, 34). The NF-κB2 pathway is slow to initiate but then is sustained (hours) compared with the rapid induction and short duration of activating NF-κB1/relA. The slow kinetics is attributed in part to a transcriptional and cotranslational processing needed by p100. That p100 synthesis is dependent on NF-κB1/relA inextricably links these two pathways together, suggesting an additional mechanism of cooperation between LTβR and TNFR1 signaling.

The phenotypes of mice deleted for various NF-κB members are complex, affecting development and immune functions. Some are lethal, no doubt due to the roles this family plays in controlling genes that determine cell survival or death. Additionally, NF-κB deficiency prominently affects responses of stromal cells coincident with the expression of LTβR. For instance, deletion of relA in mice is embryonic lethal unless crossed onto a mouse deficient in TNF-TNFR1, which results in an animal with a phenotype similar to that of a LTβR-deficient mouse: no secondary lymphoid organs and disrupted architecture (40). The complexity of protein interactions within the TNF pathway was revealed in a proteomics approach that used tandem affinity purification to isolate protein complexes associated with TNFR or known signaling molecules and identification by tandem mass spectrometry (41). As many as 241 molecular contacts were identified within the TNF pathway, confirming many basic aspects of TNF/LT signaling outlined above and adding several new components. For instance, a TRAF homologue (TRAF7) was identified as a modulator of MEKK3, a protein necessary for NF-κB1/relA activation. In the near future, the convergence of proteomic and genetic analyses should yield a comprehensive outline of the TNF/LT signaling network.

NETWORK DYNAMICS

Changes in the expression of the LT/TNF ligands and receptors among various cell types will determine the dynamics of this intercellular communication network. LTαβ, TNF, and LIGHT are all induced following activation of lymphocytes and monocytes via their respective recognition systems, which gave rise to the concept that these cytokines are inducibly expressed. However, more recent examination of gene expression profiles in naive mice revealed that these cytokines are constitutively expressed on lymphocytes within lymphoid organs, perhaps contributing to the homeostasis of the tissue (42, 43). Antigen-specific and -nonspecific activation of T and B lymphocytes and NK cells from peripheral blood induces LTα and LTβ transcription and protein expression (44, 45). A recent histological study revealed LTβ expressed not only in chronic inflammatory tissue on T cells and plasma cells but also on epitheloid histiocytes and multinucleated giant cells (46). LTαβ expression is regulated by cytokines, including Interleukin (IL)-2, which induces LTαβ expression on human T cells from peripheral blood (44); in mice

IL-4 and IL-7 cytokines and the chemokines CCL19 and CCL21 can induce LTαβ expression on splenic T cells (47) (Figure 3A). In the spleen of naive mice, LTαβ is constitutively expressed on most follicular B lymphocytes, controlled in part by CXCL13 (B lymphocyte chemoattractant); CD40-CD40L can induce expression of LTα in B cells (48) but CD4 T cells also constitutively express LTαβ. By contrast, the LTβR is not expressed on T or B lymphocytes or NK cells but is constitutively expressed on fibroblasts (stroma), epithelial cells, and myeloid cells (monocytes, dendritic, and mast cells) (49–51), suggesting that LTαβ-LTβR allows unidirectional communication between lymphocytes and the surrounding stromal and parenchymal cells. By contrast, TNF is produced by a wide array of cells, especially in response to inflammatory stimuli, but substantially by cells of the myeloid lineage. TNFR1 is broadly distributed, whereas TNFR2 is inducible on T and B lymphocytes but constitutively expressed on monocytes. Both receptors are rapidly shed from the cell surface, accumulating in plasma to significant levels during inflammatory processes. LIGHT is inducibly expressed in T cells yet is constitutively expressed by myeloid cells, primarily immature DC, a pattern intermediate to LTαβ and TNF (7, 52). HVEM is broadly distributed within the lymphoid and nonlymphoid compartment, although a systematic study has not been performed (53).

The physical location of these ligands may also contribute to the network dynamics. LTβ is not cleaved into a soluble form, and thus the LTαβ complex remains cell-associated, which dictates that signaling via the LTαβ-LTβR system will require cell-to-cell contact. TNF, LIGHT, and LTα are active in their membrane-anchored and secreted positions, theoretically acting at locations distant from the site of production. However, an additional control mechanism, the presence of soluble decoy receptors including shed forms of TNFR1, TNFR2, and DcR3, may limit the bioavailability of TNF, LTα, and LIGHT. The dynamics of these regulatory controls will depend on the concentrations and relative avidity of the ligand receptor pair. TNF and LTα bind cellular receptors with high affinity (K_d = mid-pM), whereas engineered soluble forms of LTαβ and LIGHT interact with their cell-bound receptors with moderate avidity (K_d = low nM), suggesting that even moderate avidity for a diffusion-restricted ligand is sufficient to form stable signaling complexes. By contrast, the avidity of LTα for HVEM is low (mid-nM), suggesting that physiological levels of these reactants may not be sufficient to initiate signaling, although high local concentrations may conceivably achieve levels above the threshold required for signaling.

Regulatory mechanisms affecting transcriptional induction and stability, and restricted cellular patterns of expression, among other mechanisms, also contribute to signaling specificity (reviewed in 54). The regulation of TNF transcription requires a multicomponent enhancesome that varies with the specific stimulus (55, 56). The molecular regulation of LTα, LTβ, and LIGHT gene expression is just beginning to be dissected (57, 58), but will become crucial if their polymorphic alleles are linked to disease pathogenesis.

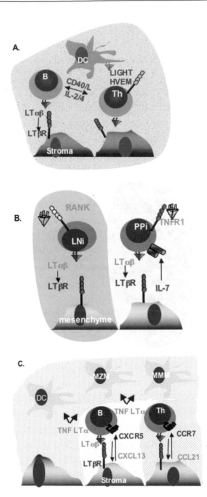

Figure 3   Lymphotoxin and TNF networks form between multiple cell types. (*A*) T and B cell expression of LTαβ is regulated via interleukins 2 and 4 and the CD40 system. LIGHT is constitutively expressed on DC by an unknown mechanism. T and B cells engage stroma expressing the LTβR, which forms appropriate microenvironments. (*B*) The development of lymph nodes and PP require distinct progenitors: the LN inducer requires RANK ligand to induce LTαβ expression, whereas the PP inducer expresses LTαβ in response to IL7 or TNF. The inducer cells interact with LTβR expressing lymphoid-specific mesenchymal cell. (*C*) Chemokine circuits form between lymphocytes and stroma. Depicted are cellular interactions in the architecture of white pulp in the spleen dependent on LT/TNF signaling. The marginal zone (*green*) contains marginal zone macrophages (MZM) and metallophilic macrophages (MMM). Dendritic cells (DC) require LT signaling for emigration to the spleen. B and T lymphocytes are compartmentalized in discrete areas in the white pulp [B cell follicle (*yellow*) and T cell zone (*blue*)] through the reciprocal induction of LT expression on lymphocytes by chemokines and chemokine expression by stromal cells via the LTβR.

THE NETWORK IN ACTION

Lymphatic Organ Formation

The formation of secondary lymphoid organs is instructive of a signaling pathway involved in mammalian organ development that includes the LT signaling network. The development and homeostasis of microenvironments in secondary lymphoid tissue are absent in mice deficient in $LT\alpha$, $LT\beta$, and $LT\beta R$ (reviewed in 59, 60). At least two cell types are necessary for secondary lymphoid organ formation, the $LT\alpha\beta$ expressing "inducer" cell (a $CD4^+CD3^-$ $IL7R\alpha^+$ mononuclear cell) and an embryonic stroma organizer cell expressing the $LT\beta R$ (reviewed in 59) (Figure 3B). The PP inducer is distinct from the LN inducer cell in respect to the requirement for IL-7 and the RANK system (26, 61). The LN- or PP-deficient phenotype is observed in several other knockout mice, delineating the framework of a signaling pathway involved in lymphoid organ development. Ikaros, ID2, and $ROR\gamma$ are transcriptional regulators essential for lymphocyte progenitors to develop, and recent results indicate that $ROR\gamma t$ is specifically expressed in the inducer cells (62). Fox 1 is needed for $LT\beta R$ expression in PP (63). Mice deficient in certain members of the NF-κB activation pathway, including NIK, IKKα and Rel B, have deficient lymphoid organogenesis (64).

An interesting but perplexing discordance between genetic and biochemical evidence arose with the TRAF adaptors. TRAF2-, 3-, or 5-deficient mice have secondary lymphoid organs, yet, unexpectedly, LN deficiency was found in TRAF6$^{-/-}$ mice even though $LT\beta R$ does not utilize TRAF6. Moreover, the TRANCE/RANK (TNFSF11A) system, which utilizes TRAF6 as an adaptor, when genetically deleted, also revealed an LN-deficient phenotype (26, 65). In this case, the experimental results obtained by Yoshida and colleagues indicated that the RANK/TRAF6 pathway was required for the induction of $LT\alpha\beta$ on the LN inducer cell, thus accounting in part for the discordance with the biochemical data ($LT\beta R$ does not bind TRAF6) (61). IL-7 and TNF were also shown to induce $LT\alpha\beta$ on PP inducer cells, which may explain why some TNF/TNFR1 mice have defects in PP development (66). These results provide another example of the concatenation of the LT network with other members of the TNF superfamily.

LT-Chemokine Circuits in Tissue Architecture

The spleen (60), nasal lymphoid tissue (67), and uterine aggregates (68) develop independently of the $LT\alpha\beta$-$LT\beta R$ network, yet the organization of the microarchitecture in these secondary lymphoid tissues depends on LT signaling. LT-dependent microarchitecture includes the integrity of the marginal zone and the presence of MZ macrophages, the function of stromal cells that allow recruitment and clustering of B cells in the follicle, T cell migration into the T cell zone, creation of follicular dendritic cell (FDC) networks, and the formation of germinal centers during immune responses (reviewed in 60, 69). In the spleen, the tissue-organizing chemokines intersect with the LT/TNF network to form a signaling amplification circuit between lymphocytes and stroma. The tissue-organizing chemokines include CXCL13 (B lymphocyte chemoattractant), CCL21 (secondary lymphoid chemokine), and CCL19 (EBV-like chemokine), where expression levels are decreased in LT-null mice (42). B cells play a vital role in forming the FDC network as well as the T cell zone, compartmentalizing lymphocytes in the splenic white pulp. A circuit is initiated by CXCR5$^+$ B cells sensing CXCL13 produced by LTβR$^+$ stromal cells, which induces LT$\alpha\beta$ expression on B cells. B cell-to-stromal cell contact then promotes stromal secretion of CXCL13 via LT$\alpha\beta$ and LTβR, thereby completing the circuit (42, 47) (Figure 3C). As B cells emigrate to the blood the expression of LT$\alpha\beta$ is lost, but as they reenter the B cell areas in response to CXCL13 they regain surface expression (42).

Similar circuits may be involved in maintaining the T cell zone through the action of the CCR7-binding chemokines, CCL19 and CCL21, produced by gp38 expressing stromal cells (47, 70). Recent results revealed that LTβR signaling induces CCL20 expression in mucosal cells (71), suggesting that a parallel circuit could be formed between LT$\alpha\beta$/LIGHT-LTβR and CCL20-CCR6 (72, 73). Moreover, these tissue-organizing chemokines are expressed in nonlymphoid tissues, including tumor and pancreatic tissue, upon initiation of LTβR signaling (16, 43).

Cyster and colleagues identified the LT-chemokine circuit as a homeostatic mechanism that maintains the microarchitecture of the spleen (42, 47, 74), yet some of the associated phenotypes may be intertwined with neonatal developmental/maturational processes. Cellular reconstitution of LT-deficient mice with LT-sufficient wild-type bone marrow restores FDC differentiation but fails to restore chemokine levels (75). Conditional deletion of LTβ from B or T cells provided another approach in distinguishing developmental from homeostatic processes (15). Lymph nodes and PP develop in the conditional knockout (14) owing to the separate lineage of the inducer cell from B and T cell lineages (59). LTβ expression by B lymphocytes is important for proper marginal zone structure and FDC networks, yet when LTβ was conditionally deleted in both B and T cells, disruption of the splenic microarchitecture became even more exaggerated (14). Enforced expression of LIGHT in T cells in LT$\alpha^{-/-}$ mice restored CCL21 but not CXCL13 expression, yet corrected T and B cell segregation (76). Thus, B and T cell expression of LT$\alpha\beta$, TNF, LIGHT, and perhaps others may contribute to the regulation of the tissue-organizing chemokines that impart selected features of lymphoid tissue microarchitecture.

Work by Ruddle et al. helped to establish the idea that sites of lymphocyte aggregates in chronically inflamed tissue, termed lymphoid organ neogenesis, is controlled in part by TNF/LTα and LT$\alpha\beta$ signaling (16, 74). TNF and LT$\alpha\beta$ are needed for the formation of granulomas that contain persistent bacterial pathogens (46, 77–80). These results suggest that modulation of the TNF/LT$\alpha\beta$/LIGHT network can be used to manipulate chemokine networks affecting inflammation and immune responses.

Deficiency in LT/TNF network in mice affects several other components of the innate and adaptive immune systems, including DC, NK cells, NKT cells, as well as differentiation of T and B cells. The differentiation of DC from bone marrow precursors requires the TNF/LTα-TNFR1 system, whereas DC recruitment to secondary lymphoid organs requires LTβR signaling (81, 82). In LT$\alpha^{-/-}$ mice, NK cells fail to differentiate into effector cells capable of restricting metastasis of transplanted tumor cells (83–85). The differentiation of NKT cells is dependent on LTβR signaling via the NIK-NF-κB2/relB pathway (86). The functions of T and B cells are altered by deprivation of LTβR signaling; however, LTβR is not expressed on T or B cells, indicating the mechanisms are indirect, presumably via stromal cell functions. This presumption is supported by results showing that FDC networks are dependent upon continuous LT$\alpha\beta$-LTβR signaling (87, 88), which can be disrupted by LTβR-Fc decoy (89). The disruption of FDC networks influences the ability of B cells to form germinal centers, affecting antibody production to specific T cell–dependent antigens. Although T and B cells appear to differentiate to normal numbers and appropriate subclasses, recent evidence is teasing out the influence of LTβR signaling on thymic medullary epithelial cell differentiation (90). In part, the control of thymic autoimmune regulator (AIRE) expression through LTβR signaling provides a critical pathway for the development of central tolerance (91). These findings reiterate the concept that LT$\alpha\beta$-LTβR signaling provides essential lines of communication between lymphocytes and stromal cells in forming crucial tissue microenvironments.

NETWORK SUBVERSION BY PATHOGENS

It has long been recognized that viruses interfere with cytokine communication pathways. Several viral families including herpes-, adeno-, papova-, and poxviradae have evolved strategies specifically targeting the LT/TNF network. Undoubtedly, the cellular survival and apoptotic pathways regulated by the TNF superfamily provide strong selective pressures for pathogens to evolve specific counter strategies that aid pathogen replication and dissemination (reviewed in 92–95).

Molecular Strategies

The most obvious viral regulators of the TNF/LT network include structural homologues from large DNA viruses, including poxviridae and herpesviruses. Historically, the first example of a viral gene product inhibiting TNF was gleaned from the genome of rabbit poxvirus, which contains an orf encoding a type II TNFR ortholog (96). A dramatically attenuated infection occurs following deletion of the MX-T2 gene, establishing the relevance of this mechanism to viral pathogenesis (96). The diversity and conservation of TNF inhibitors found in poxvirus imply an important role in pathogenesis, yet poxviruses target many cytokine signaling pathways, such as IFN and chemokines, as part of their seemingly global attack on signaling pathways of the innate and adaptive defense systems (97).

Herpesviruses cause lifelong infections and establish latent states maintained by competent immunity, although they sporadically reemerge in immune-competent host and become virulent opportunistic pathogens in the immune suppressed. The genomes of herpesvirus also contain a collection of immune modulators, including several that target the LT/TNF network. HSV (αherpesvirus) enters cells through binding of viral envelope glycoprotein D (gD) to HVEM (6), one of several HSV entry receptors (98). Crystallographic analysis of the gD-HVEM complex reveals that gD binds to a discrete region in the first cysteine-rich domain near the N terminus, albeit on the opposite face of the receptor predicted to engage the cellular ligand LIGHT or LTα (99), yet gD can compete for HVEM binding to membrane-anchored LIGHT (7). The Epstein Barr virus (γ-herpesvirus)–encoded latent membrane protein 1 (LMP1) binds TRAF adaptors (100) and activates both NF-κB1 and NF-κB2 complexes (101), behaving like a constitutively activated receptor (e.g., CD40, BAFFR) that promotes B cell survival and differentiation. Conversely, HHV8 and related γ-herpesvirus contain orthologs of FLIP, which disrupt Caspase 8 activation but also mediate NF-κB activation (102). A β-herpesvirus, human cytomegalovirus (CMV), expresses a TNFR ortholog (UL144 orf), which is closest in sequence to the extracellular domain of human HVEM and TRAIL-R2, although none of the known cellular ligands bind UL144 (103). Antibodies to UL144 ectodomain are detected in the serum from CMV-positive patients, although hypervariability in UL144 sequences does not directly correlate with virulence in humans (104); to date a functional role has not been uncovered.

Collectively, these examples represent viral mechanisms targeted specifically at the LT/TNF network. These specific mechanisms are set within a broader strategy evolved by herpesvirus that targets many other aspects of innate and adaptive immunity, necessary in order for the pathogen to successfully occupy a niche in the vertebrate host without causing overt disease. Multiple strategies targeted at NK and T cell recognition systems, effector molecules, and cytokine signaling pathways are known for cytomegalovirus (for example, see 105). The persistence of CMV and other herpesviruses in immunocompetent hosts suggests that the balance of resistance and countermeasures must be critically maintained. The molecular processes involved in the maintenance of host-virus coexistence are anything but passive, as all herpesviruses readily reactivate in patients with compromised immune systems and result in increased morbidity.

The LT/TNF-Interferon Axis

The mechanisms controlling host-virus coexistence are not well defined, but recent evidence suggests a role for interferons (106) and LT/TNF systems (107), potentially functioning as a cytokine axis. TNFR1 and LTβR signaling efficiently arrests CMV replication in human dermal fibroblasts without inducing cell death, whereas activation of Fas and TRAILR are completely ineffective at inducing death of infected cells or restricting virus replication (107). The mechanism underlying the arrest of CMV replication involves the cooperative induction of IFNβ mRNA, which inhibits virus replication after immediate early viral gene expression but before virion release. Virus spread to adjacent cells is also blocked. HCMV infection normally suppresses the IFNβ response, eventually inducing cytopathic effects that lead to cell death. However, LTβR or TNFR1 activation of an NF-κB-dependent pathway precedes or overcomes the virus imposed IFNβ blockade. IFNβ blocks virus replication and protects the cell from cytopathic effects, yet the viral genome remains in the cell. Upon cessation of IFN signaling, virion production reinitiates. This observation may represent a molecular mechanism of cooperation between host and pathogen that may help establish persistence. It is not known if this pathway is important in controlling reactivation from latency. Nonetheless, the LTβR/TNFR connection to the IFNβ system may have important implications in interpreting clinical outcomes of TNF inhibitors in human autoimmune diseases.

Experimental Animal Models

The role of the LT network in host defense against viral, bacterial, and parasitic infections in animal models depends in part on the specific pathogen (Table 2). In LT$\alpha^{-/-}$ mice, for instance, the ability to control infection with mouse γ-herpesvirus (MHV68) is not overtly compromised (108), whereas a modest increase in susceptibility to HSV-1 was observed with an underlying reduction in the ability of CD8$^+$ T cells to differentiate into effector cells (109). By contrast, LTα-deficient mice were highly susceptible to mouse CMV owing to the inability to control the initial infection, suggesting compromised innate defenses (107). Host defense may be compromised in LT-deficient mice from a general inadequacy due to structural defects in lymphoid organs or from a lack of signaling required during infection (effector responses), or both.

Bacterial defenses also require the LT signaling network. Host responses to pulmonary infection with *Mycobacterium tuberculosis* were significantly impaired in LTβR$^{-/-}$ mice but not in LIGHT$^{-/-}$ mice, indicating LT$\alpha\beta$-LTβR signaling is crucial in host defenses to this intracellular organism (80). This study by Ehlers et al. pointed to a defect in macrophage-expressed nitric oxide synthetase as a potential mechanism missing in LTβR$^{-/-}$ mice. In slight contrast, LT$\beta^{-/-}$ mice were not significantly impaired to *M. tuberculosis*, although LT$\alpha^{-/-}$ mice were susceptible (79). Chimeric mice constructed with LT$\alpha^{-/-}$ bone marrow revealed that lung granulomas were abnormal and lacked T cells normally required to corral infected macrophages (79). This result implies that LTα is required during the response to the infection and that developmentally determined lymphoid tissues are less important for this organism. Using a pharmacologic approach, Lucas et al. (78) demonstrated that LTβR-Fc increased susceptibility of mice to *Mycobacterium bovis* and that this treatment exacerbated the susceptibility with concurrent with TNFR-Fc decoy treatment, indicating independent but cooperating action of these ligands in host defense to this bacterial pathogen. Effective defenses to some pathogens depend upon LT-dependent architecture [such as lymphocytic choriomeningitis virus (LCMV)] (110), whereas the absence of lymph

TABLE 2 Lymphotoxins in host defense: mouse models

Pathogen[a]	Mouse model[b]	Susceptibility	Mechanism	Reference
Herpesvirus:				
MHV68	$LT\alpha^{-/-}$	Minimal	Nd[c]	(108)
HSV-1	$LT\alpha^{-/-}$	Increased	Decreased effector CD8$^+$ T cells	(109)
MCMV	$LT\alpha^{-/-}$	Increased	Nd	(107)
MCMV	$LT\beta$R-Fc Tg	Increased	Poor innate defenses	(107)
LCMV	$LT\beta^{-/-}$; $LT\alpha^{-/-}$	Increased	Defective architecture	(110, 176)
LCMV	$LT\beta$R-Fc	Decreased	Decreased CD8$^+$/IFNγ	(177)
Theiler's virus	$LT\alpha^{-/-}$; $LT\beta$R-Fc	Increased	Defective architecture	(178)
Influenza	$LT\alpha^{-/-}$	Minimal	Nd	(111)
M. tuberculosis	$LT\beta$R$^{-/-}$	Increased	NO$_2$ synthase decreased	(80)
M. tuberculosis	$LT\alpha^{-/-}$	Increased	No T cells in granuloma	(79)
M. bovis	$LT\beta$R-Fc	Increased	Poor granuloma formation	(78)
Listeria m.	$LT\beta$R$^{-/-}$	Increased	Nd	(80)
Leishmania m.	$LT\beta^{-/-}$	Increased	Defective architecture	(179)
Toxoplasma g	$LT\alpha^{-/-}$	Increased	NO$_2$ synthase decreased	(180)
Plasmodium b.	$LT\alpha^{-/-}$	Decreased	Decreased $LT\alpha$-dependent inflammation	(181)

[a]Virus: mouse γ-herpesvirus-68 (MHV68); herpes simplex virus (HSV1, α-herpesvirus); mouse cytomegalovirus (MCMV); lymphocytic choriomeningitis virus, (LCMV). Bacteria: *Mycobacterium*; *Listeria* monocytogenes. Parasite: *Leishmania* major; *Toxoplasma gondii*; *Plasmodium berghei*.

[b]Studies conducted in gene-deficient mice ($^{-/-}$); LTβR-Fc Tg, mice expressing LTβR-Fc as a transgene; LTβR-Fc, mice injected protein.

[c]Nd, no data.

nodes and splenic architecture seem largely unimportant for others (influenza) (111).

TNF- or TNFR1-deficient mice show a pronounced susceptibility to bacterial pathogens (112) but surprisingly minimal deficiency to several viruses (113). The TNF system in resistance to LCMV is complex. TNFR1 participates in the clearance of virus, but it is also necessary for down-modulation of effector T cells and inflammation in the lung and liver following recovery (114). The ability of TNF-TNFR1 and Fas-Fas ligand systems in controlling the persistence of effector T cells (antiinflammatory) in tissues following herpesvirus infections may be particularly relevant to anti-TNF therapies in autoimmune diseases with a potential underlying infectious etiology. Although the influence of the LIGHT system on host defenses has not been systematically studied, it is reasonable to predict that unique roles may be revealed by a specific pathogen. LT-deficient mice are not globally impaired in their immune responses to all pathogens; rather, specific pathogens during their coevolution with a vertebrate host have developed specific niches that may be dependent on the LT/TNF/LIGHT signaling network. In clinical situations where TNF/LT inhibitors are administered, specific pathogens might be expected to predominate as side effects to such therapy.

NETWORK CENSORING

Blockade of the TNF/LT/LIGHT network can modulate autoimmune diseases in mice and humans. In mice, collagen-induced arthritis (CIA), inflammatory bowel disease (IBD), and experimental autoimmune encephalomyelitis (EAE) represent three antigen-specific T cell–mediated inflammatory conditions often used as models for human diseases. The immunoregulatory roles of the $LT\alpha\beta$/LIGHT network have been investigated in several experimental animal models, with somewhat differing outcomes (recently reviewed in 115).

Collagen-Induced Arthritis

CIA, a disease with similarities to human RA, is initiated following immunization with chick type II collagen, which results in the forced recognition of self antigen. Arthritis did not develop in mice treated with $LT\beta$R-Fc several weeks prior to immunization with collagen (116). Milder disease developed if animals were treated with $LT\beta$R-Fc at the time of immunization, and some disease-modifying results were seen in established disease (116). The mechanism for reduced pathogenesis of disease following $LT\beta$R treatment may lie in alteration of the lymphoid microenvironment within the draining lymph node because, in both the lymph nodes and spleen, FDC networks were eliminated, resulting in decreased autoantibodies to collagen-II. However, $LT\alpha\beta$ and LIGHT could also be affecting other parameters of pathogenesis, including innate components of early recognition, T cell differentiation, and chemokine production required for the generation of an immune response.

Inflammatory Bowel Disease

The $LT\alpha\beta$/LIGHT-$LT\beta$R network is emerging as a critical signaling pathway in the gut and highly relevant to intestinal inflammatory disease in humans, including Crohn's disease (reviewed in 117). The biologic functions of $LT\beta$R are critical to mucosal immune responses and emerged as a key element in IgE (118) and IgA production (73, 119). Treatment of mice with $LT\beta$R-Fc or TNFR-Fc decoys blocked T cell–driven intestinal inflammation in mouse models of IBD, such as

CD45RBhi CD4$^+$ T cell–reconstituted SCID and the bone marrow–transplanted tg26 models (120), Th2-induced inflammatory response to hapten (121) and DSS-induced colitis models (122). Constitutive expression of LIGHT as transgene in mouse T cells induced chronic inflammation that specifically targets the intestine and presents with patterns of tissue destruction similar to those of human Crohn's disease (123, 124). In addition, although absent in the wild-type mice, transgenic expression of DcR3, a soluble regulator of LIGHT, TL1A, and Fas ligand, protected against diabetes (125). In humans, LIGHT is a candidate for the Crohn's disease susceptibility locus found on chromosome 19p13.3 (126); it was recently reported to be differentially regulated in the intestinal compartment and capable of inducing proinflammatory cytokine production by gut T cells (127). Thus, both human data and animal models suggest that TNFR/LTβR signaling systems may be important regulators of mucosal inflammation and immune function.

Experimental Autoimmune Encephalomyelitis

EAE is a T cell–mediated demyelinating disease that is induced in animals by immunization with myelin-basic protein in adjuvant. A role for the LT/LIGHT system in EAE has been controversial (128). Pertussis toxin, often used to induce blood-brain barrier permeability in some animal models of EAE, also blocks G protein–coupled chemokine receptor signaling, thus potentially disrupting the LT-chemokine circuit and nullifying the effect of the LTβR-Fc decoy. To circumvent such potential masking, Gommerman et al. employed models of EAE independent of the pertussis toxin, which revealed significant efficacy of LTβR-Fc in preventing paralysis (129). At the cellular level, treatment of mice with LTβR-Fc resulted in impaired secondary T cell responses to EAE autoepitopes, but there was no inhibition of T cell priming or clonal expansion, suggesting a role for LT$\alpha\beta$ in peripheral T cell differentiation (129). However, the regulatory effects of LT$\alpha\beta$/LIGHT on T cell function may also include additional indirect mechanisms, given the distribution of receptors and the complexity of dependent functions such as chemokine-directed migration and maintenance of lymphoid architecture.

IN THE CLINIC

The TNF/LTα system is now well established as an effective target to control inflammatory processes in certain human autoimmune diseases, such as rheumatoid arthritis (RA), but not others, such as MS (reviewed in 130–132). Although generally safe, TNF therapy is not without side effects, which include a small but increased risk of infectious diseases. The issue of increased incidence of non-Hodgkin's lymphoma is debated but occurs near the levels expected in patients with RA, who have a higher incidence than the general population (133). Moreover, differences in the efficacy of several TNF inhibitors (e.g., IBD) suggest multiple mechanisms of action. To a certain degree, the clinical results reaffirm prevailing paradigms in which the TNF/LT network functions in inflammation; however, some clinical experiences with these inhibitors were unexpected and may challenge current paradigms envisioned for some autoimmune diseases. Our current paradigms see RA, IBD, and MS as multifactorial, immunological diseases with significant T cell–driven inflammation. All three human conditions have unknown etiologies, with underlying genetic factors that contribute in poorly defined ways to pathogenesis. However, the use of molecularly defined drugs with well-understood mechanisms of action provides a reasonable real world experimental database of information with which to examine the role of TNF and $LT\alpha$ in the pathology of these human autoimmune diseases.

Two major types of drugs—anti-TNF neutralizing antibody (134), generically known as infliximab, and a chimera decoy receptor comprised of the TNFR2 ectodomain and the Fc of human IgG1, etanercept (135)—show dramatic efficacy and are approved for use in treating patients with RA (Table 3). These drugs competitively inhibit receptor binding by the respective antigen or ligand constituting distinct yet overlapping mechanisms of action. Infliximab recognizes an antigenic epitope on human TNF in either membrane or soluble form, but does not cross-react with $LT\alpha$. Likewise, etanercept binds both membrane and soluble TNF, but also engages with high affinity to $LT\alpha$ in its secreted homotrimeric form, a feature distinguishing it from infliximab. Neither drug binds to the membrane $LT\alpha1\beta2$ or LIGHT, although the $LT\alpha2\beta1$ complex, which is a minor form expressed by T cells, can bind to either TNFR1 or TNFR2, and thus can interact with etanercept (7, 136, 137).

At least theoretically, the differences in ligand specificity between infliximab and etanercept could distinguish roles for $LT\alpha$ and TNF in human disease pathogenesis. However, evaluating the clinical results is not so straightforward because these reagents may have additional mechanisms of action in vivo. Infliximab has been shown to activate complement and engage cellular Fc receptor–bearing cells when bound to TNF-expressing cells (138–140). Thus, in vivo the monoclonal

TABLE 3   Features of TNF inhibitors used in the clinic

Name	Trade name	Molecular form	Target	Mechanism
Infliximab	Remicade™	IgG1 mouse-human chimera	Human TNF	Competitive antagonist; cell elimination
Adalimumab	Humira™	Human IgG1	Human TNF	Competitive antagonist; cell elimination
Etanercept	Enbrel™	TNFR2 (p75)-Fc IgG1 chimera	TNF/$LT\alpha$	Competitive antagonist
Lenercept		TNFR1(p55)-Fc IgG1 chimera	TNF/$LT\alpha$	Competitive antagonist

antibody to TNF can also eliminate cells expressing membrane TNF, including activated T cells or macrophages; etanercept does not appear to have these secondary interactions. Additional considerations include intrinsic binding affinities and avidity of the drugs for their ligands, competing endogenously produced soluble receptors; and antibodies directed to the drugs themselves, as well as pharmacologic parameters associated with biologicals (half-life, bioavailablity, etc.) and concurrent immunomodulating therapy. Significant clinical experience using these TNF/LTα inhibitors has accumulated over the past few years and has generated an informative literature and database. The clinical data originate from a variety of sources, ranging from controlled clinical trials with statistical significance to those with less statistically robust sources, including open-label extension studies, case reports, and spontaneous adverse event reporting (141).

Most strikingly, the results of controlled clinical trials indicate that antibodies to TNF and the decoy receptor beneficially impact human RA through control of inflammation, tissue destruction, and improvement of function (142, 143). These results are certainly consistent with various animal models demonstrating TNF as a major cytokine in regulating inflammation and that blockade of TNF prevents joint destruction in experimental animals (144). However, in about one third of patients with RA neither of these drugs has efficacy (for review see 130). The basis underlying this nonresponsiveness in some populations is unclear, but the implication that other TNF family members may be involved has not been overlooked. Preclinical investigations of LT$\alpha\beta$ and LIGHT are in fact in progress. Given the foregoing assumptions surrounding the clinical evidence, the overall results implicate TNF as a significant factor in RA, and perhaps a less important role for LTα. However, a recent case report of a patient refractory to treatment with infliximab but responsive to LTα and TNF-blocking etanercept challenges that conclusion (145). Furthermore, LTα expression was present in biopsied joint tissue, suggesting that LTα may have a role in some cases of RA.

Perhaps more telling is the evidence arising from diseases and side effects where these TNF inhibitors differ from each other, as in iIBD (Table 4). Anti-TNF antibody is approved for use in treating Crohn's disease and is beneficial for a subset of

TABLE 4   Response of human autoimmune diseases to cytokine biologicals

Disease	Treatment[a]		
	Anti-TNF (infliximab)	**TNFR2-Fc (etanercept)**	**IFNβ (IFNβ-1b)**
Rheumatoid arthritis	+	+	−
Crohn's disease	+	−	−
Multiple sclerosis	CI	CI	+

[a] +, approved for use; −, no efficacy reported; CI, contraindicated.

Crohn's patients, but leaves another substantial nonresponsive subset, reminiscent of the response profile in RA (146). In contrast, the decoy receptor has not shown significant efficacy in IBD (147), although one early report indicated etanercept mediated a decrease in C-reactive protein, a biological marker for inflammation in some patients with Crohn's disease (148). Is the difference between these drugs in Crohn's disease due to differences in TNF and LTα biological activities in the mucosa, or are the mechanisms of drug action distinct? Secondary mechanisms other than TNF-blocking activity are reported for infliximab including activating complement, FcR, and apoptosis (139, 140), which could eliminate specific subsets of effector cells expressing TNF and would undoubtedly have a profound antiinflammatory action. However, similar anti-TNF antibody constructs, which do not induce apoptosis, can still effectively abrogate disease (147).

TNF is also required to suppress inflammation, likely by elimination of activated T cells (see 149, 150 for discussion). Hence, another plausible explanation is that neutralizing TNF disrupts the antiinflammatory action of TNF, which may outweigh its proinflammatory action in the intestine. Thus, etanercept may lose efficacy in this context, whereas infliximab specifically eliminates an "activated" lymphocyte subset and thereby augments the antiinflammatory action of TNF. An alternate hypothesis suggests that LTα may be involved in attenuating TNF function in the intestine. Here, tissue culture models indicate that LTα acts as a partial agonist when compared with TNF (151) and also has the potential to engage another receptor (HVEM), although the molecular mechanism for LTα partial agonist effect is not yet defined. Of interest is the discordance with mouse models of intestinal inflammatory disease, where both TNFR and LTβR decoys were able to suppress T cell–mediated inflammation (152). This discordance with the animal models suggests that the mechanism(s) of action of infliximab, other than TNF blockade, may underlie this difference with etanercept. However, the clinical results do not rule out other contributing factors, such as bioavailability and additional pharmacologic parameters, which might account for the differences in efficacy between the antibody and decoy receptor.

Another clinical situation that distinguishes antibody from decoy receptor is reactivation of *M. tuberculosis*. Although both etanercept and infliximab therapies are associated with increased incidence of some infectious diseases, there is a stronger link between infliximab treatment and reactivation of latent tuberculosis (153). Animal models strongly indicate that the TNF-TNFR1 system plays a role in controlling granuloma formation crucial for preventing *Mycobacterium* reactivation (154). Antibody-dependent elimination of TNF-expressing effectors cells (macrophages and T cells) would incur loss of several other effector mechanisms that may participate in controlling granuloma formation (such as LTαβ system), and thus higher rates of mycobacterium reactivation might be expected. The finding that both drugs show increased incidence of infectious diseases including *Mycobacterium* and some other organisms associated with chronic/persistent infections is consistent with the roles of TNF and LTα in host defenses. Fortunately, prescreening patients for latent tuberculosis and antibiotic treatment can alleviate this side effect of TNF therapy.

Anti-TNF therapy does not improve survival in patients with acute bacterial sepsis (155), although animal models showed that endotoxin shock was controlled by TNF inhibitors (156), a distinction attributed to infection with a replicating pathogen versus treatment with sterile toxin. Both infliximab and etanercept are contraindicated for patients with MS, based in part on the unexpected symptoms of demyelinating disease (paresthesia, optic neuritis, and confusion) developing in people with quiescent MS and new-onset cases of demyelinating disease, which reversed upon drug removal (157) (Table 4). Another TNF decoy receptor, lenercept (composed of TNFR1-Fc decoy) exacerbated symptoms in patients with MS. In a controlled phase II study, patients with relapsing-remitting MS who were treated with lenercept showed a significant exacerbation of brain lesions when compared with placebo (158). These clinical results stand in contrast to that predicted from experimental animal models examining the acute phase of EAE, which showed that TNF inhibitors could effectively block antigen-induced inflammation, although the antiinflammatory properties of TNF may be compromised simultaneously (159). That three inhibitors of TNF/LTα are linked to exacerbation of demyelinating disease in humans suggests that their common mechanism of action, blockade of TNF, is influencing pathogenesis.

What plausible mechanisms might account for this discordance in human and experimental animal models? An important finding is the efficacy of the IFN system in the treatment of MS (160). Human IFN-β-1b, (Betaferon^{TM}; Betaseron^{TM}) is effective in treating patients with relapsing-remitting forms of MS (161). The mechanism of action of IFNβ in MS is not understood, although its antiviral actions remain a highly plausible explanation. From tissue culture and experimental animal models, IFNβ is recognized as the sentinel mediator of innate defenses, primarily to viral pathogens, that induces a generalized nonpermissive state for viral replication (106, 162). IFNβ is also essential for amplification of the IFNα cascade, as well as hundreds of other genes with potent antipathogen and immunomodulatory activities (163).

The evidence that TNF/LT network forms a crucial link to the IFN responses system that effects host defense (107) provides an intriguing hypothesis in view of the findings that TNF/LT inhibitors can exacerbate MS. This hypothesis necessarily raises the issue of whether an infectious agent plays a significant role in MS, a hypothesis long considered but unproven because of the lack of definitive results. Accumulating evidence has identified human herpesvirus 6 (HHV6, a β-herpesvirus) as a possible causative agent, although causality remains a controversial issue because of the ubiquitous prevalence of HHV6 (prevalence in the population may as high as >90%) (see reviews 164–167). Evidence for HHV6 in MS includes increased frequency of detection of viral genomes in MS plaques and blood (168–171) and decrease in new lesions in MS patients treated with antiherpesvirus drug (172). Moreover, T cells crossreactive to myelin basic protein peptides and HHV6 antigens have been identified (173), and differential antibody responses to HHV6 are detected in MS patients (174). HHV6 is sensitive to IFNβ in tissue culture models (175), suggesting that the regulation of IFNβ by LTα/TNF observed with human CMV may be operative with HHV6.

These clinical results are consistent with the notion that TNF/LT and IFN systems are important cytokines modulating the pathogenesis of MS. Plainly, MS could be exacerbated if TNF/LTα inhibitors disrupt the production of IFNβ in response to HHV6, allowing the virus to transiently escape immune control. However, other significant disposing factors must contribute to the control of HHV6 because the prevalence of HHV6 is high, although demyelinating syndrome is rare in patients treated with infliximab or etanercept. Disruption of the TNF/LT pathway may expose such host predisposition, leading to enhanced viral reactivation and antigen expression in the brain, and thus increasing the probability of tissue damage and consequent loss of tolerance. Concurrent IFN treatment would inhibit viral functions and potentially restore a balanced host-pathogen interaction.

Perspective

The clinical trials and experiences directed at altering the TNF/LTα network provide real world data upon which the accuracy of our paradigms of immune function can be tested. The dramatic clinical results with TNF inhibitors are inspiring and continue to drive development of additional disease-modifying drugs by manipulating cytokine pathways, although the results are equally sobering given that a significant fraction of patients are not responsive to TNF inhibitors. Likewise, situations in which TNF/LTα inhibitors are inadequate offer challenges for the immunopathological paradigms currently employed and can rationally offer new directions toward clinical relevance.

APPENDIX

Abbreviations used: CMV, human cytomegalovirus; DC, dendritic cells; DD, death domain; FDC, follicular dendritic cell; HHV6, human herpesvirus 6; HSV, herpes simplex virus; IκB, Inhibitors of κB; IKK, IκB kinase complex; IL, interleukin; LCMV, lymphocytic choriomeningitis virus; LIGHT, LT-related inducible ligand that competes for glycoprotein D binding to herpesvirus entry mediator on T cells; LMP1, latent membrane protein 1; LT, lymphotoxins; MMM, metallophilic macrophages; MS, multiple sclerosis; MZM, marginal zone macrophages; PP, Peyer's patches; TNF, tumor necrosis factor; TRADD, TNFR associated DD; TRAFs, TNFR receptor-associated factors.

ACKNOWLEDGMENTS

The dedicated efforts of colleagues and lab members including Paula Norris, Karen Potter, Kirsten Schneider, Ian Humphreys, Offer Cohavy, Chris Benedict, and Theresa Banks are greatly appreciated. This work is supported by grants from the National Institutes of Health.

The *Annual Review of Immunology* is online at
http://immunol.annualreviews.org

LITERATURE CITED

1. Locksley RM, Killeen N, Lenardo MJ. 2001 The TNF and TNF receptor superfamilies: integrating mammalian biology. *Cell* 104:487–501

2. Bodmer JL, Schneider P, Tschopp J. 2002. The molecular architecture of the TNF superfamily. *Trends Biochem. Sci.* 27:19–26

3. Ware CF. 2003. The TNF superfamily. *Cytokine Growth Factor Rev.* 14:181–84

4. Granger SW, Ware CF. 2001. Commentary: turning on LIGHT. *J. Clin. Invest.* 108:1741–42

5. Collette Y, Gilles A, Pontarotti P, Olive D. 2003. A co-evolution perspective of the TNFSF and TNFRSF families in the immune system. *Trends Immunol.* 24:387–94

6. Montgomery RI, Warner MS, Lum B, Spear PG. 1996. Herpes simplex virus 1 entry into cells mediated by a novel member of the TNF/NGF receptor family. *Cell* 87:427–36

7. Mauri DN, Ebner R, Montgomery RI, Kochel KD, Cheung TC, et al. 1998. LIGHT, a new member of the TNF superfamily and lymphotoxin α are ligands for herpesvirus entry mediator. *Immunity* 8:21–30

8. Harrop JA, McDonnell PC, Brigham-Burke M, Lyn SD, Minton J, et al. 1998. Herpesvirus entry mediator ligand (HVEM-L), a novel ligand for HVEM/TR2, stimulates proliferation of T cells and inhibits HT29 cell growth. *J. Biol. Chem.* 273:27548–56

9. Zhai Y, Guo R, Hsu T-L, Yu G-L, Ni J, et al. 1998. LIGHT, a novel ligand for lymphotoxin β receptor and TR2/HVEM induces apoptosis and suppressess in vivo tumor formation via gene transfer. *J. Clin. Invest.* 102:1142–51

10. Yu KY, Kwon B, Ni J, Zhai Y, Ebner R, Kwon BS. 1999. A newly identified member of tumor necrosis factor receptor superfamily (TR6) suppresses LIGHT-mediated apoptosis. *J. Biol. Chem.* 274: 13733–36

11. Pfeffer K. 2003. Biological functions of tumor necrosis factor cytokines and their receptors. *Cytokine Growth Factor Rev.* 14:185–91

12. Tumanov AV, Kuprash DV, Nedospasov SA. 2003. The role of lymphotoxin in development and maintenance of secondary lymphoid tissues. *Cytokine Growth Factor Rev.* 14:275–88

13. Kuprash DV, Alimzhanov MB, Tumanov AV, Grivennikov SI, Shakhov AN, et al. 2002. Redundancy in tumor necrosis factor (TNF) and lymphotoxin (LT) signaling in vivo: mice with inactivation of the entire TNF/LT locus versus single-knockout mice. *Mol. Cell. Biol.* 22:8626–34

14. Tumanov A, Kuprash D, Lagarkova M, Grivennikov S, Abe K, et al. 2002. Distinct role of surface lymphotoxin expressed by B cells in the organization of secondary lymphoid tissues. *Immunity* 17:239–50

15. Tumanov AV, Grivennikov SI, Shakhov AN, Rybtsov SA, Koroleva EP, et al. 2003. Dissecting the role of lymphotoxin in lymphoid organs by conditional targeting. *Immunol. Rev.* 195:106–16

16. Drayton DL, Ying X, Lee J, Lesslauer W, Ruddle NH. 2003. Ectopic LT$\alpha\beta$ directs lymphoid organ neogenesis with concomitant expression of peripheral node addressin and a HEV-restricted sulfotransferase. *J. Exp. Med.* 197:1153–63

17. Schneider P, Tschopp J. 2000. Apoptosis induced by death receptors. *Pharm. Acta Helv.* 74:281–86

18. Micheau O, Tschopp J. 2003. Induction

of TNF receptor I-mediated apoptosis via two sequential signaling complexes. *Cell* 114:181–90

19. Zapata JM, Pawlowski K, Haas E, Ware CF, Godzik A, Reed JC. 2001. A diverse family of proteins containing tumor necrosis factor receptor-associated factor domains. *J. Biol. Chem.* 276:24242–52

20. Deng L, Wang C, Spencer E, Yang L, Braun A, et al. 2000. Activation of the IκB kinase complex by TRAF6 requires a dimeric ubiquitin-conjugating enzyme complex and a unique polyubiquitin chain. *Cell* 103:351–61

21. Force WR, Cheung TC, Ware CF. 1997. Dominant negative mutants of TRAF3 reveal an important role for the coiled coil domains in cell death signaling by the lymphotoxin-β receptor (LTβR). *J. Biol. Chem.* 272:30835–40

22. Li C, Norris PS, Ni CZ, Havert ML, Chiong EM, et al. 2003. Structurally distinct recognition motifs in lymphotoxin-β receptor and CD40 for tumor necrosis factor receptor-associated factor (TRAF)-mediated signaling. *J. Biol. Chem.* 278:50523–29

23. So T, Salek-Ardakani S, Nakano H, Ware CF, Croft M. 2004. TNF receptor-associated factor 5 limits the induction of Th2 immune responses. *J. Immunol.* 172:4292–97

24. Janeway CA Jr, Medzhitov R. 2002. Innate immune recognition. *Annu. Rev. Immunol.* 20:197–216

25. Takeda K, Kaisho T, Akira S. 2003. Toll-like receptors. *Annu. Rev. Immunol.* 21:335–76

26. Walsh MC, Choi Y. 2003. Biology of the TRANCE axis. *Cytokine Growth Factor Rev.* 14:251–63

27. Caamano J, Hunter CA. 2002. NF-κB family of transcription factors: central regulators of innate and adaptive immune functions. *Clin. Microbiol. Rev.* 15:414–29

28. Karin M, Lin A. 2002. NF-κB at the cross-roads of life and death. *Nat. Immunol.* 3:221–27

29. Li Q, Verma IM. 2002. NF-κB regulation in the immune system. *Nat. Rev. Immunol.* 2:725–34

30. Pahl HL. 1999. Activators and target genes of Rel/NF-κB transcription factors. *Oncogene* 18:6853–66

31. Coope HJ, Atkinson PG, Huhse B, Belich M, Janzen J, et al. 2002. CD40 regulates the processing of NF-κB2 p100 to p52. *EMBO J.* 21:5375–85

32. Kayagaki N, Yan M, Seshasayee D, Wang H, Lee W, et al. 2002. BAFF/BLyS receptor 3 binds the B cell survival factor BAFF ligand through a discrete surface loop and promotes processing of NF-κB2. *Immunity* 17:515–24

33. Dejardin E, Droin NM, Delhase M, Haas E, Cao Y, et al. 2002. The lymphotoxin-β receptor induces different patterns of gene expression via two NF-κB pathways. *Immunity* 17:525–35

34. Muller JR, Siebenlist U. 2003. Lymphotoxin β receptor induces sequential activation of distinct NF-κB factors via separate signaling pathways. *J. Biol. Chem.* 278:12006–12

35. Derudder E, Dejardin E, Pritchard LL, Green DR, Korner M, Baud V. 2003. RelB/p50 dimers are differentially regulated by tumor necrosis factor-α and lymphotoxin-β receptor activation: critical roles for p100. *J. Biol. Chem.* 278:23278–84

36. Senftleben U, Cao Y, Xiao G, Greten FR, Krahn G, et al. 2001. Activation by IKKα of a second, evolutionary conserved, NF-κB signaling pathway. *Science* 293:1495–99

37. Yin L, Wu L, Wesche H, Arthur CD, White JM, et al. 2001 Defective lymphotoxin-β receptor-induced NF-κB transcriptional activity in NIK-deficient mice. *Science* 291:2162–65

38. Miyawaki S, Nakamura Y, Suzuka H, Koba M, Yasumizu R, et al. 1994. A new mutation, aly, that induces a generalized

lack of lymph nodes accompanied by immunodeficiency in mice. *Eur. J. Immunol.* 24:429–34

39. Hochman PS, Majeau GR, Mackay F, Browning JL. 1995–1996. Proinflammatory responses are efficiently induced by homotrimeric but not heterotrimeric lymphotoxin ligands. *J. Inflam.* 46:220–34

40. Alcamo E, Hacohen N, Schulte LC, Rennert PD, Hynes RO, Baltimore D. 2002. Requirement for the NF-κB family member RelA in the development of secondary lymphoid organs. *J. Exp. Med.* 195:233–44

41. Bouwmeester T, Bauch A, Ruffner H, Angrand PO, Bergamini G, et al. 2004. A physical and functional map of the human TNF-α/NF-κB signal transduction pathway. *Nat. Cell. Biol.* 6:97–105

42. Ansel KM, Ngo VN, Hyman PL, Luther SA, Forster R, et al. 2000. A chemokine-driven positive feedback loop organizes lymphoid follicles. *Nature* 406:309–14

43. Lo JC, Chin RK, Lee Y, Kang HS, Wang Y, et al. 2003. Differential regulation of CCL21 in lymphoid/nonlymphoid tissues for effectively attracting T cells to peripheral tissues. *J. Clin. Invest.* 112:1495–505

44. Ware CF, Crowe PD, Grayson MH, Androlewicz MJ, Browning JL. 1992. Expression of surface lymphotoxin and tumor necrosis factor on activated T, B, and natural killer cells. *J. Immunol.* 149:3881–88

45. Gramaglia I, Mauri DN, Miner KT, Ware CF, Croft M. 1999. Lymphotoxin αβ is expressed on recently activated naive and Th1-like CD4 cells but is downregulated by IL-4 during TH2 differentiation. *J. Immunol.* 162:1333–38

46. Agyekum S, Church A, Sohail M, Krausz T, Van Noorden S, et al. 2003. Expression of lymphotoxin-β (LT-β) in chronic inflammatory conditions. *J. Pathol.* 199:115–21

47. Luther SA, Bidgol A, Hargreaves DC, Schmidt A, Xu Y, et al. 2002. Differing activities of homeostatic chemokines CCL19, CCL21, and CXCL12 in lymphocyte and dendritic cell recruitment and lymphoid neogenesis. *J. Immunol.* 169:424–33

48. Worm MM, Tsytsykova A, Geha RS. 1998. CD40 ligation and IL-4 use different mechanisms of transcriptional activation of the human lymphotoxin α promoter in B cells. *Eur. J. Immunol.* 28:901–6

49. Murphy M, Walter BN, Pike-Nobile L, Fanger NA, Guyre PM, et al. 1998. Expression of the lymphotoxin β receptor on follicular stromal cells in human lymphoid tissues. *Cell Death Differ.* 5:497–505

50. Browning JL, French LE. 2002. Visualization of lymphotoxin-β and lymphotoxin-β receptor expression in mouse embryos. *J. Immunol.* 168:5079–87

51. Stopfer P, Mannel DN, Hehlgans T. 2004. Lymphotoxin-β receptor activation by activated T cells induces cytokine release from mouse bone marrow-derived mast cells. *J. Immunol.* 172:7459–65

52. Morel Y, Schiano de Colella JM, Harrop J, Deen KC, Holmes SD, et al. 2000 Reciprocal expression of the TNF family receptor herpes virus entry mediator and its ligand LIGHT on activated T cells: LIGHT down-regulates its own receptor. *J. Immunol.* 165:4397–404

53. Kwon BS, Tan KB, Ni J, Oh KO, Lee ZH, et al. 1997. A newly identified member of the tumor necrosis factor receptor superfamily with a wide tissue distribution and involvement in lymphocyte activation. *J. Biol. Chem.* 272:14272–76

54. Dempsey PW, Doyle SE, He JQ, Cheng G. 2003. The signaling adaptors and pathways activated by TNF superfamily. *Cytokine Growth Factor Rev.* 14:193–209

55. Falvo JV, Uglialoro AM, Brinkman BM, Merika M, Parekh BS, et al. 2000. Stimulus-specific assembly of enhancer complexes on the tumor necrosis factor α gene promoter. *Mol. Cell. Biol.* 20:2239–47

56. Tsytsykova AV, Goldfeld AE. 2002. Inducer-specific enhanceosome formation controls tumor necrosis factor α gene expression in T lymphocytes. *Mol. Cell. Biol.* 22:2620–31

57. Voon DC, Subrata LS, Karimi M, Ulgiati D, Abraham LJ. 2004. TNF and phorbol esters induce lymphotoxin-β expression through distinct pathways involving Ets and NF-κB family members. *J. Immunol.* 172:4332–41

58. Castellano R, Van Lint C, Peri V, Veithen E, Morel Y, et al. 2002. Mechanisms regulating expression of the tumor necrosis factor-related light gene: role of calcium-signaling pathway in the transcriptional control. *J. Biol. Chem.* 277:42841–51

59. Nishikawa S, Honda K, Vieira P, Yoshida H. 2003. Organogenesis of peripheral lymphoid organs. *Immunol. Rev.* 195:72–80

60. Fu Y-X, Chaplin D. 1999. Development and maturation of secondary lymphoid tissues. *Annu. Rev. Immunol.* 17:399–433

61. Yoshida H, Naito A, Inoue J, Satoh M, Santee-Cooper SM, et al. 2002. Different cytokines induce surface lymphotoxin-$\alpha\beta$ on IL-7 receptor-α cells that differentially engender lymph nodes and Peyer's patches. *Immunity* 17:823–33

62. Eberl G, Marmon S, Sunshine MJ, Rennert PD, Choi Y, Littman DR. 2004. An essential function for the nuclear receptor RORγ(t) in the generation of fetal lymphoid tissue inducer cells. *Nat. Immunol.* 5:64–73

63. Fukuda K, Yoshida H, Sato T, Furumoto TA, Mizutani-Koseki Y, et al. 2003. Mesenchymal expression of Foxl1, a winged helix transcriptional factor, regulates generation and maintenance of gut-associated lymphoid organs. *Dev. Biol.* 255:278–89

64. Weih F, Caamano J. 2003. Regulation of secondary lymphoid organ development by the nuclear factor-κB signal transduction pathway. *Immunol. Rev.* 195:91–105

65. Kim D, Mebius RE, MacMicking JD, Jung S, Cupedo T, et al. 2000. Regulation of peripheral lymph node genesis by the tumor necrosis factor family member TRANCE. *J. Exp. Med.* 192:1467–78

66. Neumann B, Luz A, Pfeffer K, Holzmann B. 1996. Defective Peyer's patch organogenesis in mice lacking the 55-kD receptor for tumor necrosis factor. *J. Exp. Med.* 184:259–64

67. Harmsen A, Kusser K, Hartson L, Tighe M, Sunshine MJ, et al. 2002. Cutting edge: Organogenesis of nasal-associated lymphoid tissue (NALT) occurs independently of lymphotoxin-α (LT α) and retinoic acid receptor-related orphan receptor-γ, but the organization of NALT is LTα dependent. *J. Immunol.* 168:986–90

68. Kather A, Chantakru S, He H, Minhas K, Foster R, et al. 2003. Neither lymphotoxin α nor lymphotoxin β receptor expression is required for biogenesis of lymphoid aggregates or differentiation of natural killer cells in the pregnant mouse uterus. *Immunology* 108:338–45

69. Cyster JG. 2003. Lymphoid organ development and cell migration. *Immunol. Rev.* 195:5–14

70. Ngo VN, Cornall RJ, Cyster JG. 2001. Splenic T zone development is B cell dependent. *J. Exp. Med.* 194:1649–60

71. Schutyser E, Struyf S, Van Damme J. 2003. The CC chemokine CCL20 and its receptor CCR6. *Cytokine Growth Factor Rev.* 14:409–26

72. Kunkel EJ, Campbell DJ, Butcher EC. 2003. Chemokines in lymphocyte trafficking and intestinal immunity. *Microcirculation* 10:313–23

73. Rumbo M, Sierro F, Debard N, Kraehenbuhl JP, Finke D. 2004. Lymphotoxin β receptor signaling induces the chemokine CCL20 in intestinal epithelium. *Gastroenterology* 127:213–23

74. Luther SA, Lopez T, Bai W, Hanahan D, Cyster JG. 2000. BLC expression in pancreatic islets causes B cell recruitment and lymphotoxin-dependent lymphoid neogenesis. *Immunity* 12:471–81

75. Yu P, Wang Y, Chin RK, Martinez-Pomares L, Gordon S, et al. 2002. B cells control the migration of a subset of dendritic cells into B cell follicles via CXC chemokine ligand 13 in a lymphotoxin-dependent fashion. *J. Immunol.* 168:5117–23

76. Wang J, Foster A, Chin R, Yu P, Sun Y, et al. 2002. The complementation of lymphotoxin deficiency with LIGHT, a newly discovered TNF family member, for the restoration of secondary lymphoid structure and function. *Eur J. Immunol.* 32:1969–79

77. Chen CY, Cohen SA, Zaleski MB, Albini B. 1992. Genetic control of streptococcus-induced hepatic granulomatous lesions in mice. *Immunogenetics* 36:28–32

78. Lucas R, Tacchini-Cottier F, Guler R, Vesin D, Jemelin S, et al. 1999. A role for lymphotoxin β receptor in host defense against *Mycobacterium bovis* BCG infection. *Eur. J. Immunol.* 29:4002–10

79. Roach DR, Briscoe H, Saunders B, France MP, Riminton S, Britton WJ. 2001. Secreted lymphotoxin-α is essential for the control of an intracellular bacterial infection. *J. Exp. Med.* 193:239–46

80. Ehlers S, Holscher C, Scheu S, Tertilt C, Hehlgans T, et al. 2003. The lymphotoxin β receptor is critically involved in controlling infections with the intracellular pathogens *Mycobacterium tuberculosis* and *Listeria monocytogenes*. *J. Immunol.* 170:5210–18

81. Wu Q, Wang Y, Wang J, Hedgeman EO, Browning JL, Fu Y-X. 1999. The requirement of membrane lymphotoxin for the presence of dendritic cells in lymphoid tissue. *J. Exp. Med.* 190:629–38

82. Abe K, Yarovinsky FO, Murakami T, Shakhov AN, Tumanov AV, et al. 2003. Distinct contributions of TNF and LT cytokines to the development of dendritic cells in vitro and their recruitment in vivo. *Blood* 101:1477–83

83. Yokota Y, Mansouri A, Mori S, Sugawara S, Adachi S, et al. 1999. Development of peripheral lymphoid organs and natural killer cells depends on the helix-loop-helix inhibitor Id2. *Nature* 397:702–6

84. Iizuka K, Chaplin DD, Wang Y, Wu Q, Pegg LE, et al. 1999. Requirement for membrane lymphotoxin in natural killer cell development. *Proc. Natl. Acad. Sci. USA* 96:6336–40

85. Wu Q, Sun Y, Wang J, Lin X, Wang Y, et al. 2001. Signal via lymphotoxin-β R on bone marrow stromal cells is required for an early checkpoint of NK cell development. *J. Immunol.* 166:1684–89

86. Elewaut D, Shaikh RB, Hammond KJ, De Winter H, Leishman AJ, et al. 2003. NIK-dependent RelB activation defines a unique signaling pathway for the development of V α 14i NKT cells. *J. Exp. Med.* 197:1623–33

87. Fu Y-X, Molina H, Matsumoto M, Huang G, Min J, Chaplin DD. 1997. Lymphotoxin-α (LTα) supports development of splenic follicular structure that is required for IgG responses. *J. Exp. Med.* 185:2111–20

88. Endres R, Alimzhanov MB, Plitz T, Futterer A, Kosco-Vilbois MH, et al. 1999. Mature follicular dendritic cell networks depend on expression of lymphotoxin β receptor by radioresistant stromal cells and of lymphotoxin β and tumor necrosis factor by B cells. *J. Exp. Med.* 189:159–68

89. Mackay F, Browning JL. 1998. Turning off follicular dendritic cells. *Nature* 395:26–27

90. Boehm T, Scheu S, Pfeffer K, Bleul CC. 2003. Thymic medullary epithelial cell differentiation, thymocyte emigration, and the control of autoimmunity require lympho-epithelial cross talk via LTβR. *J. Exp. Med.* 198:757–69

91. Chin RK, Lo JC, Kim O, Blink SE, Christiansen PA, et al. 2003. Lymphotoxin pathway directs thymic Aire expression. *Nat. Immunol.* 4:1121–27

92. Tortorella D, Gewurz BE, Furman MH, Schust DJ, Ploegh HL. 2000. Viral

subversion of the immune system. *Annu. Rev. Immunol.* 18:861–926

93. Everett H, McFadden G. 2002. Poxviruses and apoptosis: a time to die. *Curr. Opin. Microbiol.* 5:395–402

94. Burgert HG, Ruzsics Z, Obermeier S, Hilgendorf A, Windheim M, Elsing A. 2002. Subversion of host defense mechanisms by adenoviruses. *Curr. Topics Microbiol. Immunol.* 269:273–318

95. Benedict CA, Banks TA, Ware CF. 2003. Death and survival: viral regulation of TNF signaling pathways. *Curr. Opin. Immunol.* 15:59–65

96. Upton C, Macen J, Schreiber M, McFadden G. 1991. Myxoma virus expresses a secreted protein with homology to the tumor necrosis factor receptor gene family that contributes to viral virulence. *Virology* 184:370–82

97. Seet BT, Johnston JB, Brunetti CR, Barrett JW, Everett H, et al. 2003. Poxviruses and immune evasion. *Annu. Rev. Immunol.* 21:377–423

98. Spear PG. 2004. Herpes simplex virus: receptors and ligands for cell entry. *Cell. Microbiol.* 6:401–10

99. Carfi A, Willis SH, Whitbeck JC, Krummenacher C, Cohen GH, et al. 2001. Herpes simplex virus glycoprotein D bound to the human receptor HveA. *Mol. Cell* 8:169–79

100. Xie P, Hostager BS, Bishop GA. 2004. Requirement for TRAF3 in signaling by LMP1 but not CD40 in B lymphocytes. *J. Exp. Med.* 199:661–71

101. Luftig M, Yasui T, Soni V, Kang MS, Jacobson N, et al. 2004. Epstein-Barr virus latent infection membrane protein 1 TRAF-binding site induces NIK/IKKα-dependent noncanonical NF-κB activation. *Proc. Natl. Acad. Sci. USA* 101:141–46

102. Matta H, Chaudhary PM. 2004. Activation of alternative NF-κB pathway by human herpes virus 8-encoded Fas-associated death domain-like IL-1β-converting enzyme inhibitory protein

(vFLIP). *Proc. Natl. Acad. Sci. USA* 101:9399–404

103. Benedict C, Butrovich K, Lurain N, Corbeil J, Rooney I, et al. 1999. Cutting Edge: a novel viral TNF receptor superfamily member in virulent strains of human cytomegalovirus. *J. Immunol.* 162:6967–70

104. Lurain NS, Kapell KS, Huang DD, Short JA, Paintsil J, et al. 1999. Human cytomegalovirus UL144 open reading frame: sequence hypervariability in low-passage clinical isolates. *J. Virol.* 73:10040–50

105. Yokoyama WM, Plougastel BF. 2003. Immune functions encoded by the natural killer gene complex. *Nat. Rev. Immunol.* 3:304–16

106. Sen GC. 2001. Viruses and interferons. *Annu. Rev. Microbiol.* 55:255–81

107. Benedict CA, Banks TA, Senderowicz L, Ko M, Britt WJ, et al. 2001 Lymphotoxins and cytomegalovirus cooperatively induce interferon-β, establishing host-virus détente. *Immunity* 15:617–26

108. Lee BJ, Santee S, Von Gesjen S, Ware CF, Sarawar SR. 2000. Lymphotoxin $\alpha^{-/-}$ mice can clear a productive infection with murine γ−herpesvirus-68 (MHV-68) but fail to develop splenomegaly or lymphocytosis. *J. Virol.* 74:2786–92

109. Kumaraguru U, Davis IA, Deshpande S, Tevethia SS, Rouse BT. 2001 Lymphotoxin $\alpha^{-/-}$ mice develop functionally impaired CD8[+] T cell responses and fail to contain virus infection of the central nervous system. *J. Immunol.* 166:1066–74

110. Suresh M, Lanier G, Large MK, Whitmire JK, Altman JD, et al. 2002. Role of lymphotoxin α in T-cell responses during an acute viral infection. *J. Virol.* 76:3943–51

111. Lund FE, Partida-Sanchez S, Lee BO, Kusser KL, Hartson L, et al. 2002. Lymphotoxin-α-deficient mice make delayed, but effective, T and B cell responses to influenza. *J. Immunol.* 169:5236–43

112. Pfeffer K, Matsuyama T, Kundig TM, Wakeham A, Kishihara K, et al. 1993.

Mice deficient for the 55 kd tumor necrosis factor receptor are resistant to endotoxic shock, yet succumb to *L. monocytogenes* infection. *Cell* 73:457–67

113. Fleck M, Kern ER, Zhou T, Podlech J, Wintersberger W, et al. 1998. Apoptosis mediated by Fas but not tumor necrosis factor receptor 1 prevents chronic disease in mice infected with murine cytomegalovirus. *J. Clin. Invest.* 102:1431–43

114. Suresh M, Gao X, Fischer C, Miller NE, Tewari K. 2004. Dissection of antiviral and immune regulatory functions of tumor necrosis factor receptors in a chronic lymphocytic choriomeningitis virus infection. *J. Virol.* 78:3906–18

115. Gommerman JL, Browning JL. 2003. Lymphotoxin/LIGHT, lymphoid microenvironments and autoimmune disease. *Nat. Rev. Immunol.* 3:642–55

116. Fava RA, Notidis E, Hunt J, Szanya V, Ratcliffe N, et al. 2003. A role for the lymphotoxin/LIGHT axis in the pathogenesis of murine collagen-induced arthritis. *J. Immunol.* 171:115–26

117. Spahn TW, Kucharzik T. 2004. Modulating the intestinal immune system: the role of lymphotoxin and GALT organs. *Gut* 53: 456–65

118. Kang HS, Blink SE, Chin RK, Lee Y, Kim O, et al. 2003. Lymphotoxin is required for maintaining physiological levels of serum IgE that minimizes Th1-mediated airway inflammation. *J. Exp. Med.* 198:1643–52

119. Kang HS, Chin RK, Wang Y, Yu P, Wang J, et al. 2002. Signaling via LTβR on the lamina propria stromal cells of the gut is required for IgA production. *Nat. Immunol.* 3:576–82

120. Mackay F, Browning JL, Lawton P, Shah SA, Comiskey M, et al. 1998. Both the lymphotoxin and tumor necrosis factor pathways are involved in experimental murine models of colitis. *Gastroenterology* 115:1464–75

121. Dohi T, Rennert PD, Fujihashi K, Kiyono H, Shirai Y, et al. 2001. Elimination of colonic patches with lymphotoxin β receptor-Ig prevents Th2 cell-type colitis. *J. Immunol.* 167:2781–90

122. Stopfer P, Obermeier F, Dunger N, Falk W, Farkas S, et al. 2004. Blocking lymphotoxin-β receptor activation diminishes inflammation via reduced mucosal addressin cell adhesion molecule-1 (MAdCAM-1) expression and leucocyte margination in chronic DSS-induced colitis. *Clin. Exp. Immunol.* 136:21–29

123. Shaikh R, Santee S, Granger SW, Butrovich K, Cheung T, et al. 2001. Constitutive expression of LIGHT on T cells leads to lymphocyte activation, inflammation and tissue destruction. *J. Immunol.* 167:6330–37

124. Wang J, Lo JC, Foster A, Yu P, Chen HM, et al. 2001. The regulation of T cell homeostasis and autoimmunity by T cell derived LIGHT. *J. Clin. Invest.* 108:1771–80

125. Sung HH, Juang JH, Lin YC, Kuo CH, Hung JT, et al. 2004. Transgenic expression of decoy receptor 3 protects islets from spontaneous and chemical-induced autoimmune destruction in nonobese diabetic mice. *J. Exp. Med.* 199:1143–51

126. Rioux JD, Silverberg MS, Daly MJ, Steinhart AH, McLeod RS, et al. 2000. Genomewide search in Canadian families with inflammatory bowel disease reveals two novel susceptibility loci. *Am. J. Hum. Genet.* 66:1863–70

127. Cohavy O, Zhou J, Granger SW, Ware CF, Targan SR. 2004. LIGHT expression by mucosal T cells may regulate IFN-γ expression in the intestine. *J. Immunol.* 173: 251–58

128. Steinman L. 1997. Some misconceptions about understanding autoimmunity through experiments with knockouts. *J. Exp. Med.* 185:2039–41

129. Gommerman JL, Giza K, Perper S, Sizing I, Ngam-Ek A, et al. 2003. A role for surface lymphotoxin in experimental autoimmune encephalomyelitis independent of LIGHT. *J. Clin. Invest.* 112:755–67

130. Olsen NJ, Stein CM. 2004. New drugs for rheumatoid arthritis. *N. Engl. J. Med.* 350: 2167–79

131. Feldmann M, Brennan FM, Paleolog E, Cope A, Taylor P, et al. 2004. Anti-TNFα therapy of rheumatoid arthritis: What can we learn about chronic disease? *Novartis Found. Symp.* 256:53–69; discussion 73, 106–11, 266–69

132. Khanna D, McMahon M, Furst DE. 2004. Safety of tumour necrosis factor-α antagonists. *Drug Saf.* 27:307–24

133. Ekstrom K, Hjalgrim H, Brandt L, Baecklund E, Klareskog L, et al. 2003. Risk of malignant lymphomas in patients with rheumatoid arthritis and in their first-degree relatives. *Arthritis Rheum.* 48: 963–70

134. Knight DM, Trinh H, Le J, Siegel S, Shealy D, et al. 1993. Construction and initial characterization of a mouse-human chimeric anti-TNF antibody. *Mol. Immunol.* 30:1443–53

135. Mohler KM, Torrance DS, Smith CA, Goodwin RG, Stremler KE, et al. 1993. Soluble tumor necrosis factor (TNF) receptors are effective therapeutic agents in lethal endotoxemia and function simultaneously as both TNF carriers and TNF antagonists. *J. Immunol.* 151:1548–61

136. Crowe PD, VanArsdale TL, Walter BN, Ware CF, Hession C, et al. 1994. A lymphotoxin-β-specific receptor. *Science* 264:707–10

137. Williams-Abbott L, Walter BN, Cheung T, Goh CR, Porter AG, Ware CF. 1997. The lymphotoxin-α (LTα) subunit is essential for the assembly, but not receptor specificity, of the membrane-anchored LTα1β2 heterotrimeric ligand. *J. Biol. Chem.* 272:19451–56

138. Scallon BJ, Moore MA, Trinh H, Knight DM, Ghrayeb J. 1995. Chimeric anti-TNF-α monoclonal antibody cA2 binds recombinant transmembrane TNF-α and activates immune effector functions. *Cytokine* 7:251–59

139. Lugering A, Schmidt M, Lugering N, Pauels HG, Domschke W, Kucharzik T. 2001. Infliximab induces apoptosis in monocytes from patients with chronic active Crohn's disease by using a caspase-dependent pathway. *Gastroenterology* 121:1145–57

140. Louis E, El Ghoul Z, Vermeire S, Dall'Ozzo S, Rutgeerts P, et al. 2004. Association between polymorphism in IgG Fc receptor IIIa coding gene and biological response to infliximab in Crohn's disease. *Aliment. Pharmacol. Ther.* 19:511–19

141. Food and Drug Admin. CfDEaR, Arthritis Advis. Comm. March 4, 2003. Safety update meeting on TNF blocking agents. Accessed April 26, 2004, at http://www.fda.gov/ohrms/dockets/ac/03/transcripts/3930T1.htm

142. Elliott MJ, Maini RN, Feldmann M, Long-Fox A, Charles P, et al. 1993. Treatment of rheumatoid arthritis with chimeric monoclonal antibodies to tumor necrosis factor α. *Arthritis Rheum.* 36:1681–90

143. Moreland LW, Baumgartner SW, Schiff MH, Tindall EA, Fleischmann RM, et al. 1997. Treatment of rheumatoid arthritis with a recombinant human tumor necrosis factor receptor (p75)-Fc fusion protein. *N. Engl. J. Med.* 337:141–47

144. Williams RO, Feldmann M, Maini RN. 1992. Anti-tumor necrosis factor ameliorates joint disease in murine collagen-induced arthritis. *Proc. Natl. Acad. Sci. USA* 89:9784–88

145. Buch MH, Conaghan PG, Quinn MA, Bingham SJ, Veale D, Emery P. 2004. True infliximab resistance in rheumatoid arthritis; a role for lymphotoxin-α? *Ann. Rheum. Dis.* 63:1344–46

146. Targan SR, Hanauer SB, van Deventer SJ, Mayer L, Present DH, et al. 1997. A short-term study of chimeric monoclonal antibody cA2 to tumor necrosis factor α for Crohn's disease. Crohn's Disease cA2 Study Group. *N. Engl. J. Med.* 337:1029–35

147. Sandborn WJ, Targan SR. 2002. Biologic

therapy of inflammatory bowel disease. *Gastroenterology* 122:1592–608

148. D'Haens G, Swijsen C, Noman M, Lemmens L, Ceuppens J, et al. 2001. Etanercept in the treatment of active refractory Crohn's disease: a single-center pilot trial. *Am. J. Gastroenterol.* 96:2564–68

149. Kontoyiannis D, Boulougouris G, Manoloukos M, Armaka M, Apostolaki M, et al. 2002. Genetic dissection of the cellular pathways and signaling mechanisms in modeled tumor necrosis factor-induced Crohn's-like inflammatory bowel disease. *J. Exp. Med.* 196:1563–74

150. Kollias G, Kontoyiannis D. 2002. Role of TNF/TNFR in autoimmunity: specific TNF receptor blockade may be advantageous to anti-TNF treatments. *Cytokine Growth Factor Rev.* 13:315–21

151. Andrews JS, Berger AE, Ware CF. 1990. Characterization of the receptor for tumor necrosis factor (TNF) and lymphotoxin (LT) on human T lymphocytes. TNF and LT differ in their receptor binding properties and the induction of MHC class I proteins on a human CD4$^+$ T cell hybridoma. *J. Immunol.* 144:2582–91. Erratum. 1990. *J. Immunol.* 144:4906

152. Mackay F, Browning JL, Lawton P, Shah SA, Comiskey M, et al. 1998. Both the lymphotoxin and tumor necrosis factor pathways are involved in experimental murine models of colitis. *Gastroenterology* 115:1464–75

153. Wallis RS, Broder MS, Wong JY, Hanson ME, Beenhouwer DO. 2004. Granulomatous infectious diseases associated with tumor necrosis factor antagonists. *Clin. Infect. Dis.* 38:1261–65

154. Mohan VP, Scanga CA, Yu K, Scott HM, Tanaka KE, et al. 2001. Effects of tumor necrosis factor α on host immune response in chronic persistent tuberculosis: possible role for limiting pathology. *Infect. Immun.* 69:1847–55

155. Abraham E, Anzueto A, Gutierrez G, Tessler S, San Pedro G, et al. 1998. Double-blind randomised controlled trial of monoclonal antibody to human tumour necrosis factor in treatment of septic shock. NORASEPT II Study Group. *Lancet* 351:929–33

156. Tracey KJ, Cerami A. 1993. Tumor necrosis factor: an updated review of its biology. *Crit. Care Med.* 21:S415–22

157. Mohan N, Edwards ET, Cupps TR, Oliverio PJ, Sandberg G, et al. 2001. Demyelination occurring during anti-tumor necrosis factor α therapy for inflammatory arthritides. *Arthritis Rheum.* 44:2862–69

158. The Lenercept Multiple Sclerosis Study Group and Univ. B. C. MS/MRI Anal. Group. 1999. TNF neutralization in MS: results of a randomized, placebo-controlled multicenter study. *Neurology* 53:457–65

159. Kollias G, Kontoyiannis D, Douni E, Kassiotis G. 2002. The role of TNF/TNFR in organ-specific and systemic autoimmunity: implications for the design of optimized 'anti-TNF' therapies. *Curr. Dir. Autoimmun.* 5:30–50

160. Wiendl H, Hohlfeld R. 2002. Therapeutic approaches in multiple sclerosis: lessons from failed and interrupted treatment trials. *BioDrugs* 16:183–200

161. Noseworthy JH, Lucchinetti C, Rodriguez M, Weinshenker BG. 2000. Multiple sclerosis. *N. Engl. J. Med.* 343:938–52

162. Hertzog PJ, O'Neill LA, Hamilton JA. 2003. The interferon in TLR signaling: more than just antiviral. *Trends Immunol.* 24:534–39

163. Taniguchi T, Takaoka A. 2002. The interferon-α/β system in antiviral responses: a multimodal machinery of gene regulation by the IRF family of transcription factors. *Curr. Opin. Immunol.* 14:111–16

164. Enbom M. 2001. Human herpesvirus 6 in the pathogenesis of multiple sclerosis. *Apmis* 109:401–11

165. Soldan SS, Jacobson S. 2001. Role of viruses in etiology and pathogenesis of

multiple sclerosis. *Adv. Virus Res.* 56: 517–55

166. Simmons A. 2001. Herpesvirus and multiple sclerosis. *Herpes* 8:60–63

167. Moore FG, Wolfson C. 2002. Human herpes virus 6 and multiple sclerosis. *Acta Neurol. Scand.* 106:63–83

168. Tomsone V, Logina I, Millers A, Chapenko S, Kozireva S, Murovska M. 2001. Association of human herpesvirus 6 and human herpesvirus 7 with demyelinating diseases of the nervous system. *J. Neurovirol.* 7:564–69

169. Alvarez-Lafuente R, Martin-Estefania C, de Las Heras V, Castrillo C, Picazo JJ, et al. 2002. Active human herpesvirus 6 infection in patients with multiple sclerosis. *Arch. Neurol.* 59:929–33

170. Goodman AD, Mock DJ, Powers JM, Baker JV, Blumberg BM. 2003. Human herpesvirus 6 genome and antigen in acute multiple sclerosis lesions. *J. Infect. Dis.* 187:1365–76

171. Cermelli C, Berti R, Soldan SS, Mayne M, D'Ambrosia JM, et al. 2003. High frequency of human herpesvirus 6 DNA in multiple sclerosis plaques isolated by laser microdissection. *J. Infect. Dis.* 187: 1377–87

172. Bech E, Lycke J, Gadeberg P, Hansen HJ, Malmestrom C, et al. 2002. A randomized, double-blind, placebo-controlled MRI study of anti-herpes virus therapy in MS. *Neurology* 58:31–36

173. Tejada-Simon MV, Zang YC, Hong J, Rivera VM, Zhang JZ. 2003. Cross-reactivity with myelin basic protein and human herpesvirus-6 in multiple sclerosis. *Ann. Neurol.* 53:189–97

174. Caselli E, Boni M, Bracci A, Rotola A, Cermelli C, et al. 2002. Detection of antibodies directed against human her-

pesvirus 6 U94/REP in sera of patients affected by multiple sclerosis. *J. Clin. Microbiol.* 40:4131–37

175. Hong J, Tejada-Simon MV, Rivera VM, Zang YC, Zhang JZ. 2002. Anti-viral properties of interferon beta treatment in patients with multiple sclerosis. *Mult. Scler.* 8:237–42

176. Berger DP, Naniche D, Crowley MT, Koni PA, Flavell RA, Oldstone MB. 1999. Lymphotoxin-β-deficient mice show defective antiviral immunity. *Virology* 260:136–47

177. Puglielli MT, Browning JL, Brewer AW, Schreiber RD, Shieh WJ, et al. 1999. Reversal of virus-induced systemic shock and respiratory failure by blockade of the lymphotoxin pathway. *Nat. Med.* 5:1370–74

178. Lin X, Ma X, Rodriguez M, Feng X, Zoecklein L, et al. 2003. Membrane lymphotoxin is required for resistance to Theiler's virus infection. *Int. Immunol.* 15:955–62

179. Wilhelm P, Riminton DS, Ritter U, Lemckert FA, Scheidig C, et al. 2002. Membrane lymphotoxin contributes to anti-leishmanial immunity by controlling structural integrity of lymphoid organs. *Eur. J. Immunol.* 32:1993–2003

180. Schluter D, Kwok LY, Lutjen S, Soltek S, Hoffmann S, et al. 2003. Both lymphotoxin-a and TNF are crucial for control of *Toxoplasma gondii* in the central nervous system. *J. Immunol.* 170: 6172–8

181. Engwerda CR, Mynott TL, Sawhney S, De Souza JB, Bickle QD, Kaye PM. 2002. Locally up-regulated lymphotoxin α, not systemic tumor necrosis factor α, is the principle mediator of murine cerebral malaria. *J. Exp. Med.* 195:1371–77

Annu. Rev. Immunol. 2005. 23:821–52
doi: 10.1146/annurev.immunol.23.021704.115835
Copyright © 2005 by Annual Reviews. All rights reserved
First published online as a Review in Advance on January 7, 2005

ROLE OF C5A IN INFLAMMATORY RESPONSES

Ren-Feng Guo and Peter A. Ward

*Department of Pathology, University of Michigan Medical School, Ann Arbor,
Michigan 48109-0602; email: grf@med.umich.edu; pward@umich.edu*

Key Words complement, C5a receptor, C5L2, inflammation

■ **Abstract** The complement system not only represents an effective innate immune mechanism of host defense to eradicate microbial pathogens, but it is also widely involved in many forms of acute and chronic inflammatory diseases including sepsis, acute lung injury, ischemia-reperfusion injury, and asthma, to give just a few examples. The complement-activated product, C5a, displays powerful biological activities that lead to inflammatory sequelae. C5a is a strong chemoattractant and is involved in the recruitment of inflammatory cells such as neutrophils, eosinophils, monocytes, and T lymphocytes, in activation of phagocytic cells and release of granule-based enzymes and generation of oxidants, all of which may contribute to innate immune functions or tissue damage. Accumulating data suggest that C5a provides a vital bridge between innate and adaptive immune functions, extending the roles of C5a in inflammation. Herein, we review human and animal data describing the cellular and molecular mechanisms of C5a in the development of inflammatory disorders, sepsis, acute lung injury, ischemia-reperfusion injury, and asthma.

INTRODUCTION

It has been almost a century since the complement system was discovered. In the past decade, the interest in complement research has been rekindled because of the discovery of complement receptors and new functional aspects of complement activation products. Traditionally, the complement system has been viewed as a central part of the innate immune system in host defenses against invading pathogens and in clearance of potentially damaging cell debris. However, complement activation has recently been implicated in the pathogenesis of many inflammatory and immunological diseases, including sepsis (1), acute respiratory distress syndrome (2), rheumatoid arthritis (3), glomerulonephritis (4), multiple sclerosis (5), ischemia-reperfusion injury (6), and asthma (7). Complement activation exerts its harmful roles through the generation of complement protein split products, especially C3a and C5a. Although these activation products are not necessarily the initiating factors in the inflammatory disorders, they appear to be responsible for promoting and perpetuating inflammatory reactions.

Among the complement activation products, C5a is one of the most potent inflammatory peptides, with a broad spectrum of functions. C5a is a strong chemoattractant (at 1–10 nM) for neutrophils and also has chemotactic activity for monocytes and macrophages (8). C5a causes an oxidative burst (O_2 consumption) in neutrophils and enhances phagocytosis and release of granule enzymes (9–11). C5a has also been found to be a vasodilator (12). C5a has been recently shown to be involved in modulation of cytokine expression from various cell types (13, 14), to cause reduced neutrophil apoptosis but enhanced thymocyte apoptosis (15–17), to enhance expression of adhesion molecule expression on neutrophils (18), and to activate the coagulation pathway (19). C5a exerts its effects through the high-affinity C5a receptors (C5aR and C5L2). C5aR belongs to the rhodopsin family of G-protein-coupled receptors with seven transmembrane segments (20, 21); C5L2 is similar but is not G-protein-coupled. C5a binds with high affinity to C5L2, but few biological responses have been found for this interaction (22). C5L2 is present on neutrophils and immature dendritic cells (23). C5aR expression was originally described on myeloid cells including neutrophils, eosinophils, basophils, and monocytes (20, 24–26). More recently, C5aR has also been found on a variety of nonmyeloid cells in many organs, especially in the lung and liver (27, 28). Widespread upregulation of C5aR expression occurs during onset of sepsis, suggesting the importance of C5a/C5aR signaling in the pathogenesis of sepsis-induced inflammation and outcome associated in sepsis and development of multiple organ failure (MOF) (29).

Many inflammatory diseases are attributable to the affects of C5a, and the catalog is expanding. We describe actions of C5a, focusing on its roles in innate immunity and molecular and cellular events that lead to the inflammatory sequelae. We review human and animal data, describing the potential roles of C5a in the development of acute inflammatory disorders (e.g., sepsis, acute lung injury, ischemia-reperfusion injury) and chronic inflammatory responses (e.g., asthma).

COMPLEMENT PATHWAYS AND GENERATION OF C5a

The complement system is composed of more than 30 plasma proteins and glycoproteins and soluble or membrane-bound receptors. This protein system acts as an enzymatic cascade through a variety of protein-protein interactions. Three pathways of complement activation have been recognized: the classical, alternative, and lectin-binding pathways (Figure 1). The classical pathway is activated by antigen-antibody complexes. The alternative pathway is directly initiated by surface molecules containing carbohydrates and lipids. The lectin-binding pathway is triggered by the binding of either mannose-binding lectin protein (MBL) or ficolin to bacterial/fungal carbohydrate structures, resulting in activation of MBL-associated serine proteases (MASPs), with subsequent engagement of complement proteins, such as C4 and C2. The classical pathway is activated by IgG or IgM molecules, often present as immune complexes, and by other products of the inflammatory response, such as C-reactive protein and serum amyloid protein. Membrane-bound IgG or IgM can also activate this pathway. The process begins with the binding of C1q to its ligand (e.g., Fc regions of IgG or IgM), displacing

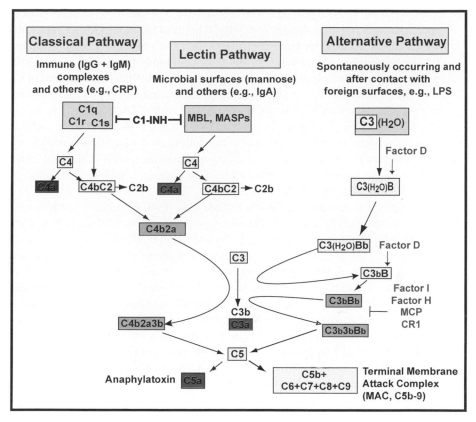

Figure 1   Complement activation pathways. The complement system can be activated through three pathways: classical, lectin, and alternative pathways.

the C1 inhibitor (C1-INH) from the complex with resultant activation of both C1r and protease, C1s. Activated C1s cleaves C4, producing C4a and C4b. C4b binds C2, which is subsequently cleaved by C1s, yielding C2b and C2a. C2b is released while C2a remains bound to C4b, forming a heterodimeric complex, C4b2a, which has C3 convertase activity, able to cleave C3 into the larger C3b and smaller C3a fragments. C5 convertase is formed by assembly of the heterotrimeric complex, C4b2a3b, which cleaves C5 into C5b and C5a. The lectin pathway is activated by contact of MBL in serum with repeating microbial surface mannose residues. Activation of MBL leads to activation of MASP-1, -2, and -3, which are analogous to C1r/C1s proteases of the classical pathway. MASPs cleave C4 and C2 precisely as occurs with C1s, leading to the formation of the classical pathway C3 and C5 convertases. The alternative pathway is activated by whole microorganisms and their products, such as lipopolysaccharide (LPS), zymosan, peptides, teichoic acid, and certain cell surfaces. Circulating C3 is continuously hydrolyzed partly to

C3(H_2O). Low grade, spontaneous hydrolysis of C3 producing C3b also serves to enhance activation of this pathway. C3(H_2O) binds to factor B to form C3(H_2O)B, which can be cleaved by factor D to form the C3 convertase, C3(H_2O)Bb, and C3 is subsequently cleaved to C3a and C3b. C3b binds factor B to form C3bB, which can be further cleaved to C3bBb by factor D. C3bBb is another form of C3 convertase to cleave C3 into C3a and C3b. This enables C3b to bind to C3bBb and form the alternative pathway C5 convertase, C3bBbC3b, which can cleave C5 into C5a and C5b. Thereafter, production of C3 and C5 products is the same as in the two other pathways. C3b can be catabolized by factor I and factor D, and by membrane-bound cofactors, such as complement receptor 1 (CR1) and membrane cofactor protein. These cofactors regulate alternative pathway activation by competitively binding to C3b.

Complement activation products include C3a, C4a, C5a, and the membrane attack complex (MAC), C5b-9. The cleavage product C5b binds to C3b to form C3b5b, which binds to C6, resulting in the formation of C5b6. Subsequent activation of C6–9 occurs in the absence of any further proteolytic cleavage and results in the formation of MAC, which can cause lysis of cells and bacteria. The complement activation products, C3a, C4a and C5a, are also known as anaphylatoxins because of their tissue-sensitizing activity. Human C5a is a 74 amino acid glycoprotein with complex antiparallel helical structures. C5a can not only be generated systemically through complement activation pathways but also may be produced locally through a phagocytic cell-related serine protease(s) containing C5 convertase activity. For instance, activated alveolar macrophages and neutrophils contain neutral proteases that can cleave C5 to produce C5a (30).

ROLE OF C5a IN SEPSIS

Sepsis was initially considered to be accompanied by the presence of bacteria in the blood (bacteremia). However, the clinical signs of sepsis frequently occur in patients without indication of bacteremia. To define sepsis properly, SIRS (systemic inflammatory response syndrome) was introduced by The Society of Critical Care Medicine and The American College of Chest Physicians in 1992 (31, 32). Patients with SIRS may display following symptoms: hypothermia ($<36°C$) or hyperthermia ($>38°C$), tachycardia (>90 beats/min), tachypnea (>20 breaths/min or $P_{CO_2} < 32$ mm Hg), and leukocytopenia ($<4 \times 10^9$ cells/liter) or leukocytosis ($>12 \times 10^9$ cells/liter). Researchers currently accept that sepsis triggers a systemic response to infection, manifested by two or more of the symptoms described above. During the onset of sepsis, the inflammatory system becomes hyperactive, involving both cellular and humoral defense mechanisms (33). Endothelial and epithelial cells, as well as neutrophils, macrophages, and lymphocytes, produce powerful proinflammatory mediators. Simultaneously, humoral defense mechanisms such as the complement system are activated, resulting in production of proinflammatory mediators, including C3a and C5a, which are powerful phlogistic mediators.

As is well known, sepsis triggers complement activation (1). Excessive activation of complement leads to high levels of complement activation products in the blood, including the potent proinflammatory peptides C3a and C5a. In humans and animals with sepsis, investigators have noted elevated plasma levels of C3a, C4a, and C5a (34–37). Engagement of alternative and classic pathways has been thought to be responsible for complement activation occurring in sepsis. A recent study has shown that the O-antigen region of LPS can activate the lectin pathway (38). Thus, in the setting of sepsis, all three complement activation pathways may be brought into play. As a result, excessive complement activation products are produced and may be responsible for organ damage and compromised innate immune systems (described below).

Linkage of C5a to Innate Immunity

Complement-mediated activation of neutrophils and monocytes causes an oxidative burst with release of reactive oxygen species (ROS), especially O_2. and H_2O_2. C5a-C5aR interaction is a critical event in *Escherichia coli*–induced upregulation of CR3 (CD11b/CD18) and the subsequent oxidative burst and phagocytosis (11). Interception of C5a/C5aR signaling in whole blood by a C5aR antagonist, the synthetic cyclic hexapeptide AcF[OpdChaWR], significantly inhibited *E. coli*–induced oxidative burst in neutrophils, markedly attenuating upregulation of CD11b on the neutrophil surface and completely abolishing both neutrophil and monocyte phagocytosis of *E. coli*. Under the same conditions, both neutrophil and monocyte phagocytosis were completely abolished by anti-CD11b antibody. These data suggest that optimal opsonization and subsequent phagocytosis of *E. coli* depend on C5a-induced upregulation of CR3. By using the same whole blood model, addition of anti-C5a to whole blood blocked *Neisseria meningitides*–induced CR3 upregulation, phagocytosis, and the oxidative burst (39). Unlike their wild-type littermates, mice deficient in C5aR were unable to clear intrapulmonary-instilled *Pseudomonas aeruginosa*, despite a marked increase in neutrophil influx. These animals eventually succumbed to bacterial pneumonia. C5aR$^{-/-}$ mice challenged with sublethal inocula of *P. aeruginosa* became superinfected with secondary bacterial strains (40). Thus, C5a/C5aR signaling is essential in host defenses in the lung and in other organs.

However, excessive C5a can be detrimental. In neutrophils, high doses of C5a can lead to nonspecific chemotactic "desensitization," thereby causing broad dysfunction. Exposure of neutrophils to C5a (at concentrations occurring in plasma of humans with sepsis) can lead to neutrophil dysfunction and paralysis of signaling pathways (41). Phorbol myristate acetate (PMA)-induced stimulation of neutrophils results in phosphorylation of cytosolic p47^{phox} and its translocation to the cell membrane, which is essential for assembly of NADPH oxidase and the subsequent production of O_2. and H_2O_2. However, preincubation of neutrophils with C5a blocks phosphorylation of p47^{phox} and its translocation to the cell membrane after addition of PMA, thereby leading to defective assembly of NADPH oxidase and a greatly depressed oxidative burst. In addition, the phosphorylation of p42/p44 mitogen-activated protein kinase (MAPK) in neutrophils in response to PMA is also impaired by prior cell contact with C5a. Because C5a is a strong activator of MAPK (including p42/p44), which is an important kinase for p47[phox] phosphorylation, the functional impairments in neutrophils exposed to C5a are likely due to paralysis in MAPK signaling cascades.

In cecal ligation and puncture (CLP)-induced sepsis, neutrophils from CLP rats display defective phagocytosis and chemotaxis (41) as well as defective assembly of NADPH oxidase. All such defects can be prevented in CLP rats after blockade of C5a or C5aR, which suggests that neutrophil innate immune functions in sepsis are seriously compromised by overproduction of C5a and excessive C5a/C5aR engagement.

C5a/C5aR Signaling in the Development of Sepsis

Apoptosis appears to play an important role in the pathogenesis of sepsis (42–44). Inhibition of lymphocyte apoptosis improves survival in experimental sepsis (45, 46). Blood lymphocyte apoptosis occurring early in humans with sepsis is associated with a poor outcome (47). Apoptosis is also an important mechanism for eliminating activated neutrophils from inflamed tissues, which prevents release of the toxic cellular products from neutrophils undergoing necrosis. Spontaneous apoptosis was significantly delayed in neutrophils obtained from patients with SIRS (8.6%) when compared with neutrophils from normal controls (34.9%) (48). Long-lived neutrophils accumulating in tissues during sepsis may be linked to development of MOF. The potential role of C5a/C5aR signaling in the development of sepsis is depicted in Figure 2. C5a/C5aR signaling in neutrophils appears to provide a survival signal for these cells. In vitro experiments have demonstrated that C5a inhibits neutrophil apoptosis in a dose- and time-dependent manner (17). The antiapoptotic effects of C5a were markedly abrogated in the presence of wortmannin, a phosphatidylinositol-3 kinase (PI3K) inhibitor, suggesting that PI3K/Akt pathway is involved in development of apoptosis, at least in neutrophils. In addition, C5a stimulation resulted in phosphorylation of Akt and Bad proteins in neutrophils, as well as decreased activity of caspase-9. These data suggest that neutrophils undergo spontaneous apoptosis via a mitochondria-dependent pathway and that this pathway can be inhibited by engagement of C5a/C5aR signaling. MAPK and protein kinase C (PKC) pathways are also likely to be involved in the antiapoptotic action of C5a because C5a is a well-known activator for MAPK and PKC, and these kinases have important functions in the regulation of neutrophil apoptosis (49). Many other inflammatory mediators have antiapoptotic effects on neutrophils, including G-CSF, GM-CSF, fMLP, ATP, leukotriene B4, IL-1β, IL-2, IL-3, IL-6, IL-15, and IFN-γ (49). As discussed above, C5a plays a pivotal role in the regulation of inflammatory mediator expression. Thus, C5a may indirectly provide survival signals to neutrophils by increasing the concentrations of antiapoptotic inflammatory mediators.

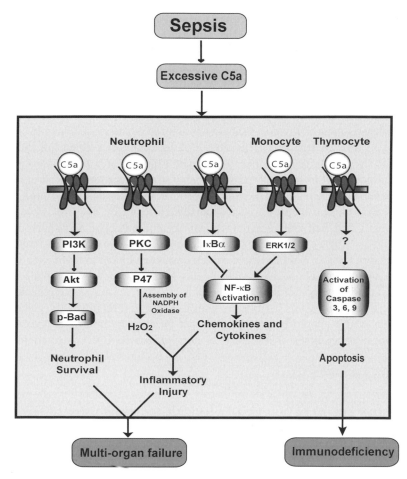

Figure 2 C5a/C5aR signaling in sepsis. C5a/C5R signaling in neutrophils leads to activation of PI3K/Akt pathways, which provide survival signals for neutrophils. Assembly of NADPH oxidase can be triggered by C5a/C5aR signaling, resulting in H_2O_2 production in organs and tissues. Increased numbers of neutrophils together with H_2O_2 generation may be linked to tissue injury and MOF. In monocytes, ERK1/2 is activated by C5a stimulation, leading to NF-κB activation and subsequent production of chemokines and cytokines, whereas in neutrophils NF-κB activation may be inhibited by C5a through induction of IκBα. C5a-induced thymocyte apoptosis may contribute to immunodeficiency in sepsis.

In a striking contrast to neutrophils, thymocytes apparently receive proapoptotic signals from C5a. Thymus atrophy due to extensive thymocyte apoptosis is well known in sepsis occurring in rodents and is considered to be a major factor that leads to decreased number of T lymphocytes in circulation and attendant immunosuppression. When C5a was generated in vivo by infusion of purified cobra venom factor (CVF), thymocyte apoptosis was significantly increased (15). In animals 12 h after induction of CLP there was an increased activity in caspase-3, -6, and -9 in thymocytes. Cytosolic cytochrome c levels increased, and Bcl-X_L expression was significantly decreased. C5a blockade in the sepsis model almost completely inhibited activation of caspase-3, -6, and -9, significantly preserved cytochrome c content in mitochondria, and preserved Bcl-X_L levels (15). These data indicate that the mitochondria-dependent cytochrome c/Apaf-1/caspase-9 pathway is involved in sepsis-induced thymocyte apoptosis and can be influenced directly or indirectly by C5a/C5aR signaling. This study did not establish a direct link between C5a and thymocyte apoptosis because in vitro exposure of normal thymocytes to C5a did not result in apoptosis. However, in a subsequent study, C5aR expression on thymocytes increased in the early stage (2–6 h) of sepsis; furthermore, C5a could directly induce apoptosis on cells obtained after CLP (16). Thus, in sepsis conditions C5a-C5aR interaction may potentiate the mitochondrial apoptotic pathway and/or enhance the expression of proapoptotic factors, such as tumor necrosis factor (TNF)-α and Fas ligand, which have been linked to thymocyte apoptosis.

As shown in Figure 2, signaling pathways employed by neutrophils and thymocytes are clearly different. During sepsis, thymocytes undergo vigorous apoptosis, whereas neutrophils became resistant to apoptosis. Interestingly, glucocorticoids can inhibit apoptosis in neutrophils but promote thymocyte apoptosis (42, 50). These data suggest that the effects elicited by C5a-C5aR interaction leading to apoptosis seem to be cell-specific, perhaps because of cell selective upregulation of C5aR during sepsis.

Protective Effects of C5a/C5aR Blockade in Sepsis

The importance of C5a/C5aR signaling for the outcome of sepsis has been highlighted by several experiments employing different animal models of sepsis. Blockade of C5a in experimental sepsis or sepsis-like conditions has proven beneficial. Infusion of monoclonal antibody against the C-terminal region of C5a improves hemodynamic parameters in pigs infused with LPS or live *E. coli* (51). In a primate model of sepsis following a 30 min infusion of liver *E. coli* (10^{10}/kg), administration of rabbit antihuman C5a polyclonal antibody to primates (*Macaca fascicularis*) improved survival rates (52). Septic animals not treated with anti-C5a antibody had 75% mortality, decreased oxygenation, severe pulmonary edema, and profound hypotension. Septic primates treated with anti-C5a antibodies had improved physiological parameters and no increased extravascular lung water. Convincing evidence for improved survival in rats treated with anti-C5a was achieved by using a rat model of sepsis induced by CLP (53). In the CLP group receiving anti-C5a antibody, the survival rate was 50% for a 10-day survival study, compared with the 9.5% survival in the reference group (53). In the same study, anti-C5a treatment reduced the levels of bacteremia and preserved the H_2O_2-producing capacity of neutrophils. In addition, anti-C5a treatment ameliorated the development of MOF in sepsis (54). The protective effects of C5a blockade appear to derive from the interception of C5a/C5aR signaling because blockade of C5aR achieved a similar level of improvement in survival in CLP animals. During the early phases of sepsis, C5aR expression was upregulated in lung, liver, kidney, and heart, and anti-C5aR treatment dramatically improved survival rate from 0% to 70% in a 7-day survival study, accompanied by a significant reduction of bacterial counts [colony forming units (CFU)] in lungs and kidneys (29).

Beneficial effects of anti-C5a treatment have been associated with reduced MOF in experimental sepsis. Progressive MOF in humans with sepsis is associated with a high mortality rate (55, 56). Development of MOF in septic patients is often with defective blood/gas exchange in lung, accompanied by activation of the clotting system and defective function of the kidneys and liver (57). The relationship between SIRS and multiple organ dysfunction syndrome has been described as progressing from sick to sicker to very sick (58). MOF is the final common pathway leading to death in modern intensive care units (57). In humans and animals, MOF is often a consequence of progressive development of tissue hypoxia, complement activation, and an unregulated production of inflammatory mediators (36, 59–61).

Accumulating evidence has established a link between C5a and MOF. Widespread upregulation of C5aR has been seen in organs (heart, liver, lungs, kidneys) from septic animals (29). Anti-C5a treatment attenuates the coagulopathy of sepsis (see below) and improves organ function (as described above). Bacteremia is an important feature of sepsis. Blood cultures from septic CLP rats showed a significant number of aerobic and anaerobic bacterial CFU (53). In the CLP group treated with anti-C5a, the CFU value was profoundly reduced (by 98%) (53). CLP rats treated with control IgG had very high CFU values (3×10^6–11×10^6/g tissue) in spleen and liver. In contrast, CFU values from the anti-C5a group decreased almost to the basal levels (53). Early respiratory alkalosis in septic animals 24 h after CLP was accompanied by the rising arterial pH from 7.47 to 7.53. Septic rats 60 h after CLP showed evidence of metabolic acidosis and lactic acidemia, with the blood pH values falling from 7.48 to 7.34 (54). In the CLP group treated with anti-C5a, all values (pH, pCO_2, HCO_3^-, pO_2) remained in the normal range, indicating that anti-C5a treatment can reverse the early respiratory alkalosis and the late-developing metabolic acidosis in septic rats (54). In septic rats, liver dysfunction was evidenced by elevations in serum bilirubin, alanine aminotransferase (ALT), aspartate aminotransferase (AST), and lactate dehydrogenase (LDH). In animals treated with anti-C5a, most of these parameters (bilirubin, ALT, AST) remained in the normal range, and the rise in LDH levels was attenuated. In addition, kidney function was protected by anti-C5a treatment, reflected in unchanged levels of serum creatinine, blood urea nitrogen, and urine protein (54).

Atrophy of the thymus associated with thymocyte apoptosis has been observed during sepsis in rodents (62–64). T cell suppression and a decreased number in total T lymphocytes are characteristic symptoms in MOF (65). The widespread lymphocyte depletion induced by apoptosis appears to cause the immunosuppression state that occurs in sepsis. In the rat model of CLP-induced sepsis, thymus atrophy occurred as early as 12 h after CLP, and reached its nadir at 24 h. C5a blockade dramatically preserved thymic weight during CLP. Anti-C5a treatment resulted in a significant decrease (by 80%) in CLP-induced thymocyte apoptosis. Anti-C5a treatment in sepsis rescued thymocytes from apoptosis via maintaining the integrity of mitochondria, preserving antiapoptotic molecule Bcl-X_L, and inhibiting activation of caspase-3, -6, and -9 (15).

Anti-C5a Treatment Attenuates SIRS

Researchers have long assumed that endogenous mediators of inflammation are important in the development of sepsis, together with microbial products such as LPS. In sepsis, the loss of the balance between proinflammatory and anti-inflammatory mediators seems to occur, producing exaggerated inflammatory responses, immunosuppression, apoptosis, and organ dysfunction. As indicated above, recent evidence suggests that C5a/C5aR signaling may influence balance in the inflammatory network. C5a stimulates the synthesis and release from human leukocytes of proinflammatory cytokines such as TNF-α, IL-β, IL-6, and IL-8 (66, 67). C5a produces a strong synergistic effect with LPS in production of TNF-α, macrophage inflammatory protein (MIP)-2, cytokine-induced neutrophil chemoattractant (CINC)-1, and IL-1β in rat alveolar epithelial cells (13). Similarly, exposure of mouse dermal endothelial cells to C5a and LPS results in enhanced production of monocyte chemoattractant protein-1 and MIP-2 compared with the effects of C5a or LPS alone. Addition of physiological concentrations of C5a (low nM range) to human umbilical vein endothelial cells (HUVEC) caused strong up-regulation of IL-8, IL-1β, and RANTES mRNA in a time- and dose-dependent manner (68). These data suggest that the C5a/C5aR signaling pathway is involved in cytokine and chemokine production in a variety of cell types. Blockade of C5a with anti-C5a in sepsis resulted in a >75% decrease in serum levels of IL-6 (67). In CLP-induced sepsis, we have demonstrated that blockade of C5aR with antibodies resulted in decreased levels of IL-6 and TNF-α in blood compared to CLP controls (29). Blockade of C5a in CLP rats significantly reduced serum levels of IL-6 during sepsis (16). The dependency of IL-6 production on C5a during sepsis was confirmed in C5aR-deficient mice. IL-6 levels in C5aR-deficient mice were significantly lower than that in control mice during sepsis. C5a stimulation of neutrophils elicited a rapid phosphorylation of p38-MAPK and p44/p42 MAPK, which are critical in IL-6 production. More recently, production of macrophage migration inhibitory factor (MIF) has been linked to C5a signaling. In vitro, C5a induced MIF release from rat and mouse neutrophils. In vivo blockade of C5aR or absence of C5aR led to significantly reduced MIF generation during the onset of sepsis. C5a-induced release in vitro of MIF from neutrophils was apparently due to upregulation of MIF in cytoplasmic granules of neutrophils via activation of the protein kinase B signaling pathway together with involvement of PI3K (69).

Surprisingly, C5a can also function as a suppressor of gene expression. C5a strongly reduced production of IL-12 in human monocytes treated with LPS or

IFN-γ (70). In HUVEC, IL-6 mRNA expression was significantly suppressed after exposure to C5a (68). We recently found that C5a can strongly suppress LPS-induced TNF-α production in neutrophils, whereas in alveolar macrophages C5a showed the opposite effect, in that LPS and C5a synergistically induced TNF-α production (71). These studies suggest that C5a/C5aR signaling can lead to totally opposite outcomes, with suppressive effects seemingly linked to induction of IκBα, correlating with an inhibitory effect on NF-κB activation. However, this is obviously not the case in monocytes, because NF-κB activation occurred within 15 min after C5a exposure (72). It is intriguing that C5a can simultaneously up- and downregulate NF-κB-dependent gene expression (such as TNF-α, IL-6, and IL-8), suggesting a complexity in C5a/C5aRs signaling. Although the understanding of C5a/C5aRs signaling for cytokine production is still in the formative stage, C5a effects in the cytokine network is not a debatable topic. Given that complement activation is an event occurring during the onset of sepsis, C5a may come into play before emergence of most of the "inflammatory cytokine storm." C5a likely plays a key role in orchestrating the performance of the cytokine network.

Involvement of C5a in Coagulation Pathways

Sepsis is a leading cause of disseminated intravascular coagulation. During sepsis, tissue factor expression occurs on the surfaces of blood monocytes and tissue macrophages, resulting in activation of the extrinsic coagulation pathway, with thrombin activation and fibrin formation (73). Simultaneously, there is inhibition of natural anticoagulant responses. All these events lead to excessive thrombin generation, fibrin formation, and consumption of clotting factors during sepsis. The clinical success of the anticoagulant, activated protein C, in septic patients underscores the importance of the coagulation pathway in the pathogenesis of sepsis. Involvement of C5a in coagulation pathways could be direct or indirect. Anti-C5a significantly ameliorated coagulation/fibrinolytic changes in sepsis, suggesting that disseminated intravascular coagulation in CLP rats is attenuated by this intervention (19). Dramatic changes in platelet counts, fibrinogen, factor VII:C, plasminogen, tissue plasminogen activator, and plasminogen activator inhibitor, as well as plasma thrombin-antithrombin complexes and D-dimer, were all markedly attenuated in CLP rats treated with anti-C5a. C5a induces tissue factor expression in endothelial cells and monocytes (74–76). In addition, the effects of C5a on coagulation pathways may be also mediated by regulating the levels of chemokines and cytokines. For instance, C5a is a strong inducer of IL-8 production, and IL-8 can promote the formation of fibrin clots and induce thrombogenesis as well as proliferation and structural reorganization of endothelial cells (77). In vitro experiments have demonstrated that the addition of LPS and/or cytokines (TNF-α) to endothelial cells increases expression of tissue factor and plasminogen activator inhibitor 1, and promotes generation of procoagulant microparticles (73). C5a can regulate the expression of many cytokines/chemokines from various cell types, thereby influencing the coagulation system.

C5a and Neutrophil Migration in Sepsis

It is known that neutrophil accumulation in organs is associated with tissue injury. C5a is not only a strong chemoattractant of neutrophils, it can, as described above, also activate endothelial and epithelial cells, setting the stage for release of neutrophil chemoattractants. C5a induced increases in both β_1 and β_2 integrin expression on blood neutrophils and enhanced adhesive interactions of neutrophils to HUVEC and to human bronchial epithelial cells (78, 79). Treatment with anti-C5a of CLP rats significantly reduced the upregulation of β_2 integrins on neutrophils (18). During sepsis, both β_1 integrin content (CD29) and β_2 integrin content (CD18) on neutrophils were elevated after the onset of sepsis following CLP (18). Under septic conditions, neutrophil accumulation in lung in response to a second insult (deposition of IgG immune complexes) was both β_2 integrin– and β_1 integrin–dependent, as opposed to the nonseptic condition in which lung neutrophil accumulation was only β_2 integrin–dependent. Anti-C5a treatment significantly attenuated β_2 integrin upregulation on neutrophils in CLP rats but had no effect on β_1 integrin expression. In vitro stimulation of neutrophils with C5a revealed that β_2 integrin expression was much more sensitive to C5a stimulation than was β_1 integrin expression. Thus, anti-C5a may protect tissue injury of various organs by limiting neutrophil sequestration through downregulating β_2 integrin expression.

Defective chemotactic responsiveness of neutrophils to C5a might be linked to significantly decreased levels on neutrophils in early sepsis (80, 81). It is well accepted that C5aR is required for chemotactic responsiveness to C5a. We have recently found that neutrophils from CLP rats display dramatically decreased levels of C5aR, associated with a concomitant decrease in chemotactic responsiveness to C5a. In septic human patients, investigators have described decreased levels of IL-8 receptors (CXCR1 and CXCR2) on neutrophils, although, surprisingly, these neutrophils display full chemotactic responsiveness to IL-8 (81). Thus, in addition to CXC chemokines, C5a may also play key roles in recruiting neutrophils into organs in sepsis. As mentioned earlier, C5a is capable of inducing CXC chemokine production from various cell types, including monocytes, epithelial cells, and endothelial cells. Thus, local production of C5a may contribute to neutrophil accumulation in organs via the induction of CXC chemokines.

C5aR Expression in Sepsis

During the onset of experimental sepsis induced by CLP, C5aR content on neutrophils drops significantly, reaching a nadir at 24 h after CLP, with a progressive but slow return thereafter (80). The dynamic pattern of C5aR expression on neutrophils during sepsis is likely due to internalization of C5a/C5aR complexes followed by surface re-expression of C5aR, given that C5aR protein and mRNA levels in neutrophils are not significantly changed at different time points of sepsis. The rapid decrease in C5aR content on neutrophils appears to be linked to elevated blood levels of C5a because intravenous blockade of C5a significantly preserved C5aR content on blood neutrophils. Previous studies have suggested that, after binding of C5a to C5aR on neutrophils, the ligand/receptor complex is rapidly internalized and C5aR is recycled to the cell surface (82–84). Other inflammatory mediators capable of causing transcriptional downregulation of C5aR may also appear in the blood during sepsis. For instance, IL-4 reduces C5aR expression on dendritic cells (85), and IL-4 is upregulated during CLP (86).

C5aR expression on neutrophils reached the lowest point 24 h after CLP, and innate immune functions (chemotaxis and oxidative burst) of neutrophils were seriously impaired (80). Beyond 24 h after CLP, blood neutrophils started to undergo a functional recovery, correlating with increased content of C5aR. This was associated with an enhanced oxidative burst as well as improved chemotaxis. Decreased surface content of C5aR on neutrophils has been noted in critically ill and anergic septic patients and in HIV patients (81, 87, 88). In the latter group, decreased levels of C5aR on neutrophils were associated with reduced chemotactic responses to C5a and elevated blood levels of C5a *des Arg*. These data establish a link between C5aR content on neutrophils and the functional capabilities of these cells in maintaining efficacious host defensive responsiveness.

Interestingly, there was a positive correlation between the level of C5aR expression on neutrophils from CLP animals and their ultimate survival (80). The correlation was such that all septic animals with C5aR levels higher than the overall median at 36 h survived, whereas 67% of animals with C5aR levels lower than the median failed to survive. Thus, C5aR levels on neutrophils may serve as a prognostic marker for clinical outcomes in sepsis. Whether the higher levels of C5aR on neutrophils of surviving animals represent animals with less C5a generation or more efficient receptor recycling pathways is currently unknown.

C5a IN ACUTE LUNG INJURY

Complement activation has been demonstrated in many forms of acute lung injury. C5a concentration increased in bronchoalveolar lavage (BAL) fluids in acute lung injury induced by acid instillation (89), and C5a concentration is also elevated in transplanted lungs in human (90). The essential role of C5a in acute lung injury has been well documented by using a model of IgG immune complex–induced alveolitis (91). In this model, C5a was required for the full development of injury and neutrophil accumulation. Neutrophil accumulation constitutes the foundation of many forms of acute lung injury. C5a, as a potent chemoattractant, can directly attract neutrophils into lung, and it can also directly activate neutrophils, macrophages, and endothelial cells. A clear confirmation of C5's role in inflammation has been defined by using C5-deficient mice and C5aR knockout mice. C5-deficient mice are more tolerant to endotoxin than are the C5-sufficient animals, and depletion of complement by bolus infusion of CVF attenuated lung injury (92). C5aR-deficient mice showed pronounced reduction of lung in the model of IgG immune complex–induced alveolitis (93). Intratracheal administration of purified rat C5a into complement-depleted rats fully restored the ability of lung to develop injury (94). Anti-C5a treatment greatly reduced injury parameters, such as vascular leakage, neutrophil influx into the alveolar space, and lung neutrophils [myeloperoxidase (MPO)] buildup. The protective role of anti-C5a was associated with drastic reductions in BAL levels of TNF-α, as well as a profound decrease in upregulation of lung vascular intercellular adhesion molecule (ICAM)-1, suggesting that C5a is essential in the foundation of the inflammatory network, regulating the expression of inflammatory mediators and expression of adhesion molecules. In the presence of a cyclic peptide antagonist (C5aRa) to the C5aR, the lung permeability index (extravascular leakage of albumin) in mice after intrapulmonary deposition of IgG immune complexes was markedly diminished, indicating the C5a-C5aR interaction provides important signals for inflammatory reactions.

Regulation of C5a on neutrophil accumulation comes from several levels, as described in Figure 3. Optimal induction of CC and CXC chemokines in lung by IgG immune complex deposition requires C5a (95). Somewhat similar to TNF-α, C5a may function as an autocrine activator to promote CXC and CC chemokine generation by alveolar macrophages. Clearly, C5a, together with other neutrophil chemoattractants, forms the chemoattracting gradient in lung and in the alveolar compartment, which appears to be essential for neutrophil recruitment. C5a can also enhance other early response cytokine production (TNF-α and IL-1) to amplify the inflammatory reaction in lung. In addition, the requirement of C5a for activation of adhesion cascade leading to tissue recruitment of neutrophils has been established. In vivo experiments have shown that recombinant C5a can increase CD11b/CD18 expression on neutrophils, inducing increased adhesion of both neutrophils and eosinophils to unstimulated HUVEC and to human bronchial epithelial cells (78, 79). C5a can activate P-selectin on endothelial cells (96), which is a critical step for tethering the neutrophils. In vivo blockade of C5a totally abolished upregulation of lung vascular P-selectin in the rat model of CVF-induced lung injury (97). Chip analyses revealed that HUVECs stimulated with C5a showed progressive increases in gene expression for cell adhesion molecules (e.g., E-selectin, especially, but also ICAM-1 and VCAM-1), cytokines/chemokines, and related receptors (e.g., VEGFC, IL-6, IL-18R) (98). High levels of lung vascular ICAM-1 were observed in rats 4 h after IgG immune complex deposition; however, complement depletion before the onset of injury completely suppressed the ICAM-1 upregulation, and intratracheal blockade of C5a resulted in 80% reduction in lung levels of ICAM-1 (94). Complement activation appears to be an upstream event in the inflammatory cascade following IgG immune complex deposition, allowing C5a to exert its inflammatory effects.

As described in Figure 3, C5a is responsible for STAT3 activation in IgG immune complex–induced lung injury (99). Anti-C5a antibody administration significantly reduces STAT3 activation after IgG immune complex deposition. Stimulation of rat alveolar macrophage cell line (NR8383) with rat C5a caused phosphorylation of STAT3 at Ser[727] but not at Thy[705]. STAT3 is a transcriptional mediator for IL-6 and IL-10. IL-10 plays an important antagonistic role to reduce the IgG immune complex–induced NF-κB activation. Thus, C5a may regulate the expression of cytokines and adhesion molecules through transcription-dependent pathways, and it may also participate in the negative feedback system in acute lung injury.

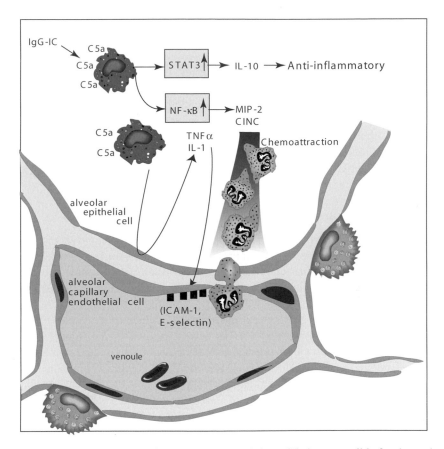

Figure 3 Regulatory role of C5a in acute lung injury. C5a is responsible for the early production of IL-1 and TNF-α in immune complex–induced acute lung injury, which leads to activation of adhesion molecules such as ICAM-1 and E-selectin on endothelial cells. C5a stimulation also results in NF-κB activation in alveolar macrophages, leading to generation of the CXC chemokines, MIP-2 and CINC. These chemokines, together with adhesion molecules, set a stage for neutrophil infiltration into lung. C5a signaling is responsible for STAT3 activation in lung after deposition of immune complexes, resulting in IL-10 production. IL-10 serves as an anti-inflammatory cytokine in this model of acute lung injury.

C5a IN I/R-MEDIATED TISSUE INJURY

Ischemia-reperfusion (I/R) injury is a common clinical event, which is characterized by the influx of neutrophils (100). During ischemia, cells and tissues undergo rapid changes that lead to perturbations in signaling pathways and surface molecule expression. In addition to ischemia caused by different types of vascular occlusion, as in most cases of myocardial infarcts, ischemic injury also appears in organ transplantation. After re-establishment or reconnection of the vasculature to the circulation, oxygen is reapplied and repair mechanisms are set into place. During reperfusion, accumulated toxic metabolites are flushed into the system, which may affect other organs and may negatively influence the process of regeneration in the ischemic organ. Under ischemic conditions, reduced oxygen supply leads to enhanced neutrophil adherence to endothelial cells owing to increased surface expression of adhesion molecules on endothelial cells (101–103). Activated neutrophils infiltrate the inflamed tissue directed by neutrophil chemoattractants. Activation of neutrophils results in a large production of ROS and the release of lysosomal enzymes in local injured organs. These toxic products lead to cell apoptosis and necrosis, resulting in loss of organ function.

Activation of Complement Pathways in I/R Injury

Complement activation and neutrophil infiltration are believed to be the most important key events in I/R injury. The requirement for the complement system in I/R-induced tissue injury has been established (6). All three pathways (classical, lectin, and alternative pathways) are activated and seem to be involved in I/R-related adverse events. C5a and the terminal MAC, C5b-9, are believed to be responsible for complement-mediated I/R-induced tissue injury. Depletion of the complement system by CVF is beneficial in liver I/R injury, accompanied by decreased polymorphonuclear leukocyte sequestration and reduced incidence of inflammatory reactions (104). Recombinant soluble complement receptor 1 (sCR1) is a complement regulatory glycoprotein that can inhibit activation of C3, thereby blocking the formation of C3a, C5a, and MAC. sCR1 showed significant beneficial effect in models of myocardial I/R (105, 106), experimental lung and liver transplantation (107–109), and intestinal I/R (110). sCR1 may also provide neuronal protection in a model of stroke and protection in I/R injury in skeletal muscle (111, 112).

Many natural and synthetic inhibitors targeting different complement activation pathways have been used to study the pathophysiology of I/R injury. Inhibition of classical pathway of complement activation by C1-INH provides protective roles in the animal models of liver, heart, and brain I/R injury (113–115). Blockade of the lectin pathway by monoclonal antibodies against rat MBL results in reduction of postischemic myocardial reperfusion injury in rats (116). More recently, factor D knockout mice have demonstrated the essential role of the alternative pathway in intestinal I/R injury (117). Factor D knockout mice display significantly less tissue damage in the intestine and lung after induction of I/R injury compared with heterozygote control animals, and also show significantly less C3 deposition in tissues. This is accompanied by less MPO activity in the intestine and lung of factor D knockout mice. Infusion of recombinant human factor D restored the tissue injury, whereas infusion of antibodies to human factor D protected mice from intestinal I/R injury again. Thus, all three complement pathways appear to be activated in I/R injury, and they may work cooperatively or independently in the development of such injury. The contribution of complement activation pathways in I/R injury could be organ-dependent. C3, C5, and C6 knockout mice were protected from kidney I/R injury, but there was no significant tissue protection in C4 knockout mice, again suggesting the importance of the alternative complement pathway (118). However, in skeletal and intestinal I/R injury experiments, both C3 and C4 knockout mice were equally protected from I/R injury, implying that the classical/lectin pathways of complement activation are important in these types of injury (119, 120).

Requirement of C5a in the Development of I/R Injury

C5 and C5a have long served as therapeutic targets in I/R injury because of their critical position in complement activation pathways. Anti-C5 treatment can inhibit both C5a production and MAC formation, thereby blocking the downstream signaling of C5a and MAC. I/R injury in intestine can be greatly attenuated by anti-C5 treatment. In the rat myocardial I/R model, anti-C5 treatment significantly reduced cell apoptosis, necrosis, and neutrophil accumulation in heart tissue (121). However, in human clinical trial studies, treatment of patients sustaining myocardial infarcts with anti-C5 monoclonal antibody did not reveal a convincing benefit in reducing infarct size (122, 123). The discrepancy between human clinical trial and animal model data remains to be resolved.

Although C5 antibody treatment blocks function of both C5a and MAC, and MAC plays an important role in maintaining immune function, blocking C5a instead of C5 may be more advantageous in the clinical setting. Therapy directed against the effects of C5a includes anti-C5a antibody and the C5aRa. A monoclonal antibody to C5a was shown to limit reperfusion injury in a pig model of myocardial infarction, as evidenced by reducing the infarct size (124). In a mouse model of renal I/R injury, C5aR expression is upregulated in tubular epithelial cells (125). Blockade of the C5aR pathway by C5aRa abrogated upregulation of CXC chemokines and infiltration of neutrophils into kidney tissue. C5aRa treatment prior to ischemia substantially reduced I/R-induced hematuria, vascular leakage, tissue levels of TNF-α and MPO, and serum levels of AST and creatinine (126). Administration of C5aRa prior to reperfusion reduced pathological markers of rat intestinal I/R, which include edema, increased blood levels at ALT, and mucosal damage (127). C3aR antagonist (C3aRa) displayed the same efficacies by ameliorating disease markers in the same model (128). However, administration of C3aRa caused a transient neutropenia and hypertension. C5aRa treatment reduced total hepatic I/R-induced mortality (129). In partial hepatic I/R rats, C5aRa treatment significantly attenuated the increases in liver enzymes, serum and tissue TNF-α, liver and lung MPO activity, and the number of infiltrating neutrophils, as well as neutrophilia and liver histopathology (129). In a rat model of limb I/R, anti-C5a antibody treatment significantly reduced lung vascular permeability, MPO content, and BAL levels of CXC chemokines (130). C5aRa treatment caused the reduction of multiple markers of local and remote organ injury following limb I/R (131). These data suggest that C5a is important in the development of I/R injury, including cardiac, renal, hepatic, intestinal, and skeletal muscle I/R injury.

As mentioned above, in I/R injury anti-C5a therapy is associated with decreased levels of neutrophil buildup in I/R organs. C5a not only serves as a powerful chemoattractant but, as indicated above, also causes activation of adhesion molecules; both functions are critical in neutrophil accumulation in organs. However, reduced I/R injury by blockade of C5a could also be neutrophil-independent. In renal I/R injury, C5aRa treatment significantly reduced the loss of renal function, abrogated CXC chemokine (KC and MIP-2) production, and reduced neutrophil infiltration by >50%. In this model, the protective role of C5aRa in renal function was neutrophil-independent (125). Although neutrophil infiltration occurred in I/R-injured kidney, depletion of neutrophils did not show any protective effect in renal dysfunction, and the beneficial effects of C5aRa were not attenuated in neutrophil-depleted mice. Thus, the role of C5a in I/R injury could be neutrophil-dependent as well as neutrophil-independent, and C5a/C5aR signaling-mediated inflammatory reactions may be sufficient to cause renal damage. In this model, C5aR expression was significantly upregulated in renal epithelial cells. C5a can activate epithelial cells to release inflammatory mediators, such as MIP-2 and TNF-α (13). Thus, the C5a/C5aR signaling seems essential in the development of I/R renal injury, probably via several mechanisms.

C5 as a Potential Target in Clinical Settings of I/R

Even though numerous experimental studies have demonstrated beneficial effects of complement inhibition for I/R-induced injury, there have been only a few clinical trials so far. sCR1 significantly inhibited postischemic myocardial inflammation and necrosis (105). These findings were extended in the rat by the use of sCR1 containing sialyl Lewis[x], emphasizing the function of sCR1 (106). Similar findings were made in cats, pigs, and rats using C1 esterase inhibitors (114, 132–134). These findings led to the first successful use of C1-inhibitors in patients receiving emergency coronary surgery for failed percutaneous transluminal coronary angioplasty in 1998 (135). In the group of patients suffering from severe reperfusion injury after coronary surgery, C1-INH seemed to be an effective adjuvant therapy to restore myocardial function. The first clinical use of anti-C5 treatment was launched in patients undergoing cardiopulmonary bypass surgery (136). In these studies, leukocyte activation, as measured by surface expression of CD11b, was reduced in patients who received anti-C5 antibody. In the group of patients treated with 2 mg/kg of antibody, there was a 40% reduction in myocardial injury, an 80% reduction in development of cognitive deficits, and a significant reduction in postoperative blood loss. In recent clinical studies, anti-C5 therapy has been combined with thrombolytic therapy and angioplasty therapy for treatment of patients with myocardial infarction (122, 123). These studies showed no measurable effect on the primary outcome (infarct size) in the anti-C5 treatment group. However, in the trial of C5 blockade in myocardial infarction associated with angioplasty, 90-day mortality was significantly reduced by 70% with bolus plus infusion of anti-C5 antibody, but the sample size was too small for statistical analysis. These data suggest that C5 inhibition may represent a novel therapeutic strategy for preventing complement-mediated inflammation and tissue injury, especially in the setting of I/R.

Data from numerous experimental studies of I/R injury in different organ systems as well as trials support the concept that inhibition of the complement system offers a therapeutic target for reducing harmful tissue injury in various clinical settings of I/R. Complement activation results in production of C5a and the MAC (C5b-9), which, in concert with neutrophils, are believed to be responsible for tissue injury during I/R. As depicted in Figure 4, MAC may directly cause cell death in tissues via induction of necrosis and/or apoptosis, and it can also trigger production of inflammatory mediators and increase adhesion molecule expression. Under such a circumstance, C5a can recruit inflammatory cells, especially neutrophils, in I/R organs. C5a stimulation of neutrophils leads to ROS production and proteinase releases, both of which may subsequently contribute to tissue damage in I/R organs. Thus, targeting C5, C5a, and C5aR may represent the most potent strategy to inhibit complement-induced organ injury during I/R.

C5a IN ALLERGY AND ASTHMA

Asthma has been recognized as an inflammatory disorder in genetically susceptible individuals, characterized by airway hyper-responsiveness (AHR) to inhaled allergens, excessive airway mucus production, lung eosinophil infiltration, and

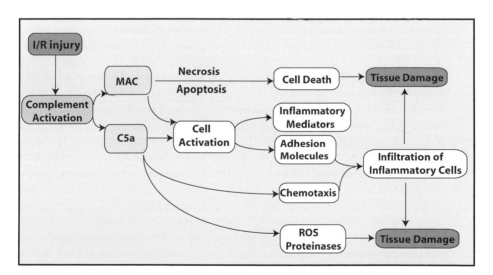

Figure 4 Complement activation contributes to the pathogenesis of I/R injury, resulting in generation of MAC and C5a. MAC may directly cause cell death in tissues via induction of necrosis and/or apoptosis, and it can also trigger production of inflammatory mediators and increase adhesion molecule expression. Expression of adhesion molecules and generation of C5a leads to infiltration of inflammatory cells, especially neutrophils, into I/R organs. ROS and proteinases released by C5-stimulated neutrophils contribute to tissue damage in I/R organs.

increased levels of serum IgE (137). In asthmatics, the airway walls and lung parenchyma contain a high level of mast cells, eosinophils, and mononuclear cells, which are mostly $CD4^+$ T cells. Another important feature of asthmatics is airway remodeling, which is triggered following local tissue damage. Airway remodeling and inflammation may result in AHR and airway obstruction. The degree of AHR is associated with the intensity of airway inflammation. Th2 cytokines (IL-4, IL-5, IL-13) released from $CD4^+$ T cells play a pivotal role in the pathogenesis of allergic asthma. Increasing evidence has suggested that activation of the complement system may be linked with the pathogenesis of asthma.

Evidence of Complement Activation in Allergy and Asthma

In atopic asthmatic patients, C5a/C5a *des Arg* was directly found in BAL fluids (138). When patients were challenged with allergen, elevated levels of C3a and C5a were found in BAL fluids, indicating that the complement system was activated in allergic inflammation of asthmatics (139). In the same study, the levels of both anaphylatoxins (C3a and C5a) were strongly correlated with eosinophil counts in BAL fluid. In a clinical setting, a nasal allergen challenge with increasing doses of pollens was performed in allergic subjects and in controls (140). In allergic subjects, allergen challenge–induced nasal symptoms is associated with increased levels of C3a *des Arg* and C5a *des Arg*, but there was no increase in the basal levels of C3a *des Arg* and C5a *des Arg* in the nonallergic controls, indicating that complement activation is accompanied by a vasculature exudative response during the immediate allergic reaction in the upper airway. Thus, complement activation occurs in the early phase of allergic reaction. Because of their potent biologic activity, these anaphylatoxins may constitute an essential part of the exudative response that promotes the ongoing inflammatory reaction. Purified C5a can initiate basophil histamine release, which is inhibited by antibody directed to the C5a receptor (141). Anti-C5a receptor antibody significantly inhibited histamine release induced by sera from patients with chronic urticaria, and the release of histamine from basophils stimulated with patient IgG was significantly enhanced by C5a, suggesting that C5a maybe responsible for the augmented release of histamine in urticaria (141).

It is reasonable to postulate that all three complement activation pathways are involved in the production of anaphylatoxins during allergic events. Allergens with carbohydrate structures may directly activate the lectin and alternative pathways, and allergen-antibody complex formation may result in classical pathway activation. Proteases from activated inflammatory cells (e.g., alveolar macrophages) may also serve as a protease source for cleavage of C3 and C5. In addition, proteases from allergens may cause cleavage of C3 and C5. For instance, house dust mite protease, Df-protease, shows strong activation of C3 and C5 in human serum, producing C3a and C5a by proteolytic cleavage of the complements (142).

The Essential Role of Complement Activation in Development of Asthma

The essential role of complement in allergic inflammation has been established in animal models. Repeated airway exposure of ovalbumin (OVA) in rats results in eosinophil and neutrophil infiltration into the bronchial submucosa, which can be suppressed by premedication with sCR1 or C5aRa (143). Although there is no systemic complement activation, C5aRa treatment before OVA exposure inhibits the late airway response, suggesting that endogenous C5a can be produced locally in lung. mRNA levels of C5aR, but not C3aR, in lung are strongly upregulated after the triple exposure to OVA. These two complement receptors are also constitutively expressed on bronchial epithelial and smooth muscle cells in both human and mouse lung (144). In a murine model of OVA-induced asthma, inhibition of complement activation by a recombinant complement inhibitor Crry-Ig (the complement receptor-related gene, fused to the IgG_1 hinge CH2 and CH3 domains) significantly prevented the development of AHR, decreased eosinophil and lymphocyte infiltration, decreased levels of IL-4, IL-5, and IL-13 in BAL, and decreased serum OVA-specific IgE and IgG_1 (145). By using chip technology, combined with quantitative trait locus analysis, the gene encoding C5 was identified as a susceptibility locus for allergen-induced AHR in a murine model of asthma (146). In the same study, the authors demonstrated that depletion of C5 in mice resulted in enhanced AHR in response to allergen challenge. Apparently, the results from the C5a inhibition experiment and C5-deficient mice do not agree in defining the role for complement activation in development of allergic inflammation, suggesting the functional complexity of complement activation products in asthma. Inhibition of complement activation during the effector phase may lead to a totally different outcome compared with inhibition of complement activation during the sensitization phase. In C5-deficient mice, C5a-initiated intracellular signaling cannot occur, but application of complement activation inhibitors may not completely shut down the C5a signaling.

Regulatory Effects of C5a in Allergic Asthma

C5a signaling is involved in both Th1 and Th2 responses via an IL-12-dependent pathway. IL-12 is a powerful cytokine that can inhibit the progression of experimental allergic asthma (147). It can elicit Th1 responses and inhibit Th2 responses, the latter being essential in the development of AHR. C5a/C5aR signaling is required for IL-12 production in human monocytes (146). Thus, the lack of IL-12 production favors Th2 responses, which may lead to the increased susceptibility to allergen-induced AHR in C5-deficient mice (146). C5aRa treatment in the rat model of OVA-induced asthma results in the suppression of IL-12, IL-4, IL-5, and eotaxin in BAL (143). These data suggest that C5a signaling is involved in both Th1 and Th2 responses. A recent review article points out that C5a/C5aR signaling plays a key role in protection from allergen-induced Th2 skewing by increasing IL-12 production, whereas C5a/C5L2 signaling inhibits IL-12 production, thereby promoting Th2 skewing (7). Thus, immune cells may adjust the expression pattern of C5aR and C5L2 to regulate Th1 and Th2 responses. This model can also explain the dual role of C5a in IL-12 production (70, 146). Interestingly, IL-4 can down-regulate the expression of C5aR on monocytes and dendritic cells (85). Therefore, decreased C5aR may serve as a feedback to limit IL-12 production and to promote Th2 skewing.

C5a has been recognized as a chemoattractant for neutrophils, monocytes, eosinophils, and T lymphocytes, and it can induce monocyte differentiation into dendritic cells (148). During allergic inflammation, C5a may activate mast cells and basophils, leading to degranulation and release of serotonin, TNF-α, and histamine (149, 150). These inflammatory cells and mediators constitute the basis for the development of AHR in asthma. Matrix metalloproteinases (MMPs) seem to be involved in tissue remodeling, and investigators have proposed that an excess of MMP-9 affects airway remodeling in chronic asthma (151). MMP-9 levels in BAL fluids clearly correlate with both acute and chronic asthma. MMP-9 might modulate airway remodeling by activating TGF-β, increasing collagen synthesis by fibroblasts, or increasing angiogenesis and airway vascular remodeling. C5a can induce MMP-9 release from human neutrophils (152). Thus, C5a may also be involved in tissue remodeling in asthma and in bronchospasm of allergic asthma. In guinea pig, C5a has been reported to stimulate airway smooth muscle contraction by inducing histamine release and production of cysteinyl leukotrienes (153).

As summarized in Figure 5, C5a regulates allergic inflammation of asthma in many ways, including proinflammatory and chemotactic activities, regulation of

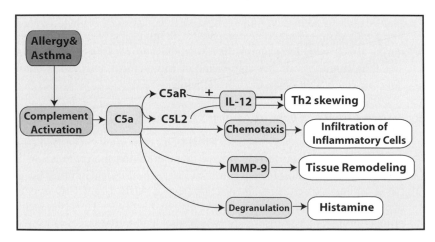

Figure 5   C5a in the pathogenesis of allergic asthma. C5a/C5aR signaling increases IL-12 production, which inhibits Th2 skewing, whereas C5a/C5L2 signaling may decrease IL-12 production, which promotes the Th2 skewing. As a chemoattractant, C5a recruits inflammatory cells, including eosinophils, into lung. C5a can stimulate mast cells and basophils to release histamine, and C5a may modulate tissue remodeling by inducing MMP-9 release from neutrophils.

Th1/Th2 responses, remodeling of damaged lung tissue, and induction of bronchospasm. These actions are likely regulated by production of C5a and expression of C5aR and C5L2. Definitive roles of C5aR and C5L2 are largely unknown. However, anti-C5a intervention appears to be an attractive strategy in treatment of asthmatic patients. In asthma, glucocorticoid therapy has been considered as a standard anti-inflammatory treatment. However, a significant number of patients fail to respond to this type of treatment. The steroid-resistant phenomena could be caused by high levels of MIF production in asthma, given that MIF can counteract the anti-inflammatory actions of glucocorticoids (154), and MIF levels in BAL fluids of asthmatic patients are significantly elevated (155). Researchers have recently recognized C5a as a strong inducer of MIF from eosinophils and neutrophils (69, 156). Therefore, anti-C5a strategy would not only be anti-inflammatory in its own action, but would also act by decreasing the potential inhibitory role of MIF on glucocorticoid therapy.

SUMMARY: C5a BLOCKING STRATEGIES IN INFLAMMATION

Complement inhibition is both advantageous and disadvantageous. An important aspect of complement inhibition therapy is to avoid disrupting the role of complement in host defenses, while effectively blocking the pathological activities of complement activation products. Interventions aimed at blocking C5a/C5aR or C5a/C5L2 signaling represent promising targets for therapeutic treatment in the inflammatory disorders discussed in this review. Targeting drug delivery to injured organs should be considered; it would minimally affect function of systemic complement activation. Small molecule antagonists for C5aR have potential application in humans. It will not be surprising to see clinical data addressing the contribution of C5a to immunopathology in the coming years.

ACKNOWLEDGMENTS

Research was supported by grants from the National Institutes of Health (GM-61656, GM-02957, and HL-31963).

The *Annual Review of Immunology* is online at
http://immunol.annualreviews.org

LITERATURE CITED

1. Ward PA. 2004. The dark side of C5a in sepsis. *Nat. Rev. Immunol.* 4:133–42

2. Robbins RA, Russ WD, Rasmussen JK, Clayton MM. 1987. Activation of the complement system in the adult respiratory distress syndrome. *Am. Rev. Respir. Dis.* 135:651–58

3. Linton SM, Morgan BP. 1999. Complement activation and inhibition in

experimental models of arthritis. *Mol. Immunol.* 36:905–14

4. Welch TR. 2002. Complement in glomerulonephritis. *Nat. Genet.* 31:333–34

5. Ffrench-Constant C. 1994. Pathogenesis of multiple sclerosis. *Lancet* 343:271–75

6. Arumugam TV, Shiels IA, Woodruff TM, Granger DN, Taylor SM. 2004. The role of the complement system in ischemia-reperfusion injury. *Shock* 21:401–9

7. Hawlisch H, Wills-Karp M, Karp CL, Kohl J. 2004. The anaphylatoxins bridge innate and adaptive immune responses in allergic asthma. *Mol. Immunol.* 41:123–31

8. Marder SR, Chenoweth DE, Goldstein IM, Perez HD. 1985. Chemotactic responses of human peripheral blood monocytes to the complement-derived peptides C5a and C5a des Arg. *J. Immunol.* 134:3325–31

9. Goldstein IM, Weissmann G. 1974. Generation of C5-derived lysosomal enzyme-releasing activity (C5a) by lysates of leukocyte lysosomes. *J. Immunol.* 113:1583–88

10. Sacks T, Moldow CF, Craddock PR, Bowers TK, Jacob HS. 1978. Oxygen radicals mediate endothelial cell damage by complement-stimulated granulocytes. An in vitro model of immune vascular damage. *J. Clin. Invest.* 61:1161–67

11. Mollnes TE, Brekke OL, Fung M, Fure H, Christiansen D, et al. 2002. Essential role of the C5a receptor in *E. coli*-induced oxidative burst and phagocytosis revealed by a novel lepirudin-based human whole blood model of inflammation. *Blood* 100:1869–77

12. Schumacher WA, Fantone JC, Kunkel SE, Webb RC, Lucchesi BR. 1991. The anaphylatoxins C3a and C5a are vasodilators in the canine coronary vasculature in vitro and in vivo. *Agents Actions* 34:345–49

13. Riedemann NC, Guo RF, Sarma VJ, Laudes IJ, Huber-Lang M, et al. 2002. Expression and function of the C5a receptor in rat alveolar epithelial cells. *J. Immunol.* 168:1919–25

14. Laudes IJ, Chu JC, Huber-Lang M, Guo RF, Riedemann NC, et al. 2002. Expression and function of C5a receptor in mouse microvascular endothelial cells. *J. Immunol.* 169:5962–70

15. Guo RF, Huber-Lang M, Wang X, Sarma V, Padgaonkar VA, et al. 2000. Protective effects of anti-C5a in sepsis-induced thymocyte apoptosis. *J. Clin. Invest.* 106:1271–80

16. Riedemann NC, Guo RF, Laudes IJ, Keller K, Sarma VJ, et al. 2002. C5a receptor and thymocyte apoptosis in sepsis. *FASEB J.* 16:887–88

17. Perianayagam MC, Balakrishnan VS, King AJ, Pereira BJ, Jaber BL. 2002. C5a delays apoptosis of human neutrophils by a phosphatidylinositol 3-kinase-signaling pathway. *Kidney Int.* 61:456–63

18. Guo RF, Riedemann NC, Laudes IJ, Sarma VJ, Kunkel RG, et al. 2002. Altered neutrophil trafficking during sepsis. *J. Immunol.* 169:307–14

19. Laudes IJ, Chu JC, Sikranth S, Huber-Lang M, Guo RF, et al. 2002. Anti-C5a ameliorates coagulation/fibrinolytic protein changes in a rat model of sepsis. *Am. J. Pathol.* 160:1867–75

20. Gerard NP, Hodges MK, Drazen JM, Weller PF, Gerard C. 1989. Characterization of a receptor for C5a anaphylatoxin on human eosinophils. *J. Biol. Chem.* 264:1760–66

21. Gerard NP, Gerard C. 1991. The chemotactic receptor for human C5a anaphylatoxin. *Nature* 349:614–17

22. Okinaga S, Slattery D, Humbles A, Zsengeller Z, Morteau O, et al. 2003. C5L2, a nonsignaling C5a binding protein. *Biochemistry* 42:9406–15

23. Ohno M, Hirata T, Enomoto M, Araki T, Ishimaru H, et al. 2000. A putative chemoattractant receptor, C5L2, is expressed in granulocyte and immature dendritic cells, but not in mature dendritic cells. *Mol. Immunol.* 37:407–12

24. Chenoweth DE, Hugli TE. 1978. Demonstration of specific C5a receptor on intact human polymorphonuclear leukocytes. *Proc. Natl. Acad. Sci. USA* 75:3943–47

25. Kurimoto Y, de Weck AL, Dahinden CA. 1989. Interleukin 3-dependent mediator release in basophils triggered by C5a. *J. Exp. Med.* 170:467–79

26. Werfel T, Oppermann M, Schulze M, Krieger G, Weber M, et al. 1992. Binding of fluorescein-labeled anaphylatoxin C5a to human peripheral blood, spleen, and bone marrow leukocytes. *Blood* 79:152–60

27. Haviland DL, McCoy RL, Whitehead WT, Akama H, Molmenti EP, et al. 1995. Cellular expression of the C5a anaphylatoxin receptor (C5aR): demonstration of C5aR on nonmyeloid cells of the liver and lung. *J. Immunol.* 154:1861–69

28. Schieferdecker HL, Schlaf G, Jungermann K, Gotze O. 2001. Functions of anaphylatoxin C5a in rat liver: direct and indirect actions on nonparenchymal and parenchymal cells. *Int. Immunopharmacol.* 1:469–81

29. Riedemann NC, Guo RF, Neff TA, Laudes IJ, Keller KA, et al. 2002. Increased C5a receptor expression in sepsis. *J. Clin. Invest.* 110:101–8

30. Huber-Lang M, Younkin EM, Sarma JV, Riedemann N, McGuire SR, et al. 2002. Generation of C5a by phagocytic cells. *Am. J. Pathol.* 161:1849–59

31. Bone RC, Balk RA, Cerra FB, Dellinger RP, Fein AM, et al. 1992. Definitions for sepsis and organ failure and guidelines for the use of innovative therapies in sepsis. The ACCP/SCCM Consensus Conference Committee. American College of Chest Physicians/Society of Critical Care Medicine. *Chest* 101:1644–55

32. Bone RC, Sprung CL, Sibbald WJ. 1992. Definitions for sepsis and organ failure. *Crit. Care Med.* 20:724–26

33. Riedemann NC, Guo RF, Ward PA. 2003. The enigma of sepsis. *J. Clin. Invest.* 112:460–67

34. de Boer JP, Creasey AA, Chang A, Roem D, Eerenberg AJ, et al. 1993. Activation of the complement system in baboons challenged with live *Escherichia coli*: correlation with mortality and evidence for a biphasic activation pattern. *Infect. Immun.* 61:4293–301

35. Smedegard G, Cui LX, Hugli TE. 1989. Endotoxin-induced shock in the rat. A role for C5a. *Am. J. Pathol.* 135:489–97

36. Bengtson A, Heideman M. 1988. Anaphylatoxin formation in sepsis. *Arch. Surg.* 123:645–49

37. Nakae H, Endo S, Inada K, Takakuwa T, Kasai T, et al. 1994. Serum complement levels and severity of sepsis. *Res. Commun. Chem. Pathol. Pharmacol.* 84:189–95

38. Zhao L, Ohtaki Y, Yamaguchi K, Matsushita M, Fujita T, et al. 2002. LPS-induced platelet response and rapid shock in mice: contribution of O-antigen region of LPS and involvement of the lectin pathway of the complement system. *Blood* 100:3233–39

39. Sprong T, Brandtzaeg P, Fung M, Pharo AM, Hoiby EA, et al. 2003. Inhibition of C5a-induced inflammation with preserved C5b-9-mediated bactericidal activity in a human whole blood model of meningococcal sepsis. *Blood* 102:3702–10

40. Hopken UE, Lu B, Gerard NP, Gerard C. 1996. The C5a chemoattractant receptor mediates mucosal defense to infection. *Nature* 383:86–89

41. Huber-Lang MS, Younkin EM, Sarma JV, McGuire SR, Lu KT, et al. 2002. Complement-induced impairment of innate immunity during sepsis. *J. Immunol.* 169:3223–31

42. Ayala A, Herdon CD, Lehman DL, DeMaso CM, Ayala CA, Chaudry IH. 1995. The induction of accelerated thymic programmed cell death during polymicrobial sepsis: control by corticosteroids but not tumor necrosis factor. *Shock* 3:259–67

43. Ayala A, Chaudry IH. 1996. Immune dysfunction in murine polymicrobial sepsis: mediators, macrophages, lymphocytes and apoptosis. *Shock* 6:S27–38

44. Ayala A, Xu YX, Chung CS, Chaudry IH. 1999. Does Fas ligand or endotoxin contribute to thymic apoptosis during polymicrobial sepsis? *Shock* 11:211–17

45. Oberholzer C, Oberholzer A, Bahjat FR, Minter RM, Tannahill CL, et al. 2001. Targeted adenovirus-induced expression of IL-10 decreases thymic apoptosis and improves survival in murine sepsis. *Proc. Natl. Acad. Sci. USA* 98:11503–8

46. Hotchkiss RS, Chang KC, Swanson PE, Tinsley KW, Hui JJ, et al. 2000. Caspase inhibitors improve survival in sepsis: a critical role of the lymphocyte. *Nat. Immunol.* 1:496–501

47. Le Tulzo Y, Pangault C, Gacouin A, Guilloux V, Tribut O, et al. 2002. Early circulating lymphocyte apoptosis in human septic shock is associated with poor outcome. *Shock* 18:487–94

48. Jimenez MF, Watson RW, Parodo J, Evans D, Foster D, et al. 1997. Dysregulated expression of neutrophil apoptosis in the systemic inflammatory response syndrome. *Arch. Surg.* 132:1263–70

49. Simon HU. 2003. Neutrophil apoptosis pathways and their modifications in inflammation. *Immunol. Rev.* 193:101–10

50. Meagher LC, Cousin JM, Seckl JR, Haslett C. 1996. Opposing effects of glucocorticoids on the rate of apoptosis in neutrophilic and eosinophilic granulocytes. *J. Immunol.* 156:4422–28

51. Mohr M, Hopken U, Oppermann M, Mathes C, Goldmann K, et al. 1998. Effects of anti-C5a monoclonal antibodies on oxygen use in a porcine model of severe sepsis. *Eur. J. Clin. Invest.* 28:227–34

52. Stevens JH, O'Hanley P, Shapiro JM, Mihm FG, Satoh PS, et al. 1986. Effects of anti-C5a antibodies on the adult respiratory distress syndrome in septic primates. *J. Clin. Invest.* 77:1812–16

53. Czermak BJ, Sarma V, Pierson CL, Warner RL, Huber-Lang M, et al. 1999. Protective effects of C5a blockade in sepsis. *Nat. Med.* 5:788–92

54. Huber-Lang M, Sarma VJ, Lu KT, McGuire SR, Padgaonkar VA, et al. 2001. Role of C5a in multi-organ failure during sepsis. *J. Immunol.* 166:1193–99

55. Deitch EA. 1992. Multiple organ failure. Pathophysiology and potential future therapy. *Ann. Surg.* 216:117–34

56. Baue AE, Durham R, Faist E. 1998. Systemic inflammatory response syndrome (SIRS), multiple organ dysfunction syndrome (MODS), multiple organ failure (MOF): Are we winning the battle? *Shock* 10:79–89

57. Baue AE. 2000. Multiple organ failure—the discrepancy between our scientific knowledge and understanding and the management of our patients. *Langenbecks Arch. Surg.* 385:441–53

58. Baue AE. 2003. Sepsis, systemic inflammatory response syndrome, multiple organ dysfunction syndrome, and multiple organ failure: Are trauma surgeons lumpers or splitters? *J. Trauma* 55:997–98

59. Ebong SJ, Call DR, Bolgos G, Newcomb DE, Granger JI, et al. 1999. Immunopathologic responses to non-lethal sepsis. *Shock* 12:118–26

60. Faist E, Wichmann MW. 1997. Immunology in the severely injured. *Chirurg* 68:1066–70 (In German)

61. Nakae H, Endo S, Inada K, Yoshida M. 1996. Chronological changes in the complement system in sepsis. *Surg. Today* 26:225–29

62. Wang SD, Huang KJ, Lin YS, Lei HY. 1994. Sepsis-induced apoptosis of the thymocytes in mice. *J. Immunol.* 152:5014–21

63. Ayala A, Herdon CD, Lehman DL, Ayala CA, Chaudry IH. 1996. Differential induction of apoptosis in lymphoid tissues during sepsis: variation in onset, frequency, and the nature of the mediators. *Blood* 87:4261–75

64. Barke RA, Roy S, Chapin RB, Charboneau R. 1994. The role of programmed cell death (apoptosis) in thymic involution following sepsis. *Arch. Surg.* 129:1256–62

65. Papathanassoglou ED, Moynihan JA, Ackerman MH. 2000. Does programmed cell death (apoptosis) play a role in the development of multiple organ dysfunction in critically ill patients? A review and a theoretical framework. *Crit. Care Med.* 28:537–49

66. Strieter RM, Kasahara K, Allen RM, Standiford TJ, Rolfe MW, et al. 1992. Cytokine-induced neutrophil-derived interleukin-8. *Am. J. Pathol.* 141:397–407

67. Hopken U, Mohr M, Struber A, Montz H, Burchardi H, et al. 1996. Inhibition of interleukin-6 synthesis in an animal model of septic shock by anti-C5a monoclonal antibodies. *Eur. J. Immunol.* 26:1103–9

68. Monsinjon T, Gasque P, Chan P, Ischenko A, Brady JJ, et al. 2003. Regulation by complement C3a and C5a anaphylatoxins of cytokine production in human umbilical vein endothelial cells. *FASEB J.* 17:1003–14

69. Riedemann NC, Guo RF, Gao H, Sun L, Hoesel M, et al. 2004. Regulatory role of C5a on macrophage migration inhibitory factor release from neutrophils. *J. Immunol.* 173:1355–59

70. Wittmann M, Zwirner J, Larsson VA, Kirchhoff K, Begemann G, et al. 1999. C5a suppresses the production of IL-12 by IFN-γ-primed and lipopolysaccharide-challenged human monocytes. *J. Immunol.* 162:6763–69

71. Riedemann NC, Guo RF, Bernacki KD, Reuben JS, Laudes IJ, et al. 2003. Regulation by C5a of neutrophil activation during sepsis. *Immunity* 19:193–202

72. Pan ZK. 1998. Anaphylatoxins C5a and C3a induce nuclear factor κB activation in human peripheral blood monocytes. *Biochim. Biophys. Acta* 1443:90–98

73. Aird WC. 2003. The role of the endothelium in severe sepsis and multiple organ dysfunction syndrome. *Blood* 101:3765–77

74. Ikeda K, Nagasawa K, Horiuchi T, Tsuru T, Nishizaka H, et al. 1997. C5a induces tissue factor activity on endothelial cells. *Thromb. Haemost.* 77:394–98

75. Muhlfelder TW, Niemetz J, Kreutzer D, Beebe D, Ward PA, et al. 1979. C5 chemotactic fragment induces leukocyte production of tissue factor activity: a link between complement and coagulation. *J. Clin. Invest.* 63:147–50

76. Carson SD, Johnson DR. 1990. Consecutive enzyme cascades: complement activation at the cell surface triggers increased tissue factor activity. *Blood* 76:361–67

77. Horuk R. 1994. The interleukin-8-receptor family: from chemokines to malaria. *Immunol. Today* 15:169–74

78. Molad Y, Haines KA, Anderson DC, Buyon JP, Cronstein BN. 1994. Immunocomplexes stimulate different signalling events to chemoattractants in the neutrophil and regulate L-selectin and β2-integrin expression differently. *Biochem. J.* 299(Pt. 3):881–87

79. Jagels MA, Daffern PJ, Hugli TE. 2000. C3a and C5a enhance granulocyte adhesion to endothelial and epithelial cell monolayers: epithelial and endothelial priming is required for C3a-induced eosinophil adhesion. *Immunopharmacology* 46:209–22

80. Guo RF, Riedemann NC, Bernacki KD, Sarma VJ, Laudes IJ, et al. 2003. Neutrophil C5a receptor and the outcome in a rat model of sepsis. *FASEB J.* 13:1889–91

81. Seely AJ, Naud JF, Campisi G, Giannias B, Liu S, et al. 2002. Alteration of chemoattractant receptor expression regulates human neutrophil chemotaxis in vivo. *Ann. Surg.* 235:550–59

82. Van Epps DE, Simpson S, Bender JG, Chenoweth DE. 1990. Regulation of C5a and formyl peptide receptor expression on human polymorphonuclear leukocytes. *J. Immunol.* 144:1062–68

83. Naik N, Giannini E, Brouchon L, Boulay

F. 1997. Internalization and recycling of the C5a anaphylatoxin receptor: evidence that the agonist-mediated internalization is modulated by phosphorylation of the C-terminal domain. *J. Cell Sci.* 110:2381–90

84. Gilbert TL, Bennett TA, Maestas DC, Cimino DF, Prossnitz ER. 2001. Internalization of the human N-formyl peptide and C5a chemoattractant receptors occurs via clathrin-independent mechanisms. *Biochemistry* 40:3467–75

85. Soruri A, Kiafard Z, Dettmer C, Riggert J, Kohl J, et al. 2003. IL-4 down-regulates anaphylatoxin receptors in monocytes and dendritic cells and impairs anaphylatoxin-induced migration in vivo. *J. Immunol.* 170:3306–14

86. Song GY, Chung CS, Chaudry IH, Ayala A. 2000. IL-4-induced activation of the Stat6 pathway contributes to the suppression of cell-mediated immunity and death in sepsis. *Surgery* 128:133–38

87. Tellado JM, McGowen GC, Christou NV. 1993. Decreased polymorphonuclear leukocyte exudation in critically ill anergic patients associated with increased adhesion receptor expression. *Crit. Care Med.* 21:1496–501

88. Meddows-Taylor S, Pendle S, Tiemessen CT. 2001. Altered expression of CD88 and associated impairment of complement 5a-induced neutrophil responses in human immunodeficiency virus type 1-infected patients with and without pulmonary tuberculosis. *J. Infect. Dis.* 183:662–65

89. Ishii Y, Kobayashi J, Kitamura S. 1989. Chemotactic factor generation and cell accumulation in acute lung injury induced by endotracheal acid instillation. *Prostaglandins Leukot Essent. Fatty Acids* 37:65–70

90. Winter SM, Paradis IL, Dauber JH, Griffith BP, Hardesty RL, et al. 1989. Proteins of the respiratory tract after heart-lung transplantation. *Transplantation* 48:974–80

91. Guo RF, Ward PA. 2002. Mediators and regulation of neutrophil accumulation in inflammatory responses in lung: insights from the IgG immune complex model. *Free Radic. Biol. Med.* 33:303–10

92. Czermak BJ, Lentsch AB, Bless NM, Schmal H, Friedl HP, et al. 1998. Role of complement in in vitro and in vivo lung inflammatory reactions. *J. Leukoc. Biol.* 64:40–48

93. Bozic CR, Lu B, Hopken UE, Gerard C, Gerard NP. 1996. Neurogenic amplification of immune complex inflammation. *Science* 273:1722–25

94. Mulligan MS, Schmid E, Beck-Schimmer B, Till GO, Friedl HP, et al. 1996. Requirement and role of C5a in acute lung inflammatory injury in rats. *J. Clin. Invest.* 98:503–12

95. Czermak BJ, Sarma V, Bless NM, Schmal H, Friedl HP, et al. 1999. In vitro and in vivo dependency of chemokine generation on C5a and TNF-α. *J. Immunol.* 162:2321–25

96. Foreman KE, Vaporciyan AA, Bonish BK, Jones ML, Johnson KJ, et al. 1994. C5a-induced expression of P-selectin in endothelial cells. *J. Clin. Invest.* 94:1147–55

97. Mulligan MS, Schmid E, Till GO, Hugli TE, Friedl HP, et al. 1997. C5a-dependent up-regulation in vivo of lung vascular P-selectin. *J. Immunol.* 158:1857–61

98. Albrecht EA, Chinnaiyan AM, Varambally S, Kumar-Sinha C, Barrette TR, et al. 2004. C5a-induced gene expression in human umbilical vein endothelial cells. *Am. J. Pathol.* 164:849–59

99. Gao H, Guo RF, Speyer CL, Reuben J, Neff TA, et al. 2004. Stat3 activation in acute lung injury. *J. Immunol.* 172:7703–12

100. Carden DL, Granger DN. 2000. Pathophysiology of ischaemia-reperfusion injury. *J. Pathol.* 190:255–66

101. Milhoan KA, Lane TA, Bloor CM. 1992. Hypoxia induces endothelial cells to increase their adherence for neutrophils:

role of PAF. *Am. J. Physiol. Heart Circ.* 263:H956–62

102. Goldman G, Welbourn R, Klausner JM, Valeri CR, Shepro D, et al. 1991. Thromboxane mediates diapedesis after ischemia by activation of neutrophil adhesion receptors interacting with basally expressed intercellular adhesion molecule-1. *Circ. Res.* 68:1013–19

103. Jerome SN, Dore M, Paulson JC, Smith CW, Korthuis RJ. 1994. P-selectin and ICAM-1-dependent adherence reactions: role in the genesis of postischemic noreflow. *Am. J. Physiol. Heart Circ.* 266: H1316–21

104. Jaeschke H, Bautista AP, Spolarics Z, Spitzer JJ. 1991. Superoxide generation by Kupffer cells and priming of neutrophils during reperfusion after hepatic ischemia. *Free Radic. Res. Commun.* 15: 277–84

105. Weisman HF, Bartow T, Leppo MK, Marsh HC Jr, Carson GR, et al. 1990. Soluble human complement receptor type 1: in vivo inhibitor of complement suppressing post-ischemic myocardial inflammation and necrosis. *Science* 249:146–51

106. Zacharowski K, Otto M, Hafner G, Marsh HC Jr, Thiemermann C. 1999. Reduction of myocardial infarct size with sCR1sLe^x, an alternatively glycosylated form of human soluble complement receptor type 1 (sCR1), possessing sialyl Lewis x. *Br. J. Pharmacol.* 128:945–52

107. Stammberger U, Hamacher J, Hillinger S, Schmid RA. 2000. sCR1sLe ameliorates ischemia/reperfusion injury in experimental lung transplantation. *J. Thorac. Cardiovasc. Surg.* 120:1078–84

108. Lehmann TG, Koeppel TA, Kirschfink M, Gebhard MM, Herfarth C, et al. 1998. Complement inhibition by soluble complement receptor type 1 improves microcirculation after rat liver transplantation. *Transplantation* 66:717–22

109. Lehmann TG, Koeppel TA, Munch S, Heger M, Kirschfink M, et al. 2001. Impact of inhibition of complement by sCR1 on hepatic microcirculation after warm ischemia. *Microvasc. Res.* 62:284–92

110. Hill J, Lindsay TF, Ortiz F, Yeh CG, Hechtman HB, et al. 1992. Soluble complement receptor type 1 ameliorates the local and remote organ injury after intestinal ischemia-reperfusion in the rat. *J. Immunol.* 149:1723–28

111. Huang J, Kim LJ, Mealey R, Marsh HC J Jr, Zhang Y, Tenner AJ, et al. 1999. Neuronal protection in stroke by an sLex-glycosylated complement inhibitory protein. *Science* 285:595–99

112. Kyriakides C, Wang Y, Austen WG J Jr, Favuzza J, Kobzik L, et al. 2001. Moderation of skeletal muscle reperfusion injury by a sLe^x-glycosylated complement inhibitory protein. *Am. J. Physiol. Cell. Physiol.* 281:C224–30

113. Bergamaschini L, Gobbo G, Gatti S, Caccamo L, Prato P, et al. 2001. Endothelial targeting with C1-inhibitor reduces complement activation in vitro and during ex vivo reperfusion of pig liver. *Clin. Exp. Immunol.* 126;412–20

114. Horstick G, Berg O, Heimann A, Gotze O, Loos M, et al. 2001. Application of C1-esterase inhibitor during reperfusion of ischemic myocardium: dose-related beneficial versus detrimental effects. *Circulation* 104:3125–31

115. De Simoni MG, Storini C, Barba M, Catapano L, Arabia AM, et al. 2003. Neuroprotection by complement (C1) inhibitor in mouse transient brain ischemia. *J. Cereb. Blood Flow Metab.* 23:232–39

116. Jordan JE, Montalto MC, Stahl GL. 2001. Inhibition of mannose-binding lectin reduces postischemic myocardial reperfusion injury. *Circulation* 104:1413–18

117. Stahl GL, Xu Y, Hao L, Miller M, Buras JA, et al. 2003. Role for the alternative complement pathway in ischemia/reperfusion injury. *Am. J. Pathol.* 162:449–55

118. Zhou W, Farrar CA, Abe K, Pratt JR, Marsh JE, et al. 2000. Predominant role

for C5b-9 in renal ischemia/reperfusion injury. *J. Clin. Invest.* 105:1363–71

119. Weiser MR, Williams JP, Moore FD J Jr, Kobzik L, Ma M, et al. 1996. Reperfusion injury of ischemic skeletal muscle is mediated by natural antibody and complement. *J. Exp. Med.* 183:2343–48

120. Williams JP, Pechet TT, Weiser MR, Reid R, Kobzik L, et al. 1999. Intestinal reperfusion injury is mediated by IgM and complement. *J. Appl. Physiol.* 86:938–42

121. Vakeva AP, Agah A, Rollins SA, Matis LA, Li L, et al. 1998. Myocardial infarction and apoptosis after myocardial ischemia and reperfusion: role of the terminal complement components and inhibition by anti-C5 therapy. *Circulation* 97:2259–67

122. Mahaffey KW, Granger CB, Nicolau JC, Ruzyllo W, Weaver WD, et al. 2003. Effect of pexelizumab, an anti-C5 complement antibody, as adjunctive therapy to fibrinolysis in acute myocardial infarction: the COMPlement inhibition in myocardial infarction treated with thromboLYtics (COMPLY) trial. *Circulation* 108:1176–83

123. Granger CB, Mahaffey KW, Weaver WD, Theroux P, Hochman JS, et al. 2003. Pexelizumab, an anti-C5 complement antibody, as adjunctive therapy to primary percutaneous coronary intervention in acute myocardial infarction: the COMplement inhibition in Myocardial infarction treated with Angioplasty (COMMA) trial. *Circulation* 108:1184–90

124. Tofukuji M, Stahl GL, Agah A, Metais C, Simons M, et al. 1998. Anti-C5a monoclonal antibody reduces cardiopulmonary bypass and cardioplegia-induced coronary endothelial dysfunction. *J. Thorac. Cardiovasc. Surg.* 116:1060–68

125. de Vries B, Kohl J, Leclercq WK, Wolfs TG, van Bijnen AA, et al. 2003. Complement factor C5a mediates renal ischemia-reperfusion injury independent from neutrophils. *J. Immunol.* 170:3883–89

126. Arumugam TV, Shiels IA, Strachan AJ, Abbenante G, Fairlie DP, et al. 2003. A small molecule C5a receptor antagonist protects kidneys from ischemia/reperfusion injury in rats. *Kidney Int.* 63:134–42

127. Arumugam TV, Shiels IA, Woodruff TM, Reid RC, Fairlie DP, et al. 2002. Protective effect of a new C5a receptor antagonist against ischemia-reperfusion injury in the rat small intestine. *J. Surg. Res.* 103:260–67

128. Proctor LM, Arumugam TV, Shiels I, Reid RC, Fairlie DP, et al. 2004. Comparative anti-inflammatory activities of antagonists to C3a and C5a receptors in a rat model of intestinal ischaemia/reperfusion injury. *Br. J. Pharmacol.* 142:756–64

129. Arumugam TV, Woodruff TM, Stocks SZ, Proctor LM, Pollitt S, et al. 2004. Protective effect of a human C5a receptor antagonist against hepatic ischaemia-reperfusion injury in rats. *J. Hepatol.* 40:934–41

130. Bless NM, Warner RL, Padgaonkar VA, Lentsch AB, Czermak BJ, et al. 1999. Roles for C-X-C chemokines and C5a in lung injury after hindlimb ischemia-reperfusion. *Am. J. Physiol.* 276:L57–63

131. Woodruff TM, Arumugam TV, Shiels IA, Reid RC, Fairlie DP, et al. 2004. Protective effects of a potent C5a receptor antagonist on experimental acute limb ischemia-reperfusion in rats. *J. Surg. Res.* 116:81–90

132. Horstick G, Heimann A, Gotze O, Hafner G, Berg O, et al. 1997. Intracoronary application of C1 esterase inhibitor improves cardiac function and reduces myocardial necrosis in an experimental model of ischemia and reperfusion. *Circulation* 95:701–8

133. Buerke M, Prufer D, Dahm M, Oelert H, Meyer J, et al. 1998. Blocking of classical complement pathway inhibits endothelial adhesion molecule expression and preserves ischemic myocardium from reperfusion injury. *J. Pharmacol. Exp. Ther.* 286:429–38

134. Buerke M, Murohara T, Lefer AM. 1995. Cardioprotective effects of a C1 esterase inhibitor in myocardial ischemia and reperfusion. *Circulation* 91:393–402

135. Bauernschmitt R, Bohrer H, Hagl S. 1998. Rescue therapy with C1-esterase inhibitor concentrate after emergency coronary surgery for failed PTCA. *Intensive Care Med.* 24:635–38

136. Fitch JC, Rollins S, Matis L, Alford B, Aranki S, et al. 1999. Pharmacology and biological efficacy of a recombinant, humanized, single-chain antibody C5 complement inhibitor in patients undergoing coronary artery bypass graft surgery with cardiopulmonary bypass. *Circulation* 100:2499–506

137. Cohn L, Elias JA, Chupp GL. 2004. Asthma: mechanisms of disease persistence and progression. *Annu. Rev. Immunol.* 22:789–815

138. Teran LM, Campos MG, Begishvilli BT, Schroder JM, Djukanovic R, et al. 1997. Identification of neutrophil chemotactic factors in bronchoalveolar lavage fluid of asthmatic patients. *Clin. Exp. Allergy* 27:396–405

139. Krug N, Tschernig T, Erpenbeck VJ, Hohlfeld JM, Kohl J. 2001. Complement factors C3a and C5a are increased in bronchoalveolar lavage fluid after segmental allergen provocation in subjects with asthma. *Am. J. Respir. Crit. Care Med.* 164:1841–43

140. Andersson M, Michel L, Llull JB, Pipkorn U. 1994. Complement activation on the nasal mucosal surface—a feature of the immediate allergic reaction in the nose. *Allergy* 49:242–45

141. Kikuchi Y, Kaplan AP. 2002. A role for C5a in augmenting IgG-dependent histamine release from basophils in chronic urticaria. *J. Allergy Clin. Immunol.* 109:114–18

142. Maruo K, Akaike T, Ono T, Okamoto T, Maeda H. 1997. Generation of anaphylatoxins through proteolytic processing of C3 and C5 by house dust mite protease. *J. Allergy Clin. Immunol.* 100:253–60

143. Abe M, Shibata K, Akatsu H, Shimizu N, Sakata N, et al. 2001. Contribution of anaphylatoxin C5a to late airway responses after repeated exposure of antigen to allergic rats. *J. Immunol.* 167:4651–60

144. Drouin SM, Kildsgaard J, Haviland J, Zabner J, Jia HP, et al. 2001. Expression of the complement anaphylatoxin C3a and C5a receptors on bronchial epithelial and smooth muscle cells in models of sepsis and asthma. *J. Immunol.* 166:2025–32

145. Taube C, Rha YH, Takeda K, Park JW, Joetham A, et al. 2003. Inhibition of complement activation decreases airway inflammation and hyperresponsiveness. *Am. J. Respir. Crit. Care Med.* 168:1333–41

146. Karp CL, Grupe A, Schadt E, Ewart SL, Keane-Moore M, et al. 2000. Identification of complement factor 5 as a susceptibility locus for experimental allergic asthma. *Nat. Immunol.* 1:221–26

147. Gavett SH, O'Hearn DJ, Li X, Huang SK, Finkelman FD, et al. 1995. Interleukin 12 inhibits antigen-induced airway hyperresponsiveness, inflammation, and Th2 cytokine expression in mice. *J. Exp. Med.* 182:1527–36

148. Soruri A, Riggert J, Schlott T, Kiafard Z, Dettmer C, Zwirner J. 2003. Anaphylatoxin C5a induces monocyte recruitment and differentiation into dendritic cells by TNF-α and prostaglandin E2-dependent mechanisms. *J. Immunol.* 171:2631–36

149. el-Lati SG, Dahinden CA, Church MK. 1994. Complement peptides C3a- and C5a-induced mediator release from dissociated human skin mast cells. *J. Invest. Dermatol.* 102:803–6

150. Askenase PW, Tsuji RF. 2000. B-1 B cell IgM antibody initiates T cell elicitation of contact sensitivity. *Curr. Top. Microbiol. Immunol.* 252:171–77

151. Atkinson JJ, Senior RM. 2003. Matrix metalloproteinase-9 in lung remodeling. *Am. J. Respir. Cell Mol. Biol.* 28:12–24

152. Takafuji S, Ishida A, Miyakuni Y, Naka-gawa T. 2003. Matrix metalloproteinase-9 release from human leukocytes. *J. Investig. Allergol. Clin. Immunol.* 13:50–55

153. Stimler NP, Bach MK, Bloor CM, Hugli TE. 1982. Release of leukotrienes from guinea pig lung stimulated by C5a des Arg anaphylatoxin. *J. Immunol.* 128:2247–52

154. Calandra T, Bernhagen J, Metz CN, Spiegel LA, Bacher M, et al. 1995. MIF as a glucocorticoid-induced modulator of cytokine production. *Nature* 377:68–71

155. Sabroe I, Pease JE, Williams TJ. 2000. Asthma and MIF: innately Th1 and Th2. *Clin. Exp. Allergy* 30:1194–96

156. Rossi AG, Haslett C, Hirani N, Greening AP, Rahman I, et al. 1998. Human circulating eosinophils secrete macrophage migration inhibitory factor (MIF). Potential role in asthma. *J. Clin. Invest.* 101:2869–74

Annu. Rev. Immunol. 2005. 23:853–75
doi: 10.1146/annurev.immunol.23.021704.115811
Copyright © 2005 by Annual Reviews. All rights reserved
First published online as a Review in Advance on December 17, 2004

DNA Degradation in Development and Programmed Cell Death

Shigekazu Nagata

Laboratory of Genetics, Integrated Biology Laboratories, Graduate School of Frontier Biosciences, Osaka University; Department of Genetics, Osaka University Medical School; Solution Oriented Research for Science and Technology, Japanese Science and Technology Agency, Osaka, Japan; email: nagata@genetic.med.osaka-u.ac.jp

Key Words apoptosis, erythropoiesis, lens cell differentiation, tissue atrophy, anemia, cataract, autoimmune disease

■ **Abstract** Most mammalian cells have nuclei that contain DNA, which replicates during cell proliferation. DNA is destroyed by various developmental processes in mammals. It is degraded during programmed cell death that accompanies mammalian development. The nuclei of erythrocytes and eye lens fiber cells are also removed during their differentiation into mature cells. If DNA is not properly degraded in these processes, it can cause various diseases, including tissue atrophy, anemia, cataract, and autoimmune diseases, which indicates that DNA can be a pathogenic molecule. Here, I present how DNA is degraded during programmed cell death, erythroid cell differentiation, and lens cell differentiation. I discuss what might be or will be learned from understanding the molecular mechanisms of DNA degradation that occurs during mammalian development.

INTRODUCTION

Human DNA, consisting of 3×10^9 bases, carries at least 30,000 genes, the information of which is used to direct the synthesis of proteins that build up and characterize cells. When useless or toxic cells are generated during animal development, or cells become senescent, they are programmed to die (programmed cell death) and are actively killed by a process called apoptosis (1). During apoptotic cell death, DNA is degraded into nucleosomal units in most cases (2), a hallmark of apoptosis. Recent studies have identified DNases responsible for apoptotic DNA degradation and show that DNA degradation itself is not essential for cell death but is essential for maintaining the homeostasis of animals (3).

If DNA is degraded, cells will not survive. Yet, we have "living" or at least "functional" cells that do not carry DNA. They are red blood cells (erythrocytes) and lens fiber cells in the eyes. DNA is removed or degraded at the final stage of their differentiation to mature red blood cells or lens fiber cells. Specific DNases have recently been identified for DNA degradation in erythroid precursor cells and

0732-0582/05/0423-0853$14.00

lens fiber cells (4, 5). Mice deficient in the respective DNase develop anemia and cataract, indicating that DNA degradation is an essential step for differentiation of erythroid cells and lens fiber cells.

PROGRAMMED CELL DEATH

Programmed cell death is a crucial process for mammalian development. It is involved in morphogenic events, such as digit formation, sexual differentiation, development of the immune and nervous systems, and metamorphosis (6, 7). Many superfluous or potentially harmful cells are produced during these developmental processes, and they are programmed to die by apoptosis in most cases. In adults, billions of senescent cells undergo apoptosis every day and are replaced by newly generated cells. Virally infected and cancerous cells are also killed by the immune system through apoptosis. So, the failure of apoptotic cell death causes an abnormal accumulation of cells, which often leads to cancer. By contrast, excessive or exaggerated apoptotic cell death causes tissue injuries, as seen in autoimmune diseases and neurodegenerative disorders (8, 9).

Apoptosis is morphologically characterized by shrinking and fragmentation of cells and their nuclei; this is different from necrotic cell death, which is accompanied by swelling of cells and their organelles (1). Apoptotic bodies are recognized by professional phagocytes (macrophages and immature dendritic cells), as well as by nonprofessional phagocytes (fibroblasts and endothelial cells) (10). Engulfment of apoptotic cells is a swift process, and it is difficult to find nonengulfed dying cells, even in tissues where many cells are known to undergo apoptosis (11). Engulfment is essential for cell death and tissue remodeling (10, 12), and if apoptotic cells are left unengulfed, cellular contents will be released by dying cells and may cause autoimmune diseases (13–15).

Programmed cell death is triggered by intrinsic and extrinsic stimuli and is mediated by caspases, a family of cysteine proteases (16, 17). Caspases exist as zymogens (procaspases) in proliferating cells. When apoptosis is triggered, caspases are activated by proteolysis to form an active enzyme as an $\alpha_2\beta_2$ tetramer (18). Human and mouse genomes carry 13 caspase genes (caspases 1–12, and caspase 14), which are divided into two groups. Human caspases 3 and 6–10 belong to the same phylogenetic group and are involved in cellular apoptosis, whereas caspases 1, 4, 5, 11, 12, and 14 belong to another group and are involved in inflammation (19). Caspases that function in the apoptotic process are further divided into two subgroups, initiator (caspases 8 and 9) and executor (caspases 3, 6, and 7). Initiator caspases 8 and 9 are activated by the extrinsic and intrinsic pathways, respectively (Figure 1).

The intrinsic pathway can be triggered by anticancer drugs, γ-irradiation, antioxidants, and growth-factor or serum deprivation, and it can be blocked by the oncogene Bcl-2. In this pathway, Bcl-2 homolog (BH) 3-only proteins, such as Puma, Noxa, and Bad, are transcriptionally activated via p53 (Puma and Noxa) or

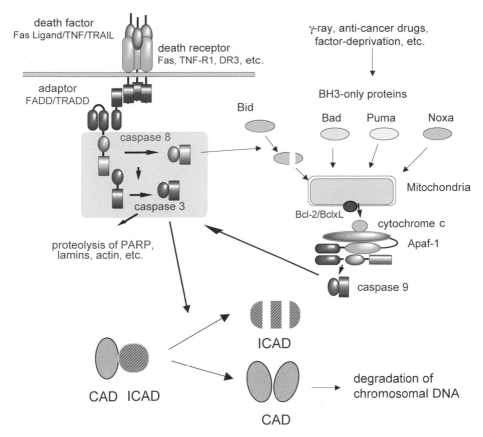

Figure 1 Apoptotic signaling pathways leading to DNA degradation. Apoptosis can be generally categorized into two pathways, extrinsic and intrinsic. In the extrinsic pathway, death factors activate caspase 8 as initiator caspases through the death receptors and adaptors. In the intrinsic pathway, anticancer drugs or growth-factor deprivation transcriptionally or post-transcriptionally activate BH3-only members of the Bcl-2 family. BH3-only members stimulate mitochondria to release cytochrome c, which can be inhibited by Bcl-2. Cytochrome c then activates caspase 9 together with an adaptor Apaf-1. Caspase 8 or caspase 9, thus activated, cleaves procaspase 3 to mature caspase 3 downstream of the caspase cascade. Caspase 3 cleaves ICAD (inhibitor of CAD) at two positions, which releases ICAD from CAD (caspase-activated DNase). CAD then forms a homodimer to become an active endonuclease.

released from their adaptor by dephosphorylation (Bad) (16, 17). These BH3-only proteins stimulate mitochondria to release cytochrome c that can activate caspase 9 together with an adaptor called apoptotic protease activating factor 1 (Apaf-1). The extrinsic pathway is triggered by death factors, such as Fas ligand (CD95 ligand), tumor necrosis factor (TNF), and TNF-related apoptosis-inducing ligand (TRAIL) (20, 21). In the extrinsic pathway, the death-inducing signaling complex (DISC), consisting of a receptor, adaptor, and procaspase 8, is formed downstream of the death receptor (21). In the DISC, procaspase 8 is autocatalytically processed to the active enzyme, which then directly activates caspase 3, an executor caspase, or cleaves a BH3-only protein Bid. Truncated Bid then induces release of cytochrome c from mitochondria (17). Executor caspases are known to cleave more than 280 nuclear and cytoplasmic proteins that are essential cell components, including kinases, transcription factors, DNA polymerases, RNA polymerase, and cytoskeletal proteins (22). Cleavage of these molecules inactivates their enzymatic activity in most cases and leads to cell death by inducing morphological and biochemical changes that characterize apoptosis.

TWO INDEPENDENT MECHANISMS FOR DNA DEGRADATION IN PROGRAMMED CELL DEATH

At the early stage of apoptosis, DNA is cleaved into large fragments (50–200 kb) (23, 24), which are subsequently cleaved into nucleosomal units (180 bp). DNA cleavage into nucleosomal units is one of the hallmarks of apoptosis (25) and is the basis for the terminal deoxynucleotidyl transferase-mediated dUTP nick end labeling (TUNEL) technique that is commonly used to detect apoptotic cells in vitro and in vivo (26). Many enzymes and factors have been proposed as responsible for DNA degradation. These factors include DNase I, DNase II, DNase γ, cyclophilin, caspase-activated DNase (CAD; also known as DNA fragmentation factor, or DFF40), and endonuclease G. Recent studies of apoptotic DNA degradation in vitro and in vivo indicate that two independent systems are involved in DNA degradation during programmed cell death (27–33). The first system is a cell-autonomous system that functions in dying cells, and the other system takes place in macrophages after dying cells are engulfed by phagocytes (Figure 2).

Cell-Autonomous DNA Degradation During Programmed Cell Death

The DNase responsible for cell-autonomous DNA degradation in dying cells is CAD because no apoptotic DNA degradation is observed in *CAD*-deficient mouse or *Drosophila* cells (3, 30, 31, 33). CAD is an endonuclease that works at neutral pH and generates double-stranded DNA breaks with a hydroxyl group at the 3′ end (34) that serve as good substrates for terminal deoxynucleotidyltransferase (TdT) (35). CAD carries histidine residues at its active site (35, 36), and the tertiary structure of mouse CAD, as shown by X-ray structure analysis, indicates that it is a homodimer that forms a scissors-like structure with a coordinating Zn ion at the active site (37) (Figure 3). It cleaves naked DNA in the cleft of the scissors. Nucleosomes cannot enter the cleft owing to structural hindrance, so CAD cleaves DNA only at the spacer regions between nucleosomes, which explains why CAD generates nucleosomal units of DNA. CAD carries a nuclear localization signal,

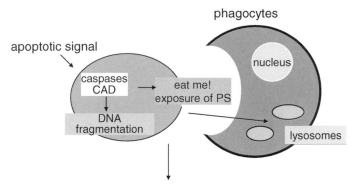

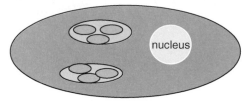

Figure 2   Apoptosis coupled with phagocytosis. When cells receive apoptotic stimuli, a cascade of caspases is activated, which leads to death by cleaving various cellular proteins, and by degrading DNA by CAD. Dying cells expose phosphatidylserine (PS) as an "eat me" signal to the surface, which is recognized by macrophages for engulfment. Engulfed dead cells go into lysosomes of macrophages, and their DNA is degraded by DNase II.

which also explains why only DNA in the nucleus, but not in mitochondria, is cleaved during apoptosis (2, 38).

CAD is a DNase with high specific activity that is potentially harmful to cells (28, 39). It cannot be synthesized alone but requires its partner, inhibitor of CAD (ICAD; also known as DFF45), for its functional folding (29, 40). ICAD has an 80 amino acid domain [CAD/CIDE (cell death–inducing DFF45-like effector) domain] at its amino-terminus that can bind to the corresponding region of CAD by a homophilic interaction (41). When CAD is synthesized on ribosomes, ICAD binds to the CAD/CIDE domain of the CAD nascent polypeptide and enhances its correct folding, together with chaperones Hsp40 and Hsp70, and CAD is released from ribosomes as a complex with ICAD (42). When cells receive apoptotic stimuli, caspase 3 cleaves ICAD at two positions (27, 29) (Figure 1). Cleaved ICAD loses its affinity for CAD, and CAD is freed to cleave chromosomal DNA in the nucleus. Accordingly, if either caspase 3 or ICAD genes are inactivated, cells cannot produce active CAD and do not undergo apoptotic DNA fragmentation (31, 33, 43).

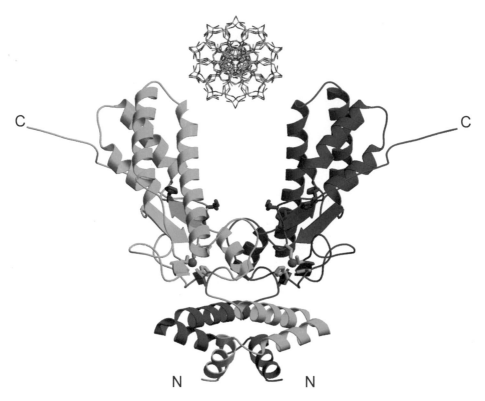

Figure 3   Tertiary structure of CAD. The active CAD dimer has a scissors-like structure, which was revealed by X-ray analysis. Each subunit is shown in green and blue. Histidine and lysine residues in the active site are in magenta and light blue, respectively, and zinc is shown as orange spheres. At the top of the cleft, a DNA strand around a nucleosome core is shown on the same scale. Reproduced from Reference 37 with permission from Elsevier.

CAD is abundantly expressed in lymphocytes that show prominent DNA fragmentation during apoptosis (44). Apoptotic DNA fragmentation is not apparent in nerve cells, hepatocytes, or embryonal fibroblasts, in which expression of CAD is low (44). When a CAD expression vector is introduced into fibroblasts together with ICAD, fibroblasts show DNA fragmentation upon exposure to apoptotic stimuli (44, 45). Exposure of *Drosophila* embryos to ultraviolet radiation makes apoptotic cell death detectable by TUNEL. However, few TUNEL-positive cells are found in *Drosophila* embryos that are deficient in ICAD (N. Mukae & S. Nagata, unpublished observations), confirming that the CAD-ICAD system plays a nonredundant role in cell-autonomous apoptotic DNA fragmentation.

DNA fragmentation is observed in most cases of apoptosis. If DNA is cleaved, cells will not proliferate and die. DNA fragmentation was therefore thought to be an essential step for cell death during apoptosis. Indeed, when recombinant, active CAD is microinjected into cells, it cleaves DNA and immediately kills the cells (46). Nonetheless, DNA degradation itself is dispensable for cell death by apoptosis (29, 44). This can be explained as follows. Caspases are activated by apoptotic stimuli upstream of CAD and cleave many cellular components, such as DNA polymerase, RNA polymerase, transcription factors, and ribosomal proteins that are essential for cell viability (22). If one of these enzymes or factors is cleaved and inactivated by caspases, the cell will not survive. Once caspases are activated in cells, there are likely dozens of ways to kill cells. This idea is supported by the fact that even enucleated cells undergo apoptotic death, showing typical morphological changes in cells (47, 48). Accordingly, mice with a *CAD* or *ICAD* (*DFF45*) deficiency develop normally (3, 31, 33) and show no abnormal phenotype. One report claims that *DFF45*-null mice exhibit an increased number of granule cells in dentate gyrus and exhibit enhanced spatial learning (49). Whether caspases are activated, and whether caspase substrates are cleaved in $DFF45^{-/-}$ granule cells, should be examined.

Among other DNases proposed for apoptotic DNA fragmentation, endonuclease G released from mitochondria during apoptosis was reported to translocate into nuclei to digest DNA (50, 51). Wang et al. (52) subsequently reported that apoptosis-inducing factor (AIF) co-operates with endonuclease G to promote DNA degradation in programmed cell death of *Caenorhabditis elegans*. However, endonuclease G is rather (dG)n/(dC)n-specific (53) and cleaves not only DNA in internucleosomal regions but also DNA within nucleosomes (54). As discussed by Wildlak et al. (54), it is unlikely that endonuclease G alone is involved in apoptotic cleavage of chromosomal DNA. The observation that the number of TUNEL-positive cells increases in an *endonuclease G*–deficient mutant of *C. elegans* (55) supports this notion. Zhang et al. (56) recently reported that *endonuclease G*–deficient mice are embryonic lethal. As discussed above, cells lacking nuclei undergo apoptosis, and DNA fragmentation is not essential for cell death. So, it is not clear how lack of *endonuclease G* causes the lethality of embryos. CAD induces condensation and fragmentation of nuclei, but apoptotic morphological change of nuclei, particularly chromatin condensation, can still be observed in cells deficient in *CAD* (57). A protein called Acinus was suggested as causing chromatin condensation in a caspase-dependent manner (58). However, Acinus was later shown to be a component of splicesome (59), and it is not clear how Acinus causes morphological changes of nuclei.

DNA Degradation of Apoptotic Cells in Macrophages

Cells that lack *CAD* or *ICAD* do not undergo DNA fragmentation in vitro in response to various apoptotic stimuli (33, 44). Accordingly, when mice are exposed to γ-rays, the number of TUNEL-positive cells in the thymus is dramatically reduced by *CAD* deficiency. The remaining TUNEL-positive thymocytes in *CAD*-deficient mice are inside macrophages in most cases. Apoptotic cells that are produced during mouse development can be detected in vivo by TUNEL staining even in *CAD*-deficient mice, and their number is similar to those found in wild-type mice. It seems that all apoptotic cells generated during mouse development are swiftly engulfed by phagocytes even when their DNA is not degraded in dying cells. However, if a large number of apoptotic cells are generated by pathological stimuli such as exposure to γ-rays, the number of apoptotic cells exceeds the capacity of the phagocytes to engulf them, and dying cells are left unengulfed, generating many TUNEL-positive cells.

Apoptotic cells in *CAD*-deficient mice have no means of digesting their own chromosomal DNA. Yet, they were TUNEL-positive inside macrophages. We therefore proposed that a DNase that is present in the lysosomes of macrophages digests the DNA of apoptotic cells after they are phagocytosed (33) (Figure 2). DNase II is a DNase that works under acidic conditions (60, 61). When apoptotic cells from *CAD*-deficient mice were cocultured with macrophages, dying cells were engulfed by macrophages, and their DNA was degraded in the macrophages (33). By contrast, when *DNase II*–deficient macrophages were used as phagocytes to engulf *CAD*-null apoptotic thymocytes, many undigested nuclei accumulated in the lysosomes of the macrophages (3).

This result was confirmed in vivo. *DNase II*–null as well as *DNase II-CAD*-double null mouse embryos contained many abnormal macrophages carrying undigested DNA (3, 62) (Figure 4). DNA that accumulated in *DNase II*–null macrophages seemed to be fragmented, but DNA in *DNase II-CAD*-double null mutant mice was intact. So, we propose that the DNA of dying cells is degraded in two steps (Figure 2). First, DNA is degraded by CAD into nucleosomal units while nucleosomes are intact. The corpses are engulfed by macrophages and transferred to their lysosomes. Lysosomal proteases digest proteins of the corpses, which includes nucleosomal proteins, and DNase II in lysosomes digests the DNA of apoptotic cells into nucleotides.

These findings also apply to *Drosophila*. *Drosophila* embryos carry nucleosomal unit DNA fragments that can be detected by ligation-mediated polymerase chain reaction (LMPCR) (63). DNA fragments are not observed in embryos that are deficient in *Drosophila ICAD*, and they are more apparent in mutants that are deficient in *DNase II* (30). This confirms that CAD in *Drosophila* also generates DNA fragments in nucleosomal units in programmed cell death, and DNase II further digests the DNA (30). *Nuc-1*, a *C. elegans* homolog of DNase II (64), is responsible for DNA degradation during programmed cell death in *C. elegans* (65). Although CAD has not been identified in *C. elegans*, the existence of strong TUNEL-positive cells in *Nuc-1* mutants (64) suggests that *C. elegans* also carries a CAD homolog or DNase that has a similar function.

ACTIVATION OF INNATE IMMUNITY BY DNA THAT ESCAPES FROM DEGRADATION DURING PROGRAMMED CELL DEATH

DNase II–deficient mice die in feto late in embryogenesis (4). The development of some tissues is impaired in *DNase II*–null embryos and is more severely impaired in *DNase II-CAD*-double null embryos (3). For example, T cell development is

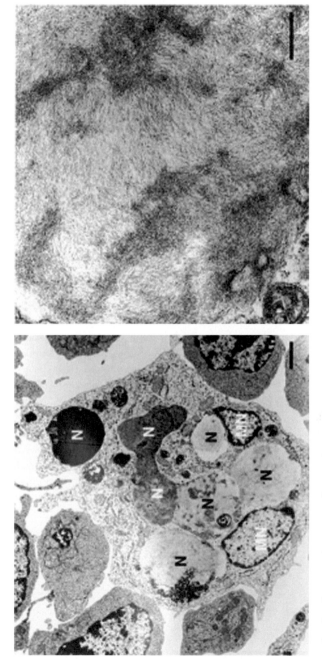

Figure 4   An electron microscope picture of macrophages in *DNase II-CAD*-double null embryos. Left panel shows a macrophage carrying many undigested nuclei (*N*). Right panel shows many long and intact strings in macrophages that could be DNA escaped from apoptotic degradation. Scale bar: 0.5 μm. Reproduced from Reference 3.

blocked at the pro-T cell stage in these mutant mice, and the number of thymocytes in double-null embryos is reduced to 15%–25% of the wild-type thymus (3). What happens when DNA is not properly degraded during programmed cell death? Among several cytokine genes examined, the interferon-β (IFN-β) gene is strongly activated in the thymus of *DNase II*–null mice (about tenfold compared with wild-type mice), and this induction is further enhanced to ~100-fold in *DNase II-CAD*-double null embryos. Type I IFNs (IFN-α and IFN-β) are used to treat patients with leukemia or hepatitis C virus, but they are known to have strong cytotoxicity, which causes tissue atrophy including of the thymus (66). Production of IFN-β in *DNase II-CAD*-double null embryos indicates that if the DNA of apoptotic cells is not properly degraded, IFN-β is produced and kills the animals.

How is the IFN-β gene activated by endogenous DNA? When mice are infected by bacteria, the nonmethylated CpG motif of bacterial DNA activates innate immunity through Toll-like receptor 9 (TLR9), which leads to induction of type I IFN genes (67). By contrast, mammalian DNA is mostly methylated and cannot activate TLR9-mediated innate immunity. It is not clear how the IFN-β gene is activated in *DNase II-CAD*-double null mice. Innate immunity in *Drosophila* is activated by two independent pathways (68). In one pathway, Gram-positive bacteria or fungi activate the antifungal peptide drosomycin gene through the Toll/Myd88 pathway. In the other pathway, Gram-negative bacteria induce expression of genes for antibacterial peptides (diptericin and attacin) by a Toll-independent immune deficiency pathway. In *DNase II-CAD*-double null flies, diptericin and attacin, but not drosomycin, genes are activated (30), which suggests that at least in *Drosophila* endogenous DNA can activate innate immunity in a Toll-independent manner.

Human patients who suffer from the autoimmune disease systemic lupus erythematosus often have a high titer of anti-DNA antibodies. Mammalian DNA, unlike bacterial DNA, cannot induce an antibody response by immunization (69), and DNA that is released from dying cells as a nuclear complex may work as autoantigens (70, 71). Production of IFN-β in *DNase II*–null mice suggests that endogenous, probably naked DNA that has escaped apoptotic DNA fragmentation can activate innate immunity. Whether this can lead to antibody production remains to be determined. In any case, understanding the molecular mechanism by which the IFN-β gene or innate immunity is activated by endogenous DNA might increase our understanding of human autoimmune diseases.

DNA DEGRADATION DURING ERYTHROPOIESIS

Mammalian red blood cells have no nuclei because they are removed at the final stage of erythroid cell differentiation (Figure 5). How nuclei are removed from red blood cells is not well understood. Early in normal mouse embryogenesis, red blood cells are produced in the yolk sac, and they are nucleated (primitive erythrocytes) (72). From E12.5 onward, erythropoiesis takes place in fetal liver instead of the yolk sac. Similar to erythroid cells produced in bone marrow in the adult, those produced in the fetal liver are enucleated; they are known as "definitive

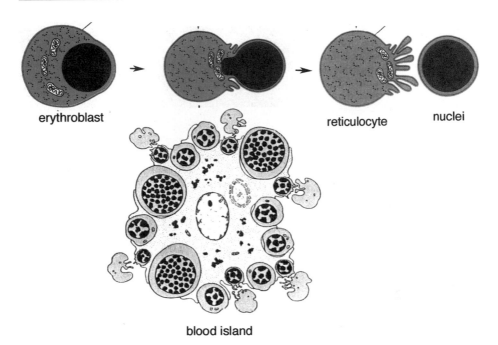

erythroblast   reticulocyte   nuclei

blood island

Figure 5   Enucleation of erythroid precursor cells and erythropoiesis in blood islands. During late erythropoiesis, cellular components of erythroblasts asymmetrically redistribute nuclei to one part and other components to the other part (*top*). At the final stage of this process, nuclei are expelled from erythroblasts, which leaves reticulocytes that later mature into erythrocytes. In bone marrow and fetal livers, erythropoiesis takes place at a specific location known as "blood islands" in which a macrophage in the center is surrounded by red blood cells of various developmental stages (*bottom*). Enucleation of erythroid precursor cells also occurs at this location. (Reprinted from Alberts B, Johnson A, Lewis J, Raff M, Roberts K, Walter P. 2002. *Molecular Biology of the Cell*, p. 1292. New York: Garland Sci., 4th ed., with permission from Taylor & Francis.)

erythrocytes." *DNase II*–null embryos suffer from severe anemia (4); the number of primitive erythrocytes at E12.5 is normal, but the number of definitive erythrocytes at E17.5 is severely reduced (less than 10% of the number in wild-type mice). This suggests that definitive erythropoiesis is specifically affected in *DNase II*–null mutants. When fetal liver cells are transferred into an irradiated host, *DNase II*–null precursor cells differentiate into mature enucleated erythrocytes, which indicates that DNase II is not necessary in erythroid cells, but is necessary in cells that support erythropoiesis.

The fetal liver of *DNase II*–null mouse has many abnormal Feulgen-positive foci, each of which consists of a macrophage that contains many undigested nucleus-like structures (Figure 6). These macrophages are surrounded by many erythroid cells at different developmental stages (erythroblast, reticulocytes, and mature enucleated erythrocytes), which indicates that these are abnormal blood

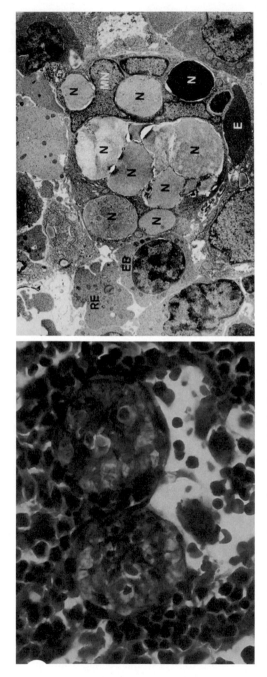

Figure 6 Macrophages carrying undigested nuclei in the fetal liver of *DNase II*–deficient embryos. The fetal liver section from *DNase II*–deficient embryos was stained with hematoxilin-eosin that detects nuclei and cytoplasm. There are many abnormal foci throughout the liver of *DNase II*–deficient embryos (*left panel*). Analysis by electron microscope indicates that these foci are macrophages in blood islands carrying numerous undigested nuclei (N) (*right panel*). RE, reticulocytes; EB, erythroblastoid cells; E, mature erythrocytes; MN, macrophage nuclei. Reproduced from Reference 4.

islands (73). Erythropoiesis takes place in these blood islands of fetal liver or bone marrow. Each island contains a macrophage in the center. The presence of undigested nuclei in macrophages suggests that these macrophages engulf the nuclei that are expelled from erythroid precursor cells and that DNase II in macrophages is responsible for digesting the DNA of these nuclei. Enucleation of erythroid precursor cells is thought to occur cell-autonomously without help from other cells (74). When mice are administered with Dichloromethylene diphosphonate (Cl_2MBP) encapsulated in liposomes, this drug is selectively incorporated into macrophages and kills them by disturbing their ion metabolism (75). But this treatment also impairs erythropoiesis (76, 77), which suggests a role for macrophages in definitive erythropoiesis. The presence of macrophages that engulf expelled nuclei may accelerate the enucleation process (78).

Macrophages engulf apoptotic but not living cells by recognizing phosphatidylserine that is exposed on apoptotic cells as an "eat me" signal (10, 79–81). During differentiation of erythroid cells, nuclei are expelled from erythroid precursors, leaving reticulocytes that further mature into red blood cells (Figure 5). Nuclei that are expelled from erythroid precursor cells are engulfed by macrophages, whereas reticulocytes are not. What molecule on nuclei is recognized for engulfment is not known. Surface markers on erythroid precursor cells are redistributed during erythroid cell maturation by an enigmatic process (74, 82, 83). The nucleus preferentially binds concanavalin A, whereas reticulocytes bind wheat germ agglutinin. Spectrin and ankyrin are also sequestered within the reticulocyte. Whether these surface markers function as the "eat me" signal of nuclei or the "do not eat me" signal of reticulocytes for macrophages needs to be clarified. In any case, it will be interesting to examine whether any of the molecules that are proposed to be involved in engulfment of apoptotic cells (10) also play a role in engulfment of nuclei that are expelled from erythroid precursor cells. Phosphatidylserine is exposed on the surface of apoptotic cells in a caspase-dependent manner. Caspase is activated during erythroid cell maturation and cleaves a set of substrates such as the GATA-1 transcription factor and lamin, which may play a role in enucleation (84, 85). Whether caspases are involved in presenting the "eat nuclei" signal to macrophages remains to be determined.

The *DNase II*–null mice do not accumulate erythroid precursor cells that contain a nucleus, which suggests that the defect is not simply at the enucleation process. IFN-β is known to inhibit erythropoiesis at the early stage (86). As discussed above for the thymus, innate immunity is likely also activated in macrophages carrying undigested DNA in fetal liver, which leads to induction of IFN-β gene expression.

DNA DEGRADATION DURING LENS CELL DIFFERENTIATION

Like erythrocytes, lens fiber cells also lack nuclei; nuclei and other cellular organelles (mitochondria and endoplasmic reticulum) are removed during differentiation into mature cells (87, 88). Elimination of cellular organelles in the lens

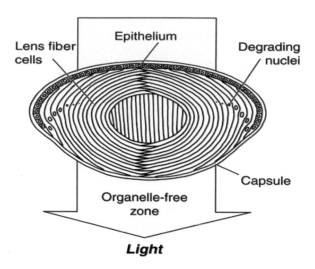

Figure 7   Differentiation from epithelial to fiber cells in the eye lens. An eye lens enclosed by a membrane-like structure (capsule) is schematically shown. At the apical part of the lens, there is a monolayer of proliferating epithelial cells. At the equator, epithelial cells move into the cortex and differentiate to fiber cells. During this process, cellular organelles such as nuclei, mitochondria, and endoplasmic reticulum are lost, forming an organelle-free zone in the center of the lens. Reproduced from Reference 112 with permission from Elsevier.

occurs during embryogenesis and after birth. In the embryonic lens, organelles are present initially throughout the lens tissues. In late embryogenesis, however, they are eliminated from the center of the lens, forming an organelle-free zone. In the neonatal lens, a monolayer of proliferating epithelial cells lies at the apical portion of the eye. At the equator of the lens, cells move toward the nucleus and start to differentiate into fiber cells (Figure 7). During this differentiation process, cells express a set of genes for crystallins that are major proteins in the eye lens. At the same time, they abruptly lose their organelles (nuclei, mitochondria, endoplasmic reticulum, and ribosomes) and housekeeping enzymes (RNA polymerase and DNA polymerase, etc.). This process is most active at the neonatal stage, but it continues throughout the life of the animal. Because there is no turnover of senescent fiber cells in the lens, the eyeball keeps growing until the animal's death.

Several groups have reported evidence for an involvement of apoptosis in lens cell differentiation (89–91). Degenerating nuclei in differentiating fiber cells are detectable by TUNEL (89). Bcl-2 and caspase 9 are expressed in the eye (92), and overexpression of Bcl-2, an inhibitor of apoptosis that is expressed in the lens, disrupts fiber cell differentiation (93). However, CAD, the endonuclease that is responsible for apoptotic DNA degradation, is not expressed in the eye, and there is no abnormality in the eye of *CAD*-null mice (5). In accord with the lack of macrophages in the lens, DNase II is not expressed in the lens either. On the other hand, DNase II–like acid DNase (DLAD; also known as DNase IIβ) (94, 95) is specifically and strongly expressed in human and murine lens cells. Mice that are deficient in the *DLAD* gene are incapable of degrading DNA during lens cell differentiation, and undigested DNA accumulates in fiber cells (Figure 8). These results indicate that DLAD is mainly responsible for degrading DNA during lens cell differentiation, and other proposed DNases, such as L-DNase II and DNase I (96, 97), might not play an important role in this process.

DLAD is active in acid conditions and is probably localized to lysosomes (94). In *DLAD*-null fiber cells, naked DNA remains in the cytoplasm, but mitochondria, the endoplasmic reticulum, and the nuclear membrane are completely lost (5). We propose that cellular organelles are degraded by autophagy in their own lysosomes during lens cell differentiation. Lysosomes contain not only DLAD but also proteases, glycosidases, and lipases. Most proteins, sugars, and lipids of cellular organelles are completely degraded in *DLAD*-deficient mice, and free DNA is left in the cytoplasm. The molecular mechanism of autophagy has been extensively studied in yeast, and several molecules that are involved in this process have been identified (98, 99). It will be interesting to examine whether these molecules are expressed in the lens, in particular in cells at the cortex, where organelles are destroyed. An in vitro differentiation system from epithelial or embryonal stem cells to lens fiber cells has been developed for chicken and monkey cells (100, 101). If this system can be applied to mouse cells, it will be useful for studies on lens cell differentiation and on the possible involvement of autophagy in this process.

DLAD-null mice develop weak cataracts, and their response to light is severely reduced (5). The development of cataracts in *DLAD*-null mice is apparently a direct effect caused by DNA accumulating in lens fiber cells, which confirms that nuclei must be lost from fiber cells to ensure the transparency of the lens. If other organelles are left undigested in the lens, they may also cause cataracts. Some human cataracts thus may be caused by a genetic defect that impairs removal of organelles during lens cell differentiation.

CONCLUSIONS

In his 1980 article (2), Dr. Andrew H. Wyllie reported for the first time apoptotic DNA fragmentation and discussed its relationship with DNA degradation during terminal differentiation of normoblasts (erythrocyte precursors) and lens fiber cells. We now know the enzymes responsible for DNA degradation that occurs during these developmental processes. As shown in Table 1, programmed cell death, erythropoiesis, and lens cell differentiation use different systems to degrade DNA. During programmed cell death, DNA is first degraded cell-autonomously by CAD through the apoptotic process, and subsequently non-cell-autonomously by DNase

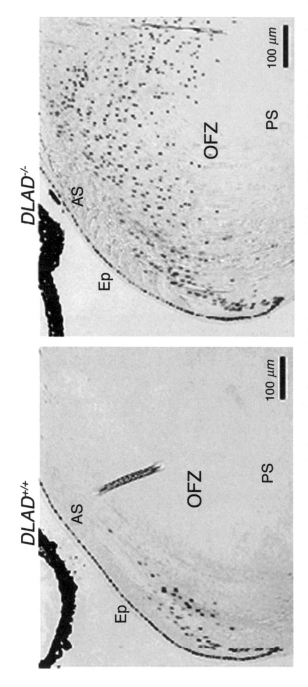

Figure 8 Accumulation of undigested DNA in fiber cells of *DLAD*-deficient mouse eyes. Staining of the *DLAD*-deficient lens section with Feulgen indicates that Feulgen-positive materials (DNA) are left undigested in fiber cells. Ep, epithelim; OFZ, organelle-free zone; AS, anterior suture; PS, posterior suture. Reproduced from Reference 5.

TABLE 1   DNases involved in mammalian developmental processes

Developmental process	Biological process	DNases	Associated diseases
Programmed cell death	Apoptosis/phagocytosis	CAD/DNase II	Tissue atrophy
Erythropoiesis	Phagocytosis	DNase II	Anemia
Lens cell differentiation	Autophagy?	DLAD	Cataract formation

II after dying cells are phagocytosed. In erythropoiesis, nuclei are expelled from erythroid precursor cells and are degraded by DNase II after they are phagocytosed by macrophages. By contrast, nuclei in lens fiber cells of the eye seem to be degraded by DLAD in their own lysosomes by autophagy. If DNA is not properly degraded during these processes, it causes tissue atrophy, anemia, and cataract formation.

Subsequent to enucleation, the mitochondria and endoplasmic reticulum are removed during differentiation of reticulocytes into mature erythrocytes. How this process occurs is poorly understood, but Pan et al. have proposed the shedding of organelles as exosomes, coupled with autophagy (102). Programmed cell death often occurs in a caspase-independent manner (103), and the involvement of autophagy in this process has been suggested (104–106). Autophagy is a process in which cells adjust their capacity to withstand starvation or other adverse conditions by degrading their own organelles and proteins (99, 107). If this process exceeds the threshold and degrades cellular components essential for their life, cells will die. In this regard, autophagic cell death may use a mechanism similar to that used for lens cell differentiation. As described here, DNA degradation during programmed cell death, erythropoiesis, and lens cell differentiation is rather simple and is mediated by specific DNases. Investigation into how the respective DNases are activated and function in these processes will help our understanding of the molecular mechanisms of these complicated developmental processes.

Lysosomal storage diseases, which are inherited genetic diseases in humans, are characterized by the gradual accumulation of undegraded substrates in lysosomes (108). Genes that are affected in these diseases code for lysosomal enzymes that are involved in the degradation of proteins, sugars, or lipids, or they are genes for lysosomal structural proteins (108–111). A mutation of lysosomal DNases (DNase II and DLAD) also causes a kind of lysosomal storage disease (3–5). It will be interesting to examine whether human patients suffering from autoimmune disease, anemia, or cataracts carry a mutation in the *CAD*, *DNase II*, or *DLAD* gene.

ACKNOWLEDGMENTS

I thank all members of my laboratory. The work in my laboratory was supported in part by grants-in-aid from the Ministry of Education, Science, Sports, and Culture in Japan.

The *Annual Review of Immunology* is online at
http://immunol.annualreviews.org

LITERATURE CITED

1. Kerr JF, Wyllie AH, Currie AR. 1972. Apoptosis: a basic biological phenomenon with wide-ranging implications in tissue kinetics. *Br. J. Cancer* 26:239–57

2. Wyllie AH. 1980. Glucocorticoid-induced thymocyte apoptosis is associated with endogenous endonuclease activation. *Nature* 284:555–56

3. Kawane K, Fukuyama H, Yoshida H, Nagase H, Ohsawa Y, et al. 2003. Impaired thymic development in mouse embryos deficient in apoptotic DNA degradation. *Nat. Immunol.* 4:138–44

4. Kawane K, Fukuyama H, Kondoh G, Takeda J, Ohsawa Y, et al. 2001. Requirement of DNase II for definitive erythropoiesis in the mouse fetal liver. *Science* 292:1546–49

5. Nishimoto S, Kawane K, Watanabe-Fukunaga R, Fukuyama H, Ohsawa Y, et al. 2003. Nuclear cataract caused by a lack of DNA degradation in the mouse eye lens. *Nature* 424:1071–74

6. Jacobson MD, Weil M, Raff MC. 1997. Programmed cell death in animal development. *Cell* 88:347–54

7. Vaux DL, Korsmeyer SJ. 1999. Cell death in development. *Cell* 96:245–54

8. Nagata S, Golstein P. 1995. The Fas death factor. *Science* 267:1449–56

9. Thompson CB. 1995. Apoptosis in the pathogenesis and treatment of disease. *Science* 267:1456–62

10. Savill J, Fadok V. 2000. Corpse clearance defines the meaning of cell death. *Nature* 407:784–88

11. Surh CD, Sprent J. 1994. T-cell apoptosis detected *in situ* during positive and negative selection in the thymus. *Nature* 372:100–3

12. Lang RA, Bishop JM. 1993. Macrophages are required for cell death and tissue remodeling in the developing mouse eye. *Cell* 74:453–62

13. Hanayama R, Tanaka M, Miyasaka K, Aozasa K, Koike M, et al. 2004. Autoimmune disease and impaired uptake of apoptotic cells in germinal centers of MFG-E8-deficient mice. *Science* 304:1147–50

14. Botto M, Dell'Agnola C, Bygrave AE, Thompson EM, Cook HT, et al. 1998. Homozygous C1q deficiency causes glomerulonephritis associated with multiple apoptotic bodies. *Nat. Genet.* 19:56–59

15. Szondy Z, Sarang Z, Molnar P, Nemeth T, Piacentini M, Mastroberardino PG, et al. 2003. Transglutaminase $2^{-/-}$ mice reveal a phagocytosis-associated crosstalk between macrophages and apoptotic cells. *Proc. Natl. Acad. Sci. USA* 100:7812–17

16. Adams JM. 2003. Ways of dying: multiple pathways to apoptosis. *Genes Dev.* 17:2481–95

17. Danial NN, Korsmeyer SJ. 2004. Cell death: critical control points. *Cell* 116:205–19

18. Nicholson DW. 1999. Caspase structure, proteolytic substrates, and function during apoptotic cell death. *Cell Death Differ.* 6:1028–42

19. Lamkanfi M, Declercq W, Kalai M, Saelens X, Vandenabeele P. 2002. Alice in caspase land. A phylogenetic analysis of caspases from worm to man. *Cell Death Differ.* 9:358–61

20. Nagata S. 1997. Apoptosis by death factor. *Cell* 88:355–65

21. Krammer PH. 2000. CD95's deadly mission in the immune system. *Nature* 407:789–95

22. Fischer U, Janicke RU, Schulze-Osthoff K. 2003. Many cuts to ruin: a comprehensive update of caspase substrates. *Cell Death Differ.* 10:76–100

23. Lagarkova MA, Iarovaia OV, Razin SV. 1995. Large-scale fragmentation of mammalian DNA in the course of apoptosis proceeds via excision of chromosomal DNA loops and their oligomers. *J. Biol. Chem.* 270:20239–41

24. Oberhammer F, Wilson JW, Dive C, Morris ID, Hickman JA, et al. 1993. Apoptotic death in epithelial cells: cleavage of DNA to 300 and/or 50 kb fragments prior to or in the absence of internucleosomal fragmentation. *EMBO J.* 12:3679–84

25. Earnshaw WC. 1995. Nuclear changes in apoptosis. *Curr. Biol.* 7:337–43

26. Gavrieli Y, Sherman Y, Ben-Sasson SA. 1992. Identification of programmed cell death in situ via specific labeling of nuclear DNA fragmentation. *J. Cell Biol.* 119:493–501

27. Liu X, Zou H, Slaughter C, Wang X. 1997. DFF, a heterodimeric protein that functions downstream of caspase-3 to trigger DNA fragmentation during apoptosis. *Cell* 89:175–84

28. Enari M, Sakahira H, Yokoyama H, Okawa H, Iwamatsu A, Nagata S. 1998. A caspase-activated DNase that degrades DNA during apoptosis, and its inhibitor ICAD. *Nature* 391:43–50

29. Sakahira H, Enari M, Nagata S. 1998. Cleavage of CAD inhibitor in CAD activation and DNA degradation during apoptosis. *Nature* 391:96–99

30. Mukae N, Yokoyama H, Yokokura T, Sakoyama Y, Nagata S. 2002. Activation of the innate immunity in *Drosophila* by endogenous chromosomal DNA that escaped apoptotic degradation. *Genes Dev.* 16:2662–71

31. Zhang J, Liu X, Scherer DC, van Kaer L, Wang X, Xu M. 1998. Resistance to DNA fragmentation and chromatin condensation in mice lacking the DNA fragmentation factor 45. *Proc. Natl. Acad. Sci. USA* 95:12480–85

32. Nagata S, Nagase H, Kawane K, Mukae N, Fukuyama H. 2003. Degradation of chromosomal DNA during apoptosis. *Cell Death Differ.* 10:108–16

33. McIlroy D, Tanaka M, Sakahira H, Fukuyama H, Suzuki M, et al. 2000. An auxiliary mode of apoptotic DNA fragmentation provided by phagocytes. *Genes Dev.* 14:549–58

34. Widlak P, Li P, Wang X, Garrard WT. 2000. Cleavage preferences of the apoptotic endonuclease DFF40 (caspase-activated DNase or nuclease) on naked DNA and chromatin substrates. *J. Biol. Chem.* 275:8226–32

35. Sakahira H, Takemura Y, Nagata S. 2001. Enzymatic active site of caspase-activated DNase (CAD) and its inhibition by inhibitor of CAD (ICAD). *Arch. Biochem. Biophys.* 388:91–99

36. Scholz SR, Korn C, Bujnicki JM, Gimadutdinow O, Pingoud A, Meiss G. 2003. Experimental evidence for a $\beta\beta\alpha$-Me-finger nuclease motif to represent the active site of the caspase-activated DNase. *Biochemistry* 42:9288–94

37. Woo E-J, Kim Y-G, Kim M-S, Han W-D, Shin S, et al. 2004. Structural mechanism for inactivation and activation of CAD/DFF40 in the apoptotic pathway. *Mol. Cell* 14:531–39

38. Murgia M, Pizzo P, Sandona D, Zanovello P, Rizzuto R, Di Virgilio F. 1992. Mitochondrial DNA is not fragmented during apoptosis. *J. Biol. Chem.* 267:10939–41

39. Halenbeck R, MacDonald H, Roulston A, Chen TT, Conroy L, Williams LT. 1998. CPAN, a human nuclease regulated by the caspase-sensitive inhibitor DFF45. *Curr. Biol.* 8:537–40

40. Sakahira H, Iwamatsu A, Nagata S. 2000. Specific chaperone-like activity of inhibitor of caspase-activated DNase for caspase-activated DNase. *J. Biol. Chem.* 275:8091–96

41. Otomo T, Sakahira H, Uegaki K, Nagata S, Yamazaki T. 2000. Structure of the heterodimeric complex between CAD domains of CAD and ICAD. *Nat. Struct. Biol.* 7:658–62

42. Sakahira H, Nagata S. 2002. Co-translational folding of caspase-activated DNase with Hsp70, Hsp40 and inhibitor of caspase-activated DNase. *J. Biol. Chem.* 277:3364–70

43. Woo M, Hakem R, Soengas MS, Duncan GS, Shahinian A, et al. 1998. Essential contribution of caspase 3/CPP32 to apoptosis and its associated nuclear changes. *Genes Dev.* 12:806–19

44. Nagase H, Fukuyama H, Tanaka M, Kawane K, Nagata S. 2003. Mutually regulated expression of caspase-activated DNase and its inhibitor for apoptotic DNA fragmentation. *Cell Death Differ.* 10:142–43

45. Mukae N, Enari M, Sakahira H, Fukuda Y, Inazawa J, et al. 1998. Molecular cloning and characterization of human caspase-activated DNase. *Proc. Natl. Acad. Sci. USA* 95:9123–28

46. Susin SA, Daugas E, Ravagnan L, Samejima K, Zamzami N, et al. 2000. Two distinct pathways leading to nuclear apoptosis. *J. Exp. Med.* 192:571–80

47. Schulze-Osthoff K, Walczak H, Droge W, Krammer PH. 1994. Cell nucleus and DNA fragmentation are not required for apoptosis. *J. Cell Biol.* 127:15–20

48. Jacobson MD, Burne JF, Raff MC. 1994. Programmed cell death and Bcl-2 protection in the absence of a nucleus. *EMBO J.* 13:1899–910

49. Slane JM, Lee HS, Vorhees CV, Zhang J, Xu M. 2000. DNA fragmentation factor 45 deficient mice exhibit enhanced spatial learning and memory compared to wild-type control mice. *Brain Res.* 867:70–79

50. van Loo G, Schotte P, van Gurp M, Demol H, Hoorelbeke B, et al. 2001. Endonuclease G: a mitochondrial protein released in apoptosis and involved in caspase-independent DNA degradation. *Cell Death Differ.* 8:1136–42

51. Li LY, Luo X, Wang X. 2001. Endonuclease G is an apoptotic DNase when released from mitochondria. *Nature* 412:95–99

52. Wang X, Yang C, Chai J, Shi Y, Xue D. 2002. Mechanisms of AIF-mediated apoptotic DNA degradation in *Caenorhabditis elegans*. *Science* 298:1587–92

53. Ruiz-Carrillo A, Renaud J. 1987. Endonuclease G: a (dG)n X (dC)n-specific DNase from higher eukaryotes. *EMBO J.* 6:401–7

54. Widlak P, Li LY, Wang X, Garrard WT. 2001. Action of recombinant human apoptotic endonuclease G on naked DNA and chromatin substrates: cooperation with exonuclease and DNase I. *J. Biol. Chem.* 276:48404–9

55. Parrish J, Li L, Klotz K, Ledwich D, Wang X, Xue D. 2001. Mitochondrial endonuclease G is important for apoptosis in *C. elegans*. *Nature* 412:90–94

56. Zhang J, Dong M, Li L, Fan Y, Pathre P, et al. 2003. Endonuclease G is required for early embryogenesis and normal apoptosis in mice. *Proc. Natl. Acad. Sci. USA* 100:15782–87

57. Sakahira H, Enari M, Ohsawa Y, Uchiyama Y, Nagata S. 1999. Apoptotic nuclear morphological change without DNA fragmentation. *Curr. Biol.* 9:543–46

58. Sahara S, Aoto M, Eguchi Y, Imamoto N, Yoneda Y, Tsujimoto Y. 1999. Acinus is a caspase-3-activated protein required for apoptotic chromatin condensation. *Nature* 401:168–73

59. Zhou Z, Licklider LJ, Gygi SP, Reed R. 2002. Comprehensive proteomic analysis of the human spliceosome. *Nature* 419:182–85

60. Bernardi G. 1971. Spleen acid deoxyribonuclease. In *The Enzymes*, ed. PD Boyer, pp. 271–87. New York and London: Academic

61. Evans CJ, Aguilera RJ. 2003. DNase II: genes, enzymes and function. *Gene* 322:1–15

62. Krieser RJ, MacLea KS, Longnecker DS, Fields JL, Fiering S, Eastman A. 2002. Deoxyribonuclease IIa is required during the phagocytic phase of apoptosis and its loss causes lethality. *Cell Death Differ.* 9:956–62

63. Staley K, Blaschke A, Chun J. 1997. Apoptotic DNA fragmentation is detected by a semi-quantitative ligation-mediated PCR of blunt DNA ends. *Cell Death Differ.* 4:66–75

64. Wu YC, Stanfield GM, Horvitz HR. 2000. NUC-1, a *Caenorhabditis elegans* DNase II homolog, functions in an intermediate step of DNA degradation during apoptosis. *Genes Dev.* 14:536–48

65. Hedgecock EM, Sulston JE, Thomson JN. 1983. Mutations affecting programmed cell deaths in the nematode *Caenorhabditis elegans. Science* 220:1277–79

66. Lin Q, Dong C, Cooper MD. 1998. Impairment of T and B cell development by treatment with a type I interferon. *J. Exp. Med.* 187:79–87

67. Krieg AM. 2002. CpG motifs in bacterial DNA and their immune effects. *Annu. Rev. Immunol.* 20:709–60

68. Hoffmann JA, Reichhart JM. 2002. *Drosophila* innate immunity: an evolutionary perspective. *Nat. Immunol.* 3:121–26

69. Gilkeson GS, Grudier JP, Karounos DG, Pisetsky DS. 1989. Induction of anti-double stranded DNA antibodies in normal mice by immunization with bacterial DNA. *J. Immunol.* 142:1482–86

70. Blatt NB, Glick GD. 1999. Anti-DNA autoantibodies and systemic lupus erythematosus. *Pharmacol. Ther.* 83:125–39

71. Hahn BH. 1998. Antibodies to DNA. *N. Engl. J. Med.* 338:1359–68

72. Russell ES. 1979. Hereditary anemias of the mouse: a review for geneticists. *Adv. Genet.* 20:357–459

73. Bernard J. 1991. The erythroblastic island: past and future. *Blood Cells* 17:5–10

74. Patel VP, Lodish HF. 1987. A fibronectin matrix is required for differentiation of murine erythroleukemia cells into reticulocytes. *J. Cell Biol.* 105:3105–18

75. Van Rooijen N, Sanders A. 1994. Liposome mediated depletion of macrophages: mechanism of action, preparation of liposomes and applications. *J. Immunol. Methods* 174:83–93

76. Sadahira Y, Yasuda T, Yoshino T, Manabe T, Takeishi T, et al. 2000. Impaired splenic erythropoiesis in phlebotomized mice injected with CL2MDP-liposome: an experimental model for studying the role of stromal macrophages in erythropoiesis. *J. Leukoc. Biol.* 68:464–70

77. Giuliani AL, Wiener E, Lee MJ, Brown IN, Berti G, Wickramasinghe SN. 2001. Changes in murine bone marrow macrophages and erythroid burst-forming cells following the intravenous injection of liposome-encapsulated dichloromethylene diphosphonate (Cl2MDP). *Eur. J. Haematol.* 66:221–29

78. Sadahira Y, Mori M. 1999. Role of the macrophage in erythropoiesis. *Pathol. Int.* 49:841–48

79. Hanayama R, Tanaka M, Miwa K, Shinohara A, Iwamatsu A, Nagata S. 2002. Identification of a factor that links apoptotic cells to phagocytes. *Nature* 417:182–87

80. Tanaka Y, Schroit AJ. 1983. Insertion of fluorescent phosphatidylserine into the plasma membrane of red blood cells. Recognition by autologous macrophages. *J. Biol. Chem.* 258:11335–43

81. Fadok VA, Voelker DR, Campbell PA, Cohen JJ, Bratton DL, Henson PM. 1992. Exposure of phosphatidylserine on the surface of apoptotic lymphocytes triggers specific recognition and removal by macrophages. *J. Immunol.* 148:2207–16

82. Geiduschek JB, Singer SJ. 1979. Molecular changes in the membranes of mouse erythroid cells accompanying differentiation. *Cell* 16:149–63

83. Schlegel RA, Phelps BM, Cofer GP, Williamson P. 1982. Enucleation eliminates a differentiation-specific surface marker from normal and leukemic murine erythroid cells. *Exp. Cell Res.* 139:321–28

84. Zermati Y, Garrido C, Amsellem S, Fishelson S, Bouscary D, et al. 2001.

Caspase activation is required for terminal erythroid differentiation. *J. Exp. Med.* 193:247–54

85. Carlile GW, Smith DH, Wiedmann M. 2004. Caspase-3 has a nonapoptotic function in erythroid maturation. *Blood* 103:4310–16

86. Ortega JA, Ma A, Shore NA, Dukes PP, Merigan TC. 1979. Suppressive effect of interferon on erythroid cell proliferation. *Exp. Hematol.* 7:145–50

87. Bassnett S. 1995. The fate of the Golgi apparatus and the endoplasmic reticulum during lens fiber cell differentiation. *Invest. Ophthalmol. Vis. Sci.* 36:1793–803

88. Bassnett S. 2002. Lens organelle degradation. *Exp. Eye Res.* 74:1–6

89. Bassnett S, Mataic D. 1997. Chromatin degradation in differentiating fiber cells of the eye lens. *J. Cell Biol.* 137:37–49

90. Wride MA. 2000. Minireview: apoptosis as seen through a lens. *Apoptosis* 5:203–9

91. Dahm R. 1999. Lens fibre cell differentiation—A link with apoptosis? *Ophthalmic Res.* 31:163–83

92. Sanders EJ, Parker E. 2002. The role of mitochondria, cytochrome c and caspase-9 in embryonic lens fibre cell denucleation. *J. Anat.* 201:121–35

93. Fromm L, Overbeek PA. 1997. Inhibition of cell death by lens-specific overexpression of Bcl-2 in transgenic mice. *Dev. Genet.* 20:276–87

94. Shiokawa D, Tanuma S. 1999. DLAD, a novel mammalian divalent cation-independent endonuclease with homology to DNase II. *Nucleic Acids Res.* 27:4083–89

95. Krieser RJ, MacLea KS, Park JP, Eastman A. 2001. The cloning, genomic structure, localization, and expression of human deoxyribonuclease IIβ. *Gene* 269:205–16

96. De Maria A, Arruti C. 2003. Bovine DNase I: gene organization, mRNA expression, and changes in the topological distribution of the protein during apoptosis in lens epithelial cells. *Biochem. Biophys. Res. Commun.* 312:634–41

97. Torriglia A, Perani P, Brossas JY, Chaudun E, Treton J, et al. 1998. L-DNase II, a molecule that links proteases and endonucleases in apoptosis, derives from the ubiquitous serpin leukocyte elastase inhibitor. *Mol. Cell. Biol.* 18:3612–19

98. Klionsky DJ, Ohsumi Y. 1999. Vacuolar import of proteins and organelles from the cytoplasm. *Annu. Rev. Cell Dev. Biol.* 15:1–32

99. Ohsumi Y. 2001. Molecular dissection of autophagy: two ubiquitin-like systems. *Nat. Rev. Mol. Cell Biol.* 2:211–16

100. Ooto S, Haruta M, Honda Y, Kawasaki H, Sasai Y, Takahashi M. 2003. Induction of the differentiation of lentoids from primate embryonic stem cells. *Invest. Ophthalmol. Vis. Sci.* 44:2689–93

101. Hirano M, Yamamoto A, Yoshimura N, Tokunaga T, Motohashi T, et al. 2003. Generation of structures formed by lens and retinal cells differentiating from embryonic stem cells. *Dev. Dyn.* 228:664–71

102. Pan BT, Johnstone RM. 1983. Fate of the transferrin receptor during maturation of sheep reticulocytes in vitro: selective externalization of the receptor. *Cell* 33:967–78

103. Golstein P, Aubry L, Levraud JP. 2003. Cell-death alternative model organisms: why and which? *Nat. Rev. Mol. Cell Biol.* 4:798–807

104. Lee CY, Clough EA, Yellon P, Teslovich TM, Stephan DA, Baehrecke EH. 2003. Genome-wide analyses of steroid- and radiation-triggered programmed cell death in *Drosophila*. *Curr. Biol.* 13:350–57

105. Gorski SM, Chittaranjan S, Pleasance ED, Freeman JD, Anderson CL, et al. 2003. A SAGE approach to discovery of genes involved in autophagic cell death. *Curr. Biol.* 13:358–63

106. Yu L, Alva A, Su H, Dutt P, Freundt E, et al. 2004. Regulation of an ATG7-beclin 1 program of autophagic cell death by caspase-8. *Science* 304:1500–2

107. Klionsky DJ, Emr SD. 2000. Autophagy

as a regulated pathway of cellular degradation. *Science* 290:1717–21

108. Neufeld EF. 1991. Lysosomal storage diseases. *Annu. Rev. Biochem.* 60:257–80

109. Tyynela J, Sohar I, Sleat DE, Gin RM, Donnelly RJ, et al. 2000. A mutation in the ovine cathepsin D gene causes a congenital lysosomal storage disease with profound neurodegeneration. *EMBO J.* 19: 2786–92

110. Nishino I, Fu J, Tanji K, Yamada T, Shimojo S, et al. 2000. Primary LAMP-2 deficiency causes X-linked vacuolar cardiomyopathy and myopathy (Danon disease). *Nature* 406:906–10

111. Tanaka Y, Guhde G, Suter A, Eskelinen EL, Hartmann D, et al. 2000. Accumulation of autophagic vacuoles and cardiomyopathy in LAMP-2-deficient mice. *Nature* 406:902–6

112. Dahm R, Gribbon C, Quinlan RA, Prescott AR. 1998. Changes in the nucleolar and coiled body compartments precede lamina and chromatin reorganization during fibre cell denucleation in the bovine lens. *Eur. J. Cell Biol.* 75:237–46

Annu. Rev. Immunol. 2005. 26:877–900
doi: 10.1146/annurev.immunol.23.021704.115742
Copyright © 2005 by Annual Reviews. All rights reserved
First published online as a Review in Advance on January 19, 2005

TOWARD AN UNDERSTANDING OF NKT CELL BIOLOGY: Progress and Paradoxes

Mitchell Kronenberg

La Jolla Institute for Allergy and Immunology, San Diego, California 92121;
email: mitch@liai.org

Key Words   T cell, natural killer, CD1d, glycolipid

■ **Abstract**   Natural killer T (NKT) cells constitute a conserved T cell sublineage with unique properties, including reactivity for a synthetic glycolipid presented by CD1d, expression of an invariant T cell antigen receptor (TCR) α chain, and unusual requirements for thymic selection. They rapidly produce many cytokines after stimulation and thus influence diverse immune responses and pathogenic processes. Because of intensive research effort, we have learned much about factors promoting the development and survival of NKT cells, regulation of their cytokine production, and the means by which they influence dendritic cells and other cell types. Despite this progress, knowledge of the natural antigen(s) they recognize and their physiologic role remain incomplete. The activation of NKT cells paradoxically can lead either to suppression or stimulation of immune responses, and we cannot predict which will occur. Despite this uncertainty, many investigators are hopeful that immune therapies can be developed based on NKT cell stimulation.

INTRODUCTION

There are several remarkable features of natural killer T (NKT) cells that have emerged from studies carried out during the previous decade. First, although they constitute less than 1% of mouse T lymphocytes, they exert a critical influence on a variety of immune responses and pathologic conditions (1–6). Second, to a surprising extent they function differently from conventional T cells. A salient feature that distinguishes NKT cells is their ability to rapidly secrete a variety of cytokines within a few hours after activation (7, 7a). Therefore, not surprisingly, this small lymphocyte subpopulation has captured the attention of many immunologists. Many excellent reviews pertain to NKT cells, including several previous ones in this series (1–6, 8). In this article, I give a brief overview of the known properties of mouse and human NKT cells, while highlighting recent findings and the important unresolved questions concerning the development, specificity, and function of these unique T lymphocytes.

0732-0582/05/0423-0877$14.00

WHAT IS AN NKT CELL?

It is important to define unambiguously what we mean by the term "NKT cell." Operationally, these lymphocytes were originally characterized in mice as cells that express both a T cell antigen receptor (TCR) and NK1.1 (NKR-P1 or CD161c), a C-lectin type NK receptor (8). This definition is not entirely satisfactory, however, and more recently NKT cells have been defined as cells that nearly always have an invariant Vα14-Jα18 rearrangement and reactivity to the glycosphingolipid α-galactosylceramide (αGalCer) (Figure 1) when presented by the class I–like molecule CD1d (9). Defined operationally in this way, NKT cells are the group of lymphocytes that can be detected by flow cytometry using tetramers of CD1d

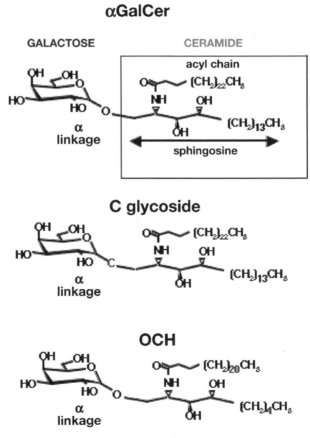

Figure 1   Structure of αGalCer and related compounds. The ceramide lipid portion of the molecule is boxed, and the aliphatic acyl chain (*upper*) and sphingosine base (*lower*) of the ceramide are indicated. How the C-glycoside and OCH differ from αGalCer is indicated in red.

loaded with αGalCer (9). They are known by several other names, including type I NKT cells, invariant (i) NKT cells, and Vα14i NKT cells (9); the latter term is used here. In many cases, Vα14i NKT cells do not express NK1.1 (9), and other T cells, including conventional, virus-specific CD8$^+$ T cells, can induce NK1.1 expression (10), hence making the earlier definition based on NK1.1 and TCR coexpression too imprecise.

Humans have a homologous population of T cells with an invariant Vα24 rearrangement (Vα24i) (11, 12) and reactivity to αGalCer when presented by human CD1d (13, 14). In humans, however, the dichotomy between CD161 expression and reactivity with CD1d tetramers is very pronounced. Most NK1.1$^+$ TCR$\alpha\beta^+$ mouse T cells are CD1d tetramer reactive (7, 15). However, although 5%–10% of human peripheral blood T cells express CD161a, only approximately 0.1% are reactive with CD1d tetramers (16–19).

DEVELOPMENT OF Vα14i NKT CELLS

Vα14i NKT Cells Are a Sublineage with Unique Requirements for their Selection

Using CD1d tetramers permits investigators to detect developing Vα14i NKT cells in a normal physiologic setting, without the potentially distorting effects on the repertoire of TCR transgenes. Investigators now agree that Vα14i NKT cells arise in the thymus in the perinatal period and do not reach significant levels until at least three weeks after birth (20–22). Their positive selection is mediated by CD1d-expressing bone marrow–derived cells rather than by cortical epithelial cells (8), a finding that helped investigators establish the distinctive nature of this T lymphocyte subset. Among the bone marrow–derived cells, CD1d$^+$ double-positive thymocytes are almost certainly the critical cell type for positive selection (23, 24). In addition to this requirement by Vα14i NKT cells for an unusual positively selecting cell type, Vα14i NKT cell development and maturation are differentially effected by a number of mutations that have relatively little effect on conventional cells (25). Several recent studies have focused on members of the NF-κB family. Vα14i NKT cell development requires the expression of NF-κB1 (p50) in a cell-autonomous manner (26, 27). NKT cell development also requires the expression of the gene for the inhibitor of κB kinase, $Ikk2$ (28). Moreover, RelB (p65) expression in an irradiation-resistant cell is required in NKT cell development (26, 29). Recently, it has been shown that, for their differentiation, Vα14i NKT cells require the transcription factor T-bet (T-box expressed in T cells) (30), a factor originally identified as important for the induction of IFN-γ synthesis and Th1 immunity in several cell types.

Why are the genetic requirements for Vα14i NKT cell development unique and complex? A few of the mutations that specifically diminish the Vα14i NKT cell population, such as those affecting AP-3 subunits and prosaposin, probably act by affecting the pathway required for the loading of endogenous glycolipids into the

CD1d groove. The adaptor protein AP-3 binds to the CD1d cytoplasmic tail and is required for CD1d trafficking to lysosomes (31, 32), where endogenous glycolipids may be processed and loaded into CD1d. Sphingolipid activator proteins, four of which are encoded by the prosaposin precursor, are lysosomal proteins that interact with CD1d molecules. They make lipids available for CD1 loading, and they apparently perform an editing or quality control function for the lipids bound to CD1d (33, 34).

In contrast to conventional thymocytes, most of the $V\alpha 14i$ NKT cells in the thymus are part of a mature, immune-competent population, capable of producing IL-4 and IFN-γ immediately after TCR stimulation (21, 22, 35). Therefore, the set of genes required for $V\alpha 14i$ NKT cell differentiation may reflect not only those required for their early maturation but also those that are required for lymphocyte expansion and differentiation to effector cells. This could explain, for example, the requirement for expression of NF-κB transcription factors in developing $V\alpha 14i$ NKT cells, as these transcription factors seem to affect the survival of the $V\alpha 14i$ NKT cells after they have expressed the TCR, undergone some expansion, and reached an intermediate stage of their differentiation (27).

Precommitment or Instruction?

The use of αGalCer-loaded CD1d tetramers has permitted several research groups to analyze the phenotype of $V\alpha 14i$ NKT cells during these later stages of their differentiation, after they have acquired a TCR. Expression of several molecules, including the IL-7 receptor, CD24, DX5, NK1.1, and Ly49 family NK receptors, occurs during later maturation steps (21, 22, 27, 36). Induction of NK1.1 expression probably can occur in the thymus, although most of the recent thymus emigrants are NK1.1 negative (21, 22), suggesting that the final maturation stages for $V\alpha 14i$ NKT cells also occur in the periphery. An unresolved issue concerns the elements that direct developing thymocytes into this sublineage. Two alternative models are illustrated in Figure 2. Investigators have presented evidence suggesting that $V\alpha 14i$ NKT cells have a double-positive precursor (20). The existence of a double-positive precursor is consistent with an instructional model in which the expression of the $V\alpha 14i$ TCR and recognition of endogenous ligands presented by CD1d commit the developing precursor to become a $V\alpha 14i$ NKT cell. A relatively high-affinity recognition of endogenous ligands presented by CD1d and/or the consequences of selection by other double-positive thymocytes may be responsible for this commitment. Other researchers have suggested that a subset of thymocytes is precommitted to become $V\alpha 14i$ NKT cells before antigen receptor rearrangement. For example, the requirement for the SRC family kinase Fyn in NKT cell development is cell autonomous (37, 38). In contrast, conventional T lymphocytes undergo relatively normal thymus differentiation in the absence of Fyn. This special requirement exhibited by of $V\alpha 14i$ NKT cells can be overcome by expression of a $V\alpha 14i$ transgene (39). In mixed bone marrow chimera experiments, in which fyn^+ and $fyn^{-/-}$ $V\alpha 14i$ transgenic precursors were cotransferred

(A) Instructional model

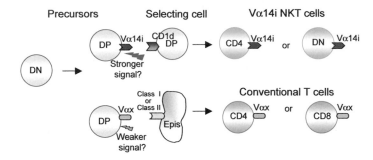

(B) Precommitment model

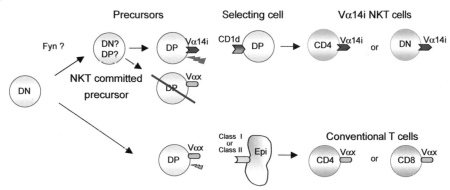

Figure 2   Models for the development of Vα14*i* NKT cells. (*A*) In the instructional model, expression of the Vα14*i* TCR instructs thymocytes to become Vα14*i* NKT cells, perhaps because of a high-affinity interaction with CD1d-presented ligands or interaction with double-positive thymocytes. Expression of other TCRs (Vαx) leads to the positive selection of conventional T cells by MHC class I– and class II–expressing epithelial cells (Epis). (*B*) According to the precommitment model, a precursor decides to become a Vα14*i* NKT cell before TCR rearrangement, as depicted.

to irradiated recipients, the *fyn*⁻/⁻ precursors contributed to the Vα14*i* NKT cell compartment as effectively as those that express Fyn (39). On the basis of these results, investigators have suggested that Vα14*i* NKT cell deficiency in *fyn*⁻/⁻ mice is not simply due to a failure to properly signal through the Vα14*i* TCR or to expand Vα14*i* NKT cell precursors. They suggest instead that *fyn* acts upstream of TCR expression, and that it in some way aids in the TCR-independent commitment of thymocytes to the Vα14*i* NKT cell sublineage, with expression of the transgene acting downstream to overcome this defect. Vα14*i* NKT cells do not have a preferential rearrangement of Vα14*i* on the unexpressed allele (40), and therefore even if a precommitment occurred, the cells precommitted to this sublineage would then also have to undergo selection on the basis of TCR specificity.

Agonist Selection of Vα14i NKT Cells?

A growing body of evidence favors the concept that the thymus does not discard all self-reactive T cells and that some potentially self-reactive T lymphocytes are preserved to carry out specialized or regulatory functions (41). Consistent with this theory, evidence suggests that TCRαβ$^+$ CD8αα intraepithelial lymphocytes (42, 43) and CD4$^+$ CD25$^+$ regulatory T cells are inherently self-reactive (44). The CD1d autoreactivity of Vα14i NKT cells has led to the suggestion that these T lymphocytes also are positively selected by self-agonist ligands (8).

The forced expression of CD8α and CD8β transgenes in T cells leads to a decrease in Vα14i NKT cells (45), suggesting that CD8-mediated enhancement of the intrinsically high affinity of the Vα14i TCR for self-antigens presented by CD1d pushes the developing Vα14i NKT cell over the threshold of negative selection. Direct evidence is lacking, however, indicating that CD8 can serve as a coreceptor for CD1d-mediated antigen recognition, and the CD8 transgenic mice have other abnormalities, including a decrease in total thymocyte numbers (45). An alternative model for the lack of CD8 expression by Vα14i NKT cells is the finding that increased or prolonged Lck signaling preferentially directs thymocytes to be CD4 positive (46, 47). Therefore, although the reason for the lack of CD8 expression by Vα14i NKT cells remains to be determined, the concept that they are positively selected by self-agonists or relatively high-avidity interactions remains an appealing one. Unlike in mice, in humans a minority of Vα24i NKT cells expresses CD8α, and some express CD8β as well (17, 19, 48, 49).

Negative Selection of Vα14i NKT Cells

Although Vα14i NKT cells may require self-agonist for their development, there must be an upper limit to the avidity window that permits their positive selection, as the results from several experiments support the concept that these cells can be negatively selected in the thymus. Addition of αGalCer to fetal thymic organ cultures causes Vα14i NKT cell negative selection (50, 51), and increased expression of CD1d in transgenic mice causes a decrease in the number of Vα14i NKT cells (50). Moreover, the remaining Vα14i NKT cells in these CD1d transgenic mice were hyporesponsive. Mouse Vα14i NKT cells tend to coexpress Vβ8.2, constituting more than 50% of the total, with Vβ7 and Vβ2 also highly represented (45). Evidence suggests that the Vβ8.2-containing Vα14i TCRs tend to have the highest affinity for αGalCer presented by CD1d (52), and in the CD1d transgenic mice, Vβ8.2 Vα14i NKT cells were underrepresented, which is consistent with the elimination of cells expressing the highest affinity TCRs (50). Chronic exposure of young adult mice to αGalCer also led to Vα14i NKT cell deletion (53). When treatment was halted, newly exported cells from the thymus reconstituted the Vα14i NKT cell population. The recovered cells were hyporesponsive, however, and they had increased expression of inhibitory NK receptors of the Ly49 family (53). This is consistent with other data indicating that the balance of signals between activating and inhibitory NK receptors, as well as TCR avidity, sets the affinity threshold and regulates the development of $V\alpha14i$ NKT cells (54).

HOMING AND HOMEOSTASIS

$V\alpha14i$ NKT cells are most prevalent in the thymus, spleen, liver, and bone marrow, with at least 5×10^5 cells generally found in each site (7, 15). They are much less abundant in lymph nodes and are rarely found in other tertiary sites such as the intestinal mucosa. They express a set of chemokine receptors consistent with tissue-seeking effector cells, with relatively little expression of CCR7 (55–57). In humans, there are differences in the chemokine receptors expressed by the $CD4^+$ and $CD4^-$ $V\alpha24i$ subsets (55), as well as functional differences in the cytokines they produce (49, 58). There is much less evidence for the existence of functional subsets or of a regional specialization of mouse $V\alpha14i$ NKT cells. Consistent with their chemokine receptor expression, mouse $V\alpha14i$ NKT cells can migrate to sites of inflammation in the lung (59–61), liver, and spleen (62).

IL-15 plays a dominant role in governing the homeostasis of $V\alpha14i$ NKT cells, including survival, turnover, and lymphopenia-induced or homeostatic proliferation (63, 64), which is the proliferation induced upon transfer to irradiated or $RAG^{-/-}$ recipients. This lymphopenia-induced proliferation does not require expression of CD1d. With respect to $V\alpha14i$ NKT cells' IL-15 requirement, and their independence from TCR signals, $V\alpha14i$ NKT cells therefore resemble conventional, $CD8^+$ memory T cells. $V\alpha14i$ NKT cells have the surface phenotype of activated cells, including expression of CD69 and high levels of CD44, even in germ-free mice (65), and they have an activated phenotype in humans when isolated from cord blood (66). This raises the question as to how $V\alpha14i$ NKT cells deal with self-antigens presented in the context of CD1d. One answer is that the self-antigens are not always expressed at levels sufficient to drive the full activation of these cells, but that their expression or presentation by CD1d may be induced upon infection, cell stress, or even apoptosis. Additionally, runaway activation of self-reactive $V\alpha14i$ NKT cells may be prevented by the expression of inhibitory NK receptors.

$V\alpha14i$ NKT cell clonal diversity can be assessed by analyzing the diversity of $TCR\beta$ complementarity-determining region (CDR) 3. Even though $V\alpha14i$ NKT cells express a limited subset of $V\beta$ segments, the $CDR3\beta$ diversity for the major $V\beta$ segments, $V\beta8.2$, $V\beta7$, and $V\beta2$, is enormous (67–69), and the likely average clone size, or number of cells with the same rearrangement, is quite small (<10 cells). Several conclusions can be drawn from these data. First, the natural antigen(s) driving the expansion of $V\alpha14i$ NKT cells likely does not contact the CDR3 region of $TCR\beta$. Furthermore, the continual turnover of these cells, measured by BrdU incorporation (23, 63), must be balanced by cell death and the export of new clones form the thymus. A puzzling finding is that the repertoire of Vβ segments in Vα14i NKT cells in different organs is distinct (69). Perhaps Vα14i NKT cells do not rapidly circulate from one organ to another, compared with the rate at which they are replenished from the thymus. Although this is a cogent explanation, analysis of adult thymectomized mice indicates that peripheral replenishment of the Vα14i NKT cell pool is possible (53). In contrast, in human adults Vα24i NKT cells have a limited Vβ diversity, although the diversity is much greater in cord blood (66). Therefore, the Vβ diversity in mouse Vα14i NKT cells may contract as a result of infection, repeated antigenic stimulation, or aging.

Following stimulation in vivo with αGalCer, anti-CD3, or IL-12, Vα14i NKT cells disappear within a few hours (7, 70). This was originally attributed to activation-induced cell death (70–74). It is now evident, however, that after αGalCer treatment many of the Vα14i NKT cells do not die, but they downregulate their TCR and NK1.1 (7, 75–77), making them undetectable. Vα14i NKT cells reexpress their TCR and expand dramatically by two days after αGalCer exposure, although many of them are NK1.1 negative (75–77). By approximately nine days after αGalCer, the number of Vα14i NKT cells returns to the level found before antigen exposure (75–77). What happens upon reexposure to αGalCer? The question of Vα14i NKT cell memory is a difficult one because Vα14i NKT cells exhibit characteristics of memory cells even before αGalCer exposure. It remains possible, however, that the behavior of Vα14i NKT cells changes after antigenic exposure. It has been reported that repeated exposure to αGalCer causes Th2 cytokine skewing of both the Vα14i NKT cell (78) and concomitant conventional T cell responses (79), but this has not been found in every study (80).

SPECIFICITY

In this review, I have treated the expression of the Vα14i TCR and reactivity to αGalCer presented by CD1d as synonymous. However, relatively rare Vα14i TCR$^+$ cells have been found that respond preferentially to phosphatidylinositol and phosphoethanolamine presented by CD1d (81, 82), and in humans αGalCer plus CD1d-reactive T cells have been identified that do not have a canonical Vα24i TCR (83). Nonetheless, equivalence of Vαi TCR expression and reactivity to αGalCer presented by CD1d remain a reasonably accurate generalization. This conclusion is supported by the results from a variety of studies, including one in which 71/73 hybridomas with a Vα14i TCR responded to αGalCer presented by CD1d (84).

Within the population of cells with a Vα14i TCR or a Vα24i TCR, subpopulations can be found that respond to other glycolipids. Given the expression of an invariant TCRα chain, these additional specificities must be based on the Vβ segment expressed or on features of the CDR3β region. For example, T cells reactive to ganglioside GD$_3$ presented by CD1d can be detected after immunization with GD$_3$ (85). The GD$_3$-reactive T cells can be depleted with αGalCer/CD1d tetramers, and they constitute a subset of the αGalCer plus CD1d-reactive cells.

Investigators generally accept that $V\alpha14i$ NKT cells are reactive to self-ligands or antigens presented by CD1d, and reactivity of these cells to microbial glycolipids has been difficult to prove unequivocally. Recently, however, Fischer et al. (86) reported that a subset of mouse $V\alpha14i$ and human $V\alpha24i$ T cells react to material purified from bacterial cell walls enriched for phosphatidylinositol tetramannoside (PIM_4). The reactive cells were a minority, consisting in some of the experiments of approximately 1% of the αGalCer/CD1d tetramer–reactive cells (86). Interestingly, PIM_2, a similar compound but with only two as opposed to four mannose sugars, was less able to stimulate NKT cells, although PIM_2 was reported earlier to have TCR-independent effects on the recruitment of $V\alpha14i$ NKT cells (62).

On the basis of the crystal structures of glycolipids with human CD1b and CD1a molecules (87–89), investigators have concluded that the aliphatic chains of αGalCer likely fill the CD1d binding groove, with the more hydrophilic portions exposed for TCR recognition. Extensive structure-function studies with compounds related to αGalCer have mapped the sites likely to be important for the TCR interaction (90–92). The most critical features are in the area around the sugar-lipid linkage, including the 2′ OH in the equatorial position in the sugar, the α linkage of the sugar to the 1 carbon of the ceramide, and the hydroxyl on the 3 carbon of the sphingosine (Figure 1). The results from several studies indicate that the $V\alpha14i$ TCR binds to complexes of αGalCer plus CD1d with a relatively high affinity and a particularly long half-life ($t_{1/2}$), on the order of minutes rather than the seconds characterizing conventional peptide plus MHC class I– or class II–reactive TCRs (93–96). Many $V\alpha14i$ NKT cells are CD4, CD8 double negative, and this strong interaction may be a requirement for activating the TCR in the absence of cooperation from CD4 or CD8 coreceptors. It remains possible, however, that synthetic αGalCer is an agonist with an exceptionally strong potency. More recently, investigators have measured the TCR affinity for a series of six αGalCer analogs, and this measurement was correlated with their antigenic potency (96). In this study, a TCR $t_{1/2}$ of at least one minute was required for effective agonist activity. $V\alpha14i$ NKT cells can also respond to signals from cytokines such as IL-12 in the absence of TCR cross-linking (97, 98), and, as suggested by one recent study (99), in the context of an inflammatory response including IL-12, the $V\alpha14i$ TCR may be activated by much weaker agonists.

Evidence strongly suggests, however, that $V\alpha14i$ NKT cells are reactive to a self-antigen bound to CD1d. $V\alpha14i$ NKT cells have an activated phenotype in cord blood (66) and in germ-free mice (65), and CD1d autoreactivity can be measured in vitro under some conditions, such as (*a*) when CD1d is overexpressed; (*b*) when the inhibitory NK receptors expressed by $V\alpha14i$ NKT cells are not expressed, as in hybridomas (100); or (*c*) when they cannot interact with their ligands on D^b-deficient antigen-presenting cells (APCs) (101). The self-ligand is likely to be a glycolipid, perhaps even a glycosphingolipid similar to αGalCer, although other types of molecules, such as lipopeptides, have been shown to be presented by different CD1 molecules (102).

CYTOKINE PRODUCTION

Activated Vα14i and Vα24i NKT cells have both perforin-dependent and FasL-dependent cytotoxic function, which is dependent upon TCR recognition of cognate antigen, as opposed to the killing of classic NK targets (103). The hallmark of the Vα14i NKT cell response, however, is the rapid and copious production of cytokines. Secretion of the prototypical Th1 and Th2 cytokines, IFN-γ and IL-4, respectively, has been most thoroughly documented, but TCR-activated NKT cells produce many other cytokines, including IL-2, tumor necrosis factor (TNF), IL-5, IL-13, and GM-CSF. The question remains as to how this mélange leads to a regulated immune response, but experimental evidence favors several possible explanations, which are not mutually exclusive.

One possibility is that there are subsets of Vα14i and Vα24i NKT cells, based on anatomic location and/or cell surface phenotype, and that the activation of one subset or the other could have a selective influence. In humans, there is evidence that the Vα24i NKT cells produce more IL-4 (49, 58), but strong evidence for functional subsets of mouse Vα14i NKT cells is lacking.

A second possibility is that the quality of the TCR signal influences the cytokine profile produced, by analogy with the effects of altered peptide ligands on conventional CD4$^+$ T cells. Consistent with this, OCH, an αGalCer analog with a shortened sphingosine (Figure 1), reportedly stimulates a higher ratio of IL-4 to IFN-γ secretion when added to total spleen cell cultures (104, 105). Promotion of Th2 cytokine secretion correlates with the reduced aliphatic chain length of OCH and related compounds (106), and evidence indicates that poor induction of the c-Rel transcription factor may be in part responsible for the reduced IFN-γ gene transcription (106). By contrast, a C-glycoside analog of αGalCer (Figure 1) has been reported to stimulate a higher ratio of IFN-γ to IL-4 (107). So far, there is no structural basis for predicting how a compound will affect the cytokines produced by activated Vα14i NKT cells. Moreover, there is recent evidence indicating that Vα14i NKT cells contain at least some mRNA for both IL-4 and IFN-γ, even before TCR activation (35, 108), although it remains to be demonstrated that these amounts are physiologically significant. However, Vα14i NKT cell cytokine production resulting from TCR stimulation is not influenced by IL-4, IL-12, or other factors that influence the cytokine production pattern of conventional T cells (108). Collectively, these data suggest that Vα14i NKT cells are poised to produce immediately both Th1 and Th2 cytokines following a TCR signal. It is possible that this immediate response, which occurs by two hours, is not sustained under some conditions, thereby allowing for Th1 or Th2 polarized cytokine production by Vα14i NKT cells (76). However, activation of Vα14i NKT cells also leads to the immediate activation of other cells types. For example, within hours of αGalCer stimulation of Vα14i NKT cells, NK cells are stimulated to secrete IFN-γ (108–110). In fact, the bulk of the systemic IFN-γ detected after αGalCer administration in vivo is due to the activity of NK cells (108). Therefore, although a direct effect of altered lipid ligands on the Vα14i NKT cell needs to be considered, the Th1 polarizing effects of a particular glycolipid on the immune response may depend more on how much it stimulates communication between $V\alpha14i$ NKT cells and NK cells or other cell types. This cell-cell communication could be a function of several factors, such as CD40L induction by the $V\alpha14i$ NKT cells, rather than alterations in the cytokine profile produced by the activated $V\alpha14i$ NKT cells themselves.

A third possibility is that cytokine production by $V\alpha14i$ NKT cells can be determined by the integration of signals from different types of receptors, and that this can influence the pattern of cytokines produced. For example, although IL-12 signals are not required for $V\alpha14i$ NKT cells to produce IFN-γ after αGalCer stimulation, IL-12 can selectively stimulate IFN-γ production by $V\alpha14i$ NKT cells in the absence of αGalCer (97, 98), and NK1.1 cross-linking has been reported to do the same (111). In a recent series of experiments, IL-12, produced by APCs stimulated with lipopolysaccharide, promotes IFN-γ but not IL-4 synthesis by $V\alpha14i$ and $V\alpha24i$ NKT cells (99). Such IFN-γ synthesis may also require a TCR signal delivered by weak agonists, however, because anti-CD1d antibodies could block the $V\alpha14i$ NKT cell response to IL-12 (99). Therefore, according to this view, integration of weak TCR signals and IL-12R-mediated signals may favor a Th1 polarized pattern of cytokine production by $V\alpha14i$ NKT cells, although stronger TCR signals favor a Th0 pattern.

A fourth possibility is that the context in which αGalCer is presented has an influence on the pattern of cytokines produced. When bone marrow–derived dendritic cells (DCs) pulsed with αGalCer were administered to mice, the response was different from the one engendered by injection of the compound itself (112). The glycolipid-pulsed DCs caused an increased and prolonged release of IFN-γ compared with the free compound. This could be due to the DC-influenced increased activation of NK cells and/or the integration of signals from other receptors on the $V\alpha14i$ NKT cells, as outlined above. Another important factor is the previous exposure to αGalCer, which, as outlined above, seems to favor Th2 responses (78, 79). In conclusion, cytokine production induced in other cells by activated $V\alpha14i$ NKT cells, and the cytokines they produce themselves, can be modulated, but they are not influenced by the same factors that determine the cytokine response of conventional CD4$^+$ T cells. In general, the pattern of cytokines produced immediately following TCR stimulation of $V\alpha14i$ NKT cells is relatively difficult to alter.

Communication with other Cell Types

Activation of $V\alpha14i$ and $V\alpha24i$ NKT cells has an effect on nearly every hematopoietic cell type, including DCs, NK cells, and B and T lymphocytes. This has usually been studied in the context of stimulation with αGalCer, however, which is a highly potent stimulus that might not reflect the outcome when these NKT cells are activated in a more physiologic way. Nevertheless, under conditions of stimulation with this synthetic antigen, DC maturation is enhanced (113–116). NK cells proliferate and secrete IFN-γ, and their cytotoxic activity is increased (103, 108–110).

B cells express activation markers, total serum Ig increases, and Vα24i NKT cells help B cells secrete Ig (78, 117, 118). Vα14i NKT cells can affect the cytokine profile elicited by CD4$^+$ T cells (79). They also provide effective help for CD8 T cells (119). Moreover, αGalCer acts as an adjuvant that can increase the magnitude of the CD8 T cell response to protein antigens (120, 121). Although it is possible that Vα14i and Vα24i NKT cells provide cognate help for CD1d-expressing B cells, many of the diverse effects of activated NKT cells may be mediated by their communication with CD1d$^+$ DC. Activated Vα14i NKT cells induce CD40L, which can interact with CD40 to stimulate release of IL-12 by DCs (122, 123).

It is appealing to speculate that physiologic activation of Vα14i NKT cells could under some circumstances be an important source of the CD4 help required during the priming of CD8 T cells, as the frequency of this population is 1% or greater than the total T cells in spleen, bone marrow, and elsewhere. During the primary response, the frequency of antigen-specific, conventional CD4$^+$ T cells might not be high enough to provide effective help, but the frequency of Vα14i NKT cells is lower in the lymph nodes, where T cell priming occurs and T cell help is needed, than in the spleen and liver.

Vα14i NKT cells are sometimes considered to be regulatory T cells. Regulation is often thought of as suppression, but in many cases Vα14i NKT cells tend to have an activating effect on immune responses, although this may be in a Th1 or a Th2 direction. In this regard, they are unlike CD4$^+$ CD25$^+$ regulatory T cells, the best-characterized regulatory population, which almost uniformly inhibit different types of immune responses. Surprisingly, there is little information as to how these two populations influence one another, but recent studies reported that activation of self-reactive CD4$^+$ CD25$^+$ regulatory T cells could inhibit the antitumor response of Vα14i NKT cells (124, 125).

Vα14i NKT Cells in the Systemic Immune Response

Vα14i NKT cells play a pivotal role in influencing a very diverse group of immune responses (1). There are controversies regarding some of these reports, which may reflect technical differences in the way the studies were carried out or differences in genetic background of the mice. For example, in a cerebral malaria model, NKT cells promoted pathogenesis in C57BL/6 mice, but they inhibited it in BALB/c mice (126). Because of these controversies, investigators should consider the experimental means by which a pivotal role for Vα14i NKT cells has been assigned. The involvement of Vα14i NKT cells has been tested in different experimental contexts by analyzing the effects of stimulation with αGalCer (1) or with related compounds such as OCH (104). As noted above, the limitation of αGalCer is that the response to this strong TCR agonist may not reflect the physiologic activation of Vα14i NKT cells. This limitation is highlighted by the results from studies of the immune response to cancers. There is a potent role for αGalCer in preventing tumor metastases (2), but in the absence of αGalCer treatment, tumor surveillance is mainly unaffected when Vα14i NKT cells are absent, although the response to methylcholanthrene-induced sarcomas (127) and GM-CSF-transfected tumors (128) constitute exceptions in which Vα14i NKT cells play an important role even in the absence of αGalCer. A second method is to analyze mice deficient for Vα14i NKT cells or their activity. Acute depletion Vα14i NKT cells can be achieved by in vivo treatment with anti-NK1.1 antibodies, but this also depletes NK cells. In vivo treatment with anti-CD1d antibodies has been used successfully to block Vα14i NKT cell activity (59). Typically, however, analysis of immune responses in the absence of Vα14i NKT cells is carried out using either CD1d$^{-/-}$ or Jα18$^{-/-}$ mice. Deletion of CD1d can have several effects, including the loss of those CD1d-reactive T cells with more diverse TCRs that are not αGalCer reactive. In the response to several viruses and in ulcerative colitis patients (129), these CD1d-reactive T cells with more diverse TCRs may be important for influencing the magnitude of the immune response (130–132).

As reviewed previously (1), the beneficial immune responses in which Vα14i NKT cells have been reported to participate include (*a*) the response to tumors; (*b*) host protection from a variety of infectious agents, including bacteria, parasites, and viruses; (*c*) the prevention of autoimmune diseases; and (*d*) the maintenance of self-tolerance. Surprisingly, however, there is no single mechanism through which they exert their influence. For example, antitumor responses (127) and the response to infectious agents (4) depend on the stimulation of IFN-γ secretion by Vα14i NKT cells, whereas the prevention of diabetes may depend on IL-4 and IL-10 secretion (133). The prevention of experimental autoimmune encephalomyelitis may depend on IL-4 secretion (104, 134). The role of Vα14i NKT cells in anterior chamber immune deviation depends on IL-10 (135). Even when there is relative agreement among researchers that Vα14i NKT cells are important, some controversy remains regarding mechanism. For example, although many studies implicate IL-4 in the protective effect of Vα14i NKT cells in diabetes (3), others do not (136). Additionally, the sources of these beneficial cytokines remain incompletely defined. Because the activation of Vα14i NKT cells results in a network of cellular activation events, it need not be the case that the Vα14i NKT cells are the sole or even the major source of the relevant cytokine, although they may be critical for the initial induction of its synthesis. Antitumor responses stimulated by αGalCer provide a model for understanding these types of interactions, as the Vα14i NKT cell–mediated stimulation of NK cells to release IFN-γ may be critical (137).

In many cases, Vα14i NKT cells are required for or participate in the development of detrimental immune responses, including the induction of airway hypersensitivity, which requires IL-4 and IL-13 (60, 61), the development of oxazalone-induced colitis, which requires IL-13 (138), and the abrogation of maternal tolerance of the fetus, dependent on TNF and IFN-γ (139). More recently, Vα14i NKT cells have been shown to play a harmful role in the atherosclerosis that develops in apolipoprotein E–deficient mice fed a high-fat diet (140, 141). This disease-promoting role for Vα14i NKT cells is consistent with the emerging view of atherosclerotic plaque as an inflammatory lesion.

Despite many studies, a consensus view has not emerged in support of the true physiologic role of $V\alpha14i$ NKT cells. This difficulty provides a stark contrast with the $CD4^+$ $CD25^+$ regulatory T cell population, which, despite some uncertainty regarding mechanism, clearly functions as a suppressive population. $V\alpha14i$ NKT cells may either suppress or activate immune responses. They may act as regulators that direct Th2 responses but may, in some cases, promote Th1 responses. Moreover, they may act as effectors as well as regulators by accumulating in sites of inflammation and by exhibiting cytotoxic activity. Furthermore, rules have not yet emerged that would allow investigators to predict the function of these cells in a particular context. One appealing speculation that can account for the myriad effects of $V\alpha14i$ NKT cell stimulation is that the main function of $V\alpha14i$ NKT cells is to condition or educate various types of DCs so that they might in turn program appropriate adaptive immune responses. Chronic stimulation of $V\alpha14i$ NKT cells might result from CD1d-mediated presentation by DCs of endogenous ligands resulting from cellular stress or danger. The DCs may take up these ligands by endocytosis, which is an effective pathway for CD1d-mediated antigen presentation. The "interpretation" of the resulting $V\alpha14i$ NKT cell response may depend on a variety factors, including the types of DCs affected, as well as the strength or quality of the TCR signal and the cytokine milieu.

Clinical Relevance of $V\alpha24i$ NKT Cells

Although basic scientists have intensely studied the unique features of NKT cell responses to lipid antigens, these cells also have fascinated more clinically oriented scientists, and clinical trials of αGalCer therapy in cancer are already underway. A number of investigators have reported decreased $V\alpha24i$ NKT cells in a variety of autoimmune diseases (142). A striking example is type I diabetes, in which the frequency of invariant $V\alpha24$-$J\alpha18$ sequences among $V\alpha24^+$ double-negative T cells was reported to be lower in diabetics than in their disease-free identical twins (143). The ability of $V\alpha24i$ NKT cell clones derived from diabetics to produce IL-4 was also impaired. These findings were especially compelling, given their similarity to those from NOD mice, but they could only be corroborated by some subsequent studies (144) and not by others (18). In addition to the generally lower frequency of $V\alpha24i$ NKT cells in humans compared with their counterparts in mice, another problem in their investigation is that study of peripheral blood NKT cells, which often is the only site accessible in human studies, may not adequately reflect the frequency and function of NKT cells in other sites. In NOD mice, the decreased numbers of $V\alpha14i$ NKT cells in organs such as the spleen are not reflected by a similar decrease in the blood (145). Moreover, there is a great range in the frequency of $V\alpha24i$ NKT cells in the peripheral blood of normal individuals, making the detection of differences between diseased and normal populations challenging.

In addition to differences in cell number, correlations between disease status and $V\alpha24i$ NKT cell function have been reported in several cases. In advanced prostate cancer patients, for example, expanded lines of $V\alpha24i$ NKT cells had a reduced capacity to produce IFN-γ upon stimulation (146). The expanded $V\alpha24i$ NKT cells from multiple sclerosis patients in remission showed a Th2 bias compared with Vα24i NKT cells obtained from healthy individuals or individuals who had undergone a relapse (147), suggesting that this Th2 bias is protective. Additionally, there is a report of an 11-year-old girl with disseminated varicella infection after vaccination who had a deficiency of NKT cells and no other detectable immune defect (148).

Despite uncertainties about Vα24i NKT cells' mode of action, modulation of Vα24i NKT cell responses remains an attractive potential target for immune therapy. Positive features of this strategy include the presence of at least some Vα24i NKT cells in all individuals, the ability to specifically target these cells by αGalCer, the relatively low toxicity of this compound (149), and the ability to expand Vα24i NKT cells in vitro in the presence of cytokines and αGalCer (13). Adoptive transfer of activated Vα24i NKT cells may be cumbersome and expensive. Thus, a more attractive strategy is direct activation of these cells in vivo. Although intravenous administration of αGalCer had only limited effects in cancer patients (150), injection of DCs pulsed with αGalCer did activate innate and acquired immunity (149), including increases in serum IFN-γ. Therefore, as evidenced in mice, transferring DCs pulsed with αGalCer could lead to a much more potent Th1 response than injecting the free compound.

CONCLUSIONS

Vα14i and Vα24i NKT cells are surprisingly different from conventional T cells in several ways, including their TCR diversity, coreceptor expression, specificity, development, homing, and cytokine production. However, they share some properties with other populations of what may be considered natural memory lymphocytes, including $\gamma\delta$ T cells, intraepithelial lymphocytes, and B-1 B cells, in that they are capable of rapid effector functions without need for priming and clonal expansion. Despite significant progress in understanding the biology of these NKT cells, their specificity and the means by which they influence immune responses remain to be defined better. Nevertheless, the manipulation of Vα24i NKT cell responses retains some promise as the possible basis for immune therapy.

NOTE ADDED IN PROOF

Recently it was shown that isoglobotrihexosylceramide, a glycosphingolipid, is recognized by both mouse and human NKT cells as an autologous antigen (151).

ACKNOWLEDGMENTS

M.K. is supported by grants from the NIH. I thank my colleagues in the lab and around the world for many helpful discussions, and Kirsten Hammond for critical reading of the manuscript. This is publication number 671 from the La Jolla Institute for Allergy and Immunology.

**The *Annual Review of Immunology* is online at
http://immunol.annualreviews.org**

LITERATURE CITED

1. Kronenberg M, Gapin L. 2002. The unconventional lifestyle of NKT cells. *Nat. Rev. Immunol.* 2:557–68
2. Smyth MJ, Crowe NY, Hayakawa Y, Takeda K, Yagita H, Godfrey DI. 2002. NKT cells—conductors of tumor immunity? *Curr. Opin. Immunol.* 14:165–71
3. Hammond KJ, Kronenberg M. 2003. Natural killer T cells: natural or unnatural regulators of autoimmunity? *Curr. Opin. Immunol.* 15:683–89
4. Skold M, Behar SM. 2003. Role of CD1d-restricted NKT cells in microbial immunity. *Infect. Immun.* 71:5447–55
5. Taniguchi M, Harada M, Kojo S, Nakayama T, Wakao H. 2003. The regulatory role of $V\alpha 14$ NKT cells in innate and acquired immune response. *Annu. Rev. Immunol.* 21:483–513
6. Brigl M, Brenner MB. 2004. CD1: antigen presentation and T cell function. *Annu. Rev. Immunol.* 22:817–90
7. Matsuda JL, Naidenko OV, Gapin L, Nakayama T, Taniguchi M, et al. 2000. Tracking the response of natural killer T cells to a glycolipid antigen using CD1d tetramers. *J. Exp. Med.* 192:741–54
7a. Yoshimoto T, Paul WE. 1994. CD4[pos], NK1.1[pos] T cells promptly produce interleukin 4 in response to in vivo challenge with anti-CD3. *J. Exp. Med.* 179:1285–95
8. Bendelac A, Rivera MN, Park SH, Roark JH. 1997. Mouse CD1-specific NK1 T cells: development, specificity, and function. *Annu. Rev. Immunol.* 15:535–62
9. Godfrey DI, MacDonald HR, Kronenberg M, Smyth MJ, Van Kaer L. 2004. NKT cells: What's in a name? *Nat. Rev. Immunol.* 4:231–37
10. Slifka MK, Pagarigan RR, Whitton JL. 2000. NK markers are expressed on a high percentage of virus-specific CD8[+] and CD4[+] T cells. *J. Immunol.* 164:2009–15
11. Porcelli S, Yockey CE, Brenner MB, Balk SP. 1993. Analysis of T cell antigen receptor (TCR) expression by human peripheral blood CD4[-]8[-] α/β T cells demonstrates preferential use of several $V\beta$ genes and an invariant $TCR\alpha$ chain. *J. Exp. Med.* 178:1–16
12. Dellabona P, Padovan E, Casorati G, Brockhaus M, Lanzavecchia A. 1994. An invariant $V\alpha 24$-$J\alpha Q/V\beta$ 11 T cell receptor is expressed in all individuals by clonally expanded CD4[-]8[-] T cells. *J. Exp. Med.* 180:1171–76
13. Brossay L, Chioda M, Burdin N, Koezuka Y, Casorati G, et al. 1998. CD1d-mediated recognition of an α-galactosylceramide by natural killer T cells is highly conserved through mammalian evolution. *J. Exp. Med.* 188:1521–28
14. Spada FM, Koezuka Y, Porcelli SA. 1998. CD1d-restricted recognition of synthetic glycolipid antigens by human natural killer T cells. *J. Exp. Med.* 188:1529–34
15. Benlagha K, Weiss A, Beavis A, Teyton L, Bendelac A. 2000. In vivo identification of glycolipid antigen-specific T cells using fluorescent CD1d tetramers. *J. Exp. Med.* 191:1895–903
16. Karadimitris A, Gadola S, Altamirano M, Brown D, Woolfson A, et al. 2001. Human CD1d-glycolipid tetramers generated by in vitro oxidative refolding chromatography. *Proc. Natl. Acad. Sci. USA* 98:3294–98
17. Kita H, Naidenko OV, Kronenberg M, Ansari AA, Rogers P, et al. 2002. Quantitation and phenotypic analysis of natural killer T cells in primary biliary cirrhosis

using a human CD1d tetramer. *Gastroenterology* 123:1031–43

18. Lee PT, Putnam A, Benlagha K, Teyton L, Gottlieb PA, Bendelac A. 2002. Testing the NKT cell hypothesis of human IDDM pathogenesis. *J. Clin. Invest.* 110:793–800

19. Rogers PR, Matsumoto A, Naidenko O, Kronenberg M, Mikayama T, Kato S. 2004. Expansion of human Vα24$^+$ NKT cells by repeated stimulation with KRN7000. *J. Immunol. Methods* 285:197–214

20. Gapin L, Matsuda JL, Surh CD, Kronenberg M. 2001. NKT cells derive from double-positive thymocytes that are positively selected by CD1d. *Nat. Immunol.* 2:971–78

21. Benlagha K, Kyin T, Beavis A, Teyton L, Bendelac A. 2002. A thymic precursor to the NK T cell lineage. *Science* 296:553–55

22. Pellicci DG, Hammond KJ, Uldrich AP, Baxter AG, Smyth MJ, Godfrey DI. 2002. A natural killer T (NKT) cell developmental pathway involving a thymus-dependent NK1.1$^-$CD4$^+$ CD1d-dependent precursor stage. *J. Exp. Med.* 195:835–44

23. Coles MC, Raulet DH. 2000. NK1.1$^+$ T cells in the liver arise in the thymus and are selected by interactions with class I molecules on CD4$^+$CD8$^+$ cells. *J. Immunol.* 164:2412–18

24. Forestier C, Park SH, Wei D, Benlagha K, Teyton L, Bendelac A. 2003. T cell development in mice expressing CD1d directed by a classical MHC class II promoter. *J. Immunol.* 171:4096–104

25. Elewaut D, Kronenberg M. 2000. Molecular biology of NK T cell specificity and development. *Semin. Immunol.* 12:561–68

26. Sivakumar V, Hammond KJ, Howells N, Pfeffer K, Weih F. 2003. Differential requirement for Rel/nuclear factor κB family members in natural killer T cell development. *J. Exp. Med.* 197:1613–21

27. Stanic AK, Bezbradica JS, Park JJ, Matsuki N, Mora AL, et al. 2004. NF-κB controls cell fate specification, survival, and molecular differentiation of immunoregulatory natural T lymphocytes. *J. Immunol.* 172:2265–73

28. Schmidt-Supprian M, Tian J, Grant EP, Pasparakis M, Maehr R, et al. 2004. Differential dependence of CD4$^+$CD25$^+$ regulatory and natural killer-like T cells on signals leading to NF-κB activation. *Proc. Natl. Acad. Sci. USA* 101:4566–71

29. Elewaut D, Shaikh RB, Hammond KJ, De Winter H, Leishman AJ, et al. 2003. NIK-dependent RelB activation defines a unique signaling pathway for the development of Vα14i NKT cells. *J. Exp. Med.* 197:1623–33

30. Townsend MJ, Weinmann AS, Matsuda JL, Salomon R, Farnham PJ, et al. 2004. T-bet regulates the terminal maturation and homeostasis of NK and Vα14i NKT cells. *Immunity* 20:477–94

31. Elewaut D, Lawton AP, Nagarajan NA, Maverakis E, Khurana A, et al. 2003. The adaptor protein AP-3 is required for CD1d-mediated antigen presentation of glycosphingolipids and development of Vα14i NKT cells. *J. Exp. Med.* 198:1133–46

32. Cernadas M, Sugita M, van der Wel N, Cao X, Gumperz JE, et al. 2003. Lysosomal localization of murine CD1d mediated by AP-3 is necessary for NK T cell development. *J. Immunol.* 171:4149–55

33. Zhou D, Cantu C 3rd, Sagiv Y, Schrantz N, Kulkarni AB, et al. 2004. Editing of CD1d-bound lipid antigens by endosomal lipid transfer proteins. *Science* 303:523–27

34. Kang SJ, Cresswell P. 2004. Saposins facilitate CD1d-restricted presentation of an exogenous lipid antigen to T cells. *Nat. Immunol.* 5:175–81

35. Stetson DB, Mohrs M, Reinhardt RL, Baron JL, Wang ZE, et al. 2003. Constitutive cytokine mRNAs mark natural killer (NK) and NK T cells poised for rapid effector function. *J. Exp. Med.* 198:1069–76

36. Gadue P, Stein PL. 2002. NK T cell precursors exhibit differential cytokine regulation and require Itk for efficient maturation. *J. Immunol.* 169:2397–406

37. Eberl G, Lowin-Kropf B, MacDonald HR. 1999. Cutting edge: NKT cell development is selectively impaired in Fyn-deficient mice. *J. Immunol.* 163:4091–94

38. Gadue P, Morton N, Stein PL. 1999. The Src family tyrosine kinase Fyn regulates natural killer T cell development. *J. Exp. Med.* 190:1189–96

39. Gadue P, Yin L, Jain S, Stein PL. 2004. Restoration of NK T cell development in *fyn*-mutant mice by a TCR reveals a requirement for Fyn during early NK T cell ontogeny. *J. Immunol.* 172:6093–100

40. Shimamura M, Ohteki T, Beutner U, MacDonald HR. 1997. Lack of directed Vα14-Jα 281 rearrangements in NK1$^+$ T cells. *Eur. J. Immunol.* 27:1576–79

41. Cheroutre H. 2004. Starting at the beginning: new perspectives on the biology of mucosal T cells. *Annu. Rev. Immunol.* 22:217–46

42. Leishman AJ, Gapin L, Capone M, Palmer E, MacDonald HR, et al. 2002. Precursors of functional MHC class I- or class II-restricted CD8$\alpha\alpha^+$ T cells are positively selected in the thymus by agonist self-peptides. *Immunity* 16:355–64

43. Yamagata T, Mathis D, Benoist C. 2004. Self-reactivity in thymic double-positive cells commits cells to a CD8$\alpha\alpha$ lineage with characteristics of innate immune cells. *Nat. Immunol.* 5:597–605

44. Jordan MS, Boesteanu A, Reed AJ, Petrone AL, Holenbeck AE, et al. 2001. Thymic selection of CD4$^+$CD25$^+$ regulatory T cells induced by an agonist self-peptide. *Nat. Immunol.* 2:301–6

45. Bendelac A, Killeen N, Littman DR, Schwartz RH. 1994. A subset of CD4$^+$ thymocytes selected by MHC class I molecules. *Science* 263:1774–78

46. Hernandez-Hoyos G, Sohn SJ, Rothenberg EV, Alberola-Ila J. 2000. Lck activity controls CD4/CD8 T cell lineage commitment. *Immunity* 12:313–22

47. Singer A. 2002. New perspectives on a developmental dilemma: the kinetic signaling model and the importance of signal duration for the CD4/CD8 lineage decision. *Curr. Opin. Immunol.* 14:207–15

48. Prussin C, Foster B. 1997. TCR Vα24 and Vβ11 coexpression defines a human NK1 T cell analog containing a unique Th0 subpopulation. *J. Immunol.* 159:5862–70

49. Gumperz JE, Miyake S, Yamamura T, Brenner MB. 2002. Functionally distinct subsets of CD1d-restricted natural killer T cells revealed by CD1d tetramer staining. *J. Exp. Med.* 195:625–36

50. Chun T, Page MJ, Gapin L, Matsuda JL, Xu H, et al. 2003. CD1d-expressing dendritic cells but not thymic epithelial cells can mediate negative selection of NKT cells. *J. Exp. Med.* 197:907–18

51. Pellicci DG, Uldrich AP, Kyparissoudis K, Crowe NY, Brooks AG, et al. 2003. Intrathymic NKT cell development is blocked by the presence of α-galactosylceramide. *Eur. J. Immunol.* 33:1816–23

52. Schumann J, Voyle RB, Wei BY, MacDonald HR. 2003. Cutting edge: influence of the TCR Vβ domain on the avidity of CD1d:α-galactosylceramide binding by invariant Vα14 NKT cells. *J. Immunol.* 170:5815–19

53. Hayakawa Y, Berzins SP, Crowe NY, Godfrey DI, Smyth MJ. 2004. Antigen-induced tolerance by intrathymic modulation of self-recognizing inhibitory receptors. *Nat. Immunol.* 5:590–96

54. Voyle RB, Beermann F, Lees RK, Schumann J, Zimmer J, et al. 2003. Ligand-dependent inhibition of CD1d-restricted NKT cell development in mice transgenic for the activating receptor Ly49D. *J. Exp. Med.* 197:919–25

55. Kim CH, Butcher EC, Johnston B. 2002. Distinct subsets of human Vα24-invariant NKT cells: cytokine responses and

chemokine receptor expression. *Trends Immunol.* 23:516–19

56. Johnston B, Kim CH, Soler D, Emoto M, Butcher EC. 2003. Differential chemokine responses and homing patterns of murine TCR $\alpha\beta$ NKT cell subsets. *J. Immunol.* 171:2960–69

57. Thomas SY, Hou R, Boyson JE, Means TK, Hess C, et al. 2003. CD1d-restricted NKT cells express a chemokine receptor profile indicative of Th1-type inflammatory homing cells. *J. Immunol.* 171:2571–80

58. Lee PT, Benlagha K, Teyton L, Bendelac A. 2002. Distinct functional lineages of human Vα24 natural killer T cells. *J. Exp. Med.* 195:637–41

59. Nieuwenhuis EE, Matsumoto T, Exley M, Schleipman RA, Glickman J, et al. 2002. CD1d-dependent macrophage-mediated clearance of *Pseudomonas aeruginosa* from lung. *Nat. Med.* 8:588–93

60. Akbari O, Stock P, Meyer E, Kronenberg M, Sidobre S, et al. 2003. Essential role of NKT cells producing IL-4 and IL-13 in the development of allergen-induced airway hyperreactivity. *Nat. Med.* 9:582–88

61. Lisbonne M, Diem S, de Castro Keller A, Lefort J, Araujo LM, et al. 2003. Cutting edge: Invariant Vα14 NKT cells are required for allergen-induced airway inflammation and hyperreactivity in an experimental asthma model. *J. Immunol.* 171:1637–41

62. Mempel M, Ronet C, Suarez F, Gilleron M, Puzo G, et al. 2002. Natural killer T cells restricted by the monomorphic MHC class 1b CD1d1 molecules behave like inflammatory cells. *J. Immunol.* 168:365–71

63. Matsuda JL, Gapin L, Sidobre S, Kieper WC, Tan JT, et al. 2002. Homeostasis of Vα14i NKT cells. *Nat. Immunol.* 3:966–74

64. Ranson T, Vosshenrich CA, Corcuff E, Richard O, Laloux V, et al. 2003. IL-15 availability conditions homeostasis of peripheral natural killer T cells. *Proc. Natl. Acad. Sci. USA* 100:2663–68

65. Park SH, Benlagha K, Lee D, Balish E, Bendelac A. 2000. Unaltered phenotype, tissue distribution and function of Vα14+ NKT cells in germ-free mice. *Eur. J. Immunol.* 30:620–25

66. D'Andrea A, Goux D, De Lalla C, Koezuka Y, Montagna D, et al. 2000. Neonatal invariant Vα24+ NKT lymphocytes are activated memory cells. *Eur. J. Immunol.* 30:1544–50

67. Apostolou I, Cumano A, Gachelin G, Kourilsky P. 2000. Evidence for two subgroups of CD4−CD8− NKT cells with distinct TCR $\alpha\beta$ repertoires and differential distribution in lymphoid tissues. *J. Immunol.* 165:2481–90

68. Ronet C, Mempel M, Thieblemont N, Lehuen A, Kourilsky P, Gachelin G. 2001. Role of the complementarity-determining region 3 (CDR3) of the TCR-β chains associated with the Vα14 semi-invariant TCRα-chain in the selection of CD4+ NK T cells. *J. Immunol.* 166:1755–62

69. Matsuda JL, Gapin L, Fazilleau N, Warren K, Naidenko OV, Kronenberg M. 2001. Natural killer T cells reactive to a single glycolipid exhibit a highly diverse T cell receptor β repertoire and small clone size. *Proc. Natl. Acad. Sci. USA* 98:12636–41

70. Eberl G, MacDonald HR. 1998. Rapid death and regeneration of NKT cells in anti-CD3ε- or IL-12-treated mice: a major role for bone marrow in NKT cell homeostasis. *Immunity* 9:345–53

71. Osman Y, Kawamura T, Naito T, Takeda K, Van Kaer L, et al. 2000. Activation of hepatic NKT cells and subsequent liver injury following administration of α-galactosylceramide. *Eur. J. Immunol.* 30:1919–28

72. Leite-de-Moraes MC, Herbelin A, Gouarin C, Koezuka Y, Schneider E, Dy M. 2000. Fas/Fas ligand interactions promote activation-induced cell death of NK T lymphocytes. *J. Immunol.* 165:4367–71

73. Hayakawa Y, Takeda K, Yagita H, Kakuta S, Iwakura Y, et al. 2001. Critical contribution of IFN-γ and NK cells, but not perforin-mediated cytotoxicity, to antimetastatic effect of α-galactosylceramide. *Eur. J. Immunol.* 31:1720–27

74. Nakagawa R, Nagafune I, Tazunoki Y, Ehara H, Tomura H, et al. 2001. Mechanisms of the antimetastatic effect in the liver and of the hepatocyte injury induced by α-galactosylceramide in mice. *J. Immunol.* 166:6578–84

75. Wilson MT, Johansson C, Olivares-Villagomez D, Singh AK, Stanic AK, et al. 2003. The response of natural killer T cells to glycolipid antigens is characterized by surface receptor down-modulation and expansion. *Proc. Natl. Acad. Sci. USA* 100:10913–18

76. Crowe NY, Uldrich AP, Kyparissoudis K, Hammond KJ, Hayakawa Y, et al. 2003. Glycolipid antigen drives rapid expansion and sustained cytokine production by NK T cells. *J. Immunol.* 171:4020–27

77. Harada M, Seino K, Wakao H, Sakata S, Ishizuka Y, et al. 2004. Down-regulation of the invariant Vα14 antigen receptor in NKT cells upon activation. *Int. Immunol.* 16:241–47

78. Burdin N, Brossay L, Kronenberg M. 1999. Immunization with α-galactosylceramide polarizes CD1-reactive NK T cells towards Th2 cytokine synthesis. *Eur. J. Immunol.* 29:2014–25

79. Singh N, Hong S, Scherer DC, Serizawa I, Burdin N, et al. 1999. Cutting edge: Activation of NK T cells by CD1d and α-galactosylceramide directs conventional T cells to the acquisition of a Th2 phenotype. *J. Immunol.* 163:2373–77

80. Cui J, Watanabe N, Kawano T, Yamashita M, Kamata T, et al. 1999. Inhibition of T helper cell type 2 cell differentiation and immunoglobulin E response by ligand-activated Vα14 natural killer T cells. *J. Exp. Med.* 190:783–92

81. Gumperz JE, Roy C, Makowska A, Lum D, Sugita M, et al. 2000. Murine CD1d-restricted T cell recognition of cellular lipids. *Immunity* 12:211–21

82. Rauch J, Gumperz J, Robinson C, Skold M, Roy C, et al. 2003. Structural features of the acyl chain determine self-phospholipid antigen recognition by a CD1d-restricted invariant NKT (iNKT) cell. *J. Biol. Chem.* 278:47508–15

83. Gadola SD, Dulphy N, Salio M, Cerundolo V. 2002. Vα24-JαQ-independent, CD1d-restricted recognition of α-galactosylceramide by human CD4$^+$ and CD8 $\alpha\beta^+$ T lymphocytes. *J. Immunol.* 168:5514–20

84. Gui M, Li J, Wen LJ, Hardy RR, Hayakawa K. 2001. TCRβ chain influences but does not solely control autoreactivity of Vα14J281 T cells. *J. Immunol.* 167:6239–46

85. Wu DY, Segal NH, Sidobre S, Kronenberg M, Chapman PB. 2003. Cross-presentation of disialoganglioside GD3 to natural killer T cells. *J. Exp. Med.* 198:173–81

86. Fischer K, Scotet E, Niemeyer M, Koebernick H, Zerrahn J, et al. 2004. Mycobacterial phosphatidylinositol mannoside is a natural antigen for CD1d-restricted T cells. *Proc. Natl. Acad. Sci. USA* 101:10685–90

87. Gadola SD, Zaccai NR, Harlos K, Shepherd D, Castro-Palomino JC, et al. 2002. Structure of human CD1b with bound ligands at 2.3 Å, a maze for alkyl chains. *Nat. Immunol.* 3:721–26

88. Zajonc DM, Elsliger MA, Teyton L, Wilson IA. 2003. Crystal structure of CD1a in complex with a sulfatide self antigen at a resolution of 2.15 Å. *Nat. Immunol.* 4:808–15

89. Batuwangala T, Shepherd D, Gadola SD, Gibson KJ, Zaccai NR, et al. 2004. The crystal structure of human CD1b with a bound bacterial glycolipid. *J. Immunol.* 172:2382–88

90. Kawano T, Cui J, Koezuka Y, Toura I, Kaneko Y, et al. 1997. CD1d-restricted and TCR-mediated activation of Vα14

NKT cells by glycosylceramides. *Science* 278:1626–29

91. Brossay L, Naidenko O, Burdin N, Matsuda J, Sakai T, Kronenberg M. 1998. Structural requirements for galactosylceramide recognition by CD1-restricted NK T cells. *J. Immunol.* 161:5124–28

92. Prigozy TI, Naidenko O, Qasba P, Elewaut D, Brossay L, et al. 2001. Glycolipid antigen processing for presentation by CD1d molecules. *Science* 291:664–67

93. Sidobre S, Naidenko OV, Sim BC, Gascoigne NR, Garcia KC, Kronenberg M. 2002. The Vα14 NKT cell TCR exhibits high-affinity binding to a glycolipid/CD1d complex. *J. Immunol.* 169:1340–48

94. Sim BC, Holmberg K, Sidobre S, Naidenko O, Niederberger N, et al. 2003. Surprisingly minor influence of TRAV11 (Vα14) polymorphism on NK T-receptor mCD1/α-galactosylceramide binding kinetics. *Immunogenetics* 54:874–83

95. Cantu C III, Benlagha K, Savage PB, Bendelac A, Teyton L. 2003. The paradox of immune molecular recognition of α-galactosylceramide: low affinity, low specificity for CD1d, high affinity for αβ TCRs. *J. Immunol.* 170:4673–82

96. Sidobre S, Hammond KJ, Benazet-Sidobre L, Maltsev SD, Richardson SK, et al. 2004. The T cell antigen receptor expressed by Vα14i NKT cells has a unique mode of glycosphingolipid antigen recognition. *Proc. Natl. Acad. Sci. USA* 101:12254–59

97. Leite-De-Moraes MC, Hameg A, Arnould A, Machavoine F, Koezuka Y, et al. 1999. A distinct IL-18-induced pathway to fully activate NK T lymphocytes independently from TCR engagement. *J. Immunol.* 163:5871–76

98. Leite-De-Moraes MC, Moreau G, Arnould A, Machavoine F, Garcia C, et al. 1998. IL-4-producing NK T cells are biased towards IFN-γ production by IL-12. Influence of the microenvironment on the functional capacities of NK T cells. *Eur. J. Immunol.* 28:1507–15

99. Brigl M, Bry L, Kent SC, Gumperz JE, Brenner MB. 2003. Mechanism of CD1d-restricted natural killer T cell activation during microbial infection. *Nat. Immunol.* 4:1230–37

100. Chiu YH, Jayawardena J, Weiss A, Lee D, Park SH, et al. 1999. Distinct subsets of CD1d-restricted T cells recognize self-antigens loaded in different cellular compartments. *J. Exp. Med.* 189:103–10

101. Ikarashi Y, Mikami R, Bendelac A, Terme M, Chaput N, et al. 2001. Dendritic cell maturation overrules H-2D-mediated natural killer T (NKT) cell inhibition: critical role for B7 in CD1d-dependent NKT cell interferon γ production. *J. Exp. Med.* 194:1179–86

102. Moody DB, Young DC, Cheng TY, Rosat JP, Roura-Mir C, et al. 2004. T cell activation by lipopeptide antigens. *Science* 303:527–31

103. Metelitsa LS, Naidenko OV, Kant A, Wu HW, Loza MJ, et al. 2001. Human NKT cells mediate antitumor cytotoxicity directly by recognizing target cell CD1d with bound ligand or indirectly by producing IL-2 to activate NK cells. *J. Immunol.* 167:3114–22

104. Miyamoto K, Miyake S, Yamamura T. 2001. A synthetic glycolipid prevents autoimmune encephalomyelitis by inducing TH2 bias of natural killer T cells. *Nature* 413:531–34

105. Stanic AK, Shashidharamurthy R, Bezbradica JS, Matsuki N, Yoshimura Y, et al. 2003. Another view of T cell antigen recognition: cooperative engagement of glycolipid antigens by Vα14Jα18 natural T (iNKT) cell receptor. *J. Immunol.* 171:4539–51. Erratum. 2004. *J. Immunol.* 172:717

106. Oki S, Chiba A, Yamamura T, Miyake S. 2004. The clinical implication and molecular mechanism of preferential

IL-4 production by modified glycolipid-stimulated NKT cells. *J. Clin. Invest.* 113:1631–40

107. Schmieg J, Yang G, Franck RW, Tsuji M. 2003. Superior protection against malaria and melanoma metastases by a C-glycoside analogue of the natural killer T cell ligand α-galactosylceramide. *J. Exp. Med.* 198:1631–41

108. Matsuda JL, Gapin L, Baron JL, Sidobre S, Stetson DB, et al. 2003. Mouse Vα14*i* natural killer T cells are resistant to cytokine polarization in vivo. *Proc. Natl. Acad. Sci. USA* 100:8395–400

109. Carnaud C, Lee D, Donnars O, Park SH, Beavis A, et al. 1999. Cutting edge: Crosstalk between cells of the innate immune system: NKT cells rapidly activate NK cells. *J. Immunol.* 163:4647–50

110. Eberl G, MacDonald HR. 2000. Selective induction of NK cell proliferation and cytotoxicity by activated NKT cells. *Eur. J. Immunol.* 30:985–92

111. Arase H, Arase N, Saito T. 1996. Interferon γ production by natural killer (NK) cells and NK1.1$^+$ T cells upon NKR-P1 cross-linking. *J. Exp. Med.* 183:2391–96

112. Fujii S, Shimizu K, Kronenberg M, Steinman RM. 2002. Prolonged IFN-γ-producing NKT response induced with α-galactosylceramide-loaded DCs. *Nat. Immunol.* 3:867–74

113. Vincent MS, Leslie DS, Gumperz JE, Xiong X, Grant EP, Brenner MB. 2002. CD1-dependent dendritic cell instruction. *Nat. Immunol.* 3:1163–68

114. Hermans IF, Silk JD, Gileadi U, Salio M, Mathew B, et al. 2003. NKT cells enhance CD4$^+$ and CD8$^+$ T cell responses to soluble antigen in vivo through direct interaction with dendritic cells. *J. Immunol.* 171:5140–47

115. Fujii S, Shimizu K, Smith C, Bonifaz L, Steinman RM. 2003. Activation of natural killer T cells by α-galactosylceramide rapidly induces the full maturation of dendritic cells in vivo and thereby acts as an adjuvant for combined CD4 and CD8 T cell immunity to a coadministered protein. *J. Exp. Med.* 198:267–79

116. Chung Y, Chang WS, Kim S, Kang CY. 2004. NKT cell ligand α-galactosylceramide blocks the induction of oral tolerance by triggering dendritic cell maturation. *Eur. J. Immunol.* 34:2471–79

117. Kitamura H, Ohta A, Sekimoto M, Sato M, Iwakabe K, et al. 2000. α-galactosylceramide induces early B-cell activation through IL-4 production by NKT cells. *Cell. Immunol.* 199:37–42

118. Galli G, Nuti S, Tavarini S, Galli-Stampino L, De Lalla C, et al. 2003. CD1d-restricted help to B cells by human invariant natural killer T lymphocytes. *J. Exp. Med.* 197:1051–57

119. Stober D, Jomantaite I, Schirmbeck R, Reimann J. 2003. NKT cells provide help for dendritic cell-dependent priming of MHC class I-restricted CD8$^+$ T cells in vivo. *J. Immunol.* 170:2540–48

120. Nishimura T, Kitamura H, Iwakabe K, Yahata T, Ohta A, et al. 2000. The interface between innate and acquired immunity: glycolipid antigen presentation by CD1d-expressing dendritic cells to NKT cells induces the differentiation of antigen-specific cytotoxic T lymphocytes. *Int. Immunol.* 12:987–94

121. Gonzalez-Aseguinolaza G, Van Kaer L, Bergmann CC, Wilson JM, Schmieg J, et al. 2002. Natural killer T cell ligand α-galactosylceramide enhances protective immunity induced by malaria vaccines. *J. Exp. Med.* 195:617–24

122. Kitamura H, Iwakabe K, Yahata T, Nishimura S, Ohta A, et al. 1999. The natural killer T (NKT) cell ligand α-galactosylceramide demonstrates its immunopotentiating effect by inducing interleukin (IL)-12 production by dendritic cells and IL-12 receptor expression on NKT cells. *J. Exp. Med.* 189:1121–28

123. Tomura M, Yu WG, Ahn HJ, Yamashita M, Yang YF, et al. 1999. A novel function of Vα14$^+$CD4$^+$NKT cells: stimulation of

IL-12 production by antigen-presenting cells in the innate immune system. *J. Immunol.* 163:93–101

124. Nishikawa H, Kato T, Tanida K, Hiasa A, Tawara I, et al. 2003. CD4$^+$ CD25$^+$ T cells responding to serologically defined autoantigens suppress antitumor immune responses. *Proc. Natl. Acad. Sci. USA* 100: 10902–6

125. Azuma T, Takahashi T, Kunisato A, Kitamura T, Hirai H. 2003. Human CD4$^+$ CD25$^+$ regulatory T cells suppress NKT cell functions. *Cancer Res.* 63:4516–20

126. Hansen DS, Siomos MA, Buckingham L, Scalzo AA, Schofield L. 2003. Regulation of murine cerebral malaria pathogenesis by CD1d-restricted NKT cells and the natural killer complex. *Immunity* 18:391–402

127. Crowe NY, Smyth MJ, Godfrey DI. 2002. A critical role for natural killer T cells in immunosurveillance of methylcholanthrene-induced sarcomas. *J. Exp. Med.* 196:119–27

128. Gillessen S, Naumov YN, Nieuwenhuis EE, Exley MA, Lee FS, et al. 2003. CD1d-restricted T cells regulate dendritic cell function and antitumor immunity in a granulocyte-macrophage colony-stimulating factor-dependent fashion. *Proc. Natl. Acad. Sci. USA* 100:8874–79

129. Fuss IJ, Heller F, Boirivant M, Leon F, Yoshida M, et al. 2004. Nonclassical CD1d-restricted NK T cells that produce IL-13 characterize an atypical Th2 response in ulcerative colitis. *J. Clin. Invest.* 113:1490–97

130. Exley MA, Bigley NJ, Cheng O, Tahir SM, Smiley ST, et al. 2001. CD1d-reactive T-cell activation leads to amelioration of disease caused by diabetogenic encephalomyocarditis virus. *J. Leukoc. Biol.* 69:713–18

131. Baron JL, Gardiner L, Nishimura S, Shinkai K, Locksley R, Ganem D. 2002. Activation of a nonclassical NKT cell subset in a transgenic mouse model of hepatitis B virus infection. *Immunity* 16:583–94

132. Durante-Mangoni E, Wang R, Shaulov A, He Q, Nasser I, et al. 2004. Hepatic CD1d expression in hepatitis C virus infection and recognition by resident proinflammatory CD1d-reactive T cells. *J. Immunol.* 173:2159–66

133. Hammond KJ, Poulton LD, Palmisano LJ, Silveira PA, Godfrey DI, Baxter AG. 1998. α/β-T cell receptor (TCR)$^+$ CD4$^-$CD8$^-$ (NKT) thymocytes prevent insulin-dependent diabetes mellitus in nonobese diabetic (NOD)/Lt mice by the influence of interleukin (IL)-4 and/or IL-10. *J. Exp. Med.* 187:1047–56

134. Singh AK, Wilson MT, Hong S, Olivares-Villagomez D, Du C, et al. 2001. Natural killer T cell activation protects mice against experimental autoimmune encephalomyelitis. *J. Exp. Med.* 194:1801–11

135. Sonoda KH, Faunce DE, Taniguchi M, Exley M, Balk S, Stein-Streilein J. 2001. NK T cell-derived IL-10 is essential for the differentiation of antigen-specific T regulatory cells in systemic tolerance. *J. Immunol.* 166:42–50

136. Beaudoin L, Laloux V, Novak J, Lucas B, Lehuen A. 2002. NKT cells inhibit the onset of diabetes by impairing the development of pathogenic T cells specific for pancreatic β cells. *Immunity* 17:725–36

137. Smyth MJ, Crowe NY, Pellicci DG, Kyparissoudis K, Kelly JM, et al. 2002. Sequential production of interferon-γ by NK1.1$^+$ T cells and natural killer cells is essential for the antimetastatic effect of α-galactosylceramide. *Blood* 99:1259–66

138. Heller F, Fuss IJ, Nieuwenhuis EE, Blumberg RS, Strober W. 2002. Oxazolone colitis, a Th2 colitis model resembling ulcerative colitis, is mediated by IL-13-producing NK-T cells. *Immunity* 17:629–38

139. Ito K, Karasawa M, Kawano T, Akasaka T, Koseki H, et al. 2000. Involvement

of decidual Vα14 NKT cells in abortion. *Proc. Natl. Acad. Sci. USA* 97:740–44

140. Tupin E, Nicoletti A, Elhage R, Rudling M, Ljunggren HG, et al. 2004. CD1d-dependent activation of NKT cells aggravates atherosclerosis. *J. Exp. Med.* 199: 417–22

141. Nakai Y, Iwabuchi K, Fujii S, Ishimori N, Dashtsoodol N, et al. 2004. Natural killer T cells accelerate atherogenesis in mice. *Blood* 104:2051–59

142. van der Vliet HJ, von Blomberg BM, Nishi N, Reijm M, Voskuyl AE, et al. 2001. Circulating V(α24$^+$) Vβ11$^+$ NKT cell numbers are decreased in a wide variety of diseases that are characterized by autoreactive tissue damage. *Clin. Immunol.* 100:144–48

143. Wilson SB, Kent SC, Patton KT, Orban T, Jackson RA, et al. 1998. Extreme Th1 bias of invariant Vα24JαQ T cells in type 1 diabetes. *Nature* 391:177–81

144. Kukreja A, Cost G, Marker J, Zhang C, Sun Z, et al. 2002. Multiple immuno-regulatory defects in type-1 diabetes. *J. Clin. Invest.* 109:131–40

145. Berzins SP, Kyparissoudis K, Pellicci DG, Hammond KJ, Sidobre S, et al. 2004. Systemic NKT cell deficiency in NOD mice is not detected in peripheral blood: implications for human studies. *Immunol. Cell. Biol.* 82:247–52

146. Tahir SM, Cheng O, Shaulov A, Koezuka Y, Bubley GJ, et al. 2001. Loss of IFN-γ production by invariant NK T cells in advanced cancer. *J. Immunol.* 167:4046–50

147. Araki M, Kondo T, Gumperz JE, Brenner MB, Miyake S, Yamamura T. 2003. Th2 bias of CD4$^+$ NKT cells derived from multiple sclerosis in remission. *Int. Immunol.* 15:279–88

148. Levy O, Orange JS, Hibberd P, Steinberg S, LaRussa P, et al. 2003. Disseminated varicella infection due to the vaccine strain of varicella-zoster virus, in a patient with a novel deficiency in natural killer T cells. *J. Infect. Dis.* 188:948–53

149. Nieda M, Okai M, Tazbirkova A, Lin H, Yamaura A, et al. 2004. Therapeutic activation of Vα24$^+$Vβ11$^+$ NKT cells in human subjects results in highly coordinated secondary activation of acquired and innate immunity. *Blood* 103:383–89

150. Giaccone G, Punt CJ, Ando Y, Ruijter R, Nishi N, et al. 2002. A phase I study of the natural killer T-cell ligand α-galactosylceramide (KRN7000) in patients with solid tumors. *Clin. Cancer Res.* 8:3702–9

151. Zhou D, Mattner J, Cantu Iii C, Schrantz N, Yin N, et al. 2004. Lysosomal glycosphingolipid recognition by NKT cells. *Science* 306:1786–89

Annu. Rev. Immunol. 2005. 23:901–44
doi: 10.1146/annurev.immunol.23.021704.115816
First published online as a Review in Advance on January 7, 2005

MACROPHAGE RECEPTORS AND IMMUNE RECOGNITION

P.R. Taylor, L. Martinez-Pomares, M. Stacey, H-H. Lin,
G.D. Brown, and S. Gordon
*Sir William Dunn School of Pathology, University of Oxford, Oxford OX1 3RE,
United Kingdom; email: siamon.gordon@path.ox.ac.uk*

Key Words pattern recognition, innate immunity, phagocytosis, micro-organisms, apoptosis

■ **Abstract** Macrophages express a broad range of plasma membrane receptors that mediate their interactions with natural and altered-self components of the host as well as a range of microorganisms. Recognition is followed by surface changes, uptake, signaling, and altered gene expression, contributing to homeostasis, host defense, innate effector mechanisms, and the induction of acquired immunity. This review covers recent studies of selected families of structurally defined molecules, studies that have improved understanding of ligand discrimination in the absence of opsonins and differential responses by macrophages and related myeloid cells.

INTRODUCTION

The surface receptors of the macrophage (MØ) and closely related myeloid cells regulate a range of functions, including differentiation, growth and survival, adhesion, migration, phagocytosis, activation, and cytotoxicity.[1] With the development of powerful immunologic and genetic tools, knowledge of membrane glycoproteins has grown rapidly, although the full repertoire of MØ surface-expressed molecules remains to be determined. Their ability to recognize a wide range of endogenous and exogenous ligands, and to respond appropriately, is central to MØ functions in homeostasis as well as host defense in innate and acquired immunity, autoimmunity, inflammation, and immunopathology (1–3). The role of classic opsonins (antibody and complement) in enhanced phagocytosis led the way; recent research into sensing of a range of microbial ligands by Toll-like receptors (TLR) and families of cytosolic proteins (e.g., NODs, NALPs) has been well documented (4–6). In this review we focus on less well-known receptor families implicated in nonopsonic recognition, mediating either cell adhesion or phagocytosis. We omit

---

[1]See Appendix for a full list of abbreviations used.

TABLE 1 Overview of MØ receptors implicated in immune recognition[a]

Receptor family	Example	Function (example)
Scavenger (collagenous)	SR-A	Phagocytosis of bacteria and apoptotic cells, endocytosis of modified LDL, adhesion
Scavenger (noncollagenous)	CD36	Phagocytosis of apoptotic cells, diacyl lipid recognition of bacteria
GPI-anchored	CD14	LPS-binding protein/interactions MD2/MyD88, TLR signaling, apoptotic cell recognition
Integrin	CR3 (CD18/11b)	Complement receptor (C3bi) mediated phagocytosis Adhesion to endothelium
Ig Superfamily	FcR (ITAM/ITIM)	Antibody-dependent binding, uptake, killing
	TREM-1 (ITAM)	Regulation of inflammation
Seven transmembrane	CCR2 C5aR EMR2 (EGF-TM7)	Receptor for MCP-1 Chemotaxis, degranulation Myeloid cell adhesion Chondroitin sulphate binding
NK-like C-type lectin-like	Dectin-1 (ITAM-like)	β-glucan receptor, fungal particle ingestion TNFα release/interaction TLR2
C-type lectin (single CTLD)	DC-SIGN	Mostly DC, pathogen recognition, ICAM adhesion
Multiple CTLD	MR	Clearance, alternative activation, antigen transport?
Toll-like receptors (Leucine-rich repeats)	TLR2 TLR4	Response to Peptidoglycan Response to LPS

[a]MØ express multiple receptors belonging to major structurally defined families. Examples shown are referred to in text.

detailed discussion of receptors for cytokines, chemokines, selectins, and integrins, which have been extensively reviewed previously. We emphasize the nature, expression, and roles of structurally diverse molecular families, loosely but not exclusively linked to particular immune recognition functions of MØ (Table 1). We consider evolving concepts of pattern recognition in relation to phagocytic uptake of microbes and apoptotic cells and summarize key findings and issues for further research. Supplemental information and references are also available; follow the Supplemental Material link from the Annual Reviews home page at http://www.annualreviews.org.

PATTERN RECOGNITION, AN EVOLVING CONCEPT

The concept of pattern recognition, proposed by Janeway and subsequently Medzhitov (7), has been extraordinarily fruitful and has stimulated research into the field of immune recognition by antigen-presenting cells (APC). It is based on the recognition of conserved microbial structures, so-called pathogen-associated molecular patterns (PAMPs), by a limited number of germ line–encoded APC pattern recognition receptors (PRR). By contrast, somatic recombination generates a large repertoire of T and B cell receptors for mainly peptide antigens. This proposal was linked to the induction of costimulatory molecules on APC, essential to stimulate lymphocyte responses. The subsequent discovery of TLR and their signaling pathways in insects and vertebrates added considerable weight to the hypothesis.

The original concept needs to be refined with advancing molecular characterization of receptor-ligand interactions. Natural ligands on microorganisms are still poorly defined and include nonessential proteins (e.g., flagellin) as well as lipopolysaccharide (LPS), peptidoglycans (PGN), and related molecules. Clearly, these molecules are also expressed by commensal and opportunistic pathogenic organisms. To take this into account, researchers have suggested anatomical sequestration of organism and host. In addition, several PRR interact with endogenous, host-derived as well as exogenous microbial ligands. This brings into question the mechanisms of sensing and intracellular signaling that generate diverse pro- or anti-inflammatory responses. What is not in doubt is that the APC repertoire is very broad, encompassing protein, carbohydrate, lipid, and nucleic acid ligands; receptor diversity is markedly increased by combinatorial expression, alternate splicing to generate multiple isoforms, post-translational glycosylation, lipid modifications and proteolysis. Comparative genomic studies in *Drosophila*, *C. elegans*, and other invertebrates have identified large numbers of lectin-like and scavenger receptor cysteine-rich (SRCR) domain-containing molecules, as well as leucine-rich domain molecules related to TLR. Although most of these putative receptors remain orphans, their abundance attests to the ancient evolutionary origins of innate recognition mechanisms.

TLRs in vertebrates are able to sense diverse, microbial, and other ligands and to transmit signals via adaptor molecules selectively, but they depend on other surface molecules such as CD14/MD2 (4) and C-type lectin-like receptors (8) for proximal ligand binding and recognition. Collaboration among different membrane receptor families, as well as with nonclassical opsonins and proteinase cascades such as complement, is likely to be an important mechanism to enhance affinity of binding and specificity. Some nonopsonic receptors display low-affinity, promiscuous binding, in the case of SR-A, to many polyanionic structures (9); however, others have high-affinity binding for specific ligands, e.g., Dectin-1. Ligand structures may themselves display considerable promiscuity in binding to multiple receptors.

Finally, cellular expression of each receptor is tightly regulated on monocyte-MØ, myeloid dendritic cells (DCs), and polymorphonuclear leukocytes (PMN) during their differentiation, migration into different tissue microenvironments, and cell activation. This increases the complexity of receptor interactions with neighboring cells, as well as with extracellular matrix and constituents of plasma and lymph.

HETEROGENEOUS ANTIGEN AND SURFACE RECEPTOR PHENOTYPE OF TISSUE MØ

Most resident MØ in the normal adult are derived from circulating bone marrow–derived monocytes. Blood monocyte-like cells also give rise to related DCs and osteoclasts (1). Studies of the expression of differentiation antigens and surface receptors with monoclonal antibodies (mAb) have shown that tissue MØ become markedly heterogeneous and express very different phenotypes, reflecting specialization of function within particular microenvironments. As well as distinct subpopulations in lymphoid organs, MØ are found in nonlymphoid organs like the liver (Kupffer cells), lung (alveolar MØ), nervous system (microglia), epidermis (Langerhans cells), reproductive organs, and serosal cavities. MØ are also found within the lamina propria of gut and the interstitium of organs such as the heart, pancreas, and kidney. In response to inflammatory and immune stimulation, additional monocytes are recruited in increased numbers to local sites, where they display different phenotypes from originally resident MØ. It is convenient to distinguish "elicited" and "immunologically activated" MØ, depending on the cytokine milieu. Newly recruited monocytes/MØ adapt to their local microenvironment and become hard to distinguish from the original resident MØ, which themselves undergo activation by local stimuli. Examples of surface heterogeneity of MØ and DCs in some of these anatomical locations are summarized in Figure 1. Antigen and receptor markers shown are described below.

MØ play a broad homeostatic role in clearance of senescent cells and in tissue remodeling and repair after injury or infection. Analysis of the receptor mechanisms involved, for example in the clearance of apoptotic cells, has implicated many receptors in the recognition process (see below). Many of the same receptors mediate uptake of modified host lipoproteins, contributing to the inflammatory and repair process implicated in atherogenesis (9, 10). Generation of mice deficient in CD47 (discussed below) shows the importance of signaling through its MØ-expressed ligand, CD172a, in suppressing inappropriate self-phagocytosis. The recent generation of mannose receptor (MR)–deficient mice has demonstrated the importance of this receptor in the maintenance of normal levels of endogenous glycoproteins and clearance of lysosomal hydrolases during steady state and inflammatory conditions (see MØ C-type lectins).

MØ are present in large numbers at portals of entry from the outside environment, for example within the lungs, which are constantly exposed to foreign particles, viruses, bacteria, and fungi. Alveolar MØ express high levels of PRR including scavenger receptors (SR), MR, and the β-glucan specific receptor,

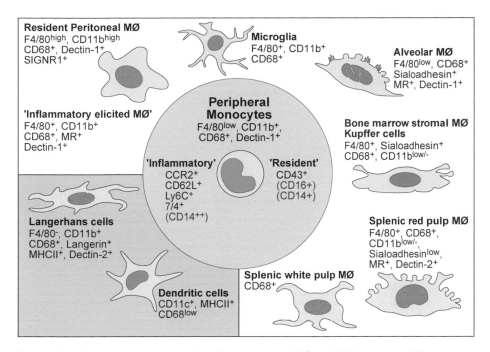

Figure 1   Phenotypic heterogeneity of monocytes/MØ and DCs during differentiation in vivo. Circulating monocytes that give rise to resident- and inflammatory-type elicited MØ already display a distinct phenotype, as do MØ and DCs in different tissue microenvironments. Differentiation antigens and membrane receptors are described subsequently in this review. Antigens listed in brackets correspond to human receptors; all other antigens refer to studies of murine cells.

Dectin-1. In such a relatively opsonin-poor environment, the expression of specific receptors for the direct recognition and uptake of microbes could play an important role in innate host defense. Exposure of MØ to microbial products and cell-derived cytokines such as IFN-γ and IL-4, in vitro and in vivo, has been shown to induce different activation states in these cells, adding to further heterogeneity (11) (Table 2). These stimuli modulate surface receptor expression, secretory and antimicrobial activities, antigen presentation and costimulation, and antigen-specific lymphocyte responses.

MØ HETEROGENEITY AND THE SPLEEN

The rodent spleen is an example of heterogeneity that underlies the potential diversity of immune recognition by MØ (Figure 2). The spleen is rich in subpopulations of MØ that differ in receptor expression, microanatomical location, life history,

TABLE 2   Macrophage activation: heterogeneity of phenotype[a]

	Innate activation	Classical activation	Alternative activation
Stimuli	*Neisseria meningitidis*[b]	IFN-γ	IL-4/13
Effects on surface antigens	↑ MARCO ↑ CD200 ↑ Co-stimulatory antigens (synergy with IFN-γ)	↑ MHC class II ↑ CD86 ↓ MR	↑ MR ↑ Dectin-1 ↑ CD23 ↓ CD14 CD163
Metabolic changes	↑ iNOS Respiratory burst	↑ iNOS Respiratory burst	↑ Arginase
Secretory responses	Synergy with IFN-γ-induced responses	Pro-inflammatory cytokine and chemokines (TNFα, IL-12, IL-1, IL-6, IP-10, MIP-1α, MCP-1) and low MW mediators	IL-1RA IL-10 Chemokines (e.g., AMAC-1) Chitinase-like proteins (Ym1/2)
Functional effects of activation	Phagocytosis (by regulation of receptors) Pro-inflammatory signaling via TLR Enhanced costimulatory antigen expression	↑ Antigen presentation ↑ Killing of intracellular pathogens Pro-inflammatory	↑ Fibronectin and matrix associated proteins. Promotes cell growth, collagen formation, and tissue repair. ↑Humoral/allergic immunity ↑Parasite killing

[a]MØ display a spectrum of distinct phenotypes associated with different forms of immune activation.

[b]*N. meningitidis* is given as an example of a direct Gram-negative microbial stimulus based on Reference 15 and unpublished observations by S. Mukhopadhyay.

and function. Individual receptors are described below. Red pulp MØ in the spleen, expressing high levels of the F4/80 antigen and the MR, include stromal-type MØ involved in hemopoiesis and are extensively involved in the clearance of senescent erythrocytes. In the marginal zone (MZ) of the spleen, which is notably lacking in F4/80 expression, two MØ populations are present within a complex mix of fibroblasts, endothelia, DCs, and subpopulations of lymphocytes. The MZ represents the interface of splenic lymphoid tissue and the circulation (12). Sialoadhesin high-expressing metallophilic MØ are found in the inner layer of the MZ adjacent to the white pulp. The existence of the metallophilic MØ is dependent on M-CSF and members of the TNF (tumor necrosis factor) receptor family, and although their function in the evolution of an immune response is still poorly understood, they appear to play a role in the initial response to systemic infection. Phagocytic marginal zone MØ (MZMØ) are found in the outer marginal zone. MZMØ

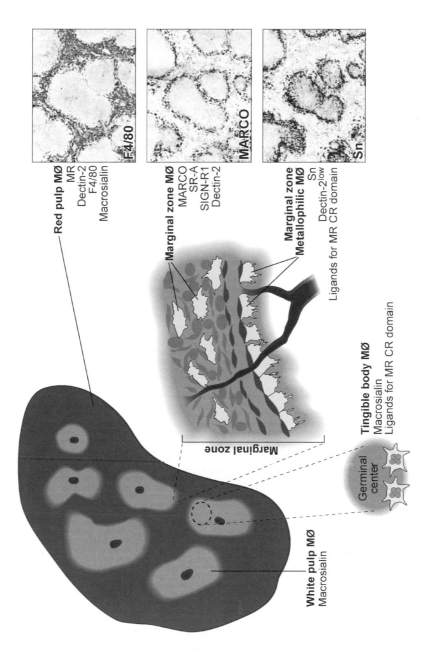

Figure 2 Heterogeneity of MØ subpopulations in mouse spleen, illustrated by use of differentiation and receptor antigens. The immunohistochemical images show clear heterogeneity of expression of F4/80, MARCO, and Sialoadhesin, exhibited by red pulp, MZ, and metallophilic MØ. Schematic diagram based on G. Kraal (12).

express an array of PRR including the scavenger receptor-A (SR-A), macrophage receptor collagenous domain (MARCO), and SIGN-related 1 (SIGNR1). These receptors allow the MZMØ to recognize and interact with soluble and particulate antigens and microorganisms within the circulation. MØ are also present within the splenic white pulp, including tingible body MØ, which phagocytose apoptotic B cells generated during germinal center reactions. These white pulp MØ express the pan MØ antigen CD68, but lack other MØ markers such as F4/80.

SCAVENGER RECEPTORS AND MICROBIAL RECOGNITION

SR-A I/II

Historically, the identification of SR-A (I,II) (referred to here as SR-A) as an important nonopsonic receptor for modified low density lipoproteins, acetylated LDL, and other selected polyanions including lipid A, drew attention to its possible role in foam cell formation and atherogenesis (13) as well as host defense (9). It was the first collagenous transmembrane receptor to be cloned, and its cysteine-rich domain (SRCR) found in the SR-A I isoform became the prototype for the presence of similar domains in a range of immune cell adhesion molecules expressed by lymphoid as well as myeloid cells (Figure 3). The SR-A ligand-binding site for polyanionic ligands is thought to be associated with the collagenous domain. In the case of CD163, a MØ-restricted endocytic receptor for hemoglobin-haptoglobin complexes, multiple SRCR domains are likely to be responsible for ligand binding (14).

The molecular cell biology of SR-A has been extensively reviewed (9, 15). We emphasize microbial recognition here, and below we consider its role in apoptotic cell clearance. The molecule is well expressed at the surface of MØ and subpopulations of DC, but not monocytes or PMN; selected endothelia also express SR-A. A large part of SR-A expression is intracellular, within the endocytic compartment. Studies by Peiser et al. (16) showed that select bacteria were taken up via SR-A; this was demonstrated in phagocytosis assays with bone marrow culture–derived MØ (BMDM) from wild-type and knockout mice. These cells express high levels of receptor owing to upregulation by M-CSF present in the culture medium. Peritoneal exudate MØ express lower levels of SR-A, as well as additional SR. *Neisseria meningitidis* (virulent and nonvirulent strains) express microbial ligands for nonopsonic uptake via SR-A. The phagocytic ligand is independent of lipid A, which is required for the induction of proinflammatory cytokine secretion. Unpublished studies have identified novel protein ligands, concentrated in outer membrane vesicles, that are bound and endocytosed via SR-A (L. Peiser, unpublished results).

Several studies with wild-type and knockout mice have implicated SR-A in microbial resistance/susceptibility to bacterial infection in vivo including *Listeria*

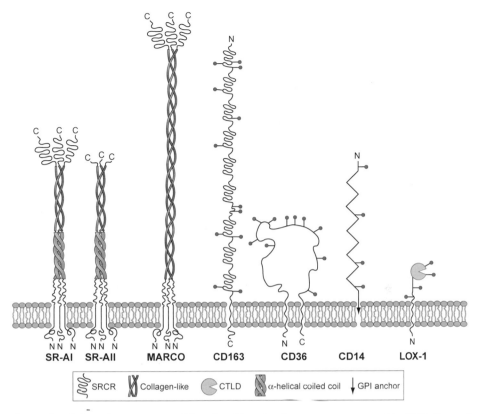

Figure 3   Selected scavenger and functionally related receptors expressed by MØ. Several have been implicated in binding of G$^+$ and G$^-$ bacteria as well as uptake of polyanionic ligands (acetylated LDL) and in the uptake of apoptotic cells. CD163 contains multiple SRCR domains and binds hemoglobin-haptoglobin complexes.

monocytogenes and *Staphylococcus aureus* (17). In other models, prior BCG infection was used to activate MØ in vivo, sensitizing the mouse to LPS challenge. SR-A protects the animal against systemic TNF release and septic shock. Table 3 summarizes phenotypic changes derived from genetic ablation of SR-A and other MØ-expressed receptors/ligands.

MARCO

MARCO is a MØ- and DC-restricted SR-A family member that resembles SR-A, but it is the product of a distinct gene, and its expression pattern is very different (18). It is constitutively present on MZ and some, but not most, tissue MØ, and it is readily induced by microbial and other stimuli, acting through various TLR. It is predominantly expressed at the cell surface, mediating adhesion to substrata and ingestion of particulates such as titanium dioxide by alveolar MØ.

TABLE 3 Phenotypes derived from receptor/ligand knockouts

Receptor	Knockout MØ phenotype summary
Scavenger and related	
SR-A	Impaired clearance of modified LDL. Impaired phagocytosis of apoptotic cells (in vitro) and select microorganisms. Altered susceptibility to endotoxic shock and atherosclerosis
CD36	Effects on clearance of apoptotic cells, atherogenesis and resistance to select bacteria
CD14	Impaired responses to endotoxin and altered responses to infection
PSR	Neonatal lethal, defective fetal liver erythropoiesis, variable effects on development and clearance of apoptotic cells
Integrins	
CD11b	Altered myeloid cell recruitment in inflammation and impaired complement-opsonized phagocytosis
Ig Superfamily	
'TREM2'	DAP12-deficient mice have Nasu-Hakola-like disease symptoms similar to DAP12/TREM2-deficient humans Symptoms: presenile dementia and bone cysts
'CD200R'	CD200-deficient mice exhibit enhanced MØ activation leading to an increase in severity of inflammatory diseases
'SIRPα'	Phagocytosis of CD47-deficient erythrocytes is not inhibited via SIRPα. CD47-SIRPα also regulates Fc and complement-mediated phagocytosis
'M-CSFR'	Osteopetrotic phenotype in mice with a natural mutation in M-CSF. Reduced numbers of monocytes and selected MØ including osteoclasts
Siglec-1	Siglec-1-deficient MØ exhibit a significant defect in *Neisseria* binding (*in vitro*)
Siglec-3	Mice are viable and fertile. No obvious phenotype described
PIRB	Impaired DC maturation with enhanced Th2 responses. Increased graft-versus-host disease
C-type-lectin-like	
CD69	Alterated B cell development. Enhanced antitumor response. Enhanced autoimmune reactivity and inflammation in experimental arthritis
C-type Lectins	
Mannose receptor	Impaired clearance of select, endogenous glycoproteins. Also reported as a lethal phenotype owing to abnormal lutropin clearance. Apparently normal control of fungal infection
Endo180	Defect in collagen binding and internalization

Non-phagocytic ligands have also been reported on B lymphocytes, which may traffic through the MZ (19). Although the polyanion-sensitive binding properties of this SR remain poorly defined, MARCO is known to bind a range of Gram-positive and Gram-negative bacteria, contributing to localization and clearance of circulating organisms in the MZ.

CD36

CD36 is a double-spanning SR (Figure 3) with a very different structure from SR-A. It is related to other SR-B molecules (20) and is thought to be associated with lipid rafts. An evolutionarily related molecule, Croquemort, is found in *Drosophila* (21). CD36 is expressed on monocytes, MØ, platelets, and selected endothelia and is best known as a SR for oxidized LDL and apoptotic cells (see below).

The role of CD36 in innate immunity was overlooked until recently, when it turned out to be the genetic target in an ENU mutagenesis program, responsible for a novel TLR-associated phenotype termed "oblivious" (K. Hoebe and B. Beutler, personal communication). Its ligand was shown to be diacyl fatty acids found in microbial walls. CD36-deficient mice are susceptible to "spontaneous" eye infections by Gram-positive organisms. CD36 has also been implicated in cytoadherence of *Plasmodium falciparum*.

Lectin-like oxidized low density lipoprotein receptor (LOX-1) (Figure 3) and other newly described SR expressed by MØ and endothelium have been reported to bind bacteria (see Supplemental Material). These and other bacterial binding receptors, e.g., CD14, expressed by MØ are considered further below. Other receptors for PGN present in both Gram-positive and Gram-negative bacteria have been described in vertebrates and *Drosophila* (22).

Although a range of bacterial recognition receptors is now known, their microbial ligands remain uncharacterized, with the exception of CD36. Ligand expression by different organisms varies greatly and multiple MØ receptors are likely to collaborate in binding of whole bacteria and in signal transduction.

RECOGNITION OF APOPTOTIC CELLS BY MØ

Apoptosis is a natural process during development, the induction of an adaptive immune response and the resolution of inflammation. The onset of apoptosis in vivo is accompanied by rapid clearance of effete cells by both professional and nonprofessional phagocytes. In a normal animal, this process is extremely efficient, and it is difficult to detect apoptotic bodies that are not associated with phagocytes in tissues. This process may be more than just "waste disposal;" the phagocytosis of apoptotic cells by MØ results in the production of anti-inflammatory mediators (23), and the failure to clear apoptotic cells efficiently may lead to exacerbation of inflammation and a predisposition to the development of autoimmunity (24). Recently, attention has therefore turned to the recognition mechanisms used by

MØ and the identification of multiple candidate receptors (25, 26). Although to date only a few of these candidates have been shown to play a physiological role in this process in vivo, this may reflect a lack of study as well as receptor redundancy.

Vitronectin Receptor (αvβ3-integrin)

The first identified receptor for the phagocytosis of apoptotic leukocytes was the vitronectin receptor (VnR, αvβ3-integrin) (reviewed by 26). Since its identification, many other candidate recognition mechanisms have been proposed. Subsequently, researchers have shown that VnR cooperates with thrombospondin and CD36, with soluble thrombospondin serving as a bridge able to bind both the apoptotic leukocyte and phagocyte, possibly via these two receptors.

Phosphatidyl Serine Receptor (PSR)

The phosphatidyl serine receptor (PSR), which recognizes phosphatidyl-L-serine but not phosphatidyl-D-serine, was first shown to play a role in the clearance of apoptotic cells by Fadok and colleagues (27). Subsequently, researchers showed that different populations of MØ were heterogeneous with regard to their dependence on the PSR or VnR. Ultimately the PSR was cloned by phage display using a mAb raised against PSR on activated MØ, and it conferred phagocytic activity for apoptotic cells on cells that were not normally phagocytic (28). More recently, abnormal development and neonatal lethality, associated with impaired clearance of apoptotic cells, have been reported in PSR-deficient mice (29), and mutation of the *C. elegans* homolog of PSR also leads to an in vivo defect in the clearance of cell corpses (30). The developmental and clearance defects associated with PSR deficiency may be variable.

Scavenger Receptors

CD36   CD36 has been implicated in the recognition of apoptotic cells in cooperation with thrombospondin and VnR. Further experiments suggest that expression of CD36 alone in the usually nonphagocytic COS-7 fibroblastic background is sufficient to confer upon transfectants the capacity to phagocytose apoptotic cells. The apoptotic cell ligand for CD36 is not defined, but because it also has the capacity to bind to anionic phospholipids, the recognition of apoptotic cells by CD36 may involve related structures.

SR-A   Blockade of SR-A on MØ, or its genetic deletion, has been shown to impair the recognition of apoptotic thymocytes by MØ (31). The observed defect in apoptotic cell recognition by blockade or deletion of SR-A applies to both thioglycollate-elicited peritoneal MØ and primary thymic MØ. However, in the thymus under steady-state conditions or in the context of experimentally increased apoptotic cell burden, a defect in in vivo apoptotic cell clearance could not be detected, supporting the idea of widespread redundancy within these recognition systems (17). The ligand on apoptotic cells that is recognized by SR-A is not known.

CD14   Characterization of a mAb that blocked the recognition of apoptotic cells by human monocyte-derived MØ led to the identification of CD14 as a candidate receptor for apoptotic cells (32). Transfection of COS cells with CD14 conferred upon these cells the capacity to interact with apoptotic cells. CD14 is known to bind to phospholipids, but investigators have suggested that this is not the mechanism by which CD14 recognizes apoptotic cells. Furthermore, intracellular adhesion molecule (ICAM)-3 expressed on the apoptotic cell may function as the ligand for CD14. CD14 is discussed in more detail later.

LOX-1   CHO cells expressing bovine LOX-1 were able to bind aged erythrocytes and apoptotic cells, and these interactions were inhibited by known LOX-1 ligands and PS liposomes (33). Because PS can block these interactions, PS was considered to be the ligand on the apoptotic cell. Additional functions of LOX-1 are discussed with other NK-like C-type lectins below.

β2-GPI Receptor

β2-glycoprotein I (β2-GPI) is a plasma protein that can bind to exposed PS on the surface of apoptotic cells. It forms a bridge between the apoptotic cell and MØ via an unidentified receptor (34). The requirement for the plasma protein in this process was shown by blockade with β2-GPI specific F(ab)$_2$ fragments, which blocked enhanced uptake by MØ, and MØ association with β_2-GPI could only occur after prior recognition of PS.

Complement Receptors 3 and 4 (CR3 and CR4)

Korb and Ahearn reported a possible role for complement in the recognition of apoptotic cells when they observed binding of C1q to apoptotic cells (reviewed by 24). A role for complement receptors in the clearance of apoptotic cells was first demonstrated by the identification of heat labile components of serum, which enhanced apoptotic cell binding to MØ. Serum-depletion studies implicated both the classical and alternative pathways of complement, and antibody blockade showed that CR3 and CR4 played a role in the clearance of opsonised apoptotic cells by human MØ. The recognition of apoptotic cells by CR3 and CR4 depends on prior opsonization, unlike most of the receptors discussed in this review. A role for the classical pathway of complement in the clearance of apoptotic cells was verified in mice using a novel in vivo clearance model.

CD91-Calreticulin Recognition of C1q, SP-A, and SP-D

After the initial observation that C1q could bind directly to apoptotic cells and the suggestion that CR3 and CR4 play a major role as MØ receptors for apoptotic cell recognition, investigations in mice led to the discovery of a differential importance of the classical pathway complement components in the clearance of apoptotic cells. C1q-deficient mice displayed a more profound defect in apoptotic cell clearance than C4-deficient mice, and more apoptotic bodies were present in the kidneys of disease-free C1q-deficient mice. A C1q receptor may play additional roles in apoptotic cell recognition to those receptors that recognized C3 activation fragments, perhaps by direct recognition through C1q receptors. Ogden and colleagues (35) identified calreticulin (also known as cC1qR) in a complex with the endocytic receptor CD91 (α-2-macroglobulin receptor) as the surface receptor for C1q. They showed that the structurally similar mannose-binding lectin (MBL) was able to facilitate apoptotic cell clearance via the same surface receptor complex.

Surfactant proteins A (SP-A) and D (SP-D) have also been implicated in recognition of apoptotic cells. The addition of either SP-A or -D to in vitro assays with isolated alveolar MØ leads to enhancement of phagocytosis of apoptotic neutrophils (36). Like C1q and MBL, both SP-A and -D were able to bind to MØ via the calreticulin:CD91 receptor complex (37). Furthermore, in clearance studies, SP-D affected the clearance of apoptotic cells in vivo.

MER and Gas6

Gas6 (growth arrest specific gene 6) is a ligand of the receptor tyrosine kinases Axl, Sky, and Mer. Gas6 exhibits Ca^{2+}-dependent binding to PS (38) and PS-containing liposomes, suggesting that Gas6 may function as a bridge between the apoptotic cell and MØ. Scott and colleagues (39) genetically deleted MER, a member of the Axl/Mer/Tyro3 receptor tyrosine kinase family. The MER-deficient mouse exhibited in vivo defects in the clearance of apoptotic cells, and in vitro MØ showed a marked impairment in their ability to internalize apoptotic cells.

Annexins

Because of the recognized role of annexins in binding to PS, Fan et al. (40) investigated the role of annexins I and II in the recognition of apoptotic cells by MØ. Not only is PS exposed on the surface of apoptotic cells, but its exposure on the surface of the phagocyte is also required for the recognition of apoptotic cells. Annexins I and II differ from the other annexins in that they are able to aggregate liposomes and therefore may simultaneously bind apoptotic cell– and phagocyte-exposed PS. Blockade of annexins I and II with mAbs impaired apoptotic cell recognition in vitro.

SEVEN TRANSMEMBRANE RECEPTORS

The seven-span membrane (TM7) receptors are the largest superfamily of cell-surface receptors, comprising >1% of the functional genes within the human genome. Found on all cell types including MØ, TM7 molecules transduce signals for an array of stimuli, including microbial products, peptides and amino acid derivatives, lipid analogues, ions, and external sensory stimuli such as light, taste, and odors, via classical G protein–coupled pathways. In addition to these signaling pathways, a variety of G protein–independent mechanisms have begun to emerge. Receptors for chemokines, including C5a and formyl peptide, have been reviewed extensively. Here we describe a subfamily of surface TM7 with large extracellular domains with putative adhesion and signaling functions in MØ.

The EGF-TM7 Family

The human EGF-TM7 family comprises CD97, EGF-module-containing mucin-like hormone receptor (EMR) 1, EMR2, EMR3, and EMR4 (41) (Figure 4). These predominantly leukocyte-restricted glycoproteins are defined by their unusual hybrid structure, which consists of a large extracellular domain containing varying numbers of epidermal growth factor (EGF)-like repeats coupled to a family B GPCR (G protein–coupled receptor)-related moiety via a region containing a GPCR proteolytic site (GPS). The majority of the genes have been shown to express multiple protein isoforms possessing various numbers and arrangement of their extracellular EGF domains. As similar EGF domains mediate protein-protein interactions in numerous other proteins and TM7 domains have the obvious potential to signal, it has long been proposed that EGF-TM7 receptors may couple extracellular recognition events to intracellular signaling in leukocytes. Extracellular ligands have been identified for several of the receptors, and roles in myeloid recognition and migration have been demonstrated. The EGF-TM7 receptors are not present in invertebrates, but they have been identified in a number of vertebrates (41). These findings, together with the absence of mouse EMR2 and EMR3 orthologs, indicate a relatively recent and rapid evolution, a phenomenon often found within the immune genes.

EMR1 (F4/80)   EMR1 possesses six EGF domains linked to a TM7 region; so far, expression data for the human molecule are restricted to RT-PCR, but results indicate high levels of expression on blood monocytes and MØ cell lines. EMR1 shows 68% homology to its murine ortholog F4/80. F4/80 has long been used as a specific marker for populations of mouse tissue MØ. F4/80 is present in the liver (Kupffer cells), lamina propria (gut), splenic red pulp, lymph nodes (medulla), brain (microglia), bone marrow stroma, and Langerhans cells in the skin (Figure 1). F4/80 is downregulated upon stimulation of Langerhans cells as they migrate to the draining lymph nodes and is absent in T cell areas of the spleen and lymph nodes, indicating a possible role in the retention/adhesion of MØ in specific tissue areas. F4/80 is also expressed by eosinophils and some DCs. Although F4/80 knockout mice do not exhibit any gross phenotype or aberrant MØ populations (42), antibody blocking studies have implicated F4/80 in MØ-dependent IFN-γ release from NK cells in response to *Listeria* and in peripheral tolerance (43, 44). Recent data obtained using F4/80-deficient mice in models of oral tolerance and

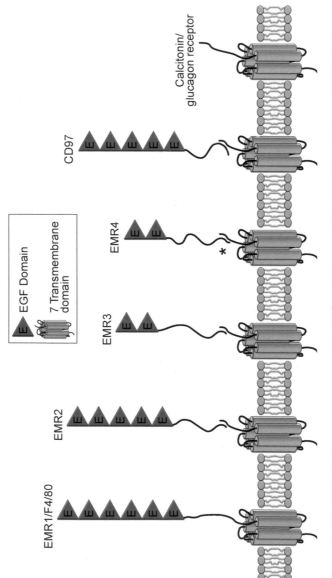

Figure 4   The EGF-TM7 receptors expressed by MØ and other myeloid cells. *The ortholog of EMR4 in human contains a deletion that results in a premature stop codon.

anterior chamber-associated immune deviation have demonstrated a role for F4/80 in tolerance (H-H. Lin, unpublished data).

EMR2   EMR2 is highly expressed on PMNs and certain tissue MØ and to a lesser extent on peripheral monocytes (45). Ligand-binding studies have shown that the largest EMR2 isoform containing five EGF domains binds specifically to a restricted population of chondroitin sulphate B species found in tissues and expressed by B cells, facilitating cell attachment in vitro (46; M. Kwakkenbos, unpublished data). As glycosaminoglycan populations are known to alter during inflammation and wound repair, chondroitin sulphate recognition by EMR2-expressing MØ and PMNs may allow the interaction with B cells and retention/migration within tissues. The signaling consequences of chondroitin sulphate binding remain to be established. Preliminary data suggest EMR2 ligation can result in cellular activation (M. Stacey, unpublished data). A mouse model is not available because a murine ortholog to EMR2 does not exist.

CD97   The EGF domains of the full-length CD97 protein are 97.5% identical to those of EMR2 (41, 45). Like EMR2, various CD97 protein isoforms are expressed, consisting of different numbers of the EGF domains. However, unlike EMR2, CD97 has a less restricted expression pattern and is found on B and T cells, smooth muscle cells, and myeloid cells. The largest 5-domain isoform of CD97 binds to chondroitin sulphate, whereas a smaller 3-domain isoform of CD97 also recognizes the complement regulatory protein, decay accelerating factor (DAF/CD55) (see below). The significance of the recognition of CD55 and chondroitin sulphate remains unclear; recently, mouse studies have shown that CD97 may play a role in neutrophil migration. In murine sodium dextran sulphate–induced experimental colitis, treatment with antimouse CD97 antibody delayed homing of neutrophils to the colon, and in *S. pneumoniae*–induced pneumonia, it caused a reduced inflammatory infiltrate in the lung after 20 h, resulting in diminished survival (47). CD97 expression has been implicated in a number of human autoimmune diseases. In rheumatoid arthritis, synovial MØ have increased levels of CD97 and are seen to be in close association with CD55+ fibroblast-like synoviocytes (48; E. Kop, unpublished data). Studies of multiple sclerosis patients showed that although white matter from healthy tissues express no CD97, microglia and infiltrating MØ and T cell in MS patients express high levels of CD97. The concomitant upregulation of CD55 on endothelium in MS (49) may play a role in migration or activation of CD97+ MØ. Studies of the CD97$^{-/-}$ mouse should shed further light on the physiological role of CD97.

EMR3   To date, expression data on EMR3 are restricted to RNA analysis. However, results show that expression is restricted to MØ and neutrophils. Ligand studies using the two EGF domains from EMR3 have demonstrated the existence of cognate receptors on culture-derived human MØ and activated neutrophils (50). Previously, the chromosomal location of EMR3, 19p3.1 has been linked to Crohn's disease, a condition associated with aberrant mucosal immune responses characterized by the dense infiltration of MØ and lymphocytes. Recent sequencing of DNA from more than 1200 patients and 700 healthy individuals has demonstrated that polymorphisms in the *EMR3* gene as well as other EMR family members are strongly linked to Crohn's disease susceptibility (D. Jewell, unpublished data).

EMR4   Mouse EMR4 is predominantly expressed on resident MØ. The expression of *mEMR4* is higher on peritoneal MØ elicited with Biogel and thioglycollate broth. Similarly, mEMR4 is overexpressed in TNF-α treated resident peritoneal MØ, whereas IL-4 reduces expression. Antibody staining revealed expression on populations of DCs. Ligand studies have demonstrated a ligand on the A20 lymphoma cell line, suggesting a possible role in the regulation of B cells by MØ and DCs. The gene encoding human EMR4 appears to be a potential pseudogene or soluble protein, owing to a deletion that inserts a premature stop codon (51). Interestingly, however, the gene is intact in both New and Old World apes, implying a rapidly evolving gene.

GLYCOSYLPHOSPHATIDYLINOSITOL (GPI)-ANCHORED MEMBRANE PROTEINS

In addition to using membrane-spanning hydrophobic residues for the association with plasma membrane, cell surface receptors can also use a phosphatidylinositol-based glycolipid (GPI) to anchor in cell membranes. As a result of their GPI anchor, the intracellular sorting and cell surface distribution of the GPI-anchored proteins is distinct from that of the transmembrane proteins. Thus, GPI-anchored proteins were found in detergent-resistant fractions located in the sphingolipid and cholesterol-enriched subdomains (lipid rafts) of cell membranes. These characteristics have been implicated in several important biological functions of GPI-anchored proteins, including intracellular signaling and receptor-mediated uptake of pathogens. Although the GPI-anchored proteins are widely expressed, we focus on two major GPI-anchored receptors that are relevant to immune recognition by MØ.

CD14

CD14 is mainly expressed on cells of the myeloid lineage, including monocytes, MØ, and granulocytes, although other cell types such as B cells, liver parenchymal cells, and gingival fibroblasts can also express CD14. With the use of antibody that prevented binding of LPS-LBP (LPS-binding protein) complex–coated erythrocytes to MØ, CD14 was identified more than a decade ago as a receptor for LPS (52). Furthermore, expression of CD14 on CD14-negative cells rendered cells responsive to LPS (53). Over the years, other microbial and endogenous ligands were identified for CD14, such as LTA (lipoteichoic acid), PGN, and apoptotic cells (54).

Because CD14 does not contain a transmembrane domain (Figure 3), accessory molecules are needed for signal transduction. In recent years, TLR4 and TLR2 were identified as coreceptors with CD14 for specific microbial ligands (55). The extracellular domain of CD14 contains 10 leucine-rich motifs (56). The N-terminal portion of the CD14 is important for LPS binding and the interaction with accessory receptors (57).

In addition to the membrane-bound form, a soluble form of CD14 (sCD14) was first observed in monocytes as the MY-4 antigen (58). TNF-α and LPS induce the release of sCD14, whereas IFN-γ and IL-4 inhibit it. In patients with septic shock, the level of sCD14 in serum was increased substantially, and the levels of sCD14 correlate with mortality (59).

CD55

Also named decay accelerating factor (DAF), CD55 is a complement regulatory protein that protects cells from complement-mediated attack (60). It enhances the decay of the C3/C5 convertases formed in the alternative and classical pathways of complement activation. CD55 is expressed on all cells exposed to plasma, including cells of hemopoietic and nonhemopoietic origins. In addition to interaction with the convertases, CD55 has been used as a cellular receptor by a range of viral and bacterial pathogens (61). Anti-CD55 antibody inhibits the binding of several echoviruses to susceptible cells (62), and transfection of CD55 in nonsusceptible cells enabled cells to bind viruses efficiently (63). CD55 is also a receptor for bacterial fimbriae and other adhesins (64–67).

CD55 belongs to the RCA (receptor of complement activation) family and contains four protein short consensus repeat (SCR) modules in the extracellular domain (60, 68). Detailed structural-functional studies, along with genetically engineered mutants and specific mAbs to distinct SCRs, have located most of the binding sites for individual viral and bacterial ligands. Different SCRs were used as binding sites for different but closely related viruses. Furthermore, most of the virus- and bacteria-binding sites are located in SCR2-4 that are also important for complement regulation (69).

In the past decade, CD97, a member of the EGF-TM7 receptor family, was identified as an endogenous cellular ligand for CD55 (70). Like most of the cell surface protein-protein interaction on leukocytes, the CD55-CD97 interaction is of low affinity (K_D of 86 μM) (71). More recently, an anti-adhesive function of CD55 in human neutrophil transmigration across mucosal epithelia has been reported, although the reciprocal cellular ligand for CD55 was not identified (72).

MEMBERS OF THE IMMUNOGLOBULIN SUPERFAMILY (IgSF)

MØ express important IgSF, such as various FcR and the receptor for M-CSF. These have been extensively reviewed elsewhere. Here we summarize data on a variety of other molecules implicated in MØ recognition (Figure 5).

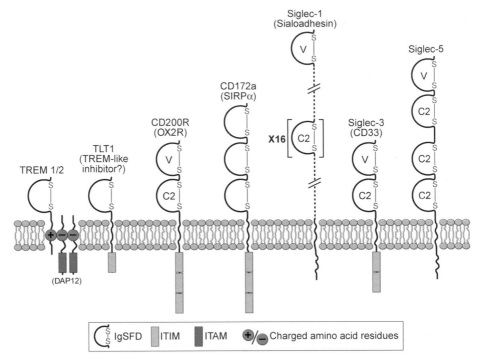

Figure 5 Selected IgSF glycoproteins expressed by MØ. Some receptors contain ITIM sequences in their cytoplasmic tails, which mediate inhibitory signals. TREM1 and TREM2 have charged residues in their transmembrane domains, which allow association with the ITAM-containing DAP12.

Triggering Receptors Expressed by Myeloid Cells (TREMs)

The TREM family of molecules consists of four myeloid transmembrane glycoprotein receptors. Little is known about the inhibitory receptor (TREM-like transcript 1, TLT1), other than that it contains an immunoreceptor tyrosine-based inhibition motif (ITIM) domain that when phosphorylated recruits SH2-domain-containing protein tyrosine phosphatase 1 (SHP1) (73). The activatory receptors TREM1 and TREM2 are functionally better characterized and are described below. A third receptor of unknown function (TREM3) also appears to be an activatory receptor, although in humans it may be a pseudogene.

TREM1   TREM1 is expressed by monocytes/MØ and neutrophils and associates with the immunoreceptor tyrosine-based activation motif (ITAM)-containing signaling molecule DAP12 (74). The use of mAb against TREM1 highlights the potential importance of TREM1 in inflammation as it induces the expression of IL-8, monocyte chemoattractant protein 1 (MCP1, CCL2), MCP3, and macrophage inflammatory protein 1α (MIP1α) (75). Anti-TREM1 mAb also enhances LPS-induced TNFα production by monocytes and stimulates myeloperoxidase release by granulocytes. The potential role of TREM1 as an amplifier of inflammation has been confirmed in vivo by blockade of its natural ligand interaction with a soluble recombinant TREM1-Fc chimeric protein. Blockade of TREM1 in vivo prevents shock and death in septic shock models, which use live *E. coli* or cecal ligation and puncture (76).

TREM2   Whereas TREM1 appears to act mainly through regulating the activation of monocytes and granulocytes, TREM2 acts on other myeloid cells (DCs, osteoclasts, and microglia). In humans, TREM2 is expressed by monocyte-derived DC, and mAb against TREM2 induces a partial maturation state in which CCR7, MHC class II, and the costimulatory molecule CD86 were upregulated (73).

A role for TREM2 in brain and bone function has recently been discovered as a result of studies of the rare human disease Nasu-Hakola disease (polycystic lipomembranous osteodysplasia with sclerosing leukoencephalopathy), which is characterized by both presenile dementia and the formation of bone cysts. Linkage analysis identified mutations in DAP12 in this disease (73), and, interestingly, DAP12-deficient mice have similar features (77). Further analysis of patients with normal DAP12 expression identified mutations in TREM2. TREM2 and DAP12 are expressed by osteoclasts, and monocytes derived from TREM2- and DAP12-deficient subjects do not differentiate in vitro into mature osteoclasts, nor do monocytes from DAP12-deficient mice. Microglia and oligodendrocytes express TREM2 and DAP12, consistent with the neural phenotype of deficient individuals. In vitro differentiation of monocytes into DCs appears to be impaired in TREM2-deficient individuals. Therefore, TREM2/DAP12 expression by myeloid precursors is required for normal maturation of DCs, osteoclasts, and microglia, although the mechanism is not clear.

TREM2 has also been reported to have SR-like properties, binding to anionic carbohydrates on bacteria and yeast, which suggests that TREM2 may play a role in pathogen recognition (reviewed by 73).

Sialic Acid–Binding Immunoglobulin-like Lectins (Siglecs)

Members of the siglec family expressed on MØ include Siglec-1 (Sialoadhesin), Siglec-3 (CD33), and Siglec-5. The siglecs are a major group of receptors involved in the recognition of sialic acid, with individual specificity for particular sialic acid linkages (78). All siglecs possess an N-terminal V-type Ig domain that binds sialic acid and between 1 and 16 C2-type Ig domains (Figure 5).

SIGLEC-1 (SIALOADHESIN)   Siglec-1, the first identified siglec, is the largest, with 17 Ig domains. It was identified as a nonphagocytic MØ sheep erythrocyte receptor (79) and is expressed at high levels on specific subsets of MØ, particularly in lymphoid tissues such as the splenic metallophilic MØ. Siglec-1 is an extended molecule, enabling it to interact with sialic acids without interference from sialic acids expressed by the same cell. The tightly regulated expression pattern and ability to bind sialic acids suggests that Siglec-1 may be involved in recognition of sialic acids on other host cells, as has been shown for granulocytes, as well as on microbes. Siglec-1$^{-/-}$ MØ display a reduced capacity to bind to *Neisseria* (80).

SIGLEC-3 (CD33) AND RELATED MOLECULES EXPRESSED BY MØ   CD33 is relatively small, with two Ig-like domains. One way it differs significantly from Siglec-1 is in the presence in its cytoplasmic tail of two ITIMs. When mAb are used to crosslink CD33 at the same time as FcγRI, the resultant Ca^{2+} flux is reduced compared with crosslinking of FcγRI alone, suggesting that CD33 could function as an inhibitory receptor (81). CD33 expressed in transfected cells is unable to rosette erythrocytes unless the transfected cell is first treated with sialidase to remove sialic acids that mask its binding potential. The existence of a series of CD33-related siglecs expressed by monocyte and MØ (Siglecs-5, -7, -9, -10, -11) (82) has clouded the issue of which receptors in mouse and human are the functional equivalents, and this can only be resolved by comparative expression and ligand binding assays. With this in mind, a CD33-deficient mouse has been generated, which currently has no ascribed phenotype (83); however, there are clear differences between human and mouse CD33, such as the lack of ITIMs in the murine molecule. Although the binding profiles of at least the human versions of the CD33-related siglecs are beginning to be characterized, there is little information so far regarding their physiological roles.

The ILT/LIR/MIR Family of Receptors

A family of receptors has acquired the names Ig-like transcripts (ILTs), monocyte/MØ Ig-like receptors (MIRs), and leukocyte Ig-like receptors (LIRs) (reviewed by 84). This family is genetically and functionally related to the killer cell Ig-like receptors (KIRs), which are a group of NK (natural killer) cell receptors for HLA class I molecules. ILT/MIR/LIR isoforms are expressed by myeloid and lymphoid cells, and some of the family members recognize HLA class I. One subset of this family (ILT2, 3, 4, 5 and LIR8) contains ITIMs and inhibits cellular activation via recruitment of SHP1. Other members of the family (ILT1, ILT1-like protein, ILT7, ILT8 and LIR6a) associate with the ITAM-containing FcR common γ-chain to transmit activatory signals into the cell. ILT6 does not fall into either of these subsets; it is expressed as a soluble molecule with no transmembrane or cytoplasmic domains.

Members of the ILT family are expressed by monocytes, MØ, and DCs (among others). ILT2 and ILT4 both recognize HLA class I molecules, as well as the trophoblast-expressed nonclassical class I molecule HLAG1 and the virally encoded class I–like molecule UL-18. Both ILT2 and ILT4 are ITIM-containing molecules. This interaction may suppress leukocyte activity at the maternal-fetal interface and may be used by viruses to suppress responses to infected cells.

The murine homologs of this family are known as paired Ig-like receptors (PIRs). Although the family structure is different between man and mouse, the study of the murine PIR family has provided some insights into the function of the family. Only one member of the PIR family, PIRB, contains ITIMs and mediates inhibition of cellular functions; the other family members (PIRAs) associate with the γ-chain. The PIRs are expressed by cells of the monocyte/MØ/DC lineages, granulocytes, and B cells. PIRB may be constitutively phosphorylated and may associate with SHP1, possibly as a consequence of direct interaction with MHC class I (85). Deletion of the inhibitory receptor PIRB in mice in vivo leads to impaired DC maturation, increased Th2 responses (86), and enhanced graft-versus-host disease (87).

OX2 (CD200) Receptor (CD200R)

CD200 (OX2) was first identified by the generation of a mAb that revealed expression by a variety of cells, including thymocytes, B cells, activated T cells, neurons, and endothelial cells, but not resting MØ (reviewed by 88). CD200 contains two Ig domains and a single transmembrane region. A low-affinity receptor (CD200R) was identified, which was phylogenetically related to CD200 and genetically linked. Like CD200, CD200R contains two Ig domains; however, CD200R has a larger cytoplasmic domain that contains tyrosines that can be phosphorylated, suggesting that CD200R may transmit an intracellular signal (Figure 5). The expression of CD200R is largely restricted to cells of the monocyte/MØ/DC lineages.

The generation of CD200-deficient mice provided the first evidence of the in vivo physiological role of CD200-CD200R interactions (89). Naive CD200-deficient mice are relatively normal, and only slightly increased numbers of some MØ and abnormal mesenteric lymph node organization were reported. However, after immunological challenge, such as experimental allergic encephalomyelitis (EAE), altered responses were evident in CD200-deficient mice. EAE could be readily induced in the CD200-deficient mice, whereas the background C57BL/6 strain is not normally very susceptible; the onset of disease was also more rapid and the lesions contained more MØ. Similarly, in a model of facial nerve transection, CD200R-expressing microglia exhibit greater activation in the CD200-deficient mice, presumably as a result of the loss of a negative signal from the CD200 expressing neurons.

These results have been verified in normal mice using CD200-Fc and CD200R-Fc fusion proteins. The CD200R-Fc prevents ligation of endogenous CD200R by blocking CD200, leading to enhanced myeloid cell activity after immunological challenge. Conversely, administration of CD200-Fc seems to induce a negative signal suppressing myeloid cell activity.

CD200R may associate with SH2-containing inositol phosphatase (SHIP), consistent with its apparent role in the downregulation of myeloid cell activity. Thus, a model has been developed in which CD200 expression at the surface of many cell types enables interaction with CD200R on myeloid cells, leading to generation of an inhibitory signal within the myeloid cell, which limits cellular activation.

SIRPα (CD172a)

SIRPα (CD172a), like CD200R, is largely restricted to myeloid cells, whereas its ligand CD47 is more broadly expressed, including on myeloid cells. CD172a contains three extracellular Ig-like domains; its intracellular domain contains several tyrosines and has been shown to interact with the tyrosine phosphatases SHP1 and SHP2. This inhibits MØ activation, such as response to growth factors or phagocytosis via Fc or complement receptors (90, 91).

CD200 is unlikely to be a signaling molecule because it possesses a short cytoplasmic domain with no obvious signaling motifs, and it transmits its negative signal to myeloid cells via the signaling CD200R. CD47, however, is a more complicated ligand for the inhibitory CD172a; it also functions as a receptor for thrombospondin family members and is a component of a complex containing integrins, heteromeric G proteins, and cholesterol (92).

CD47 has a single N-terminal IgV-like domain, five transmembrane domains, and an alternatively spliced intracellular domain. The Ig-like domain is required for interaction with CD172a. Expression of CD47 on erythrocytes functions as a signal of "self" to MØ by ligation of CD172a, which inhibits phagocytosis (93). As a consequence, CD47-deficient erythrocytes are rapidly phagocytosed by MØ.

Interestingly, Gardai and colleagues (94) have identified SP-A and -D as ligands for CD172a. The globular heads of these molecules bind to CD172a, transmitting an inhibitory signal to alveolar MØ in the lung under steady-state conditions. However, when alternative surfactant protein ligands such as microbes or dying cells are present, bound surfactant proteins expose their collagenous domains and bind to alternative MØ receptors. This provides an interesting model in which recognition of surfactant protein by CD172a provides a regulatory signal unless other surfactant protein ligands are present.

NK-LIKE C-TYPE LECTIN RECEPTORS ON MØ

NK-like C-type lectin receptors (NKCL) are type II transmembrane receptors possessing an extracellular carbohydrate binding domain (CTLD), a stalk region of variable length, a transmembrane region, and a cytoplasmic tail that may or may not contain signaling motifs (Figure 6). The CTLD of these receptors shares structural similarity with the domains found in classical C-type lectin receptors, consisting of approximately 120 amino acids with at least 3 disulfide bonds, generated through 6 conserved cysteine residues. However, these domains generally lack the residues involved in calcium binding, which are required for carbohydrate binding in the classical C-type lectins. Many of these receptors also possess extra cysteines in their stalk regions, which are involved in homo- or heterodimerization.

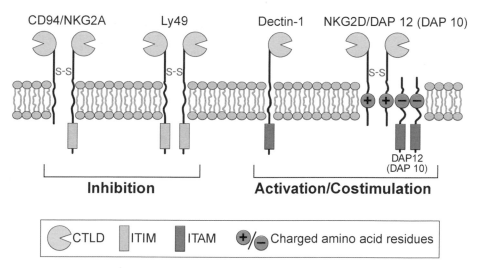

Figure 6   Examples of homo- and heterodimerized NKCL receptors and their signaling motifs. The inhibitory NKCLs possess ITIM sequences in their cytoplasmic tails, whereas the activatory receptors possess charged residues that allow association with the ITAM-containing DAP12. Charged residues can also allow association with the PI3K-binding DAP10, thought to function in costimulation. Dectin-1 is unique in that it is a single chain receptor possessing its own ITAM-like sequence.

The NKCLs consist of a number of families of highly related receptors that are often encoded by linked gene clusters, including the NKG2, NKRP1, and Ly49 families, as well as a number of other related molecules, such as CD69, CD94, Dectin-1, and LOX-1. These genes are mostly located within a single region, the NK complex, on human chromosome 12 and in a syntenic region on mouse chromosome 6. While many of the genes in this complex are orthologous, such as CD69 or CD94, there is significant interspecies diversity in the organization and complexity of this region. For example, there are 16 Ly49 genes in mouse, although only one has been identified in human. The structure of these genes is very similar, with three exons encoding the CRD and one exon for each of the remaining regions of these receptors. Many of the NKCL genes, such as NKG2D, are also alternatively spliced, often in a stimulus or cell-type specific manner, resulting in receptors that can possess different functional abilities.

Many NKCLs, including most members of the NKG2 and Ly49 families, appear to be expressed exclusively by NK cells and certain subsets of T cells. However, a limited number have also been identified on other cells, including a related subgroup that appears to be predominantly expressed in myeloid and endothelial cells. Expression of NKCLs can be regulated by the stage of cellular differentiation and activation and by cytokines and other agents. In addition, individual cells may express different receptor combinations, giving rise to diverse cellular populations.

The NKCLs can be broadly categorized as activatory or inhibitory. Most inhibitory receptors, such as MICL, possess one or more ITIMs in their cytoplasmic tails that become tyrosine phosphorylated upon ligation. This leads to the recruitment of phosphatases, such as SHP1 or SHP2, which mediate the downstream inhibitory effects. Activatory NKCLs, such as NKG2D, generally lack cytoplasmic signaling motifs, but they contain charged residues in their transmembrane domains that allow association with signaling partners, including DAP10 or DAP12. DAP12 contains a cytoplasmic ITAM that induces cellular activation through Syk, whereas the cytoplasmic tail of DAP10 contains a consensus motif for phosphatidylinositol 3-kinase. Other NKCLs, such as Dectin-1, induce intracellular signals through unique, and mostly unknown, mechanisms.

The signals generated by the NKCL receptors, especially members of the Ly49, NKG2, and NKRP1 families, are involved in the regulation of cytotoxicity, through recognition of MHC class I (or related molecules) or C-type lectin-like receptors. Others, including those in the subgroup expressed in myeloid and endothelial cells, appear to have more diverse ligands and cellular functions. However, many NKCLs are "orphan" receptors with no known functions or ligands. Here we focus in more detail on those NKCLs that are expressed by MØ and have defined functions, e.g., Dectin-1, LOX-1, and CD69. Those receptors expressed by MØ with no known functions are listed in Table 4 (95–99). Although NKG2D, the subject of review elsewhere (100), was originally described on MØ, recent evidence suggests that this molecule is not expressed by these cells (101), and so this receptor is not discussed further here.

Dectin-1

Murine Dectin-1 was originally isolated as a receptor that recognized an unidentified ligand on T cells, but it was later reidentified as a receptor for β-glucan polysaccharides (8, 102). Dectin-1 does not appear to oligomerize, but it associates

TABLE 4   Selected orphan NK-like C-type lectins expressed by MØ

Receptor	Abbrev.	Relevant expression	Signaling
Ly49Q	Ly49Q	Monocytes and MØ	ITIM via SHP1/2
Myeloid inhibitory C-type lectin receptor	MICL	Monocytes and granulocytes	ITIM via SHP1/2
CLEC-1/2	CLEC-1/2	DCs and monocytes	Non-typical Tyr-based motifs
Killer cell lectin-like receptor-1	KLRF1	Monocytes	Non-typical Tyr-based motifs
Myeloid DAP12-associating lectin-1	MDL-1	Monocytes, MØ, and DC	Associates with DAP12

with the tetraspanin receptor CD63, although the functional significance of this is unclear (103). Dectin-1 is expressed predominantly on myeloid cells, including MØ and neutrophils, and can be regulated by cytokines and other agents, including microbial stimuli (102, 104). Human Dectin-1 differs from the mouse receptor in that it is alternatively spliced, giving rise to a number of different cell-specific isoforms, of which only two are functional. Dectin-1 recognizes a variety of plant, bacterial, and fungal β-1,3 and/or β-1,6 glucan-linked carbohydrates, in a Ca^{2+}-independent manner, in both soluble and particulate form. This receptor can also recognize intact fungi such as *Saccharomyces cerevisiae*, *Candida albicans*, and *Pneumocystis carinii* (102, 105).

Dectin-1 possesses a cytoplasmic ITAM-like sequence that is involved in mediating proinflammatory cytokine production in response to β-glucan particles, in cooperation with TLR2 (106, 107). Dectin-1 can stimulate the oxidative burst in response to β-glucans, independently of the TLR pathway (106). Dectin-1 is also a phagocytic receptor, a process mediated by the cytoplasmic motif, but occurring through a novel, unidentified, Syk-independent pathway (108).

In addition to the exogenous ligands, Dectin-1 recognizes an endogenous ligand on T cells (102). The receptor can act as a costimulatory molecule, inducing the proliferation of both $CD4^+$ and $CD8^+$ T cells in vitro, and Dectin-1 expression has been observed on DCs in T cell areas of the spleen and lymph nodes (109), consistent with a role in T cell activation. Dectin-1 is present on subpopulations of MØ and DCs in the medullary and corticomedullary regions of the thymus, suggesting an additional role in thymocyte development (109). The endogenous ligand of Dectin-1 has yet to be identified.

LOX-1

LOX-1 (Figure 3) was originally isolated from a bovine aortic endothelial cDNA expression library screened for receptors for oxidized LDL (OxLDL) (110). LOX-1 is an N-glycosylated dimer that can be cleaved at the membrane proximal region of the extracellular domain, producing a soluble form whose function is unknown (111). This receptor is expressed on vascular endothelial cells, platelets, smooth muscle cells, fibroblasts, and MØ. Expression of LOX-1 can be regulated by a variety of proinflammatory, oxidative, and mechanical stimuli, and its expression is upregulated in pathological conditions in vivo, including diabetes, hyperlipidemia, atherosclerosis, and hypertension.

In addition to recognizing OxLDL, LOX-1 recognizes a variety of other ligands, including modified lipoproteins, aged/ apoptotic cells, activated platelets, hsp70, and bacteria (110, 112). The CTLD domain of this receptor mediates the ligand recognition, probably through electrostatic interactions of positively charged residues with negatively charged regions in the ligands, in a manner reminiscent of other SR.

Although lacking any conserved signaling motif in its cytoplasmic tail, LOX-1 can mediate endocytosis of OxLDL and phagocytosis of aged/apoptotic cells; it modulates cytokine production and induces superoxide anion production, NF-κB activation, and apoptosis. In addition, LOX-1 acts as a cell-adhesion molecule involved in leukocyte recruitment in inflammation, and through its interactions with hsp70, LOX-1 has been implicated in DC-mediated antigen cross-presentation (112, 113).

LOX-1 is present in atherosclerotic lesions and is thought to play a role in this disease through its ability to recognize and respond to OxLDL. Although this receptor can induce pathological changes in endothelial cells, its role in MØ and the formation of foam cells is unclear.

CD69

Cebrian and colleagues (114) identified CD69, or activation inducer molecule (AIM), as a marker on lymphocytes that was rapidly induced following cellular activation. The receptor is widely expressed on cells of hemopoietic origin, including neutrophils, monocytes, and MØ, which could be induced by cytokines and various other agents, including microbial stimuli (115). CD69 is a disulfide-linked, differentially glycosylated homodimer with a typical NKCL structure (116). Although the physiological ligands for CD69 are unknown, it binds selected carbohydrates in a novel Ca^{2+}-dependent manner (117).

CD69 is an activating receptor that has been shown in antibody cross-linking experiments to induce a wide variety of cellular responses. In monocytes and MØ, CD69 triggering induced extracellular Ca^{2+} influx, nitric oxide production, cytotoxicity, phospholipase A2 activation, and cytokine production (118). Triggering of CD69 induced MØ/monocyte apoptosis, in conjunction with LPS, and aided in the killing of *Leishmania* in infected MØ. Although lacking any conserved motifs, the cytoplasmic tail of CD69 can become phosphorylated and, in NK cells, its cellular functions depend on src-mediated Syk activation (119).

The generation of CD69-deficient mice has given additional insights into the physiological role of this receptor. Although hemopoietic cell development was mostly normal in CD69$^{-/-}$ mice, alterations in B cell development were apparent (120). More recently, these mice have revealed a role for CD69 as a negative regulator of antitumor responses and of autoimmune reactivity and inflammation, through induction of TGF-β (121, 122).

CLR

Researchers have identified a family of seven C-type lectin-related (CLRa-g) molecules that, although similar to the NKCLs, lack at least one of the conserved cysteines thought to form disulfide bridges in the CRD (123). The various members of this family have distinct expression patterns in tissues. CLRb is the best studied and is expressed on most hemopoietic cells, including MØ and DCs, and is regulated by cytokines and other agents, including calciotropic agents (124). CLRb, also known as OCIL (osteoclast-derived inhibitory lectin), CLRd (OCILrP1), and CLRg (OCILrP2), which is also expressed in MØ and DCs (125), are involved in the regulation of osteoclastogenesis in vitro, although the mechanism is unknown (126). Despite the unusual CTLD, CLRb can also recognize certain glycosamino-glycans in a Ca^{2+}-independent manner (127). Recently, the CLR family of proteins has been identified as ligands for the NK-specific NKRP1 family of NKCLs. The interaction between CLR and NKRP1 appears to be specific for each family member and results in modulation of NK cell function (124, 125). Although conserved motifs have been identified in the cytoplasmic tails of the CLRs (126), there is no evidence of any intracellular signaling.

RECEPTORS IN MACROPHAGES CONTAINING C-TYPE LECTIN DOMAINS

Receptors included in this section contain C-type lectin-like domains (CTLD) in which, in addition to a particular protein conformation containing two α-helices and two antiparallel β-sheets, Ca^{2+} coordination enables carbohydrate recognition. Two major groups can be distinguished: type II membrane molecules containing a single C-type lectin domain and type I receptors with several CTLDs, which have been generated through domain duplication.

Type II Membrane Receptors Containing a Single C-Type Lectin Domain

Table 5 lists a range of molecules expressed by MØ in mouse and human (128–137). Selected receptors are considered in more detail here.

DC-SIGN AND RELATED MOLECULES   DC-SIGN is a type II membrane molecule with a cytoplasmic domain containing an internalization motif, a transmembrane domain, stalk region, and CTLD (Figure 7). It was first characterized as an HIV gp120-binding protein, which was able to mediate the LFA-1-independent interaction of DCs with ICAM-3, a molecule highly expressed by naive T cells (134, 135). DC-SIGN is highly expressed by immature and mature DCs and DCs in the lung, dermis, mucosal tissue, T cell areas of the tonsil, lymph node, and spleen, as well as by subpopulations of MØ in the lung (alveolar) and placenta. DC-SIGN binds ICAM-2, and therefore a role in DC trafficking has been suggested (138). DC-SIGN functions as an endocytic receptor and enhances antigen internalization and presentation by DCs to T cells. A related protein with similar functional characteristics and liver and lymph node–restricted expression has been characterized and named DC-SIGNR/L-SIGN. Binding to a wide variety of microbes and viruses has now been demonstrated (e.g., *Candida albicans*, hepatitis C virus, dengue virus, Ebola virus, *Schistosoma* mansoni egg antigens, feline immunodeficiency virus and alphaviruses, *Leishmania*, and mycobacterium via recognition of ManLam).

Five DC-SIGN and DC-SIGNR/L-SIGN homologs have been detected in mouse (139): DC-SIGN (gene located next to CD23, as is human DC-SIGN, and highly

TABLE 5   Group II animal lectins in macrophages. Type II membrane receptors containing a single CTLD[a]

Protein(s)[b]	Comments	Expression
DCAR, DC immunoactivaing receptor	Associates with Fc receptor γ-chain. DCAR and DCIR (see below) are considered putative paired immunoreceptors	RT-PCR: strong in lung and spleen, weak in skin and LN BMDC. Exact cellular distribution remains to be clarified
DCIR, DC immunoreceptor (CLECFSF6)	Functional ITIM	Northern blot: PBL > BM, spleen, and LN Mo, granulocytes, DC, and B cells
DC-SIGN, DC-specific intercellular adhesion molecule 3-grabbing nonintegrin.	Endocytic receptor. Ca^{2+}-dependent recognition of mannose oligosaccharides on self and nonself: e.g., ICAM-2 and -3, HIV gp120, Man-LAM, fungi, etc.	Human: MoDC, MoMØ. DC and MØ populations in situ Mouse: RT-PCR: CD11c$^+$ DC > B cells Northern blot: spleen > lung $\gg$ kidney
Dectin-2, DC-associated lectin-2 (CLECSF10/NKCL)	Soluble Dectin-2 prevented UV-induced immunosupression, and the induction of tolerance. May exhibit Ca^{2+}-dependent mannose binding	Northern blot: Spleen and thymus RT-PCR: mRNA expression in epidermal cells sensitive to depletion of MHC class II$^+$ cells Myeloid progenitors
MCL, MØ C-type lectin (CLECSF8)	Endocytic	Mouse: Peritoneal MØ (MØ $\gg$ BM > spleen = lung > LN by Northern blot) Human: Northern blot: BM, PBL, spleen RT-PCR: Mo and MØ
MGL1 and 2, MØ galactose/N-acetylgalactosamine specific C-type lectins 1 and 2	pH and Ca^{2+}-dependent binding to α- and β-GalNAc (MGL1) and Lewis-X (MGL2). Dermal MGL1/2$^+$ MØ migrate to draining lymph nodes during the sensitisation phase of contact sensitivity	mAb LOM14 mAb recognizes both mouse MGL1 and 2 on tumoricidal peritoneal MØ, connective tissue MØ, and BMDC In humans: MGL1 expressed by Mo at an intermediate state during their differentiation into MØ immature MoDC, and cells in human dermis (90% CD68$^+$)
Mincle, MØ inducible C-type lectin (CLECSF9)	Expression strongly induced in response to IFN-γ, TNFα, IL-6, and LPS	Elicited peritoneal MØ
SIGNR-1, SIGN-related-1	A murine homolog of DC-SIGNR. Endocytic receptor. Ca^{2+} dependent sugar recognition of self and nonself: e.g., human ICAM-2 and -3, mouse ICAM-2, HIV gp120, mouse ICAM-2, *M. tuberculosis*, fungi, etc.	Splenic marginal zone MØ LN medullary and subcapsular sinus MØ Liver sinusoid endothelial cells

[a]Mo, monocyte; MØ, macrophage; MoMØ, monocyte derived MØ (human); MoDC, monocyte derived DC (human); BMDC, bone marrow derived MØ (mouse); LN, lymph nodes; BM, bone marrow; PBL, peripheral blood leukocytes; RT-PCR, reverse transcriptase-polymerase chain reaction.

[b]Alternate names given in parentheses.

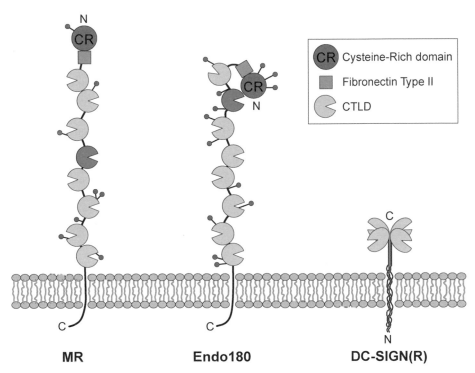

Figure 7   Selected Ca^{2+}-dependent C-type lectins expressed by MØ. Structural studies with Endo180 show its CR domain close to the mannose binding CTLD2. It is not known if the mannose binding CTLD4 of MR exhibits similar juxtaposition to its CR domain. DC-SIGNR forms tetrameric structures.

expressed in DCs, it is considered the mouse ortholog). Others include SIGNR1, 2, 3, and 4. Mouse DC-SIGN is expressed in spleen and lung and at lower levels in kidney, heart, thymus, and lymph nodes. Of the other four homologs, attention has mostly focused on SIGNR1. SIGNR1 is expressed in lymph nodes and at lower levels in spleen. SIGNR1 has been identified as the antigen on MZ MØ recognized by mAb ERTR9, a reagent that had previously been shown specifically to label MZ MØ in spleen and to block binding of neutral polysaccharides (dextran) to the MZ in vivo (136, 137). Additionally, SIGNR1 has been detected in liver endothelial sinusoidal cells, but not on Kupffer cells, and in medullary and subcapsular sinus MØ in lymph nodes. SIGNR1 binds hICAM-2, hICAM-3 and HIV gp-120, and mouse ICAM-2, and confers on transfected cells the ability to internalize dextran and bind zymosan and *Candida albicans*. Recognition of capsular polysaccharide from *S. pneumoniae* by SIGNR1 has also been reported both in vivo (using a novel mAb 22D1 that mediates specific downmodulation of the receptor on MZMØ) and in vitro (140).

DC-ASSOCIATED LECTIN-2 (DECTIN-2)   Two groups identified Dectin-2 independently: Fernandes et al. (141), through the analysis of genes overexpressed in a mouse model of chronic myelogenous leukemia blast crisis, and Ariizumi et al. (142), through a subtractive cDNA cloning strategy for genes selectively expressed by the DC-like murine cell line XS52, but not by the monocyte-like cells J774. Dectin-2 is a type II membrane protein with a single C-type lectin domain (which retains the residues for Ca^{2+}-dependent carbohydrate binding) on a short stalk, a transmembrane domain, and a cytoplasmic tail with no obvious signaling motifs. Dectin-2 is predominantly expressed in spleen and thymus, and RT-PCR analysis of epidermal cells suggested expression by Langerhans cells. The existence of lectin activity for Dectin-2 is unclear. Interestingly, Dectin-2 has been implicated in UV radiation-induced tolerance; administration of soluble bacterial-derived Dectin-2 was able to prevent UV-induced immunosuppression and the induction of tolerance and apparently restored the antigen response in already tolerized animals (143). Further work is required to understand the underlying mechanism.

Type I Membrane Receptors Containing Several C-Type Lectin Domains

The mannose receptor (MR) (CD206) was the first reported member of a family of four endocytic receptors that share the same overall structure: a cysteine-rich (CR) domain, a domain-containing fibronectin type II (FNII) repeats and multiple CTLD in the extracellular region, a transmembrane domain, and a short cytoplasmic tail (144, 145) (Figure 7). Other members of this family include DEC205 (CD205), a receptor mostly restricted to DCs that contains 10 CTLD, the Phospholipase A_2 (PLA$_2$) receptor, and Endo180, which, together with MR, contains 8 CTLD. Sequence analysis and sugar binding studies have demonstrated that only MR and Endo180 contain CTLD that could act as C-type lectin domains. For this reason, MR and Endo180 will be the only molecules discussed in this review.

MANNOSE RECEPTOR   The MR has been identified from different sources as a 175 kDa protein by its selective binding to mannose. The MR is expressed by most MØ populations, but is also expressed by hepatic and lymphatic endothelia, mesangial cells in kidneys, tracheal smooth muscle cells, and retinal pigment epithelium. The MR was first identified because of its suggested role in removal of lysosomal hydrolases from the circulation (144). It is a recycling receptor present in the endocytic compartment, and its cytoplasmic tail contains two internalization motifs. Physiological clearance seems to be a major role of the MR; MR-deficient mice have increased circulating levels of most lysosomal hydrolases tested, as well as COOH-terminal propeptide domains of the proalpha 1 and 2 chains of type 1 procollagen and the proalpha 1 chain of type III procollagen (146).

MR recognizes mannose, fucose, and N-acetylglucosamine in a Ca^{2+}-dependent manner via CTLD4, with CTLD4-8 sufficient to provide similar high-affinity binding to the full-length receptor (147). Endogenous ligands for the CTLD of MR have been described in mouse thyroid gland (thyroglobulin), salivary glands, and exocrine pancreas (148). Other endogenous ligands for which MR could mediate clearance are tissue plasminogen activator and neutrophil-derived myeloperoxidase. Glycoprotein hormones from the anterior pituitary are efficiently cleared by the liver, and a hepatic-specific form of the MR may mediate this uptake (149). The CR domain of MR is also a lectin and binds to SO_4-4-GalNAc, which is found in glycoprotein pituitary hormones. This activity may work in conjunction with the CTLD to facilitate recognition of these hormones by the MR (148). Ligands for the CR domain (CRL) have been detected on the surface of select MØ subpopulations in secondary lymphoid organs: MZ metallophilic MØ in spleen and subcapsular sinus MØ in lymph nodes in naive animals. Further analysis of this interaction demonstrated binding to cell-specific glycoforms of sialoadhesin and CD45. The importance of the presence and location of these specific ligands is unclear, but they appear to label cells involved in the presentation of antigen. These CRL-expressing cells could potentially interact with a soluble form of the MR (see below) or with cells expressing MR; however, this requires further study. The FNII domain is the most conserved domain between the members of the MR family and is predicted to bind collagen. Although this property has been demonstrated in the case of PLA_2R and Endo180 (see below), no information is available in regard to MR.

In addition to the clearance of endogenous glycoproteins, many other functions have been ascribed to MR. The two best-studied functions are in pathogen recognition and antigen presentation. A wide range of potential microbial ligands has been reported, such as fungi and viruses (see Supplemental Material), many of which are also now being reported as ligands for other mannose recognition receptors such as DC-SIGN. Despite the relatively poor expression observed on DCs in vivo, DCs in vitro express high levels of the MR and use mannose receptors for enhanced antigen internalization and presentation. In human lymph node, MR has been implicated in lymphocyte binding to lymphatic endothelium through a novel interaction with L-selectin. This interaction may be important for lymphocyte exit from lymph node.

MR expression is upregulated by IL-4/13 and IL-10 and is downregulated by IFN-γ. Surface expression is also affected by proteolytic cleavage of the extracellular domain, which generates a functional soluble form of the MR (sMR) that has been observed in mouse serum.

Endo180   Endo180 is a constitutively recycling endocytic receptor that is predominantly expressed in vivo and in vitro on fibroblasts, endothelial cells, and MØ. Dermal $CD14^+$ MØ and cells that resemble Hofbauer cells in placenta expressed Endo180. Unlike MR, no expression of Endo180 has been observed in the thymus or in the liver. Like MR, Endo180 binds to mannose, fucose, and N-acetylglucosamine in a Ca^{2+}-dependent manner through CTLD2, but not to galactose (150). Endo180 binds to both native and denatured collagens, and this binding seems to be mediated by the FNII domain. In cell culture systems, expression of Endo180 results in the rapid uptake of soluble collagens for delivery to the lysosomal compartments. Endo180 has also been identified as uP-ARAP (urokinase-type plasminogen activator receptor associated protein), which forms a complex on the cell surface with pro-uPA and its receptor (reviewed by 151).

Endo180 is a general promoter of random cell migration and has a more specific function in cell chemotaxis in a uPA gradient. Endo180 expression enhanced uPA-mediated filopodia production and promoted rapid activation of Cdc42 and Rac. Mice have been generated with a targeted deletion in Endo180, which results in a truncated Endo180 protein that lacks the cysteine-rich domain, the FNII domain, and CTLD1 (152). Analysis of embryonic fibroblasts revealed that this mutation did not disrupt the C-type lectin activity mediated by CTLD2 but resulted in cells with a defect in collagen binding and internalization and an impaired migratory phenotype.

CONCLUSION

A great deal remains to be learned about the nature, ligands, interactions, and functions of the receptors described in this review. Their ability to discriminate among different classes of organisms, as well as modified host cells, remains poorly understood. Microbial specificity of ligand expression is unexplored, and may not fit with the earlier concept of pattern recognition of conserved structures; nevertheless, organisms have diversified, under evolutionary pressure from the innate as well as the adaptive immune system, and may be able to avoid recognition, e.g., by masking surface expression of wall constituents. Our knowledge of bacterial and fungal recognition and sensing is most advanced because their surfaces may be most foreign. Much less is known about viral recognition, except for host-derived carbohydrates. Multicellular parasites may also express host molecules on their surface and have other means to avoid recognition. Modified host components that are expressed by apoptotic cells are under intense study, but almost nothing is known about modifications associated with development of tumors, which may escape surveillance by APC.

The differential responses to exogenous and endogenous ligands (signaling, gene expression, induction or suppression of acquired immunity) are of great interest. Considerable progress has been made in the analysis of TLR-adaptor-NF-κB/interferon pathways, but the question remains: How do the same receptors generate such different outcomes to truly foreign and abnormal modified host ligands? These outcomes could be due to different interactions of multi-receptor complexes at the cell surface, differential expression of receptors by MØ and DCs (themselves markedly heterogeneous as a result of differentiation), or activation and responses to their local microenvironments, or they could result from intracellular mechanisms that remain obscure.

The first stage of cataloging receptors and their potential ligands and functions in immune recognition is well advanced. Integrating this information with studies of surface expression and secretory and endocytic traffic will require more emphasis on the cell biology of APC. Interactions of receptors with extracellular matrix and plasma will further modulate recognition by APC as a fundamental aspect of the immune response.

APPENDIX

Abbreviations used: APC, antigen-presenting cell; AIM, activation inducer molecule; β_2GPI, β_2 glycoprotein I; BMDM, bone marrow culture–derived macrophages; CLR, C-type lectin related; CR, cysteine-rich domain of macrophage mannose receptor; CR3, complement receptor 3; CR4, complement receptor 4; CRD, carbohydrate recognition domain; CRL, ligands for the CR domain; CTLD, C-type lectin carbohydrate-binding domain; CTR, C-type lectin-related receptor; DC-SIGN, DC-specific integrin grabbing nonintegrin; DAF, decay acceleration factor; DAP, DNAX activation protein; EAE, experimental autoimmune encephalomyelitis; EGF, epidermal growth factor; EMR, EGF-like module containing mucin-like hormone receptor; FNII, fibronectin type II; Gas6, growth arrest specific gene 6; GPCR, G protein–coupled receptor; GPI, glycosylphosphatidylinositol; GPS, GPCR proteolytic site; ICAM, intercellular adhesion molecule; IgSF, immunoglobulin superfamily; ILT, immunoglobulin-like transcript; ITAM, immunoreceptor tyrosine-based activation motif; ITIM, immunoreceptor tyrosine-based inhibitory motif; KIR, killer cell immunoglobulin-like receptor; LDL, low-density lipoprotein; LIR, leukocyte immunoglobulin-like receptor; LOX-1, lectin-like oxidized low-density lipoprotein receptor; LPS, lipopolysaccharide; LTA, lipoteichoic acid; MØ, macrophage; mAb, monoclonal antibody; MARCO, macrophage receptor with collagenous domain; MBL, mannose-binding lectin; MCP-1, monocyte chemoattractant protein-1; M-CSF, macrophage colony stimulating factor; MIP-1α, macrophage inflammatory protein-1α; MIR, monocyte/macrophage immunoglobulin-like receptor; MR, mannose receptor; MZ, marginal zone; NKCL, NK-like C-type lectin-like receptor; OCIL, osteoclast-derived inhibitory lectin; OxLDL, oxidized LDL; PAMP, pathogen-associated molecular pattern; PGN, peptidoglycans; PLA$_2$, phospholipase A$_2$; PMN, polymorphonuclear leukocyte; PIR, paired immunoglobulin-like receptor; PRR, pattern recognition receptor; PS, phosphatidyl serine; RCA, receptor of complement activation; SCR, short consensus repeat; SHIP, SH2-containing inositol phosphatase; SHP1, SH2-domain-containing protein tyrosine phosphatase 1; Siglec, sialic acid–binding immunoglobulin-like lectin; SIGNR1, SIGN-related 1; SIRP1α, signal regulatory protein 1α; SP-A, surfactant protein A; SP-D, surfactant protein D; SR, scavenger receptor; SRCR, scavenger receptor cysteine-rich domain; TM7, seven transmembrane; TLT1, TREM-like transcript 1; TLR, Toll-like receptor; TNF, tumor necrosis factor; TREM, triggering receptor on myeloid cells; uPARAP, urokinase-type plasminogen activator receptor associated protein; VnR, vitronectin receptor.

ACKNOWLEDGMENTS

We thank colleagues for their contributions, the Medical Research Council (UK), The Wellcome Trust, Arthritis Research Campaign (UK), British Heart Foundation, and Histiocytosis Association of America for grant support, and Christine Holt for help in preparing the manuscript.

The *Annual Review of Immunology* is online at
http://immunol.annualreviews.org

LITERATURE CITED

1. Gordon S. 2003. Macrophages and the immune response. In *Fundamental Immunology*, ed. W Paul, pp. 481–95. Philadelphia: Lippincott Raven
2. Gordon S. 2002. Pattern recognition receptors: doubling up for the innate immune response. *Cell* 111:927–30
3. Kaufmann SHE, Medzhitov R, Gordon S, eds. 2004. *The Innate Immune Response to Infection*. Washington, DC: ASM Press. 465 pp.
4. Akira S, Takeda K, Kaisho T. 2001. Toll-like receptors: critical proteins linking innate and acquired immunity. *Nat. Immunol.* 2:675–80
5. Inohara N, Nunez G. 2003. NODs: intracellular proteins involved in inflammation and apoptosis. *Nat. Rev. Immunol.* 3:371–82
6. Tschopp J, Martinon F, Burns K. 2003. NALPs: a novel protein family involved in inflammation. *Nat. Rev. Mol. Cell Biol.* 4:95–104
7. Janeway CA Jr, Medzhitov R. 2002. Innate immune recognition. *Annu. Rev. Immunol.* 20:197–216
8. Brown GD, Gordon S. 2003. Fungal beta-glucans and mammalian immunity. *Immunity* 19:311–15
9. Krieger M. 1997. The other side of scavenger receptors: pattern recognition for host defense. *Curr. Opin. Lipidol.* 8:275–80
10. Glass CK, Witztum JL. 2001. Atherosclerosis: the road ahead. *Cell* 104:503–16
11. Gordon S. 2003. Alternative activation of macrophages. *Nat. Rev. Immunol.* 3:23–35
12. Kraal G. 1992. Cells in the marginal zone of the spleen. *Int. Rev. Cytol.* 132:31–74
13. Brown MS, Goldstein JL. 1983. Lipoprotein metabolism in the macrophage: implications for cholesterol deposition in atherosclerosis. *Annu. Rev. Biochem.* 52:223–61
14. Kristiansen M, Graversen JH, Jacobsen C, Sonne O, Hoffman HJ, et al. 2001. Identification of the haemoglobin scavenger receptor. *Nature* 409:198–201
15. Mukhopadhyay S, Gordon S. 2004. The role of scavenger receptors in pattern recognition and innate immunity. *Immunobiology*. In press
16. Peiser L, De Winther MP, Makepeace K, Hollinshead M, Coull P, et al. 2002. The class A macrophage scavenger receptor is a major pattern recognition receptor for Neisseria meningitidis which is independent of lipopolysaccharide and not required for secretory responses. *Infect. Immun.* 70:5346–54
17. Platt N, Haworth R, Darley L, Gordon S. 2002. The many roles of the class A macrophage scavenger receptor. *Int. Rev. Cytol.* 212:1–40
18. Kraal G, van der Laan LJ, Elomaa O, Tryggvason K. 2000. The macrophage receptor MARCO. *Microbes Infect.* 2:313–16
19. Karlsson MC, Guinamard R, Bolland S,

Sankala M, Steinman RM, Ravetch JV. 2003. Macrophages control the retention and trafficking of B lymphocytes in the splenic marginal zone. *J. Exp. Med.* 198:333–40

20. Febbraio M, Hajjar DP, Silverstein RL. 2001. CD36: a class B scavenger receptor involved in angiogenesis, atherosclerosis, inflammation, and lipid metabolism. *J. Clin. Invest.* 108:785–91

21. Franc NC, Dimarcq JL, Lagueux M, Hoffmann J, Ezekowitz RA. 1996. Croquemort, a novel *Drosophila* hemocyte/macrophage receptor that recognizes apoptotic cells. *Immunity* 4:431–43

22. Rainet M, Pearson A, Baksa K, Harikrishna A. 2003. Pattern recognition on receptors in *Drosophila*. In *Innate Immunity*, ed. RA Ezekowitz, JA Hoffmann, pp. 127–35. Totona, NJ: Human

23. Fadok VA, Bratton DL, Konowal A, Freed PW, Westcott JY, Henson PM. 1998. Macrophages that have ingested apoptotic cells in vitro inhibit proinflammatory cytokine production through autocrine/paracrine mechanisms involving TGF-β, PGE2, and PAF. *J. Clin. Invest.* 101:890–98

24. Pickering MC, Botto M, Taylor PR, Lachmann PJ, Walport MJ. 2000. Systemic lupus erythematosus, complement deficiency, and apoptosis. *Adv. Immunol.* 76:227–324

25. Henson PM, Bratton DL, Fadok VA. 2001. Apoptotic cell removal. *Curr. Biol.* 11:R795–805

26. Savill J, Dransfield I, Gregory C, Haslett C. 2002. A blast from the past: clearance of apoptotic cells regulates immune responses. *Nat. Rev. Immunol.* 2:965–75

27. Fadok VA, Voelker DR, Campbell PA, Cohen JJ, Bratton DL, Henson PM. 1992. Exposure of phosphatidylserine on the surface of apoptotic lymphocytes triggers specific recognition and removal by macrophages. *J. Immunol.* 148:2207–16

28. Fadok VA, Bratton DL, Rose DM, Pearson A, Ezekewitz RA, Henson PM.

2000. A receptor for phosphatidylserine-specific clearance of apoptotic cells. *Nature* 405:85–90

29. Li MO, Sarkisian MR, Mehal WZ, Rakic P, Flavell RA. 2003. Phosphatidylserine receptor is required for clearance of apoptotic cells. *Science* 302:1560–63

30. Wang X, Wu YC, Fadok VA, Lee MC, Gengyo-Ando K, et al. 2003. Cell corpse engulfment mediated by *C. elegans* phosphatidylserine receptor through CED-5 and CED-12. *Science* 302:1563–66

31. Platt N, Suzuki H, Kurihara Y, Kodama T, Gordon S. 1996. Role for the class A macrophage scavenger receptor in the phagocytosis of apoptotic thymocytes in vitro. *Proc. Natl. Acad. Sci. USA* 93:12456–60

32. Devitt A, Moffatt OD, Raykundalia C, Capra JD, Simmons DL, Gregory CD. 1998. Human CD14 mediates recognition and phagocytosis of apoptotic cells. *Nature* 392:505–9

33. Oka K, Sawamura T, Kikuta K, Itokawa S, Kume N, et al. 1998. Lectin-like oxidized low-density lipoprotein receptor 1 mediates phagocytosis of aged/apoptotic cells in endothelial cells. *Proc. Natl. Acad. Sci. USA* 95:9535–40

34. Balasubramanian K, Schroit AJ. 1998. Characterization of phosphatidylserine-dependent β2-glycoprotein I macrophage interactions. Implications for apoptotic cell clearance by phagocytes. *J. Biol. Chem.* 273:29272–77

35. Ogden CA, deCathelineau A, Hoffmann PR, Bratton D, Ghebrehiwet B, et al. 2001. C1q and mannose binding lectin engagement of cell surface calreticulin and CD91 initiates macropinocytosis and uptake of apoptotic cells. *J. Exp. Med.* 194:781–95

36. Schagat TL, Wofford JA, Wright JR. 2001. Surfactant protein A enhances alveolar macrophage phagocytosis of apoptotic neutrophils. *J. Immunol.* 166:2727–33

37. Vandivier RW, Ogden CA, Fadok VA, Hoffmann PR, Brown KK, et al. 2002.

Role of surfactant proteins A, D, and C1q in the clearance of apoptotic cells in vivo and in vitro: calreticulin and CD91 as a common collectin receptor complex. *J. Immunol.* 169:3978–86

38. Nakano T, Ishimoto Y, Kishino J, Umeda M, Inoue K, et al. 1997. Cell adhesion to phosphatidylserine mediated by a product of growth arrest-specific gene 6. *J. Biol. Chem.* 272:29411–14

39. Scott RS, McMahon EJ, Pop SM, Reap EA, Caricchio R, et al. 2001. Phagocytosis and clearance of apoptotic cells is mediated by MER. *Nature* 411:207–11

40. Fan X, Krahling S, Smith D, Williamson P, Schlegel RA. 2004. Macrophage Surface Expression of Annexins I and II in the Phagocytosis of Apoptotic Lymphocytes. *Mol. Biol. Cell* 15:2863–72

41. Kwakkenbos MJ, Kop EN, Stacey M, Matmati M, Gordon S, et al. 2004. The EGF-TM7 family: a postgenomic view. *Immunogenetics* 55:655–66

42. Schaller E, Macfarlane AJ, Rupec RA, Gordon S, McKnight AJ, Pfeffer K. 2002. Inactivation of the F4/80 glycoprotein in the mouse germ line. *Mol. Cell. Biol.* 22: 8035–43

43. Warschkau H, Kiderlen AF. 1999. A monoclonal antibody directed against the murine macrophage surface molecule F4/80 modulates natural immune response to *Listeria* monocytogenes. *J. Immunol.* 163:3409–16

44. Wang Y, Goldschneider I, O'Rourke J, Cone RE. 2001. Blood mononuclear cells induce regulatory NK T thymocytes in anterior chamber-associated immune deviation. *J. Leukoc. Biol.* 69:741–46

45. Lin H-H, Stacey M, Hamann J, Gordon S, McKnight AJ. 2000. Human EMR2, a novel EGF-TM7 molecule on chromosome 19p13.1, is closely related to CD97. *Genomics* 67:188–200

46. Stacey M, Chang GW, Davies JQ, Kwakkenbos MJ, Sanderson RD, et al. 2003. The epidermal growth factor-like domains of the human EMR2 receptor mediate cell attachment through chondroitin sulphate glycosaminoglycans. *Blood* 102:2916–24

47. Leemans JC, te Velde AA, Florquin S, Bennink RJ, de Bruin K, et al. 2004. The epidermal growth factor-seven transmembrane (EGF-TM7) receptor CD97 is required for neutrophil migration and host defense. *J. Immunol.* 172:1125–31

48. Hamann J, Wishaupt JO, van Lier RA, Smeets TJ, Breedveld FC, Tak PP. 1999. Expression of the activation antigen CD97 and its ligand CD55 in rheumatoid synovial tissue. *Arthritis Rheum.* 42:650–58

49. Visser L, de Vos AF, Hamann J, Melief MJ, van Meurs M, et al. 2002. Expression of the EGF-TM7 receptor CD97 and its ligand CD55 (DAF) in multiple sclerosis. *J. Neuroimmunol.* 132:156–63

50. Stacey M, Lin HH, Hilyard KL, Gordon S, McKnight AJ. 2001. Human epidermal growth factor (EGF) module-containing mucin-like hormone receptor 3 is a new member of the EGF-TM7 family that recognizes a ligand on human macrophages and activated neutrophils. *J. Biol. Chem.* 276:18863–70

51. Hamann J, Kwakkenbos MJ, de Jong EC, Heus H, Olsen AS, van Lier RA. 2003. Inactivation of the EGF-TM7 receptor EMR4 after the Pan-Homo divergence. *Eur. J. Immunol.* 33:1365–71

52. Wright SD, Ramos RA, Tobias PS, Ulevitch RJ, Mathison JC. 1990. CD14, a receptor for complexes of lipopolysaccharide (LPS) and LPS binding protein. *Science* 249:1431–33

53. Lee JD, Kato K, Tobias PS, Kirkland TN, Ulevitch RJ. 1992. Transfection of CD14 into 70Z/3 cells dramatically enhances the sensitivity to complexes of lipopolysaccharide (LPS) and LPS binding protein. *J. Exp. Med.* 175:1697–705

54. Van Amersfoort ES, Van Berkel TJ, Kuiper J. 2003. Receptors, mediators, and mechanisms involved in bacterial sepsis and septic shock. *Clin. Microbiol. Rev.* 16:379–414

55. Triantafilou M, Triantafilou K. 2002. Lipopolysaccharide recognition: CD14, TLRs and the LPS-activation cluster. *Trends Immunol.* 23:301–4

56. Ferrero E, Hsieh CL, Francke U, Goyert SM. 1990. CD14 is a member of the family of leucine-rich proteins and is encoded by a gene syntenic with multiple receptor genes. *J. Immunol.* 145:331–36

57. Juan TS, Hailman E, Kelley MJ, Busse LA, Davy E, et al. 1995. Identification of a lipopolysaccharide binding domain in CD14 between amino acids 57 and 64. *J. Biol. Chem.* 270:5219–24

58. Bazil V, Horejsi V, Baudys M, Kristofova H, Strominger JL, et al. 1986. Biochemical characterization of a soluble form of the 53-kDa monocyte surface antigen. *Eur. J. Immunol.* 16:1583–89

59. Landmann R, Zimmerli W, Sansano S, Link S, Hahn A, et al. 1995. Increased circulating soluble CD14 is associated with high mortality in gram-negative septic shock. *J. Infect Dis.* 171:639–44

60. Lublin DM, Atkinson JP. 1989. Decay-accelerating factor: biochemistry, molecular biology, and function. *Annu. Rev. Immunol.* 7:35–58

61. Lindahl G, Sjobring U, Johnsson E. 2000. Human complement regulators: a major target for pathogenic microorganisms. *Curr. Opin. Immunol.* 12:44–51

62. Ward T, Pipkin PA, Clarkson NA, Stone DM, Minor PD, Almond JW. 1994. Decay-accelerating factor CD55 is identified as the receptor for echovirus 7 using CELICS, a rapid immuno-focal cloning method. *EMBO J.* 13:5070–74

63. Bergelson JM, Mohanty JG, Crowell RL, St. John NF, Lublin DM, Finberg RW. 1995. Coxsackievirus B3 adapted to growth in RD cells binds to decay-accelerating factor (CD55). *J. Virol.* 69:1903–6

64. Nowicki B, Labigne A, Moseley S, Hull R, Hull S, Moulds J. 1990. The Dr hemagglutinin, afimbrial adhesins AFA-I and AFA-III, and F1845 fimbriae of uropathogenic and diarrhea-associated Escherichia coli belong to a family of hemagglutinins with Dr receptor recognition. *Infect. Immun.* 58:279–81

65. Pham T, Kaul A, Hart A, Goluszko P, Moulds J, et al. 1995. *dra*-related X adhesins of gestational pyelonephritis-associated *Escherichia coli* recognize SCR-3 and SCR-4 domains of recombinant decay-accelerating factor. *Infect. Immun.* 63:1663–68

66. Nowicki B, Selvarangan R, Nowicki S. 2001. Family of Escherichia coli Dr adhesins: decay-accelerating factor receptor recognition and invasiveness. *J. Infect. Dis.* 183(Suppl. 1):24–27

67. Le Bouguenec C, Lalioui L, du Merle L, Jouve M, Courcoux P, et al. 2001. Characterization of AfaE adhesins produced by extraintestinal and intestinal human Escherichia coli isolates: PCR assays for detection of Afa adhesins that do or do not recognize Dr blood group antigens. *J. Clin. Microbiol.* 39:1738–45

68. Caras IW, Davitz MA, Rhee L, Weddell G, Martin DW Jr, Nussenzweig V. 1987. Cloning of decay-accelerating factor suggests novel use of splicing to generate two proteins. *Nature* 325:545–49

69. Lea S. 2002. Interactions of CD55 with non-complement ligands. *Biochem. Soc. Trans.* 30:1014–19

70. Hamann J, Vogel B, van Schijndel GM, van Lier RA. 1996. The seven-span transmembrane receptor CD97 has a cellular ligand (CD55, DAF). *J. Exp. Med.* 184:1185–89

71. Lin HH, Stacey M, Saxby C, Knott V, Chaudhry Y, et al. 2001. Molecular analysis of the epidermal growth factor-like short consensus repeat domain-mediated protein-protein interactions: dissection of the CD97-CD55 complex. *J. Biol. Chem.* 276:24160–69

72. Lawrence DW, Bruyninckx WJ, Louis NA, Lublin DM, Stahl GL, et al. 2003. Antiadhesive role of apical decay-accelerating factor (CD55) in human

neutrophil transmigration across mucosal epithelia. *J. Exp. Med.* 198:999–1010

73. Colonna M. 2003. TREMs in the immune system and beyond. *Nat. Rev. Immunol.* 3: 445–53

74. Colonna M, Facchetti F. 2003. TREM-1 (triggering receptor expressed on myeloid cells): a new player in acute inflammatory responses. *J. Infect. Dis.* 187(Suppl. 2): S397–401

75. Bleharski JR, Kiessler V, Buonsanti C, Sieling PA, Stenger S, et al. 2003. A role for triggering receptor expressed on myeloid cells-1 in host defense during the early-induced and adaptive phases of the immune response. *J. Immunol.* 170:3812–18

76. Bouchon A, Facchetti F, Weigand MA, Colonna M. 2001. TREM-1 amplifies inflammation and is a crucial mediator of septic shock. *Nature* 410:1103–7

77. Kaifu T, Nakahara J, Inui M, Mishima K, Momiyama T, et al. 2003. Osteopetrosis and thalamic hypomyelinosis with synaptic degeneration in DAP12-deficient mice. *J. Clin. Invest.* 111:323–32

78. Crocker PR. 2002. Siglecs: sialic-acid-binding immunoglobulin-like lectins in cell-cell interactions and signalling. *Curr. Opin. Struct. Biol.* 12:609–15

79. Crocker PR, Gordon S. 1986. Properties and distribution of a lectin-like hemagglutinin differentially expressed by murine stromal tissue macrophages. *J. Exp. Med.* 164:1862–75

80. Jones C, Virji M, Crocker PR. 2003. Recognition of sialylated meningococcal lipopolysaccharide by siglecs expressed on myeloid cells leads to enhanced bacterial uptake. *Mol. Microbiol.* 49:1213–25

81. Paul SP, Taylor LS, Stansbury EK, McVicar DW. 2000. Myeloid specific human CD33 is an inhibitory receptor with differential ITIM function in recruiting the phosphatases SHP-1 and SHP-2. *Blood* 96:483–90

82. Crocker PR, Varki A. 2001. Siglecs, sialic acids and innate immunity. *Trends Immunol.* 22:337–42

83. Brinkman-Vander Linden ECM, Angata T, Reynolds SA, Powell LD, Hedrick SM, Varki A. 2003. CD33/Siglec-3 binding specificity, expression pattern, and consequences of gene deletion in mice. *Mol. Cell. Biol.* 23:4199–206

84. Colonna M, Nakajima H, Cella M. 2000. A family of inhibitory and activating Ig-like receptors that modulate function of lymphoid and myeloid cells. *Semin. Immunol.* 12:121–27

85. Ho LH, Uehara T, Chen CC, Kubagawa H, Cooper MD. 1999. Constitutive tyrosine phosphorylation of the inhibitory paired Ig-like receptor PIR-B. *Proc. Natl. Acad. Sci. USA* 96:15086–90

86. Ujike A, Takeda K, Nakamura A, Ebihara S, Akiyama K, Takai T. 2002. Impaired dendritic cell maturation and increased T(H)2 responses in PIR-B$^{-/-}$ mice. *Nat. Immunol.* 3:542–48

87. Nakamura A, Kobayashi E, Takai T. 2004. Exacerbated graft-versus-host disease in Pirb$^{-/-}$ mice. *Nat. Immunol.* 5:623–29

88. Barclay AN, Wright GJ, Brooke G, Brown MH. 2002. CD200 and membrane protein interactions in the control of myeloid cells. *Trends Immunol.* 23:285–90

89. Hoek RM, Ruuls SR, Murphy CA, Wright GJ, Goddard R, et al. 2000. Down-regulation of the macrophage lineage through interaction with OX2 (CD200). *Science* 290:1768–71

90. Kharitonenkov A, Chen ZJ, Sures I, Wang HY, Schilling J, Ullrich A. 1997. A family of proteins that inhibit signalling through tyrosine kinase receptors. *Nature* 386:181–86

91. Oldenborg PA, Gresham HD, Lindberg FP. 2001. CD47-signal regulatory protein α (SIRP α) regulates Fc γ and complement receptor-mediated phagocytosis. *J. Exp. Med.* 193:855–62

92. Brown EJ, Frazier WA. 2001. Integrin-associated protein (CD47) and its ligands. *Trends Cell Biol.* 11:130–35

93. Oldenborg PA, Zheleznyak A, Fang YF, Lagenaur CF, Gresham HD, Lindberg FP. 2000. Role of CD47 as a marker of self on red blood cells. *Science* 288:2051–54

94. Gardai SJ, Xiao YQ, Dickinson M, Nick JA, Voelker DR, et al. 2003. By binding SIRP α or calreticulin/CD91, lung collectins act as dual function surveillance molecules to suppress or enhance inflammation. *Cell* 115:13–23

95. Toyama-Sorimachi N, Tsujimura Y, Maruya M, Onoda A, Kubota T, et al. 2004. Ly49Q, a member of the Ly49 family that is selectively expressed on myeloid lineage cells and involved in regulation of cytoskeletal architecture. *Proc. Natl. Acad. Sci. USA* 101:1016–21

96. Roda-Navarro P, Arce I, Renedo M, Montgomery K, Kucherlapati R, Fernandez-Ruiz E. 2000. Human KLRF1, a novel member of the killer cell lectin-like receptor gene family: molecular characterization, genomic structure, physical mapping to the NK gene complex and expression analysis. *Eur. J. Immunol.* 30:568–76

97. Marshall AS, Willment JA, Lin HH, Williams DL, Gordon S, Brown GD. 2004. Identification and characterization of a novel human myeloid inhibitory C-type lectin-like receptor (MICL) that is predominantly expressed on granulocytes and monocytes. *J. Biol. Chem.* 279:14792–802

98. Colonna M, Samaridis J, Angman L. 2000. Molecular characterization of two novel C-type lectin-like receptors, one of which is selectively expressed in human dendritic cells. *Eur. J. Immunol.* 30:697–704

99. Bakker AB, Baker E, Sutherland GR, Phillips JH, Lanier LL. 1999. Myeloid DAP12-associating lectin (MDL)-1 is a cell surface receptor involved in the activation of myeloid cells. *Proc. Natl. Acad. Sci. USA* 96:9792–96

100. Raulet DH. 2003. Roles of the NKG2D immunoreceptor and its ligands. *Nat. Rev. Immunol.* 3:781–90

101. Diefenbach A, Tomasello E, Lucas M, Jamieson AM, Hsia JK, et al. 2002. Selective associations with signaling proteins determine stimulatory versus costimulatory activity of NKG2D. *Nat. Immunol.* 3:1142–49

102. Herre J, Gordon S, Brown GD. 2004. Dectin-1 and its role in the recognition of beta-glucans by macrophages. *Mol. Immunol.* 40:869–76

103. Mantegazza AR, Barrio MM, Moutel S, Bover L, Weck M, et al. 2004. CD63 Tetraspanin slows down cell migration and translocates to the endosomal/lysosomal/MIICs route after extracellular stimuli in human immature dendritic cells. *Blood* 104:1183–90

104. Willment JA, Lin HH, Reid DM, Taylor PR, Williams DL, et al. 2003. Dectin-1 expression and function are enhanced on alternatively activated and GM-CSF-treated macrophages and are negatively regulated by IL-10, dexamethasone, and lipopolysaccharide. *J. Immunol.* 171:4569–73

105. Steele C, Marrero L, Swain S, Harmsen AG, Zheng M, et al. 2003. Alveolar macrophage-mediated killing of *Pneumocystis carinii* f. sp. muris involves molecular recognition by the Dectin-1 beta-glucan receptor. *J. Exp. Med.* 198:1677–88

106. Gantner BN, Simmons RM, Canavera SJ, Akira S, Underhill DM. 2003. Collaborative induction of inflammatory responses by dectin-1 and Toll-like receptor 2. *J. Exp. Med.* 197:1107–17

107. Brown GD, Herre J, Williams DL, Willment JA, Marshall AS, Gordon S. 2003. Dectin-1 mediates the biological effects of beta-glucans. *J. Exp. Med.* 197:1119–24

108. Herre J, Marshall AS, Caron E, Edwards AD, Williams DL, et al. 2004. Dectin-1 uses novel mechanisms for yeast phagocytosis in macrophages. *Blood* 104:4038–45

109. Reid DM, Montoya M, Taylor PR, Borrow P, Gordon S, et al. 2004. Expression of the beta-glucan receptor, Dectin-1, on murine leukocytes in situ correlates with its function in pathogen recognition and reveals potential roles in leukocyte interactions. *J. Leukoc. Biol.* 76:86–94

110. Chen M, Masaki T, Sawamura T. 2002. LOX-1, the receptor for oxidized low-density lipoprotein identified from endothelial cells: implications in endothelial dysfunction and atherosclerosis. *Pharmacol. Ther.* 95:89–100

111. Xie Q, Matsunaga S, Niimi S, Ogawa S, Tokuyasu K, et al. 2004. Human lectin-like oxidized low-density lipoprotein receptor-1 functions as a dimer in living cells. *DNA Cell Biol.* 23:111–17

112. Delneste Y, Magistrelli G, Gauchat J, Haeuw J, Aubry J, et al. 2002. Involvement of LOX-1 in dendritic cell-mediated antigen cross-presentation. *Immunity* 17:353–62

113. Honjo M, Nakamura K, Yamashiro K, Kiryu J, Tanihara H, et al. 2003. Lectin-like oxidized LDL receptor-1 is a cell-adhesion molecule involved in endotoxin-induced inflammation. *Proc. Natl. Acad. Sci. USA* 100:1274–79

114. Cebrian M, Yague E, Rincon M, Lopez-Botet M, de Landazuri MO, Sanchez-Madrid F. 1988. Triggering of T cell proliferation through AIM, an activation inducer molecule expressed on activated human lymphocytes. *J. Exp. Med.* 168:1621–37

115. Marzio R, Mauel J, Betz-Corradin S. 1999. CD69 and regulation of the immune function. *Immunopharmacol. Immunotoxicol.* 21:565–82

116. Lopez-Cabrera M, Santis AG, Fernandez-Ruiz E, Blacher R, Esch F, et al. 1993. Molecular cloning, expression, and chromosomal localization of the human earliest lymphocyte activation antigen AIM/CD69, a new member of the C-type animal lectin superfamily of signal-transmitting receptors. *J. Exp. Med.* 178:537–47

117. Pavlicek J, Sopko B, Ettrich R, Kopecky V Jr, Baumruk V, et al. 2003. Molecular characterization of binding of calcium and carbohydrates by an early activation antigen of lymphocytes CD69. *Biochemistry* 42:9295–306

118. Marzio R, Jirillo E, Ransijn A, Mauel J, Corradin SB. 1997. Expression and function of the early activation antigen CD69 in murine macrophages. *J. Leukoc. Biol.* 62:349–55

119. Pisegna S, Zingoni A, Pirozzi G, Cinque B, Cifone MG, et al. 2002. Src-dependent Syk activation controls CD69-mediated signaling and function on human NK cells. *J. Immunol.* 169:68–74

120. Lauzurica P, Sancho D, Torres M, Albella B, Marazuela M, et al. 2000. Phenotypic and functional characteristics of hematopoietic cell lineages in CD69-deficient mice. *Blood* 95:2312–20

121. Esplugues E, Sancho D, Vega-Ramos J, Martinez C, Syrbe U, et al. 2003. Enhanced antitumor immunity in mice deficient in CD69. *J. Exp. Med.* 197:1093–106

122. Sancho D, Gomez M, Viedma F, Esplugues E, Gordon-Alonso M, et al. 2003. CD69 downregulates autoimmune reactivity through active transforming growth factor-β production in collagen-induced arthritis. *J. Clin. Invest.* 112:872–82

123. Plougastel B, Dubbelde C, Yokoyama WM. 2001. Cloning of Clr, a new family of lectin-like genes localized between mouse Nkrp1a and Cd69. *Immunogenetics* 53:209–14

124. Carlyle JR, Jamieson AM, Gasser S, Clingan CS, Arase H, Raulet DH. 2004. Missing self-recognition of Ocil/Clr-b by inhibitory NKR-P1 natural killer cell receptors. *Proc. Natl. Acad. Sci. USA* 101:3527–32

125. Iizuka K, Naidenko OV, Plougastel BF, Fremont DH, Yokoyama WM. 2003. Genetically linked C-type lectin-related

ligands for the NKRP1 family of natural killer cell receptors. *Nat. Immunol.* 4:801–7

126. Zhou H, Kartsogiannis V, Quinn JM, Ly C, Gange C, Elliott J, et al. 2002. Osteoclast inhibitory lectin, a family of new osteoclast inhibitors. *J. Biol. Chem.* 277:48808–15

127. Gange CT, Quinn JM, Zhou H, Kartsogiannis V, Gillespie MT, Ng KW. 2004. Characterization of sugar binding by osteoclast inhibitory lectin. *J. Biol. Chem.* 279:29043–49

128. Kanazawa N, Tashiro K, Inaba K, Miyachi Y. 2003. Dendritic cell immunoactivating receptor, a novel C-type lectin immunoreceptor, acts as an activating receptor through association with Fc receptor γ chain. *J. Biol. Chem.* 278:32645–52

129. Bates EE, Fournier N, Garcia E, Valladeau J, Durand I, et al. 1999. APCs express DCIR, a novel C-type lectin surface receptor containing an immunoreceptor tyrosine-based inhibitory motif. *J. Immunol.* 163:1973–83

130. Balch SG, McKnight AJ, Seldin MF, Gordon S. 1998. Cloning of a novel C-type lectin expressed by murine macrophages. *J. Biol. Chem.* 273:18656–64

131. Mizuochi S, Akimoto Y, Imai Y, Hirano H, Irimura T. 1997. Unique tissue distribution of a mouse macrophage C-type lectin. *Glycobiology* 7:137–46

132. Tsuiji M, Fujimori M, Ohashi Y, Higashi N, Onami TM, et al. 2002. Molecular cloning and characterization of a novel mouse macrophage C-type lectin, mMGL2, which has a distinct carbohydrate specificity from mMGL1. *J. Biol. Chem.* 277:28892–901

133. Matsumoto M, Tanaka T, Kaisho T, Sanjo H, Copeland NG, et al. 1999. A novel LPS-inducible C-type lectin is a transcriptional target of NF-IL6 in macrophages. *J. Immunol.* 163:5039–48

134. Geijtenbeek TB, Kwon DS, Torensma R, van Vliet SJ, van Duijnhoven GC, et al. 2000. DC-SIGN, a dendritic cell-specific HIV-1-binding protein that enhances trans-infection of T cells. *Cell* 100:587–97

135. Geijtenbeek TB, Torensma R, van Vliet SJ, van Duijnhoven GC, Adema GJ, et al. 2000. Identification of DC-SIGN, a novel dendritic cell-specific ICAM-3 receptor that supports primary immune responses. *Cell* 100:575–85

136. Geijtenbeek TB, Groot PC, Nolte MA, van Vliet SJ, Gangaram-Panday ST, et al. 2002. Marginal zone macrophages express a murine homologue of DC-SIGN that captures blood-borne antigens in vivo. *Blood* 100:2908–16

137. Kang YS, Yamazaki S, Iyoda T, Pack M, Bruening SA, et al. 2003. SIGN-R1, a novel C-type lectin expressed by marginal zone macrophages in spleen, mediates uptake of the polysaccharide dextran. *Int. Immunol.* 15:177–86

138. Geijtenbeek TB, Krooshoop DJ, Bleijs DA, van Vliet SJ, van Duijnhoven GC, et al. 2000. DC-SIGN-ICAM-2 interaction mediates dendritic cell trafficking. *Nat. Immunol.* 1:353–57

139. Park CG, Takahara K, Umemoto E, Yashima Y, Matsubara K, et al. 2001. Five mouse homologues of the human dendritic cell C-type lectin, DC-SIGN. *Int. Immunol.* 13:1283–90

140. Kang YS, Kim JY, Bruening SA, Pack M, Charalambous A, et al. 2004. The C-type lectin SIGN-R1 mediates uptake of the capsular polysaccharide of Streptococcus pneumoniae in the marginal zone of mouse spleen. *Proc. Natl. Acad. Sci. USA* 101:215–20

141. Fernandes MJ, Finnegan AA, Siracusa LD, Brenner C, Iscove NN, Calabretta B. 1999. Characterization of a novel receptor that maps near the natural killer gene complex: demonstration of carbohydrate binding and expression in hematopoietic cells. *Cancer Res.* 59:2709–17

142. Ariizumi K, Shen GL, Shikano S, Ritter R 3rd, Zukas P, et al. 2000. Cloning of a second dendritic cell-associated C-type lectin

(dectin-2) and its alternatively spliced isoforms. *J. Biol. Chem.* 275:11957–63

143. Aragane Y, Maeda A, Schwarz A, Tezuka T, Ariizumi K, Schwarz T. 2003. Involvement of dectin-2 in ultraviolet radiation-induced tolerance. *J. Immunol.* 171:3801–7

144. Pontow SE, Kery V, Stahl PD. 1992. Mannose receptor. *Int. Rev. Cytol.* 137B:221–44

145. East L, Isacke CM. 2002. The mannose receptor family. *Biochim. Biophys. Acta* 1572:364–86

146. Lee SJ, Evers S, Roeder D, Parlow AF, Risteli J, et al. 2002. Mannose receptor-mediated regulation of serum glycoprotein homeostasis. *Science* 295:1898–901

147. Taylor ME, Drickamer K. 1993. Structural requirements for high affinity binding of complex ligands by the macrophage mannose receptor. *J. Biol. Chem.* 268:399–404

148. Martinez-Pomares L, Linehan SA, Taylor PR, Gordon S. 2001. Binding properties of the mannose receptor. *Immunobiology* 204:527–35

149. Roseman DS, Baenziger JU. 2000. Molecular basis of lutropin recognition by the mannose/GalNAc-4-SO4 receptor. *Proc. Natl. Acad. Sci. USA* 97:9949–54

150. Sheikh H, Yarwood H, Ashworth A, Isacke CM. 2000. Endo180, an endocytic recycling glycoprotein related to the macrophage mannose receptor is expressed on fibroblasts, endothelial cells and macrophages and functions as a lectin receptor. *J. Cell Sci.* 113:1021–32

151. Engelholm LH, Nielsen BS, Dano K, Behrendt N. 2001. The urokinase receptor associated protein (uPARAP/endo180): a novel internalization receptor connected to the plasminogen activation system. *Trends Cardiovasc. Med.* 11:7–13

152. East L, McCarthy A, Wienke D, Sturge J, Ashworth A, Isacke CM. 2003. A targeted deletion in the endocytic receptor gene Endo180 results in a defect in collagen uptake. *EMBO Rep.* 4:710–16

Annu. Rev. Immunol. 2005. 23:945–74
doi: 10.1146/annurev.immunol.23.021704.115747
First published online as a Review in Advance on January 7, 2005

REGULATION OF LYMPHOID DEVELOPMENT, DIFFERENTIATION, AND FUNCTION BY THE NOTCH PATHWAY

Ivan Maillard,[1,2] Terry Fang,[2] and Warren S. Pear[2,3,4]

[1]Division of Hematology-Oncology, [2]Abramson Family Cancer Research Institute, [3]Department of Pathology and Laboratory Medicine, [4]Institute for Medicine and Engineering, University of Pennsylvania, Philadelphia, Pennsylvania 19104-6160; email: ivan.maillard@uphs.upenn.edu, tfang@mail.med.upenn.edu, wpear@mail.med.upenn.edu

Key Words Notch, T lymphocytes, B lymphocytes, thymus, hematopoietic stem cells

■ **Abstract** The Notch pathway is gaining increasing recognition as a key regulator of developmental choices, differentiation, and function throughout the hematolymphoid system. Notch controls the generation of hematopoietic stem cells during embryonic development and may affect their subsequent homeostasis. Commitment to the T cell lineage and subsequent stages of early thymopoiesis is critically regulated by Notch. Recent data indicate that Notch can also direct the differentiation and activity of peripheral T and B cells. Thus, the full spectrum of Notch effects is just beginning to be understood. In this review, we discuss this explosion of knowledge as well as current controversies and challenges in the field.

INTRODUCTION: OVERVIEW OF NOTCH SIGNALING

Notch signaling regulates many aspects of cellular differentiation in multicellular organisms (1). Notch was first identified in strains of haploinsufficient flies exhibiting notching at their wing edges (2). Subsequent analyses in *Drosophila* showed that Notch signals regulate cell fates, cell numbers via effects on proliferation and survival, and cell position. These effects depend on dose, timing, and context of the Notch signal. Nearly all aspects of invertebrate Notch signaling are recapitulated in mammals in which this pathway plays multiple roles in normal development and disease.

The diverse functions of Notch are mediated through a conserved signaling pathway in which transmembrane Notch receptors undergo regulated proteolysis and nuclear translocation to activate transcription (Figure 1). The four mammalian Notch receptors contain conserved protein domains (3). The extracellular portion of Notch consists of 29–36 tandem epidermal growth factor (EGF-like)

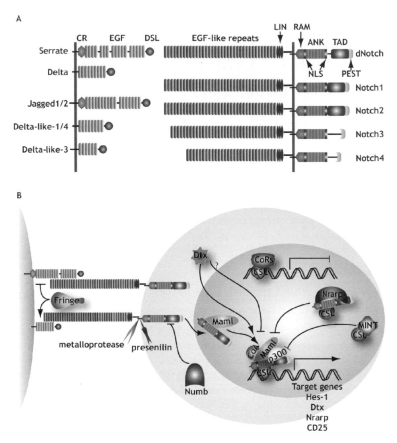

Figure 1   The Notch signaling pathway. (*A*) Structure of Notch receptors and ligands. Notch ligands are transmembrane proteins that contain a large extracellular region with a DSL domain and EGF-like repeats. Mice have five DSL family members. Jagged1 and 2 are Serrate homologs, while Delta-like-1, -3, and -4 are homologous to Delta. Notch is a heterodimeric transmembrane receptor. The extracellular domain contains EGF-like repeats and LIN/Notch repeats. The intracellular domain contains a RAM domain, nuclear localization sequences, seven ankyrin repeats, a transactivation domain (TAD), and a PEST sequence. Mice have four Notch receptors that differ mainly in the number of EGF-like repeats and C-terminal sequences located between the ankyrin repeats and PEST sequences. (*B*) Notch signaling. Upon ligand binding, two sequential cleavages occur. A metalloprotease cleaves at an extracellular site and subsequently a γ-secretase complex cleaves within the transmembrane region. This liberates ICN, allowing its translocation to the nucleus, where it binds the transcription factor CSL/RBP-J. Together with Mastermind, ICN and CSL/RBP-J form a large multiprotein complex and recruit coactivators such as p300, converting CSL/RBP-J from a transcriptional repressor to a transcriptional activator. Notch is regulated by Deltex (Dtx), Numb, MINT, Notch-related ankyrin repeat protein (Nrarp), Fringe, and others.

repeats, which bind DSL ligands (Delta-Serrate-Lag2), and three LIN12/Notch repeats, which prevent ligand-independent signaling. The intracellular domain of Notch (ICN, intracellular Notch) contains domains that mediate signal transduction. These domains include the RAM domain and ankyrin repeats, which interact with downstream effector proteins, nuclear localization sequences, and a C-terminal PEST domain regulating protein stability.[1]

During transit to the membrane, Notch receptors undergo cleavage by a furin-like protease at a site (S1) just external to the transmembrane subunit (4) (Figure 1). This creates a heterodimeric receptor with noncovalently associated extracellular and transmembrane subunits. Ligand binding initiates two cleavage events that release ICN from the membrane. The first cleavage is metalloprotease-dependent and occurs extracellularly close to the transmembrane domain (S2), creating a short-lived membrane-bound form of the Notch transmembrane subunit. The second cleavage occurs within the transmembrane domain (S3) and is mediated by a multiprotein complex with γ-secretase activity containing presenilin, nicastrin, APH-1, and PEN-2 proteins (5). γ-secretase inhibitors and loss of presenilin or nicastrin function prevent Notch signaling (6).

Following cleavage, ICN translocates to the nucleus, where it binds the helix-loop-helix transcription factor CSL/RBP-J (for CBF1/RBP-Jk in mammals, Suppressor of Hairless in *Drosophila*, Lag-1 in *C. elegans*) through its RAM and ankyrin repeat domains. ICN also recruits Mastermind-like proteins (MAMLs) through ankyrin repeat interactions (3, 7). The three mammalian MAMLs recruit transcriptional coactivators, such as p300 (8, 9), creating a high molecular weight complex capable of transcriptional activation (8–10). Inhibiting the ability of MAMLs to recruit coactivators creates a complex that cannot activate transcription in vitro and in vivo (11, 12). Genetic and biochemical data show that, in the absence of ICN, CSL/RBP-J binds corepressors and inhibits transcription, whereas interaction with ICN displaces corepressors and recruits coactivators, leading to transcriptional activation. Surprisingly, analysis of RBP-J knockout mice has not yet revealed phenotypes reflecting loss of CSL/RBP-J repression (13–15). Thus, the precise role of CSL/RBP-J mediated repression awaits further studies.

To date, few targets of Notch signaling have been identified. A frequent target in *Drosophila* and mammals is the family of bHLH-type transcriptional repressors, known as Hairy/Enhancer of Split (HES) (16). Notch signaling activates HES transcription, which leads to repression of HES target genes. Many other tissue-specific targets probably exist. How specificity is achieved within a signaling pathway that appears to be stereotyped, yet is able to deliver widely divergent signals, is poorly understood.

The Notch activation complex is short-lived, as nuclear ICN is targeted for destruction through its C-terminal PEST domain, probably by members of the SEL-10 family (17). Thus, it is difficult to detect nuclear Notch, and indirect methods are required to determine the presence of active Notch signaling. These include evidence of Notch receptor cleavage and expression of direct transcriptional targets.

---

[1]See Appendix for a full list of abbreviations used.

The latter is not always reliable, as expression of some Notch targets may occur in a CSL-dependent, yet Notch-independent fashion (18). An additional level of complexity is that Notch signaling may occur in a CSL/RBP-J-independent fashion (19). The physiological role of this type of signaling is unknown.

Flies have a single Notch receptor and two ligands, Serrate and Delta, whereas mammals possess two Serrate-like ligands (Jagged 1 and 2) and three Delta-like ligands (Dll-1, -3, and -4) (Figure 1). These ligands are transmembrane proteins whose extracellular domain contains EGF-like repeats and an N-terminal DSL domain. The intracellular domains of the ligands are poorly conserved but have important functions because their deletion leads to loss-of-function phenotypes. Although there are multiple receptors and ligands, the determinants of specificity are poorly understood.

Notch signaling is modulated by extracellular, cytoplasmic, and nuclear proteins. One type of extracellular regulator, Fringe, may influence ligand specificity by modifying the Notch extracellular domain so that Delta, but not Jagged/Serrate, can initiate signaling (20). Cytoplasmic Notch regulators include Numb and Deltex. Numb is thought to act upstream of Notch and suppress its activity, perhaps by preventing nuclear translocation of Notch (21). Deltex is another primarily cytoplasmic protein that, unlike Numb, is a positive modifier of Notch activity in *Drosophila* (22). In contrast, recent studies suggest that, in some circumstances, Deltex can inhibit Notch signaling (23). Nuclear regulators of Notch include proteins such as SEL-10, that regulate its turnover, and unidentified kinases marking Notch for degradation (24). Cdk8 was recently suggested to perform the latter function (24a).

Notch signaling can regulate a variety of events, including cell fate decisions, apoptosis, proliferation, and border formation. Relevant to hematopoiesis is Notch's ability to regulate lineage specification at developmental branch points. For example, during peripheral neurogenesis in flies, an equipotent precursor gives rise to alternative cell fates, depending on whether it expresses Notch (capable of Notch signaling) or its ligand (incapable of Notch signaling). In other circumstances, Notch signaling maintains cells in undifferentiated states. This was demonstrated in hematopoietic progenitors in which Notch preserved a pluripotential state while allowing *ex vivo* expansion (25). In other contexts, such as keratinocyte differentiation, Notch signals promote differentiation (26). These examples illustrate that, despite a seemingly stereotyped signaling pathway, the outcome of Notch signaling is diverse and is likely to depend on timing, signal strength, and developmental context.

NOTCH IN HEMATOPOIETIC AND LYMPHOID DEVELOPMENT

Notch and Hematopoietic Stem Cells

The Notch pathway is linked to early hematopoiesis during embryonic development and to the control of hematopoietic stem cell (HSC) self-renewal. Notch1 plays a critical role in the generation of the earliest embryonic HSCs required for definitive hematopoiesis (27) (Table 1). Hirai's group (27) found a marked impairment in the ability of Notch1$^{-/-}$ embryos to generate hematopoietic colonies from structures including the aorta-gonad-mesonephros region, an important site of early hematopoietic activity where HSCs likely arise from hemangioblast precursors. Reconstitution of conditioned newborn recipients was defective, strongly suggesting a defect in HSC numbers or function. Importantly, Notch1 seemed critical during a narrow time window, after which the HSC pool could be maintained without Notch. The molecular mechanisms by which Notch controls the generation of embryonic HSCs is unknown, but the effect is cell autonomous (28). Interactions with other key factors in this process, such as LMO2, GATA-2, AML1, and SCL/Tal-1, need to be explored.

Ligand-mediated Notch stimulation, or expression of constitutively active forms of Notch, can promote self-renewal of adult HSCs (25, 29, 30). Recent data suggest that osteoblasts, a critical cell type in HSC niches, upregulate Jagged1 when activated by parathyroid hormone (PTH) or PTH-related protein, which may activate the Notch pathway in resident HSCs (31). However, it is unclear if this translates into a physiological role for Notch in the maintenance of HSCs. To date, no genetic models of Notch inactivation have shown clearcut evidence for such a role. In particular, bone marrow (BM) from conditional Notch1 or CSL/RBP-J knockout mice can compete with wild-type BM in trilineage hematopoiesis of mixed BM chimeras, which is strong evidence against a major HSC deficiency in the absence of Notch1 or CSL/RBP-J (13, 32). More definitive answers may come from careful studies of HSC function in genetic models of Notch inactivation, including systems in which CSL/RBP-J-independent activities can be blocked. Because HSC self-renewal is controlled through multiple pathways, it is critical to understand the relative importance and interactions of Notch and other factors, such as Wnt, HoxB4, and Sonic Hedgehog (33–35).

Notch and T Cell Development

T LINEAGE COMMITMENT   The best-established function of Notch during lymphoid development is its role in T lineage commitment (Figure 2). As first shown by Radtke's group, Notch1's loss of function results in a marked decrease in the size of the thymus that lacks T cells and contains an excess of B cells (13, 32). These B cells resemble BM B cells and develop intrathymically (36). Conversely, expression of constitutively active Notch1 in HSCs results in extrathymic T cell development and suppression of BM B cell development (37). In culture, expression of Notch ligands of the Delta-like family (Dll-1 or Dll-4) in BM stromal cell lines is sufficient to drive multipotent hematopoietic progenitors, or even embryonic stem cells, to the T cell lineage, while suppressing B cell development (38–41).

Notch1 inactivation causes a complete block in T lineage development, indicating that other Notch family members cannot compensate for the loss of Notch1 in vivo (32). The unique requirement for Notch1 during thymopoiesis is not well

TABLE 1   Genetic models of Notch signaling

A. Knockouts

Gene	Non-hematolymphoid phenotype	Hematolymphoid defect	Reference
notch1$^{-/-}$	Embryonic lethality <E11.5; defects in somitogenesis and vasculogenesis	Defective formation of embryonic HSCs	(27, 105–107)
notch1$^{+/-}$	—	Reduced $\alpha\beta$ and to a lesser extent $\gamma\delta$ T cells in mixed BM chimeras	(71)
notch2$^{-/-}$	Embryonic lethality <E11.5	—	(108)
notch2^{del1} (hypomorphic)	Perinatal lethality; defects in kidney, heart, and eye development	—	(109)
notch2$^{+/-}$	—	Reduced MZ and B1 B cells	(100)
notch3$^{-/-}$	—	—	(110)
notch4$^{-/-}$	—	—	(111)
csl/rbpj$^{-/-}$	Embryonic lethality <E10.5; defects in placenta formation, somitogenesis, and neurogenesis; and growth retardation	—	(112)
jagged1$^{-/-}$	Embryonic lethality <E11.5; defects in vasculogenesis	—	(113)
jagged2$^{-/-}$	Perinatal death; cranio-facial and limb defects	Reduced $\gamma\delta$ T cells in perinatal thymus	(73)
dll-1$^{-/-}$	Embryonic lethality E10–E12; defects in somite borders and mesoderm segmentation	—	(114)
dll-3$^{-/-}$	Defects in early somite formation resulting in vertebral and rib deformities	—	(115, 116)
dll-4$^{+/-}$	Embryonic lethality <E11.5; defects in vasculogenesis	—	(116a)
hes1$^{-/-}$	Embryonic lethality E12.5-birth; neural tube defects and premature neurogenesis	Normal T cell development in HES-1$^{-/-}$ FTOCs and decreased efficiency of T cell reconstitution from HES-1$^{-/-}$ FL cells	(64, 65, 117)

(Continued)

TABLE 1   (*Continued*)

Gene	Non-hematolymphoid phenotype	Hematolymphoid defect	Reference
mint$^{-/-}$	Embryonic lethality <E14.5; abnormalities in pancreas and heart	Increase in MZ B cells in RAG2$^{-/-}$ mice reconstituted with MINT$^{-/-}$ FL cells	(118)
lfng$^{-/-}$	Defects in somite boundary formation and reduced viability owing to skeletal deformities of the trunk	—	(119, 120)

B. Conditional knockouts

Gene	Cre	Phenotype	Reference
notch1	Mx	Block in T cell development; development of intrathymic B cells	(32)
notch1	lck	Block in T cell development at DN3-DN4 transition	(72)
notch1	CD4	Normal T cell development	(63)
notch2	Mx	Normal T cell development	(63)
notch2	CD19	No MZB cells	(46)
csl/rbpj	lck	Block in T cell development at DN3-DN4 transition and increased $\gamma\delta$ T cells	(15)
csl/rbpj	CD4	Normal T cell development and defects in peripheral CD4$^+$ T cell proliferation and IL-4/IFN-γ production	(15, 85)
csl/rbpj	Mx	Block in T cell development; development of intrathymic B cells	(13)

(*Continued*)

TABLE 1   (*Continued*)

Gene	Cre	Phenotype	Reference
csl/rbpj	CD19	No MZB cells	(14)
dll-1	Mx	Normal T cell development and no MZB cells	(40)
dll-1	CD19	Normal MZB cell development	(40)
numb$^{-/-}$	β-actin	Embryonic lethality <E11.5; defects in cranial neural tube closure and premature neurogenesis	(121)

C. Transgenic/overexpression systems

Gene	System	Phenotype	Reference
icn1	Retrovirus/BM reconstitution	Block in early B cell development; thymic-independent T cell development in the BM; inhibition of DP to SP transition; development of T cell lymphomas	(37, 83)
icn1	Lck driven transgene	Increased numbers of CD8$^+$ T cells; suppressed CD4$^+$ T cell development; development of T cell lymphomas	(66, 81, 82)
icn3	Lck driven transgene	Failure to downregulate CD25; high incidence of T cell lymphomas; failure to develop induced autoimmune diabetes	(43, 99)
dll-4	Retrovirus/BM reconstitution	Development of T cell lymphomas; block in B cell development	(122, 123)
deltex	Retrovirus/BM reconstitution	Block in T cell development; development of intrathymic B cells	(23, 49)

(*Continued*)

TABLE 1   (*Continued*)

Gene	System	Phenotype	Reference
lnfg	Lck driven transgene	Block in T cell development; development of intrathymic B cells	(48)
dnmaml	Retrovirus/BM reconstitution	Block in T cell and MZB cell development; development of intrathymic B cells	(12)
nrarp	Retrovirus/BM reconstitution	Block in T cell development	(49)
numb	Lck driven transgene	Normal lymphocyte development	(124)

understood. It is not due to an intrinsic inability of Notch2-4 to drive T cell development because ICN2-4 expression leads to extrathymic T cell development (42–44; J.C. Aster and W.S. Pear, unpublished) and because Notch2-4 can rescue T cell development in the absence of Notch1 signals (I. Maillard and W.S. Pear, unpublished). In addition to Notch1, Notch2 is expressed in hematopoietic progenitors (45), and the expression pattern of Notch3 is similar to Notch1 in developing thymocytes (46), although it is possible that rare relevant thymic progenitors express only Notch1. The distinctive functions of Notch family members could be related to the activation of different downstream signals or to a variable binding efficiency with different Notch ligands. However, Delta-like family members seem to be relevant Notch ligands for T lineage commitment, and Notch2 can productively interact with Dll-1 in vivo as demonstrated by the specific requirement for a Dll-1/Notch2 interaction during marginal zone B (MZB) cell development (40, 46).

Inhibitors of the Notch pathway acting through different molecular mechanisms were characterized through their effect on Notch1-dependent T lineage commitment. Constitutive expression of Fringe, Deltex, Nrarp, and a dominant negative Mastermind mutant were shown to inhibit Notch1 signals and T cell development in vivo (12, 23, 48, 49). In the case of Fringe, the interaction occurred extracellularly through a non-cell-autonomous mechanism. Deltex and Nrarp were inhibitory despite being downstream targets of Notch, suggesting that temporal and quantitative expression of these genes must be precisely controlled. For Deltex, the inhibition was Notch1-specific because inhibition of Notch2-mediated MZB cell development was not observed (12). Inhibition of Notch1 through interference with Mastermind was the first confirmation that MAMLs are critical components of the Notch pathway in vivo.

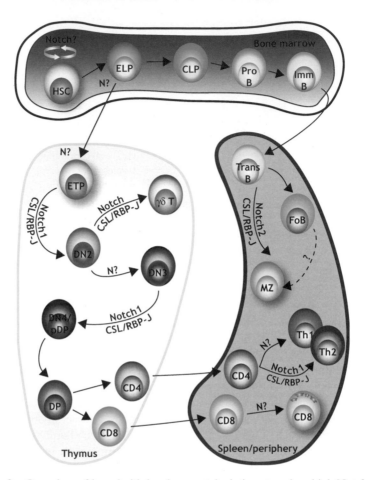

Figure 2   Overview of lymphoid development depicting steps in which Notch plays an important role. Question marks indicate developmental steps where the role of Notch remains to be clarified. Abbreviations: HSC, hematopoietic stem cell; ELP, early lymphoid progenitor; CLP, common lymphoid progenitor; MZB, marginal zone B cell; ETP, early T lineage progenitor; DN, double negative; (p)DP, pre-double positive; Th, T helper.

The role of Notch in T lineage commitment is well established; however, neither the precise identity of the cells receiving the Notch signal nor the precise location where the signal is received is known. Multiple studies suggest that Notch-mediated T lineage commitment occurs in the thymus, where incoming multipotent progenitors encounter Notch ligands and undergo T lineage specification. In particular, Notch overexpression and loss-of-function studies have been widely interpreted to support the existence of a multipotent, or at least bipotent, progenitor with T lineage and B lineage potential that enters the thymus, undergoes

Models for Notch-dependent T cell development

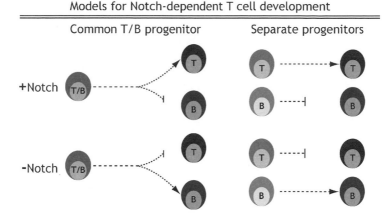

Figure 3   Models for Notch-dependent T lineage commitment.

T lineage development after receiving a Notch signal, and gives rise to intrathymic B cells in the absence of such signal (Figure 3). However, the nature of the earliest intrathymic T cell progenitors remains debated, largely because the small number of progenitors seeding the thymus are difficult to identify directly. Despite these shortcomings, evidence increasingly suggests that common lymphoid progenitors (CLPs), defined as $Lin^-IL7R\alpha^+Sca-1^{lo}c-kit^{lo}$ (50) or $Lin^-IL7R\alpha^+AA4.1^+Sca-1^{lo}$ (51), are not physiological T cell progenitors. CLPs are inefficient at generating T cells, and cells with a CLP phenotype cannot be identified at a detectable frequency in the thymus or blood of normal mice (52, 53). In contrast, potent T lineage potential has been detected in a population referred to as early T lineage progenitors (ETPs) that are found within the DN1 ($Lin^-CD44^+CD25^-$) fraction of thymocyte progenitors. ETPs express high c-kit levels and share many characteristics with multipotent BM progenitors (52). Recently, investigators also identified cells with similar characteristics in the blood, providing a likely reservoir to recruit the earliest thymocyte progenitors (53).

At the population level, ETPs can generate T, NK, B, myeloid, and dendritic cells. It is tempting to speculate that multipotent progenitors in the ETP fraction receive a Notch signal after thymic colonization, which would commit them to the T cell lineage and suppress alternative lineage potentials. However, the existence of such a multipotent progenitor is not established at the single cell level, and the thymus may be colonized in parallel by different progenitors with different lineage potentials, including some that could be committed to the T cell lineage (Figure 3). Recent data by Petrie's group (54) suggest that T and B lineage potentials can be segregated into different subfractions of DN1 prothymocytes. In this study, the authors used combinatorial staining for c-kit and CD24 to resolve five different DN1 populations. When assayed on Dll-1-transduced OP9 cells, two fractions, termed DN1a and DN1b, expressing high c-kit levels and low levels of CD24, showed the robust T lineage expansion potential expected of *bona fide* ETPs. These fractions had the concomitant ability to generate NK cells, but no detectable B potential. In contrast, B lineage potential was detected only in a population referred to as DN1c, which expressed high levels of CD24 and slightly lower levels of c-kit and lacked potent T lineage expansion potential. These data suggest that ETPs lose B lineage potential either very early after thymic entry or in a prethymic location.

Altogether, these data from Petrie's group suggest that the earliest steps of T lineage commitment may occur very early after thymic entry or prethymically, possibly within the BM. Prethymic T cell commitment has been studied in detail during fetal development. Rodewald et al. (55) reported the presence of circulating, T cell–committed progenitors in murine fetal blood. Katsura's group (56) published multiple reports using a clonal assay of lineage development, the multilineage progenitor assay, to characterize the lineage potential of individual fetal progenitors from liver, blood, and thymus. These studies have identified T lineage–restricted progenitors in the fetal liver as early as day 11–12 of gestation. Interestingly, these progenitors coexist with cells that have bipotent T and myeloid potential, or B and myeloid potential, whereas progenitors with T and B but not myeloid potential could not be identified. T lineage–committed progenitors were found to circulate in fetal blood between days 12 and 15 of embryonic development. In addition, many of the earliest thymocyte progenitors had restricted potential, either for T or B lineage. These data strongly suggest that, at least during fetal development, T cell commitment can occur extrathymically, probably within the fetal liver. Whether this process requires a Notch signal, or whether it can happen through alternative pathways, is not known. Expression of Notch ligands occurs in the fetal liver (57), and hematopoietic progenitors express several Notch family members, suggesting a possible Notch-dependent process. Conversely, additional factors, such as GATA-3, could account for prethymic T lineage commitment (58).

Low and/or transient Notch signaling may be sufficient to suppress B lineage potential. Thus, the earliest T committed progenitors may not necessarily bear detectable hallmarks of Notch signaling. Harman and collaborators (59) carefully studied evidence of Notch signaling by RT-PCR in migrant lymphoid progenitors in and around the fetal thymus. Their results indicate that high levels of Notch downstream targets were only detected in cells isolated from within the fetal thymus, and not from the perithymic mesenchyme or from fetal liver progenitors. Although these findings were interpreted as evidence for an exclusive intrathymic location of Notch activation, they do not rule out significant transient and/or low-level Notch activation before thymic entry.

In culture, ligands of the Delta-like family (Dll-1 or Dll-4) are sufficient to drive T lineage development (38–41). In vivo overexpression of Dll-4 results in extrathymic T cell development and tumorigenesis. Dll-1 is widely expressed in the thymic stroma, particularly around the cortico-medullary junction, a site where incoming progenitors enter the thymus (54, 60). This expression pattern is consistent with a critical role for Dll-1 early after thymic entry and during subsequent migration of thymocyte progenitors through the thymic cortex, a process that occurs in tight association with stromal cells (61, 62). However, conditional inactivation of Dll-1 in thymic stromal cells does not impair T cell development (40). Whether Dll-1 and Dll-4 are used in a redundant fashion during thymopoiesis requires analysis of compound Dll-1/Dll-4 knockout mice.

In terms of the relevant Notch-mediated intracellular signals for T lineage commitment, conditional inactivation of CSL/RBP-J results in a developmental block similar to the block observed in Notch1-deficient mice (13, 63), indicating that relevant Notch-dependent signals are mediated by CSL/RBP-J during T cell commitment. Whether CSL/RBP-J-independent pathways play a role during other stages of hematolymphoid development remains to be determined. Comparisons of mice lacking CSL/RBP-J with mice lacking individual Notch receptors, or combinations thereof, will be informative in exploring the existence of such pathways.

Limited information is available on relevant Notch downstream targets activated downstream of Notch1 and CSL/RBP-J during T lineage commitment. In part, this is due to technical difficulties in studying rare cell populations undergoing T lineage commitment. The basic helix-loop-helix transcription factor HES-1, which is upregulated by Notch in many organs, is neither necessary nor sufficient for T lineage commitment. Indeed, HES-1 knockout mice have abnormalities in thymopoiesis that can be overcome by injecting increasing numbers of progenitors (64, 65). Furthermore, expression of HES-1 in the absence of canonical Notch signals in fetal thymic organ cultures does not rescue T cell development (I. Maillard and W.S. Pear, unpublished). Thus, HES-1 may influence the efficiency of T lineage commitment, but it does not replace all the effects of Notch1, perhaps not a surprising finding for a transcriptional repressor. Among other Notch targets, Deltex1 is regulated by Notch during T cell development. Although the effects of Deltex1 at physiological levels are unknown, overexpression of Deltex1 inhibits rather than rescues Notch1 during T lineage commitment (23). Finally, CD25 and pre-Tα were also reported to be Notch targets, but their biological function and their expression pattern are not consistent with a major role during initial steps of T cell commitment (66, 67).

NOTCH AND NK CELL DEVELOPMENT   Emerging data show that continuous delivery of Notch signals is critical during early thymocyte development and that it contributes to suppressing NK potential after B cell potential has been lost. Using their OP9 coculture system, Zuniga-Pflucker and collaborators (62) recently showed that suppression of alternative B or NK lineage potential in multipotent progenitors requires different levels of Notch signaling. In this work, hematopoietic progenitors were cultured on Dll-1-expressing stromal cells in the presence of increasing amounts of γ-secretase inhibitors to titrate the intensity of Notch signaling. At low inhibitor concentrations, an increase in the generation of NK cells was observed, while increased B cell development was not, presumably because residual levels of Notch signaling were sufficient to suppress B but not NK development. Interestingly, the residual NK potential of DN2 thymocytes was more apparent in the absence of Dll-1, suggesting that continuous Notch signaling maintains T cell commitment at this stage. A similar effect of Notch inhibition on NK cell development was reported in rat fetal thymic organ cultures (68).

That NK cell accumulation has not been reported in the thymus of various Notch-deficient murine models suggests several possibilities. First, the thymus may be inhospitable for NK development, perhaps because key cytokines such as IL-15 are not present at sufficient levels. Another possibility is that low levels of Notch signaling are important for the generation, thymic localization, and/or expansion of thymic progenitors with T/NK potential. In the total absence of Notch signals, these progenitors may be affected and intrathymic NK cell development may thus not be observed.

$\alpha\beta$ VERSUS $\gamma\delta$ LINEAGE DECISION   Beyond initial T lineage commitment, developing thymocytes undergo the decision to become either $\alpha\beta$ or $\gamma\delta$ lineage T cells. An instructive model of $\alpha\beta$ versus $\gamma\delta$ development suggests that the nature of the first successful T cell receptor (TCR) gene rearrangement dictates the lineage decision, so that cells first producing a functional β chain together with pre-TCRα (pTα) commit to the $\alpha\beta$ lineage, and cells rearranging both γ and δ genes are instructed to the $\gamma\delta$ lineage. However, $\alpha\beta$ versus $\gamma\delta$ lineage decisions may be determined in part prior to TCR rearrangement. For example, the reduced number of $CD4^+CD8^+$ DP cells that develop in TCRβ-deficient mice seems to be selected by $\gamma\delta$ TCRs (69). Conversely, TCR$\alpha\beta$ transgenic mice have an abnormal population of $CD4^-CD8^-$ TCR$\alpha\beta^+$ cells with functional characteristics of $\gamma\delta$ T cells (70).

A role for Notch1 in the $\alpha\beta$ versus $\gamma\delta$ lineage decision was first suggested by Robey's group (71). These investigators generated mixed BM chimeras with Notch1$^{+/-}$ and Notch1$^{+/+}$ progenitors (71). In the thymus of these mice, a decreased proportion of $\alpha\beta$ lineage cells was derived from the Notch1$^{+/-}$ progenitors in competition with the Notch1$^{+/+}$ cells, whereas the reduction in $\gamma\delta$ T cells was much less dramatic. These data suggest that higher levels of Notch signaling can favor the $\alpha\beta$ lineage. It is unclear from these data if $\gamma\delta$ development is the default cell fate and increasing Notch signaling plays an inductive role toward the $\alpha\beta$ lineage, or if Notch controls a true binary cell fate decision from a common progenitor.

Additional results from Robey's group and others indicate that Notch can probably influence $\gamma\delta$ versus $\alpha\beta$ lineage choice independently of the expression of pre-TCR or TCR$\gamma\delta$. Indeed, the thymus of lck-ICN1 transgenic mice showed an increased number of $CD8^+$ TCR$\gamma\delta^+$ cells but not $CD4^-CD8^-$ TCR$\gamma\delta^+$ cells. Lck-ICN1 transgenic mice crossed to a TCR$\gamma\delta$ transgenic strain had a significant increase in $CD8^+$ TCR$\gamma\delta^+$ cells but a decrease in the percentage of $CD4^-CD8^-$ TCR$\gamma\delta^+$ cells, suggesting that the increased $CD8^+$ TCR$\gamma\delta^+$ cells may actually be $\alpha\beta$ lineage cells selected through the expression of TCR$\gamma\delta$. Moreover, expression of transgenic ICN1 in a TCRβ-deficient background increased the generation of $CD4^+CD8^+$ cells expressing TCR$\gamma\delta$ with functional rearrangements at the TCRδ locus, suggesting that Notch could increase the development of $\alpha\beta$ lineage cells even when pre-TCR components are deficient and $\alpha\beta$ lineage cells are selected through the expression of TCR$\gamma\delta$.

Because these data were primarily generated using overexpression systems, with the exception of mixed BM chimeras, it was important to evaluate the physiological role of Notch in the $\alpha\beta$ versus $\gamma\delta$ lineage decision using loss-of-function systems as well. Honjo's group (15) reported the phenotype of CSL/RBP-J conditional knockout mice crossed to lck-Cre, in which the CSL/RBP-J-dependent activity of all four Notch family members is abolished. These mice had a modest (about twofold) increase in the absolute number of thymic $\gamma\delta$ T cells. BrdU labeling experiments showed both accelerated appearance and disappearance of BrdU$^+$ cells in the knockout mice, suggesting that inactivation of Notch pathway increases both the intrathymic generation of $\gamma\delta$ T cells and their emigration to the periphery. This binary effect also indicates that the effect of the Notch pathway would be underestimated by merely assessing the total numbers of $\gamma\delta$ T cells in the thymus of the knockout mice. In contrast, a normal absolute number of thymic $\gamma\delta$ T cells was observed in Notch1 conditional knockout mice crossed to lck-Cre, suggesting that Notch1 by itself does not play a major role in the regulation of this lineage decision, or that deletion of the Notch1 gene occurs too late to affect the decision process (72). Differences between these results and observations from Honjo's group are most likely explained by the effect of Notch family members other than Notch1, most likely Notch2 and Notch3, although a direct comparison of the two mouse strains is needed. Alternatively, loss of CSL/RBP-J repressor functions could account for the phenotype. Finally, a modest decrease in thymic $\gamma\delta$ T cells was reported in Jagged2 knockout mice (73). Because these mice die perinatally owing to other defects, the analysis was limited to the neonatal thymus. However, this phenotype may point to a specific role of Jagged in the thymus. Thus, despite intense study, the role of Notch in $\gamma\delta$ development remains unsettled.

PRE-TCR CHECKPOINT   The pre-TCR checkpoint or β selection is a highly regulated process that selects for successful expression of a functional TCRβ chain paired to pTα. Selection requires RAG-mediated recombination and intact pre-TCR signaling. A critical role for Notch1 during this checkpoint was first reported by Radtke's group (72) in conditional Notch1 knockout crossed to lck-Cre mice, where inactivation of Notch1 starts at the DN2 stage of development. Decreased but not abolished generation of DP thymocytes was observed, resulting in a smaller thymus containing a higher percentage of DN cells. The phenotype at the DN3-DN4 transition was complex, with accumulation of an abnormal population of CD25^{bright} DN3 cells and an aberrant population of cells that had downregulated CD25, thus appearing as DN4 thymocytes. Fewer of these cells expressed intracellular TCRβ, indicating that many were not normal DN4 cells. The presence of CD25^{bright} cells was reminiscent of mouse strains with defective pre-TCR function, such as pT$\alpha^{-/-}$, TCR$\beta^{-/-}$, or RAG-1$^{-/-}$ mice. Levels of pTα were normal, but decreased VDJ recombination was reported in DN3 cells, suggesting that Notch could influence rearrangement of the TCRβ gene and thus expression of a functional pre-TCR, although this phenomenon could not easily explain the abnormal population of DN4 cells.

A similar thymic phenotype was observed by Honjo and collaborators studying CSL/RBP-J knockout mice crossed to lck-Cre (15), indicating that the phenomenon is Notch1-dependent and CSL/RBP-J-mediated. This study also identified an abnormal DN4 population lacking expression of intracellular TCRβ or TCRγ, but unlike Radtke and collaborators, the Honjo study did not show reduced expression of TCRβ in DN3 cells. Furthermore, although an abnormal CD25[bright] population was identified, pre-TCR components appeared intact as shown by normal intracellular levels of CD3 and TCRβ in DN3 cells and unchanged pTα mRNA in total DN thymocytes. This raises the possibility that the effect of Notch1 at the pre-TCR checkpoint is not due to defective expression of pre-TCR components. This hypothesis was recently tested by Zuniga-Pflucker's group (74) using the OP9 coculture system. In this elegant study, introduction of either a functional TCRβ chain or constitutively active downstream components of the pre-TCR signaling machinery into RAG-deficient DN3 cells was insufficient to restore progression to the DP stage in the absence of Notch signaling. Furthermore, DN3 cells cultured in the absence of Notch signaling died, suggesting that Notch functions as a survival factor at this stage of development. These results suggest a role for Notch during β selection that could be completely independent of pre-TCR signaling. It remains to be shown whether this is true in vivo. There is only an incomplete block in the generation of DP thymocytes in lck-Cre x Notch1[flox/flox] or lck-Cre x CSL/RBP-J[flox/flox] mice, which could indicate a less stringent requirement for Notch in vivo. Alternatively, the partial block may also be explained by the precise timing of Notch or CSL/RBP-J inactivation in vivo, which could allow cells expressing Cre at a later time to survive the pre-TCR checkpoint.

The critical intracellular signals mediated by Notch during β selection are currently unknown, as is the potential interaction of Notch with other factors such as E2A, GATA-3, or cyclin D3, which were shown to regulate β selection (75–77). Furthermore, NF-κB is another potential hub for interaction with the Notch pathway because NF-κB activation plays an important role downstream of pre-TCR signals (78, 79), and Notch upregulates NF-κB activity (43, 80).

NO PHYSIOLOGICAL ROLE FOR NOTCH IN THE CD4 VERSUS CD8 DECISION   The role of Notch in the CD4 versus CD8 lineage decision has been a longstanding controversy. Several gain-of-function approaches showed that constitutive Notch signaling could affect DP thymocytes in a number of ways, including effects on differentiation, survival, and proliferation (66, 81–83). Several studies suggested a promotion of the CD8 fate at the expense of CD4. Nevertheless, interpretation of these results was difficult because the gain-of-function Notch allele also induced a block in differentiation and either leukemia or a preleukemic state. Furthermore, there was never an adequate explanation for the low basal levels of Notch expression and signaling in DP thymocytes. Now, two loss-of-function approaches provide compelling data that Notch does not influence the CD4 versus CD8 decision. Radtke's group (63) reported that conditional Notch1 knockout mice crossed to CD4-Cre transgenic mice did not show any abnormality in the CD4:CD8 ratio, or in the rate of generation of these populations. Honjo's group (15) obtained similar findings in conditional CSL/RBP-J knockout mice crossed to CD4-Cre mice, in which CSL/RBP-J-mediated signals from all four Notch receptors are inhibited. These results rule out the hypothesis that compensatory signaling through Notch2-4 explains the normal CD4/CD8 differentiation seen in the absence of Notch1, and they provide a definitive demonstration that Notch signals, at least when mediated through CSL/RBP-J, are not physiological regulators of the CD4 versus CD8 decision. The molecular mechanisms for the various effects observed in gain-of-function systems remain unclear at this point.

NOTCH IN THE PERIPHERAL IMMUNE SYSTEM

Notch and Peripheral T Cells

Although CD4$^+$ and CD8$^+$ T cells are considered mature upon exit from the thymus, additional signals drive differentiation into effector T cells. TCR-mediated antigen recognition initiates differentiation in collaboration with signals from the microenvironment. Differentiation is linked to the expression of transcription factors that act as master regulators of genetic programs. However, the upstream events leading to the expression of these master regulators are unclear. Emerging data suggest a role for the Notch pathway in these functions.

EXPRESSION OF NOTCH LIGANDS AND RECEPTORS   Key components of the Notch pathway are expressed by relevant cellular partners during peripheral immune responses. Naive CD4$^+$ and CD8$^+$ T cells express Notch1 and Notch2 (84–86). Relative levels of Notch1-4 mRNA increase significantly after antigenic stimulation of naive CD4$^+$ T cells (87), suggesting that all four Notch family members can potentially play a role in peripheral T cells and that interference with only one Notch family member may be insufficient to block the effects of Notch in T cells. Dendritic cells (DCs) express Notch1, Notch2, Jagged1, Jagged2, Dll-1, and Dll-4 (85, 88). Furthermore, recent data by Flavell's group (85) indicate that the expression of Delta-like and Jagged ligands on DCs is dynamically regulated in response to innate stimuli. These data situate Notch ligands and receptors at the interface between the innate immune system and the adaptive T cell response. Here, we discuss recent data supporting a role for Notch in regulating T cell activation, helper T cell differentiation, and tolerance induction (Figure 4).

T CELL ACTIVATION   Several studies have recently linked the Notch pathway with TCR-mediated T cell activation. Adler et al. (87) showed that upon TCR stimulation, expression of all four Notch receptors is upregulated in CD4$^+$ T cells. Furthermore, detection of the cleaved activated form of Notch1 and upregulation of the Notch target HES-1 indicate ongoing Notch signaling in stimulated

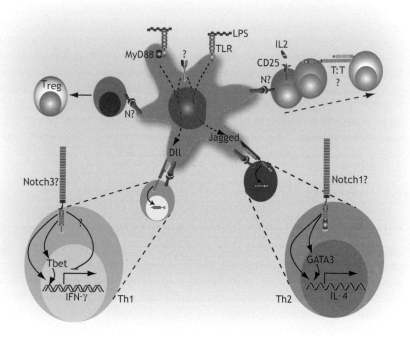

Figure 4 Proposed roles for Notch in peripheral CD4$^+$ T cells. Notch can affect TCR-mediated stimulation. Stimuli that activate different Toll-like receptor (TLR) pathways can upregulate specific Notch ligands on antigen-presenting cells (APCs), which bind to Notch receptors on CD4$^+$ T cells and skew T helper differentiation. A Jagged-Notch1 signal may lead to transcriptional activation of the IL-4 gene and to upregulation of GATA3, promoting Th2 differentiation. Delta-Notch3 signals may regulate IFN-γ production, although positive and negative regulation has been proposed. The generation of regulatory T cells via Notch may occur through multiple ligands and possibly through Notch3. Expression of ligands on T cells suggests the potential for T-T interactions.

T cells (87, 89). Inhibiting Notch signaling with γ-secretase inhibitors results in decreased proliferation and decreased production of IL-2 and IFN-γ (87, 89). This effect is limited to suboptimal TCR stimulation, suggesting that Notch delivers costimulatory signals in these conditions. The opposite phenotype is seen in CD4$^+$ DO11.10 T cells upon overexpression of ICN1, which results in enhanced expression of CD25 and increased proliferation in response to low doses of peptide. These complementary studies suggest that Notch signals can enhance responsiveness to TCR stimulation. The molecular mechanisms of this effect remain to be clarified.

Although these studies suggest a role for Notch in T cell activation, loss-of-function experiments were based mainly on γ-secretase inhibitors, which inhibit the proteolytic processing of a number of molecules besides Notch (e.g., CD44, N-cadherin, Notch ligands). In addition, their use in antigen-presenting cell (APC)–T cell cocultures could lead to non-cell-autonomous effects because APCs express Notch receptors. Thus, the relevance of these findings was unclear, especially because peripheral T cells in conditional Notch1 knockout mice crossed to CD4-Cre failed to show defective T cell proliferation and activation (90). Important confirmatory findings have now come from the study of conditional CSL/RBP-J knockout mice. These studies showed decreased proliferation of CSL/RBP-J knockout peripheral CD4$^+$ T cells after TCR stimulation in the presence of APCs, a finding that parallels in vitro findings with γ-secretase inhibitors and indicates that other Notch family members can compensate for Notch1 deficiency in peripheral T cells (15).

A recent study by Bluestone's group (91) adds complexity to the emerging role of Notch in peripheral T cells. In this study, immobilized ligands were used to stimulate Notch receptors on naive CD4$^+$ T cells. When CD4$^+$ cells were stimulated with anti-CD3 in the presence of a B cell line engineered to express Dll-1, a profound proliferation block was observed. This could be recapitulated using a Jagged-myc fusion protein and an agonistic anti-Notch1 antibody. The proliferation block was reversed by γ-secretase inhibitors, suggesting Notch specificity. Interestingly, γ-secretase inhibitors alone resulted in increased proliferation of purified T cells in response to anti-CD3/CD28 stimulation, whereas a modest decrease in proliferation was seen in cultures containing APCs.

These data apparently contradict results from other investigators (15, 87, 89). Although the reasons for this discrepancy remain to be clarified, activation of the Notch pathway may result in different effects on naive versus activated T cells, and may depend on cellular context, as evidenced by several groups reporting different results when experiments are performed in the presence or absence of APCs (15, 91). In part, this may be due to variable levels and/or to the nature of Notch ligands encountered by T cells during T-T or T-APC interactions. Another concern is that the level of Notch activation achieved by ligand stimulation may be markedly above the levels reached in physiological settings. In this regard, Maekawa and collaborators (92) have used a Dll-1-Fc fusion protein to stimulate naive CD4$^+$ T cells. A broad concentration range of Dll-1-Fc did not have any effect on T cell proliferation, whereas very high amounts inhibited T cell proliferation, which is similar to the findings reported by Eagar et al. (91). Therefore, assessing the physiological relevance of the effects described by Bluestone's group will require confirmation in genetic models of Notch inactivation.

CYTOKINE GENE REGULATION AND HELPER T CELL DIFFERENTIATION   Differentiation of CD4$^+$ T cells into Th1 or Th2 cells is influenced by many factors, including cytokines such as IL-12 for Th1 and IL-4 for Th2 development. However, other signals from the lymphoid microenvironment, in particular from APCs, are likely involved, and key transcriptional regulators such as T-bet and GATA3 expressed downstream of signals transmitted from APCs to naive T cells have important roles in controlling activation or silencing of Th1- or Th2-specific genes (93).

Data have now accumulated supporting a role for the Notch pathway as a regulator of the crosstalk between APCs and T cells during CD4$^+$ T cell differentiation. In an important recent study, Flavell's group (85) demonstrated that APCs upregulate Jagged or Delta-like ligands in response to different innate stimuli. Stimuli that normally induce a Th1 response, such as LPS, resulted in upregulation of both Jagged and Delta-like ligands, whereas type 2 stimuli such as cholera toxin and PGE$_2$ induced Jagged2 but not Dll-4. Interestingly, LPS-induced upregulation of Dll-4, but not of Jagged1, was dependent on Myd88, a TLR adaptor molecule that is critical for a Th1 response. Antigenic stimulation of naive CD4$^+$ T cells in the context of APCs engineered to express Dll-1 led to the secretion of Th1 cytokines, whereas Jagged1 promoted a Th2 cytokine profile. Importantly, Jagged1-expressing APCs were able to induce IL-4 production even in STAT6-deficient CD4$^+$ T cells. Similarly IL-4 production and GATA3 expression in STAT6$^{-/-}$ CD4$^+$ cells were rescued by retroviral transduction of ICN1. Consistent with an important physiological role for this process, CSL/RBP-J-deficient CD4$^+$ T cells had impaired IL-4 production, and this impairment could not be rescued with exogenous IL-4. Reporter assays provided evidence that Notch may be acting directly on the IL-4 locus, as mutation of a conserved CSL/RBP-J binding site in a 3′ enhancer element resulted in loss of Notch responsiveness. Altogether, these data situate the Jagged/Notch axis in the position to trigger direct and early upregulation of IL-4 and possibly GATA3 in response to Th2-promoting innate stimuli. In contrast, the Delta-like/Notch axis was capable of upregulating IFN-γ and T-bet, although the mechanisms of this effect have not been characterized.

Different Notch receptors may also exert distinct effects on CD4$^+$ T cells, as suggested by a study from Yasutomo's group (92) reporting a specific role for Notch3 in peripheral T cells. In this study, stimulation of CD4$^+$ T cells with an agonistic Dll-1-Fc fusion protein resulted in increased amounts of IFN-γ even when the cells were polarized in Th2 conditions. Increased levels of T-bet mRNA were observed, although it is not clear if this was a direct consequence of Dll-1-mediated stimulation. Interestingly, the effect of Dll-1 was abrogated in cells carrying a Notch3 antisense construct, whereas overexpression of ICN3 but not ICN1 was able to parallel the induction of IFN-γ by Dll-1. Finally, Notch pathway stimulation through Dll-1-Fc in vivo conferred protection against *Leishmania major* infection in normally susceptible BALB/c mice, in which resistance to *L. major* is largely governed by the host's ability to produce IFN-γ in the setting of a potent Th1 response. Collectively, these data suggest that a specific Dll-1-Notch3 interaction can promote IFN-γ in CD4$^+$ T cells, and that this effect may be functionally relevant. To date, the molecular basis for the specific effects of distinct Notch ligands and receptors is unknown. This could be related to differential ligand-receptor binding or differential activation of signal transduction pathways. The possibility of CSL/RBP-J-independent effects must also be considered.

The ultimate effect of the Notch pathway on Th1 versus Th2 differentiation may depend on the balance between Jagged and Delta-like ligands, as well as on the balance between different Notch family members. Thus, the overall effect is difficult to predict, and it would not be surprising if different experimental models lead to different conclusions. In contrast to the key role of Notch1 during T cell development, redundancy appears to occur in peripheral CD4$^+$ T cells. Indeed, normal in vitro Th1 and Th2 polarization was reported in conditional Notch1 knockout mice, in contrast to CSL/RBP-J knockout mice in which the activity of all Notch receptors is affected (15, 94). Detailed analysis of CSL/RBP-J knockout mice so far has shown reduced production of IL-4 and increased production of IFN-γ, although the relative importance of these findings varied in different experimental settings (15, 85). When the distribution of immunoglobulin isotypes in CD4-Cre $\times$ CSL/RBP-J$^{f/f}$ mice was analyzed as a reflection of global T helper cell function, basal levels of the IL-4-dependent isotypes IgG1 and IgE were reduced, while IFN-γ-dependent IgG2a, IgG2b and IgG3 isotypes were essentially unchanged (15). In contrast, antigen-specific Ig isotypes after ovalbumin immunization showed more modest decreases in IgG1/IgE and significant increases in IgG2a/2b. These data confirm that the Notch pathway is physiologically important to promoting IL-4 and limiting IFN-γ production, but they also indicate that the Notch pathway's effects differ in the setting of spontaneous class switching or of a T-dependent humoral immune response. Notably, no loss-of-function counterpart to the Notch-mediated increase in IFN-γ production described by Yasutomo's group (92) has been reported so far in CSL/RBP-J knockout mice. Although this may be related to experimental conditions, it is also possible that CSL/RBP-J deficiency results in the loss of Notch-independent repressive functions of CSL/RBP-J and thus of Notch-independent phenotypes. On the other hand, Notch-dependent but CSL/RBP-J-independent mechanisms are possible.

T CELL TOLERANCE   Several reports suggest a role for Notch signaling in tolerance through increased generation of regulatory T cells (Tregs). Human CD4$^+$CD25$^+$ T cells express Notch4 mRNA, and a high proportion of mouse CD4$^+$CD25$^+$ T cells express Notch3 mRNA (43, 95). Several groups have shown that overexpression of Notch ligands on APCs could induce the development of Tregs. Mice immunized with peptide-pulsed DCs overexpressing Jagged1 developed tolerance against subsequent peptide rechallenge, and CD4$^+$ T cells from these mice transferred tolerance to third-party recipients (86). Similarly, human Epstein-Barr virus–transformed lymphoblastoid cell lines transduced with Jagged1 inhibited proliferation and cytotoxicity of EBV-reactive allogeneic or autologous T cells (96, 97). Suppression correlated with production of the anti-inflammatory cytokines IL-10 and TGFβ. In another system, mice immunized with allogeneic L cells transduced with Dll-1 became tolerant against rechallenge with lymph node cells expressing the allogeneic MHC while maintaining the ability to respond to an alternative alloantigen (98).

Screpanti's group (99) examined lck-Notch3 transgenic mice for Tregs. These investigators (43) had previously reported a progressive accumulation of thymocytes that fail to downregulate CD25 and a high incidence of T cell lymphomas in these mice. They observed a high percentage of CD4$^+$CD25$^+$ T cells that suppressed proliferation of CD4$^+$CD25$^-$ T cells in vitro. The mice failed to develop autoimmunity in a streptozotocin model of diabetes. Although the investigators used young mice to avoid interference with emerging tumors, they did not analyze T cell clonality. Moreover, regulatory cells may arise in these mice because of tumor-related immunosuppression. Whether expression of Notch3 contributes to development of Tregs requires further studies. Currently, there is no report about Notch3 or other Notch knockout mice with any deficiencies in Tregs or autoimmunity.

Notch and Peripheral B Cells

Although Notch1 is the key Notch receptor during T cell development, evolution seems to have selected Notch2 to fulfill functions in B cells. Notch2 is the predominant Notch family member expressed in developing and mature B cells (46). Several recent reports indicate that Notch2 is critical for the generation of MZB cells, and that this is mediated through a specific interaction with Dll-1 in a CSL/RBP-J-dependent manner (12, 14, 40, 46, 100). MZB cells are noncirculating peripheral B cells that reside in the marginal zone of the spleen and function in early T-independent antibody responses to blood-derived antigens, as reviewed elsewhere (101). The precise ontogeny of MZB cells remains controversial. One hypothesis is that MZB cells are derived from transitional B cell subsets, a pool of immature splenic B cells that has recently emigrated from the BM. However, it is also possible that MZB cells are recruited from other mature B cell subsets because the size of the MZB cell pool is tightly controlled and adjusted in the periphery (102, 103). When Notch2-mediated signaling is disrupted, MZB cells are drastically decreased in parallel to another population of splenic B cells with similar immunophenotypic characteristics (sIgM^{hi} CD21^{hi}), but expressing higher levels of CD23 (12, 46, 100). This population probably represents MZB precursors that also depend on Notch signaling. Understanding how Notch signaling is regulated in these cells and how they relate to other B cell subsets is important to understanding the generation of MZB cells.

The essential role of Dll-1 as a ligand for Notch2 during MZB cell development provides insights into the cellular partners interacting during this process (40). Clearly, the ligand must be expressed by a heterologous cell type because a CD19-Cre transgene did not inhibit MZB cell development when introduced into the Dll-1$^{flox/flox}$ background (40). Because splenic DCs are known to express Dll-1, it is tempting to speculate that they are the relevant Dll-1-expressing cell type. Because these cells are located throughout the spleen, the question arises as to where relevant Dll-1-Notch2 interactions occur. This question was indirectly addressed by Cyster's group (104) when they studied the function of sphingosine-1-phosphate (S1P) receptors, a class of molecules controlling responsiveness to blood-derived lysophospholipids. They found that MZB cells express high levels of these receptors and that disruption of S1P1 prevents localization of splenic B cells to the MZ, while preserving their differentiation. These findings dissociate the generation of MZB cells from their MZ localization and suggest that the

Dll-1-Notch2 interaction driving MZB cell development may not occur in the MZ itself, but elsewhere in the spleen. Alternatively, it is possible that MZB precursors still must pass through the MZ even if they are not retained there.

Beyond its now well-established role in MZB development, Notch signaling may also contribute to the generation of B1 B cells, although data so far are controversial (14, 46, 100). By analogy to the emerging role of Notch in peripheral T cells, the potential role of Notch in the differentiation and function of mature B cells will be interesting to explore.

CONCLUDING REMARKS

The Notch pathway is increasingly recognized as a key regulator of developmental choices, differentiation, and function throughout the hematolymphoid system. Recent knowledge builds on a longstanding interest in the physiological role of Notch in multicellular organisms, both in normal and pathological conditions. Better biochemical understanding of the Notch pathway as well as expanding genetic models of Notch inactivation have now started to generate exciting new developments.

We should remember that when constitutively active Notch molecules were first expressed in murine HSCs, investigators were surprised that a single molecule could drive T cell development outside of the thymus (37). Together with loss-of-function studies, this finding identified the central role of Notch proteins during T lineage commitment (13, 32). With the development of BM stromal cell lines that express Notch ligands and that can support T cell development, Zuniga-Pflucker and collaborators (39) have moved one step further by showing that the process can occur entirely in vitro. This finding provides a powerful tool for evaluating the complex regulation of T lineage development. However, it is important to validate new findings using in vivo models of T lineage development. This should be facilitated by using different genetic models of Notch pathway inactivation, either through disruption of single Notch family members, inactivation of the transcription factor CSL/RBP-J, or interference with the assembly of the Notch transcriptional activation complex. The diverse roles played by Notch suggest potential therapeutic applications in a wide variety of areas related to the immune system. The recent explosion in knowledge will set the stage for utilizing this information for therapeutic benefit.

APPENDIX

Abbreviations used: APC, antigen-presenting cell; BM, bone marrow; CLP, common lymphoid progenitor; CSL, CBF1/RBP-Jk in mammals, Suppressor of Hairless in *Drosophila*, Lag-1 in *C. elegans*; DC, dendritic cell; Dll, Delta-like; DN, double negative; DP, double positive; DSL, Delta-Serrate-Lag2; EBV, Epstein-Barr virus; EGF, epidermal growth factor; ETP, early T lineage progenitor; HES, Hairy/Enhancer of Split; HSC, hematopoietic stem cell; ICN, intracellular Notch; MAML, Mastermind-like; MZB cell, marginal zone B cell; NK, natural killer; Nrarp, Notch-related ankyrin repeat protein; PEST, proline/glutamic acid/serine/

threonine; PTH, parathyroid hormone; pTα, pre-TCRα; RAM, RBP-J-association motif; S1P, sphingosine-1-phosphate; TAD, transactivation domain; TCR, T cell receptor; TLR, Toll-like receptor; Treg, regulatory T cell.

ACKNOWLEDGMENTS

We thank Avinash Bhandoola, Benjamin Schwarz, and members of the Pear lab for helpful discussions and critical review of the manuscript. We apologize to authors whose work could not be cited because of space limitations.

**The *Annual Review of Immunology* is online at
http://immunol.annualreviews.org**

LITERATURE CITED

1. Lai EC. 2004. Notch signaling: control of cell communication and cell fate. *Development* 131:965–73

2. Morgan TH. 1917. The theory of the gene. *Am. Nat.* 51:513–44

3. Lubman OY, Korolev SV, Kopan R. 2004. Anchoring Notch genetics and biochemistry; structural analysis of the ankyrin domain sheds light on existing data. *Mol. Cell* 13:619–26

4. Selkoe D, Kopan R. 2003. Notch and Presenilin: regulated intramembrane proteolysis links development and degeneration. *Annu. Rev. Neurosci.* 26:565–97

5. Fortini ME. 2002. γ-secretase-mediated proteolysis in cell-surface-receptor signalling. *Nat. Rev. Mol. Cell Biol.* 3:673–84

6. Wolfe MS. 2001. γ-secretase inhibitors as molecular probes of presenilin function. *J. Mol. Neurosci.* 17:199–204

7. Nam Y, Weng AP, Aster JC, Blacklow SC. 2003. Structural requirements for assembly of the CSL · intracellular Notch1 · Mastermind-like 1 transcriptional activation complex. *J. Biol. Chem.* 278:21232–39

8. Fryer CJ, Lamar E, Turbachova I, Kintner C, Jones KA. 2002. Mastermind mediates chromatin-specific transcription and turnover of the Notch enhancer complex. *Genes Dev.* 16:1397–411

9. Wallberg AE, Pedersen K, Lendahl U, Roeder RG. 2002. p300 and PCAF act cooperatively to mediate transcriptional activation from chromatin templates by Notch intracellular domains in vitro. *Mol. Cell. Biol.* 22:7812–19

10. Jeffries S, Robbins DJ, Capobianco AJ. 2002. Characterization of a high-molecular-weight Notch complex in the nucleus of Notch(ic)-transformed RKE cells and in a human T-cell leukemia cell line. *Mol. Cell. Biol.* 22:3927–41

11. Weng AP, Nam Y, Wolfe MS, Pear WS, Griffin JD, et al. 2003. Growth suppression of pre-T acute lymphoblastic leukemia cells by inhibition of Notch signaling. *Mol. Cell. Biol.* 23:655–64

12. Maillard I, Weng AP, Carpenter AC, Rodriguez CG, Sai H, et al. 2004. Mastermind critically regulates Notch-mediated lymphoid cell fate decisions. *Blood* 104:1696–702

13. Han H, Tanigaki K, Yamamoto N, Kuroda K, Yoshimoto M, et al. 2002. Inducible gene knockout of transcription factor recombination signal binding protein-J reveals its essential role in T versus B lineage decision. *Int. Immunol.* 14:637–45

14. Tanigaki K, Han H, Yamamoto N, Tashiro K, Ikegawa M, et al. 2002. Notch-RBP-J signaling is involved in

cell fate determination of marginal zone B cells. *Nat. Immunol.* 3:443–50

15. Tanigaki K, Tsuji M, Yamamoto N, Han H, Tsukada J, et al. 2004. Regulation of $\alpha\beta/\gamma\delta$ T cell lineage commitment and peripheral T cell responses by Notch/RBP-J signaling. *Immunity* 20:611–22

16. Davis RL, Turner DL. 2001. Vertebrate hairy and Enhancer of split related proteins: transcriptional repressors regulating cellular differentiation and embryonic patterning. *Oncogene* 20:8342–57

17. Lai EC. 2002. Protein degradation: four E3s for the Notch pathway. *Curr. Biol.* 12:74–78

18. Barolo S, Walker RG, Polyanovsky AD, Freschi G, Keil T, Posakony JW. 2000. A Notch-independent activity of suppressor of hairless is required for normal mechanoreceptor physiology. *Cell* 103:957–69

19. Martinez Arias A, Zecchini V, Brennan K. 2002. CSL-independent Notch signalling: a checkpoint in cell fate decisions during development? *Curr. Opin. Genet. Dev.* 12:524–33

20. Moloney DJ, Panin VM, Johnston SH, Chen J, Shao L, et al. 2000. Fringe is a glycosyltransferase that modifies Notch. *Nature* 406:369–75

21. Berdnik D, Torok T, Gonzalez-Gaitan M, Knoblich JA. 2002. The endocytic protein α-Adaptin is required for numb-mediated asymmetric cell division in *Drosophila*. *Dev. Cell* 3:221–31

22. Matsuno K, Diederich RJ, Go MJ, Blaumueller CM, Artavanis-Tsakonas S. 1995. Deltex acts as a positive regulator of Notch signaling through interactions with the Notch ankyrin repeats. *Development* 121:2633–44

23. Izon DJ, Aster JC, He Y, Weng A, Karnell FG, et al. 2002. Deltex1 redirects lymphoid progenitors to the B cell lineage by antagonizing Notch1. *Immunity* 16:231–43

24. Wu G, Lyapina S, Das I, Li J, Gurney M,

et al. 2001. SEL-10 is an inhibitor of Notch signaling that targets Notch for ubiquitin-mediated protein degradation. *Mol. Cell. Biol.* 21:7403–15

24a. Fryer C, White B, Jones K. 2004. Mastermind recruits CycC:CDK8 to phosphorylate the Notch ICD and coordinate activation with turnover. *Mol. Cell* 16:509–20

25. Varnum-Finney B, Xu L, Brashem-Stein C, Nourigat C, Flowers D, et al. 2000. Pluripotent, cytokine-dependent, hematopoietic stem cells are immortalized by constitutive Notch1 signaling. *Nat. Med.* 6:1278–81

26. Rangarajan A, Talora C, Okuyama R, Nicolas M, Mammucari C, et al. 2001. Notch signaling is a direct determinant of keratinocyte growth arrest and entry into differentiation. *EMBO J.* 20:3427–36

27. Kumano K, Chiba S, Kunisato A, Sata M, Saito T, et al. 2003. Notch1 but not Notch2 is essential for generating hematopoietic stem cells from endothelial cells. *Immunity* 18:699–711

28. Hadland BK, Huppert SS, Kanungo J, Xue Y, Jiang R, et al. 2004. A requirement for Notch1 distinguishes two phases of definitive hematopoiesis during development. *Blood* 104:3097–105

29. Varnum-Finney B, Brashem-Stein C, Bernstein ID. 2003. Combined effects of Notch signaling and cytokines induce a multiple log increase in precursors with lymphoid and myeloid reconstituting ability. *Blood* 101:1784–89

30. Stier S, Cheng T, Dombkowski D, Carlesso N, Scadden DT. 2002. Notch1 activation increases hematopoietic stem cell self-renewal in vivo and favors lymphoid over myeloid lineage outcome. *Blood* 99:2369–78

31. Calvi LM, Adams GB, Weibrecht KW, Weber JM, Olson DP, et al. 2003. Osteoblastic cells regulate the hematopoietic stem cell niche. *Nature* 425:841–46

32. Radtke F, Wilson A, Stark G, Bauer M, van Meerwijk J, et al. 1999. Deficient T cell fate specification in mice with an induced inactivation of Notch1. *Immunity* 10:547–58

33. Reya T, Duncan AW, Ailles L, Domen J, Scherer D, et al. 2003. A role for Wnt signalling in self-renewal of haematopoietic stem cells. *Nature* 423:409–14

34. Antonchuk J, Sauvageau G, Humphries RK. 2002. HOXB4-induced expansion of adult hematopoietic stem cells ex vivo. *Cell* 109:39–45

35. Bhardwaj G, Murdoch B, Wu D, Baker DP, Williams KP, et al. 2001. Sonic hedgehog induces the proliferation of primitive human hematopoietic cells via BMP regulation. *Nat. Immunol.* 2:172–80

36. Wilson A, MacDonald HR, Radtke F. 2001. Notch 1-deficient common lymphoid precursors adopt a B cell fate in the thymus. *J. Exp. Med.* 194:1003–12

37. Pui JC, Allman D, Xu L, DeRocco S, Karnell FG, et al. 1999. Notch1 expression in early lymphopoiesis influences B versus T lineage determination. *Immunity* 11:299–308

38. Jaleco AC, Neves H, Hooijberg E, Gameiro P, Clode N, et al. 2001. Differential effects of Notch ligands Delta-1 and Jagged-1 in human lymphoid differentiation. *J. Exp. Med.* 194:991–1002

39. Schmitt TM, Zuniga-Pflucker JC. 2002. Induction of T cell development from hematopoietic progenitor cells by Delta-like-1 in vitro. *Immunity* 17:749–56

40. Hozumi K, Negishi N, Suzuki D, Abe N, Sotomaru Y, et al. 2004. Delta-like 1 is necessary for the generation of marginal zone B cells but not T cells in vivo. *Nat. Immunol.* 5:638–44

41. Schmitt TM, de Pooter RF, Gronski MA, Cho SK, Ohashi PS, Zuniga-Pflucker JC. 2004. Induction of T cell development and establishment of T cell competence from embryonic stem cells differentiated in vitro. *Nat. Immunol.* 5:410–17

42. Witt CM, Hurez V, Swindle CS, Hamada Y, Klug CA. 2003. Activated Notch2 potentiates CD8 lineage maturation and promotes the selective development of B1 B cells. *Mol. Cell. Biol.* 23:8637–50

43. Bellavia D, Campese AF, Alesse E, Vacca A, Felli MP, et al. 2000. Constitutive activation of NF-κB and T-cell leukemia/lymphoma in Notch3 transgenic mice. *EMBO J.* 19:3337–48

44. Vercauteren SM, Sutherland HJ. 2004. Constitutively active Notch4 promotes early human hematopoietic progenitor cell maintenance while inhibiting differentiation and causes lymphoid abnormalities in vivo. *Blood* 104:2315–22

45. Varnum-Finney B, Purton LE, Yu M, Brashem-Stein C, Flowers D, et al. 1998. The Notch ligand, Jagged-1, influences the development of primitive hematopoietic precursor cells. *Blood* 91:4084–91

46. Saito T, Chiba S, Ichikawa M, Kunisato A, Asai T, et al. 2003. Notch2 is preferentially expressed in mature B cells and indispensable for marginal zone B lineage development. *Immunity* 18:675–85

47. Deleted in proof

48. Koch U, Lacombe TA, Holland D, Bowman JL, Cohen BL, et al. 2001. Subversion of the T/B lineage decision in the thymus by Lunatic Fringe-mediated inhibition of Notch-1. *Immunity* 15:225–36

49. Yun TJ, Bevan MJ. 2003. Notch-regulated ankyrin-repeat protein inhibits Notch1 signaling: multiple Notch1 signaling pathways involved in T cell development. *J. Immunol.* 170:5834–41

50. Kondo M, Weissman IL, Akashi K. 1997. Identification of clonogenic common lymphoid progenitors in mouse bone marrow. *Cell* 91:661–72

51. Miller JP, Izon D, DeMuth W, Gerstein R, Bhandoola A, Allman D. 2002. The earliest step in B lineage differentiation from common lymphoid progenitors is critically dependent upon interleukin 7. *J. Exp. Med.* 196:705–11

52. Allman D, Sambandam A, Kim S, Miller JP, Pagan A, et al. 2003. Thymopoiesis independent of common lymphoid progenitors. *Nat. Immunol.* 4:168–74

53. Schwarz BA, Bhandoola A. 2004. Circulating hematopoietic progenitors with T lineage potential. *Nat. Immunol.* 5:953–60

54. Porritt HE, Rumfelt LL, Tabrizifard S, Schmitt TM, Zuniga-Pflucker JC, Petrie HT. 2004. Heterogeneity among DN1 prothymocytes reveals multiple progenitors with different capacities to generate T cell and non-T cell lineages. *Immunity* 20:735–45

55. Rodewald HR, Kretzschmar K, Takeda S, Hohl C, Dessing M. 1994. Identification of pro-thymocytes in murine fetal blood: T lineage commitment can precede thymus colonization. *EMBO J.* 13:4229–40

56. Katsura Y. 2002. Redefinition of lymphoid progenitors. *Nat. Rev. Immunol.* 2:127–32

57. Walker L, Carlson A, Tan-Pertel HT, Weinmaster G, Gasson J. 2001. The Notch receptor and its ligands are selectively expressed during hematopoietic development in the mouse. *Stem Cells* 19:543–52

58. Ting CN, Olson MC, Barton KP, Leiden JM. 1996. Transcription factor GATA-3 is required for development of the T-cell lineage. *Nature* 384:474–78

59. Harman BC, Jenkinson EJ, Anderson G. 2003. Entry into the thymic microenvironment triggers Notch activation in the earliest migrant T cell progenitors. *J. Immunol.* 170:1299–303

60. Lind EF, Prockop SE, Porritt HE, Petrie HT. 2001. Mapping precursor movement through the postnatal thymus reveals specific microenvironments supporting defined stages of early lymphoid development. *J. Exp. Med.* 194:127–34

61. Prockop SE, Palencia S, Ryan CM, Gordon K, Gray D, Petrie HT. 2002. Stromal cells provide the matrix for migration of early lymphoid progenitors through the thymic cortex. *J. Immunol.* 169:4354–61

62. Schmitt TM, Ciofani M, Petrie HT, Zuniga-Pflucker JC. 2004. Maintenance of T cell specification and differentiation requires recurrent Notch receptor-ligand interactions. *J. Exp. Med.* 200:469–79

63. Wolfer A, Bakker T, Wilson A, Nicolas M, Ioannidis V, et al. 2001. Inactivation of Notch 1 in immature thymocytes does not perturb CD4 or CD8T cell development. *Nat. Immunol.* 2:235–41

64. Kaneta M, Osawa M, Sudo K, Nakauchi H, Farr AG, Takahama Y. 2000. A role for pref-1 and HES-1 in thymocyte development. *J. Immunol.* 164:256–64

65. Tomita K, Hattori M, Nakamura E, Nakanishi S, Minato N, Kageyama R. 1999. The bHLH gene Hes1 is essential for expansion of early T cell precursors. *Genes Dev.* 13:1203–10

66. Deftos ML, Huang E, Ojala EW, Forbush KA, Bevan MJ. 2000. Notch1 signaling promotes the maturation of CD4 and CD8 SP thymocytes. *Immunity* 13:73–84

67. Reizis B, Leder P. 2002. Direct induction of T lymphocyte-specific gene expression by the mammalian Notch signaling pathway. *Genes Dev.* 16:295–300

68. van den Brandt J, Voss K, Schott M, Hunig T, Wolfe MS, Reichardt HM. 2004. Inhibition of Notch signaling biases rat thymocyte development towards the NK cell lineage. *Eur. J. Immunol.* 34:1405–13

69. Kang J, Coles M, Cado D, Raulet DH. 1998. The developmental fate of T cells is critically influenced by TCR$\gamma\delta$ expression. *Immunity* 8:427–38

70. Terrence K, Pavlovich CP, Matechak EO, Fowlkes BJ. 2000. Premature expression of T cell receptor (TCR)$\alpha\beta$ suppresses TCR$\gamma\delta$ gene rearrangement but permits development of $\gamma\delta$ lineage T cells. *J. Exp. Med.* 192:537–48

71. Washburn T, Schweighoffer E, Gridley T, Chang D, Fowlkes BJ, et al. 1997. Notch activity influences the $\alpha\beta$ versus

$\gamma\delta$ T cell lineage decision. *Cell* 88:833–43

72. Wolfer A, Wilson A, Nemir M, MacDonald HR, Radtke F. 2002. Inactivation of Notch1 impairs VDJβ rearrangement and allows pre-TCR-independent survival of early $\alpha\beta$ lineage thymocytes. *Immunity* 16:869–79

73. Jiang R, Lan Y, Chapman HD, Shawber C, Norton CR, et al. 1998. Defects in limb, craniofacial, and thymic development in Jagged2 mutant mice. *Genes Dev.* 12:1046–57

74. Ciofani M, Schmitt TM, Ciofani A, Michie AM, Cuburu N, et al. 2004. Obligatory role for cooperative signaling by pre-TCR and Notch during thymocyte differentiation. *J. Immunol.* 172:5230–39

75. Engel I, Johns C, Bain G, Rivera RR, Murre C. 2001. Early thymocyte development is regulated by modulation of E2A protein activity. *J. Exp. Med.* 194:733–45

76. Pai SY, Truitt ML, Ting CN, Leiden JM, Glimcher LH, Ho IC. 2003. Critical roles for transcription factor GATA-3 in thymocyte development. *Immunity* 19:863–75

77. Sicinska E, Aifantis I, Le Cam L, Swat W, Borowski C, et al. 2003. Requirement for cyclin D3 in lymphocyte development and T cell leukemias. *Cancer Cell* 4:451–61

78. Voll RE, Jimi E, Phillips RJ, Barber DF, Rincon M, et al. 2000. NF-κB activation by the pre-T cell receptor serves as a selective survival signal in T lymphocyte development. *Immunity* 13:677–89

79. Aifantis I, Gounari F, Scorrano L, Borowski C, von Boehmer H. 2001. Constitutive pre-TCR signaling promotes differentiation through Ca^{2+} mobilization and activation of NF-κB and NFAT. *Nat. Immunol.* 2:403–9

80. Oakley F, Mann J, Ruddell RG, Pickford J, Weinmaster G, Mann DA. 2003. Basal expression of IκBα is controlled by the mammalian transcriptional repressor RBP-J (CBF1) and its activator Notch1. *J. Biol. Chem.* 278:24359–70

81. Fowlkes BJ, Robey EA. 2002. A reassessment of the effect of activated Notch1 on CD4 and CD8 T cell development. *J. Immunol.* 169:1817–21

82. Robey E, Chang D, Itano A, Cado D, Alexander H, et al. 1996. An activated form of Notch influences the choice between CD4 and CD8 T cell lineages. *Cell* 87:483–92

83. Izon DJ, Punt JA, Xu L, Karnell FG, Allman D, et al. 2001. Notch1 regulates maturation of CD4$^+$ and CD8$^+$ thymocytes by modulating TCR signal strength. *Immunity* 14:253–64

84. Ohishi K, Varnum-Finney B, Flowers D, Anasetti C, Myerson D, Bernstein ID. 2000. Monocytes express high amounts of Notch and undergo cytokine specific apoptosis following interaction with the Notch ligand, Delta-1. *Blood* 95:2847–54

85. Amsen D, Blander JM, Lee GR, Tanigaki K, Honjo T, Flavell RA. 2004. Instruction of distinct CD4 T helper cell fates by different Notch ligands on antigen-presenting cells. *Cell* 117:515–26

86. Hoyne GF, Le Roux I, Corsin-Jimenez M, Tan K, Dunne J, et al. 2000. Serrate1-induced Notch signalling regulates the decision between immunity and tolerance made by peripheral CD4$^+$ T cells. *Int. Immunol.* 12:177–85

87. Adler SH, Chiffoleau E, Xu L, Dalton NM, Burg JM, et al. 2003. Notch signaling augments T cell responsiveness by enhancing CD25 expression. *J. Immunol.* 171:2896–903

88. Yamaguchi E, Chiba S, Kumano K, Kunisato A, Takahashi T, Hirai H. 2002. Expression of Notch ligands, Jagged1, 2 and Delta1 in antigen presenting cells in mice. *Immunol. Lett.* 81:59–64

89. Palaga T, Miele L, Golde TE, Osborne BA. 2003. TCR-mediated Notch signaling regulates proliferation and IFN-γ

production in peripheral T cells. *J. Immunol.* 171:3019–24

90. Radtke F, Wilson A, Ernst B, MacDonald HR. 2002. The role of Notch signaling during hematopoietic lineage commitment. *Immunol. Rev.* 187:65–74

91. Eagar TN, Tang Q, Wolfe M, He Y, Pear WS, Bluestone JA. 2004. Notch 1 signaling regulates peripheral T cell activation. *Immunity* 20:407–15

92. Maekawa Y, Tsukumo S, Chiba S, Hirai H, Hayashi Y, et al. 2003. Delta1-Notch3 interactions bias the functional differentiation of activated CD4+ T cells. *Immunity* 19:549–59

93. Murphy KM, Reiner SL. 2002. The lineage decisions of helper T cells. *Nat. Rev. Immunol.* 2:933–44

94. Tacchini-Cottier F, Allenbach C, Otten LA, Radtke F. 2004. Notch1 expression on T cells is not required for CD4+ T helper differentiation. *Eur. J. Immunol.* 34:1588–96

95. Ng WF, Duggan PJ, Ponchel F, Matarese G, Lombardi G, et al. 2001. Human CD4+CD25+ cells: a naturally occurring population of regulatory T cells. *Blood* 98:2736–44

96. Vigouroux S, Yvon E, Wagner HJ, Biagi E, Dotti G, et al. 2003. Induction of antigen-specific regulatory T cells following overexpression of a Notch ligand by human B lymphocytes. *J. Virol.* 77:10872–80

97. Yvon ES, Vigouroux S, Rousseau RF, Biagi E, Amrolia P, et al. 2003. Over expression of the Notch ligand, Jagged-1 induces alloantigen-specific human regulatory T cells. *Blood* 102:3815–21

98. Wong KK, Carpenter MJ, Young LL, Walker SJ, McKenzie G, et al. 2003. Notch ligation by Delta1 inhibits peripheral immune responses to transplantation antigens by a CD8+ cell-dependent mechanism. *J. Clin. Invest.* 112:1741–50

99. Anastasi E, Campese AF, Bellavia D, Bulotta A, Balestri A, et al. 2003. Expression of activated Notch3 in transgenic mice enhances generation of T regulatory cells and protects against experimental autoimmune diabetes. *J. Immunol.* 171:4504–11

100. Witt CM, Won WJ, Hurez V, Klug CA. 2003. Notch2 haploinsufficiency results in diminished B1 B cells and a severe reduction in marginal zone B cells. *J. Immunol.* 171:2783–88

101. Martin F, Kearney JF. 2002. Marginal-zone B cells. *Nat. Rev. Immunol.* 2:323–35

102. Hao Z, Rajewsky K. 2001. Homeostasis of peripheral B cells in the absence of B cell influx from the bone marrow. *J. Exp. Med.* 194:1151–64

103. Vinuesa CG, Sze DM, Cook MC, Toellner KM, Klaus GG, et al. 2003. Recirculating and germinal center B cells differentiate into cells responsive to polysaccharide antigens. *Eur. J. Immunol.* 33:297–305

104. Cinamon G, Matloubian M, Lesneski MJ, Xu Y, Low C, et al. 2004. Sphingosine 1-phosphate receptor 1 promotes B cell localization in the splenic marginal zone. *Nat. Immunol.* 5:713–20

105. Swiatek PJ, Lindsell CE, Franco del Amo F, Weinmaster G, Gridley T. 1994. Notch1 is essential for postimplantation development in mice. *Genes Dev.* 8:707–19

106. Conlon RA, Reaume AG, Rossant J. 1995. Notch1 is required for the coordinate segmentation of somites. *Development* 121:1533–45

107. Huppert SS, Le A, Schroeter EH, Mumm JS, Saxena MT, et al. 2000. Embryonic lethality in mice homozygous for a processing-deficient allele of Notch1. *Nature* 405:966–70

108. Hamada Y, Kadokawa Y, Okabe M, Ikawa M, Coleman JR, Tsujimoto Y. 1999. Mutation in ankyrin repeats of the mouse Notch2 gene induces early embryonic lethality. *Development* 126:3415–24

109. McCright B, Gao X, Shen L, Lozier J, Lan Y, et al. 2001. Defects in development of the kidney, heart and eye vasculature in mice homozygous for a hypomorphic Notch2 mutation. *Development* 128:491–502

110. Krebs LT, Xue Y, Norton CR, Sundberg JP, Beatus P, et al. 2003. Characterization of Notch3-deficient mice: normal embryonic development and absence of genetic interactions with a Notch1 mutation. *Genesis* 37:139–43

111. Krebs LT, Xue Y, Norton CR, Shutter JR, Maguire M, et al. 2000. Notch signaling is essential for vascular morphogenesis in mice. *Genes Dev.* 14:1343–52

112. Oka C, Nakano T, Wakeham A, de la Pompa JL, Mori C, et al. 1995. Disruption of the mouse RBP-Jκ gene results in early embryonic death. *Development* 121:3291–301

113. Xue Y, Gao X, Lindsell CE, Norton CR, Chang B, et al. 1999. Embryonic lethality and vascular defects in mice lacking the Notch ligand Jagged1. *Hum. Mol. Genet.* 8:723–30

114. Hrabe de Angelis M, McIntyre J 2nd, Gossler A. 1997. Maintenance of somite borders in mice requires the Delta homologue Dll1. *Nature* 386:717–21

115. Kusumi K, Sun ES, Kerrebrock AW, Bronson RT, Chi DC, et al. 1998. The mouse pudgy mutation disrupts Delta homologue Dll3 and initiation of early somite boundaries. *Nat. Genet.* 19:274–78

116. Dunwoodie SL, Clements M, Sparrow DB, Sa X, Conlon RA, Beddington RS. 2002. Axial skeletal defects caused by mutation in the spondylocostal dysplasia/pudgy gene Dll3 are associated with disruption of the segmentation clock within the presomitic mesoderm. *Development* 129:1795–806

116a. Gale NW, Dominguez MG, Noguera I, Pan L, Hughes V, et al. 2004. Haploinsufficiency of delta-like 4 ligand results in embryonic lethality due to major defects in arterial and vascular development. *Proc. Natl. Acad. Sci. USA* 101:15949–54

117. Ishibashi M, Ang SL, Shiota K, Nakanishi S, Kageyama R, Guillemot F. 1995. Targeted disruption of mammalian hairy and Enhancer of split homolog-1 (HES-1) leads to up-regulation of neural helix-loop-helix factors, premature neurogenesis, and severe neural tube defects. *Genes Dev.* 9:3136–48

118. Kuroda K, Han H, Tani S, Tanigaki K, Tun T, et al. 2003. Regulation of marginal zone B cell development by MINT, a suppressor of Notch/RBP-J signaling pathway. *Immunity* 18:301–12

119. Zhang N, Gridley T. 1998. Defects in somite formation in Lunatic Fringe-deficient mice. *Nature* 394:374–77

120. Evrard YA, Lun Y, Aulehla A, Gan L, Johnson RL. 1998. Lunatic Fringe is an essential mediator of somite segmentation and patterning. *Nature* 394:377–81

121. Zhong W, Jiang MM, Schonemann MD, Meneses JJ, Pedersen RA, et al. 2000. Mouse numb is an essential gene involved in cortical neurogenesis. *Proc. Natl. Acad. Sci. USA* 97:6844–49

122. Yan XQ, Sarmiento U, Sun Y, Huang G, Guo J, et al. 2001. A novel Notch ligand, Dll4, induces T-cell leukemia/lymphoma when overexpressed in mice by retroviral-mediated gene transfer. *Blood* 98:3793–99

123. Dorsch M, Zheng G, Yowe D, Rao P, Wang Y, et al. 2002. Ectopic expression of Delta4 impairs hematopoietic development and leads to lymphoproliferative disease. *Blood* 100:2046–55

124. French MB, Koch U, Shaye RE, McGill MA, Dho SE, et al. 2002. Transgenic expression of numb inhibits Notch signaling in immature thymocytes but does not alter T cell fate specification. *J. Immunol.* 168:3173–80

Annu. Rev. Immunol. 2005. 23:975–1028
doi: 10.1146/annurev.immunol.22.012703.104538
Copyright © 2005 by Annual Reviews. All rights reserved
First published online as a Review in Advance on January 7, 2005

CELL BIOLOGY OF ANTIGEN PROCESSING IN VITRO AND IN VIVO

E. Sergio Trombetta and Ira Mellman

*Department of Cell Biology and Section of Immunobiology, Ludwig Institute for Cancer Research, Yale University School of Medicine, New Haven, Connecticut 06520-8002;
email: sergio.trombetta@yale.edu, ira.mellman@yale.edu*

Key Words   dendritic cells, antigen presentation, endocytosis, proteolysis

■ **Abstract**   The conversion of exogenous and endogenous proteins into immunogenic peptides recognized by T lymphocytes involves a series of proteolytic and other enzymatic events culminating in the formation of peptides bound to MHC class I or class II molecules. Although the biochemistry of these events has been studied in detail, only in the past few years has similar information begun to emerge describing the cellular context in which these events take place. This review thus concentrates on the properties of antigen-presenting cells, especially those aspects of their overall organization, regulation, and intracellular transport that both facilitate and modulate the processing of protein antigens. Emphasis is placed on dendritic cells and the specializations that help account for their marked efficiency at antigen processing and presentation both in vitro and, importantly, in vivo. How dendritic cells handle antigens is likely to be as important a determinant of immunogenicity and tolerance as is the nature of the antigens themselves.

INTRODUCTION

Despite our advanced understanding of the molecular interactions between peptide ligands, MHC molecules, and their receptors on T cells, the factors that determine the immunogenicity of proteins remain poorly understood. This situation reflects the fact that the cells and intracellular pathways leading to the formation of peptide-MHC complexes (pMHC) are intricate and variable, but essential to determining how antigens are processed and presented. Although these events have been characterized in general terms, they cannot yet be studied with the precision of the structural and biophysical approaches used to study peptide-MHC interactions.

The situation is further complicated by the fact that the cells responsible for antigen processing and presentation are proving richly diverse, perhaps reflecting the diversity of antigens and circumstances that the immune system is capable of dealing with. Thus, what is true concerning the response to one antigen may not hold true for others, and even the response to any given antigen can be quite variable. Processing and presentation are affected by several factors, including the

0732-0582/05/0423-0975$14.00   **975** physical form of the antigen at time of delivery, the site and method of delivery, the nature of the antigen-presenting cell (APC) that first encounters the antigen, and the inflammatory status or adjuvant used. As a result, current approaches to inducing antigen-specific immunity remain largely empirical. For antigens that induce undesirable autoimmune or inflammatory responses, we still do not know the precise reasons for their immunogenicity, or why their repertoire is so limited.

The past several years have yielded great advances in our understanding of the cell biology and biochemistry of antigen processing and presentation. Much of what has been learned derives from in vitro studies that rely increasingly on cultured primary APCs. These efforts have begun to identify and characterize the various types of APCs involved, as well as mechanisms of action. A major challenge is to understand how these mechanisms are modified, controlled, and differentially applied to the diverse antigens, cell types, and conditions that mediate the immune response. Even more important is to determine how principles defined in vitro apply in vivo. Understanding APC function more fully is likely to rationalize the role of antigen in guiding the immune response (1).

This review assesses what we have learned thus far about the functional attributes of APCs, placing special emphasis on dendritic cells (DCs). The capture and processing of antigen by DCs plays a primary role in immunity, enabling T cells to detect their cognate peptide-MHC complexes in virtually all other settings, such as helping B cells, activating macrophages, and focusing cytokines and cytotoxic activities even on nonhematopoietic cells. For APCs to perform their functions, not only their activities but also their anatomical distributions are key. Accordingly, throughout the review we try to integrate how in vitro insights can help us understand antigen presentation in vivo.

ANTIGEN-PRESENTING CELLS: ON THE IMPORTANCE OF BEING PROFESSIONAL

The demonstration that virtually any cell type expressing cell surface MHC class II α/β heterodimers was able to engage T cells in an antigen-specific manner (2) initiated a long series of studies in which surrogate APCs and model antigens could be studied under defined conditions in culture. Such approaches established some basic pathways for the loading of peptides onto MHC class I and class II (MHC-I and MHC-II) molecules (3–11). One important lesson that has emerged, however, is that different cell types can process and present antigens at vastly different efficiencies (12–14). This finding has led investigators to consider certain cells as "professional" APCs, a group that typically includes B lymphocytes, macrophages (MØ), and especially dendritic cells (DCs).

The Cellular Basis of Antigen Presentation: Properties of Professional APCs In Vitro and In Vivo

B LYMPHOCYTES   If B cells are not the most professional of all APCs, they are certainly the most focused. Their need to present antigen is intimately linked to their primary function in antibody secretion, rather than the need to promulgate T cell responses (as is true for DCs). B cells are very poor at internalizing antigen except via their surface Ig receptors, which allows them to focus on generating pMHC-II that stimulates (and in turn receives help from) T cells, linking the specificity of the humoral and T cell responses.

Several factors contribute to their exquisite efficiency at presenting antigens on MHC-II (15, 16). Despite their modest capacity for endocytosis, binding of antigen to surface Ig induces internalization of the receptor, accelerates delivery to endocytic compartments, and possibly modulates expression of MHC-II (15, 16). Thus, B cells might be able to regulate their capacity for antigen presentation in response to external stimuli, analogous to the alterations exhibited by DCs during maturation (17).

B cells also constitutively express exceptionally high levels of MHC-II. B cell blasts, for example, express a higher density of MHC-II than even DCs (J. Unternaehrer & I. Mellman, in preparation). They also express abundant costimulatory and adhesion molecules needed for T cell interactions. B cells also express the chaperones human leukocyte antigen (HLA)-DM and HLA-DO, which contribute to peptide loading onto MHC-II molecules. Although B cells can present endogenous antigens on MHC-I, presentation of exogenous antigens on MHC-I is poorly described in B cells and probably quite limited.

MACROPHAGES   Macrophages (MØ) have long been considered prototypical APCs, in part owing to the fact that they have been associated with innate immune responses to microorganisms for over a century. Their role as APCs was further emphasized by their extraordinary capacity for endocytosis, enabling them to internalize up to 50% of their cell surface area in a single round of particle phagocytosis or up to 200% of their surface area per hour during constitutive fluid uptake (18). MØ can internalize virtually any form of antigen, cell-associated or soluble, either nonspecifically or via specific receptors (FcγR, lectins, etc.), allowing them to stimulate T cells of various specificities, a fact attested to by years of in vitro study.

MØ express MHC-I, MHC-II, and costimulatory molecules, upregulating their levels upon activation by inflammatory cytokines or bacterial products. However, compared with B cells or DCs, the levels of MHC-II and costimulators expressed even by activated MØ are substantially lower (Figure 1). These low levels of MHC-II in part explain why MØ are generally less efficient at antigen presentation and T cell stimulation than either B cells or DCs, both ex vivo and in vivo (14, 19–23). MØ are nevertheless present in great numbers at sites of infection and chronic inflammation where they may contribute to T cell stimulation.

In addition, despite MØ's profound capacity for endocytosis, the organization and properties of the endocytic organelles found in MØ may be suboptimal for efficient antigen presentation (14). Lysosomal compartments in MØ are perhaps better adapted for digestion of internalized material, contributing to what may be a major function for MØ in innate immunity: the clearance of invading microorganisms (see below) (24, 25).

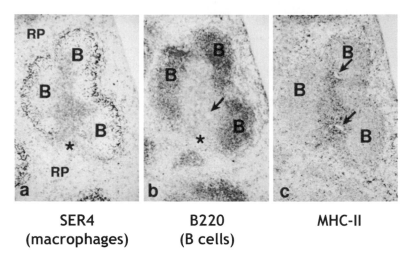

| SER4 | B220 | MHC-II |
| (macrophages) | (B cells) | |

Figure 1 High-level expression of MHC-II in DC in lymphoid organs. Low-magnification views of splenic white pulp nodule labeled for CD4 (in *blue*) marks the T cell areas relative to the SER4-positive MØ (*left*) and B220-positive B cells (*center*), both revealed in brown. MHC-II, also brown, was visualized using the M5/114 monoclonal antibody (*right*). Follicular B cell areas (B) are surrounded by red pulp (RP). Arrowheads mark central arteries of the T cell areas. The marginal zone of SER4-positive MØ is interrupted where T cells enter the white pulp (*). The greatest MHC-II staining was due to DCs in the T cell area, greatly in excess of the MHC-II staining associated with MØ in the marginal zone. (Reproduced from Reference 65.)

DENDRITIC CELLS: GENERAL AND DISTINCTIVE FEATURES   Dendritic cells (DCs) are unique among all APCs in the adult immune system in many critical ways. Unlike MØ or B cells, DCs' primary function appears to be antigen presentation. Both DCs and MØ differentiate from circulating bone marrow–derived precursors and complete their differentiation upon leaving the blood stream and taking residence in peripheral tissues. Nearly all tissues contain both DCs and MØ at the steady state, although the two cell types differ in important ways. DCs have a unique distribution within lymphoid organs, accumulating in regions where MØ and B cells are generally excluded. DCs are enriched in the areas where naive T cells are activated, in an optimal position to be interrogated by a continuously moving swarm of T cells seeking their cognate pMHC complexes (26–29) (Figure 1). DCs have unique surveillance and migratory properties (30), enabling them to carry antigens captured in the periphery to secondary lymphoid organs, or to internalize them directly from the lymph (31). This includes, for example, the sampling of commensal bacteria, which are ingested and rapidly destroyed by MØ but conveyed by DCs to lymph nodes where they induce IgA responses (32). Similarly, apoptotic cells contained within migratory DCs can be observed in the afferent lymphatics of the gut (33) en route to lymph nodes, probably to assist in the maintenance of self-tolerance (34).

These observations have interesting implications for how and where APCs may present antigen. MØ may present antigen in vivo, especially at sites of inflammation where the cytokine environment enhances their expression of MHC-II and costimulatory molecules, and where T cells are already present (35). However, DCs are significantly more efficient at T cell stimulation (14, 19–23) and are distinguished by their ability to stimulate immunologically naive T cells (19, 23). Mice deficient in some MØ populations genetically [op/op mice (36, 37)] or depleted using toxic liposomes (38) do not exhibit substantial defects in initiating adaptive immune responses, whereas the opposite is true in mice lacking DCs (39). Moreover, MHC-II expression on DCs is sufficient to initiate CD4 T cell responses (40, 41). The preeminence of DCs in initiating immune responses is likely to reflect a combination of basic features of DC biology: a greater inherent efficiency for antigen presentation, and the capacity to accumulate within the T cell areas of lymphoid organs. Although B cells might, at least in vitro, also accomplish these functions, the possibility that they do so in vivo is relatively insignificant given that B cells are mostly restricted to single antigenic specificities. Although it is beyond the scope of this review to consider the function of DCs in initiating and regulating the immune response in any detail, it must be mentioned that DCs also instruct T cell responses, being capable of polarizing T cell development (42) or inducing T cell tolerance (34). Regulatory T cells can also be uniquely stimulated to proliferate by DC, enhancing their suppressor capacity (43, 44). DCs can also perform some "innate" functions, such as secreting IL-12 and type I interferons, as well as mobilizing NK and NKT cells (23).

DCs endocytose avidly and present virtually any form of protein antigen on MHC-I or MHC-II molecules. Indeed, the ability of DCs to "cross-present" exogenous antigens on MHC-I molecules is arising as a distinguishing feature; MØ are also capable of cross-presentation, but with efficiencies that are orders of magnitude lower (45, 46). In addition to their distinct antigen handling and homing properties, DCs exhibit a variety of other features that greatly enhance their capacity as APCs. Among these are exceptionally high levels of MHC-II and costimulatory molecules, certainly as compared with MØ in most tissues (Figure 1). DCs also express CD86 at a greater than fivefold higher density than B cells (J. Unternaehrer & I. Mellman, in preparation). In addition, the extensive folds and dendritic extensions characteristic of DCs enables them to form close contact with multiple T cells simultaneously (47–49). MHC-II molecules on the DC plasma membrane also appear to be laterally clustered, which may further facilitate the efficiency of T cell scanning by increasing the effective local density of MHC molecules at contact sites, even in the absence of antigen-specific recognition (50–53; J. Unternaehrer & I. Mellman, in preparation).

CELLULAR SPECIALIZATIONS OF DCs: MATURATION   One of the most complex and intriguing specializations of DCs is the process of maturation. Maturation was a term originally used to describe the acquisition of antigen-presenting activity by cultured DCs after isolation from tissues. Epidermal Langerhans cells (LCs), for example, do not effectively present antigen when first isolated from skin explants, but they do after 1–2 days in culture (54). Over the past several years, this phenomenon has been extensively studied in vitro using DC cultures, illuminating some general principles and features of DC maturation. It is now clear that virtually all activities mediated by DCs are linked to and regulated by maturation.

First and foremost, maturation induces a dramatic structural reorganization (17), or "phenotypic maturation" (Figure 2). Functionally immature DCs, like the ones freshly isolated from tissues or that first arise from bone marrow cultures, express relatively low levels of surface MHC-II and costimulatory molecules. Instead, abundant MHC-II is accumulated within their lysosomal compartment, together with antigens internalized by the marked endocytic activity characteristic of most

Immature DC

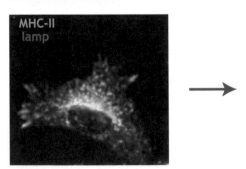

Peripheral and lymphoid tissues
Highly endocytic
Low surface MHC-II and costimulators

Antigen accumulation

Mature DC

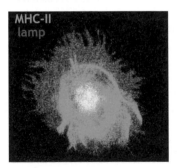

Lymphoid tissues
Endocytosis reduced
High surface MHC-II and costimulators

T cell stimulation

Figure 2 DC maturation is accompanied by a dramatic reorganization of form and function. Immunofluorescence images of mouse bone marrow–derived immature DC (*left*) and mature DC (*right*) expressing MHC-II-GFP are shown in green, and the resident lysosomal membrane protein Lamp is shown in red. Maturation was triggered in vitro by LPS. Under steady-state conditions, phenotypically immature DCs can be found in peripheral tissues and in secondary lymphoid organs. They are highly endocytic and accumulate most of their MHC-II molecules inside the cell in lysosomal compartments (Lamp$^+$). Upon maturation, DCs become less endocytic, and MHC-II is transported to the plasma membrane, where it accumulates together with high levels of costimulatory molecules. Mature DCs are generally restricted to secondary lymphoid organs.

immature DCs (55, 56). DCs begin to mature immediately after receiving adequate stimulus [Toll-like receptor (TLR) ligands, inflammatory cytokines, T cell ligands (e.g., CD40 ligand), NK cells, or disruption of homotypic contacts between immature DCs]. First, there is a transient increase in macropinocytic uptake (57), followed rapidly by its nearly complete downregulation (58–61). Second, MHC-II molecules escape from the lysosomal compartment and are transported to the plasma membrane (62, 63). Finally, the overall levels of MHC-II, costimulatory molecules, and MHC-I increase at the surface, which also begins to extend the DC's characteristic "dendritic" extensions and membrane folds. Concomitant with these events, the cells also enhance their ability to form and to accumulate pMHC-II complexes, even using antigen internalized before the maturation stimulus (55, 56). The mechanistic details of how this occurs are considered below.

While such observations define a useful general paradigm, they are almost certainly an oversimplification of the actual situation. DCs of multiple maturation phenotypes (immature DCs, mature DCs, and cells exhibiting intermediate to high levels of MHC molecules with or without high expression of costimulatory molecules) can be detected in lymph nodes at the steady state (64–68). Although some of these may be DCs still in the process of maturation, an intriguing possibility is that they represent distinct functional states, reflecting the qualitatively different modes of T cell stimulation that DCs are capable of effecting.

There is now considerable evidence that DCs serve not only to initiate immunity but also to maintain peripheral tolerance, deleting self-reactive T lymphocytes and/or expanding regulatory T cells, encouraging them to become more suppressive in an antigen-specific manner (34, 43, 44). Because the induction of T cell tolerance was classically thought to result from the presentation of pMHC in the absence of costimulatory molecules, one idea is that immature DCs present in lymph nodes comprise a tolerogenic population. It is possible that immature DCs do make sufficient pMHC to perform this function. However, maturation (or the onset of an inflammatory state in vivo) may enhance the absolute number, and possibly the repertoire, of MHC-II and pMHC complexes manyfold. Thus, optimal tolerance induction may require the antigen processing activity of a mature DC to ensure that self-pMHC are made at the same efficiency under tolerogenic conditions as under conditions leading to immunity; this is important lest an immunogenic mature DC present a self-antigen to which tolerance has not been assured.

Some DCs with "intermediate" maturation phenotypes (e.g., high MHC-II, low or moderate CD86) (64, 65) may represent tolerogenic populations. However, the actual characteristics of tolerogenic DCs remain unknown (34, 44). Reconciling the function versus the phenotype of mature DCs is further complicated by the fact that different maturation stimuli may produce qualitatively different outcomes: mature DCs that are immunostimulatory in distinct ways, selectively polarizing Th1 versus Th2 responses (42). Such effects may reflect differential production of cytokines or alterations in the expression of surface molecules, but they demonstrate that not all DCs that appear phenotypically mature are functionally equivalent. Even though the terminology used to describe DC maturation is clearly inadequate, we limit our use of the concept here to denote the general phenotypic and biochemical changes triggered by classical maturation stimuli in vitro.

DENDRITIC CELL HETEROGENEITY   Apart from their maturation state, several classes of DCs can be distinguished in vivo on the basis of their progenitors, tissue distribution, and surface markers (69–71). In the mouse, up to five distinct populations have been proposed (72). DCs expressing CD8α, for example, have been associated with the cross-presentation of exogenous antigens on MHC-I. Whether this reflects a fundamental difference or simply the enhanced phagocytic activity of this particular population is unknown (73). In general, the extent to which each of these populations represent functionally distinct entities is unclear.

Nevertheless, it has proved practical to use defined cell culture systems and assess their properties to analyze the cell biological basis of DC function. Four DC types have been most often studied in culture: (*a*) nonproliferating human CD14$^+$ monocyte-derived DCs (differentiated in GM-CSF and IL-4), (*b*) mouse myeloid DCs differentiated from proliferating bone marrow progenitors, (*c*) human LC-like DCs derived from proliferating CD34$^+$ stem cells, and (*d*) human (or mouse) plasmacytoid DCs (pDCs). Monocyte- and bone marrow–derived cells have many features in common, and indeed our general understanding of DC organization, maturation, and function derive from these systems. At the same time, the two are likely to have some important differences. pDCs, however, are quite distinct and in some respects are closer to B lymphocytes and plasma cells than to monocyte- and bone marrow–derived DCs (70). Although they do not secrete antibody, pDCs contain abundant endoplasmic reticulum (ER), express less MHC-II than myeloid DCs, and are distinguished by a marked capacity for releasing type I interferons, even without exposure to infectious virus. pDCs have thus been associated with viral immunity and autoimmune disorders (74). Other DC populations can be distinguished (LCs, blood DCs), and it will be important to establish how many of these recapitulate the general principles established thus far. It is now important to relate these basic insights obtained with DC cultures to DC function in vivo; that the two are related is without doubt, but identifying the connections is not always easy. By allowing comparisons of underlying mechanisms, differences are instructive and help provide insights into in vivo function.

THE AMATEUR HOUR   Although high-level expression of MHC-II molecules is largely restricted to professional APCs described above, other cell types also express MHC-II molecules under normal and/or pathological condition, including endothelial cells (75, 372), some epithelial cells (76), and tumor cells (77). Together with MHC-II, these cell types express variable levels of costimulatory molecules and accessory factors (invariant chain, HLA-DM, HLA-DO), giving rise to heterogeneous capacity for antigen processing and presentation, and consequently to a variable repertoire of peptides selected, which are often derived from endogenous proteins (78, 79). Presentation of endogenous proteins by these "nonprofessional"

APCs can mediate tissue damage in autoimmune conditions or may alter immuno-surveillance of tumors, but their precise contribution is not yet clear.

THE MECHANISTIC BASIS OF ANTIGEN PROCESSING

Having considered the cellular basis of antigen processing and presentation, we now turn to a more mechanistic consideration of how APCs perform their tasks. Interestingly, both MHC-I- and MHC-II-restricted antigen processing pathways rely on ancient proteolytic mechanisms (proteasomes, lysosomes) that in the vast majority of cell types are used simply for catabolic and homeostatic purposes. Rather than develop dedicated mechanisms, evolution chose to modify preexisting ones for use in the immune response.

Until recently, MHC-I and MHC-II were thought to focus on the presentation of peptides derived from distinct sources. MHC-I ligands were derived from endogenous cytosolic proteins, whereas MHC-II ligands were exogenous, encountering MHC-II molecules following endocytosis. Although this paradigm remains largely correct, we now know that both boundaries can be crossed: MHC-I can present peptides derived from exogenous antigens, and MHC-II can present intracellular antigens that do not come from the extracellular space. Although virtually all nucleated cells, not just professional or amateur APCs, can present endogenous proteins on MHC-I, DCs (and to a far lesser extent MØ) can efficiently use exogenously obtained peptides for this purpose: an event referred to as "cross-presentation." Moreover, it is important to remember that only DCs can prime naive CD8$^+$ T cell responses, regardless of antigen source. We consider both the various sources and fates of antigens sampled and presented by APCs.

SOURCES OF ANTIGENS IN THE MHC-I PATHWAY

Endogenous Proteins

Endogenous proteins destined for presentation on MHC-I molecules are ubiquitinated in the cytosol and fed to the proteasome to initiate fragmentation for MHC-I presentation. However, the source of proteasomal substrates is quite varied (Figure 3). Peptide ligands for MHC-I can be derived from cryptic transcription products, such as open reading frames contained within 5' and 3' untranslated regions, alternative open reading frames, introns, or intron-exon junctions (80–89). Defective ribosomal products (DRiPs) are also a source of proteasomal substrates, offering a broad sample of the cellular and viral proteins synthesized by the APC (90). In DCs, DRiPs can accumulate transiently as aggregates in the cytosol during maturation and are believed to affect the repertoire of endogenous proteins available for proteasomal digestion (91, 92).

MHC-I ligands are also obtained from "stable" proteins, as evidenced by presentation of several species of posttranslationally modified peptides: N-glycosylated

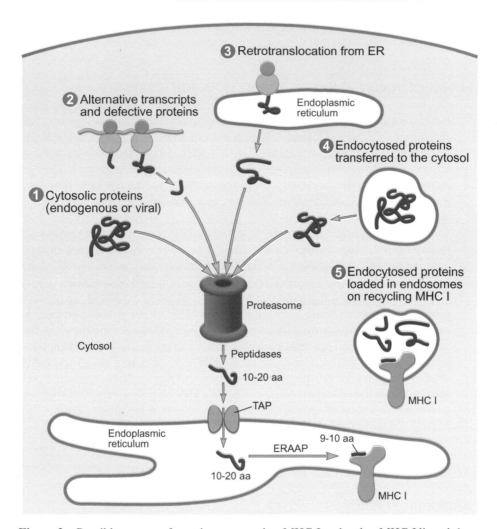

Figure 3   Possible sources of proteins presented on MHC-I molecules. MHC-I ligands have been shown to derive from various sources, including (*1*) cytosolic proteins (endogenous or viral), (*2*) alternative translation products and defective ribosomal products, (*3*) proteins retrotranslocated to the cytosol from the ER, and (*4*) internalized proteins transferred to the cytosol and imported into the ER in a TAP-dependent fashion. In each of these routes, proteins are ultimately degraded in the cytosol by the proteasome and further trimmed by cytosolic peptidases. The resulting peptides are transported into the lumen of the ER for loading on newly synthesized MHC-I products. There is also evidence for another pathway (*5*) in which internalized proteins are processed and loaded in the endocytic pathway onto MHC-I molecules that recycle from the plasma membrane, independently of TAP. For detailed reviews concerning the biochemical steps involved in the MHC-I pathway, see, for example, References 3–7, 82.

peptides (93), phosphopeptides (94), de-amidated peptides (e.g., Asn to Asp) (93), or peptides with modified cysteine residues (95). Also, for some antigens the efficiency of presentation correlates with the abundance of the mature protein (96–98).

Proteins synthesized on membrane-bound ribosomes destined for the secretory pathway appear to be segregated from the proteasome and therefore ineligible for the conventional pathway. However, secretory and membrane proteins can still gain access to the cytosol after being retrotranslocated from the ER, in a process that typically results in ubiquitination and proteasomal degradation (82, 99–102). This process was first believed to involve retrograde transport through the Sec61 channel (103). However, it now seems more likely that other proteins (e.g., Derlin-1, VIMP) play this role, together with the cytosolic ATPase p97 (104, 105). The system is opportunistically targeted by viruses, which encode proteins that downregulate surface MHC-I, helping infected cells evade T cell killing (106–108). Many peptides derived from membrane or secretory proteins correspond to sequences derived either from the transmembrane regions or signal sequences (109–112), although it is unclear how such peptides are derived.

It was recently reported that MHC-I ligands can contain sequences that are not contiguous in the original protein but are spliced together from neighboring peptides (113, 114). These findings suggest that if there are no major restrictions to the splicing reaction, the number of potential MHC-I epitopes could be considerably larger than anticipated. Peptide splicing was previously described in bacteria, plants, and protozoans, but these cases may not be mechanistically related.

Exogenous Proteins

Exogenous proteins (i.e., not synthesized by the APC) constitute a critical source of peptide ligands for MHC-I, and they are quite prevalent in priming CD8$^+$ T cell responses (Figure 4). Indeed, cross-presentation may be the main way MHC-I-restricted responses to tumor antigens or microbes that do not infect DCs can be generated: DCs could ingest infected cells or cancer cells and derive antigens from these sources (72, 115). The "exogenous" pathway also provides a unique opportunity for APCs to present internalized antigens simultaneously on MHC-I, MHC-II, and CD1. However, presentation of exogenous proteins in the absence of their coding sequences is not able to present cryptic epitopes derived from alternative genomic transcripts, which are recognized in certain antiviral, antitumor, and autoimmune responses (83–89).

To some extent, exogenous antigens can be presented on MHC-I in a TAP-independent manner, indicating that they do not require transport to the cytosol and can thus be loaded in the endocytic pathway (116–120) (pathway 5 in Figure 3). Exogenous antigens can also be transferred to the cytosol, where they are digested by proteasomes and loaded onto MHC-I in a TAP-dependent manner (120–124) (pathway 4 in Figure 3).

DCs can apparently modulate their capacity for presentation of exogenous antigens during maturation (45, 125–127), at least in part independently of their capacity to load endogenous proteins on MHC-I or to regulate MHC-II presentation

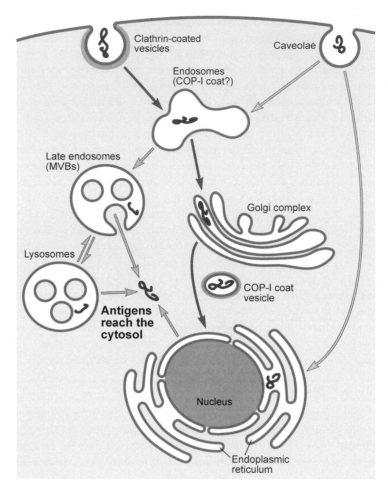

Figure 4 Cross-presentation: possible routes of access to the cytosol for internalized proteins to be presented on MHC-I. Exogenous antigens can gain access to MHC class I molecules following endocytosis. It remains unclear, however, what the mechanisms are by which they traverse the endosomal membrane that comprises the compartment barrier separating the antigens from the proteasome (120). Indirect evidence suggests that antigens egress from endosomes or lysosomes, although it is unknown if this occurs by transient physical rupture of the endosomal membrane or if it reflects the existence of a specific channel or translocator. Alternatively, antigens might make use of an established retrograde pathway leading from endosomes to the Golgi and then to the ER (*purple arrows*), or following internalization in caveolae, a fraction of which fuse with the ER (*blue arrows*). From the ER lumen, antigens may reach the cytosol using a translocation channel that is involved in retrotranslocation during protein degradation (103). The identity of this channel is uncertain (104, 105). Elements of the ER can conceivably gain access to endosomal compartments by normal recycling or possibly by fusion of ER with endosomal or phagosomal membranes (see text for details).

(45). CD40 ligand induced cross-presentation in bone marrow–derived DCs (45), although in vivo loading of exogenous proteins on MHC-I in DCs was not dependent on CD40, indicating that other signals must also be capable of activating this pathway (67).

The Elusive Mechanism of Cross-Presentation

The pathway of "cross-presentation" introduces a remarkable problem in membrane topology: How are antigens contained in the lumen of endocytic vesicles transferred across membranes for proteasomal proteolysis in the cytosol? Cross-presentation occurs with greatest efficiency in DCs, although MØ and other cell types may be partially capable of this activity as well (120). To be cross-presented, antigens can be internalized by multiple mechanisms, including receptor-mediated endocytosis via clathrin-coated vesicles [FcγR (45, 124), the lectin DEC-205 (128)], macropinocytosis, or phagocytosis (120, 129, 130). In fact, mice injected with a small amount of soluble antigen targeted to the antigen receptor DEC-205 show a strong and persistent activation of $CD8^+$ T cells by cross-presentation (128).

Regardless of the efficiency, the topology problem remains: How do proteins reach the cytosol from whichever endocytic organelle they reside after internalization? One possibility is egress from endosomal compartments, as exploited by several bacterial toxins (131, 133). Endocytic compartments appear to "leak" part of their content or to contain specific channels or translocators that permit egress of proteins or peptides to the cytosol by means of size-limited channels or leak pathways (120, 122, 124, 373), but their biochemical basis has proved difficult to establish.

Another possibility is that a fraction of internalized antigens may be delivered to the ER where escape to the cytosol could capitalize on the ER's ability to mediate protein transfer across membranes (103) (Figure 4). Although delivery to the ER after endocytosis is a rare event, there is good evidence that internalized proteins can reach the ER in a number of ways. Several bacterial toxins use this strategy to penetrate into the cytosol (131, 133). Similarly, some viruses (e.g., SV40) internalized via caveolae are delivered to the ER (134–136). Proteins containing the KDEL ER retrieval signal can be detected and returned to the ER following endocytosis via clathrin coated pits (137). COPI proteins normally involved in traffic between the ER and the Golgi have been shown to play a functional role at the level of endosomes (138–140). Thus, an intersection between the endocytic and early secretory pathways is well documented.

Cross-presentation was recently proposed as involving the ER in phagocytic process. Proteomic analysis of isolated phagosomes suggested that several ER components, including TAP and tapasin, may be components of the phagosome membrane (141), suggesting that exogenous proteins may already gain access to the ER-based MHC-I loading machinery in phagosomes (142–145). Recent experiments have shown that a viral-derived TAP antagonist (CMV US6) added to the outside of DCs inhibits cross-presentation (120) and may impede even endogenous presentation (P. Cresswell, personal communication). Such findings are consistent with a functional intersection between the endocytic or phagocytic pathways with the ER, but they do not define how or from what compartment antigen egress itself occurs. Functional fusion between the ER and the phagosomal or plasma membrane is difficult to demonstrate (141), although there is functional evidence for endosomal fusion at sites of phagocytosis (146), under conditions in which an appreciable contribution from the ER cannot be detected (147). Certain bacteria (e.g., *Legionella*) encode proteins required to recruit ER during phagocytosis to avoid transfer to lysosomes; otherwise, conventional phagocytosis occurs in their absence (148). A similar situation has been observed during phagocytosis in Dictyostelium: ER elements associate (but do not necessarily fuse) with forming phagosomes containing *Legionella* but not *E. coli* (149). It is critical to attempt a visualization and selective disruption of individual membrane transport steps of the possible pathways involved in cross-presentation to firmly elucidate the mechanisms of cross-presentation.

One further consideration pertains to the traffic of the MHC-I molecules that are loaded with exogenous peptides. Elimination of a tyrosine residue in the cytoplasmic domain of murine MHC-I reduced entry of at least a subpopulation of MHC-I into late endocytic compartments and also reduced their capacity for cross-presentation (150). This observation is consistent with the idea that loading of MHC-I for cross-presentation occurs within endocytic compartments, but further work is required to demonstrate this directly and to establish the source of the peptides used for loading.

SOURCES OF ANTIGENS IN THE MHC-II PATHWAY

Antigens loaded on MHC-II are typically exogenous proteins internalized by the APC or endogenous proteins resident in the endosomal system. However, antigens presumably excluded from the endosomal system, such as proteins localized in the cytosol or the nucleus, can also be presented by MHC-II molecules (151–162). In fact, a fraction of the peptides bound to MHC-II are derived from proteins normally resident in the cytosol (163–170). Thus, the presence of endogenous cellular proteins on MHC-II is not restricted to a few select antigens (171).

In principle, these cytosolic antigens could be recaptured as exogenous material by endocytosis of antigen liberated from apoptotic cells, or by phagocytosis of apoptotic bodies. However, in many cases the cytosolic epitopes were isolated from cell lines in culture, which are not highly phagocytic. Also, a high rate of cell death and phagocytosis would be necessary to account for the abundance of some cytosolic epitopes. A more likely source of peptides derived from cytosolic antigens is the transfer of material from the cytosol into lysosomes, or autophagy (172) (Figure 5). The sampling of cytosolic proteins for MHC-II presentation may be relevant for (*a*) viruses that fuse at the plasma membrane, releasing most of their

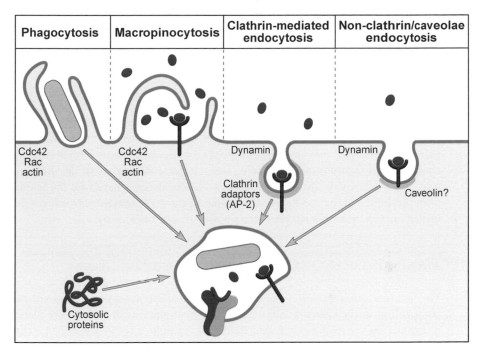

Figure 5 Types of endocytosis used for antigen accumulation. APCs internalize exogenous antigens using, to variable extents, the same mechanisms of endocytosis found in other cell types and organisms. Phagocytosis involves the ingestion of large particles or cells >1 μm in diameter. Particle binding to specific receptors signals actin assembly and drives pseudopod extension and particle engulfment. It has recently been proposed that the ER fuses with the cell surface to supply the extra membrane for this event, although this suggestion still awaits direct support (374). Macropinocytosis is constitutive in MØ and immature DCs, but it can also be triggered by growth factors or certain pathogenic bacteria (e.g., Salmonella). Macropinocytosis is also actin-dependent and can account for the uptake of large quantities of extracellular fluid and fluid-dissolved antigens. Soluble receptor-ligand complexes are typically internalized by clathrin-coated vesicles or (to a lesser extent) by caveolin-containing invaginations designated "caveolae." It is unclear if DCs exhibit this mode of uptake, but they may exhibit a related form of endocytosis that involves neither clathrin nor caveolin. Proteins internalized by any of these mechanisms eventually reach endosomal/lysosomal compartments, where they can be processed by resident proteases and loaded onto MHC-II, typically newly synthesized, but also recycled from the plasma membrane. Endogenous proteins in the cytosol or other organelles can also be imported into lysosomes by autophagy, or perhaps by TAP, for loading onto MHC-II. (For more detailed overviews of endocytic mechanisms see, for example, 188, 189. For more detailed views of the MHC-II pathway see, for example, 8, 9, 364.)

proteins directly in the cytosol; (*b*) viruses that establish persistent latent infections and constitutively express low levels of cytosolic antigens (173); and perhaps even (*c*) tolerogenic presentation of endogenous cytosolic proteins. Proteins from other compartments (e.g., the nucleus) might similarly be presented on MHC-II following autophagy. Furthermore, there is evidence for presentation on MHC-II after cytoplasmic processing (158, 174) and TAP-dependent translocation of cytosolic as well as exogenous antigens (L. Eisenlohr, personal communication).

The results summarized above indicate a lack of absolute topological restrictions on MHC-I and MHC-II, implying that in principle, any protein can potentially be presented on MHC-I or MHC-II (Figures 4 and 5). The differences between MHC-I and MHC-II may thus be distinguished more on the basis of their binding characteristics and physiological role. The relative contribution of the different routes in vivo is still unknown. Their prevalence likely depends on the nature of the antigen and the mechanisms available in the APC involved, which can be further altered by host-microbe interactions (107, 108, 175, 176).

MECHANISMS OF EXOGENOUS ANTIGEN CAPTURE

The fact that different APCs capture antigens in different ways makes a critical contribution to the heterogeneity of what they can present. It is therefore worth reconsidering the relative contributions of the multiple ways in which APCs can capture antigens, again both in vitro and in vivo.

Extracellular Loading

The simplest way of loading peptides on MHC-I and MHC-II is by direct binding of isolated peptides to MHC molecules exposed at the cell surface. Experimentally, loading MHC extracellularly with defined peptides is broadly employed in epitope mapping studies and in clinical trials that use "peptide pulsed" APCs. Direct peptide loading can conceivably occur in vivo if the required peptide ligand is available at sufficient concentration in the extracellular space. Perhaps in support of this possibility, empty or peptide-receptive MHC-II (177, 178) and H2-M (179, 180) have been detected at the surface of APCs. Furthermore, in vitro studies suggest that APCs can sometimes present peptides generated and released by neighboring cells. However, the contribution of peptide exchange at the cell surface in vivo remains unknown. The abundance of Ii-derived peptides in cells deficient in H2-M (181) suggests that this exchange mechanism may not be very prevalent. Peptide exchange at the cell surface is unlikely to be highly dependent on H2-M given its rather strict requirement for acid pH (182, 183).

pMHC formed from direct binding of free peptides to MHC-II may have a different conformation and specificity for T cell stimulation than the same pMHC formed by the same peptide extracted from the intact protein by intracellular processing (184, 185). Although demonstrated as yet for only a restricted number of examples, if this consideration applies more generally, it has implications for epitope mapping studies and peptide-based vaccines. A dual conformation for a peptide bound to MHC-I (HLA-B*2705) but not for HLA-B*2709 (differing from HLA-B*2705 in a single amino acid) was observed by X-ray crystallography (186). Interestingly, the HLA allele that gives rise to a dual conformation is associated with autoimmunity. The biochemical basis for why alternative conformations might exist remains unknown, making it difficult to decide the phenomenon's physiological or pathological significance.

Mechanisms of Antigen Uptake for Intracellular Loading: Overview of Endocytosis

Although peptide exchange can occur at the cell surface, conversion of internalized antigens (or endogenous antigens for MHC-I) into pMHC is almost certainly more prevalent, and ironically more efficient. The relative use by APCs of alternative endocytic routes (Figure 5) dictates not only their capacity for antigen uptake, but also that different endocytic routes may have different functional consequences (25, 187). For example, the ingestion of microbes is generally accompanied by inflammatory responses, whereas the opposite may occur after uptake of apoptotic or necrotic cells. TLRs appear not only to signal the presence of pathogens but also to modulate early events during phagocytic uptake and the kinetics of lysosomal fusion (188, 189). In DCs, endocytosis is upregulated shortly after maturation is induced (57) and is subsequently downregulated (59–61), but not all forms of endocytosis may be affected in the same way.

Four general types of endocytosis can be distinguished on the basis of the size of cargo internalized and/or the mechanism of internalization: phagocytosis, macropinocytosis, clathrin-dependent receptor-mediated endocytosis, and caveolae-mediated endocytosis (190, 191) (Figure 5). Some forms of entry may involve an as-yet-uncharacterized non-clathrin/non-caveolar pathway. Furthermore, some pathogens (e.g., *Toxoplasma gondii*) gain entry by helping to form their own parasitophorous vacuoles *de novo* (192). Under normal conditions, the common fate for internalized solutes is delivery to hydrolase-rich lysosomes. In some cases, however, delivery to the Golgi complex or ER is also possible (131, 193, 194).

Macropinocytosis

One of the most common ways of studying antigen presentation ex vivo has been to expose APCs to large concentrations of soluble model antigens for various periods (1 h to 1 day). In the case of immature DCs and probably MØ, the bulk of these antigens are internalized via macropinocytosis (60, 61, 195). This form of endocytosis in DCs is downregulated upon maturation, but there seems to be little effect on clathrin-mediated pathway (61). Thus, even in mature DCs, antigen (at least when targeted to specific receptors), might still be internalized and thus in principle available for processing and representation.

The impact of antigen uptake via macropinocytosis in vivo is not clear. It may certainly apply to those cells encountering antigens present in fluids, but many antigen encounters probably occur in tissues, where extracellular fluid is not abundant. Furthermore, pathogens release few soluble antigens, with most proteins integrated in membranes, cell walls, or cytoplasmic compartments that would need to be taken up as particles (i.e., by phagocytosis).

Under conditions in which antigens are indeed available in soluble forms, especially after experimental injections of antigen, MØ and immature DCs use their well-developed macropinocytic activity for capture. In fact, MØ and DCs are the main cell types found to carry injected soluble antigens to lymph nodes after intravenous, intraperitoneal, or intradermal injections (25, 196, 197). In contrast, B cells have very low macropinocytic activity. If they are incubated ex vivo for long periods with high concentrations of soluble antigens, B cells manage to present them on MHC-II or MHC-I (16). These conditions are unlikely to occur in vivo, where B cells are mostly limited to the capture of trace amounts of antigens for which they carry specific cell surface receptors (see below). After intravenous injection of a high dose of hen egg lysozyme (HEL), most B cells display HEL-derived pMHC in vivo (198), although the pathway leading to presentation of nonspecific antigens by B cells is decidedly different than that responsible for receptor-mediated presentation (199). Moreover, when mice are injected with lower doses of antigen, no antigen internalization or pMHC formation is detected in B cells (31).

Mechanisms and Functions of Receptor-Mediated Endocytosis in Antigen Presentation

The immune system uses a broad range of cell surface receptors to capture extracellular material more efficiently (15, 200). Receptor-mediated antigen uptake has at least two important consequences for the immune system. First, the concentrating effect has clear quantitative advantages, making antigen capture by APCs both faster and more efficient because they can present antigen found at much lower concentrations, usually by several orders of magnitude (15). Even highly macropinocytic cells like MØ and DCs benefit from receptor-mediated uptake mechanisms: At least a fraction of the uptake of typical fluid phase markers (dextran, HRP) can be accounted for by mannose receptor binding in DCs (61, 195).

Second, qualitative aspects of receptor-mediated antigen uptake can contribute to functional diversity among different APCs, by selective expression of receptors or by functionally different consequences upon ligand engagement. An example of how expression of certain antigen receptors on select APCs can have profound effects on the immune response was provided by the study of DEC-205, a lectin-like receptor preferentially expressed by DCs that is internalized by clathrin coated vesicles (201–203). Targeting antigens to DEC-205 (using monoclonal antibodies against DEC-205 as surrogate ligands) resulted in a 100- to 1000-fold more efficient antigen capture and presentation than soluble antigen, inducing either tolerogenic responses (under noninflammatory conditions) or strong immunity (under activating conditions, co-administered with CD40L). Antigens delivered via DEC-205 were presented on both MHC-II and MHC-I, leading to strong activation of CD4 and CD8 T cells (128, 204, 205). These results indicate how targeting select APCs in situ via specific antigen receptors can be exploited successfully to manipulate antigen presentation and immunogenicity. The nature of the receptor and subsequent endosomal targeting pathways may also be key. DEC-205, for example, is more effective than mannose receptor in mediating antigen presentation in vitro (203); this may contribute to its efficacy in vivo.

An example of functional differences between APCs and their endocytic abilities is provided by Fcγ receptors (FcγR), which highlight how the immune system can use similar capture mechanisms for qualitatively different results. Antigens bound to soluble Ig can follow different fates depending on the cell type that captures them. Inhibitory, endocytosis-incompetent FcγR splice variants on B cells prevent receptor-mediated uptake of antibody-antigen complex (206), whereas endocytosis-competent FcγR on MØ and DCs foster antigen capture and presentation (15, 207). B cell type FcγR are also expressed on "follicular DCs" in B cell follicles, where they may help retain antigen for B cell recognition (208, 209). Finally, the MHC-I-related neonatal Fc receptor (FcRn) expressed on epithelial cells can capture IgG-antigen complexes, but instead of delivering their cargo to lysosomal compartments, they transcytose the immune complexes to the lamina propia, where they can then be recaptured by resident DCs (210).

Antigen receptors can be highly specific and selective for unique antigens, like the surface Ig on B cells. Their affinity for the antigen can sometimes be quite high, allowing B cells to capture antigens present at minute concentrations (15). Depending on the affinity of the bound antibodies, they can affect the release of antigen in endosomal compartments and even help sculpt the action of lysosomal proteases on the antigen. Such an "imprinting" effect of the bound antibody can mediate the selective pairing of B and T cells (16, 211, 212). Ligation of the B cell receptor also seems to induce rearrangement of endosomal compartments and is thought to promote pMHC formation (213).

Some APCs also express receptors for antigen-derived fragments bound to endogenous heat shock proteins, resulting in re-presentation of the internalized peptide (214, 215). Certain TLRs (e.g., TLR5) can bind directly to microbial antigens, and conceivably could also result in presentation (216).

Many other endocytic receptors on APCs (complement receptors, scavenger receptors, lectins) are not specific for individual protein antigens and do not recognize protein determinants directly. Many of them are related to similar receptors found in invertebrates and even in some unicellular organisms. These receptors are often implicated in adsorption of microbes, and are sometimes shown to be involved in their uptake, processing, and presentation. The lectin DC-SIGN, for example, interacts with HIV, although the immediate consequence is to sequester the virus from immune recognition rather than trigger a presentation response (217). The abundance of receptors, particularly lectins, on DCs and other APCs will likely provide an array of specificities that facilitate antigen uptake.

Phagocytosis

The uptake of particulate antigens is a very prevalent form of antigen uptake in vivo for both pathogen-derived and endogenous antigens. From an evolutionary perspective, it is probably also the first pathway associated with host defense. A number of the endocytic receptors that can recognize ligands free in solution also contribute to the phagocytic process by recognizing their ligands on the surface of microbes. These include FcγRs, complement receptors, and a variety of lectins. Even in the eventual absence of strong adsorptive receptors, some microbes can actively promote their own entry into cells (218) or shed vesicles that may be internalized (219).

APCs vary widely in their capacity for phagocytosis. B cells are very poorly phagocytic (220–222). Presentation of particulate antigens by some B cell lines has been described, but it was weaker and more limited than MØ and was significantly lower with B cells isolated from spleen (223). Other APCs like MØ and immature DCs can avidly phagocytose a broad range of particulates, including apoptotic cells, microbes, inert particles, or liposomes.

The engulfment of apoptotic cells provides antigenic material that can be readily converted into pMHC. DCs can actually produce pMHC-II complexes (YAe antigen) more efficiently from apoptotic splenocytes than from preprocessed peptide (224). The phagocytosis by APCs of endogenous cells that have died during microbial infections is emerging as an important way of sampling pathogens present in the engulfed cells, especially for microbes that may not infect APCs (33, 72, 225–228). The ingestion of apoptotic cells is also believed to play a key role in sampling self-antigens in the steady state for the maintenance of tolerance (73, 229, 230). When captured by APC, apoptotic cells have the potential to serve up a "complete meal" of self-antigens, in principle without regard to their intracellular localization or solubility, although it is not yet established that antigens in different intracellular localizations are equivalently processed. In fact, the intracellular location of antigen may affect presentation (96, 231, 232).

The capture of apoptotic bodies by DC was first described in cell culture, but DCs have been shown to acquire self-antigens from apoptotic cells and present them in situ (33, 233). It is not clear whether capture of apoptotic cells by DCs in vivo takes place before, during, or after cell death. If the lessons from model organisms apply to mammals, apoptosis and engulfment should be highly synchronized, favoring "local" engulfment triggered by death (24, 234).

DCs have been found to contain viral antigens shortly after infection under conditions in which DCs themselves do not appear infected, indicating that DCs capture viral antigens from neighboring infected cells (225). Also, DCs may not always wait for other cells to die before sampling them, since DCs could conceivably "bite" pieces of live neighboring cells (235, 236). There is evidence that T cells (237), B cells (223, 238), and DCs (239) nibble pieces of contacting live cells. Even infective viruses can be transferred between living cells without requiring cell death (240–244). The transfer of cell fragments between live neighboring cells has been described in several other systems, such as the transfer of melanin from melanocytes to keratinocytes in the skin (245) or the capture of membrane-bound ligands in invertebrates (246, 247).

Having considered the mechanisms of antigen uptake, we now turn to the mechanisms of antigen processing.

ANTIGEN PROCESSING IN THE MHC-I PATHWAY

It is now well established that the proteasome plays a critical role in initiating protein breakdown to generate most peptide ligands for MHC-I (82, 248–250). The subunit composition of the proteasome and the expression of modulatory cofactors can vary between tissues and also in response to an inflammatory environment, affecting the repertoire of peptides produced (251–254). The proteasome has also recently been implicated in the splicing of peptides to create MHC-I ligands that are not contiguous in the original protein sequence (114).

Proteasome digestion products usually require N-terminal trimming by cytosolic peptidases (255–257). A delicate balance must be maintained because excess trimming by cytosolic peptidases can also destroy MHC-I epitopes. Cytosolic chaperones are thought to protect peptides from exhaustive degradation in the cytosol (258). After peptides are transported into the ER, there is even further trimming by an amino peptidase resident in the ER (designated ERAAP or ERAP1) (259–262) (Figure 3). These final trimming steps, thought to be influenced by binding to MHC-I, are critical for proper peptide loading (82, 263, 264). For some epitopes, the residues flanking the core MHC-I ligand can influence processing (82), and mutations in such regions can result in immune evasion (265). These examples emphasize that the selection of antigenic peptides does not follow strict universal rules, contributing to our relative inability to predict immunogenicity.

Those antigens that are presented on MHC-I via the exogenous pathway in a proteasome and TAP-independent fashion are believed to be processed by lysosomal proteases. In fact, the lysosomal protease cathepsin S may be involved in the generation of MHC-I ligands from ovalbumin cross-presented via the TAP-independent vacuolar pathway (266).

ANTIGEN PROCESSING IN THE MHC-II PATHWAY

The processing of exogenous antigens for presentation on MHC-II molecules occurs within the endocytic pathway. However, our views of how pMHC-II are formed and loaded are still evolving as new regulatory mechanisms continue to emerge, particularly in DCs. One continuing problem has been the identification of the site(s) where antigen processing and peptide loading occur (Figure 6). Lysosomes (or late endosomes) have long been considered obvious candidates from the point of view that they favor digestion of internalized antigens. However, in most

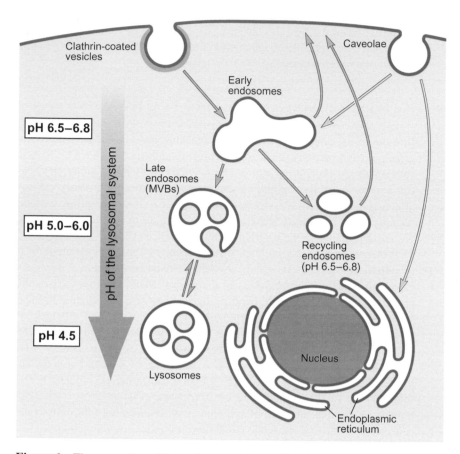

Figure 6   The organelles of the endocytic pathway. This figure illustrates the types of common endocytic organelles found in all cell types, including APCs. Most receptor recycling occurs rapidly (t1/2 1–2 min) via recycling endosomes, although a small fraction of recycling receptors (25%) reaches recycling endosomes from which the return to the plasma membrane occurs more slowly (20–30 min). Some transport from recycling endosomes to the Golgi complex may also occur. Ligands and receptors are targeted to lysosomes by being sorted from recycling receptors at the level of early endosomes. They are taken to late endosomes, which accumulate characteristic membrane inclusions (multivesicular bodies or MVBs) and then to lysosomes. This pathway exposes internalized cargo to a progressively lower pH and to higher concentrations of lysosomal hydrolases. Late endosomes and lysosomes probably are in continuous equilibrium with each other, with lysosomes fusing with late endosomes and being regenerated following complete degradation of digestible content. Caveolae mediate internalization to endosomes or to the ER (*blue arrows*).

cells, lysosomes rapidly cleave protein substrates to amino acids (267). Moreover, membrane transport from lysosomes to the plasma membrane is ordinarily inefficient or slow (268). Endosomes (early or recycling endosomes) provide for efficient recycling, but MHC-II molecules do not normally accumulate in these organelles, where most membrane proteins reside only briefly, perhaps not long enough to permit efficient peptide loading (190).

Work in B cell lines and MØ led to the idea that APCs overcome these problems by adaptations of the endocytic pathway, yielding putative specialized loading compartments first designated MIIC (for MHC-II compartments). However, MHC-II-containing compartments in these APCs were found to represent conventional endosomes and lysosomes and are simply the sites to which the bulk of MHC-II and HLA-DM accumulate (269, 270). Although these remain open issues, recent work suggests that DCs also utilize conventional endosomes and lysosomes but regulate their activities to optimize antigen processing (see below) (62). Before considering the sites of antigen processing, however, we should consider the event itself.

The Order of Events in Antigen Processing: Peptide Generation Versus Peptide Loading

A key question concerning antigen processing in the MHC-II pathway remains unresolved: Are peptides generated first and then loaded, as in the MHC-I pathway, or are peptides generated after binding of intact antigen to MHC-II molecules? Although the first model is widely presumed to be prevalent (in textbooks and nearly all diagrams), it is inherently problematic. Ten- to 15-mer peptides rarely accumulate in endocytic compartments, and certainly not at the concentrations and for the length of time presumably required to bind at equilibrium to MHC-II. Although this may occur, intermediate proteolytic fragments are rare and short lived in the terminal degradative environment of lysosomes.

An alternative model proposes that epitopes could be protected from destruction by binding as large proteins to MHC-II before lysosomal proteases have a chance to degrade them (271–274) (Figure 7). The open binding groove in MHC-II allows the binding to whole proteins or long polypeptides (275–281), and the protruding ends unprotected by MHC-II could be trimmed by endo- and exopeptidases, while the peptides in the MHC-II groove are protected from degradation (276, 282). Some support for this model comes from studies in which long polypeptides were found to co-precipitate with MHC-II molecules, at least in cells whose lysosomes were inactivated by treatment with acidification inhibitors (278, 283). These large polypeptides could then disappear, but whether they were actually the precursors of immunogenic peptides remains unknown.

Thus, the extent to which antigens bind to MHC-II before or after being cleaved remains unclear. A range of possible scenarios exists in which some proteins predominantly bind intact to MHC-II, others require fragmentation before they can bind to MHC-II, and still others experience a bit of both (Figure 7). In fact, examples can be found of proteins that apparently have to be cleaved before they can bind

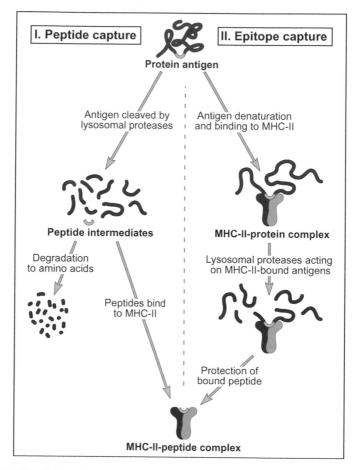

Figure 7 Possible pathways for generation of peptide-MHC-II complexes. Pathway I, "peptide capture," is perhaps the most commonly assumed. It is imagined that protein antigens are first cleaved by lysosomal proteases, and the resulting peptides then bind to MHC-II. In pathway II, "epitope capture," antigens would bind to MHC-II first, and the protruding ends unprotected by MHC-II would be subsequently trimmed by lysosomal proteases. These two pathways are not necessarily mutually exclusive, and antigens can follow a combination of both pathways I and II. (For further discussions on antigen processing mechanisms, see 15, 274.)

(284). For instance, the epitope 48–60 in HEL presented by I-A^b is blocked when Arg 61 is present (as in 48–61). This Arg 61 is efficiently removed in the C3H.SW mouse strain but not in the C57BL/6 strain, resulting in its unresponsiveness to HEL48-60, arguing for a role of cleavage at Arg61 before binding to I-A^b (285).

Although several considerations favor the model in which proteins are trimmed after binding to MHC-II, testing this model directly has been difficult (274).

However, if the "capture" model is indeed prevalent, then lysosomal proteases in APCs may simply be charged with a trimming function, which may not require much specificity. Therefore, the proteases could be quite redundant, raising the question of whether any lysosomal protease is indeed critical for MHC-II presentation. Truly APC-specific proteases have not yet been identified. The lysosomal proteases that have been implicated in the MHC-II pathway (e.g., cathepsins S, L, B, D, and AEP) are often expressed in other tissues at higher levels (197, 286, 287). Most lysosomal proteases are relatively nonspecific, reflecting their primary role in catabolism.

Biochemistry and Cell Biology of the Processing of the Invariant Chain Versus the Processing of Protein Antigens

The critical role of the invariant chain (Ii) in the MHC-II pathway raised significant interest in elucidating the proteolytic events leading to its degradation, which provides the opportunity to study the cleavage of a substrate common to all APCs (Figure 8). The results are often sought to argue for critical roles for selected proteases, but they could also be taken to indicate a fair amount of

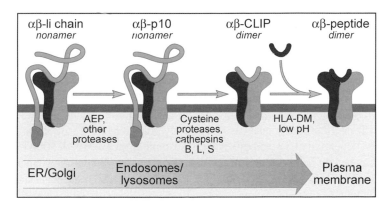

Figure 8   Overview of MHC-II-invariant chain processing. The cleavage of the nonameric Ii-MHC-II complex is typically initiated in endosomes by the cleavage of Ii chain by AEP (legumain) or other unidentified proteases to yield a ∼10 kD amino terminal Ii chain fragment termed p10. This fragment, which still contains the endosome-lysosome targeting signal in its cytoplasmic domain, remains as a trimer and interacts with three $\alpha\beta$ dimers. Further cleavage (involving various cathepsins including B, S, or L, depending on the cell types) results in a minimal class II–associated Ii-derived peptide (CLIP) bound to MHC-II. This cleavage is accompanied by the dissociation of the Ii chain-$\alpha\beta$ nonamer to yield three $\alpha\beta$ dimers. CLIP is subsequently exchanged for antigenic peptides, in a reaction favored by acidic pH and facilitated by the MHC-II-like chaperone HLA-DM.

redundancy (16, 288–292). For example, although Ii degradation can be initiated by asparagine-specific endopeptidase (AEP), other proteases can do it as well (293). The redundancy in initiating Ii cleavage is consistent with the difficulty in blocking these early steps using protease inhibitors (16, 288–292) or in $AEP^{-/-}$ mice (H. Ploegh, personal communication).

A large body of work has evaluated the role of individual proteases in the final steps of Ii degradation using knockout mice deficient in cathepsins B, S, L, and D. These studies found that complete Ii cleavage is affected in the thymus in the absence of cathepsin L (294), or in B cells and DCs in the absence of cat S (295, 296). The processing of Ii in MØ appeared qualitatively normal in mice deficient in cat L, cat S, or both (297), highlighting how different proteases can participate in cleaving the same substrate. Furthermore, the effects of cat L or cat S deficiency on MHC-II function can be haplotype specific (290). Finally, the accumulation of a nested set of Ii-derived peptides bound to MHC-II in cells lacking H2-M further suggests that in a single cell type the cleavage of Ii is not strictly site specific (181).

These results highlight the difficulties in evaluating the roles of individual lysosomal proteases in antigen processing using protease knockout mice. Even if an antigen is a preferred substrate for a genetically deleted protease, in the absence of that protease the next most likely enzyme might compensate. Also, phenotypes observed in the absence of a protease could be indirect. The lack of a particular protease can affect the stability and maturation of other enzymes. This may further affect the lysosomal environment, for example, by altering the steady-state levels of Ii, which is known to affect antigen presentation (298) and the endocytic system (299).

The apparent lack of specific cleavage requirements for Ii may also extend to the generation of MHC-II ligands. Indeed, Ii is also a good example of how different MHC-II molecules (mouse or human) can bind to the same peptide (CLIP), with different flanking sequences and slightly altered MHC-II topology, and then can be sequentially trimmed by several lysosomal proteases (274, 300). Some antigens may benefit from one or more proteolytic cleavages before they can bind to MHC-II, and in these cases, individual proteases may be important. One such example is the tetanus toxoid C-fragment, which depends on initial Asn-specific cleavage by AEP (301). These results have a straightforward interpretation because they were obtained by modifying cleavage sites in the antigen, without affecting proteolysis in the APC. Legumain (AEP) is an interesting protease for this purpose because it acts well on intact proteins. However, AEP is very specific for cleavage after accessible Asn. Furthermore, surface exposed Asn are often N-glycosylated in eukaryotes, making them resistant to AEP cleavage (302). Certain antigens can use other "unlocking" proteases: the introduction of a dibasic (Arg-Arg) motif (which is not expected to be a substrate for AEP) enhanced the presentation of HEL (303). Finally, at least for some antigens, denaturation at acid pH or reduction of disulfide bonds in lysosomes may cause sufficient unfolding to permit MHC-II binding without previous cleavage.

Lysosomal Proteolysis and Peptide-MHC-II Formation: Less is More?

Recent evidence indicates that different APCs can exhibit markedly different capacities for lysosomal degradation. Both in culture and in vivo, MØ express high levels of many lysosomal proteases, resulting in a high capacity for lysosomal digestion and allowing MØ to rapidly degrade internalized material (S. Trombetta, unpublished). Such remarkable capacity for lysosomal degradation may be used by MØ to destroy ingested microbes rapidly, serving a key role as a first line of defense. Indeed, such high proteolytic potential is shared by MØ in *Drosophila* (197), suggesting that avid ingestion and digestion by MØ may be evolutionary conserved as a feature of innate immunity.

In contrast, cells expressing high levels of MHC-II, like B cells and DCs, contain much lower levels of lysosomal proteases than MØ, and consequently have a much lower capacity for lysosomal degradation (S. Trombetta, unpublished). This finding may seem counterintuitive because APCs are usually thought to require highly proteolytic lysosomes to ensure cleavage of a broad range of substrates. However, this seemingly counterintuitive finding may actually account for a number of previous observations. Protection from premature lysosomal proteolysis enhanced pMHC-II formation for HEL, ovalbumin, RNase (304), and possibly peptides (185). Low lysosomal proteolysis may also provide better opportunities for modulation of pMHC-II formation by lysosomal pH or protease inhibitors, at least in DCs (see below).

A reduced capacity for lysosomal proteolysis may help to explain early in vitro observations (referred to as "antigenic memory") that were indeed one of the functional criteria used to identify DCs (19). In several different systems, DCs can generate pMHC complexes, both MHC-II and MHC-I, from antigens internalized up to three days earlier (19–21, 52, 55, 56, 305–308). Low lysosomal proteolysis allows DCs to preserve and disseminate internalized material during their migration to lymphoid organs (197), which may be related to the fact that several days may be required for DCs to journey from peripheral tissues to lymphoid organs (26, 31). If antigens were degraded too rapidly, they might be consumed prematurely or the resultant pMHC complexes might be turned over long before antigens had a chance for presentation to T cells. Furthermore, the reduced capacity for lysosomal proteolysis may play a role in the capacity of DCs to store and subsequently spread HIV (309) and other microbes, both pathological and beneficial (32). This characteristic is not shared by MØ.

DCs can further limit their capacity for proteolysis by expressing various protease inhibitors. These include the Ii p41 isoform (containing a protease inhibitor domain) (310) and members of the cystatin family, especially cystatin C, an exceptionally potent inhibitor of cathepsin S and L, but also of other cysteine proteases (311–313). From proteomic and microarray analysis, cystatin C appears to be a major component of immature DC lysosomes. Mixing experiments have shown the presence of functional protease inhibitors in DC extracts, which are sufficient to attenuate the lysosomal proteolytic potential from other cell types, including MØ (S. Trombetta, unpublished).

REGULATION OF ANTIGEN PROCESSING AND PRESENTATION IN THE MHC-II PATHWAY

Recent evidence indicates that pMHC-II formation by DCs can be regulated under physiological conditions. Inflammatory stimuli promote the formation and accumulation of HEL-derived pMHC in vivo (314) and in bone marrow–derived DCs (52, 55, 315). The induction of pMHC-II formation upon DC maturation is accompanied by a generalized activation of lysosomal function (56). The degradation of two different model antigens, HEL and HRP, is enhanced upon DC maturation, suggesting that the general proteolytic capacity in lysosomes is augmented, rather than a few specific cleavage steps of a select antigen. These observations suggest that lysosomal proteolysis could potentially be regulated independently of upregulation of co-stimulation, creating putative immature but active tolerogenic DCs (34).

When analyzed in vitro, both immature and mature DCs exhibited similar capacities for lysosomal proteolysis, indicating that lysosomes in immature DCs maintain conditions in vivo that attenuate their capacity for lysosomal proteolysis (56). The precise mechanism by which proteolysis is activated is unclear, but certain lysosomal proteases are converted to their mature forms (56, 316) or redistributed (316, 317) upon DC maturation. Lysosomal proteases can also be recruited in an orderly manner to maturing phagosomes (318, 319).

However, not all DC populations may exhibit each of these features. Human monocyte-derived DCs, for example, may not induce pMHC-II formation during maturation as much as they stabilize pMHC-II complexes formed at similar rates (308, 320). This stabilization may reflect the greatly reduced rate of MHC-II internalization that occurs in these cells concomitant with the cessation of macropinocytosis upon receipt of a maturation stimulus. Interestingly, monocyte-derived DCs may have protease contents more similar to MØ than to other DC populations (N. McCurley, E.S. Trombetta & I. Mellman, unpublished), suggesting that their lysosomes may not be amenable to as careful regulation and that these cells may have other distinct functional properties.

The Contribution of Lysosomal pH to the MHC-II Pathway and Its Regulation in APCs

Acidification of endosomes/lysosomes has long been known to be required for efficient antigen processing. Indeed, regulated activation of lysosomal acidification appears to be an important element controlling antigen presentation during DC maturation. The induction of maturation lowers lysosomal pH by ~1 pH unit, from ~pH 5.5 (suboptimal for proteolysis) to pH 4.5 (more adequate pH for proteolysis and peptide loading) (56), providing an attractive explanation for how maturation stimuli might enhance pMHC-II formation by DCs.

Lysosomal acidification can modulate antigen degradation and peptide loading in several ways besides optimizing proteolysis. Lower lysosomal pH may also favor other aspects of pMHC formation, such as binding of peptides or large fragments to MHC-II (321, 322), dissociation of Ii (181, 183, 323, 324), peptide editing by HLA-DM, and enzymatic disulfide reduction by GILT (325). The regulation of lysosomal pH is also a target for some pathogens, such as *Helicobacter* (326) and *Mycobacterium* (327, 328), which raise phagosomal pH, a feature expected to hinder MHC-II presentation.

Elucidating the signaling pathways that regulate acidification in DCs will be interesting because these signals may regulate lysosomal function separately from other hallmarks of DC maturation, such as the upregulation of costimulatory molecules. Such uncoupling may also be effected by alterations in cytokine environment, which has been proposed to affect lysosomal pH (329–331).

The control of lysosomal pH depends on many factors and is primarily due to the influx of H^+ into the lysosome (332) mediated by the vacuolar ATPase (V-ATPase) (333, 334). Modulation of lysosomal pH can thus be achieved by regulating the activity of the V-ATPase, which can occur in multiple ways and has been observed from unicellular eukaryotes to mammals (333, 334). One mechanism of V-ATPase activation involves the recruitment of the cytoplasmic sector (V1) onto the membrane bound V0 sector, resulting in a higher proportion of assembled and functional H^+ pumps (Figure 9). The regulated assembly and activity of the V-ATPase observed in developing DCs (56) has been described in yeast, insects, and vertebrates (335–340). The signals controlling V-ATPase assembly in any of these examples, much less in DCs, are unknown.

Other Factors Affecting pMHC Formation

Finally, a variety of posttranslational modifications are known to affect antigen processing or T cell recognition. Although the physiological relevance of these may not always be apparent, they do comprise a rich source of heterogeneity that must be considered to understand the immunogenicity of protein antigens.

Tumor cells, for example, can modulate the antigens they present in at least two ways. Downregulation of GILT in melanoma cells, for example, alters the presentation of disulfide-containing peptides on MHC-II (341). In the MHC-I pathway, alterations in the proteasome expression are also used by tumor cells to destroy specific T cell epitopes (85).

In some instances, T cell responses are specific for modified peptides including acetylation (342), isoaspartylation (343), deamidation (344, 345), citrullination (346), phosphorylation (347), glycosylation (342, 348–352), and possibly metal-coordination (353). Identifying the APCs capable of processing the modified proteins, as well as the mechanisms used, will be important (354). For example, DCs may not remove certain glycans, hindering T cell recognition of glycosylated peptides (355).

Thus, a variety of factors affecting the biochemistry of antigen processing and peptide modification contribute to the diversity of pMHC-II complexes. Most of

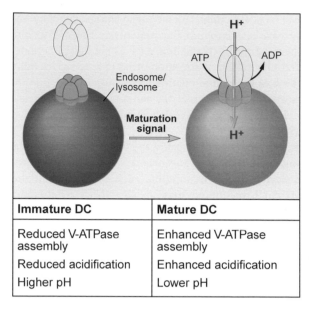

Immature DC	Mature DC
Reduced V-ATPase assembly	Enhanced V-ATPase assembly
Reduced acidification	Enhanced acidification
Higher pH	Lower pH

Figure 9   Schematic representation of regulated proton pump assembly. The pH inside endosomal/lysosomal compartments is regulated primarily by the action of an ATP-dependent proton pump or V-ATPase, a multisubunit complex containing membrane-bound (represented in *blue*) and peripheral components (represented in *yellow*) (326, 327). The activity of the V-ATPase can be regulated by multiple mechanisms. In DCs, induction of V-ATPase activity was found to correlate with enhanced assembly triggered by maturation.

these are as yet without known mechanisms and therefore are difficult to predict. Chaperones such as HLA-DO play some, but apparently contradictory, roles at this level (356, 357). It is also clear that specificity and predictability cannot be attributed to specialized protease mechanisms in either the MHC-II or the MHC-I pathways. Understanding antigen processing will likely require a more detailed understanding of its underlying cell biology, where DCs clearly excel at generating specialized or modified mechanisms to handle both antigens and MHC molecules.

CELL BIOLOGY OF MHC-II FUNCTION IN DENDRITIC CELLS

Like other APCs, DCs do not appear to have cell type–specific endocytic compartments devoted to antigen processing or peptide loading. Rather, they appear to modify the features of otherwise conventional organelles to overcome their inherent limitations (62). We have already considered how alterations in maturation or cytokine environment can control lysosomal acidification and antigen processing. Another important and unique feature, however, is how highly regulated the traffic of MHC-II molecules is from lysosomal compartments to the plasma membrane (17). This change reflects the contribution of multiple factors, the relative importance of each being likely to vary among different types of DCs.

In mouse bone marrow–derived DCs, newly synthesized MHC-II is largely transported according to the classical pathway first defined in lymphoblastoid and melanoma cells: After leaving the Golgi complex, $\alpha\beta$-Ii complexes are diverted from the constitutive secretory pathway (leading to the surface) and targeted to endocytic organelles, owing to the endosome-lysosome targeting signal found in the Ii cytoplasmic domain. Quantitative surface biotinylation studies suggest that only a minority of each new MHC-II cohort reaches the plasma membrane, but those molecules that do are rapidly internalized and arrive at endosomes as well (307, 358). Endosomes (especially early endosomes; see Figure 6) serve as sorting sites for membrane proteins, and continuously interrogate their cargo to determine which should proceed to the surface, be targeted to the Golgi complex, or be left to proceed to late endosomes/multivesicular bodies (MVBs) and lysosomes. For reasons that are not entirely understood, the latter pathway predominates in immature DCs (Figure 10A). Complete Ii cleavage and dissociation from $\alpha\beta$ dimers is affected in the absence of cathepsin S in DCs (and B cells). The activity of this enzyme (and other proteases) is suppressed in immature DCs both by the presence of abundant cystatin C and by the elevated pH found in the endocytic pathway. Indeed, although Ii chain cleavage still occurs, it occurs more slowly (311), with even a slight delay in its removal, probably explaining why the complex is sorted to late endocytic compartments (190). Regulation of cytosolic factors influencing membrane traffic might further promote this pathway.

Upon maturation, newly synthesized MHC-II is targeted directly to the plasma membrane, where it accumulates (Figure 10A). This could easily reflect an increased kinetic efficiency of Ii degradation due to an increase in cathepsin S and lysosomal protease activity in general (56, 311). Indeed, inhibiting cathepsin S activity (pharmacologically or by cystatin C overexpression) redirects new MHC-II to lysosomes, even in fully mature bone marrow–derived DCs. Clearly, however, other factors can be expected to play a role, especially given the dramatic overall reorganization exhibited by maturing DCs. For example, the decrease in macropinocytosis would tend to retain MHC-II at the surface, although some endocytosis might still be expected because of the continued activity of the clathrin-mediated pathway (61).

Human monocyte-derived DCs may use a different mechanism to achieve the same end. Perhaps because protease levels in these cells more closely approximate the higher levels found in MØ (see above), regulating MHC-II traffic by controlling Ii processing may be ineffective. Therefore, it appears that a greater cohort of new MHC-II reaches the surface even in immature cells, with the dramatic cessation of endocytosis possibly primarily responsible for achieving the increase in plasma membrane MHC-II at equilibrium (308). This difference may affect the nature of the peptides presented and may also reduce the ability of monocyte-derived DCs to sequester undigested antigen relative to other DC types, as discussed above.

In general, immature DCs contain abundant MVBs (359–362), classically defined as late endosomes or lysosomes containing internal vesicular inclusions. Interestingly, much of the MHC-II (>75%) found in MVBs is localized to these vesicular inclusions, a priori unexpected because in other cell types this

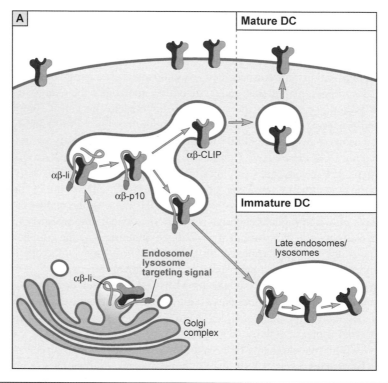

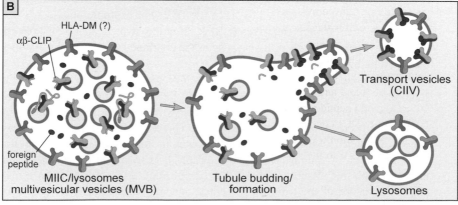

localization is generally reserved for receptors that are marked for degradation and downregulation (363). Thus, it is remarkable that DCs are capable of recovering even a portion of these MHC-II molecules upon maturation, by triggering the formation of tubular extensions from late endocytic compartments that carry MHC-II to the surface (320, 362), visible by live cell imaging experiments (63, 364) (Figure 10*B*). Indeed, the MHC-II becomes loaded with immunogenic peptide before activation of this previously unidentified retrograde pathway (52). That the tubules actually fuse with the plasma membrane has been directly demonstrated by total internal reflectance microscopy (63).

The source of the MHC-II molecules in these tubules, however, remains a bit uncertain. Maturation correlates with an apparent reduction in MVB profiles, leading to the suggestion that the internal vesicles fuse with the limiting membrane (362). They may also simply be degraded upon activation of lysosomal protease activity; MVB inclusions are indeed highly sensitive to such digestion in yeast, where they can only be seen in mutant strains affected in lysosomal proteolysis. MVB fusion has been suggested as a trigger for peptide loading because HLA-DM was at first thought to be present predominantly on the late endosome/lysosome limiting membrane (362); however, recent observations suggest that HLA-DM may be equally present on internal and limiting membranes (M. Ebersold, M. Pypaert, S. Trombetta, I. Mellman, unpublished).

In some cases, the pMHC-II-containing MVB compartments could also fuse directly with the plasma membrane of DCs (or other APCs, in this case), releasing the internal inclusions as "exosomes" (365, 366). These vesicles seem to contain many of the components required for T cell stimulation (367, 368) and prime immune responses in vitro and in vivo (369, 370). Exosomes can be released by many cell types, and probably reflect a normal process of lysosomal exocytosis which, in the case of cells such as NK and cytotoxic T cells, controls the release of the lysosome-like granules containing important effector elements (371).

Figure 10   Overview of MHC-II transport in DC. (*A*) Newly synthesized MHC II-Ii complexes are transported to late endosomes/lysosomes, where they accumulate in immature DCs. At this stage, lysosomes are poorly degradative, owing to the contribution of several factors, including (and most likely not limited to) elevated lysosomal pH and the accumulation of protease inhibitors (such as cystatin C and the p41 form of Ii). Upon maturation, the pH drops, lysosomal proteolysis is increased, and consequently cleavage of Ii and antigens is augmented, resulting in enhanced Ii removal, antigen processing, and peptide loading, followed by transport of MHC-II to the cell surface. (*B*) Immature DCs contain abundant MVBs, with MHC-II enriched in their internal vesicles. Maturation triggers the formation of tubular extensions from these MVBs that carry MHC-II to the cell surface. The MHC-II-rich internal vesicles either contribute to the process by fusing with the lysosome's limiting membrane (as proposed but as yet unproved) or are degraded upon the activation of lysosomal hydrolases upon maturation.

PERSPECTIVES

The demonstration of a regulated lysosome-to-plasma membrane pathway solved a major problem in DC biology, and in our understanding of antigen presentation in general. By using the lysosomal compartment as a primary site for antigen processing and peptide loading, DCs use lysosomes' ability to accumulate antigens and other molecules. At the same time, they limit the proteolytic potential of their lysosomes, and even further attenuate it prior to maturation. This arrangement not only ensures sufficient time for the biochemical events associated with pMHC-II formation, but also does so under conditions that are not so harsh as to result in the wanton destruction of potentially rare antigens. The final key was to provide an efficient mode of exit from this compartment, a pathway not commonly found in other cell types. Indeed, lysosome to plasma membrane transport probably does occur in other cell types, even if infrequently. However, the event remained undetected because of the lack of synchrony provided by DC maturation.

Our *leitmotiv* throughout has been considering the importance of applying in vitro results for understanding APC function in vivo. One can anticipate rich heterogeneity among different APC types, and even among different populations of DCs. Such a situation prevents inflexible generalizations, but it does provide insights that will be useful when considering how immune responses are initiated in vivo. Thus, we can now rationalize DC function knowing that they capture and retain antigen, degrading it slowly enough so that individual DCs can generate diverse and stable pMHC complexes that can be carried from the periphery to secondary lymphoid organs. Once there, the cells can then persist or their antigens can be captured by other APCs that might phagocytose incoming DCs or bind the exosomes they release. As a result, the DC has the dual role of not only presenting captured antigens but also disseminating them throughout the immune system. Combined with DCs' exceptional capacities for migration, homing, and expression of costimulatory, adhesion, and immunomodulatory molecules, their role as antigen conveyor is perhaps the most important general element describing their efficiency as initiators of antigen-dependent immunity.

DCs are therefore special in their ability to capture and present antigens. One potential qualitative difference is their capacity for cross-presentation, a feature that enables the DC to present antigens from microbes that may not infect DCs or from differentiated cells that express self-proteins not made by DCs. Apart from this, however, they are not fundamentally different from other APCs. Indeed, the entire logic of the immune response depends on the DC's ability to generate T lymphocytes that can go on to recognize pMHC complexes expressed by other cells, such as B cells, pathogen-infected cells, or tumor cells. DC specializations therefore relate to their unique ability to provide a controlling influence in the immune system, not to accomplish tasks that reflect entirely novel mechanisms in cell biology.

ACKNOWLEDGMENTS

The authors are most grateful to Ralph Steinman, Ona Bloom, and Mia Yun for reading early versions of the manuscript and for their incisive and helpful comments. We also thank Hidde Ploegh, Laurence Eisenlohr, and Peter Cresswell, among others, for so generously sharing unpublished information with us, and Graham Warren, members of the Mellaren lab, and many, many others for stimulating discussions. Finally, we are indebted to the American Heart Association, the National Institutes of Health, and the Ludwig Institute for Cancer Research for their continuing support and encouragement.

**The *Annual Review of Immunology* is online at
http://immunol.annualreviews.org**

LITERATURE CITED

1. Zinkernagel RM, Hengartner H. 2001. Regulation of the immune response by antigen. *Science* 293:251–53
2. Malissen B, Price MP, Goverman JM, McMillan M, White J, et al. 1984. Gene transfer of H-2 class II genes: antigen presentation by mouse fibroblast and hamster B-cell lines. *Cell* 36:319–27
3. Rock KL, Goldberg AL. 1999. Degradation of cell proteins and the generation of MHC class I-presented peptides. *Annu. Rev. Immunol.* 17:739–79
4. Jackson MR, Peterson PA. 1993. Assembly and intracellular transport of MHC class I molecules. *Annu. Rev. Cell Biol.* 9:207–35
5. Pamer E, Cresswell P. 1998. Mechanism of MHC classI-restricted antigen processing. *Annu. Rev. Immunol.* 16:323–58
6. Heemels MT, Ploegh H. 1995. Generation, translocation, and presentation of MHC class I-restricted peptides. *Annu. Rev. Biochem.* 64:463–91
7. York IA, Rock KL. 1996. Antigen processing and presentation by the class I major histocompatibility complex. *Annu. Rev. Immunol.* 14:369–96
8. Cresswell P. 1994. Assembly, transport, and function of MHC class II molecules. *Annu. Rev. Immunol.* 12:259–93
9. Wolf P, Ploegh H. 1995. How MHC class II molecules acquire peptide cargo: biosynthesis and trafficking through the endocytic pathway. *Annu. Rev. Cell Dev. Biol.* 11:267–306
10. Germain RN. 1994. MHC-dependent antigen processing and peptide presentation: providing ligands for T lymphocyte activation. *Cell* 76:287–99
11. Bryant P, Ploegh H. 2004. Class II MHC peptide loading by the professionals. *Curr. Opin. Immunol.* 16:96–102
12. Robadey C, Wallny HJ, Demotz S. 1996. Cell type-specific processing of the I-Ed-restricted hen egg lysozyme determinant 107–116. *Eur. J. Immunol.* 26:1656–59
13. Schneider SC, Sercarz EE. 1997. Antigen processing differences among APC. *Hum. Immunol.* 54:148–58
14. Mellman I, Turley SJ, Steinman RM. 1998. Antigen processing for amateurs and professionals. *Trends Cell Biol.* 8:231–37
15. Lanzavecchia A. 1990. Receptor-mediated antigen uptake and its effect on antigen presentation to class II-restricted T lymphocytes. *Annu. Rev. Immunol.* 8:773–93
16. Watts C. 1997. Capture and processing of exogenous antigens for presentation on MHC molecules. *Annu. Rev. Immunol.* 15:821–50

17. Mellman I, Steinman RM. 2001. Dendritic cells: specialized and regulated antigen processing machines. *Cell* 106:255–58

18. Steinman RM, Mellman IS, Muller WA, Cohn ZA. 1983. Endocytosis and the recycling of plasma membrane. *J. Cell Biol.* 96:1–27

19. Steinman RM. 1991. The dendritic cell system and its role in immunogenicity. *Annu. Rev. Immunol.* 9:271–96

20. Inaba K, Metlay JP, Crowley MT, Steinman RM. 1990. Dendritic cells pulsed with protein antigens in vitro can prime antigen-specific, MHC-restricted T cells in situ. *J. Exp. Med.* 172:631–40. Erratum. 1990. *J. Exp. Med.* 172(4): 1275

21. Crowley M, Inaba K, Steinman RM. 1990. Dendritic cells are the principal cells in mouse spleen bearing immunogenic fragments of foreign proteins. *J. Exp. Med.* 172:383–86

22. Steinman R, Inaba K. 1989. Immunogenicity: role of dendritic cells. *BioEssays* 10:145–52

23. Banchereau J, Steinman RM. 1998. Dendritic cells and the control of immunity. *Nature* 392:245–52

24. Lauber K, Blumenthal SG, Waibel M, Wesselborg S. 2004. Clearance of apoptotic cells; getting rid of the corpses. *Mol. Cell* 14:277–87

25. Aderem A, Underhill DM. 1999. Mechanisms of phagocytosis in macrophages. *Annu. Rev. Immunol.* 17:593–623

26. Itano AA, Jenkins MK. 2003. Antigen presentation to naive CD4 T cells in the lymph node. *Nat. Immunol.* 4:733–39

27. von Andrian UH, Mempel TR. 2003. Homing and cellular traffic in lymph nodes. *Nat. Rev. Immunol.* 3:867–78

28. Catron DM, Itano AA, Pape KA, Mueller DL, Jenkins MK. 2004. Visualizing the first 50 hr of the primary immune response to a soluble antigen. *Immunity* 21:341–47

29. Mempel TR, Henrickson SE, Von Andrian UH. 2004. T-cell priming by dendritic cells in lymph nodes occurs in three distinct phases. *Nature* 427:154–59

30. Randolph GJ. 2001. Dendritic cell migration to lymph nodes: cytokines, chemokines, and lipid mediators. *Semin. Immunol.* 13:267–74

31. Itano AA, McSorley SJ, Reinhardt RL, Ehst BD, Ingulli E, et al. 2003. Distinct dendritic cell populations sequentially present antigen to CD4 T cells and stimulate different aspects of cell-mediated immunity. *Immunity* 19:47–57

32. Macpherson AJ, Uhr T. 2004. Induction of protective IgA by intestinal dendritic cells carrying commensal bacteria. *Science* 303:1662–65

33. Huang FP, Platt N, Wykes M, Major JR, Powell TJ, et al. 2000. A discrete subpopulation of dendritic cells transports apoptotic intestinal epithelial cells to T cell areas of mesenteric lymph nodes. *J. Exp. Med.* 191:435–44

34. Steinman RM, Hawiger D, Nussenzweig MC. 2003. Tolerogenic dendritic cells. *Annu. Rev. Immunol.* 21:685–711

35. Unanue ER, Askonas BA. 1968. The immune response of mice to antigen in macrophages. *Immunology* 15:287–96

36. Chang MD, Stanley ER, Khalili H, Chisholm O, Pollard JW. 1995. Osteopetrotic (op/op) mice deficient in macrophages have the ability to mount a normal T-cell-dependent immune response. *Cell. Immunol.* 162:146–52

37. Wiktor-Jedrzejczak W, Ansari AA, Szperl M, Urbanowska E. 1992. Distinct in vivo functions of two macrophage subpopulations as evidenced by studies using macrophage-deficient op/op mouse. *Eur. J. Immunol.* 22:1951–54

38. Delemarre FG, Kors N, van Rooijen N. 1990. The in situ immune response in popliteal lymph nodes of mice after macrophage depletion. Differential effects of macrophages on thymus-dependent and thymus-independent immune responses. *Immunobiology* 180:395–404

39. Jung S, Unutmaz D, Wong P, Sano G, de los Santos K, et al. 2002. In vivo depletion of CD11c⁺ dendritic cells abrogates priming of CD8⁺ T cells by exogenous cell-associated antigens. *Immunity* 17:211–20

40. Lemos MP, Fan L, Lo D, Laufer TM. 2003. CD8α⁺ and CD11b⁺ dendritic cell-restricted MHC class II controls Th1 CD4⁺ T cell immunity. *J. Immunol.* 171:5077–84

41. Lemos MP, Esquivel F, Scott P, Laufer TM. 2004. MHC class II expression restricted to CD8α⁺ and CD11b⁺ dendritic cells is sufficient for control of *Leishmania major. J. Exp. Med.* 199:725–30

42. Lanzavecchia A, Sallusto F. 2001. Regulation of T cell immunity by dendritic cells. *Cell* 106:263–66

43. Yamazaki S, Iyoda T, Tarbell K, Olson K, Velinzon K, et al. 2003. Direct expansion of functional CD25⁺ CD4⁺ regulatory T cells by antigen-processing dendritic cells. *J. Exp. Med.* 198:235–47

44. Tarbell KV, Yamazaki S, Olson K, Toy P, Steinman RM. 2004. CD25⁺ CD4⁺ T cells, expanded with dendritic cells presenting a single autoantigenic peptide, suppress autoimmune diabetes. *J. Exp. Med.* 199:1467–77

45. Delamarre L, Holcombe H, Mellman I. 2003. Presentation of exogenous antigens on major histocompatibility complex (MHC) class I and MHC class II molecules is differentially regulated during dendritic cell maturation. *J. Exp. Med.* 198:111–22

46. Albert ML, Pearce SF, Francisco LM, Sauter B, Roy P, et al. 1998. Immature dendritic cells phagocytose apoptotic cells via ανβ5 and CD36, and cross-present antigens to cytotoxic T lymphocytes. *J. Exp. Med.* 188:1359–68

47. Inaba K, Steinman RM. 1986. Accessory cell-T lymphocyte interactions. Antigen-dependent and -independent clustering. *J. Exp. Med.* 163:247–61

48. Inaba K, Romani N, Steinman RM. 1989. An antigen-independent contact mechanism as an early step in T cell-proliferative responses to dendritic cells. *J. Exp. Med.* 170:527–42

49. Steinman RM, Inaba K. 1988. The binding of antigen presenting cells to T lymphocytes. *Adv. Exp. Med. Biol.* 237:31–41

50. Kropshofer H, Spindeldreher S, Rohn TA, Platania N, Grygar C, et al. 2002. Tetraspan microdomains distinct from lipid rafts enrich select peptide-MHC class II complexes. *Nat. Immunol.* 3:61–68

51. Rohn TA, Boes M, Wolters D, Spindeldreher S, Muller B, et al. 2004. Upregulation of the CLIP self peptide on mature dendritic cells antagonizes T helper type 1 polarization. *Nat. Immunol.* 5:909–18

52. Turley SJ, Inaba K, Steinman RM, Mellman I. 2000. Transport of peptide-MHC class II complexes in developing dendritic cells. *Science* 288:522–27

53. Bertho N, Cerny J, Kim YM, Fiebiger E, Ploegh H, Boes M. 2003. Requirements for T cell-polarized tubulation of class II+ compartments in dendritic cells. *J. Immunol.* 171:5689–96

54. Larsen CP, Steinman RM, Witmer PM, Hankins DF, Morris PJ, Austyn JM. 1990. Migration and maturation of Langerhans cells in skin transplants and explants. *J. Exp. Med.* 172:1483–93

55. Inaba K, Turley S, Iyoda T, Yamaide F, Shimoyama S, et al. 2000. The formation of immunogenic major histocompatibility complex class II-peptide ligands in lysosomal compartments of dendritic cells is regulated by inflammatory stimuli. *J. Exp. Med.* 191:927–36

56. Trombetta ES, Ebersold M, Garrett W, Pypaert M, Mellman I. 2003. Activation of lysosomal function during dendritic cell maturation. *Science* 299:1400–3

57. West MA, Wallin RP, Matthews SP, Svensson HG, Zaru R, et al. 2004. Enhanced dendritic cell antigen capture via Toll-like receptor-induced actin remodeling. *Science* 305:1153–57

58. Steinman RM, Swanson J. 1995. The endocytic activity of dendritic cells. *J. Exp. Med.* 182:283–88

59. Sallusto F, Lanzavecchia A. 1994. Efficient presentation of soluble antigen by cultured human dendritic cells is maintained by granulocyte/macrophage colony-stimulating factor plus interleukin 4 and downregulated by tumor necrosis factor α. *J. Exp. Med.* 179:1109–18

60. West MA, Prescott AR, Eskelinen EL, Ridley AJ, Watts C. 2000. Rac is required for constitutive macropinocytosis by dendritic cells but does not control its downregulation. *Curr. Biol.* 10:839–48

61. Garrett WS, Chen LM, Kroschewski R, Ebersold M, Turley S, et al. 2000. Developmental control of endocytosis in dendritic cells by Cdc42. *Cell* 102:325–34

62. Chow A, Mellman I. 2005. Old lysosomes, new tricks: dynamics of MHC class II transport in dendritic cells. *Trends Immunol.* In press

63. Chow A, Toomre D, Garrett W, Mellman I. 2002. Dendritic cell maturation triggers retrograde MHC class II transport from lysosomes to the plasma membrane. *Nature* 418:988–94

64. Inaba K, Pack M, Inaba M, Sakuta H, Isdell F, Steinman RM. 1997. High levels of a major histocompatibility complex II-self peptide complex on dendritic cells from the T cell areas of lymph nodes. *J. Exp. Med.* 186:665–72

65. Steinman RM, Pack M, Inaba K. 1997. Dendritic cells in the T-cell areas of lymphoid organs. *Immunol. Rev.* 156:25–37

66. Liu K, Iyoda T, Saternus M, Kimura Y, Inaba K, Steinman RM. 2002. Immune tolerance after delivery of dying cells to dendritic cells in situ. *J. Exp. Med.* 196:1091–97

67. Fujii S, Liu K, Smith C, Bonito AJ, Steinman RM. 2004. The linkage of innate to adaptive immunity via maturing dendritic cells in vivo requires CD40 ligation in addition to antigen presentation and CD80/86 costimulation. *J. Exp. Med.* 199:1607–18

68. Wilson NS, El-Sukkari D, Belz GT, Smith CM, Steptoe RJ, et al. 2003. Most lymphoid organ dendritic cell types are phenotypically and functionally immature. *Blood* 102:2187–94

69. Shortman K, Liu YJ. 2002. Mouse and human dendritic cell subtypes. *Nat. Rev. Immunol.* 2:151–61

70. Banchereau J, Briere F, Caux C, Davoust J, Lebecque S, et al. 2000. Immunobiology of dendritic cells. *Annu. Rev. Immunol.* 18:767–811

71. Liu Y. 2001. Dendritic cell subsets and lineages, and their functions in innate and adaptive immunity. *Cell* 106:259–62

72. Carbone F, Heath W. 2003. The role of dendritic cell subsets in immunity to viruses. *Curr. Opin. Immunol.* 15:416–20

73. Iyoda T, Shimoyama S, Liu K, Omatsu Y, Akiyama Y, et al. 2002. The CD8+ dendritic cell subset selectively endocytoses dying cells in culture and in vivo. *J. Exp. Med.* 195:1289–302

74. Banchereau J, Pascual V, Palucka AK. 2004. Autoimmunity through cytokine-induced dendritic cell activation. *Immunity* 20:539–50

75. Choi J, Enis DR, Koh KP, Shiao SL, Pober JS. 2004. T lymphocyte-endothelial cell interactions. *Annu. Rev. Immunol.* 22:683–709

76. Bottazzo GF, Pujol-Borrell R, Hanafusa T, Feldmann M. 1983. Role of aberrant HLA-DR expression and antigen presentation in induction of endocrine autoimmunity. *Lancet* 2:1115–19

77. Ostrand-Rosenberg S. 1994. Tumor immunotherapy: the tumor cell as an antigen-presenting cell. *Curr. Opin. Immunol.* 6:722–27

78. Muntasell A, Carrascal M, Serradell L, van Veelen P, Verreck F, et al. 2002. HLA-DR4 molecules in neuroendocrine epithelial cells associate to a heterogeneous repertoire of cytoplasmic and

surface self peptides. *J. Immunol.* 169:5052–60

79. Muntasell A, Carrascal M, Alvarez I, Serradell L, van Veelen P, et al. 2004. Dissection of the HLA-DR4 peptide repertoire in endocrine epithelial cells: strong influence of invariant chain and HLA-DM expression on the nature of ligands. *J. Immunol.* 173:1085–93

80. Boon T, Van Pel A. 1989. T cell-recognized antigenic peptides derived from the cellular genome are not protein degradation products but can be generated directly by transcription and translation of short subgenic regions. A hypothesis. *Immunogenetics* 29:75–79

81. Mayrand SM, Green WR. 1998. Nontraditionally derived CTL epitopes: exceptions that prove the rules? *Immunol. Today* 19:551–56

82. Shastri N, Schwab S, Serwold T. 2002. Producing nature's gene-chips: the generation of peptides for display by MHC class I molecules. *Annu. Rev. Immunol.* 20:463–93

83. Bullock TN, Eisenlohr LC. 1996. Ribosomal scanning past the primary initiation codon as a mechanism for expression of CTL epitopes encoded in alternative reading frames. *J. Exp. Med.* 184:1319–29

84. Saeterdal I, Bjorheim J, Lislerud K, Gjertsen MK, Bukholm IK, et al. 2001. Frameshift-mutation-derived peptides as tumor-specific antigens in inherited and spontaneous colorectal cancer. *Proc. Natl. Acad. Sci. USA* 98:13255–60

85. Probst-Kepper M, Stroobant V, Kridel R, Gaugler B, Landry C, et al. 2001. An alternative open reading frame of the human macrophage colony-stimulating factor gene is independently translated and codes for an antigenic peptide of 14 amino acids recognized by tumor-infiltrating CD8 T lymphocytes. *J. Exp. Med.* 193:1189–98

86. Wang RF, Parkhurst MR, Kawakami Y, Robbins PF, Rosenberg SA. 1996. Utilization of an alternative open reading frame of a normal gene in generating a novel human cancer antigen. *J. Exp. Med.* 183:1131–40

87. Rimoldi D, Rubio-Godoy V, Dutoit V, Lienard D, Salvi S, et al. 2000. Efficient simultaneous presentation of NY-ESO-1/LAGE-1 primary and nonprimary open reading frame-derived CTL epitopes in melanoma. *J. Immunol.* 165:7253–61

88. Saulquin X, Scotet E, Trautmann L, Peyrat MA, Halary F, et al. 2002. +1 Frameshifting as a novel mechanism to generate a cryptic cytotoxic T lymphocyte epitope derived from human interleukin 10. *J. Exp. Med.* 195:353–58

89. Cardinaud S, Moris A, Fevrier M, Rohrlich PS, Weiss L, et al. 2004. Identification of cryptic MHC I-restricted epitopes encoded by HIV-1 alternative reading frames. *J. Exp. Med.* 199:1053–63

90. Yewdell JW, Schubert U, Bennink JR. 2001. At the crossroads of cell biology and immunology: DRiPs and other sources of peptide ligands for MHC class I molecules. *J. Cell Sci.* 114:845–51

91. Lelouard H, Gatti E, Cappello F, Gresser O, Camosseto V, Pierre P. 2002. Transient aggregation of ubiquitinated proteins during dendritic cell maturation. *Nature* 417:177–82

92. Lelouard H, Ferrand V, Marguet D, Bania J, Camosseto V, et al. 2004. Dendritic cell aggresome-like induced structures are dedicated areas for ubiquitination and storage of newly synthesized defective proteins. *J. Cell Biol.* 164:667–75

93. Mosse CA, Meadows L, Luckey CJ, Kittlesen DJ, Huczko EL, et al. 1998. The class I antigen-processing pathway for the membrane protein tyrosinase involves translation in the endoplasmic reticulum and processing in the cytosol. *J. Exp. Med.* 187:37–48

94. Zarling AL, Ficarro SB, White FM, Shabanowitz J, Hunt DF, Engelhard VH. 2000. Phosphorylated peptides are naturally processed and presented by

major histocompatibility complex class I molecules in vivo. *J. Exp. Med.* 192:1755–62

95. Chen W, Yewdell JW, Levine RL, Bennink JR. 1999. Modification of cysteine residues in vitro and in vivo affects the immunogenicity and antigenicity of major histocompatibility complex class I-restricted viral determinants. *J. Exp. Med.* 189:1757–64

96. Shen L, Rock KL. 2004. Cellular protein is the source of cross-priming antigen in vivo. *Proc. Natl. Acad. Sci. USA* 101:3035–40

97. Norbury CC, Basta S, Donohue KB, Tscharke DC, Princiotta MF, et al. 2004. CD8$^+$ T cell cross-priming via transfer of proteasome substrates. *Science* 304:1318–21

98. Wolkers MC, Brouwenstijn N, Bakker AH, Toebes M, Schumacher TN. 2004. Antigen bias in T cell cross-priming. *Science* 304:1314–17

99. Bacik I, Snyder HL, Anton LC, Russ G, Chen W, et al. 1997. Introduction of a glycosylation site into a secreted protein provides evidence for an alternative antigen processing pathway: transport of precursors of major histocompatibility complex class I-restricted peptides from the endoplasmic reticulum to the cytosol. *J. Exp. Med.* 186:479–87

100. Bonifacino JS, Weissman AM. 1998. Ubiquitin and the control of protein fate in the secretory and endocytic pathways. *Annu. Rev. Cell Dev. Biol.* 14:19–57

101. Ellgaard L, Molinari M, Helenius A. 1999. Setting the standards: quality control in the secretory pathway. *Science* 286:1882–88

102. Trombetta ES, Parodi AJ. 2003. Quality control and glycoprotein folding in the secretory pathway. *Annu. Rev. Cell Dev. Biol.* 19:649–76

103. Tsai B, Ye Y, Rapoport TA. 2002. Retrotranslocation of proteins from the endoplasmic reticulum into the cytosol. *Nat. Rev. Mol. Cell Biol.* 3:246–55

104. Lilley BN, Ploegh HL. 2004. A membrane protein required for dislocation of misfolded proteins from the ER. *Nature* 429:834–40

105. Ye Y, Shibata Y, Yun C, Ron D, Rapoport TA. 2004. A membrane protein complex mediates retro-translocation from the ER lumen into the cytosol. *Nature* 429:841–47

106. Furman MH, Ploegh H. 2002. Lessons from viral manipulation of protein disposal pathways. *J. Clin. Invest.* 110:875–79

107. Tortorella D, Gewurz BE, Furman MH, Schust DJ, Ploegh HL. 2000. Viral subversion of the immune system. *Annu. Rev. Immunol.* 18:861–926

108. Yewdell JW, Hill AB. 2002. Viral interference with antigen presentation. *Nat. Immunol.* 3:1019–25

109. Wei ML, Cresswell P. 1992. HLA-A2 molecules in an antigen-processing mutant cell contain signal sequence-derived peptides. *Nature* 356:443–46

110. Henderson RA, Michel H, Sakaguchi K, Shabanowitz J, Appella E, et al. 1992. HLA-A2.1-associated peptides from a mutant cell line: a second pathway of antigen presentation. *Science* 255:1264–66

111. Hombach J, Pircher H, Tonegawa S, Zinkernagel RM. 1995. Strictly transporter of antigen presentation (TAP)-dependent presentation of an immunodominant cytotoxic T lymphocyte epitope in the signal sequence of a virus protein. *J. Exp. Med.* 182:1615–19

112. Braciale TJ, Braciale VL, Winkler M, Stroynowski I, Hood L, et al. 1987. On the role of the transmembrane anchor sequence of influenza hemagglutinin in target cell recognition by class I MHC-restricted, hemagglutinin-specific cytolytic T lymphocytes. *J. Exp. Med.* 166:678–92

113. Hanada K, Yewdell JW, Yang JC. 2004. Immune recognition of a human renal cancer antigen through post-translational protein splicing. *Nature* 427:252–56

114. Vigneron N, Stroobant V, Chapiro J, Ooms A, Degiovanni G, et al. 2004. An antigenic peptide produced by peptide splicing in the proteasome. *Science* 304:587–90

115. Sigal LJ, Crotty S, Andino R, Rock KL. 1999. Cytotoxic T-cell immunity to virus-infected non-haematopoietic cells requires presentation of exogenous antigen. *Nature* 398:77–80

116. Pfeifer JD, Wick MJ, Roberts RL, Findlay K, Normark SJ, Harding CV. 1993. Phagocytic processing of bacterial antigens for class I MHC presentation to T cells. *Nature* 361:359–62

117. Bachmann MF, Oxenius A, Pircher H, Hengartner H, Ashton-Richardt PA, et al. 1995. TAP1-independent loading of class I molecules by exogenous viral proteins. *Eur. J. Immunol.* 25:1739–43

118. Kleijmeer MJ, Escola JN, UytdeHaag FG, Jakobson E, Griffith JM, et al. 2001. Antigen loading of MHC class I molecules in the endocytic tract. *Traffic* 2:124–37

119. Berwin B, Rosser MF, Brinker KG, Nicchitta CV. 2002. Transfer of GRP94(Gp96)-associated peptides onto endosomal MHC class I molecules. *Traffic* 3:358–66

120. Ackerman AL, Cresswell P. 2004. Cellular mechanisms governing cross-presentation of exogenous antigens. *Nat. Immunol.* 5:678–84

121. Harding CV, Song R. 1994. Phagocytic processing of exogenous particulate antigens by macrophages for presentation by class I MHC molecules. *J. Immunol.* 153:4925–33

122. Norbury CC, Hewlett LJ, Prescott AR, Shastri N, Watts C. 1995. Class I MHC presentation of exogenous soluble antigen via macropinocytosis in bone marrow macrophages. *Immunity* 3:783–91

123. Kovacsovics-Bankowski M, Rock KL. 1995. A phagosome-to-cytosol pathway for exogenous antigens presented on MHC class I molecules. *Science* 267:243–46

124. Rodriguez A, Regnault A, Kleijmeer M, Ricciardi-Castagnoli P, Amigorena S. 1999. Selective transport of internalized antigens to the cytosol for MHC class I presentation in dendritic cells. *Nat. Cell Biol.* 1:362–68

125. den Haan JM, Bevan MJ. 2002. Constitutive versus activation-dependent cross-presentation of immune complexes by CD8$^+$ and CD8$^-$ dendritic cells in vivo. *J. Exp. Med.* 196:817–27

126. Reis e Sousa C, Germain RN. 1995. Major histocompatibility complex class I presentation of peptides derived from soluble exogenous antigen by a subset of cells engaged in phagocytosis. *J. Exp. Med.* 182:841–51

127. Gil-Torregrosa BC, Lennon-Dumenil AM, Kessler B, Guermonprez P, Ploegh HL, et al. 2004. Control of cross-presentation during dendritic cell maturation. *Eur. J. Immunol.* 34:398–407

128. Bonifaz LC, Bonnyay DP, Charalambous A, Darguste DI, Fujii S, et al. 2004. In vivo targeting of antigens to maturing dendritic cells via the DEC-205 receptor improves T cell vaccination. *J. Exp. Med.* 199:815–24

129. Rock KL. 1996. A new foreign policy: MHC class I molecules monitor the outside world. *Immunol. Today* 17:131–37

130. Steinman RM, Inaba K, Turley S, Pierre P, Mellman I. 1999. Antigen capture, processing, and presentation by dendritic cells: recent cell biological studies. *Hum. Immunol.* 60:562–67

131. Sandvig K, Van Deurs B. 2002. Membrane traffic exploited by protein toxins. *Annu. Rev. Cell Dev. Biol.* 18:1–24

132. Falguieres T, Mallard F, Baron C, Hanau D, Lingwood C, et al. 2001. Targeting of Shiga toxin B-subunit to retrograde transport route in association with detergent-resistant membranes. *Mol. Biol. Cell* 12:2453–68

133. Smith DC, Lord JM, Roberts LM, Tartour E, Johannes L. 2002. 1st class ticket to class I: protein toxins as pathfinders

for antigen presentation. *Traffic* 3:697–704

134. Anderson HA, Chen Y, Norkin LC. 1996. Bound simian virus 40 translocates to caveolin-enriched membrane domains, and its entry is inhibited by drugs that selectively disrupt caveolae. *Mol. Biol. Cell* 7:1825–34

135. Pelkmans L, Kartenbeck J, Helenius A. 2001. Caveolar endocytosis of simian virus 40 reveals a new two-step vesicular-transport pathway to the ER. *Nat. Cell Biol.* 3:473–83

136. Norkin LC, Anderson HA, Wolfrom SA, Oppenheim A. 2002. Caveolar endocytosis of simian virus 40 is followed by brefeldin A-sensitive transport to the endoplasmic reticulum, where the virus disassembles. *J. Virol.* 76:5156–66

137. Miesenbock G, Rothman JE. 1995. The capacity to retrieve escaped ER proteins extends to the trans-most cisterna of the Golgi stack. *J. Cell Biol.* 129:309–19

138. Gu F, Aniento F, Parton RG, Gruenberg J. 1997. Functional dissection of COP-I subunits in the biogenesis of multivesicular endosomes. *J. Cell Biol.* 139:1183–95

139. Whitney JA, Gomez M, Sheff D, Kreis TE, Mellman I. 1995. Cytoplasmic coat proteins involved in endosome function. *Cell* 83:703–13

140. Daro E, Sheff D, Gomez M, Kreis T, Mellman I. 1997. Inhibition of endosome function in CHO cells bearing a temperature-sensitive defect in the coatomer (COPI) component ε-COP. *J. Cell Biol.* 139:1747–59

141. Gagnon E, Duclos S, Rondeau C, Chevet E, Cameron PH, et al. 2002. Endoplasmic reticulum-mediated phagocytosis is a mechanism of entry into macrophages. *Cell* 110:119–31

142. Desjardins M. 2003. ER-mediated phagocytosis: a new membrane for new functions. *Nat. Rev. Immunol.* 3:280–91

143. Houde M, Bertholet S, Gagnon E, Brunet S, Goyette G, et al. 2003. Phagosomes are competent organelles for antigen cross-presentation. *Nature* 425:402–6

144. Guermonprez P, Saveanu L, Kleijmeer M, Davoust J, Van Endert P, Amigorena S. 2003. ER-phagosome fusion defines an MHC class I cross-presentation compartment in dendritic cells. *Nature* 425:397–402

145. Ackerman AL, Kyritsis C, Tampe R, Cresswell P. 2003. Early phagosomes in dendritic cells form a cellular compartment sufficient for cross presentation of exogenous antigens. *Proc. Natl. Acad. Sci. USA* 100:12889–94

146. Bajno L, Peng XR, Schreiber AD, Moore HP, Trimble WS, Grinstein S. 2000. Focal exocytosis of VAMP3-containing vesicles at sites of phagosome formation. *J. Cell Biol.* 149:697–706

147. Henry RM, Hoppe AD, Joshi N, Swanson JA. 2004. The uniformity of phagosome maturation in macrophages. *J. Cell Biol.* 164:185–94

148. Roy CR. 2002. Exploitation of the endoplasmic reticulum by bacterial pathogens. *Trends Microbiol.* 10:418–24

149. Fajardo M, Schleicher M, Noegel A, Bozzaro S, Killinger S, et al. 2004. Calnexin, calreticulin and cytoskeleton-associated proteins modulate uptake and growth of *Legionella pneumophila* in *Dictyostelium discoideum*. *Microbiology* 150:2825–35

150. Lizee G, Basha G, Tiong J, Julien JP, Tian M, et al. 2003. Control of dendritic cell cross-presentation by the major histocompatibility complex class I cytoplasmic domain. *Nat. Immunol.* 4:1065–73

151. Michalek MT, Benacerraf B, Rock KL. 1992. The class II MHC-restricted presentation of endogenously synthesized ovalbumin displays clonal variation, requires endosomal/lysosomal processing, and is up-regulated by heat shock. *J. Immunol.* 148:1016–24

152. Jacobson S, Sekaly RP, Jacobson CL, McFarland HF, Long EO. 1989. HLA class II-restricted presentation of cytoplasmic

measles virus antigens to cytotoxic T cells. *J. Virol.* 63:1756–62

153. Nuchtern JG, Biddison WE, Klausner RD. 1990. Class II MHC molecules can use the endogenous pathway of antigen presentation. *Nature* 343:74–76

154. van Binnendijk RS, Poelen MC, de Vries P, Voorma HO, Osterhaus AD, Uytdehaag FG. 1989. Measles virus-specific human T cell clones. Characterization of specificity and function of CD4$^+$ helper/cytotoxic and CD8$^+$ cytotoxic T cell clones. *J. Immunol.* 142:2847–54

155. Malnati MS, Marti M, LaVaute T, Jaraquemada D, Biddison W, et al. 1992. Processing pathways for presentation of cytosolic antigen to MHC class II-restricted T cells. *Nature* 357:702–4

156. Brooks AG, McCluskey J. 1993. Class II-restricted presentation of a hen egg lysozyme determinant derived from endogenous antigen sequestered in the cytoplasm or endoplasmic reticulum of the antigen presenting cells. *J. Immunol.* 150:3690–97

157. Jaraquemada D, Marti M, Long EO. 1990. An endogenous processing pathway in vaccinia virus-infected cells for presentation of cytoplasmic antigens to class II-restricted T cells. *J. Exp. Med.* 172:947–54

158. Mukherjee P, Dani A, Bhatia S, Singh N, Rudensky AY, et al. 2001. Efficient presentation of both cytosolic and endogenous transmembrane protein antigens on MHC class II is dependent on cytoplasmic proteolysis. *J. Immunol.* 167:2632–41

159. Oxenius A, Bachmann MF, Ashton-Rickardt PG, Tonegawa S, Zinkernagel RM, Hengartner H. 1995. Presentation of endogenous viral proteins in association with major histocompatibility complex class II: on the role of intracellular compartmentalization, invariant chain and the TAP transporter system. *Eur. J. Immunol.* 25:3402–11

160. Oxenius A, Bachmann MF, Mathis D, Benoist C, Zinkernagel RM, Hengartner H. 1997. Functional in vivo MHC class II loading by endogenously synthesized glycoprotein during viral infection. *J. Immunol.* 158:5717–26

161. Oukka M, Colucci-Guyon E, Tran PL, Cohen-Tannoudji M, Babinet C, et al. 1996. CD4 T cell tolerance to nuclear proteins induced by medullary thymic epithelium. *Immunity* 4:545–53

162. Sant AJ. 1994. Endogenous antigen presentation by MHC class II molecules. *Immunol. Res.* 13:253–67

163. Hunt DF, Michel H, Dickinson TA, Shabanowitz J, Cox AL, et al. 1992. Peptides presented to the immune system by the murine class II major histocompatibility complex molecule I-Ad. *Science* 256:1817–20

164. Nelson CA, Roof RW, McCourt DW, Unanue ER. 1992. Identification of the naturally processed form of hen egg white lysozyme bound to the murine major histocompatibility complex class II molecule I-Ak. *Proc. Natl. Acad. Sci. USA* 89:7380–83

165. Engelhard VH. 1994. Structure of peptides associated with class I and class II MHC molecules. *Annu. Rev. Immunol.* 12:181–207

166. Rudensky A, Preston-Hurlburt P, Hong SC, Barlow A, Janeway CA Jr. 1991. Sequence analysis of peptides bound to MHC class II molecules. *Nature* 353:622–27

167. Chicz RM, Urban RG, Lane WS, Gorga JC, Stern LJ, et al. 1992. Predominant naturally processed peptides bound to HLA-DR1 are derived from MHC-related molecules and are heterogeneous in size. *Nature* 358:764–68

168. Chicz RM, Urban RG, Gorga JC, Vignali DA, Lane WS, Strominger JL. 1993. Specificity and promiscuity among naturally processed peptides bound to HLA-DR alleles. *J. Exp. Med.* 178:27–47

169. Newcomb JR, Cresswell P. 1993. Characterization of endogenous peptides bound to purified HLA-DR molecules and their

absence from invariant chain-associated α β dimers. *J. Immunol.* 150:499–507

170. Dongre AR, Kovats S, deRoos P, McCormack AL, Nakagawa T, et al. 2001. In vivo MHC class II presentation of cytosolic proteins revealed by rapid automated tandem mass spectrometry and functional analyses. *Eur. J. Immunol.* 31:1485–94

171. Lechler R, Aichinger G, Lightstone L. 1996. The endogenous pathway of MHC class II antigen presentation. *Immunol. Rev.* 151:51–79

172. Nimmerjahn F, Milosevic S, Behrends U, Jaffee EM, Pardoll DM, et al. 2003. Major histocompatibility complex class II-restricted presentation of a cytosolic antigen by autophagy. *Eur. J. Immunol.* 33:1250–59

173. Munz C. 2004. Epstein-Barr virus nuclear antigen 1: from immunologically invisible to a promising T cell target. *J. Exp. Med.* 199:1301–4

174. Lich JD, Elliott JF, Blum JS. 2000. Cytoplasmic processing is a prerequisite for presentation of an endogenous antigen by major histocompatibility complex class II proteins. *J. Exp. Med.* 191:1513–24

175. Harding CV, Ramachandra L, Wick MJ. 2003. Interaction of bacteria with antigen presenting cells: influences on antigen presentation and antibacterial immunity. *Curr. Opin. Immunol.* 15:112–19

176. Sacks D, Sher A. 2002. Evasion of innate immunity by parasitic protozoa. *Nat. Immunol.* 3:1041–47

177. Santambrogio L, Sato AK, Carven GJ, Belyanskaya SL, Strominger JL, Stern LJ. 1999. Extracellular antigen processing and presentation by immature dendritic cells. *Proc. Natl. Acad. Sci. USA* 96:15056–61

178. Santambrogio L, Sato AK, Fischer FR, Dorf ME, Stern LJ. 1999. Abundant empty class II MHC molecules on the surface of immature dendritic cells. *Proc. Natl. Acad. Sci. USA* 96:15050–55

179. Andersson T, Patwardhan A, Emilson A, Carlsson K, Scheynius A. 1998. HLA-DM is expressed on the cell surface and colocalizes with HLA-DR and invariant chain in human Langerhans cells. *Arch. Dermatol. Res.* 290:674–80

180. Arndt SO, Vogt AB, Markovic-Plese S, Martin R, Moldenhauer G, et al. 2000. Functional HLA-DM on the surface of B cells and immature dendritic cells. *EMBO J.* 19:1241–51

181. Riberdy JM, Newcomb JR, Surman MJ, Barbosa JA, Cresswell P. 1992. HLA-DR molecules from an antigen-processing mutant cell line are associated with invariant chain peptides. *Nature* 360:474–77

182. Denzin LK, Cresswell P. 1995. HLA-DM induces CLIP dissociation from MHC class II α β dimers and facilitates peptide loading. *Cell* 82:155–65

183. Sloan VS, Cameron P, Porter G, Gammon M, Amaya M, et al. 1995. Mediation by HLA-DM of dissociation of peptides from HLA-DR. *Nature* 375:802–6

184. Pu Z, Carrero JA, Unanue ER. 2002. Distinct recognition by two subsets of T cells of an MHC class II-peptide complex. *Proc. Natl. Acad. Sci. USA* 99:8844–49

185. Pu Z, Lovitch SB, Bikoff EK, Unanue ER. 2004. T cells distinguish MHC-peptide complexes formed in separate vesicles and edited by H2-DM. *Immunity* 20:467–76

186. Hulsmeyer M, Fiorillo MT, Bettosini F, Sorrentino R, Saenger W, et al. 2004. Dual, HLA-B27 subtype-dependent conformation of a self-peptide. *J. Exp. Med.* 199:271–81

187. Underhill DM, Ozinsky A. 2002. Phagocytosis of microbes: complexity in action. *Annu. Rev. Immunol.* 20:825–52

188. Blander JM, Medzhitov R. 2004. Regulation of phagosome maturation by signals from Toll-like receptors. *Science* 304:1014–18

189. Doyle SE, O'Connell RM, Miranda GA, Vaidya SA, Chow EK, et al. 2004. Toll-like receptors induce a phagocytic gene

program through p38. *J. Exp. Med.* 199:
81–90

190. Mellman I. 1996. Endocytosis and molecular sorting. *Annu. Rev. Cell Dev. Biol.*
12:575–625

191. Conner SD, Schmid SL. 2003. Regulated portals of entry into the cell. *Nature*
422:37–44

192. Sinai AP, Joiner KA. 1997. Safe haven: the cell biology of nonfusogenic pathogen vacuoles. *Annu. Rev. Microbiol.* 51:415–62

193. Montesano R, Roth J, Robert A, Orci L. 1982. Non-coated membrane invaginations are involved in binding and internalization of cholera and tetanus toxins. *Nature* 296:651–53

194. Pelkmans L, Helenius A. 2003. Insider information: what viruses tell us about endocytosis. *Curr. Opin. Cell Biol.* 15:414–22

195. Sallusto F, Cella M, Danieli C, Lanzavecchia A. 1995. Dendritic cells use macropinocytosis and the mannose receptor to concentrate macromolecules in the major histocompatibility complex class II compartment: downregulation by cytokines and bacterial products. *J. Exp. Med.* 182:389–400

196. Silverstein SC, Steinman RM, Cohn ZA. 1977. Endocytosis. *Annu. Rev. Biochem.* 46:669–722

197. Delamarre L, Pack M, Chang H, Mellman I, Trombetta S. 2005. Differential lysosomal proteolysis in antigen presenting cells determines antigen fate in vivo. *Science.* In press

198. Zhong G, Reis e Sousa C, Germain RN. 1997. Antigen-unspecific B cells and lymphoid dendritic cells both show extensive surface expression of processed antigen-major histocompatibility complex class II complexes after soluble protein exposure in vivo or in vitro. *J. Exp. Med.* 186:673–82

199. Lazzarino DA, Blier P, Mellman I. 1998. The monomeric guanosine triphosphatase rab4 controls an essential step on the path-

way of receptor-mediated antigen processing in B cells. *J. Exp. Med.* 188:1769–74

200. Lanzavecchia A. 1985. Antigen-specific interaction between T and B cells. *Nature* 314:537–39

201. Jiang W, Swiggard WJ, Heufler C, Peng M, Mirza A, et al. 1995. The receptor DEC-205 expressed by dendritic cells and thymic epithelial cells is involved in antigen processing. *Nature* 375:151–55

202. Inaba K, Swiggard WJ, Inaba M, Meltzer J, Mirza A, et al. 1995. Tissue distribution of the DEC-205 protein that is detected by the monoclonal antibody NLDC-145. I. Expression on dendritic cells and other subsets of mouse leukocytes. *Cell. Immunol.* 163:148–56

203. Mahnke K, Guo M, Lee S, Sepulveda H, Swain SL, et al. 2000. The dendritic cell receptor for endocytosis, DEC-205, can recycle and enhance antigen presentation via major histocompatibility complex class II-positive lysosomal compartments. *J. Cell Biol.* 151:673–84

204. Hawiger D, Inaba K, Dorsett Y, Guo M, Mahnke K, et al. 2001. Dendritic cells induce peripheral T cell unresponsiveness under steady state conditions in vivo. *J. Exp. Med.* 194:769–79

205. Bonifaz L, Bonnyay D, Mahnke K, Rivera M, Nussenzweig MC, Steinman RM. 2002. Efficient targeting of protein antigen to the dendritic cell receptor DEC-205 in the steady state leads to antigen presentation on major histocompatibility complex class I products and peripheral CD8+ T cell tolerance. *J. Exp. Med.* 196:1627–38

206. Amigorena S, Bonnerot C, Drake JR, Choquet D, Hunziker W, et al. 1992. Cytoplasmic domain heterogeneity and functions of IgG Fc receptors in B lymphocytes. *Science* 256:1808–12

207. Regnault A, Lankar D, Lacabanne V, Rodriguez A, Thery C, et al. 1999. Fcγ receptor-mediated induction of dendritic

cell maturation and major histocompatibility complex class I-restricted antigen presentation after immune complex internalization. *J. Exp. Med.* 189:371–80

208. Heyman B. 2000. Regulation of antibody responses via antibodies, complement, and Fc receptors. *Annu. Rev. Immunol.* 18:709–37

209. Tew JG, Wu J, Fakher M, Szakal AK, Qin D. 2001. Follicular dendritic cells: beyond the necessity of T-cell help. *Trends Immunol.* 22:361–67

210. Yoshida M, Claypool SM, Wagner JS, Mizoguchi E, Mizoguchi A, et al. 2004. Human neonatal Fc receptor mediates transport of IgG into luminal secretions for delivery of antigens to mucosal dendritic cells. *Immunity* 20:769–83

211. Simitsek PD, Campbell DG, Lanzavecchia A, Fairweather N, Watts C. 1995. Modulation of antigen processing by bound antibodies can boost or suppress class II major histocompatibility complex presentation of different T cell determinants. *J. Exp. Med.* 181:1957–63

212. Jaume JC, Parry SL, Madec AM, Sonderstrup G, Baekkeskov S. 2002. Suppressive effect of glutamic acid decarboxylase 65-specific autoimmune B lymphocytes on processing of T cell determinants located within the antibody epitope. *J. Immunol.* 169:665–72

213. Lankar D, Vincent-Schneider H, Briken V, Yokozeki T, Raposo G, Bonnerot C. 2002. Dynamics of major histocompatibility complex class II compartments during B cell receptor-mediated cell activation. *J. Exp. Med.* 195:461–72

214. Berwin B, Hart JP, Rice S, Gass C, Pizzo SV, et al. 2003. Scavenger receptor-A mediates gp96/GRP94 and calreticulin internalization by antigen-presenting cells. *EMBO J.* 22:6127–36

215. Becker T, Hartl FU, Wieland F. 2002. CD40, an extracellular receptor for binding and uptake of Hsp70-peptide complexes. *J. Cell Biol.* 158:1277–85

216. Hayashi F, Smith KD, Ozinsky A, Hawn TR, Yi EC, et al. 2001. The innate immune response to bacterial flagellin is mediated by Toll-like receptor 5. *Nature* 410:1099–103

217. Geijtenbeek TBH, van Vliet SJ, Engering A, 't Hart BA, van Kooyk Y. 2004. Self- and nonself-recognition by C-type lectins on dendritic cells. *Annu. Rev. Immunol.* 22:33–54

218. Cossart P, Sansonetti PJ. 2004. Bacterial invasion: the paradigms of enteroinvasive pathogens. *Science* 304:242–48

219. Wai SN, Lindmark B, Soderblom T, Takade A, Westermark M, et al. 2003. Vesicle-mediated export and assembly of pore-forming oligomers of the enterobacterial ClyA cytotoxin. *Cell* 115:25–35

220. Dal Monte P, Szoka FC Jr. 1989. Effect of liposome encapsulation on antigen presentation in vitro. Comparison of presentation by peritoneal macrophages and B cell tumors. *J. Immunol.* 142:1437–43

221. Stockinger B. 1992. Capacity of antigen uptake by B cells, fibroblasts or macrophages determines efficiency of presentation of a soluble self antigen (C5) to T lymphocytes. *Eur. J. Immunol.* 22:1271–78

222. Galelli A, Charlot B, Deriaud E, Leclerc C. 1993. B cells do not present antigen covalently linked to microspheres. *Immunology* 79:69–76

223. Vidard L, Kovacsovics-Bankowski M, Kraeft SK, Chen LB, Benacerraf B, Rock KL. 1996. Analysis of MHC class II presentation of particulate antigens of B lymphocytes. *J. Immunol.* 156:2809–18

224. Inaba K, Turley S, Yamaide F, Iyoda T, Mahnke K, et al. 1998. Efficient presentation of phagocytosed cellular fragments on the major histocompatibility complex class II products of dendritic cells. *J. Exp. Med.* 188:2163–73

225. Fleeton MN, Contractor N, Leon F, Wetzel JD, Dermody TS, Kelsall BL. 2004. Peyer's patch dendritic cells process viral antigen from apoptotic epithelial cells in

the intestine of reovirus-infected mice. *J. Exp. Med.* 200:235–45

226. Ravichandran KS. 2003. "Recruitment signals" from apoptotic cells: invitation to a quiet meal. *Cell* 113:817–20

227. Larsson M, Fonteneau JF, Bhardwaj N. 2001. Dendritic cells resurrect antigens from dead cells. *Trends Immunol.* 22:141–48

228. Fonteneau JF, Larsson M, Bhardwaj N. 2002. Interactions between dead cells and dendritic cells in the induction of antiviral CTL responses. *Curr. Opin. Immunol.* 14:471–77

229. Steinman RM, Turley S, Mellman I, Inaba K. 2000. The induction of tolerance by dendritic cells that have captured apoptotic cells. *J. Exp. Med.* 191:411–16

230. Savill J, Dransfield I, Gregory C, Haslett C. 2002. A blast from the past: clearance of apoptotic cells regulates immune responses. *Nat. Rev. Immunol.* 2:965–75

231. Ferry H, Jones M, Vaux DJ, Roberts IS, Cornall RJ. 2003. The cellular location of self-antigen determines the positive and negative selection of autoreactive B cells. *J. Exp. Med.* 198:1415–25

232. Golovina TN, Wherry EJ, Bullock TN, Eisenlohr LC. 2002. Efficient and qualitatively distinct MHC class I-restricted presentation of antigen targeted to the endoplasmic reticulum. *J. Immunol.* 168:2667–75

233. Mougneau E, Hugues S, Glaichenhaus N. 2002. Antigen presentation by dendritic cells in vivo. *J. Exp. Med.* 196:1013–16

234. Reddien PW, Horvitz HR. 2004. The engulfment process of programmed cell death in *Caenorhabditis elegans. Annu. Rev. Cell Dev. Biol.* 20:193–221

235. Harshyne LA, Watkins SC, Gambotto A, Barratt-Boyes SM. 2001. Dendritic cells acquire antigens from live cells for cross-presentation to CTL. *J. Immunol.* 166:3717–23

236. Joly E, Hudrisier D. 2003. What is trogocytosis and what is its purpose? *Nat. Immunol.* 4:815

237. Huang JF, Yang Y, Sepulveda H, Shi W, Hwang I, et al. 1999. TCR-mediated internalization of peptide-MHC complexes acquired by T cells. *Science* 286:952–54

238. Batista FD, Iber D, Neuberger MS. 2001. B cells acquire antigen from target cells after synapse formation. *Nature* 411:489–94

239. Valdez Y, Mah W, Winslow MM, Xu L, Ling P, Townsend SE. 2002. Major histocompatibility complex class II presentation of cell-associated antigen is mediated by CD8α^+ dendritic cells in vivo. *J. Exp. Med.* 195:683–94

240. Jolly C, Kashefi K, Hollinshead M, Sattentau QJ. 2004. HIV-1 cell to cell transfer across an Env-induced, actin-dependent synapse. *J. Exp. Med.* 199:283–93

241. Sornasse T, Flamand V, De Becker G, Bazin H, Tielemans F, et al. 1992. Antigen-pulsed dendritic cells can efficiently induce an antibody response in vivo. *J. Exp. Med.* 175:15–21

242. Wykes M, Pombo A, Jenkins C, MacPherson GG. 1998. Dendritic cells interact directly with naive B lymphocytes to transfer antigen and initiate class switching in a primary T-dependent response. *J. Immunol.* 161:1313–19

243. MacPherson G, Kushnir N, Wykes M. 1999. Dendritic cells, B cells and the regulation of antibody synthesis. *Immunol. Rev.* 172:325–34

244. Colino J, Shen Y, Snapper CM. 2002. Dendritic cells pulsed with intact *Streptococcus pneumoniae* elicit both protein- and polysaccharide-specific immunoglobulin isotype responses in vivo through distinct mechanisms. *J. Exp. Med.* 195: 1–13

245. Seiberg M. 2001. Keratinocyte-melanocyte interactions during melanosome transfer. *Pigment Cell Res.* 14:236–42

246. Cagan RL, Kramer H, Hart AC, Zipursky SL. 1992. The bride of sevenless and sevenless interaction: internalization of a transmembrane ligand. *Cell* 69:393–99

247. Henderson ST, Gao D, Lambie EJ, Kimble J. 1994. *lag-2* may encode a signaling ligand for the GLP-1 and LIN-12 receptors of *C. elegans. Development* 120:2913–24

248. York IA, Goldberg AL, Mo XY, Rock KL. 1999. Proteolysis and class I major histocompatibility complex antigen presentation. *Immunol. Rev.* 172:49–66

249. Niedermann G, Geier E, Lucchiari-Hartz M, Hitziger N, Ramsperger A, Eichmann K. 1999. The specificity of proteasomes: impact on MHC class I processing and presentation of antigens. *Immunol. Rev.* 172:29–48

250. Voges D, Zwickl P, Baumeister W. 1999. The 26S proteasome: a molecular machine designed for controlled proteolysis. *Annu. Rev. Biochem.* 68:1015–68

251. Hill CP, Masters EI, Whitby FG. 2002. The 11S regulators of 20S proteasome activity. *Curr. Top. Microbiol. Immunol.* 268:73–89

252. Whitby FG, Masters EI, Kramer L, Knowlton JR, Yao Y, et al. 2000. Structural basis for the activation of 20S proteasomes by 11S regulators. *Nature* 408:115–20

253. Goldberg AL, Cascio P, Saric T, Rock KL. 2002. The importance of the proteasome and subsequent proteolytic steps in the generation of antigenic peptides. *Mol. Immunol.* 39:147–64

254. Cascio P, Call M, Petre BM, Walz T, Goldberg AL. 2002. Properties of the hybrid form of the 26S proteasome containing both 19S and PA28 complexes. *EMBO J.* 21:2636–45

255. Kessler B, Hong X, Petrovic J, Borodovsky A, Dantuma NP, et al. 2003. Pathways accessory to proteasomal proteolysis are less efficient in major histocompatibility complex class I antigen production. *J. Biol. Chem.* 278:10013–21

256. Kessler BM, Glas R, Ploegh HL. 2002. MHC class I antigen processing regulated by cytosolic proteolysis-short cuts that alter peptide generation. *Mol. Immunol.* 39:171–79

257. Rock KL, York IA, Goldberg AL. 2004. Post-proteasomal antigen processing for major histocompatibility complex class I presentation. *Nat. Immunol.* 5:670–77

258. Kunisawa J, Shastri N. 2003. The group II chaperonin TRiC protects proteolytic intermediates from degradation in the MHC class I antigen processing pathway. *Mol. Cell* 12:565–76

259. Eisenlohr LC, Bacik I, Bennink JR, Bernstein K, Yewdell JW. 1992. Expression of a membrane protease enhances presentation of endogenous antigens to MHC class I-restricted T lymphocytes. *Cell* 71:963–72

260. Snyder HL, Yewdell JW, Bennink JR. 1994. Trimming of antigenic peptides in an early secretory compartment. *J. Exp. Med.* 180:2389–94

261. Serwold T, Gonzalez F, Kim J, Jacob R, Shastri N. 2002. ERAAP customizes peptides for MHC class I molecules in the endoplasmic reticulum. *Nature* 419:480–83

262. York IA, Chang SC, Saric T, Keys JA, Favreau JM, et al. 2002. The ER aminopeptidase ERAP1 enhances or limits antigen presentation by trimming epitopes to 8–9 residues. *Nat. Immunol.* 3:1177–84

263. Falk K, Rotzschke O, Rammensee HG. 1990. Cellular peptide composition governed by major histocompatibility complex class I molecules. *Nature* 348:248–51

264. Brouwenstijn N, Serwold T, Shastri N. 2001. MHC class I molecules can direct proteolytic cleavage of antigenic precursors in the endoplasmic reticulum. *Immunity* 15:95–104

265. Draenert R, Le Gall S, Pfafferott KJ, Leslie AJ, Chetty P, et al. 2004. Immune selection for altered antigen processing leads to cytotoxic T lymphocyte escape in chronic HIV-1 infection. *J. Exp. Med.* 199:905–15

266. Shen L, Sigal LJ, Boes M, Rock KL. 2004. Important role of cathepsin S in generating peptides for TAP-independent MHC class I crosspresentation in vivo. *Immunity* 21:155–65

267. De Duve C, Wattiaux R. 1966. Functions of lysosomes. *Annu. Rev. Physiol.* 28:435–92

268. Kornfeld S, Mellman I. 1989. The biogenesis of lysosomes. *Annu. Rev. Cell Biol.* 5:483–525

269. Pierre P, Denzin LK, Hammond C, Drake JR, Amigorena S, et al. 1996. HLA-DM is localized to conventional and unconventional MHC class II-containing endocytic compartments. *Immunity* 4:229–39

270. Kleijmeer MJ, Morkowski S, Griffith JM, Rudensky AY, Geuze HJ. 1997. Major histocompatibility complex class II compartments in human and mouse B lymphoblasts represent conventional endocytic compartments. *J. Cell Biol.* 139:639–49

271. Werdelin O. 1986. Determinant protection. A hypothesis for the activity of immune response genes in the processing and presentation of antigens by macrophages. *Scand. J. Immunol.* 24: 625–36

272. Deng H, Apple R, Clare-Salzler M, Trembleau S, Mathis D, et al. 1993. Determinant capture as a possible mechanism of protection afforded by major histocompatibility complex class II molecules in autoimmune disease. *J. Exp. Med.* 178:1675–80

273. Sercarz EE, Lehmann PV, Ametani A, Benichou G, Miller A, Moudgil K. 1993. Dominance and crypticity of T cell antigenic determinants. *Annu. Rev. Immunol.* 11:729–66

274. Sercarz EE, Maverakis E. 2003. MHC-guided processing: binding of large antigen fragments. *Nat. Rev. Immunol.* 3:621–29

275. Lee P, Matsueda GR, Allen PM. 1988. T cell recognition of fibrinogen. A determinant on the A alpha-chain does not require processing. *J. Immunol.* 140:1063–68

276. Donermeyer DL, Allen PM. 1989. Binding to Ia protects an immunogenic peptide from proteolytic degradation. *J. Immunol.* 142:1063–68

277. Sette A, Adorini L, Colon SM, Buus S, Grey HM. 1989. Capacity of intact proteins to bind to MHC class II molecules. *J. Immunol.* 143:1265–67

278. Castellino F, Zappacosta F, Coligan JE, Germain RN. 1998. Large protein fragments as substrates for endocytic antigen capture by MHC class II molecules. *J. Immunol.* 161:4048–57

279. Jensen PE. 1993. Acidification and disulfide reduction can be sufficient to allow intact proteins to bind class II MHC. *J. Immunol.* 150:3347–56

280. Lindner R, Unanue ER. 1996. Distinct antigen MHC class II complexes generated by separate processing pathways. *EMBO J.* 15:6910–20

281. Streicher HZ, Berkower IJ, Busch M, Gurd FR, Berzofsky JA. 1984. Antigen conformation determines processing requirements for T-cell activation. *Proc. Natl. Acad. Sci. USA* 81:6831–35

282. Mouritsen S, Meldal M, Werdelin O, Hansen AS, Buus S. 1992. MHC molecules protect T cell epitopes against proteolytic destruction. *J. Immunol.* 149: 1987–93

283. Villadangos JA, Driesen C, Shi G, Chapman HA, Ploegh H. 2000. Early endosomal maturation of MHC class II molecules independently of cysteine proteases and H-2M. *EMBO J.* 19:882–91

284. Davidson HW, Reid PA, Lanzavecchia A, Watts C. 1991. Processed antigen binds to newly synthesized MHC class II molecules in antigen-specific B lymphocytes. *Cell* 67:105–16

285. Grewal IS, Moudgil KD, Sercarz EE. 1995. Hindrance of binding to class II major histocompatibility complex molecules by a single amino acid residue contiguous to a determinant leads to crypticity of the

determinant as well as lack of response to the protein antigen. *Proc. Natl. Acad. Sci. USA* 92:1779–83

286. Barrett A, Rawlings N, Woessner J, eds. 2003. *Handbook of Proteolytic Enzymes.* New York: Academic Press. 2nd ed.

287. Shi GP, Webb AC, Foster KE, Knoll JH, Lemere CA, et al. 1994. Human cathepsin S: chromosomal localization, gene structure, and tissue distribution. *J. Biol. Chem.* 269:11530–36

288. Villadangos JA, Ploegh HL. 2000. Proteolysis in MHC class II antigen presentation: Who's in charge? *Immunity* 12:233–39

289. Lennon-Dumenil AM, Bakker AH, Wolf-Bryant P, Ploegh HL, Lagaudriere-Gesbert C. 2002. A closer look at proteolysis and MHC-class-II-restricted antigen presentation. *Curr. Opin. Immunol.* 14:15–21

290. Honey K, Rudensky AY. 2003. Lysosomal cysteine proteases regulate antigen presentation. *Nat. Rev. Immunol.* 3:472–82

291. Driessen C, Lennon-Dumenil AM, Ploegh HL. 2001. Individual cathepsins degrade immune complexes internalized by antigen-presenting cells via Fcγ receptors. *Eur. J. Immunol.* 31:1592–601

292. Honey K, Nakagawa T, Peters C, Rudensky A. 2002. Cathepsin L regulates CD4$^+$ T cell selection independently of its effect on invariant chain: a role in the generation of positively selecting peptide ligands. *J. Exp. Med.* 195:1349–58

293. Manoury B, Mazzeo D, Li DN, Billson J, Loak K, et al. 2003. Asparagine endopeptidase can initiate the removal of the MHC class II invariant chain chaperone. *Immunity* 18:489–98

294. Nakagawa T, Roth W, Wong P, Nelson A, Farr A, et al. 1998. Cathepsin L: critical role in Ii degradation and CD4 T cell selection in the thymus. *Science* 280:450–53

295. Nakagawa TY, Brissette WH, Lira PD, Griffiths RJ, Petrushova N, et al. 1999.

Impaired invariant chain degradation and antigen presentation and diminished collagen-induced arthritis in cathepsin S null mice. *Immunity* 10:207–17

296. Driessen C, Bryant RA, Lennon-Dumenil AM, Villadangos JA, Bryant PW, et al. 1999. Cathepsin S controls the trafficking and maturation of MHC class II molecules in dendritic cells. *J. Cell Biol.* 147:775–90

297. Shi GP, Bryant RA, Riese R, Verhelst S, Driessen C, et al. 2000. Role for cathepsin F in invariant chain processing and major histocompatibility complex class II peptide loading by macrophages. *J. Exp. Med.* 191:1177–86

298. Sant AJ, Miller J. 1994. MHC class II antigen processing: biology of invariant chain. *Curr. Opin. Immunol.* 6:57–63

299. Romagnoli P, Layet C, Yewdell J, Bakke O, Germain RN. 1993. Relationship between invariant chain expression and major histocompatibility complex class II transport into early and late endocytic compartments. *J. Exp. Med.* 177:583–96

300. Zhu Y, Rudensky AY, Corper AL, Teyton L, Wilson IA. 2003. Crystal structure of MHC class II I-A^b in complex with a human CLIP peptide: prediction of an I-A^b peptide-binding motif. *J. Mol. Biol.* 326:1157–74

301. Antoniou AN, Blackwood SL, Mazzeo D, Watts C. 2000. Control of antigen presentation by a single protease cleavage site. *Immunity* 12:391–98

302. Manoury B, Hewitt E, Morrice N, Dando P, Barrett A, Watts C. 1998. An asparaginyl endopeptidase processes a microbial antigen for class II MHC presentation. *Nature* 396:695–99

303. Schneider SC, Ohmen J, Fosdick L, Gladstone B, Guo J, et al. 2000. Cutting edge: Introduction of an endopeptidase cleavage motif into a determinant flanking region of hen egg lysozyme results in enhanced T cell determinant display. *J. Immunol.* 165:20–23

304. Harding CV, Collins DS, Slot JW,

Geuze HJ, Unanue ER. 1991. Liposome-encapsulated antigens are processed in lysosomes, recycled, and presented to T cells. *Cell* 64:393–401

305. Pure E, Inaba K, Crowley MT, Tardelli L, Witmer PM, et al. 1990. Antigen processing by epidermal Langerhans cells correlates with the level of biosynthesis of major histocompatibility complex class II molecules and expression of invariant chain. *J. Exp. Med.* 172:1459–69

306. Romani N, Koide S, Crowley M, Witmer PM, Livingstone AM, et al. 1989. Presentation of exogenous protein antigens by dendritic cells to T cell clones. Intact protein is presented best by immature, epidermal Langerhans cells. *J. Exp. Med.* 169:1169–78

307. Pierre P, Turley SJ, Gatti E, Hull M, Meltzer J, et al. 1997. Developmental regulation of MHC class II transport in mouse dendritic cells. *Nature* 388:787–92

308. Cella M, Engering A, Pinet V, Pieters J, Lanzavecchia A. 1997. Inflammatory stimuli induce accumulation of MHC class II complexes on dendritic cells. *Nature* 388:782–87

309. Cameron PU, Freudenthal PS, Barker JM, Gezelter S, Inaba K, Steinman RM. 1992. Dendritic cells exposed to human immunodeficiency virus type-1 transmit a vigorous cytopathic infection to CD4$^+$ T cells. *Science* 257:383–87

310. Kampgen E, Koch N, Koch F, Stoger P, Heufler C, et al. 1991. Class II major histocompatibility complex molecules of murine dendritic cells: synthesis, sialylation of invariant chain, and antigen processing capacity are down-regulated upon culture. *Proc. Natl. Acad. Sci. USA* 88:3014–18

311. Pierre P, Mellman I. 1998. Developmental regulation of invariant chain proteolysis controls MHC class II trafficking in mouse dendritic cells. *Cell* 93:1135–45

312. Ni J, Fernandez MA, Danielsson L, Chillakuru RA, Zhang J, et al. 1998. Cystatin F is a glycosylated human low molecular weight cysteine proteinase inhibitor. *J. Biol. Chem.* 273:24797–804

313. Halfon S, Ford J, Foster J, Dowling L, Lucian L, et al. 1998. Leukocystatin, a new class II cystatin expressed selectively by hematopoietic cells. *J. Biol. Chem.* 273:16400–8

314. Manickasingham S, Reis e Sousa C. 2000. Microbial and T cell-derived stimuli regulate antigen presentation by dendritic cells in vivo. *J. Immunol.* 165:5027–34

315. Veeraswamy RK, Cella M, Colonna M, Unanue ER. 2003. Dendritic cells process and present antigens across a range of maturation states. *J. Immunol.* 170:5367–72

316. Li DN, Matthews SP, Antoniou AN, Mazzeo D, Watts C. 2003. Multistep autoactivation of asparaginyl endopeptidase in vitro and in vivo. *J. Biol. Chem.* 278:38980–90

317. Lautwein A, Burster T, Lennon-Dumenil AM, Overkleeft HS, Weber E, et al. 2002. Inflammatory stimuli recruit cathepsin activity to late endosomal compartments in human dendritic cells. *Eur. J. Immunol.* 32:3348–57

318. Desjardins M, Huber LA, Parton RG, Griffiths G. 1994. Biogenesis of phagolysosomes proceeds through a sequential series of interactions with the endocytic apparatus. *J. Cell Biol.* 124:677–88

319. Lennon-Dumenil AM, Bakker AH, Maehr R, Fiebiger E, Overkleeft HS, et al. 2002. Analysis of protease activity in live antigen-presenting cells shows regulation of the phagosomal proteolytic contents during dendritic cell activation. *J. Exp. Med.* 196:529–40

320. Barois N, de Saint-Vis B, Lebecque S, Geuze HJ, Kleijmeer MJ. 2002. MHC class II compartments in human dendritic cells undergo profound structural changes upon activation. *Traffic* 3:894–905

321. Jensen PE. 1990. Regulation of antigen presentation by acidic pH. *J. Exp. Med.* 171:1779–84

322. Jensen PE. 1991. Enhanced binding of peptide antigen to purified class II major histocompatibility glycoproteins at acidic pH. *J. Exp. Med.* 174:1111–20

323. Avva RR, Cresswell P. 1994. In vivo and in vitro formation and dissociation of HLA-DR complexes with invariant chain-derived peptides. *Immunity* 1:763–74

324. Weber DA, Evavold BD, Jensen PE. 1996. Enhanced dissociation of HLA-DR-bound peptides in the presence of HLA-DM. *Science* 274:618–20

325. Phan UT, Arunachalam B, Cresswell P. 2000. Gamma-interferon-inducible lysosomal thiol reductase (GILT). Maturation, activity, and mechanism of action. *J. Biol. Chem.* 275:25907–14

326. Molinari M, Salio M, Galli C, Norais N, Rappuoli R, et al. 1998. Selective inhibition of Ii-dependent antigen presentation by *Helicobacter pylori* toxin VacA. *J. Exp. Med.* 187:135–40

327. Sturgill-Koszycki S, Schlesinger PH, Chakraborty P, Haddix PL, Collins HL, et al. 1994. Lack of acidification in Mycobacterium phagosomes produced by exclusion of the vesicular proton-ATPase. *Science* 263:678–81

328. Hackam DJ, Rotstein OD, Zhang W, Gruenheid S, Gros P, Grinstein S. 1998. Host resistance to intracellular infection: Mutation of natural resistance-associated macrophage protein 1 (Nramp1) impairs phagosomal acidification. *J. Exp. Med.* 188:351–64

329. Brisseau GF, Grinstein S, Hackam DJ, Nordstrom T, Manolson MF, et al. 1996. Interleukin-1 increases vacuolar-type H^+-ATPase activity in murine peritoneal macrophages. *J. Biol. Chem.* 271:2005–11

330. Fiebiger E, Meraner P, Weber E, Fang IF, Stingl G, et al. 2001. Cytokines regulate proteolysis in major histocompatibility complex class II–dependent antigen presentation by dendritic cells. *J. Exp. Med.* 193:881–92

331. Drakesmith H, O'Neil D, Schneider SC,

Binks M, Medd P, et al. 1998. In vivo priming of T cells against cryptic determinants by dendritic cells exposed to interleukin 6 and native antigen. *Proc. Natl. Acad. Sci. USA* 95:14903–8

332. Mellman I, Fuchs R, Helenius A. 1986. Acidification of the endocytic and exocytic pathways. *Annu. Rev. Biochem.* 55:663–700

333. Stevens TH, Forgac M. 1997. Structure, function and regulation of the vacuolar (H^+)-ATPase. *Annu. Rev. Cell Dev. Biol.* 13:779–808

334. Nishi T, Forgac M. 2002. The vacuolar (H^+)-ATPases—nature's most versatile proton pumps. *Nat. Rev. Mol. Cell Biol.* 3:94–103

335. Kane PM. 2000. Regulation of V-ATPases by reversible disassembly. *FEBS Lett.* 469:137–41

336. Sumner JP, Dow JA, Earley FG, Klein U, Jager D, Wieczorek H. 1995. Regulation of plasma membrane V-ATPase activity by dissociation of peripheral subunits. *J. Biol. Chem.* 270:5649–53

337. Mallya SK, Partin JS, Valdizan MC, Lennarz WJ. 1992. Proteolysis of the major yolk glycoproteins is regulated by acidification of the yolk platelets in sea urchin embryos. *J. Cell Biol.* 117:1211–21

338. Fagotto F. 1995. Regulation of yolk degradation, or how to make sleepy lysosomes. *J. Cell Sci.* 108:3645–47

339. Fagotto F, Maxfield FR. 1994. Changes in yolk platelet pH during *Xenopus laevis* development correlate with yolk utilization. A quantitative confocal microscopy study. *J. Cell Sci.* 107:3325–37

340. Barasch J, Gershon MD, Nunez EA, Tamir H, al-Awqati Q. 1988. Thyrotropin induces the acidification of the secretory granules of parafollicular cells by increasing the chloride conductance of the granular membrane. *J. Cell Biol.* 107:2137–47

341. Haque MA, Li P, Jackson SK, Zarour HM, Hawes JW, et al. 2002. Absence of γ-interferon-inducible lysosomal thiol

reductase in melanomas disrupts T cell recognition of select immunodominant epitopes. *J. Exp. Med.* 195:1267–77

342. Zamvil SS, Mitchell DJ, Moore AC, Kitamura K, Steinman L, Rothbard JB. 1986. T-cell epitope of the autoantigen myelin basic protein that induces encephalomyelitis. *Nature* 324:258–60

343. Mamula MJ, Gee RJ, Elliott JI, Sette A, Southwood S, et al. 1999. Isoaspartyl post-translational modification triggers autoimmune responses to self-proteins. *J. Biol. Chem.* 274:22321–27

344. Sollid LM. 2000. Molecular basis of celiac disease. *Annu. Rev. Immunol.* 18: 53–81

345. Cirrito TP, Pu Z, Deck MB, Unanue ER. 2001. Deamidation of asparagine in a major histocompatibility complex-bound peptide affects T cell recognition but does not explain type B reactivity. *J. Exp. Med.* 194:1165–70

346. Cao L, Sun D, Whitaker JN. 1998. Citrullinated myelin basic protein induces experimental autoimmune encephalomyelitis in Lewis rats through a diverse T cell repertoire. *J. Neuroimmunol.* 88:21–29

347. van Stipdonk MJ, Willems AA, Amor S, Persoon-Deen C, Travers PJ, et al. 1998. T cells discriminate between differentially phosphorylated forms of αB-crystallin, a major central nervous system myelin antigen. *Int. Immunol.* 10:943–50

348. Dudler T, Altmann F, Carballido JM, Blaser K. 1995. Carbohydrate-dependent, HLA class II-restricted, human T cell response to the bee venom allergen phospholipase A2 in allergic patients. *Eur. J. Immunol.* 25:538–42

349. Corthay A, Backlund J, Broddefalk J, Michaelsson E, Goldschmidt TJ, et al. 1998. Epitope glycosylation plays a critical role for T cell recognition of type II collagen in collagen-induced arthritis. *Eur. J. Immunol.* 28:2580–90

350. Haurum JS, Arsequell G, Lellouch AC, Wong SY, Dwek RA, et al. 1994. Recognition of carbohydrate by major histocompatibility complex class I-restricted, glycopeptide-specific cytotoxic T lymphocytes. *J. Exp. Med.* 180:739–44

351. Glithero A, Tormo J, Haurum JS, Arsequell G, Valencia G, et al. 1999. Crystal structures of two H-2Db/glycopeptide complexes suggest a molecular basis for CTL cross-reactivity. *Immunity* 10:63–74

352. Speir JA, Abdel-Motal UM, Jondal M, Wilson IA. 1999. Crystal structure of an MHC class I presented glycopeptide that generates carbohydrate-specific CTL. *Immunity* 10:51–61

353. Lu L, Vollmer J, Moulon C, Weltzien HU, Marrack P, Kappler J. 2003. Components of the ligand for a Ni^{++} reactive human T cell clone. *J. Exp. Med.* 197:567–74

354. Engelhard VH, Brickner AG, Zarling AL. 2002. Insights into antigen processing gained by direct analysis of the naturally processed class I MHC associated peptide repertoire. *Mol. Immunol.* 39:127–37

355. Vlad AM, Muller S, Cudic M, Paulsen H, Otvos L Jr, et al. 2002. Complex carbohydrates are not removed during processing of glycoproteins by dendritic cells: processing of tumor antigen MUC1 glycopeptides for presentation to major histocompatibility complex class II-restricted T cells. *J. Exp. Med.* 196:1435–46

356. Alfonso C, Karlsson L. 2000. Nonclassical MHC class II molecules. *Annu. Rev. Immunol.* 18:113–42

357. Brocke P, Garbi N, Momburg F, Hammerling GJ. 2002. HLA-DM, HLA-DO and tapasin: functional similarities and differences. *Curr. Opin. Immunol.* 14:22–29

358. Villadangos JA, Cardoso M, Steptoe RJ, van Berkel D, Pooley J, et al. 2001. MHC class II expression is regulated in dendritic cells independently of invariant chain degradation. *Immunity* 14:739–49

359. Steinman RM, Kaplan G, Witmer MD, Cohn ZA. 1979. Identification of a novel cell type in peripheral lymphoid organs of mice. V. Purification of spleen dendritic

cells, new surface markers, and maintenance in vitro. *J. Exp. Med.* 149:1–16

360. Stossel H, Koch F, Kampgen E, Stoger P, Lenz A, et al. 1990. Disappearance of certain acidic organelles (endosomes and Langerhans cell granules) accompanies loss of antigen processing capacity upon culture of epidermal Langerhans cells. *J. Exp. Med.* 172:1471–82

361. Kleijmeer MJ, Oorschot VM, Geuze HJ. 1994. Human resident Langerhans cells display a lysosomal compartment enriched in MHC class II. *J. Invest. Dermatol.* 103:516–23

362. Kleijmeer M, Ramm G, Schuurhuis D, Griffith J, Rescigno M, et al. 2001. Reorganization of multivesicular bodies regulates MHC class II antigen presentation by dendritic cells. *J. Cell Biol.* 155:53–63

363. Katzmann DJ, Odorizzi G, Emr SD. 2002. Receptor downregulation and multivesicular-body sorting. *Nat. Rev. Mol. Cell Biol.* 3:893–905

364. Boes M, Cerny J, Massol R, Opden Brouw M, Kirchhausen T, et al. 2002. T-cell engagement of dendritic cells rapidly rearranges MHC class II transport. *Nature* 418:983–88

365. Thery C, Zitvogel L, Amigorena S. 2002. Exosomes: composition, biogenesis and function. *Nat. Rev. Immunol.* 2:569–79

366. Denzer K, Kleijmeer MJ, Heijnen HF, Stoorvogel W, Geuze HJ. 2000. Exosome: from internal vesicle of the multivesicular body to intercellular signaling device. *J. Cell Sci.* 113(Part 19):3365–74

367. Thery C, Boussac M, Veron P, Ricciardi-Castagnoli P, Raposo G, et al. 2001. Proteomic analysis of dendritic cell-derived exosomes: a secreted subcellular compartment distinct from apoptotic vesicles. *J. Immunol.* 166:7309–18

368. Thery C, Regnault A, Garin J, Wolfers J, Zitvogel L, et al. 1999. Molecular characterization of dendritic cell-derived exosomes. Selective accumulation of the heat shock protein hsc73. *J. Cell Biol.* 147:599–610

369. Zitvogel L, Regnault A, Lozier A, Wolfers J, Flament C, et al. 1998. Eradication of established murine tumors using a novel cell-free vaccine: dendritic cell-derived exosomes. *Nat. Med.* 4:594–600

370. Wolfers J, Lozier A, Raposo G, Regnault A, Thery C, et al. 2001. Tumor-derived exosomes are a source of shared tumor rejection antigens for CTL cross-priming. *Nat. Med.* 7:297–303

371. Stinchcombe J, Bossi G, Griffiths GM. 2004. Linking albinism and immunity: the secrets of secretory lysosomes. *Science* 305:55–59

372. Fehling H, Viville S, van Ewijk W, Benoist C, Mathis D. 1989. Fine-tuning of MHC class II gene expression in defined microenvironments. *Trends Genet.* 5:342–47

373. Meier O, Boucke K, Hammer SV, Keller S, Stidwill RP, et al. 2002. Adenovirus triggers macropinocytosis and endosomal leakage together with its clathrin-mediated uptake. *J. Cell Biol.* 158:1119–31

374. Touret N, Paroutis P, Grinstein S. 2005. The nature of the phagosomal membrane: endoplasmic reticulum vs. plasmalemma. *J. Leuk. Biol.* In press

SUBJECT INDEX

CUMULATIVE INDEXES

CONTRIBUTING AUTHORS, VOLUMES 13–23

A

Abel L, 20:581–620
Abraham RT, 14:483–510
Acha-Orbea H, 13:459–86
Acuto O, 18:165–84
Aderem A, 17:593–623
Adorini L, 16:495–521
Afkarian M, 18:451–94
Aguet M, 15:563–91
Akira S, 21:335–76
Alberola-Ila J, 15:125–54
Alexander WS, 22:503–29
Alfonso C, 18:113–42
Allen P, 19:375–96
Allen PM, 14:1–27
Allison JP, 19:565–94
Alt FW, 14:459–81
Altman A, 20:761–94
Amigorena S, 20:621–67
Anderson AC, 20:101–23
Anderson AO, 14:155–77
Anderson G, 14:73–99
Anderson KV, 22:457–83
Anderson MK, 17:109–47
Anderson MS, 23:447–85
Apasov S, 22:657–82
Arden B, 16:523–44
Arend WP, 16:27–55
Aruffo A, 14:591–617
Asao H, 14:179–205
Ashwell JD, 18:309–45
Asnagli H, 18:451–94
Auchincloss H Jr, 16:433–70
Avitahl N, 15:155–76

B

Baccala R, 23:307–35
Bach EA, 15:563–91
Bach J, 19:131–61

Bachmann MF, 14:333–67;
  15:235–70; 17:829–74
Baggioline M, 15:675–705
Bajorath J, 14:591–617
Baldwin AS, 14:649–83
Banchereau J, 18:767–811
Barouch DH, 20:73–99
Barrett JW, 21:377–423
Bastone A, 23:337–66
Beavil AJ, 21:579–628
Beavil RL, 21:579–628
Beilhack GF, 21:759–806
Bendelac A, 15:535–62
Ben-Neriah Y, 18:621–63
Bennink JR, 17:51–88
Bentley GA, 14:563–90
Berg LJ, 23:549–600
Berger EA, 17:657–700
Berland R, 20:253–300
Bettelli E, 20:101–23
Beutler B, 23:307–35
Bevan MJ, 13:93–126
Biassoni R, 14:619–48;
  19:197–223
Biragyn A, 22:181–215
Biron CA, 17:189–220
Bluestone JA, 14:233–58;
  19:225–52; 23:447–85
Blumberg RS, 20:495–549
Boehm U, 15:749–95
Boerth NJ, 17:89–108
Boldin MP, 17:331–67
Bolen JB, 15:371–404
Bolland S, 19:275–90
Boman HG, 13:61–92
Boniface JJ, 16:523–44
Bottazzi B, 23:337–66
Bottino C, 14:619–48;
  19:197–223

Botto M, 22:431–56
Bottomly K, 15:279–322
Boyle WJ, 20:795–823
Bradley LM, 16:201–23
Brennan CA, 22:457–83
Brennan FM, 14:397–440
Brenner MB, 22:817–90
Briére F, 18:767–811
Brigl M, 22:817–90
Bromley SK, 19:375–96
Brown GD, 23:901–44
Brown PO, 18:829–59
Browning JL, 21:231–64
Buckley RH, 22:625–55
Brugge JS, 15:371–404
Brunetti CR, 21:377–423
Buhlmann JE, 14:591–617
Burack WR, 19:375–96
Burki K, 14:207–32
Burmester GR, 13:229–50
Burton DR, 19:253–74
Busslinger M, 22:55–79
Byers DE, 15:851–79

C

Cahalan MD, 13:623–53
Calame K, 16:163–200
Calame KL, 21:205–30
Caldwell C, 22:657–82
Call ME, 23:101–25
Cameron C, 21:377–423
Cantoni C, 19:197–223
Cantrell D, 14:259–74;
  18:165–84
Carbone FR, 19:47–64
Cariappa A, 23:161–96
Carreno BM, 20:29–53
Carroll MC, 16:545–68;
  18:393–422

1065

CHAPTER TITLES, VOLUMES 13–23

T Lymphocyte and NK Cell Receptors

Lymphocyte Surface Antigens and Activation Mechanisms

Tolerance

Regulation of the Immune Response

Cytotoxic Cells

Autoimmunity

Immunodeficiency

HIV, AIDS and Other Retroviral Infections